PREVENTIVE CARDIOLOGY

Notice

Medicine is an ever-changing science. As new research and clinical experience broaden our knowledge, changes in treatment and drug therapy are required. The authors and the publisher of this work have checked with sources believed to be reliable in their efforts to provide information that is complete and generally in accord with the standards accepted at the time of publication. However, in view of the possibility of human error changes in medical sciences, neither the editors nor the publisher nor any other party who has been involved in the preparation or publication of this work warrants that the information contained herein is in every respect accurate or complete, and they disclaim all responsibility for any errors or omissions or for the results obtained from use of the information contained in this work. Readers are encouraged to confirm the information contained herein with other sources. For example and in particular, readers are advised to check the product information sheet included in the package of each drug they plan to administer to be certain that the information contained in this work is accurate and that changes have not been made in the recommended dose or in the contraindications for administration. This recommendation is of particular importance in connection with new or infrequently used drugs.

PREVENTIVE CARDIOLOGY
A Practical Approach

Second edition

EDITOR-IN-CHIEF

Nathan D. Wong, PhD, FACC, FAHA
Professor and Director
Heart Disease Prevention Program
Division of Cardiology
College of Medicine, University of California, Irvine;
Adjunct Professor
Department of Epidemiology
School of Public Health,
University of California, Los Angeles

Associate Editors

Henry R. Black, MD, FACP, FAHA
Associate Vice-President for Research
Associate Dean for Research
Charles J. and Margaret Roberts Professor and Chairman
Department of Preventive Medicine
Rush University Medical Center
Chicago, Illinois

Julius M. Gardin, MD, FACC, FAHA, FACP, FSGC
St. John Guild Distinguished Chair in Cardiovascular Diseases
Chief, Division of Cardiology
St. John Hospital and Medical Center
Professor of Internal Medicine
Wayne State University School of Medicine
Detroit, Michigan

McGraw-Hill
Medical Publishing Division

New York   Chicago   San Francisco   Lisbon   London   Madrid
Mexico City   Milan   New Delhi   San Juan   Seoul   Singapore   Sydney   Toronto

The **McGraw·Hill** Companies

Preventive Cardiology: A Practical Approach

1 2 3 4 5 6 7 8 9 0 DOC/DOC 0 9 8 7 6 5 4

ISBN: 0-07-140996-3

This book was set in Garamond by Pine Tree Composition.
The editors were Darlene Cooke, Shelley Reinhardt, Christie Naglieri, and Patrick Carr.
The production supervisor was Cheryl Souffrance.
The cover designer was Elizabeth Pisacreta.
The indexer was Michael Ferreira.
R.R. Donnelley was the printer and binder.

This book is printed on acid-free paper.

Library of Congress Cataloging-in-Publication Data

Preventive cardiology: a practical approach/editor-in-chief, Nathan D. Wong; associate editors, Henry R. Black, Julius M. Gardin.—2nd ed.
  p. ; cm.
Includes bibliographical references and index.
ISBN 0-07-140996-3 (hardcover)
1. Heart—Diseases—Prevention. 2. Heart—Disease—Risk factors.   I. Wong, Nathan D.
II. Black, Henry R. (Henry Richard), 1942-III. Gardin, Julius M.
[DNLM: 1. Cardiovascular Diseases—prevention & control. WG 120 P9445 2004]
RC262.P687 2004
616.1'205–dc22

2004042669

To all of our colleagues, whose work on understanding the causes of and
treatments for cardiovascular disease have done so much to reduce
its burden. And to the hundreds of thousands of volunteers who
participated in the studies described in this book. Without their efforts,
courage, and altruism, this book could not exist.
The Editors

To Mia, my loving wife, David, my cherished son, and Don and Lunny,
my devoted parents.
NDW

To my wife Benita: the love of my life, my partner, and my friend, and to
Dana, Matt, Becky and Sabrina, who help give life real meaning.
HRB

To our children–Adam, Tova, and Margot–our precious legacy.
JMG

Contents

Contributors

Wilbert S. Aronow, MD
Clinical Professor of Medicine and Chief, Cardiac
    Clinic, New York Medical College; Adjunct
    Professor of Geriatrics and Adult Development,
    Mount Sinai School of Medicine, New York,
    New York
Seniors

David R. Baines, MD
Faculty, Alaska Family Practice Residency, Anchorage,
    Alaska; Assistant Clinical Professor, University of
    Washington School of Medicine, Seattle,
    Washington
Native Americans

Stanley L. Bassin, EdD
Clinical Professor, Division of Cardiology, Department
    of Medicine, University of California, Irvine;
    California State Polytechnic University,
    Pomona, California; Professor Faculty Emeritus,
    Department of Kinesiology and Health Promotion,
    Pomona California
Physical Activity; Hispanic Americans

Ronny A. Bell, PhD, MS
Associate Professor, Department of Public Health
    Sciences, Wake Forest University School of
    Medicine, Winston-Salem, North Carolina
Global Trends in Cardiovascular Disease

Gary G. Bennett, PhD
Faculty, Alaska Family Practice Residency, Anchorage,
    Alaska; Assistant Assistant Professor, Department of
    Society, Human Development and Health, Harvard
    School of Public Health and Center for
    Community-Based Research, Dana-Farber Cancer
    Institute, Boston, Massachusetts
Psychosocial Factors

Lisa F. Berkman, PhD
Thomas D. Cabot Professor of Public Policy,
    Departments of Society, Human Development, and
    Health and Epidemiology, Harvard School of Public
    Health, Boston, Massachusetts
Psychosocial Factors

Henry R. Black, MD
Associate Vice-President for Research; Associate Dean
    for Research; Charles J. and Margaret Roberts
    Professor and Chairman, Department of Preventive
    Medicine, Rush University Medical Center,
    Chicago, Illinois
*Hypertension; Establishing a Preventive Cardiology
    Program*

George L. Blackburn, MD, PhD
S. Daniel Abraham Associate Professor of Nutrition;
    Associate Director, Division of Nutrition, Harvard
    Medical School; Director, Center for the Study of
    Nutrition Medicine, Beth Israel Deaconess Medical
    Center, Boston, Massachusetts
Obesity and Weight Control

Robert D. Brook, MD
Assistant Professor of Medicine, Division of
    Cardiovascular Medicine, Vascular Medicine and
    Hypertension Program, University of Michigan
    School of Medicine, Ann Arbor, Michigan
Secondary Prevention

Gregory L. Burke, MD, MS
Professor and Chair, Department of Public Health
    Sciences, Wake Forest University School of
    Medicine, Winston-Salem, North Carolina
Global Trends in Cardiovascular Disease

Michael H. Criqui, MD, MPH
Professor and Vice Chair, Department of Family and
    Preventive Medicine; Professor, Department of
    Medicine, University of California, San Diego
    School of Medicine
Surrogate Measures of Atherosclerosis

Dennis M. Davidson, MD, PhD
Clinical Professor of Medicine, Division of Cardiology,
    University of California, Irvine,
    College of Medicine
Children and Adolescents

Prakash C. Deedwania, MD
Professor of Medicine, University of California,
San Francisco School of Medicine; Chief,
Cardiology Section, Director, Cardiovascular
Research, UCSF Program, Fresno Clinical Professor
of Medicine, Stanford University, Palo Alto,
California
*East Asians, South Asians, and Asian and Pacific-Islander
Americans*

Omar F. Duenes, BS, PA-S
California Polytechnic University,
Pomona, California
Hispanic Americans

William J. Elliott, MD, PhD
Professor of Preventive Medicine, Internal Medicine,
and Pharmacology, Rush Medical College of Rush
University at Rush University Medical Center;
Attending Physician, Rush University Medical
Center, Chicago, Illinois
Hypertension

Gregg C. Fonarow, MD
Eliot Corday Professor of Cardiovascular Medicine and
Science, University of California, Los Angeles
Division of Cardiology; Director,
Ahmanson-University of California, Los Angeles
Cardiomyopathy Center & Co-Director, University
of California, Los Angeles Preventative Cardiology
Program, David Geffen School of Medicine at
University of California, Los Angeles
Implementing Preventive Cardiology Guidelines

Charles K. Francis, MD
Rudin Scholar in Urban Health
Director, Office of Health Disparities
New York Academy of Medicine
New York, New York

Julius M. Gardin, MD
St. John Guild Distinguished Chair In Cardiovascular
Diseases; Chief, Division of Cardiology, St. John
Hospital and Medical Center; Professor of Internal
Medicine, Wayne State University School of
Medicine, Detroit, Michigan
*Noninvasive Ultrasonographic Assessment of
Cardiovascular Disease; Establishing a Preventive
Cardiology Program*

Philip Greenland, MD
Harry W. Dingman Professor and Chair, Department
of Preventive Medicine, Professor of Medicine
(Cardiology), The Feinberg School of Medicine,
Northwestern University Medical School, Chicago,
Illinois
Secondary Prevention

Rajeev Gupta, MD
Consultant Physician and Professor of Medicine,
Monilek Hospital and Research Centre and
Mahatma Gandhi National Institute of Medical
Sciences, Jaipur, India
*East Asians, South Asians, and Asian and Pacific-Islander
Americans*

William L. Haskell, PhD
Professor, Stanford University School of Medicine,
Stanford, California
Physical Activity

Denise D. Hermann, MD
Associate Professor of Medicine; Assistant Director,
Heart Failure/Cardiac Transplantation Program,
University of California, San Diego
Naturoceuticals and Other Complementary Therapies

Kirsten F. Hilpert, BS
Pennsylvania State University, University Park,
Pennsylvania
Nutrition

Paul N. Hopkins, MD
Professor of Internal Medicine, Cardiovascular Genetics
Research Clinic, University of Utah School of
Medicine, Salt Lake City, Utah
Family History and Genetic Factors

Steven C. Hunt, PhD
Professor, Cardiovascular Genetics Division, University
of Utah School of Medicine, Salt Lake City, Utah
Family History and Genetic Factors

Mahtab Jafari, PharmD
Associate Clinical Professor, College of Medicine,
University of California, Irvine
Establishing a Preventive Cardiology Program

William B. Kannel, MD, MPH
Professor of Medicine and Public Health, Boston
University School of Medicine, Boston,
Massachusetts
Global Cardiovascular Risk Evaluation

Jennifer Kaseta, MD
Clinical Instructor, Department of Internal Medicine,
Division of Endocrinology and Metabolism,
University of Michigan School of Medicine, Ann
Arbor, Michigan
Diabetes and the Metabolic Syndrome

Moti L. Kashyap, MD
Director, Atherosclerosis Research Center, VA Medical
Center, Long Beach, California; Professor of
Medicine, University of California, Irvine
Dyslipidemia

Tony Kendrick, MS
Medical Researcher/Writer/Editor and Public Relations
Consultant, Gaithersburg, Maryland
Native Americans

Ronald M. Krauss, MD
Senior Scientist and Director, Atherosclerosis Research,
Children's Hospital Oakland Research Institute,
Oakland, California; Guest Senior Scientist,
Department of Genome Sciences, Lawrence
Berkeley National Laboratory; Adjunct Professor,
Department of Nutritional Sciences, University of
California, Berkeley
Nutrition

Penny M. Kris-Etherton, PhD, RD
Distinguished Professor of Nutritional Sciences,
Pennsylvania State University, University Park,
Pennsylvania
Nutrition

Harry A. Lando, PhD
Division of Epidemiology, School of Public Health,
University of Minnesota, Minneapolis,
Minnesota
Tobacco Use, Passive Smoking, and Smoking Cessation

Russell V. Luepker, MD
Mayo Professor, Division of Epidemiology, University
of Minnesota School of Public Health, Minneapolis,
Minnesota
Tobacco Use, Passive Smoking, and Smoking Cessation

Shaista Malik, MD, MPH
Cardiology Fellow, Division of Cardiology, Department
of Medicine University of California,
Irvine
Dyslipidemia

Karen C. McCowen, MD, MRCPI
Assistant Professor of Medicine, Harvard Medical
School, Beth Israel Deaconess Medical Center,
Boston, Massachusetts
Obesity and Weight Control

Cheryl K. Nordstrom, PhD
Center for Social Epidemiology & Population Health,
School of Public Health; University of Michigan,
Ann Arbor, Michigan
*Noninvasive Ultrasonographic Assessment of
Cardiovascular Disease*

Keith C. Norris, MD
Professor of Medicine, Associate Dean for Research,
Charles R. Drew University of Medicine and
Science, Los Angeles, California
African-Americans

Thomas A. Pearson, MD, PhD, MPH
Albert D. Kaiser Professor and Chair, Department of
Community and Preventive Medicine, University of
Rochester School of Medicine, Rochester,
New York
Primary Prevention

Paul M. Ridker, MD
Eugene Braunwald Professor of Medicine, Harvard
Medical School; Director, Center for Cardiovascular
Disease Prevention, Brigham and Women's Hospital,
Boston, Massachusetts
Thrombosis, Inflammation, and Infection

James R. Sowers, MD
Thomas W. and Joan F. Burns Missouri Chair in
Diabetology; Director of the University of Missouri
Diabetes and Cardiovascular Center; Associate Dean
for Clinical Research; Professor of Medicine,
Physiology and Pharmacology, Department of
Internal Medicine, University of Missouri,
Columbia
Diabetes and the Metabolic Syndrome

Karol E. Watson, MD, PhD
Co-Director, University of California, Los Angeles Program in Preventive Cardiology, David Geffen School of Medicine at University of California, Los Angeles
Women

Thomas K. Welty, MD, MPH
Clinical Assistant Professor, Native Elder Research Center, Department of Psychiatry, University of Colorado School of Medicine, Denver, Colorado
Native Americans

Matthew A. Wilson, MD
Preventive Cardiology Fellow, Department of Community and Preventive Medicine, University of Rochester Medical Center, Rochester, New York
Primary Prevention

Nathan D. Wong, PhD
Professor and Director, Heart Disease Prevention Program, Division of Cardiology, College of Medicine, University of California, Irvine, and Adjunct Professor, Department of Epidemiology, School of Public Health, University of California, Los Angeles
Noninvasive Ultrasonographic Assessment of Cardiovascular Disease; Surrogate Measures of Atherosclerosis; Dyslipidemia; Physical Activity; Thrombosis, Inflammation, and Infection; Establishing a Preventive Cardiology Program

Lily L. Wu, PhD
Associate Professor of Medicine, Cardiovascular Genetics Research Clinic, University of Utah School of Medicine, Salt Lake City, Utah
Family History and Genetic Factors

Foreword to the First Edition, 2000

This comprehensive text, *Preventive Cardiology,* is indeed timely. It can help meet an important challenge, fundamentally strategic in nature. The decades-long effort to control the epidemic of coronary heart disease (CHD) in the United States has apparently stalled after years of progress. It seems we are at a watershed, and the outcome for the next phase remains to be determined.

From the mid-1960s through the 1980s, CHD (and stroke) mortality rates declined steadily and substantially. This advance involved all adult age strata, men and women, all regions of the country, and all ethnic and socioeconomic groups (although it was smaller among the less educated and affluent). Correspondingly, since the major cardiovascular diseases (CVD) have been responsible for a majority of all adult deaths, the CVD downtrend produced a decline in all causes of mortality and an increase in life expectancy.

But in the 1990s the favorable CHD mortality trend slowed, and the decline in stroke mortality ceased. Will this adverse pattern of the 1990s persist? Even get worse? Will the CHD-CVD death rates increase again, as they did earlier in the century? Or can the interruption in the downtrend be halted and the declines be made to resume and accelerate? This is the strategic challenge in the new century—to get this trend back on track, and keep it there.

This is vital for the decade ahead, both to achieve national health goals for the year 2010 and to position us to tackle the "bottom line" objective of not only curbing but also ending the CHD-CVD epidemic well before midcentury. Population-wide practical and effective CHD-CVD prevention, particularly primary prevention, and most particularly primordial prevention—the primary prevention of the major risk factors responsible for the epidemic—is of the essence in regard to these goals. Hence the relevance and potential importance of this text.

The unfavorable CHD-CVD mortality trend of the 1990s developed despite multiple advances in clinical treatment for patients with acute CHD or with major CHD risk factors (e.g., high blood pressure, hypercholesterolemia)—coronary artery bypass surgery, coronary angioplasty, antithrombotic and thrombolytic drugs, antihypertensives, statins, etc. Trials have demonstrated that these interventions improve prognosis for CHD patients and for the coronary-prone, and the results have been widely applied by practitioners. Interventional cardiology has become a new subspecialty. And it has been implied that in this high-tech era, further development and application of these secondary preventive, high-risk strategies are all that is needed to curb the CHD epidemic, i.e., the basic concept of the 1960s and 1970s—population-wide primary prevention is an essential strategic thrust to control epidemic CHD—may now be "old hat."

But critical scrutiny of recent data compels a different conclusion: First of all, despite all the progress, sudden death (usually out-of-hospital and unattended) with first heart attack remains a common problem resistant to high-tech approaches. And acute death (30-day mortality) with first heart attacks in persons not dying suddenly has proven to be only partially amenable to modern treatment. In fact, review of data from treatment trials in patients at high risk or with CHD reveals a downside generally left unmentioned amidst the emphasis on favorable effects of the newer interventions: Invariably, despite the benefits from the newer treatments, morbidity and mortality risks for these patients remain greater, and years of life expectancy remain fewer, than for people at low risk thanks to favorable status for all major CHD-CVD risk factors. This is the case, for example, for long-term prognosis of myocardial infarction (MI) patients treated in-hospital with thrombolytics, for patients with high blood pressure treated with antihypertensives, and for patients with above-optimal serum cholesterol treated with statins. The problem is not with the interventions, all of them important advances. The problem is the pathobiology of the underlying disease, severe atherosclerosis. Once the heart is damaged, there is no cure, no return to *status quo ante*; there is only palliation, amelioration, and slowing and avoidance of further progression. Even for higher-risk persons without clinical evidence yet of CHD-CVD, it is not possible fully to overcome the decades-long adverse effects of exposure to above-optimal blood pressure, above-optimal serum cholesterol, the adverse lifestyles—especially dietary patterns—playing a major causative role in the epidemic occurrence of these established major risk factors. And, correspondingly, long-term adverse effects of smoking, sedentary habits, diabetes, and obesity are also reversible only in part by the interventions for high-risk and already-afflicted adults. Valuable though they are, these interventions—given the pathobiology of the disease—are at that point little and late, however high tech.

Thus, the fundamental strategy—set down 30 years ago—remains valid and critically important:

. . . a strategy of primary prevention of premature atherosclerotic diseases be adopted as long-term national policy for the United States and to implement this strategy adequate resources of money and manpower be committed to accomplish:

a.   Changes in diet to prevent or control hyperlipidemia, obesity, hypertension and diabetes.

b. Elimination of cigarette smoking.

c. Pharmacologic control of elevated blood pressure.

(Recommendations for the Primary Prevention of the Atherosclerotic Diseases, Inter-Society Commission for Heart Disease Resources, *Circulation* 1970.[1])

That strategy has been U.S. policy for many years. Three comments are in order here, by way of update, based on experiences in the effort to implement this strategy, and relevant research data accrued since 1970:

1. Epidemic CHD-CVD is absent among the small proportion (<10 percent) of young adult and middle-aged Americans with favorable levels for *all* quickly measurable major risk factors, i.e., men and women with serum cholesterol <200 mg/dL and systolic/diastolic blood pressure (SBP/DBP) <120/80 mmHg, who are also non-smokers, not diabetic, and free of prior MI history.[2] Their long-term CHD-CVD mortality rates are a small proportion of mortality from all causes; all causes of death rates are low, i.e., about half those of all other persons of corresponding age and gender; their life expectancy is greater by several years.

    These facts underscore and refine the foregoing strategy: The need is not only to prevent and control high levels of the major risk factors, but it is also to achieve favorable levels of all these traits concurrently for more and more people, so that low-risk status becomes commonplace throughout the population. That is, the need is for primordial prevention of all the adverse lifestyles and lifestyle-related risk factors producing the CHD-CVD epidemic—primordial prevention from conception and weaning on, by mass improvement in lifestyles.

    While the national policy is population-wide primary prevention, there is as yet no commitment to population-wide primordial prevention—by the federal government, the American Heart Association, the American College of Cardiology, or other professional organizations. This policy matter—on the key component of strategy for ending the CHD-CVD epidemic—needs attention and action.

2. Scientifically, all the essential knowledge is in hand to enable adoption and implementation of this policy. Thus, for decades, it has been known that population serum cholesterol-lipid levels can be favorably influenced by nutritional-hygienic means, i.e., lower intake of saturated fats and cholesterol; higher intake of unsaturated fats (mono-and poly-) and water-soluble fiber; favorable calorie balance (to prevent and correct obesity). Public and professional education, particularly on dietary lipid composition, has led to favorable population-wide trends in this area, and average serum cholesterol of adults has declined from 1950 to 1960 levels of about 235 to 240 mg/dL to 200 to 205 mg/dL nowadays, i.e., within hailing distance of the national goal of no more than 200 mg/dL, showing what can be done. (All this, despite a steady increase in population body mass—a challenge for preventive cardiology.)

    Research advances of the late 1980s and 1990s on nutrition and blood pressure make clear that multiple improvements in dietary pattern can favorably influence this major risk factor as well. These encompass lower salt intake, avoidance of high alcohol consumption, increased potassium ingestion, favorable calorie balance, and the several components of the Dietary Approaches to Stop Hypertension (DASH) clinical trial combination diet, i.e., increased intake of fruits, vegetables, fat-free and low-fat dairy products, and reduced consumption of total fat, saturated fat, and cholesterol. Note the concordance between the dietary recommendations for favorable plasma cholesterol-lipid and blood pressure levels.

    With effective implementation and adoption of these recommendations, it is reasonable to expect lower population-wide average levels of serum cholesterol and SBP/DBP in youth and young adulthood, and little or no rise with age (contrary to the present situation). That is, with improved norms of human behavior, favorable levels—low-risk levels—can become the rule throughout adulthood, for all strata of the population, rather than the exception. The same holds for the other traits contributing to the epidemic—obesity, sedentary habits, and smoking.

3. To achieve these goals, both the long-term policy commitment and mobilization of resources are needed, as the 1970 statement noted.[1] To date, "resources of money and manpower" for population-wide CHD-CVD primary prevention, particularly primordial prevention, have been modest. This is so when the reckoning includes the total commitment of all agencies (official, voluntary, professional). Given the present-day challenge, the opportunities, and the potential benefits for all population strata, it is reasonable to say at this juncture that they are insufficient, by several orders of magnitude. This is a key aspect of policy also requiring attention.

    This is being written on the eve of an NHLBI-sponsored "National Conference on CVD Prevention: Meeting the Healthy People Objectives for Cardiovascular Health"–a Conference mandated by the U.S. Congress—aiming to address these matters, overall, and in regard to the socioeconomic and ethnic strata of the population with more adverse lifestyles, risk factor patterns, and CHD-CVD rates. So this is indeed a "right" moment for *Preventive Cardiology*.

REFERENCES

1. Inter-Society Commission for Heart Disease Resources, Atherosclerosis Study Group and Epidemiology Study Group: Primary prevention of the atherosclerotic diseases. *Circulation* 1970;42:A55–A95.
2. Stamler J, Stamler R, Neaton JD, et al: Relationship of baseline low risk factor profile to long-term cardiovascular and non-cardiovascular mortality and to life expectancy: findings for five large cohorts of young adult and middle-aged men and women. *JAMA* 1999;282: 2012–2018.

Jeremiah Stamler, M.D.

Professor Emeritus, Department of Preventive Medicine

Feinberg School of Medicine

Northwestern University, Chicago, Illinois

Foreword to the Second Edition, 2004

Publication of the second edition of *Preventive Cardiology*—only a few years after the first—is a positive event. It reflects the recognition by a significant cadre of health professionals that preventive strategies are essential for ending the epidemic of coronary/cardiovascular diseases (CHD/CVD).

Since the first edition went to press, there have been important developments, favorable and otherwise. On the positive side, research findings have enriched the database demonstrating the preventive efficacy of low risk (LR) status (see Foreword to the First Edition, 2000). We now know that LR status—defined in a variety of ways—results in freedom from the mass onslaught of CHD/CVD over decades into older age for young adult and middle-aged women and men of all major ethnic strata (including African-Americans, Hispanic-Americans, and non-Hispanic whites), both less and more affluent, less and more educated. Death from CHD/CVD is rare (endemic, not epidemic) among LR cohorts; mortality from non-cardiovascular diseases (including cancers) and from all causes is much lower. Life expectancy is much longer. CHD/CVD and other morbidity are less frequent well into older age. During older age (from age 65 on), the Medicare costs of LR people—average annual costs, cumulative costs (e.g., to age 80 or to demise), and costs during the last year or two of life—are lower. Women and men assessed as low risk in young adulthood and middle age also register more favorable scores on multiple indices of quality of life in older age.

Given all these facts about the value of being low risk and its crucial relevance for prevention of epidemic CHD/CVD, the National Heart Lung and Blood Institute (NHLBI) a few years ago appropriately designated the need to progressively increase the proportion of the population at low risk as a key strategy for CHD/CVD prevention, with particular emphasis on primordial prevention of all lifestyle and lifestyle-related major risk factors– that is, their prevention especially from conception, birth, and weaning, as well as during childhood, youth, and adulthood. And data from NHLBI research and successive National Health and Nutrition Examination Surveys (NHANES) during the last four decades of the twentieth century show that it is possible to increase the percentage of the population at low risk. This is possible across-the-board—for women and men, for all adult age groups, for all major ethnic and socioeconomic status (SES) strata.

But—on the downside—only a small minority of adult Americans were at low risk in 1990 and 2000 despite the upward trend nationally in this proportion during the preceding decades. And LR status was less common among men than women, less common among African-Americans than whites, and less common among lower than higher SES strata. And from 1990 to 2000, no increase was registered in the proportion at low risk. And the obesity epidemic continues unabated in these first few years of the new century. And—probably related to the higher prevalence rate of overweight/obesity—the estimated proportions of the population with high blood pressure and/or diabetes are up, not down. And tens of millions of people have been and are being lured by special commercial interests down a diet path—the high-fat low-carbohydrate "panacea"—never before trod long-term by any sizeable population group. Basic lessons on healthy nutrition—from decades of epidemiologic, metabolic ward, clinical, animal experimental, and anthropologic research—have been and are being bypassed, glossed over, or obscured. And resources remain all too small and inadequate for a successful, sustained struggle to end these adverse trends and get America back on the sound track of progressive, substantial increases in the proportion of the population at low risk—and thereby achieve substantial declines in CHD/CVD, so that well before mid-century, our morbidity/disability/mortality rates become low, and the war against the terror of the CHD/CVD epidemic is won.

So the second edition of *Preventive Cardiology* is even more timely than the first edition—to help all of us meet the imminent strategic challenges at every level, national to local.

Jeremiah Stamler, M.D.

Professor Emeritus, Department of Preventive Medicine

Feinberg School of Medicine

Northwestern University, Chicago, Illinois

Preface

In the second edition of *Preventive Cardiology: A Practical Approach,* we seek to provide the reader with a practical approach toward understanding the etiology of atherosclerotic cardiovascular disease, as well as standard and novel clinical approaches to its early identification and prevention. As was true for the first edition, this second edition comprises a wealth of information for the health care provider relating to the identification and management of key risk factors and to the development of a preventive cardiology clinic. Dietary, physical activity, behavioral, and pharmacologic strategies to risk factor management are highlighted.

Distinctive aspects of the book include its detailed discussion of screening for risk factors for atherosclerotic cardiovascular disease, the most current clinical guidelines for the management of these risk factors, and noninvasive techniques for measuring subclinical disease—a modifiable state beyond the presence of risk factors, but prior to clinical manifestations. Other chapters provide detailed discussions of nutritional approaches and counseling, physical activity recommendations, evaluation and management of psychosocial factors, and screening for genetic factors that may predispose to cardiovascular risk. The book also provides separate chapters regarding the prevention of heart disease in special populations—women, the elderly, children and adolescents, and specific ethnic groups—including African-Americans, Hispanic Americans, Asian and Pacific Islanders, and Native Americans. The last section of the book concentrates on practical strategies for the primary and secondary prevention of cardiovascular diseases and approaches to setting up a preventive cardiology clinic, as well as a discussion of strategies for implementation of guidelines.

In this second edition, we provide significantly updated material regarding recent trends in cardiovascular disease, new methods for risk assessment and screening, the latest findings from clinical trials and their implications for prevention, as well as recently released guidelines for control of hypertension, dyslipidemia, and other risk factors.

We give special thanks to our contributors, many renowned in their respective areas of specialization, for their devoted efforts, without which this text would not be possible. We also thank our colleagues for their inspiration, and our students among whom will emerge tomorrow's leaders of the field.

This text would not have been possible without the considerable efforts and dedication of Shelley Reinhardt, Patrick Carr, Darlene B. Cooke, and Martin Wonsiewicz of McGraw-Hill.

Finally, we wish to acknowledge the support of our families and the many sacrifices they have made to make this text possible. Our wives remain our greatest support and strength: Mia K. Wong, Benita Black, and Dr. Susan Gardin.

PART I

Epidemiology

Global cardiovascular risk evaluation **1**

William B. Kannel

KEY POINTS

- *A number of major risk factors for atherosclerotic cardiovascular disease have been delineated and their importance confirmed. These include: dyslipidemia, glucose intolerance, insulin resistance, hypertension, cigarette smoking, adiposity, physical inactivity, left ventricular hypertrophy, atrial fibrillation, and cardiomegaly. A number of these have been selected to formulate disease-specific multivariable risk profiles.*

- *Because cardiovascular disease risk factors usually cluster, and the cardiovascular disease risk imposed by any particular risk factor varies widely in relation to this, multivariable cardiovascular disease risk assessment has become a necessity, especially now that near-average blood pressure and blood lipids are recommended for treatment.*

- *Although novel risk factor evaluation deserves attention, one or more of the standard cardiovascular disease risk factors appear to account for as much as 85% of cardiovascular disease arising in the population.*

- *Multivariable risk formulations are available to facilitate office evaluation of the risk of each of the major atherosclerotic cardiovascular disease outcomes including coronary heart disease, stroke, peripheral artery disease, and heart failure, using ordinary office procedures and readily available blood tests.*

- *Because of shared modifiable risk factors, measures taken to prevent any one cardiovascular disease outcome can be expected also to benefit the others.*

- *Further improvement in the detection, evaluation, and control of the major risk factors identified is needed, particularly in the high-risk segment of the population. We need to improve implementation of recommended guidelines for primary and secondary atherosclerotic cardiovascular disease.*

INTRODUCTION

Epidemiologic research conducted over the past five decades has contributed to the explosive expansion of knowledge regarding the natural history of cardiovascular disease (CVD). This research has provided significant information that has helped public health workers, scientists, and physicians increase their understanding of the factors predisposing to the occurrence of CVD. These have come to be known as *risk factors*, a term coined by the Framingham Heart Study.[1] Identification of these modifiable risk factors helped stimulate an interest in preventive cardiology worldwide and has made cardiovascular epidemiology the basic science of preventive cardiology. The increased awareness of the major cardiovascular risk factors promulgated by the Framingham Heart Study and corroborated by other investigators encouraged public health initiatives against smoking in the 1960s, hypertension in the 1970s, and hypercholesterolemia in the 1980s.[2]

Epidemiological research exploring the evolution of CVD was stimulated by the mounting epidemic of CVD from the 1930s through the 1950s. By 1949, CVD had become the leading cause of death in the United States, accounting for half of all deaths. The US Public Health Service decided to explore the problem, seeking out modifiable predisposing conditions using an epidemiologic approach, which, at the time, was a novel concept.[3] This entailed long-term prospective observational investigation of suspected host and environmental factors that might be expected to promote CVD in a representative general population sample.

The population approach used provided a less distorted appraisal of the evolution of CVD than was obtained from clinical studies subject to selection bias. It soon became apparent that coronary heart disease (CHD) is an extremely common and highly lethal disease that attacks one in five persons before 60 years of age, that women lag men in incidence by 20 years, and that sudden death is a prominent feature of CHD. One in every six coronary attacks was found to have sudden death as the first, last, and only symptom.[4] It also became evident that the disease can be asymptomatic in its most severe form, with one in three myocardial infarctions not being recognized because of their silent or atypical nature.[5] Because of this clinical profile, a preventive approach seemed essential. Fortunately, epidemiologic research was able to identify a number of modifiable predisposing factors, making it possible to identify high-risk candidates for preventive measures long in advance of the appearance of symptoms. Because the Framingham Study cohort had been followed for more than five decades, it was possible to ascertain that the lifetime risk of coronary events is 48.6% for 40-year-old men and 31.7% for women of that age.[6] This rate for women is three times that for developing breast cancer, which they fear more.

MISCONCEPTIONS CORRECTED

Before epidemiologic researchers examined the relationship between hypertension and CVD, it was believed that common hypertension was a benign condition and that it was essential that blood pressure rise with age to ensure adequate perfusion of the tissues as the arterioles narrowed.[7,8] The cardiovascular sequelae of increased blood pressure were thought to derive from the diastolic blood pressure, and it was held that the disproportionate rise in systolic blood pressure with advancing age was an innocuous accompaniment of arterial stiffening.[7,8] Further, it was believed that treatment of isolated systolic hypertension would not only be fruitless, but also produce intolerable and dangerous side effects. Women were thought to tolerate hypertension well, and it was believed that *normal* blood pressures in both sexes were substantially higher in the elderly than in the middle-aged.

It took epidemiologic research to convince skeptics that serum cholesterol is a true risk factor for CHD, that the lipoprotein-cholesterol fractions were fundamental to atherogenesis, and that diets rich in saturated fat and cholesterol—presumed to be healthy—promoted dyslipidemia and its cardiovascular sequelae.[9] Population research established that HDL cholesterol was actually a strong independent risk factor inversely related to the development of CHD.[10,11]

Epidemiologic research was required to demonstrate that cigarette smoking was not only a carcinogen for, but also a substantial risk factor, for atherosclerotic CVD. Population research established that smoking is a major risk factor for CHD, precipitating heart attacks and sudden deaths, especially in high-risk coronary candidates. Epidemiologic research has shown that the risk of heart attacks could be promptly halved in smokers who quit, regardless of how long or how much they previously smoked.[12,13]

Before epidemiologic investigation, physical exercise was considered dangerous for CHD candidates. Population research established that physical activity is actually protective. There was skepticism about the importance of obesity as a risk factor for CVD, but this has been dispelled by epidemiologic research demonstrating that obesity promotes all of the major cardiovascular risk factors. Left ventricular hypertrophy was shown to be an ominous harbinger of CVD rather than an incidental compensatory response to hypertension, CHD, and heart valve deformity.[14]

Before prospective epidemiologic investigation was performed to determine how those who developed atherosclerotic CVD differed from those who did not, it was held that a single etiology would be found to be essential and, in most instances, sufficient to produce the pathology. However, five decades of epidemiologic research indicates that atherosclerotic disease is distinctly multifactorial, giving rise to the risk factor concept. Certain living habits promote atherogenic traits in genetically susceptible persons. After prolonged exposure, these traits result in a compromised circulation, leading to clinical events. Thus, atherosclerotic cardiovascular disease is now regarded as a multifactorial process involving a variety of predisposing risk factors, each of which is best considered as an ingredient of a cardiovascular risk profile.[15–19]

Although it has frequently been suggested that more than 50% of patients with CHD lack conventional risk factors, recent reports, including one comprising more than 120,000 patients enrolled in clinical trials of CHD, indicated at least one major risk factor to be present in 85% of men and 81% of women,[20] and another report involving nearly 400,000 individuals enrolled in three US cohort studies showed that among those with fatal CHD, 87 to 100% had had at least one clinically elevated major risk factor.[21]

CARDIOVASCULAR RISK PROFILES

A preventive approach to atherosclerotic CVD is feasible and is crucial because, once clinically manifest, the disease is apt to progress with lethal consequences, and treatment can seldom cure or restore the patient to full function. Prevention is now feasible because epidemiologic research has identified a number of modifiable predisposing lifestyles and personal attributes that, when corrected, have been shown to reduce the likelihood of the development of clinical atherosclerotic CVDs.[22–24] To evaluate cost-effectively those at risk for major cardiovascular events, multivariable risk profiles have been formulated to facilitate targeting of preventive measures.[15–19] The American Heart Association Task Force on Risk Reduction recently emphasized the importance of these risk profiles in motivating and reassuring patients, and in assisting in selection of therapy.[25] They concluded that these scores direct health care professionals to look at the whole patient and to recognize the cumulative nature of risk factors.

A half-century of epidemiologic research by the Framingham Heart Study and others has identified a number of major cardiovascular risk factors that have a strong independent impact on the rate of development of atherosclerotic CVD.[23] These risk factors can be readily ascertained from ordinary office procedures and formulated into a predictive risk profile.[15–19] The Framingham Heart Study and others have identified and quantified several classes of cardiovascular risk factors, including atherosclerotic personal attributes, lifestyles that promote risk, signs of organ damage, and innate susceptibility. Those easy to ascertain during an office visit are a cigarette smoking history, blood lipids, glucose intolerance, blood pressure, and left ventricular hypertrophy as seen on the electrocardiogram.[23,24]

These major established risk factors contribute powerfully and significantly to CHD risk (Table 1-1). For stroke, the relevant factors are hypertension, left ventricular hypertrophy, and diabetes, but dyslipidemia appears to play a minor role (Table 1-2). For peripheral artery disease, glucose intolerance, cigarette smoking, and left ventricular hypertrophy are the most influential factors (Table 1-3). For heart failure, important factors are hypertension, diabetes, and reduced vital capacity, whereas serum total cholesterol appears unrelated (Table 1-4).

TABLE 1-1   Risk of Coronary Heart Disease According to Standard Risk Factors: Framingham Heart Study—36-Year Follow-up

| | Ages 35–64 y | | | | Ages 65–94 y | | | |
| | Rate/1000 | | Risk ratio | | Rate/1000 | | Risk ratio | |
Risk factor	Men	Women	Men	Women	Men	Women	Men	Women
Cholesterol ≥240 mg/dL	34	15	1.9*	1.8†	59	39	1.2‡	2.0*
Blood pressure ≥140/90 mm Hg	45	21	2.0*	2.2*	73	44	1.6†	1.9*
Diabetes	39	42	1.5*	3.7*	79	62	1.6†	2.1*
ECG-LVH	79	55	3.0*	4.6*	134	94	2.7*	3.0*
Smoking	33	13	1.5†	1.1	53	38	1.0	1.2

*P < .001, †P < .01, ‡P < .05. Biennial rates and risk ratios age adjusted.

SOURCE: Reproduced, with permission, from Kannel WB, et al. Comparison of risk profiles for cardiovascular events: implications for prevention. Adv Intern Med 1997;42:39–66.

TABLE 1-2 Risk of Stroke According to Standard Risk Factors: Framingham Heart Study—36-Year Follow-up

| | Ages 35–64 y | | | | Ages 65–94 y | | | |
| | Rate/1000 | | Risk ratio | | Rate/1000 | | Risk ratio | |
Risk factor	Men	Women	Men	Women	Men	Women	Men	Women
Cholesterol ≥240 mg/dL	3	2	1.0	1.1	10	12	1.0	1.0
Blood pressure ≥140/90 mm Hg	7	4	5.7*	4.0*	20	17	2.0*	2.6*
Diabetes	7	4	3.0†	2.4‡	20	28	1.6	2.9*
ECG-LVH	13	13	5.1*	8.1*	44	51	3.6*	5.0*
Smoking	4	1	2.5	1.0	17	20	1.4	1.9*

*P < .001, †P < .01, ‡P < .05. Biennial rates and risk ratios age adjusted. Risk ratio for those with a given trait vs. those without it.

SOURCE: Reproduced, with permission, from Kannel WB, et al. Comparison of risk profiles for cardiovascular events: implications for prevention. *Adv Intern Med* 1997;42:39–66.

TABLE 1-3 Risk of Peripheral Artery Disease by Standard Risk Factors: Framingham Heart Study—36-Year Follow-up

| | Ages 35–64 y | | | | Ages 65–94 y | | | |
| | Rate/1000 | | Risk ratio | | Rate/1000 | | Risk ratio | |
Risk factor	Men	Women	Men	Women	Men	Women	Men	Women
Cholesterol ≥240 mg/dL	8	4	2.0†	1.9	18	8	1.4	1.0
Blood pressure ≥140/90 mm Hg	10	7	2.0*	3.7*	17	10	1.6‡	2.0†
Diabetes	18	18	3.4*	6.4*	21	16	9.7‡	2.6†
ECG-LVH	16	17	2.7	5.3*	36	14	23.7†	2.2
Smoking	9	5	2.5*	2.0†	18	11	8.5†	1.8‡

*P < .001, †P < .01, ‡P < .05. Biennial rates and risk ratios age adjusted. Risk ratio for those with a given trait vs. those without it.

SOURCE: Reproduced, with permission, from Kannel WB, Wilson PWF. Comparison of risk profiles for cardiovascular events: implications for prevention. *Adv Intern Med* 1997;42:39–66.

TABLE 1-4 Risk of Heart Failure by Standard Risk Factors: Framingham Heart Study—36-Year Follow-up

| | Ages 35–64 y | | | | Ages 65–94 y | | | |
| | Rate/1000 | | Risk ratio | | Rate/1000 | | Risk ratio | |
Risk factor	Men	Women	Men	Women	Men	Women	Men	Women
Cholesterol ≥240 mg/dL	7	4	1.2	1.1	21	18	1.0	1.0
Blood pressure ≥140/90 mm Hg	14	6	4.0*	3.0*	33	24	1.9*	1.9*
Diabetes	23	21	4.4†	8.0*	40	51	2.0*	3.6*
ECG-LVH	71	36	15.0*	13.0*	99	84	4.9*	5.4*
Smoking	7	3	1.5*	1.1	23	22	1.0	1.3‡

*P < .001, ‡P < .01, ‡P < .05. Biennial rates and risk ratios adjusted for age. Risk ratio for those with a given trait vs. those without it.

SOURCE: Reproduced, with permission, from Kannel WB, Wilson PWF. Comparison of risk profiles for cardiovascular events: implications for prevention. *Adv Intern Med* 1997;42:39–66.

The standard risk factors were shown to influence CVD rates with different strengths in men and women. Diabetes was shown to operate more powerfully in women, eliminating their advantage over men for most atherosclerotic cardiovascular events.[26,27] Cigarette smoking was found to be more influential in men.

Some of the standard risk factors, including glucose intolerance, smoking, dyslipidemia, and hypertension, tend to have lower risk ratios in advanced age, causing some to question the relevance of risk factors in later life. However, this reduced relative risk is offset by a higher absolute incidence of disease and a large excess risk in advanced age. Thus, the standard risk factors continue to be important in the elderly. Atherosclerotic cardiovascular events in the heart, brain, and limbs can now be predicted from epidemiologic data.[15–19]

Clinical categorical risk assessments according to the number of arbitrarily defined abnormalities present can identify persons at high risk, but epidemiologic research points out that this approach tends to overlook those at high risk because of multiple marginal abnormalities. Identification of persons with several borderline risk factor values for treatment is important because such persons are at high risk and experience most of the cardiovascular events in the general population.

Epidemiologic research has shown that prevention based on *individual* risk factor assessment and treatment is inefficient and misleading. This approach often falsely reassures or needlessly alarms potential candidates for cardiovascular disease, because the risk of such events associated with any particular risk factor varies widely depending on the burden of associated risk factors. An-other reason for quantitative multivariable risk assessment is the epidemiologically established fact that all the standard risk factors tend to cluster together because they are metabolically linked (Table 1-5). Clusters of three or more risk factors occur at four to five times the expected rate.

Multivariable analysis of risk factors is undertaken to identify those at high risk for CVD who need aggressive preventive measures and to seek clues to pathogenesis of the disease. The set of risk factors employed for the former is driven by practical considerations, and those for the latter, by the hypothesis being tested. Efficient methods for combining the predictive information from a number of risk factors are now available, making it possible to estimate the probability that persons with certain characteristics will develop CVD in a specified interval. This methodology implicitly recognizes that no known risk factor either inevitably leads to development of disease or confers absolute immunity. In considering multivariable risk formulations, one must understand that there is no unconditional probability of disease development, nor any conditional probability that will not alter if other factors are entered into consideration. Adding variables ordinarily increases ability to estimate risk by designating more people at very high or low risk, but the three best risk factors usually perform almost as well as a larger set, even though all may be independent predictors. How many risk factors to include depends on the purpose for assigning risk and the costs entailed. It must be anticipated that a regression estimate will fit the data from which it is derived better than it will fit another data set.

TABLE 1-5   Risk Factor Clustering in Framingham Offspring, Aged 18 to 74 Years, by Index Quintile Risk Factor Variable (Sex-Specific)

	Sex	n	Distribution of RF scores (percent in top quintile)					
			None	One	Two	Three	Four	Five
High cholesterol	Men	505	29	28	23	15	4	1
	Women	519	26	26	23	17	5	2
Low HDL* cholesterol	Men	501	27	27	26	14	4	1
	Women	544	38	26	18	11	5	2
High BMI	Men	497	23	29	27	15	5	1
	Women	533	15	31	27	18	7	2
High systolic blood pressure	Men	530	25	29	24	16	5	1
	Women	545	19	28	26	18	7	2
High triglycerides	Men	491	11	28	33	21	6	1
	Women	522	20	29	23	18	7	2
High glucose	Men	477	23	31	22	17	5	1
	Women	608	29	26	21	15	6	2
Expected			33	41	20	5	0.6	0.03

*HDL, high-density lipoprotein; BMI, body mass index; RF, risk factor.

TABLE 1-6 Incidence of Major Atherosclerotic Cardiovascular Events by Age and Sex: Framingham Heart Study 44-Year Follow-up*

| | *Age-adjusted average annual rate per 1000* | | | | | | | | | |
| | All CVD[†] | | CHD | | Stroke CHF | | | PAD | | |
Age	Men	Women	Men	Women	Men	Women	Men	Women	Men	Women
36–64	17	9	12	5	2	2	2	1	3	2
65–94	44	30	27	16	13	11	12	9	8	5
Risk ratio[‡]	2.6	3.3	2.3	3.2	6.5	5.5	6.0	9.0	2.7	2.5

*Includes 20-year follow-up of Framingham offspring cohort.
[†]CHD, coronary heart disease; CHF, congestive heart failure; PAD, peripheral artery disease.
[‡]Risk ratio comparing incidences in older (age 65–94) vs. younger (age 36–64) persons.

Framingham Study risk profiles have been tested in a variety of population samples and found to be reasonably accurate, except for those in areas where the coronary heart disease rates are very low.[28–31] However, even in these areas, persons at high risk can be distinguished from those at low risk, and by adjusting the intercept, the true absolute risk can be estimated.[32]

CORONARY RISK PROFILE

Prevention of CHD by risk factor control deserves high priority because the incidence of CHD equals that of all the other major clinical manifestations of atherosclerosis combined (Table 1-6). Age gradients in incidence are greatest for stroke and heart failure. Multivariable formulations for quantifying risk of CHD have been developed

from Framingham Heart Study data that enable physicians to estimate their patients' probability of an event from a set of established independent risk factors.[15–19] A simplified version of the Framingham Heart Study profile for CHD risk allows for classification based on Joint National Committee (JNC)-V blood pressure and National Cholesterol Education Program (NCEP) cholesterol designated treatment categories in addition to age, HDL cholesterol, diabetes, and smoking.[19] The risk of developing CHD increases with the burden of these risk factors, depending on the intensity of exposure to them (Figure 1-1). The risk-factor score corresponds to the probability of a coronary event over a specified interval. These estimated event rates, when compared with the average risk for persons of the same age, provide absolute and relative risk estimates. Persons estimated to be

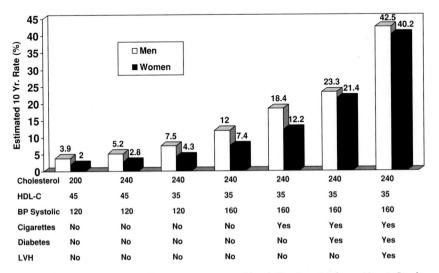

FIGURE 1-1 Incidence of CHD in 42-year-old adults, Framingham Heart Study, 1972–1984. *Key:* HDL-C, high-density lipoprotein cholesterol; BP, blood pressure; LVH, left ventricular hypertrophy.

Age	Points
20-34	−9
35-39	−4
40-44	0
45-49	3
50-54	6
55-59	8
60-64	10
65-69	11
70-74	12
75-79	13

Total Cholesterol	Points				
	Age 20-39	Age 40-49	Age 50-59	Age 60-69	Age 70-79
<160	0	0	0	0	0
160-199	4	3	2	1	0
200-239	7	5	3	1	0
240-279	9	6	4	2	1
≥280	11	8	5	3	1

	Points				
	Age 20-39	Age 40-49	Age 50-59	Age 60-69	Age 70-79
Nonsmoker	0	0	0	0	0
Smoker	8	5	3	1	1

HDL (mg/dL)	Points
≥60	−1
50-59	0
40-49	1
<40	2

Systolic BP (mmHg)	If Untreated	If Treated
<120	0	0
120-129	0	1
130-139	1	2
140-159	1	2
≥160	2	3

Point Total	10-Year Risk %
<0	<1
0	1
1	1
2	1
3	1
4	1
5	2
6	2
7	3
8	4
9	5
10	6
11	8
12	10
13	12
14	16
15	20
16	25
≥17	≥30

FIGURE 1-2 Calculation of estimated 10-year risk of coronary heart disease events in men. (From the Third Report of the National Cholesterol Education Program (NCEP) Adult Treatment Panel (ATP III) Executive Summary, National Institutes of Health, NIH publication 01-3670, 2001).

Age	Points
20-34	−7
35-39	−3
40-44	0
45-49	3
50-54	6
55-59	8
60-64	10
65-69	12
70-74	14
75-79	16

Total Cholesterol	Points				
	Age 20-39	Age 40-49	Age 50-59	Age 60-69	Age 70-79
<160	0	0	0	0	0
160-199	4	3	2	1	1
200-239	8	6	4	2	1
240-279	11	8	5	3	2
≥280	13	10	7	4	2

	Points				
	Age 20-39	Age 40-49	Age 50-59	Age 60-69	Age 70-79
Nonsmoker	0	0	0	0	0
Smoker	9	7	4	2	1

HDL (mg/dL)	Points
≥60	−1
50-59	0
40-49	1
<40	2

Systolic BP (mmHg)	If Untreated	If Treated
<120	0	0
120-129	1	3
130-139	2	4
140-159	3	5
≥160	4	6

Point Total	10-Year Risk %
<9	<1
9	1
10	1
11	1
12	1
13	2
14	2
15	3
16	4
17	5
18	6
19	8
20	11
21	14
22	17
23	22
24	27
≥25	≥30

FIGURE 1-3 Calculation of estimated 10-year risk of coronary heart disease events in women. (From Adult Treatment Panel III, Women (from the Third Report of the National Cholesterol Education Program (NCEP) Adult Treatment Panel (ATP III) Executive Summary, National Institutes of Health, NIH publication 01-3670, 2001).

at high risk of a coronary event are also likely to be at increased risk of all the other CVD outcomes.

Most recently, a modified point system has been developed based on the NCEP Adult Treatment Panel (ATP) III guidelines, where the probability of a hard CHD event (myocardial infarction or death) in 10 years is predicted on the basis of categories of age, systolic blood pressure, total and HDL cholesterol (HDL-C), and cigarette smoking status for men and women separately. Calculation of 10-year risk is recommended for those with two or more established CHD risk factors (including male age 45 and older and female age 55 and older), and a calculated 10-year risk of >20% is now defined as a CHD risk equivalent. These calculations are not performed in those with known CHD or other CHD risk equivalents (eg, diabetes, peripheral arterial disease, abdominal aortic aneurysm, symptomatic carotid disease), where secondary prevention risk factor management is already recommended[33] (Figures 1-2 and 1-3). Framingham Study data additionally suggest that electrocardiographic evidence of left ventricular hypertrophy should also be designated as a CHD equivalent because it carries the same risk as electrocardiographic evidence of a myocardial infarction (Table 1-1).

STROKE PROFILE

Epidemiologic research has also yielded a risk profile for estimating the risk of developing an atherothrombotic brain infarction, the most common variety of stroke and the most feared atherosclerotic sequela of identified risk factors. The predisposing risk factors and cardiac conditions include the standard risk factors plus atrial fibrillation, CHD, and heart failure (Table 1-7). These independent risk factors have been formulated into a stroke risk profile based on Framingham Heart Study data and made available by the American Heart Association (AHA).[17] Risk of stroke in persons with any one of these risk factors varies widely depending on the number of accompanying risk factors) (Figure 1-4). The risk profile tables that have been developed enable estimation of the joint effect of any combination of the predisposing factors, providing estimates of absolute and relative risks of developing a stroke (Table 1-8).

PERIPHERAL ARTERY DISEASE PROFILE

Population research at the Framingham Heart Study has also produced multivariable risk profiles for estimation of occurrence of intermittent claudication, the cardinal clinical manifestation of peripheral artery disease.[18] The major cardiovascular risk factors have been shown to predict intermittent claudication better than they predict CHD.[34] Modification of these independent risk factors may reduce the probability of developing peripheral artery disease and, in turn, improve cardiovascular morbidity and mortality. Using this risk formulation, an individual's probability of developing intermittent claudication can be readily assessed on routine examination and laboratory analysis performed in a physician's office. The information needed, aside from age and sex, are blood pressure, cholesterol, blood glucose level, history of cigarette smoking, and presence of CHD. As for other atherosclerotic cardiovascular disease outcomes, the risk of intermittent claudication varies over a wide range depending on the burden of the aforementioned risk factors. Cigarette smoking substantially escalates the risk at any level of other risk factors (Figure 1-5). Multivariate risk formulation scores enable physicians to easily estimate the probability of developing peripheral

TABLE 1-7 Multivariate Risk Factors for Stroke from the Framingham Heart Study: Subjects Aged 55 to 84 Years*

Risk factor	Multivariate risk ratio	
	Men	**Women**
Age (10 years)	1.66	1.93
Systolic blood pressure (10 mm Hg)	1.91	1.68
Antihypertensive medication	1.39	—
Diabetes	1.40	1.72
Cigarette smoking	1.67	1.70
Cardiovascular disease	1.68	1.54
Atrial fibrillation	1.83	3.16
Left ventricular hypertrophy	2.32	2.34

*Each relative risk is adjusted for the effects of the other risk factors.

SOURCE: Adapted, with permission, from Wolf et al.[17]

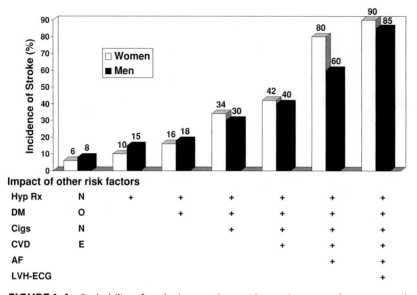

FIGURE 1-4 Probability of stroke (percent) over 10 years in men and women aged 70 years, systolic blood pressure, 160 mm Hg. *Key:* Hyp Rx, under antihypertensive therapy; CVD, cardiovascular disease; AF, atrial fibrillation; ECG-LVH, left ventricular hypertrophy by electrocardiogram. Reproduced, with permission, from Kannel WB. Blood pressure as a contributor to stroke. *Fed Pract* 1995;Nov(suppl):14–20.

artery disease based on data collected as part of a routine examination (Table 1-9). The risk profile can also be used to motivate patients to modify risk factors to avoid not only intermittent claudication, but also CHD, heart failure, and stroke.

HEART FAILURE PROFILE

Epidemiologic research pointed out that cardiac failure is a terminal condition with a survival experience little better than that of cancer. Once clinically overt, the median survival for Framingham Heart Study subjects with heart failure was only 1.7 years in men and 3.2 years in women, and sudden death was a common feature of this mortality.[35] Major independent contributors to the occurrence of heart failure have been identified and quantified by population research.[36] The relevant risk factors include electrocardiographic left ventricular hypertrophy, cardiac enlargement on chest x-ray, rapid heart rate, reduced vital capacity, presence of significant heart murmurs, CHD, and systolic blood pressure. Multivariate risk formulations for estimating the probability of developing heart failure from the burden of these risk factors were devised, based on Framingham Heart Study data.[36] By means of such multivariate risk assessments, it is possible to identify high-risk candidates for heart failure among those with either normal or impaired left ventricular function (Table 1-10).

REFINEMENTS IN RISK ASSESSMENT

Stimulated by epidemiologic research, further refinements in risk factor assessment for predicting and controlling atherosclerotic CVD have evolved. The atherogenic aspect of serum total cholesterol is now known to be its low-density lipoprotein component, and high-density lipoprotein, involved in removal of cholesterol from the tissues and inversely related to the incidence of CHD, is now an established protective factor.[37–39] The strength of the association between total cholesterol (TC) and CHD was found to decline with advancing age in men, but the TC/HDL-C ratio has been demonstrated to be a reliable predictor of CHD at all ages in both sexes (Table 1-11).[37,40] This ratio predicts equally well at TC values above and below 240 mg/dL. It is thus far the most efficient lipid profile predictor of CHD. A high triglyceride level accompanied by a reduced HDL-C often indicates the presence of atherogenic small, dense LDLs. Recently developed Framingham risk algorithms for short-term CHD risk show triglycerides to be an integral part of the risk prediction equation for women.[32] Assessment of hypertension now places greater emphasis on the systolic

TABLE 1-8   Stroke Risk Factor Prediction Chart

Men and Women		Points for each risk factor						
Age	SBP*		HYP Rx	Diabetes	Cigs	CVD	AF	LVH-ECG
		Men	No = 0	No = 0	No = 0	No = 0	No = 0	No = 0
54–56 = 0	95–105 = 0		Yes = 2	Yes = 2	Yes = 3	Yes = 3	Yes = 4	Yes = 6
57–59 = 1	106–116 = 1	Women	No = 0	No = 0	No = 0	No = 0	No = 0	No = 0
60–62 = 2	117–126 = 2		Yes = see below	Yes = 3	Yes = 3	Yes=2	Yes = 6	Yes = 4
63–65 = 3	127–137 = 3							
66–68 = 4	138–148 = 4							
69–71 = 5	149–159 = 5							
72–74 = 6	160–170 = 6							

For women, add points depending on SBP:

SBP	95–104	105–114	115–124	125–134	135–144	145–154
Points	6	5	5	4	3	3
SBP	155–164	165–174	175–184	185–194	195–204	
Points	2	1	1	0	0	

10-yr probability of stroke for point total

Men						Women						Average 10-y % probability		
Points	% Prob.	Points	% Prob.	Points	% Prob.	Points	% Prob.	Points	% Prob.	Points	% Prob.	Age	M	F
1	2.6	11	11.2	21	41.7	1	1.1	11	7.6	21	43.3	55–59	5.9	3.0
2	3.0	12	12.9	22	46.6	2	1.3	12	9.2	22	50.0	60–64	7.8	4.7
3	3.5	13	14.8	23	51.8	3	1.6	13	11.1	23	57.0	65–69	11.0	7.2
4	4.0	14	17.0	24	57.3	4	2.0	14	13.3	24	64.2	70–74	13.7	10.9
5	4.7	15	19.5	25	62.8	5	2.4	15	16.0	25	71.4	75–79	18.0	15.5
6	5.4	16	22.4	26	68.4	6	2.9	16	19.1	26	78.2	80–84	22.3	23.9
7	6.3	17	25.5	27	73.8	7	3.5	17	22.8	27	84.4			
8	7.3	18	29.0	28	79.0	8	4.3	18	27.0					
9	8.4	19	32.9	29	83.7	9	5.2	19	31.9					
10	9.7	20	37.1	30	87.9	10	6.3	20	37.3					

*SBP, systolic blood pressure; HYP Rx, under antihypertensive therapy; Diabetes, history of diabetes; Cigs, smokes cigarettes; CVD, history of myocardial infarction, angina pectoris, coronary insufficiency, intermittent claudication, or congestive heart failure; AF, history of atrial fibrillation; LVH-ECG, left ventricular hypertrophy on ECG.

SOURCE: From the Framingham Heart Study and the American Heart Association.

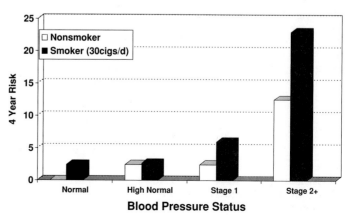

FIGURE 1-5   Estimated 4-year probability of intermittent claudication in 70-year-old men, Framingham Heart Study. *Key:* BP, blood pressure; NL, normal; Stg 1, stage 1 hypertension; Stg 2+, stage 2 or greater hypertension; CHD, coronary heart disease; cigs, cigarettes. (Reproduced, with permission, from Murabito J, et al.[18])

TABLE 1-9 4-Year Probability of Intermittent Claudication for Persons Aged 45 to 84 Years: Framingham Heart Study

Point Score	0	1	2	3	4	5	6	7
Age (y)	45–49	50–54	55–59	60–64	65–69	70–74	75–79	80–84
Sex	Female			Male				
Cholesterol (mg/dL)	<170	170–209	210–249	250–289	>289			
Blood pressure	Normal	High–normal	Stage 1		Stage 2+			
Cigarettes per day	0	1–5	6–10	11–20	>20			
Diabetes	No					Yes		
CHD	No					Yes		

4-y probability of intermittent claudication by point score total

Points	% Prob.	Points	% Prob.		Average	4-y	% Prob.
					Age	Men	Women
10–12	1	23	10		45–54	0.9	0.4
13–15	2	24	11		55–64	2.1	1.2
16–17	3	25	13		65–74	2.5	1.5
18	4	26	16		75–84	1.9	1.1
19	5	27	18				
20	6	28	21				
21	7	29	24				
22	8	30	28				

SOURCE: Reproduced, with permisson, from Murabito et al.[18]

TABLE 1-10 Heart Failure Risk Profile: Global Risk Assessment of Men with Hypertension, Coronary or Valvular Heart Disease: Framingham Study 38-year Follow-up*

Risk Factor	Points									
	0	1	2	3	4	5	6	7	8	9
Age (y)	45–49	50–54	55–59	60–64	65–69	70–74	75–79	80–84	85–89	90–94
Systolic BP (mm Hg)	<120	120–139	140–169	170–189	190–219	>219				
Heart rate (BPM)	<55	55–64	65–79	80–89	90–104	>104				
LVH-ECG	No				Yes					
Coronary disease	No								Yes	
Valve disease	No					Yes				
Diabetes	No	Yes								

Points	4-y Prob.	Points	4-y Prob.	Points	4-y Prob.	Points	4-y Prob.	4-y Incidence per 100 person-exams		
								Age	Men	Women
5	1	16	8	24	30	28	49	45–54	1.97	1.02
10	2	18	11	25	34	29	54	55–64	3.14	1.76
12	3	20	16	26	39	30	59	65–74	4.80	3.04
14	5	22	22	27	44			75–84	9.45	5.29
								85–94	12.95	9.87

*Age regression: 37% increment/decade.

SOURCE: Reproduced, with permission, from Kannel WB, et al.[36]

TABLE 1-11   Development of CHD by Total/HDL-C Ratio According to Age: Framingham Heart Study 16-Year Follow-up

	Total/HDL-C ratio (Quintile 5/Quintile 1)			Total cholesterol (≥240 mg/dL vs <200 mg/dL)	
	49–59 y	60–69 y	70–81 y	35–64 y	65–94 y
Men	3.4*	2.9*	2.3*	1.9†	1.2
Women	3.7*	6.7*	3.3*	1.8‡	2.0

*.01 < P < .05.
†P < .001.
‡.001 < P < .01.

blood pressure and isolated systolic hypertension as a hazard for all cardiovascular sequelae of hypertension.[41] The additional potential utility of pulse pressure,[42] ambulatory blood pressure monitoring, and circadian blood pressure variation is currently under investigation.

Interest in diabetes now focuses on lesser degrees of glucose intolerance and the influence of this condition as an ingredient of an insulin resistance syndrome.[43] Epidemiologic obesity research now emphasizes the importance of patterns of obesity and, in particular, abdominal obesity.[44] It is now regarded as a component of an insulin resistance or *metabolic* syndrome comprising dyslipidemia, hypertension, abnormal lipoprotein lipase, hyperinsulinemia, and abdominal obesity. A high triglyceride to HDL-C ratio in obese persons usually indicates the presence of insulin resistance. A clinically useful definition of the metabolic syndrome has recently been proposed by the NCEP-ATP-III[33] and is described in more detail in Chapter 9. Although measures of general obesity (eg, body mass index), abdominal obesity, triglycerides, physical activity, and family history of premature CHD are not included in most of these risk algorithms, the clinician should be reminded that this does not negate their potential significance in contributing to CHD risk, nor negate the importance of their control.

The Framingham Study data were recently used to develop a simplified coronary disease prediction model building on the blood pressure and lipid categories recommended for risk assessment and treatment by JNC-V and NCEP-ATP-II.[19,35] The utility and accuracy of the blood pressure, cholesterol, and LDL-C recommended categories for multivariable CHD prediction was evaluated. The accuracy of this more categorical approach was comparable to that of CHD prediction using the variables in a continuous graded fashion. Electrocardiogram-detectable left ventricular hypertrophy (ECG-LVH) was not included in this risk formulation because of the variation in criteria used for its detection. New guidelines for risk assessment and treatment designate as CHD equivalents: diabetes, other atherosclerotic CVD, and multiple risk factors imposing a 20% or greater 10-year risk of CHD.[35]

NEWER RISK FACTORS

There is general agreement on the established cardiovascular risk factors (Table 1-12), and epidemiologic research continues to identify or evaluate additional risk factors that contribute to the occurrence of atherosclerotic CVD and warrant further clarification (Table 1-13).[45] A variety of lipid measurements now available to researchers await long-term evaluation to determine whether they should be included in vascular disease risk formulations. Subgroups of HDLs and LDLs have been shown to be associated with CHD, but the utility of these refinements over the standard lipoprotein determinations is not established.[43–46] Similarly, increased lipoprotein (a) has been shown to be associated with greater risk of CHD and stroke in some, but not all studies.[50–52] Though elevated triglyceride has

TABLE 1-12   Established Cardiovascular Disease Risk Factors

Nonmodifiable factors	Modifiable risk factors	
Age	Cigarette smoking	Inactivity
Sex	Obesity	Diabetes
Family history	Hypertension	Total cholesterol
	HDL-C	LDL-C

SOURCE: Adapted from Hoeg.[45]

TABLE 1-13 Proposed Cardiovascular Disease Risk Factors

Proatherogenic	Prothrombogenic	Antiatherogenic
LDL-C	Plasminogen	HDL-C
Hypertension	Fibrinogen	Apolipoprotein A1
Insulin resistance	Factor VII	Lecithin-cholesterol
Acyl transferase		
Liporotein particle subspecies	PAI-1	Hepatic lipase
Homocysteine	Lipoprotein(a)	LDL receptor
Lipoprotein particle oxidation		VLDL receptor
		Apolipoprotein E

SOURCE: Adapted from Hoeg.[45]

consistently been found to be associated with an increased risk of coronary disease, the predictive power is often attenuated or lost when HDL-C and diabetes are taken into account. However, a recent meta-analysis of 17 studies by Hokanson and co-workers strongly suggests an independent incremental risk of CHD in relation to triglyceride.[53] It appears that this relationship is strongest when the LDL-C/HDL-C or TC/HDL-C ratio is high.[54]

The antioxidants vitamins E and C and β-carotene have been found in observational studies to be associated with reduced risk of CHD.[55–57] However, clinical trials have not always confirmed the observational data.[55] Homocysteine, an amino acid regulated by vitamins B_{12}, B_6, and folate, is another factor that has been associated with CHD and atherosclerosis, and higher concentrations of homocysteine were found in 29% of Framingham Heart Study participants and in 5% of subjects in the Physicians' Health Study.[58–60] Although elevated homocysteine has been found to be associated with an increased risk of CVD, no clinical trials have thus far tested whether reducing homocysteine by supplementation with these vitamins decreases the risk of atherosclerotic events.

Inflammatory mechanisms are now believed to be important in atherogenesis and precipitation of clinical coronary events.[61] C-reactive protein (CRP), an acute-phase reactant, known for decades to increase markedly in response to inflammation, has been shown to predict cardiovascular events in patients with CHD.[62] High-sensitivity testing for minor elevations suggests that CRP elevation within the "normal range" may not only be a marker for chronic inflammation, but also may be involved in atherogenesis. There is the possibility that CRP testing may enhance CHD prediction because it has been reported to be a stronger predictor of CHD events than is LDL-C, and adds prognostic information to that conveyed by the Framingham multivariable risk

score.[62] However, the predictive power of CRP has been shown in some studies to be markedly diminished when adjusted for other risk factors.[61]

In addition to *diabetes*, insulin resistance, hyperinsulinemia, and glucose intolerance are reported to be atherogenic.[43,63] In the Framingham Study, diabetes is associated with a doubled CHD risk in men and a tripled CHD risk in women.[64] A greater proportion of the general population has impaired glucose tolerance, the prevalence of which increases with age. Glycosylated hemoglobin, which reflects glycemic status over 6 weeks, is related to the prevalence of CVD in Framingham Study men and women.[65] A few prospective investigations have reported that insulin levels, fasting or 2 hours after a standard oral glucose load, may help predict CHD over and above traditional risk factors.[66–68] Diabetes has been designated as a CHD equivalent in guidelines for treatment of dyslipidemia.[33]

Hematologic factors such as the leukocyte count and plasma fibrinogen may indicate active, fissuring atherosclerotic lesions that are undergoing an inflammatory response to cholesterol deposition and subintimal hemorrhage.[69–70] Prospective epidemiologic investigation indicates that CHD incidence is related to the antecedent leukocyte count within what is regarded as its normal range.[66,68] In the Framingham Study, a one-standard-deviation increment in the leukocyte count in men was associated with a 42% increase in CHD incidence that in men, but not women, was confined to nonsmokers.[71] The impact on risk rivals that of other major risk factors.

Fibrinogen, within the normal range, is another well-documented major independent risk factor in several population studies, including Framingham.[72,73] The occurrence of CVD, including coronary disease, stroke, and peripheral artery disease, is increased in men and women with high-normal fibrinogen. The excess risk persists on adjustment for the standard risk factors, and fibrinogen adds to the risk of diabetes, hypertension, blood lipids, and cigarette smoking.[74]

Other hematologic factors have been linked to the development of CHD. These include factor VII and von Willebrand factor antigen, but their utility is not clear.[75,76] Fibrinolytic mechanisms are also under investigation because decreased fibrinolysis may promote fibrin deposition, unstable plaques, and increased CHD rates in persons with advanced lesions. Among these are PAI-1 and tPA antigen, which have been reported to be associated with development of myocardial infarction and angina.[77] The disproportionate rate of myocardial infarction that occurs between 6 AM and noon may be related to transiently increased blood coagulability and platelet aggregation.[78,79]

EPIDEMIOLOGIC PITFALLS

Epidemiologic investigation can suggest guilt only by association. Hence it should come as no surprise that clinical trial results sometimes differ from those of observational population studies. An identified risk factor is not necessarily causal, even if biologically plausible.

Clinical and epidemiologic investigations have documented that the risk of coronary disease increases substantially after menopause, and this was attributed largely to the loss of the cardioprotective effects of estrogen. In a review of the epidemiologic evidence in 1991, Stampfer and Colditz pointed out that five *hospital-based* case–control studies yielded largely null results, whereas six *population-based* studies found a decreased relative risk of myocardial infarction for hormone users, and one that was statistically significant. Of 16 *prospective* studies, least subject to selection bias, 15 found decreased relative risks, in most instances statistically significant.[80] The Framingham Study alone in 1985 showed no benefit and a possible increased risk for stroke among women reporting estrogen use, despite a more favorable initial cardiovascular risk profile.[81] Increased myocardial infarction rates were observed in this observational study, particularly in those who smoked: and in nonsmokers, estrogen use was associated only with excess stroke incidence. The Framingham Study investigators concluded, "the potential drawbacks of postmenopausal estrogen therapy should be considered carefully before recommending widespread use." Stampfer and Colditz concluded that, overall, the bulk of the evidence strongly supports a protective effect of estrogens that is unlikely to be explained by confounding factors, and they estimated a relative risk of 0.50–0.56.[80]

Two recent trials of the efficacy of hormone replacement therapy have challenged our understanding of the alleged protective role of estrogen against cardiovascular disease in postmenopausal women. It came as a surprise to most when the first large-scale randomized trial, the Heart and Estrogen/Progestin Replacement Study (HERS), reported that hormone replacement therapy did not reduce the risk of recurrent coronary disease events.[82] Based on the negative findings, the AHA recommended that hormone replacement therapy not be initiated solely for secondary prevention of CVD.[83] In 2002, the Women's Health Initiative Randomized Controlled Trial tested the risks and benefits of the most commonly used combined estrogen/progestin hormone preparation in a *primary* prevention trial.[84] After 5.2 years of follow-up, the trial was stopped because of excessive occurrence of breast cancer and evidence of risks exceeding benefits for CHD, stroke, pulmonary embolism, colorectal cancer, hip fracture, and death from other causes. There was a 29% excess risk of CHD and 41% excess of stroke, and a twofold excess of pulmonary embolism. It was concluded that this hormone therapy should not be used for primary prevention of CHD.

After it was determined that vitamins C, E, and β-carotene have antioxidant properties, observational epidemiologic investigations in the Nurses Health Study and Health Associates Study were undertaken to examine their relationship to the rate of development of coronary heart disease.[55–57] Greater vitamin E intake among participants of the Health Professionals Study was found to be significantly associated with a reduced risk of CHD.[57] However, a trial of low-dose vitamin E supplementation in Finnish smokers did not reduce the CHD rate and two large trials of β-carotene supplementation gave no indication of cardioprotection.[85]

Overweight and obesity are highly prevalent metabolic disorders in the United States that have increased to epidemic proportions. Epidemiologists in the 1960s concluded, on the basis of prospective epidemiologic data, that the role of obesity in CVD was equivocal.[86,87] In the 1970s, it was commonly held that obesity per se did not contribute to development of CVD.[88] After longer periods of observation and consideration of patterns of obesity, corpulence is no longer considered innocent. The clear and consistent demonstration that changes in weight are accompanied by corresponding changes in atherogenic risk factors revealed the true role of adiposity as a cardiovascular hazard.[89] Recent prospective epidemiologic investigation demonstrates a continuous, graded influence of the body mass index (BMI) on CHD incidence, even at below-average weights. Central, abdominal, or visceral adiposity has been shown to be a predictor of CVD, independent of the general level of obesity. This variety of obesity promotes a cluster of atherogenic risk factors by inducing insulin resistance.

GLOBAL RISK ASSESSMENT AND PREVENTION

The risk major of atherosclerotic CVD can now be estimated conditional on the level of a set of modifiable risk factors that can be objectively and conveniently determined from ordinary office procedures and simple laboratory tests. Categorical risk assessment according to the number of arbitrarily defined risk factors can identify persons at high risk, but they often falsely reassure persons who are at high risk because of multiple marginal abnormalities. The segment of the population with such clusters of "borderline" abnormalities yields most of the cardiovascular events, so it is important not to overlook them. Global risk formulations facilitate quantified estimation of the probability of an event that can be compared with the average for persons of the same age.

Epidemiologic data demonstrating the hazards of even mild degrees of hypertension, dyslipidemia, and glucose intolerance have prompted trials to determine the benefits of treating these levels of risk factors for primary and secondary prevention.[23,25,90–94] The effectiveness of antihypertensive treatment for stroke and coronary disease is now well substantiated for persons with isolated systolic hypertension, and the efficacy of treatment of dyslipidemia, including low HDL-C and elevated LDL-C, is well documented for lipid abnormalities extending down into the high-normal range.[90–94]

Controlled clinical trial evidence of the benefits of exercise, weight control, and smoking abatement in CVD risk reduction is lacking. However, these interventions are likely to be worthwhile in helping to control the major risk factors. Optimal preventive management, as well as risk assessment, should be multifactorial. Preventive population strategies should include public health measures that improve the distribution of risk factors to more favorable average values, health education to enable people to protect their own health, and preventive medicine for high-risk candidates for CVD requiring drugs. Implementation of preventive measures such as diet modification, exercise, smoking abatement, and weight control requires behavior modification and community efforts to promote healthy lifestyles.

Despite the variety of therapies available and trial evidence of the benefit of treating hypertension and diabetes, these conditions remain highly prevalent and undertreated. In the United States, the compliance rate for statin therapy of dyslipidemia can be as low as 40% at 3 years.[95] Physicians are reported to obtain an LDL-C value on their high-risk CHD patients only 50% of the time.[96] Among the 51 million Americans who qualify for treatment of dyslipidemia, fewer than 18 million actually receive treatment.[97] Among those being treated 32 to 82% are reported to fail to achieve NCEP-recommended LDL-C goals due to noncompliance and inadequate therapy.[97,98]

More than 30% of hypertensive Americans are unaware of their problem, more than 40% remain untreated, and approximately 40% of men and 50% of women with known hypertension have pressures that exceed recommended values.[92] Among diabetics, 81% are not at the recommended systolic blood pressure goal. Consistent with data from elsewhere, control of systolic blood pressure (<140 mm Hg) in the Framingham Study participants on treatment (49%) is particularly poor compared with diastolic pressure (<90 mm Hg) control (83%). This poor control of systolic blood pressure in the Framingham Study was associated with obesity, older age, and left ventricular hypertrophy.[99] A general practice survey confirms that isolated systolic hypertension is the variety least likely to be treated[100] and, even when treated, is seldom reduced to the recommended goal.[101] This failure to reach the recommended goal is attributable, in part, to faulty selection and titration of medication and, in part, to difficulty in reaching recommended targets with standard therapy.[102] Unfortunately, more than one antihypertensive agent is usually required to adequately control blood pressure. About one half of patients prescribed antihypertensive medication stop taking it by the end of the first year.[103] Combination medication to control hypertension and dyslipidemia-correcting medication should help make comprehensive global risk reduction more feasible. Poor control of hypertension and dyslipidemia derives from several factors. The need for long-term adherence to treatment of an asymptomatic condition is always a problem. Patients seek a cure rather than control of their health problems. Occurrence or fear of adverse side effects in healthy persons is often a barrier to compliance. The high cost of medications is frequently a problem for the elderly living on small, fixed incomes. Patients are often on a number of other medications that may interfere or increase the burden of taking the recommended medications. There is fear that vigorous control of lipids and blood pressure may be dangerous or cause intolerable side effects.

Preventive cardiology is presently only obliquely recognized by reimbursement through Medicare. There are no comprehensive primary prevention programs offered through Medicare, and secondary prevention is provided through cardiac rehabilitation programs that are limited to symptomatic patients and those with a recent myocardial infarction or coronary artery bypass surgery. The benefits offered by HMOs derive from these Medicare guidelines. Awaiting overt evidence of cardiovascular disease before initiating treatment of hypertension, dyslipidemia, or glucose intolerance is no longer justified. In some respects, occurrence of symptoms may be more properly regarded as a medical failure than the first indication for treatment. As suggested by Dean Chobanian of Boston University, "[i]ntensified efforts to alter modifiable cardiovascular risk factors such as blood pressure, lipoprotein levels, smoking, blood glucose levels, weight and physical activity levels must become a national priority."[104]

CHALLENGES FOR THE TWENTY-FIRST CENTURY

Whereas CHD and stroke mortality have declined in the past several decades, the incidences of initial occurrence of these diseases and of heart failure have not shown a similar decrease. The result of these trends is an increasing pool of persons with established CHD, stroke, and heart failure. The long-term outlook of persons with any one of these conditions is guarded because they are at high risk of atherosclerotic disease in other vascular territories.[105] Persons with intermittent claudication are at a two- to fourfold increased risk of CHD, stroke, or heart failure. After initial myocardial infarction, there is a three- to sixfold increased risk of heart failure and stroke. After a stroke, the risk of heart failure and CHD is increased twofold.[105] In view of this, we need a better understanding of the reason for the difference in the impact of the major risk factors on the various clinical atherosclerotic disease outcomes. It seems evident, however, that the measures taken to prevent one CVD outcome should carry a bonus in preventing the others.

We need to seek ways to maintain the rate of decline in coronary and stroke mortality that has been observed since 1968 but seems to be slackening lately. There is also a need to reverse the upward trend in CHD mortality in Eastern Europe and the former Soviet Union and to prevent the almost inevitable rise in CHD mortality in Asia as Asian nations westernize their diet and lifestyle.

Campaigns focusing on improving awareness and treatment of major risk factors are needed. An investigation of population awareness and control of hypercholesterolemia in 1995 found that only 42% of hypercholesterolemic subjects were aware of their condition and only 4% were both treated and controlled.[106] With respect to high blood pressure, the most recent data indicate that 69% are aware of their condition, 58% are on treatment, but only about 60% of men and less than 50% of women on treatment are adequately controlled.[92,107] After the recent implementation of the NCEP, the levels of treatment and control of hyperlipidemia have improved, but they are substantially lower than those for hypertension.[108] Further improvement in the detection and control of these and other major risk factors, such as diabetes and cigarette smoking, especially in younger persons, is clearly needed, particularly in populations where cardiovascular risk is high or in those whose access to preventive services and health care is inadequate.

During this first decade of the twenty-first century, we are facing an emerging epidemic of diabetes. Although improved medications for controlling glucose levels, dyslipidemia, hypertension, and proteinuria are being introduced, we must find a way to control the epidemic of obesity, which substantially contributes to the risk of diabetes and its CVD sequelae. We need better methods to prevent unwanted weight gain and to achieve sustained weight reduction safely in those who have become obese. Abdominal obesity is an important feature of the insulin resistance or *metabolic* syndrome that appears to be an important determinant of the tendency for multiple atherogenic risk factors to cluster. We need a validated operational definition of this syndrome, so that its prevalence, determinants, and cardiovascular hazards can be better understood. There is a need to determine whether drug-specific correction of insulin resistance improves the cardiovascular risk profile and, in turn, the atherosclerotic CVD outlook.

With an aging population of increased size, it will be necessary to keep the elderly healthy enough to remain in the work force. More attention needs to be focused on the efficacy and cost effectiveness of risk factor control in the older segment of the population. More information is needed on the benefits of exercise in the elderly so as to determine the optimal frequency and duration of exercise and the minimal threshold for cardiovascular benefit in this age group.

Epidemiologic data have established that women undergoing menopause promptly face a threefold escalation in their risk of CHD over that of women who remain premenopausal at the same age. Although results from observational studies suggest a protective role for estrogen replacement therapy for CVD, trials such as the Women's Health Initiative and HERS indicate no benefit and possibly some harm. At present, vigorous control of the risk factors known to reduce the female CVD advantage over men is indicated for women undergoing menopause.

Clinical trials have demonstrated the efficacy of correcting dyslipidemia in persons with CHD and those at high risk of developing it. Aggressive reduction of LDL-C levels in high-risk individuals holds promise in reducing morbidity and mortality from CHD in the twenty-first century. The reduction in clinical events has far exceeded expectations from the amount of regression of lesions induced, suggesting that lipid-lowering drugs may be stabilizing lesions that would otherwise be likely to undergo thrombotic occlusion. More research is needed to gain insight into the ways to stabilize lesions. There is also a need to further clarify the role of small, dense LDLs, lipoprotein (a), oxidized LDLs, and triglycerides in atherogenesis and the value of correcting these lipid abnormalities.

There is a continuing need to identify additional risk factors that could explain those CVD events occurring in patients whose predicted risk of CVD may be low and/or who do not exhibit one of the established risk factors. Approximately one fourth of patients with premature CVD do not exhibit one of the standard risk factors. More investigation is needed to establish the role of newly discovered risk factors, such as homocysteine, lipoprotein oxidation, antioxidant vitamins, infectious agents such as *Chlamydia*, acute-phase reactants, lipoprotein (a), apoprotein E isoforms, and insulin resistance, in accelerating atherogenesis and to determine the preventive efficacy of correcting them. Clotting factors, indicators of inflammation, and other infectious agents also deserve more attention. The importance of genetic determinants of risk factors and susceptibility to their influence need further investigation. Further research is needed to determine whether left ventricular hypertrophy, an ominous harbinger of cardiovascular events, can be better reversed by specific antihypertensive agents and by correction of ischemia and valve deformity and to determine the clinical benefit of such reversals.

Although multivariate risk assessment is vital, its effectiveness may also be enhanced with better screening modalities, particularly for subclinical atherosclerosis. The potential use of measurements from echocardiography and carotid ultrasound to further stratify risk needs to be reviewed, as do emerging technologies such as computed tomography and magnetic resonance imaging, although the initial investment, procedural costs, and practical application of all these vary substantially.

Enough information is available about major correctable risk factors for CVD to implement effective public health and physician-administered preventive measures designed to continue the decline in cardiovascular mortality. We have done well in establishing guidelines for most risk factors and disease conditions, but have failed to adequately implement these guidelines in our health care settings. Reorganization of the health care delivery system is needed to place more emphasis on prevention, with reward structures in place for providers who are successful in identifying and controlling their patients at risk. More effort is needed to alter the ecology to one more favorable to cardiovascular health, so that the average blood pressures, lipid values, body weights, and glucose values are at more optimal levels. To achieve this, it will be necessary to alter the national diet, engineer physical activity back into daily life, curb unrestrained weight gain, and get rid of the cigarette. The less affluent segment of the public needs to be better educated about risk factors so that they can take measures to protect their own health.

A major challenge for the future is to implement cost-effective comprehensive preventive programs for initial and recurrent CVD events using multivariate risk assessment to target high-risk candidates so that fewer have to be treated to prevent one event. Because indiscriminate therapy focused on single risk factors requires that hundreds must be treated to prevent one event, we must find better ways to promote multifactorial risk assessment to target hypertensive, dyslipidemic, and glucose-intolerant persons for long-term drug therapy. Only in this way will it be possible to avoid needlessly alarming or falsely reassuring possible candidates for atherosclerotic CVD. Because all atherosclerotic CVD events share most risk factors, and the fact that one cardiovascular event frequently leads to another, it is desirable to formulate a general cardiovascular risk profile. This was attempted in 1976 based on Framingham Study data then available and strongly suggested that atherosclerotic CVD in aggregate could be predicted with a standard set of risk factors.[15] One general CVD risk formulation could identify persons at high risk of coronary disease, stroke, peripheral artery disease, and heart failure as efficiently as the disease-specific risk profiles.

Adoption of the multifactorial approach to risk evaluation and reduction will offer the best opportunity for primary and secondary prevention of CVD. Risk factor modification in the public at large and among those at high risk offers the best chance for reducing the prevalence of CHD. Although the concept of cardiovascular risk factors is well established in clinical practice, the emergence of more sensitive and specific screening methods for atherosclerosis, as well as newer risk factors, will further refine our ability to accurately identify and manage those at increased risk for CHD. There is clearly more to be learned about the evolution of atherosclerotic disease, but we must press on, applying more vigorously the valuable information we already have which should enable us to further curb the epidemic of atherosclerotic CVD. We must come to regard the occurrence of an overt atherosclerotic event as a medical failure, rather than the first indication for treatment.

REFERENCES

1. Kannel WB, Dawber TR, Kagan A, et al. Factors of risk in development of coronary heart disease—six year follow-up experience: the Framingham Study. *Ann Intern Med* 1961;55: 33–50.

2. Report of Intersociety Commission for Heart Disease: Resources for primary prevention of atherosclerotic disease. *Circulation* 1984;70(suppl A):155A–205A.

3. Dawber TR. *The Framingham Study: The Epidemiology of Atherosclerotic Disease.* Cambridge. MA: Harvard University Press; 1980:14–29.

4. Gordon T, Kannel WB. Premature mortality from coronary heart disease: the Framingham Study. *JAMA* 1971;215:1617–1625.

5. Kannel WB, Abbott RD. Incidence and prognosis of unrecognized myocardial infarction: an update on the Framingham Study. *N Engl J Med* 1984;311:1144–1147.

6. Lloyd-Jones DM, Larson MG, Beiser A, Levy D. Lifetime risk of developing coronary heart disease. *Lancet* 1999;353:89–92.

7. Wilking SVB, Belanger AJ, Kannel WB, et al. Determinants of isolated systolic hypertension. *JAMA* 1988;260:3451–3455.

8. Kannel WB, Gordon T, Schwartz MJ. Systolic versus diastolic blood pressure and risk of coronary heart disease: the Framingham Study. *Am J Cardiol* 1971;27:335–345.

9. Gotto AM Jr, LaRosa JC, Hunninghake D, et al. The cholesterol facts: a summary of the evidence relating dietary fats, serum cholesterol and coronary heart disease. A joint statement by the American Heart Association and the National Heart, Lung and Blood Institute. *Circulation* 1990;81:1721–1733.

10. Grundy SM, Goodman DS, Rifkind BM, et al. The place of HDL in cholesterol management: a perspective from the National Cholesterol Education Program. *Arch Intern Med* 1989;149:505–510.

11. Castelli WP, Garrison RJ, Wilson PWF, et al. Coronary heart disease incidence and lipoprotein levels: the Framingham study. *JAMA* 1986;256:2835–2838.

12. Rosenberg L, Kaufman DW, Helmrich SP, et al. The risk of myocardial infarction after quitting smoking in men under 55 years of age. *N Engl J Med* 1985;313:1511–1514.

13. Kannel WB, McGee DL, Castelli WP. Latest perspectives on cigarette smoking and cardiovascular disease: the Framingham Study. *J Cardiac Rehab* 1984;4:267–277.

14. Kannel WB, Dannenberg AL, Levy D. Population implications of left ventricular hypertrophy. *Am J Cardiol* 1987;60:851–931.

15. Kannel WB, McGee DL, Gordon T. A general cardiovascular risk profile: the Framingham Study. *Am J Cardiol* 1976;38:46–51.

16. Anderson KM, Wilson PWF, Odell PM, et al. An updated coronary risk profile: a statement for health professionals. *Circulation* 1991;83:357–363.

17. Wolf PA, D'Agostino RB, Belanger AJ, et al. Probability of stroke: a risk profile from the Framingham study. *Stroke* 1991;3:312–318.

18. Murabito JM, D'Agostino RB, Silberschatz H, Wilson PWF. Intermittent claudication: a risk profile from the Framingham Heart Study. *Circulation* 1997;96:44–49.

19. Wilson PWF, D'Agostino RB, Levy D, et al. Prediction of coronary heart disease using risk factor categories. *Circulation* 1998;97:1837–1847.

20. Khot UN, Khot MB, Bajzer CT, et al. Prevalence of conventional risk factors in patients with coronary heart disease. *JAMA* 2003;290:898–904.

21. Greenland P, Knoll MD, Stamler J, et al. Major risk factors as antecedents of fatal and nonfatal coronary heart disease events. *JAMA* 2003;290:891–897.

22. Manson JE, Tosteson H, Ridker PM, et al. The primary prevention of myocardial infarction. *N Engl J Med* 1992;326:1406–1416.

23. Kannel WB. Contribution of the Framingham study to preventive cardiology. *J Am Coll Cardiol* 1990;15:206–211.

24. Kannel WB, Sytkowski PA. Atherosclerosis risk factors. *Pharmacol Ther* 1987;32:207–235.

25. Grundy SM, Galady GJ, Criqui MH, et al: AHA Scientific Statement: primary prevention of coronary heart disease: guidance from Framingham. *Circulation* 1998;97:1876–1887.

26. Kannel WB, McGee DL: Diabetes and glucose tolerance as risk factors for cardiovascular disease: the Framingham Study. *Diabetes Care* 1979;2:120–126.

27. Manson JE, Colditz GA, Stampfer MJ, et al: A prospective study of maturity-onset diabetes and risk of coronary heart disease and stroke in women. *Arch Intern Med* 1991;151:1141–1147.

28. Brand RJ, Rosenman RH, Sholz RI, Friedman M. Multivariate prediction of coronary heart disease in the Western Collaborative Group Study compared to the findings of the Framingham Study. *Circulation* 1976;53:348–355.

29. Leaverton PE, Sorlie PD, Kleinman JC, et al. Representativeness of the Framingham risk model for coronary heart disease mortality: a comparison with a national cohort study. *J Chronic Dis* 1987;40:775–784.

30. McGee D, Gordon. The results of the Framingham Study applied to four other S.S.-based studies of cardiovascular disease. In: Kannel WB, Gordon, eds. *The Framingham Study: An Epidemiological Investigation of Cardiovascular Disease.* Section 31. U.S. Dept of Health Education and Welfare publication 76-1083. Bethesda, MD: U.S. Government Printing Office; 1976.

31. The Multiple Risk Factor Intervention Trial Group. Statistical design considerations in the Multiple Risk Factor Intervention Trial (MRFIT). *J Chronic Dis* 1977;30:261–275.

32. D'Agostino RB, Grundy S, Sullivan LM, Wilson P, for the CHD Risk Prediction Group. Validation of the Framingham risk prediction scores: results of a multiple ethnic group investigation. *JAMA* 2001;286:180–187.

33. Executive Summary of the Third Report of the National Cholesterol Education Program (NCEP) Expert Panel on Detection, Evaluation, and Treatment of High Blood Cholesterol in Adults (Adult Treatment Panel III). *JAMA* 2001;285:2486–2497.

34. Kannel WB, McGee DL. Update on some epidemiologic features of intermittent claudication: the Framingham Study. *J Am Geriatr Soc* 1985;33:13–18.

35. Ho KK, Anderson KM, Kannel WB, et al. Survival after the onset of congestive heart failure in Framingham Heart Study subjects. *Circulation* 1993;88:107–115.

36. Kannel WB, D'Agostino RB, Silbershatz H, et al. Profile for estimating risk of heart failure. *Arch Intern Med* 1999;159:1197–1204.

37. Kannel WB. High-density lipoproteins: epidemiologic profile and risks of coronary artery disease. *Am J Cardiol* 1983;52:9B–12B.

38. Expert Panel on Detection, Evaluation and Treatment of High Blood Cholesterol in Adults: summary of the second report of the NCEP Expert Panel (Adult Treatment Panel II). *JAMA* 1993;269:3015–3023.

39. NIH Consensus Development Panel. Triglyceride, high-density lipoprotein and coronary heart disease. *JAMA* 1993;269:505–510.

40. Wilson PWF, Kannel WB. Hypercholesterolemia and coronary risk in the elderly: the Framingham Study. *Am J Geriatr Cardiol* 1993;2:52–56.

41. Kannel WB, Dawber TR, McGee DL, et al. Perspectives on systolic hypertension: the Framingham Study. *Circulation* 1980;61:1179–1182.

42. Franklin SS, Gustin W, Wong ND, et al. Hemodynamic patterns of age-related change in blood pressure: the Framingham Heart Study. *Circulation* 1997;96:308–315.

43. Reaven GM. Banting Lecture 1988: role of insulin resistance in human disease. *Diabetes* 1988;37:1595–1607.

44. Bjorntorp P. Regional patterns of fat distribution. *Ann Intern Med* 1985;103:994–995.

45. Hoeg JM. Evaluating coronary heart disease risk: tiles in the mosaic. *JAMA* 1997;277:1387–1390.

46. Buring JE, O'Conner GT, Goldhaber SZ, et al. Decreased HDL$_2$ and HDL$_3$ cholesterol, Apo A-I and Apo A-II and increased risk of myocardial infarction. *Circulation* 1992;85:22–29.

47. Wilson PWF. Relation of high-density lipoprotein subfractions and apolipoprotein isoforms to coronary disease. *Clin Chem* 1995;41:165–169.

48. Austin MA, Hokanson JE, Brunzell JD. Characterization of low-density lipoprotein subclasses: methodologic approaches and clinical relevance. *Curr Opin Lipid* 1994;5:395–403.

49. Campos H, Genest JJ Jr, Blijlevens E, et al. Low-density lipoprotein particle size and coronary artery disease. *Arterioscler Thromb* 1992;12:187–195.

50. Ridker PM, Stampfer MJ, Hennekens CH. Plasma concentration of plasma lipoprotein (a) and the risk of future stroke. *JAMA* 1995;273:1269–1273.

51. Ridker PM, Hennekens CH. Lipoprotein (a) and risks of cardiovascular disease. *Ann Epidemiol* 1994;4:360–362.

52. Schaefer EJ, Lamon-Fava S, Jenner JL, et al. Lipoprotein (a) levels and risk of coronary heart disease in men: the Lipid Research Clinics Coronary Primary Prevention Trial. *JAMA* 1994;272:999–1003.

53. Hokanson JE, Austin MA, Edwards KL. Hypertriglyceridemia as a cardiovascular risk factor independent of high-density lipoprotein: a meta-analysis of population-based prospective studies. *J Cardiovasc Risk* 1996;3:213–219.

54. Ginsberg HN. Hypertriglyceridemia: new insights and new approaches to pharmacologic therapy [editorial]. *Am J Cardiol* 2001;87:1174–1180.

55. Hennekens CH, Buring JE, Peto R. Antioxidant vitamins: benefits not yet proved [editorial]. *N Engl J Med* 1994; 330:1080–1081.

56. Stampfer MJ, Hennekens CH, Manson JE, et al. Vitamin E consumption and risk of coronary heart disease in women. *N Engl J Med* 1993;328:1444–1449.

57. Rimm EB, Stampfer MJ, Aschero A. Vitamin E consumption and risk of coronary heart disease in men. *N Engl J Med* 1993; 328:1450–1456.

58. Genest JJ Jr, McNamara JR, Salem DN, et al. Plasma homocysteine levels in men with premature coronary artery disease. *J Am Coll Cardiol* 1990;16;1114–1119.

59. Selhub J, Jacques PF, Boston AG, et al. Association between plasma homocysteine and extracranial carotid stenosis. *N Engl J Med* 1995;332:286–291.

60. Stampfer MJ, Malinow MR, Willett WC, et al. A prospective study of plasma homocysteine and risk of myocardial infarction in US physicians. *JAMA* 1992;268:877–881.

61. Mosca L. C-reactive protein–to screen or not to screen. *N Engl J Med* 2002;347:1615–1616.

62. Ridker PM, Rifai N, Rose L, et al. Comparison of C-reactive protein and low density lipoprotein cholesterol levels in the prediction of first coronary events. *N Engl J Med* 2002;347:1557–1565.

63. Zavaroni I, Bonora E, Pagliara M, et al. Risk factors for coronary artery disease in healthy persons with hyperinsulinemia and normal glucose tolerance. *N Engl J Med* 1989;320:702–706.

64. Wilson PWF, Kannel WB. Epidemiology of hyperglycemia and atherosclerosis. In: Ruderman N, Williamson J, Brownlee M, eds. *Hyperglycemia, Diabetes, and Vascular Disease.* New York: Oxford University Press, 1992:21–29.

65. Singer DE, Nathan DM, Anderson KM, et al. Association of HbA1c with prevalent cardiovascular disease in the original cohort of the Framingham Heart Study. *Diabetes* 1992; 41:202–208.

66. Pyorala K. Relationship of glucose tolerance and plasma insulin to the incidence of coronary heart disease: results from two population studies in Finland. *Diabetes Care* 1979;2:131–141.

67. Fontbonne AM, Eschwege EM. Insulin and cardiovascular disease: Paris Prospective Study. *Diabetes Care* 1991;14:461–469.

68. Stout RW. Insulin and atheroma: 20-year perspective. *Diabetes Care* 1990;13:631–654.

69. Ernst E, Hammerschmidt DE, Bagge U, et al. Leukocytes and risk of ischemic diseases. *JAMA* 1987;257:2318–2324.

70. Fuster V, Badimon L, Badimon JJ, et al. The pathogenesis of coronary artery disease and the acute coronary syndromes (Part 1). *N Engl J Med* 1992;326:242–250.

71. Kannel WB, Anderson KM, Wilson PWF. White blood cell count and cardiovascular disease: insights from the Framingham Study. *JAMA* 1992;267:1253–1256.

72. Ernst E, Resch KL. Fibrinogen as a cardiovascular risk factor: a meta-analysis and review of the literature. *Ann Intern Med* 1993;118:956–963.

73. Kannel WB, Wolf PA, Castelli WP, et al. Fibrinogen and risk of cardiovascular disease: the Framingham Study. *JAMA* 1987;258:1183–1186.

74. Kannel WB, D'Agostino RB, Wilson PWF, et al. Diabetes, fibrinogen and cardiovascular disease: the Framingham experience. *Am Heart J* 1990;120:672–676.

75. Folsom AR, Wu KK, Shahar E, et al, for the Atherosclerosis Risk in Communities (ARIC) Study Investigators. Association of hemostatic variables with prevalent cardiovascular disease and asymptomatic carotid artery atherosclerosis. *Arterioscler Thromb* 1993;13:1829–1836.

76. Thompson SG, Kienast J, Pyke SD, et al, for the European Concerted Action on Thrombosis and Disabilities Angina Pectoris Study Group. Hemostatic factors and the risk of myocardial infarction or sudden death in patients with angina pectoris. *N Engl J Med* 1995; 332:635–641.

77. Ridker PM, Vaughan DE, Stampfer MJ, et al. Endogenous tissue-type plasminogen activator and risk of myocardial infarction. *Lancet* 1993;341:1165–1168.

78. Muller JE, Tofler GH. Circadian variation and cardiovascular disease. *N Engl J Med* 1991;325:1038–1039.

79. Tofler GH, Brezinski D, Schaefer AI, et al. Concurrent morning increase in platelet aggregability and the risk of myocardial infarction and sudden death. *N Engl J Med* 1987; 316:1514–1518.

80. Stampfer M, Colditz G. Estrogen replacement therapy for coronary heart disease: a quantitative assement of the epidemiologic evidence. *Prev Med* 1991;20:47–63.

81. Wilson PWF, Garrison RJ, Castelli WP. Postmenopausal estrogen use, cigarette smoking and cardiovascular disease. *N Engl J Med* 1985;313:1038–1043.

82. Hulley S, Grady D, Bush T, et al, for the Heart and Estrogen/progestin Replacement Sudy (HERS) Reserch Group. Randomized trial of estrogen plus progestin for secondary prevention of coronary heart disease in postmenopausal women. *JAMA* 1998;280:605–613.

83. Mosca L, Collins P, Heerington DM, et al. Hormone replacement therapy and cardiovascular disease: a statement for health care professionals from the American Heart Association. *Circulation* 2001;104:499–503.

84. Risks and benefits of estrogen plus progestin in healthy postmenopausal women: principal results from the Women's Health Initiative Randomized Controlled Trial Writing Group for the Women's Health Initiative investigators. *JAMA* 2002;288:321–333.

85. Hennekens CH, Buring JE, Manson JE, et al. Lack of effect of long-term supplementation with beta carotene on the incidence of malignant neoplasms and cardiovascular disease. *N Engl J Med* 1996;334:1145–1149.

86. Keys A. Overweight, obesity coronary heart disease and mortality. *Nutr Rev* 1980;38:297–307.

87. Mann GV. The influence of body weight on health (second of 2 parts). *N Engl J Med* 1974;291:226–232.

88. Barrett-Conner EL. Obesity, atherosclerosis and cardiovascular disease. *Ann Intern Med* 1985;103:1010–1019.

89. Ashley FW Jr, Kannel WB. Relation of weight change to changes in atherogenic traits: the Framingham Study. *J Chronic Dis* 1974;27:103–114.

90. Sacks FM, Pfeffer MA, Moye LA, et al, for the Cholesterol and Recurrent Events Trail Investigators. The effect of pravastatin on coronary events after myocardial infarction in patients with average cholesterol levels. *N Engl J Med* 1996;335:1001–1009.

91. Downs JR, Clearfield M, Weis S, et al, for the AFCAPS/TexCAPS Reseach Group. Primary prevention of acute coronary events with lovastatin in men and women with average cholesterol levels: results of AFCAPS/TexCAPS. *JAMA* 1998;279:1615–1622.

92. Hajjar I, Kotchen TA. Trends in prevalence, awareness, treatment, and control of hypertension in the United States, 1988–2000. *JAMA* 2003;290:199–206.

93. SHEP Cooperative Research Group. Prevention of stroke by antihypertensive drug treatment in older persons with isolated systolic hypertension: final results of the Systolic Hypertension in the Elderly Program (SHEP). *JAMA* 1991;265:3255–3264.

94. Staessen JA, Fagard R, Thijs L, et al. Randomized double-blind comparison of placebo and active treatment for older persons with isolated systolic hypertension. *Lancet* 1997;350:757–767.

95. Muhlstein J, Horne B, Blair T, et al. Usefulness of in-hospital prescription of statin agents after angiographic diagnosis of coronary artery disease in improving continued compliance and reduced mortality. *Am J Cardiol* 2001:257–261.

96. Frolkis JP, Zyzanski SJ, Schwarz JM, Suhan PS. Physician noncompliance with the 1993 National Cholesterol Education Program (NCEP-ATPII) guidelines. *Circulation* 1998;98: 851–855.

97. Hoerger TJ, Bala MV, Bray JW, et al. Treatment patterns and distribution of low-density lipoprotein cholesterol levels in treatment-eligible United States adults. *Am J Cardiol* 1998; 82:61–65.

98. Pearson TA, Laurora I, Chu H, Kafonek S. The Lipid Treatment Assessment Project (L-TAP): a multicenter survey to evaluate the percentages of dyslipidemic patients receiving lipid-lowering therapy and achieving low-density lipoprotein cholesterol goals. *Arch Intern Med* 2000;160:459–467.

99. Lloyd-Jones DM, Evans JC, Larson MG, et al. Differential control of systolic and diastolic blood pressure: factors associated with lack of blood pressure control in the community. *Hypertension* 2000;36:504–509.

100. Coppola WG, Whincup PH, Walker M, et al. Identification and management of stroke risk in older people: a national survey of current practice in primary care. *J Hum Hypertens* 1997;11:185–191.

101. Berlowitz DR, Ash AS, Hickey EC, et al. Inadequate management of high blood pressure in a hypertensive population. *N Engl J Med* 1998;339:1957–1963.

102. Bakris GL. Maximizing cardiorenal benefit in the management of hypertension: achieving blood pressure goals. *J Clin Hypertens* 1999;1:141–147.

103. Bloom BS. Continuation of initial antihypertensive medication after one year of therapy. *Clin Ther* 1998;20:671–681.

104. Chobanian AV. Control of hypertension-an important national priority. *N Engl J Med* 2001;345:534–535.

105. Cupples LA, D'Agostino RB, Kiely D. *The Framingham Heart Study. Section 35: An Epidemiological Investigation of Cardiovascular Disease. Survival Following Cardiovascular Events: 30-Year Follow-Up.* Bethesda, MD: National Heart Lung and Blood Institute; 1988.

106. Nieto FJ, Alonso J, Chambliss LE, et al. Population awareness and control of hypertension and hypercholesterolemia: the Atherosclerosis in Communities Study. *Arch Intern Med* 1995;155:677–684.

107. Chobanian AV, Bakris GL, Black HR, et al. The seventh report of the Joint National Committee on Prevention, Detection, Evaluation, and Treatment of High Blood Pressure: the JNC 7 Report. *JAMA* 2003;289:2560–2572.

108. Grundy SM. Cholesterol and coronary heart disease: the 21st century. *Arch Intern Med* 1997;157:1177–1784.

Global trends in cardiovascular disease: incidence and risk factors

2

Gregory L. Burke
Ronny A. Bell

KEY POINTS

- *Cardiovascular disease (CVD) is the leading cause of death in the United States and other countries, accounting for approximately 40% of all deaths. Evidence indicates that the burden of CVD is increasing among developing countries.*

- *Significant geographic variation exists in CVD morbidity, mortality, and risk factors as evidenced by data from World Health Organization Multinational Monitoring of Trends and Determinants in Cardiovascular Disease (WHO MONICA) Project.*

- *CVD mortality has been declining substantially in most countries, whereas Eastern European and Asian nations have had increases in CVD mortality.*

- *CVD risk factors such as hypertension, hypercholesterolemia, cigarette smoking, obesity, physical inactivity, and diabetes are very common in adult populations worldwide.*

- *Many CVD risk factors have been declining, consistent with improved awareness and medical care for these conditions, whereas other risk factors, such as physical inactivity, obesity, and diabetes are rapidly increasing.*

- *Primary and secondary prevention strategies by the medical care system in the United States and other developed countries have contributed to the recent decline in CVD mortality rates. A particular area of concern for the future is congestive heart failure.*

- *Future projections indicate that CVD will be the leading cause of death in both developed and developing regions of the world by the year 2020.*

- *In Western developed countries, specific steps should be taken to deal with the existing high burden of CVD. Primordial prevention should be emphasized, including increased physical activity, promotion of a heart-healthy diet, and a decreased prevalence of obesity*

Cardiovascular disease (CVD) continues to be the leading cause of death in the United States and other developed countries. More recently, evidence points toward an increasing burden from CVD in developing countries. Current projections suggest that overall CVD rates will continue to increase, and CVD will be the leading cause of death in both the developed and the developing world. The large global burden of CVD exists despite the availability of proven primary and secondary preventive strategies that have not been effectively disseminated. However, prior to implementing a large-scale CVD prevention program, it is imperative that key decision makers are aware of the scope of the problem. The purpose of this chapter is to provide an overview of the data on differences between populations and secular trends in CVD risk factors, morbidity, and mortality. Specifically, we present data across age, gender, and geographic entities, as well as provide a brief overview of recent time trends in CVD incidence and risk factors.

CVD MORBIDITY AND MORTALITY: RATES AND TRENDS IN THE UNITED STATES AND OTHER COUNTRIES

In the following section, we review recent, existing national and international data on CVD mortality and morbidity. The focus of this section is the current burden from CVD and recent trends in CVD events. The bulk of the US data were obtained from published reports of the National Center for Health Statistics (NCHS), the American Heart Association (AHA), and region-specific surveillance studies. International data were extracted primarily from World Health Organization (WHO) reports, as well as the World Health Organization Multinational Monitoring of Trends and Determinants in Cardiovascular Disease (WHO MONICA) Project.[1–6]

International comparisons of CVD morbidity and mortality

CVD (ICD-9 codes 390–450) is the leading cause of death in most countries, particularly in economically developed countries. Significant international variation in CVD mortality and morbidity has been documented from nation-specific data and in WHO MONICA communities. Figure 2-1 shows 1999 mortality rates for coronary heart disease (CHD) in 15 countries.[1] CHD death rates (per 100,000 population) among men aged 35 to 74 in these populations were highest in Eastern Europe and lowest in Asia, with an approximately eightfold variation

between the two regions. Among women aged 35 to 74, a similar picture of CVD death rates was observed, with an approximately sevenfold variation between the highest rates observed in Eastern Europe and lowest rates observed in Asia. Among these countries, the United States ranks seventh worst of the 15 for men and fifth worst for women.

Figure 2-2 shows 1999 mortality rates for stroke in 15 countries.[1] Stroke death rates (per 100,000 population) among men and women aged 35 to 74 in these populations were highest in Eastern Europe and Asia and lowest in Australia and the United States, with an approximately sixfold variation between the two regions. Among these countries, the United States ranks second best of the 15 countries for both men and women.

Data, including CVD morbidity from 36 WHO MONICA population sites in 1985 to 1987,[2] are presented in Figure 2-3 to describe the geographic variation of CVD events (defined as "definite" fatal, "probable" fatal, "unclassified," and "definite" nonfatal). For all sites, CVD event rates of 456 per 100,000 for men and 101 per 100,000 for women were observed. Population-specific event rates ranged from 915 per 100,000 in North Karelia, Finland, to 76 per 100,000 in Beijing, China, for men and from 256 in Glasgow, United Kingdom, to 30 in Catalonia, Spain, for women. Importantly, these data indicate an even greater heterogeneity in CVD burden across populations when nonfatal events are included.

CVD mortality in the United States

In the United States, about 1.4 million people died from CVD in 2000, representing approximately 40% of all deaths.[3] CVD is the overall leading cause of death in

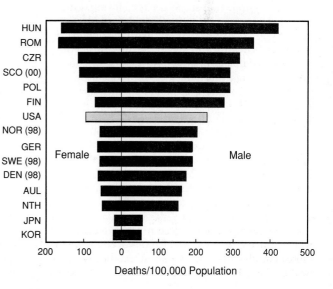

FIGURE 2-1 Age-adjusted death rates for coronary heart disease by country and sex, ages 35 to 74, 1999. SOURCE: National Heart, Lung, and Blood Institute.[1]

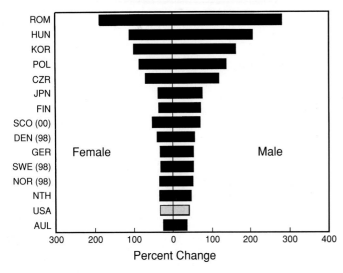

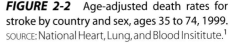

FIGURE 2-2 Age-adjusted death rates for stroke by country and sex, ages 35 to 74, 1999. SOURCE: National Heart, Lung, and Blood Insititute.[1]

the United States and is the leading cause of death in men greater than 45 years of age and in women greater than 65 years of age. In addition, CVD is the leading cause of death for all race/gender groups in the United States. Approximately 62 million Americans, or about 20% of the population, have some form of CVD, which accounted for about 6.3 million hospital discharges in 2000. More than half of CVD deaths are due to CHD and 18% to stroke. The economic costs of CVD in the United States are enormous, estimated to be $352 billion in 2000.[3]

Table 2-1 summarizes 2000 US data for all-cause and CVD mortality rates and years of potential life lost (YPLL) before the age of 75 by race/ethnicity group.[4] Overall, heart disease contributed to 253 deaths and 1271 YPLL lost prior to age 75 per 100,000 population, while stroke was associated with 61 deaths and 226 YPLL per 100,000 population. The greatest CVD burden in the United States was observed in the African-American population, with rates of heart disease mortality approximately 27% higher than those of non-Hispanic whites. This gap was even greater for stroke mortality rates, with rates for African-Americans 39% higher than those for non-Hispanic whites. Heart disease mortality rates were lowest for Asians/Pacific Islanders (145/100,000). Stroke mortality rates were lowest in American Indians/Alaska Natives (40 per 100,000) and Hispanics (39 per 100,000) (NCHS). YPLL lost prior to age 75 mirrored the mortality data, with African-Americans having the greatest amount of productive life lost from CHD and Asian-Americans having the least. YPLL lost prior to age 75 for stroke was highest for African-Americans and lowest in non-Hispanic whites (1.8-fold difference). Thus, substantial differences in CVD burden were observed across race/ethnic groups in the United States.

There are also substantial differences in CVD, ischemic heart disease, and stroke mortality within the United States. Table 2-2 summarizes 1999 death rates ranked by state from the highest to lowest incidence.[3] For CVD mortality, Mississippi had the highest rate (449.6/100,000), more than 66% higher than the rate of the lowest ranked state, Utah (269.8/100,000). For CHD, New York had the highest rate (247.8/100,000), more than double the rate of the lowest ranked state, Utah (117.6/100,000). South Carolina ranked the highest in stroke death rates (85.6/100,000), more than double that of New York (42.1/100,000), the lowest ranking state for stroke deaths. Although the specific factors responsible for the great variation in ischemic heart disease and stroke rates are unclear, these data may suggest where statewide prevention programs are most needed.

Secular trends in CVD mortality

Most industrialized nations have observed substantial reductions in CVD mortality since the 1960s, congruent with changes in major CVD risk factors (discussed in the next section). Among 15 countries (Figure 2-4), mortality rates for CHD in men and women aged 35 to 74 declined in 12 of the 15 countries from 1990 to 1999; this included an approximately 3% reduction per year for the United States.[1] Two Eastern European countries (Hungary and Romania) and Korea observed *increases* in CHD mortality, up to 13%.

Stroke mortality rates have also steadily declined in recent years.[1] Among 15 countries, 13 had average annual reductions in stroke mortality among men aged 35 to 74 from 1990 to 1999; only one country (Romania) had an increase in average annual stroke mortality during this period (approximately 6.0%) (Figure 2-5).

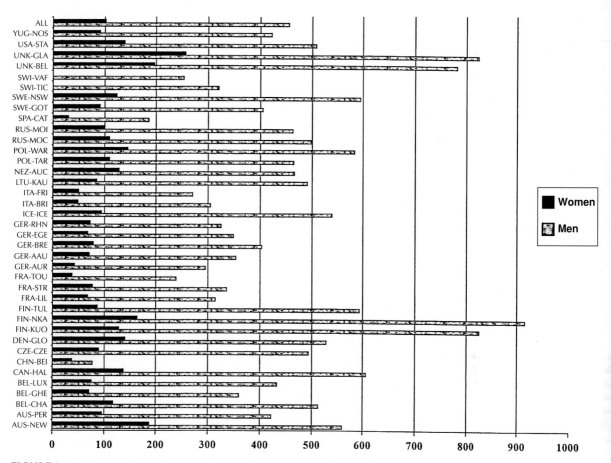

FIGURE 2-3 Coronary heart disease event rate (per 100,000 population) for 36 WHO MONICA communities. (Reproduced with permission from WHO Monica Project.[2]) *Key:* AUS-NEW, AUS-PER, Australia; BEL-CHA, BEL-GHE; BEL-LUX; Belgium; CAN-HAL, Canada; CHN-BEI, China; CZE-CZE, Czech Republic; DEN-GLO, Denmark; FIN-KUO, FIN-NKA, FIN-TUL, Finland; FRA-LIL, FRA-STR, FRA-TOU, France; GER-AUR, GER-AUU, GER-BRE, GER-EGE, GER-RHN, Germany; HUM-BUD, HUN-PEC, Hungary; ICE-ICE, Iceland; ITA-BRI, ITA-FRI, Italy; LTU-KAU, Lithuania; NEZ-AUC, New Zealand; POL-TAR, POL-WAR, Poland; RUS-MOC, RUS-MOI, RUS-NOC, RUS-NOI, Russia; SPA-CAT, Spain; SWE-GOT, SWE-NSW, Sweden; SWI-TIC, SWI-VAF, Switzerland; UNK-BEL,UNK-GLA, UK; USA-STA, USA; YUG-NOS, Yugoslavia.

TABLE 2-1 US Mortality Rate and Years of Potential Life Lost Before Age 75 for Heart Disease and Stroke, 2000

Race/gender group	All causes		Diseases of the heart		Cerebrovascular disease	
	Mortality rate*	YPLL[†]	Mortality rate	YPLL	Mortality rate	YPLL
All Persons	872	7695	253	1271	61	226
American Indian/Alaska Native	697	9472	165	1244	40	239
Asian/Pacific Islander	507	3929	145	596	53	209
Black	1130	13177	327	2302	82	513
Hispanic	586	6284	165	816	39	208
Non-Hispanic white	362	6972	258	1184	59	185

*Age-adjusted mortality rate per 100,000 population.
[†]Years of potential life lost before age 75 per 100,000 population under 75 years of age.

SOURCE: Adapted from *Health, United States, 2002*, Hyattsville, Md: National Center for Health Statistics; 2002.

TABLE 2-2 Age-Adjusted Death Rates for Total Cardiovascular Disease, Coronary Heart Disease, and Stroke by State in 1999

State	Rank	Total CVD Death rate	Percent change, 1989–1999	Rank	CHD Death rate	Percent change, 1989–1999	Rank	Stroke Death rate	Percent change, 1989–1999
Alabama	46	401.7	−12.9	20	171.6	−24.3	46	72.4	−17.2
Alaska	4	282.1	−22.6	3	125.8	−36.9	43	70.7	−3.6
Arizona	15	308.6	−14.5	25	179.0	−20.3	10	56.1	−2.3
Arkansas	45	401.1	−7.5	32	195.1	−18.8	51	80.0	−4.2
California	28	339.3	−19.2	34	198.3	−24.7	29	63.3	−19.3
Colorado	6	284.0	−17.3	7	136.4	−34.9	11	57.0	−5.8
Connecticut	16	311.2	−15.7	21	171.6	−22.8	4	50.1	−12.6
Delaware	30	345.3	−20.8	42	208.9	−26.6	6	50.4	−21.5
District of Columbia	38	368.5	−16.7	28	186.7	−2.9	8	52.2	−24.9
Florida	22	325.5	−13.9	36	200.2	−19.6	7	51.5	−11.8
Georgia	42	390.8	−14.2	19	171.1	−28.5	47	73.6	−15.4
Hawaii	3	280.9	−13.0	2	122.4	−26.5	28	63.2	−9.8
Idaho	11	307.1	−16.5	11	156.4	−25.4	36	67.3	−9.0
Illinois	33	364.0	−18.6	40	203.0	−26.9	33	63.9	−10.1
Indiana	41	378.3	−14.8	35	198.3	−24.1	38	69.4	−12.5
Iowa	24	330.3	−14.1	33	195.8	−16.9	25	62.7	−6.7
Kansas	23	327.7	−14.8	13	158.8	−26.3	21	61.7	−6.0
Kentucky	48	407.6	−11.6	45	212.8	−20.9	45	71.0	−11.4
Louisiana	47	403.0	−17.7	38	202.4	−29.4	39	69.7	−12.5
Maine	25	331.4	−16.4	24	178.2	−25.9	31	63.4	−4.1
Maryland	29	344.8	−17.8	31	191.9	−21.4	26	63.1	−5.4
Massachusetts	8	299.6	−20.8	10	153.1	−31.5	5	50.3	−17.7
Michigan	40	376.9	−15.7	46	215.4	−27.1	30	63.3	−9.6
Minnesota	2	279.3	−22.4	4	129.7	−37.2	16	60.1	−15.6
Mississippi	52	449.6	−11.4	48	223.7	−21.7	44	70.8	−16.8
Missouri	44	392.8	−7.7	47	221.1	−14.7	34	66.1	−3.7
Montana	7	297.8	−15.3	5	129.9	−29.1	24	62.3	−5.6
Nebraska	19	321.1	−16.1	9	143.0	−31.8	18	60.6	−9.5
Nevada	34	364.2	−14.7	26	181.1	−23.1	19	60.7	2.6
New Hampshire	21	322.6	−15.5	27	186.0	−17.6	15	58.6	−7.9
New Jersey	27	338.4	−18.4	41	206.0	−24.9	2	47.5	−19.8
New Mexico	9	301.9	−14.9	16	167.6	−20.5	9	54.5	−1.9
New York	37	366.7	19.3	52	247.4	:22.1	1	42.1	−26.3
North Carolina	36	365.5	−16.9	29	190.4	−27.3	49	78.1	−11.4
North Dakota	20	321.7	−12.9	18	169.8	−19.0	32	63.4	−1.6
Ohio	39	372.3	−15.3	43	209.2	−24.1	23	62.1	−8.4
Oklahoma	51	416.5	−6.9	51	237.2	−9.4	40	69.8	−7.8
Oregon	13	308.0	−17.2	8	140.8	−34.3	50	78.6	5.9

(continued)

TABLE 2-2   (continued)

State	Total CVD			CHD			Stroke		
	Rank	Death rate	Percent change, 1989–1999	Rank	Death rate	Percent change, 1989–1999	Rank	Death rate	Percent change, 1989–1999
Pennsylvania	35	364.2	−16.4	39	202.6	−26.9	13	58.0	−10.3
Puerto Rico	5	283.8	—	6	133.2	—	14	58.5	—
Rhode Island	17	311.8	−20.7	44	211.2	−18.7	3	49.9	−13.6
South Carolina	43	392.7	−16.1	30	191.2	−25.3	52	85.6	−11.9
South Dakota	14	308.2	−19.7	23	174.0	−27.4	20	60.7	−6.0
Tennessee	49	408.1	−8.6	49	227.4	−15.6	48	78.0	−8.6
Texas	32	360.2	−12.5	37	201.4	−15.8	35	66.3	−8.1
Utah	1	269.8	−21.6	1	117.6	−34.8	17	60.2	−11.9
Vermont	10	304.5	−17.2	17	169.3	−24.7	12	57.7	−5.6
Virginia	31	347.4	−18.2	15	165.5	−28.1	41	69.8	−10.9
Washington	12	307.9	−19.0	14	162.8	−27.6	42	69.8	−5.1
West Virginia	50	413.4	−12.2	50	233.1	−19.8	27	63.1	−7.3
Wisconsin	26	333.9	−17.0	22	171.8	−31.1	37	67.9	−4.8
Wyoming	18	315.6	−11.9	12	158.1	−18.9	22	61.7	2.8
Total US		352.4	−15.7		195.6	−24.0		61.8	−9.5

*Total cardiovascular disease is defined as ICD-10 100-199, Coronary heart disease as ICD-10 120-125, and Stroke as ICD-10 160-169. (Reproduced with permission from the American Heart Association.[3])

Reductions during this period were greatest in the Czech Republic. Among women in this age group, 12 of the 15 countries observed reductions in average annual stroke mortality, ranging from an approximately 8.0% decline in the Czech Republic to an approximately 4% increase in Romania. In the United States, average annual reductions in stroke mortality during this period were less than 1% for both men and women.[1]

Changes in stroke attack rates for the 17 WHO-MONICA sites are illustrated in Figure 2-6. Among men aged 35 to 64, 13 sites observed reductions in average annual stroke attack rates (fatal and nonfatal) over 5- or 6-year periods from 1982 to1990.[5] Fifteen of seventeen sites reported average annual reductions in stroke attack rates for women. For men, the greatest decreases in stroke rates were observed in Novosibirsk, Russia (−6.5%), and Glostrup, Denmark (−4.6%). For women, even larger reductions were observed in some sites (Moscow, Russia, −13.8%; Kuopio Province, Finland, −9.4%; and Halle County, Germany, −8.3%). Five of the fifteen sites with reductions in annual stroke attack rates for women observed reductions of 4.0% or greater, whereas only two sites observed similar reductions for men.[5]

Table 2-3 summarizes the age-adjusted cause-specific mortality rates and the change from 1970 to 2000. There was a 52% overall reduction in CHD mortality from

1970 (698.9/100,000) to 2000 (341/100,000).[1] Even greater reductions were observed for stroke mortality during these periods (62% reduction).

Rosemond and colleagues examined trends in heart disease incidence and mortality across four race/gender groups (white men and women, black men and women) in four US communities (Forsyth County, NC; Jackson, MS; suburbs of Minneapolis, MN; Washington County, MD) from 1987 to 1994.[7] While all four groups had reductions in CHD mortality, the largest decreases in CHD mortality were observed among white males (average annual rate change of −4.7%), and the smallest decline in CHD mortality was observed for black men (average annual rate change of −2.5%). Average annual rates of hospitalization for first myocardial infarction actually increased during this period for black women (7.4%) and black men (2.9%) while remaining essentially unchanged for white men (−0.3%) or lower for white women (−2.5%). There was also evidence of an overall decrease in rates of recurrent myocardial infarction and improvement in survival after myocardial infarction.[7]

To summarize the CVD morbidity and mortality data, although most economically developed nations have had major reductions in CVD mortality and morbidity in the latter part of the twentieth century, there was still substantial heterogeneity in CVD rates and in

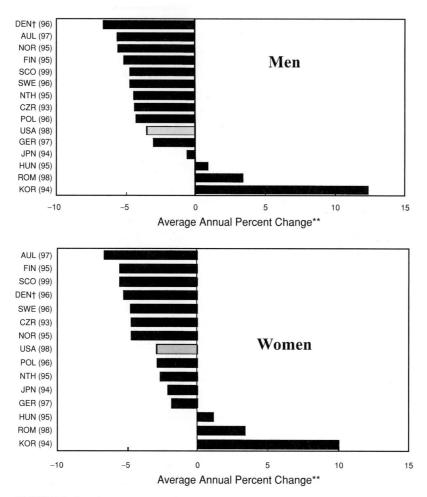

SOURCE: National Heart, Lung and Blood Insititute.[1]

the rates of reduction of CVD mortality between nations. Eastern European and Asian nations have had increases in CVD mortality. In the United States, rates of CVD mortality and morbidity continue to decline, although there is still significant variation between regions (states) and among race/ethnic groups in the burden of CVD, with African-Americans-bearing the greatest burden from CVD. These data suggest high-risk groups and at which preventive efforts and programs may be best targeted.

CVD RISK FACTORS: NATIONAL AND INTERNATIONAL RATES AND TRENDS

In this section, we present data on the prevalence of and trends in selected CVD risk factors (ie, cigarette smok-

ing, obesity, high blood pressure, high serum cholesterol, diabetes). These data are presented for both the United States and other countries as potential mediating factors for the previously described trends in CVD morbidity and mortality.

High blood pressure

Elevated systolic ($\geq$140 mm Hg) and diastolic ($\geq$90 mm Hg) blood pressure, or hypertension, greatly increases the risk of heart disease and stroke. The recently published Seventh Report of the Joint National Committee on Prevention, Detection, Evaluation, and Treatment of High Blood Pressure (JNC-7) recognizes an additional category of "prehypertension" (systolic blood pressure

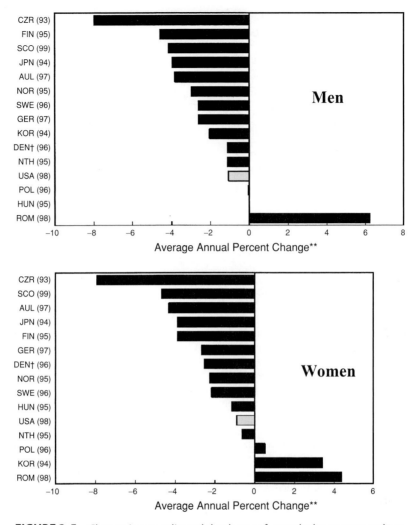

FIGURE 2-5   Change in age-adjusted death rates for stroke by country and sex, ages 35 to 74, 1990–1999. SOURCE: National Heart, Lung, and Blood Institute.[1]

120–139 mm Hg or diastolic blood pressure 80–89 mm Hg) to emphasize the role of increased risk of CVD associated with blood pressure elevated above 115/75 mm Hg.[8]

International data indicate a great deal of geographic variation in blood pressure.[9] Table 2-4 shows that, among adults aged 35 to 64 from WHO MONICA communities in the final wave of the survey, systolic blood pressure ranged, on average, from 121.1 mm Hg (Catalonia, Spain) to 142.2 mm Hg (North Karelia, Finland) among men, and from 117.0 mm Hg (Toulouse, France) to 138.5 mm Hg (Kuopio Province, Finland). During the approximately 10-year period from the initial to the final WHO MONICA surveys, the vast majority

of participating communities observed reductions in systolic blood pressure. The downward trends were greater for women than men, with nearly three fourths of the communities showing significant reductions for women. Only one of these communities had a significant increase in systolic blood pressure (Halifax, Canada).[10]

In the United States, approximately 50 million individuals have hypertension. Substantial reductions in hypertension were made from 1976–1980 to 1999–2000; prevalence rates among all persons declined from 39% in 1976–1980 to 24% in 1988–1994 (Table 2-5).[11] Percentage reductions were greatest during this period for non-Hispanic white men (45%) and lowest for African-American men and women (28% for both).

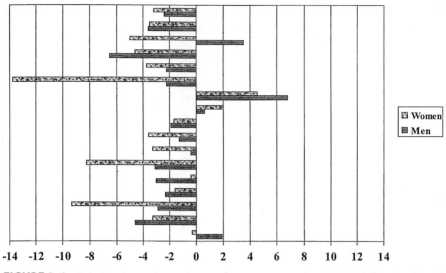

FIGURE 2-6 Relative change in stroke attack rates per year (per 100,000) for 17 selected WHO MONICA communities. (Reproduced with permission from WHO Monica Project.[5])

Slight increases in the prevalence of hypertension among Mexican-American men and women were observed during this period, although the prevalence of hypertension in this population remains lower than in other racial groups. More recently, however, a slight increase in hypertension has been observed. According to data from the National Health and Nutrition Examination Survey (NHANES) 1999–2000, the prevalence of hypertension among adults increased to approximately 29% in 1999–2000, an increase of about 4.0% from 1988–1994.[12] The most significant increases in this recent period are among older adults (+7.9%) and among women (+5.6%). Across the United States, there is significant variation in the prevalence of self-reported hypertension, ranging from 14.2% in Arizona to 33.5% in Mississippi (Table 2-6).[13]

Significant improvements in hypertension awareness, treatment, and control have been achieved in the United States since the mid-1970s.[8] Seventy percent of adults aged 18 to 74 were aware of hypertension in 1999–2000, up from 51% in 1976–1980. During the same period, treatment for hypertension increased from 31 to 59%, and control of hypertension increased from 10 to 34% (albeit much lower than the Healthy People 2010 goal of 50% of persons with hypertension being in control) (Figure 2-7). Improvements in treatment, however, have been due exclusively to improvements in men, and no significant improvements in treatment have been seen in

TABLE 2-3 Age-Adjusted Death Rates and Percent Change for All Causes and Cardiovascular Diseases, United States 1970 and 2000

Cause of death	Deaths/100,000 population		1970–2000 difference	Percent change
	1970	2000		
All causes	1222.6	872.4	−350.2	−28.6
CVD*	698.9	341.0	−357.9	−51.2
CHD	448.0	186.6	−261.4	−58.3
CHF	8.3	19.1	10.8	130.1
Stroke	147.7	56.8	−90.9	−61.5
Other CVD	94.9	78.5	−16.4	−17.3
Non-CVD	523.7	531.4	7.7	1.5

*Excludes congenital anomalies of the circulatory system.

SOURCE: *NHLBI 2002 Chart Book on Cardiovascular, Lung, and Blood Diseases.*[1]

TABLE 2-4 Prevalence of Major Cardiovascular Risk Factors for Men and Women Aged 35 to 64 Across WHO MONICA Communities

Country	Daily smokers (%) Men	Women	Systolic blood pressure (mm Hg) Men	Women	Total cholesterol (mmol) Men	Women	Mean BMI (kg/m^2) Men	Women
Australia								
Newcastle	21.8	16.5	130.9	127.1	5.76	5.58	27.9	27.3
Perth	24.2	12.5	134.0	125.4	5.53	5.36	26.4	26.1
Belgium								
Charteroi	48.3	29.3	130.7	124.9	6.18	6.10	27.1	26.8
Ghent	42.9	26.8	129.0	121.5	6.03	5.96	26.4	26.1
Canada, Halifax	31.7	24.9	129.5	125.7	5.64	5.77	27.5	27.6
China, Beijing	63.5	9.0	131.5	130.2	4.52	4.49	24.1	24.5
Czech Republic	38.7	23.0	137.2	133.8	6.17	6.14	27.6	27.8
Denmark, Glostrup	43.5	44.7	125.8	121.1	5.96	5.82	26.0	24.7
Finland								
Kuopio Province	30.4	13.4	140.2	138.5	6.01	5.75	27.3	27.1
North Karelia	27.0	11.5	142.2	137.2	6.03	5.75	27.5	27.1
Turku/Loimaa	29.4	18.7	139.5	135.1	5.88	5.72	27.1	26.2
France								
Lille	32.8	16.7	134.8	128.7	5.84	5.82	26.4	26.4
Strasbourg	23.3	14.9	135.3	127.0	6.03	5.91	27.3	26.2
Toulouse	24.2	21.6	124.9	117.0	5.82	5.65	26.1	24.5
Germany								
Augsburg (Rural)	24.3	15.7	135.6	128.8	6.09	5.93	27.8	26.8
Augsburg (Urban)	35.4	24.9	136.8	130.7	6.19	5.92	27.1	26.5
Breman	44.8	30.0	132.3	128.3	6.05	5.85	26.8	26.3
East Germany	31.7	16.8	140.3	138.0	6.16	6.03	26.7	26.4
Iceland Reykjavik	20.9	30.8	125.9	121.6	6.22	5.99	26.9	26.5
Italy								
Area Brianza	34.0	22.8	130.6	126.8	5.93	5.89	26.4	25.5
Fruili	29.0	22.2	139.5	134.3	5.87	5.66	26.9	25.8
Lithuania, Kaunas	34.9	4.4	137.4	134.2	5.96	6.19	27.1	28.0
New Zealand, Auckland	17.0	14.2	126.1	122.4	5.70	5.56	26.7	25.6
Poland								
Tarnobrzeg Voivodship	54.4	20.7	133.8	133.9	5.58	5.51	25.9	28.5
Warsaw	51.5	33.9	132.4	128.1	5.75	5.65	27.1	27.5
Russia								
Moscow (Control)	47.1	13.6	130.0	132.7	5.26	5.55	25.2	26.5
Moscow (Intervention)	41.8	14.2	133.4	132.9	5.38	5.51	25.6	26.3
Spain, Catalonia	41.2	15.0	121.1	118.3	N/A*	N/A	N/A	N/A
Sweden								
Gothenburg	25.5	28.6	133.9	129.5	5.57	5.44	26.2	24.9
Northern Sweden	21.0	28.2	130.0	125.9	6.28	6.12	26.4	25.7
Switzerland								
Ticino	35.5	26.2	131.7	124.0	6.54	6.19	26.5	25.3
Vaud/Fribourg	26.7	24.8	132.4	124.4	6.31	6.06	26.5	24.7
United Kingdom								
Belfast	28.8	24.6	134.9	129.5	5.90	5.91	26.3	25.6
Glasgow	41.1	41.0	132.6	126.2	6.05	6.08	26.8	26.9
USA, Stanford	23.0	18.7	128.6	119.4	5.40	5.31	26.9	26.6
Yugoslavia Novi Sad	48.6	29.8	136.1	137.0	6.37	6.19	27.3	27.8

* N/A not available.

SOURCE: Data reported for final WHO MONICA survey conducted in 1991–1997. Data available on the WHO MONICA website at www.ktl.fi/publications/MONICA.

TABLE 2-5 Estimated Prevalence of Overweight, Obesity, Hypercholesterolemia and Hypertension (Systolic > 140 mm Hg or Diastolic > 90 mm Hg) by Race/Ethnicity and Gender, NHANES II and NHANES III*

	Men			Women		
Group	NHANES II (1976–1980)	NHANES III (1988–1994)	% Change	NHANES II (1976–1980)	NHANES III (1988–1994)	% Change
Non-Hispanic whites						
Overweight	51.5	59.6	15.7	37.4	45.5	21.7
Obesity	12.0	20.0	66.6	14.8	22.4	51.4
High cholesterol	24.7	17.3	−30.0	28.3	20.2	−28.7
Hypertension	43.9	24.4	−44.5	32.1	19.3	−39.9
Non-Hispanic African-Americans						
Overweight	48.9	57.5	17.6	60.2	66.5	10.5
Obesity	15.0	21.3	42.0	30.0	37.4	24.7
High cholesterol	24.0	15.7	−34.6	24.9	19.8	−20.5
Hypertension	48.7	35.0	−28.2	47.6	34.2	−28.2
Mexican-American						
Overweight	59.7	67.1	12.4	60.1	67.6	12.5
Obesity	15.4	23.1	50.0	25.4	34.2	34.6
High cholesterol	18.8	17.8	−5.4	20.0	17.5	−12.5
Hypertension	25.0	25.2	0.8	21.8	22.0	0.9
All race-ethnic groups						
Overweight	51.4	59.3	15.4	40.8	49.6	21.6
Obesity	12.3	19.9	61.8	16.5	24.9	50.9
High cholesterol	24.6	17.5	−28.9	27.6	20.0	−27.6
Hypertension	44.0	25.3	−42.5	34.0	20.8	−38.9

*The following definitions were used: overweight (BMI $\geq$25 kg/m^2); obesity (BMI >30 kg/m^2); hypercholesterolemia ($\geq$6.2 mmol/L); hypertension (SBP $\geq$40 or DBP $\geq$90 mm Hg)

SOURCE: Adapted, with permission, from Flegal et al[14] and from National Center for Health Statistics.[11]

women during the past decade. Also, improvements in control of hypertension have been exclusively in non-Hispanic white men.[11,12]

Cholesterol

Elevated serum cholesterol is an established risk factor for CVD among middle-aged adults. International data from WHO-MONICA indicate significant geographic variation in mean cholesterol values, ranging from 4.5 mmol/L (173 mg/dL) in men and women in Beijing, China, to 6.4 mmol/L (246 mg/dL) and 6.2 mmol/L (239 mg/dL) among men and women in Ticino, Switzerland. The difference between the highest and lowest centers in mean cholesterol values is approximately 40 to 45% (Table 2–4).[9] The prevalence of diagnosed hypercholesterolemia ranges from 1 and 2.1% for men and women in Kaunus, Lithuania, to 42.4 and 35.0%, respectively, in North Karelia, Finland.

There have been consistent declines in population cholesterol levels in recent years in the WHO MONICA populations. From the initial to the final survey

periods, mean cholesterol values significantly declined in about half of the centers for both men and women, with the greatest of these differences observed in Lille, France, for men (a reduction of 0.7 mmol/L [27 mg/dL]), and Gothenburg, Sweden, for women (a reduction of 0.8 mmol/L [31 mg/dL]). The greatest increases during this period for both men and women were observed in Ticino, Switzerland (+0.97 mmol/L [37 mg/dL] for men, +0.76 mmol/L [29 mg/dL] for women).[10]

In the United States, approximately 105 million adults aged 20 years and older have high cholesterol (total cholesterol $\geq$200 mg/dL). The mean serum cholesterol value in the United States is approximately 203 mg/dL.[3] The prevalence of elevated serum cholesterol is slightly higher among women (20.0%) than men (17.5%), with very little variation across race/ethnic group. About 10% of US adolescents have elevated serum cholesterol. In the United States, the overall prevalence of elevated serum cholesterol declined by 28 to 29% from 1976 to 1994 (Table 2–5). Self-reported hypercholesterolemia in the US adult population ranges from 21.2% in Oklahoma to 37.1% in West Virginia (Table 2–6).[13]

TABLE 2-6   State-specific Prevalence of Risk Factors for Cardiovascular Disease Among Adults

State	High blood pressure*	Diabetes*	Obesity[†]	High cholesterol*	Cigarette smoking[‡]	Physical inactivity[§]
Alabama	31.2	9.6[#]	24.5	33.2	23.8	31.2
Alaska	21.3	4.0	22.1	29.0	26.2	21.1
Arizona	14.2	6.1	18.5	25.0	21.5	21.9
Arkansas	28.4	7.8	22.4	32.7	25.5	31.5
California	23.0	6.5	21.9	30.0	17.2	26.6
Colorado	22.2	4.6	14.9	25.9	22.3	19.2
Connecticut	20.4	6.3	17.9	28.0	20.6	24.0
Delaware	25.5	7.1	20.8	31.6	25.0	25.7
Florida	27.7	8.2	18.8	33.0	22.4	27.7
Georgia	26.3	6.9	22.7	29.2	23.7	27.3
Hawaii	22.7	6.2	17.9	27.6	20.5	18.9
Idaho	23.0	5.4	20.5	30.1	19.6	21.0
Illinois	26.7	6.6	21.0	31.8	23.7	26.5
Indiana	25.7	6.5	24.5	31.6	27.4	26.2
Iowa	24.2	5.7	22.5	31.7	22.1	25.9
Kansas	21.4	5.8	21.6	27.1	22.2	26.7
Kentucky	27.5	6.7	24.6	32.5	30.9	33.4
Louisiana	26.0	7.6	24.0	26.5	24.6	35.6
Maine	26.7	6.7	19.5	31.2	23.9	23.2
Maryland	24.5	6.9	20.5	30.6	21.1	24.2
Massachusetts	21.8	5.6	16.6	29.3	19.5	22.8
Michigan	25.2	7.2	25.0	32.9	25.6	23.4
Minnesota	22.0	4.4	19.9	31.3	22.2	17.1
Mississippi	33.5	9.3	26.5	30.1	25.3	33.4
Missouri	24.6	6.6	23.2	30.2	25.9	27.5
Montana	23.2	5.6	18.8	30.5	21.9	21.9
Nebraska	22.0	5.2	20.7	27.4	20.2	31.4
Nevada	29.1	5.7	19.5	35.1	26.9	22.6
New Hampshire	23.4	5.4	19.4	33.2	24.1	19.5
New Jersey	23.5	7.1	19.6	27.1	21.1	26.6
New Mexico	21.0	6.2	19.7	27.3	23.8	25.8
New York	22.9	6.6	20.3	28.6	23.2	28.7
North Carolina	24.1	6.7	22.9	31.2	25.7	26.4
North Dakota	26.1	5.1	20.4	30.6	22.1	23.2
Ohio	27.4	7.2	22.4	32.5	27.6	26.2
Oklahoma	20.9	7.7	22.6	21.2	28.7	32.8
Oregon	22.3	5.7	21.1	29.0	20.5	20.8
Pennsylvania	23.9	6.7	22.1	28.2	24.5	24.7
Rhode Island	22.9	6.4	17.7	28.6	23.9	24.9

(continued)

TABLE 2-6 (continued)

State	High blood pressure*	Diabetes*	Obesity†	High cholesterol*	Cigarette smoking‡	Physical inactivity§
South Carolina	25.2	8.1	22.5	27.3	26.0	26.4
South Dakota	23.8	6.1	21.2	29.4	22.3	25.4
Tennessee	28.6	7.7	23.4	29.1	24.4	35.1
Texas	24.2	7.1	24.6	30.9	22.4	27.1
Utah	21.3	4.3	19.1	28.4	**13.2**	**16.5**
Vermont	21.0	5.1	17.6	26.7	22.4	20.3
Virginia	23.5	6.0	20.9	31.1	22.5	23.2
Washington	22.1	5.7	19.3	28.3	22.5	17.1
West Virginia	31.0	8.8	25.1	37.1	28.2	31.7
Wisconsin	25.0	5.6	22.4	31.6	23.6	20.7
Wyoming	22.0	4.5	19.7	30.9	22.2	21.2

* Physician diagnosed.
†Obesity defined as BMI $\geq$30 kg/m^2.
‡Current smokers.
§No reported leisure time physical activity during previous month.
#Highest and lowest rates for each risk factor category in boldface.
SOURCE: 1999 (Hypertension and High Cholesterol) and 2001 (Obesity, Current Smoking, Physical Inactivity) Behavioral Risk Factor Surveillance System. Atlanta, Ga: Centers for Disease control and prevention.

Cigarette smoking

Tobacco use has been linked to CVD mortality and subclinical CVD. Data from WHO-MONICA populations indicate very high rates of cigarette smoking across the world[9] (Table 2–4). Population percentages of regular smokers (those reporting smoking cigarettes every day) for men aged 35 to 64 ranged from 17.0% in Auckland, New Zealand, to 63.5% in Beijing, China; in women the percentages ranged from 3.0% in Beijing, China, to 44.7% in Glostrup, Denmark. An additional 20 to 35%

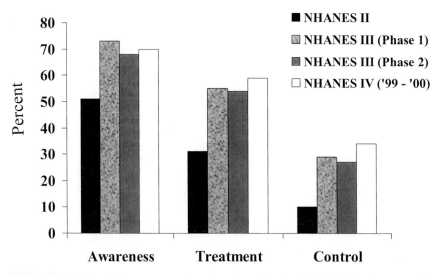

FIGURE 2-7 Trends in awareness, treatment, and control of high blood pressure in adults aged 18 to 74. (Data adapted from the National High Blood Pressure Education Program.[8])

of the populations in most of these sites were identified as occasional smokers and ex-smokers.

International data on secular trends in smoking prevalence in the WHO MONICA populations indicate significant declines in most areas.[10] For men, more than half of the communities observed significant reductions in smoking prevalence, with another one third observing nonsignificant reductions. Only one community, Beijing, China, observed a significant increase for men from baseline to final survey period. For women, only about one third of the communities observed a significant decline in smoking prevalence, whereas more than half had some degree of increase. For men and women, the greatest declines were observed in the Stanford, California, community (absolute decreases of −13.4% for men and −15.3% for women).

In the United States, approximately 49 million adults (25.7% of men and 21.0% of women) are considered current smokers.[3] Cigarette use is more common among persons of lower socioeconomic status across all race/ethnic groups for men and women. Between states, there is roughly a twofold variation in adult smoking prevalence, ranging from 13.2% in Utah to 30.9% in Kentucky. California, having an active tobacco prevention program funded by tobacco tax monies, reports a smoking prevalence of 17.2%, which is consistent with the declines observed in the Stanford cohort participating in the WHO MONICA survey (Table 2–6).[13]

Cigarette smoking has been declining in the United States over the last three decades. According to data from the National Health Interview Survey (Figure 2-8),[11] in 1974 the prevalence of current cigarette smoking among adults ≥25 years was 36.9%, a rate that is 63% higher than the 2000 estimate of 22.6%. Declines were greatest among black males; 53.4% of adult black men smoked in 1974, compared with 26.5% in 2000, a decrease of approximately 50%.

Obesity

Obesity is a well-established risk factor for CVD, and contributes to an increased prevalence of other CVD risk factors, such as hypertension, hypercholesterolemia, and diabetes mellitus. In the final wave of WHO MONICA surveys, mean body mass index (BMI) for men and women ranged from lows of 25.2 and 23.5 for men and women, respectively, in Moscow, Russia, and Gothenburg, Sweden, to highs of 27.9 and 28.5 for men and women, respectively, in Newcastle, Australia, and Tarnobrzeg Voivodship, Poland.[9]

Unlike some other CVD risk factors, BMI has been increasing in most communities across the world. Only three WHO MONICA communities observed reductions in BMI for men from initial to final survey periods, and about half showed significant increases. For women, about one half of the communities observed increases and one half showed decreases, and about half of each of these on both sides were significant.[10] The greatest increases for men and women were observed in Newcastle, Australia, and Halifax, Canada, respectively (+1.8 kg/m^2 in both communities).

In the United States, approximately 130 million adults are overweight (BMI 25.0–29.9) or obese (BMI ≥30). Obesity is more common among persons of lower socioeconomic status and among some ethnic minority

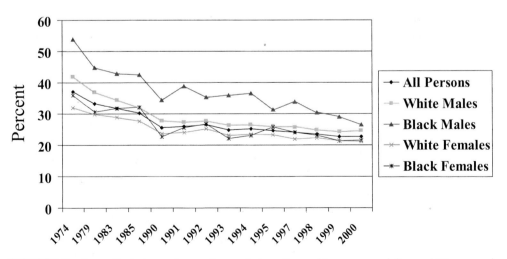

FIGURE 2-8   Age-adjusted prevalence of current cigarette smoking among adults aged 25 years and older, by race and sex, 1974–1995. SOURCE: *Health,* United States, 1998.[11]

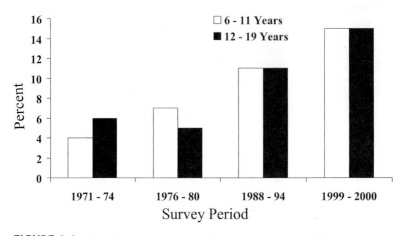

FIGURE 2-9 Prevalence and trends of overweight among US adolescents. (Adapted with permission from Ogden et al.[16])

groups. According to data from NHANES-III, the prevalence of overweight, varied across race/gender groups from 45.5% (white women) to 67.6% (Mexican-American women).[14] The prevalence of obesity, defined as BMI ≥30.0, ranged from 20% for non-Hispanic white men to 37.4% for African-American women. Among states, the prevalence of obesity ranges from 14.9% in Colorado to 26.5% in Mississippi. Similarly, there are great variations in the prevalence of no leisure time physical activity (during the past month), ranging from 16.5% in Utah to 36.5% in Louisiana (Table 2–6).[13]

These data also show that the prevalence of overweight and obesity is increasing. Flegal and colleagues observed an increase in the prevalence of overweight from 46.0 to 54.4% (an 18% increase) from NHANES-II (1976–1980) to NHANES-III (1988–1994),[14] while the prevalence of obesity increased from 14.5 to 22.5% (an increase of 55%) during the same period. The greatest increase in overweight was observed for white women (22% increase), and the greatest increase in obesity was observed for white men (66% increase) (Table 2–5).

In NHANES 1999–2000, the prevalence of obesity among adults increased to 31% and the prevalence of overweight or obesity increased to 64.5%.[15] These data also showed that rates of extreme obesity (BMI ≥40) increased from 2.9% in 1988–1994 to 4.7% in 1999–2000. In the Stanford, California, community participating in the WHO MONICA survey, mean BMI increased from the initial to final survey period by 1.0 kg/m2 for men and 1.9 kg/m2 for women.[9] More alarmingly, overweight is increasing dramatically among US children; from 1971–1974 to 1999–2000, the prevalence of overweight (BMI≥95th percentile for sex-specific

growth charts) more than tripled among children aged 6 to 11 years, increasing from 4 to 15% (Figure 2-9).[16]

Diabetes mellitus

Diabetes is now recognized as an established risk factor for CVD. Diabetes is now considered a CHD "risk equivalent," indicating that the risk of CHD for persons with diabetes is equivalent to that of persons with a history of CHD, and that such persons should be treated according to secondary prevention guidelines.[17] Diabetes increases the risk of CVD two- to fourfold, and CVD accounts for 60 to 70% of deaths among persons with diabetes.[18] Risk factors for type 2 diabetes (the most common form of diabetes) include: increasing age; family history of diabetes; overweight/obesity, particularly central adiposity; being a member of certain ethnic minority groups, especially African-Americans, Native Americans, and Hispanic-Americans; and a history of gestational diabetes.[19]

Approximately 17 million Americans, or 6.2% of the population, have diabetes (fasting glucose ≥126 mg/dL or on hypoglycemic medication), the majority of whom have type 2 diabetes.[19] About the same number have "prediabetes," which is defined as impaired fasting glucose based on fasting glucose values of 110 to 125 mg/dL or impaired glucose tolerance based on glucose values of 140 to 199 mg/dL after a 2-hour oral glucose tolerance test.[19,20] Diabetes in the United States ranges from 4.0% (Alaska) to 9.6% (Alabama) (Table 2–6).[13] About one million people aged 20 and older are diagnosed with diabetes each year. In 1995, an estimated 135 million adults worldwide had diabetes.[21]

The number of adults with diabetes has increased dramatically in recent years, consistent with increases in

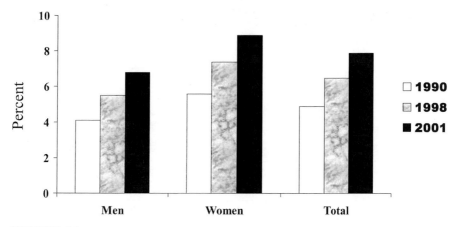

FIGURE 2-10   Time trends for diagnosed diabetes in the United States, overall and by sex, 1990, 1998, and 2001. (Adapted with permission from Mokdad et al.[22])

obesity and physical inactivity during that period. The prevalence of diabetes increased 33% from 1990 to 1998 and 61% from 1990 to 2001 (Figure 2-10).[22,23] Internationally, an estimated 300 million people will have diabetes by 2025, with a near tripling in prevalence in countries such as India, Mexico, and China.[21]

Metabolic syndrome

Some CVD risk factors (including abdominal obesity, impaired fasting glucose, low high-density lipoprotein [HDL] cholesterol, elevated triglycerides, and elevated blood pressure) occur in conjunction with each other in a condition recently referred to as the *metabolic syndrome*. This clustering greatly increases the risk of CVD. Definitions of the metabolic syndrome are provided by WHO and the Third Adult Treatment Panel (ATP-III)

(Table 2-7). An estimated 22% of the US population has metabolic syndrome.[24] The prevalence of metabolic syndrome increases with age, from approximately 6.7% among adults 20 to 29 years old to about 40 to 45% among adults older than 60. Mexican-Americans have the greatest likelihood of developing metabolic syndrome, with rates of 28.3 and 35.6% among men and women, respectively.[24]

MEDICAL CARE TRENDS

Substantial changes have occurred over the 1980s and 1990s in the medical care of CVD. Changes have occurred both in risk factor reduction in high-risk groups and in the treatment administered during and after acute CVD events. Over the past few decades, there have been

TABLE 2-7   Definitions of the Metabolic Syndrome: WHO and ATP-III

	WHO*	**ATP-III**[†]
Central adiposity	Waist-to-hip ratio >0.90 in men or >0.85 in women, or BMI >30 kg/m²	Waist circumference >102 cm in men and >88 cm in women
Lipids	Triglycerides ≥150 mg/dL, and/or HDL-C <35 mg/dL in men and <39 mg/dL in women	Triglycerides ≥150 mg/dL, HDL-C <40 mg/dL in men and <50 mg/dL in women
Blood pressure	≥160/90 mm Hg	≥130/85 mg/dL
Glucose	See below	≥110 mg/dL
Microalbuminuria	Urinary albumin excretion rate >20 μg/min, or albumin creatinine ratio >20 mg/g	N/A

*WHO defines metabolic syndrome as diabetes, impaired glucose tolerance, impaired fasting glucose, or insulin resistance plus two or more risk factors.
[†]ATP-III defines metabolic syndrome as three or more of the risk factors listed above. Hypertriglyceridemia and low HDL-C count as separate risk factors. Microalbuminuria is not included in ATP-III.

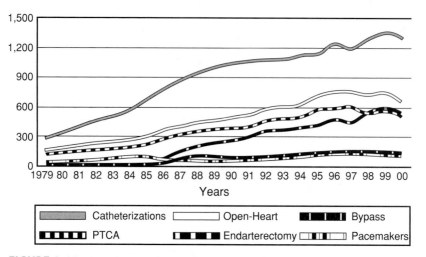

FIGURE 2-11 Trends in cardiovascular procedures in the United States. (Reproduced with permission from the American Heart Association.[3])

dramatic improvements in awareness, treatment, and control of hypertension and elevated serum cholesterol levels in the United States linked to changes in medical evaluation and treatment. Increased use of pharmacologic as well as nonpharmacologic modalities to reduce risk factors for CVD has been postulated to contribute to up to 50% of the observed decline in CHD mortality, and changes in medical care have been suggested to contribute to the remaining 50% of the decline. There remains, however, room for significant improvement regarding the identification, management, and control of those with elevated cholesterol levels[25,26] or hypertension.[27]

Substantial changes in medical care for CVD are illustrated in Figure 2-11, which documents trends in cardiovascular operations and procedures in the United States from 1979 to 2000.[3] Specifically, the number of cardiac catheterizations has increased from approximately 300,000 per year in 1979 to more than 1.3 million in 2000. Likewise, similar increases in the numbers of coronary artery bypass graft procedures, percutaneous transluminal coronary angioplasty procedures, pacemaker implantations, and carotid endarterectomies have occurred. An important area for future preventive efforts is related to the observed shifts in the manifestations of CVD. Specifically, there has been a great increase in the number of hospital discharges for congestive heart failure in the United States (Figure 2-12), from less than 100 cases per 100,000 in 1970 to nearly 600 per 100,000 in women and 400 per 100,000 in men by 2000.[3] This shift is likely due to both the increased pool of individuals surviving acute coronary events and the aging of the US population.

An important factor contributing to reductions in CVD burden in the United States is intervention targeted toward the high-risk subgroups that bear a disproportionate burden of the CVD morbidity/mortality. Thus, the adoption of primary and secondary prevention strategies by the medical care system in the United States and other developed countries has contributed to the recent decline in CVD mortality rates.

MIGRANT STUDIES

As has been shown above, substantial differences in CVD burden exist between different countries. These differences may be attributable to many factors, including country/regional differences in genotypes, gene–environment interactions, differences in health behaviors, and differences in the awareness and diagnosis of CVD. Studies of individuals that migrate from areas of low CVD prevalence to areas of higher CVD prevalence provide valuable evidence corroborating the observed ecological comparisons of countries.

Figure 2-13 shows mean cholesterol levels and corresponding CHD incidence rates among participants in the Ni-Hon-San Study, which contrasts Japanese individuals who remained in Japan with those who migrated to Hawaii and with those who migrated to the San Francisco Bay area. These data reveal that with respect to behavior leading to risk factors, migrants become more similar to the inhabitants of their newly adopted country.[28] Likewise, CVD morbidity and mortality in migrants to the US mainland were observed to approach levels observed in US Caucasian populations, rather than staying at the lower rates observed in Japanese who remained in Japan (Figure 2-13).

This information suggests that environmental factors likely play a key role in mediating some of the large

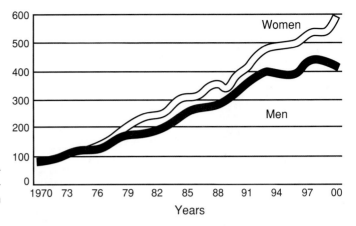

FIGURE 2-12   Hospital discharges for congestive heart failure in the United States. (Reproduced with permission from the American Heart Association.[3])

differences observed between countries. It is unlikely that individuals genetically predisposed toward an abnormal CVD risk profile and higher rates of CVD morbidity and mortality will migrate. Therefore, the adoption of new health behaviors by migrants likely mediates the majority of the increase in CVD burden. This is extremely important in the context of international CVD prevention. It suggests that increasing rates of CVD that are either currently occurring or projected to occur in countries with previously low rates of CVD are likely mediated to a great extent by the adoption of a more Westernized lifestyle.

FUTURE TRENDS IN CVD

Using currently observed trends in CVD as a predictor of subsequent trends and global disease burden is a challenging task. There are, however, a number of key points that can be elucidated with some confidence.

These include: (1) a continuing, unacceptably high burden of CVD is observed in developed countries; (2) the CVD burden is rapidly increasing in emerging economies; and (3) a large number of modifiable risk factors are known.

Projections done by Murray and Lopez indicate that CVD will be the leading cause of death in both developed and developing regions of the world by the year 2020.[29] These projections are shown in Figure 2-14, which contrasts the leading causes of death in developed and developing countries projected for 2020. In developed countries, ischemic heart disease and cerebral vascular disease are projected to account for nearly 37% of all-cause mortality, while they are projected to account for more than 25% of all-cause mortality in developing countries. Importantly, both the endemically high rates of CVD in developed countries and the rapidly increasing rates of CVD in developing

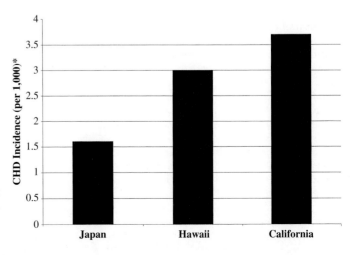

FIGURE 2-13   Incidence of coronary heart disease in middle-aged Japanese men residing in Japan, Hawaii, and California. (Adapted with permission from Robertson et al.[28])

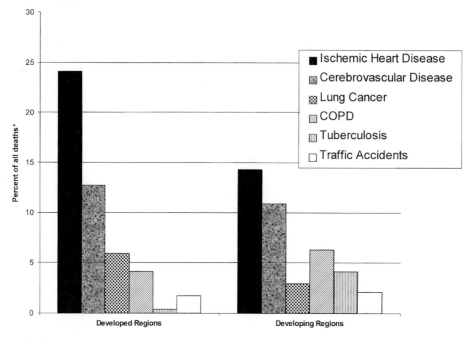

FIGURE 2-14 Projected leading causes of death in 2020 by region of the world.
SOURCE: Murray and Lopez.[29]

countries are linked to population levels of CVD risk factors.

The remarkable declines in cardiovascular mortality observed in Western countries over the last three decades are attributable in large measure to successful primary and secondary prevention of CVD. Despite these dramatic improvements in developed countries, substantial opportunities remain to reduce CVD burden further. For example, cigarette smoking continues to be a habit of more than 20 to 40% of adults in many of these countries. Further opportunities remain for identification and treatment of elevated blood pressure, dyslipidemia, and obesity. Although the prognosis following myocardial infarction and stroke has shown dramatic improvements, further advances in the early detection and early treatment of these conditions would certainly be of great benefit. Therefore, while huge improvements have been observed for CVD burden in developed countries, unacceptably large subgroups of the population remain at high risk for CVD events.

Conversely, in developing countries, less emphasis has been placed on chronic disease prevention due to economic pressures and the historically lower rates of CVD burden in these societies. Unless we are able to learn from the unfortunate lessons associated with the epidemic of CVD in developed countries, the developing countries will likely repeat the history of increasing CVD

burden that was seen in the developed countries during much of the twentieth century. As we have shown, many of these developing countries currently have high rates of cigarette smoking, increasing rates of obesity, and increasing rates of CVD risk factors. Ironically, it is the ongoing adoption of Western lifestyles that places individuals in the developing world at risk for CVD. Active efforts are required even to maintain current levels of physical activity and healthy components of traditional diets in these countries. In addition, the development of effective prevention strategies for CVD, such as risk factor screening/treatment and appropriate medical intervention for acute events, is necessary to reverse the current path toward increasing burden from CVD.

Important steps should be taken to reduce the future burden of CVD in both developing and developed countries. In Western developed countries, specific steps should be taken to deal with the existing high burden of CVD. Prevention of the development of risk factors in the first place (primordial prevention) should be emphasized, including increased physical activity, promotion of a heart-healthy diet, and a decreased prevalence of obesity. Interventions that focus on reducing the prevalence of traditional risk factors should continue to be emphasized as an important part of primary and secondary prevention efforts. Specific efforts should include: identification and treatment of hypertension; identification and treatment of dyslipidemia; and enhanced efforts to prevent smoking initiation and to encourage smoking cessation. Given the large number individuals with CVD in developed countries, secondary prevention efforts will be an important strategy to reduce subsequent CVD morbidity and mortality.

While the strategy in developing countries is similar, CVD interventions should be tailored to the specific needs of these emerging economies. In many of these settings, the current burden of CVD is relatively low but the potential for a substantially greater burden is high. In these countries, primordial prevention of CVD will be key. Encouraging the maintenance of heart-healthy habits such as physical activity, a traditional (and healthier) diet, and low rates of obesity is paramount. Given their lower prevalence of CVD, the developing countries secondary prevention efforts are minimal or nonexistent. However, secondary prevention programs need to be initiated with respect to traditional risk factors such as cigarette smoking. It is hoped the emerging economies will learn from the mistakes of developed countries and hence avoid the epidemic of CVD.

SUMMARY

Despite the fact that most countries have observed reductions in the prevalence of CVD risk factors in recent years, there remains tremendous international variation in the prevalence of major CVD risk factors as well as the incidence of CVD. Exceptions to the improving CVD risk profile are the increasing rates of obesity and diabetes, particularly in the more developed countries, which may have a deleterious impact on future trends in CVD incidence. The overall reductions in CVD risk factors may explain, in part, the concordant reductions in CVD mortality and morbidity in the United States and other developed countries.

This chapter has focused on describing recent trends in CVD in the United States and other countries. Substantial heterogeneity exists in CVD mortality between countries. Encouraging improvements have been observed over the last few decades in countries with the highest rates of CVD mortality, while less encouraging developments have occurred in regions of the world with lower rates of CVD, such as Eastern Europe. In addition, projections suggest that the burden of CVD will rapidly increase in developing countries in South Asia and the Pacific Rim. As would be expected, international trends in CVD morbidity and mortality are highly correlated with the presence or absence of health behaviors and traditional CVD risk factors.

Substantial opportunities exist to reduce further the burden in developed countries and prevent further increases in CVD in developing countries. Subsequent chapters in this book focus on effective strategies for CVD prevention in both clinical and community settings. Although implementation of these prevention and treatment strategies requires substantial allocation of human and monetary resources, the potential payoffs in reduction of death and disability make this effort essential.

REFERENCES

1. National Heart, Lung, and Blood Institute. *Morbidity and Mortality: 2002 Chartbook on Cardiovascular, Lung, and Blood Diseases.* Bethesda, Md: National Institutes of Health; 2002.

2. WHO MONICA Project. Myocardial infarction and coronary deaths in the World Health Organization MONICA Project. *Circulation* 1994;90:583–612.

3. American Heart Association. *Heart and Stroke Facts, 2003.* Dallas, Tex: American Heart Association; 2002.

4. Pastor PN, Makuc DM, Reuben C, Xia H. *Chartbook on Trends in the Health of Americans.* Health, United States, 2002. Hyattsville, Md: National Center for Health Statistics;2002.

5. WHO MONICA Project. Stroke trends in the WHO MONICA Project. *Stroke* 1997;28:500–506.

6. WHO MONICA Project. Ecological analysis of the association between mortality and major risk factors of cardiovascular disease. *Int J Epidemiol* 1994;23:505–516.

7. Rosamond WD, Chambless LE, Folsom AR, et al. Trends in the incidence of myocardial infarction and in mortality due to coronary heart disease, 1987 to 1994. *N Engl J Med* 1998;339:861–867.

8. National High Blood Pressure Education Program. *The Seventh Report of the Joint National Committee on Prevention, Detection, Evaluation, and Treatment of High Blood Pressure.* Bethesda, Md: US Department of Health and Human Services, National Institutes of Health, National Heart, Lung, and Blood Institute; May 2003. NIH publication 03-5233.

9. WHO Monica Project. Data available at: www.ktl.fi/publications/monica.

10. Evans A, Tolonen H, Hense H-W, et al, for the WHO MONICA Project. Trends in coronary risk factors in the WHO MONICA project. *Int J Epidemiol* 2001;30:S35–S40.

11. *Health, United States, 1998, with Socioeconomic Status and Health Chartbook.* Hyattsville, Md: National Center for Health Statistics; 1998.

12. Hajjar I, Kotchen TA. Trends in prevalence, awareness, treatment, and control of hypertension in the United States, 1988–2000. *JAMA* 2003;290:199–206.

13. Centers for Disease Control and Prevention. Data available at: www.cdc.gov/brfss.

14. Flegal KM, Carroll MD, Kuczmarski RJ, Johnson CL. Overweight and obesity in the United States: prevalence and trends, 1960–94. *Int J Obesity* 1998;22:39–47.

15. Flegal KM, Carroll MD, Ogden CL, Johnson CL. Prevalence and trends in obesity among US adults, 1999–2000. *JAMA* 2002;288:1723–1727.

16. Ogden CL, Flegal KM, Carroll MD, Johnson CL. Prevalence and trends in overweight among U.S. children and adolescents, 1999–2000. *JAMA* 2002;288:1728–1732.

17. Executive Summary of the Third Report of the National Cholesterol Education Program (NCEP). Expert Panel on Detection, Evaluation, and Treatment of High Blood Cholesterol in Adults (Adult Treatment Panel III). *JAMA* 2001;285:2486–2497.

18. National Diabetes Data Group. *Diabetes in America.* 2nd ed. Bethesda, Md: National Institutes of Health, National Institutes of Diabetes and Digestive and Kidney Diseases; 1995. NIH publication 95-1468.

19. Centers for Disease Control and Prevention. *National Diabetes Fact Sheet: General Information and National Estimates on Diabetes in the United States, 2000.* Atlanta, Ga: US Department of Health and Human Services, Centers for Disease Control and Prevention; 2002.

20. Benjamin SM, Valdez R, Geiss LS, et al. Estimated number of adults with prediabetes in the U.S. in 2000: opportunities for prevention. *Diabetes Care* 2003;26:645–649.

21. King H, Aubert RE, Herman WH. Global burden of diabetes, 1995–2025: prevalence, numerical estimates, and projections. *Diabetes Care* 1998;21:1414–1431.

22. Mokdad AH, Ford ES, Bowman BA, et al. Diabetes trends in the U.S.: 1990–1998. *Diabetes Care* 2000;23:1278–1283.

23. Mokdad AH, Ford ES, Bowman BA, et al. Prevalence of obesity, diabetes, and obesity-related health risk factors, 2001. *JAMA* 2003;289:76–79.

24. Ford ES, Giles WH, Dietz WH. Prevalence of the metabolic syndrome among U.S. adults: findings from the Third National Health and Nutrition Examination Survey. *JAMA* 2002;287:356–359.

25. Stafford RS, Blumenthal D, Pasternak RC. Variations in cholesterol management practices by U.S physicians. *J Am Coll Cardiol* 1997;29:139–146.

26. Danias PG, O'Mahony S, et al. Serum cholesterol levels and underevaluated and undertreated. *Am J Cardiol* 1998;81:1353–1355.

27. Joint National Committee on Prevention Detection Evaluation and Treatment of High Blood Pressure. The sixth report of the Joint National Committee on Prevention, Detection, Evaluation, and Treatment of High Blood Pressure. *Arch Intern Med* 1997;157:2413–2446.

28. Robertson TL, Kato H, Rhoads GG, et al. Epidemiologic studies of coronary heart disease and stroke in Japanese men living in Japan, Hawaii and California. *Am J Cardiol* 1977;39:239–243.

29. Murray JL, Lopez AD. *The Global Burden of Disease: A Comprehensive Assessment of Global Mortality and Disability from Diseases, Injuries and Risk Factors in 1990 and Projected to 2020.* Geneva: World Health Organization; 1996.

PART II

Screening for Cardiovascular Risk and Subclinical Disease

Noninvasive ultrasonographic assessment of cardiovascular disease

3

Julius M. Gardin
Cheryl K. Nordstrom
Nathan D. Wong

KEY POINTS

- _Ultrasound assessment of wall thickening in the carotid arteries, left ventricular dimensions and function, and brachial artery reactivity has been shown to correlate with cardiovascular risk factors and disease and has been proposed for use in cardiovascular risk stratification._

- _Carotid intimal–medial thickness is independently associated with the risk of future cardiovascular events and stroke, and has been used in clinical trials for assessing the impact of therapeutic risk-reducing interventions. Recommendations for its assessment in persons over age_ 50 at intermediate risk of coronary heart disease have been proposed; however, measures are highly dependent on the facilities and expertise of the laboratory used.

- _Ultrasonographic measures of brachial artery reactivity have been shown to be associated with cardiovascular risk factors and angiographic coronary artery disease. Standardization of measurement of this technology and additional studies regarding its incremental contribution to predicting cardiovascular events are needed before widespread utilization can be proposed._

- Left ventricular mass measured by echocardiography is independently related to the risk of future cardiovascular events. Other echocardiographic measures, including systolic and diastolic function and left ventricular dimensions and wall thicknesses, also have important prognostic implications. Echocardiographic assessment of selected patient populations, such as persons with hypertension, has been shown to improve risk stratification.

Although traditional methods of cardiac risk assessment from the physical examination, laboratory tests, and treadmill exercise testing are often used clinically in cardiovascular disease (CVD) risk stratification,[1] evaluation of subclinical disease is often not taken into account. Persons with subclinical disease, regardless of whether other risk factors are present, are at greater risk of future cardiovascular events than are those without subclinical disease.[2]

Ultrasonography of the carotid arteries and of the heart (echocardiography)[3–7] has been used for more than a decade in population-based epidemiologic follow-up studies and even longer clinically in cardiovascular risk assessment. More recently, brachial artery reactivity, as measured by ultrasound, has been shown to be highly correlated with traditional risk factors.[8,9] This chapter reviews the evidence supporting measures derived from these modalities and their relation to cardiovascular risk, as well as the appropriateness of their use at present for evaluation of subclinical disease.

CAROTID B-MODE ULTRASONOGRAPHY

Multiple studies, including observational studies and clinical trials involving anti-atherosclerotic agents, have helped to establish high-resolution B-mode ultrasound imaging as a valid and reliable technique for measuring baseline carotid wall thickness and changes in thickness.[10] Carotid artery intima–media thickness (IMT) and changes in thickness can be measured cost-effectively and conveniently in large numbers of persons (Fig. 3-1). Carotid wall thickness has been measured in large population-based epidemiologic studies over the past decade, providing significant insight into its role in cardiovascular risk assessment and as a measure of subclinical atherosclerotic disease.

Relation to cardiovascular risk factors and events

Over recent years, several studies have documented a relation of carotid atherosclerosis to the risk of coronary heart disease (CHD) events. A limited 1-year follow-up of 1257 middle-aged Finnish men revealed an association between common carotid artery IMT and cardiac events.[11] More recently, a nested case–control study within the Rotterdam Elderly Study showed an association between common carotid artery IMT and the risk of myocardial infarction (MI) and stroke.[12]

Among nearly 13,000 men and women aged 45 to 64 at baseline participating in the Atherosclerosis Risk in Communities (ARIC) study, carotid IMT, consisting of the mean of B-mode ultrasound measurements at six sites in the carotid arteries, predicted CHD over subsequent years. For a mean IMT of 1 mm or greater compared with less than 1 mm, the relative risk (RR) for incident CHD was greater in women (RR = 5.07, 95% confidence interval [CI] = 3.08–8.36) than in men (RR = 1.85, 95% CI = 1.28–2.69).[6] A closer association in this study of low-density lipoprotein cholesterol (LDL-C), compared with other lipid fractions, with carotid wall thickness suggested a particularly important role for LDL-C in earlier stages of atherosclerosis, while additional evidence suggests that other lipids may be more important in later stages.[13] Moreover, in a recent study of young adult

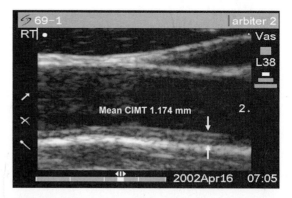

FIGURE 3-1 Example of an ultrasound image from the distal common carotid artery with quantification of intima–media thickness. CIMT, carotid intima–media thickness. (Reproduced, with permission, from Redberg et al. *J Am Coll Cardiol* 2003;41:1886–1898.)

participants in the Bogalusa Heart Study, those in the highest fifth percentile of IMT were most likely to be obese, to be hypertensive, and to have dyslipidemia, and more often had an abnormal electrocardiogram (ECG) and a history of smoking, which underscores the importance of these cardiac risk factors in youth as predictors of subclinical disease later in life.[14]

A report from the Cardiovascular Health Study incorporating 6.2 years of follow-up data in this cohort showed, after adjustment for major risk factors, increased carotid IMT to be significantly associated with risk for MI or stroke.[15] Unadjusted rates of combined MI or stroke were directly related to quintile of IMT for all three measures (maximal common carotid IMT, maximal internal carotid IMT, and combined maximal common and internal carotid artery IMT). Relative risks (and 95% CIs) for second through fifth quintiles, compared with the first quintile, were 1.54 (1.04–2.28), 1.84 (1.26–2.67), 2.01 (1.38–2.91), and 3.15 (2.19–4.52), respectively, adjusted for major risk factors. Longitudinal analysis for MI and stroke paralleled these results. Cumulative event-free rates for a combined endpoint of MI and stroke were substantially less with increasing quintile of combined standardized average values of the maximal common carotid and internal carotid artery IMT (Fig. 3-2). Furthermore, in participants who had no history of CVD, there was a closer association of internal carotid artery IMT, as opposed to common carotid artery IMT, with incident CHD.[5] Moreover, a combined index of the sum of internal carotid artery and common carotid artery IMT was more closely related to cardiovascular risk factors than was either measurement alone.

Patients with CHD have been demonstrated to have a significantly higher prevalence of atherosclerotic plaques in the carotid, femoral, and thoracic aorta, with extra-coronary plaque being a stronger predictor of CHD than conventional CHD risk factors.[16] One study showed each 0.1-mm increase in common carotid artery IMT to be associated with a 1.91-fold (95% CI = 1.46–2.50) increased risk for positive exercise tests or CHD as defined by the ECG and medical history.[17] Although significant correlations of carotid thickening with the number of coronary risk factors[18] and angiographic coronary artery disease have been shown,[19,20] reported specificity and sensitivity for identifying those with angiographically significant CHD have not always been high.[20]

Among persons with a history of previous coronary artery bypass surgery enrolled in the Cholesterol-Lowering Atherosclerosis Study (CLAS), carotid artery IMT, as well as progression in IMT, predicted the risk of coronary events independently of that predicted by angiographic arterial measures and lipid levels. Each 0.03-mm increase per year in carotid arterial IMT conferred relative risks of 2.2 (95% CI = 1.4–3.6) for nonfatal MI or coronary death and 3.1 (95% CI = 2.1–4.5) for any coronary event (both $P < .001$).[21]

Role in assessing effects of therapy

There is great interest in examining whether use of certain preventive therapies may be related to altering the degree of progression of atherosclerosis, assessed using measures of subclinical disease, particularly in asymptomatic individuals free of CHD. Practically, such a population can be studied only by using a noninvasive assessment modality, as use of more invasive coronary angiographic techniques is normally limited to those with presumed or symptomatic coronary disease. Studies involving cholesterol-lowering therapy have been most demonstrative.[22,23] For

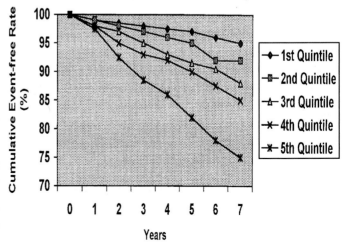

FIGURE 3-2 Unadjusted cumulative event-free rates for the combined endpoint of myocardial infarction or stroke, according to quintile of combined IMT. The estimated cumulative rate of the combined endpoint for the fifth quintile of the combined measure was more than 25% at 7 years, as compared with a cumulative rate of less than 5% for the first quintile. (Reproduced, with permission, from O'Leary et al.[15])

example, the Asymptomatic Carotid Artery Progression Study (ACAPS) showed lovastatin therapy in those aged 40 to 79 years with elevated LDL-C to be associated with actual regression in maximum IMT.[22] The Kuopio Atherosclerosis Prevention Study reported, in men 45 to 65 years of age, a 45% lower rate of progression of carotid atherosclerosis in those treated, as compared with those not treated with pravastatin, and the greater the degree of baseline IMT, the more pronounced the effects.[23] Finally, the longitudinal Cardiovascular Health Study showed current users of estrogen, as well as users of estrogen plus progestin, to have smaller internal and common carotid wall thicknesses, as compared with nonusers.[24]

Clinical implications

Although the degree of carotid atherosclerosis bears a relation to coronary atherosclerosis and the risk of CHD events and stroke, relative risks relating carotid atherosclerosis to coronary events are only modest, usually in the range of 1.5 to 3. Certain high-risk individuals with multiple risk factors or preexisting CHD may benefit from such assessment, which can be used in further risk stratification; however, a physician should determine the appropriate clinical indications before such testing is performed. Recently, the American Heart Association Prevention V Conference recommended its use, along with traditional risk factors, in evaluating asymptomatic patients over age 45 with intermediate risk.[25]

Advantages of carotid ultrasound imaging include its noninvasive nature and the relatively direct assessment it provides of parameters related to atherosclerosis; however, its principal limitation remains that measures of carotid wall thickness or progression may not directly relate to changes in coronary atherosclerotic burden.[26] In addition to its established relation to clinical event risk, promising data are emerging with respect to its utility in tracking the effects of preventive therapies through serial measurements.[22,23] Nevertheless, although epidemiologic data generally show an increased cardiovascular event risk in those with a carotid IMT 1 mm or greater, or for persons in the highest quintile of IMT,[27] no universal consensus exists as to what constitutes an abnormal test result. Furthermore, no guidelines exist on recommending follow-up above certain cutpoints or on how such recommendations should be modified according to an individual's cardiovascular risk factor profile.[28] In addition, reproducibility of the measurement is highly variable and dependent on the laboratory and staff used. Despite the existence of high-quality research laboratories, use of this technique as a screening tool is not widespread.

BRACHIAL ARTERY REACTIVITY TESTING

Background and methodology

Endothelial dysfunction is an early physiologic event in atherogenesis.[29] In vitro studies have shown that endothelium is normal in the earliest stages of atherosclerosis, before plaque buildup and before clinical detection of disease, and that endothelial injury predisposes to thrombosis, leukocyte adhesion, and proliferation of smooth muscle cells in the arterial wall.[30] An important functional consequence of endothelial dysfunction is the inability to release endothelium-derived relaxing factor (EDRF), now known as nitric oxide.[31] Coronary artery endothelial dysfunction has been demonstrated in vivo in response to various pharmacologic and physiologic stimuli, primarily in adults with symptoms of established coronary atherosclerosis.[32] These studies used invasive coronary angiography, which is not suitable either for investigation of the early development of vascular damage in younger symptom-free subjects or for serial studies of progression or reversibility in these subjects.

A noninvasive method has been developed that uses high-resolution ultrasound to measure changes in brachial or superficial femoral artery diameter in response to increased flow or to sublingual nitroglycerin.[33] Increased flow can be induced as reactive hyperemia after 4 to 5 minutes of cuff occlusion of the brachial artery.[34] In arteries lined by healthy endothelium, increased flow causes dilatation of the vessel.[35–36] However, this vasodilatory mechanism fails to operate in the presence of endothelial dysfunction.[37] In contrast, the mechanism of action of nitroglycerin, which causes vasodilatation by direct action on the smooth muscle, is independent of the presence or the state of the endothelium.

Relation to cardiovascular risk factors and disease

Of interest, a number of risk factors for CHD have been shown to produce abnormalities in flow-mediated dilatation (FMD) of the brachial artery. For example, impaired FMD has been shown, in insulin-dependent diabetes mellitus, to be related to the duration of the disease and to LDL-C levels.[8] Brachial artery FMD was found to be significantly impaired in diabetic subjects (diameter change = $5.0 \pm 3.7\%$ [mean $\pm$ SD]), as compared with control subjects ($9.3 \pm 3.8\%$, $P < .001$).

FMD has also been shown to be significantly impaired in passive smokers and active smokers compared with control subjects. There was also an inverse relation between the intensity of exposure to tobacco smoke and FMD, suggesting that passive smoking is associated with dose-related impairment of endothelium-dependent dilatation in healthy young adults. Reduced FMD of the brachial or superficial femoral artery was independently associated with cigarette smoking, older age, male gender, and larger vessel size. A composite risk factor score was independently related to FMD, suggesting risk factor interaction. These findings suggest that loss of endothelium-dependent dilatation in the systemic arteries occurs in the preclinical phase of vascular disease and is associated with an interaction of traditional risk factors for atherosclerosis.[9] Reduced flow-mediated brachial arterial dilatation is also related to older age, suggesting that aging is associated with progressive endothelial dysfunction in normal humans, and this appears to occur earlier in men than in women. A steep decline in flow-mediated endothelial function in women commences at about the time of menopause, suggesting a protective effect of estrogens on the arterial wall.[38]

Finally, a recent study revealed brachial artery wall thickness has been shown to be independently associated with angiographic coronary artery disease, after adjustment for other risk factors, in patients being evaluated for chest pain.[39]

Clinical relevance

Although the preceding data relating brachial FMD to cardiovascular risk factors are encouraging, further data, particularly those relating FMD to cardiovascular endpoints in large populations, are needed before recommendations for routine assessment of selected populations can be made. Recently, guidelines have been published in an effort to standardize the assessment of brachial FMD [40] Although this technique represents a potentially important tool for the noninvasive assessment of subclinical CVD risk, as well as for studying the effectiveness of various interventions that may affect vascular health, technical and interpretative limitations still remain that limit its widespread applicability.

ECHOCARDIOGRAPHY

Role of echocardiography in population-based studies

The role of cardiac ultrasound, in particular two-dimensionally guided M-mode echocardiography, in assessing subclinical disease risk, has been the subject of several major population-based studies over the past two decades.[41–45] The Bogalusa[41] and Muscatine[42] studies in longitudinal cohorts of youth documented a relationship between increased left ventricular mass measured by echocardiography and blood pressure. The Framingham Heart Study was the first longitudinal study to extensively document the prognostic significance of echocardiographic measures, particularly left ventricular mass.[43–45] The Coronary Artery Risk Development

in Young Adults (CARDIA) study,[46] the Cardiovascular Health Study (CHS),[4] and, most recently, the Strong Heart Study[47] have involved multiple field centers performing echocardiography using a common protocol.

In the CARDIA study[45] and CHS,[4] baseline ECGs were recorded onto super-VHS tape using a standard protocol and equipment. Echocardiographic images were digitized and measurements made at a centralized reading site using customized image-analysis software. Quality control measures included standardized training of echocardiography technicians and readers, periodic blind duplicate readings with reader review sessions, phantom studies, and quality-control audits.

Measures of interest in the CHS and CARDIA study involved those related to left ventricular anatomy and function. Specifically, two-dimensional echocardiography was used to assess left ventricular global and regional systolic function. In addition, two-dimensionally directed M-mode echocardiography was used to derive measures of left ventricular (LV) mass and its three component variables: ventricular septal thickness at end-diastole (VSTd), LV (internal) dimension at end-diastole (LVIDd), and LV posterior wall thickness at end-diastole (PWTd) (Fig. 3-3). Measurements in the CHS and CARDIA study were performed according to conventions established by the American Society of Echocardiography (ASE),[48] with LV mass determined according to the formula described by Devereux and co-workers: LV mass (in grams) = $0.80 \times 1.04 [(VSTd + LVIDd + PWTd)^3 - (LVIDd)^3] + 0.6$, where thickness and dimension measurements are expressed in centimeters.[49] Key two-dimensionally directed M-mode echocardiographic measures performed as part of the CHS Echocardiography Reading Center protocol are listed in Table 3-1.[4]

Pulsed Doppler echocardiographic measurements of LV diastolic function, including mitral peak flow velocity in early and late diastole (PFVE and PFVA, respectively), as well as the PFVE/PFVA ratio, have also been described in various populations, including Framingham, CARDIA, and CHS. For example, Xie and colleagues, in the CARDIA study, demonstrated that in Caucasian and African-American young adults, Doppler measures of LV diastolic filling were related to age, gender, body weight, blood pressure, heart rate, LV systolic function, and lung function.[50] Women tended to have significantly higher peak PFVE and PFVA than did men, independent of other variables. However, the PFVE/PFVA ratio did not differ between genders. In the Framingham Heart Study, Benjamin and co-workers also found age to be a major determinant of Doppler LV filling parameters.[51]

Although data suggesting that Doppler filling velocity patterns in healthy young adults can be used to predict subsequent cardiovascular disease (CVD) are not

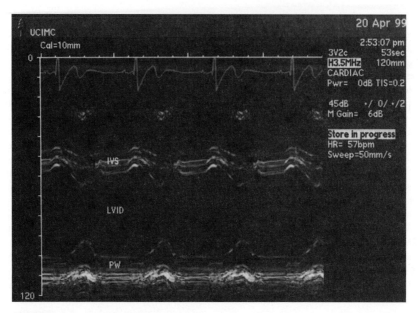

FIGURE 3-3 Two-dimensionally guided M-mode echocardiographic images demonstrating important components of the calculated left ventricular mass: LVIDd, left ventricular internal dimension at end-diastole; VSTd, ventricular septal thickness at end-diastole; PWTd, posterior wall thickness at end-diastole. These measurements were all made at the onset of the QRS complex (electrocardiogram at top). Key: IVS, VSTd; LVID, LVIDd; PW, PWTd.

available, there are data on patients who have had a previous MI or have dilated cardiomyopathies, suggesting that mitral early diastolic deceleration time, for example, can be used to predict subsequent CVD events and prognosis.[52,53] Among the elderly subjects of the CHS, men with congestive heart failure (CHF) had the highest PFVE/PFVA ratio (1.19), whereas the subgroup with hypertension had the lowest ratios (0.89 and 0.87 in females and males, respectively). The authors concluded that the hypertensive subjects most likely

TABLE 3-1 Two-Dimensionally Directed M-Mode Echocardiographic Measurements Performed in the Cardiovascular Health Study

LVIDd	Left ventricular internal dimension in diastole
LVIDs	Left ventricular internal dimension in systole
VSTd	Ventricular septal thickness in diastole
VSTs	Ventricular septal thickness in systole
LVPWTd	Left ventricular posterior wall thickness in diastole
LVPWTs	Left ventricular posterior wall thickness in systole
LA	Left atrial dimension
Ao	Aortic root dimension
LVFS	Left ventricular percentage fractional shortening (calculated)
LVESS	Left ventricular end-systolic stress (calculated)
LV	mass(g) (calculated) $= 0.80\ \{1.04[(\text{VSTd} + \text{LVIDd} + \text{PWTd})^3 - (\text{LVIDd})^3]\} + 0.6$

SOURCE: Adapted with permission from Gardin et al.[4]

exhibited an abnormal LV relaxation pattern, whereas patients with CHF had a Doppler pattern suggesting an increased early diastolic left atrial–left ventricular pressure gradient.[53]

Relation of LV mass to atherosclerosis and risk factors

Although increased LV mass may be a consequence of hypertensive heart disease, among other causes, and is not a direct measure of subclinical atherosclerosis, it does bear a relationship to atherosclerosis and the risk of CVD events. In subjects primarily free of clinical coronary disease, measures of LV mass relate to common carotid artery diameter and IMT ($r = .40$ and $.20$, respectively, $P < .01$).[54]

Further, measurements of echocardiographic LV mass are strongly related to important risk factors for CHD. In the CHS cohort of elderly men and women, factors positively associated with LV mass included body weight, male gender, systolic blood pressure, present smoking, major and minor electrocardiographic abnormalities, and treatment for hypertension, whereas diastolic blood pressure, bioresistance (a measure of adiposity), and high-density lipoprotein cholesterol (HDL-C) were inversely related to LV mass. In addition, pulse pressure was positively related to LV mass.[55] In younger adults, LV mass has been shown to be independently associated with body mass index (or subscapular skinfold thickness) and systolic blood pressure.[46]

Echocardiographic LV mass and prognosis

Increased LV mass, as well as LV hypertrophy as defined by echocardiography, has been shown to be associated with an increased incidence of subsequent CHD events and mortality. Findings from the Framingham Heart Study originally established the prognostic significance of increased LV mass.[43] In a 4-year follow-up study of 3220 subjects 40 years of age and older who were initially free of cardiovascular disease, a 50 g/m increment in LV mass divided by height, adjusted for other risk factors, was found to be associated with relative risks of new CVD events of 1.49 (95% CI = 1.20–1.85) in men and 1.57 (95% CI = 1.20–2.04) in women. Relative risks for death from all causes were 1.49 (95% CI = 1.14–1.94) in men and 2.01 (95% CI = 1.44–2.81) in women.[42] Among the subgroup of elderly subjects aged 59 to 90 years, similar increases in risk for new coronary events were seen with increased LV mass.[44] LV mass/height cutoff values of 143 g/m for men and 102 g/m for women have been used to define LV hypertrophy by the Framingham Heart Study.[45]

Preliminary data from the CHS suggest that, among elderly subjects without prevalent CVD at baseline, the highest quartile of LV mass conferred a relative risk of 3.35, compared with the lowest quartile, for incident CHF. Furthermore, eccentric and concentric LV hypertrophy, respectively, defined using a ratio of 2 × (LV diastolic wall thickness) to internal dimension, conferred adjusted hazard ratios, compared with normal LV geometry, of 2.05 and 1.61 for incident CHD and 2.95 and 3.32 for incident CHF.[56]

In a 10-year follow-up study of 151 hypertensive patients who had repeat echocardiography, Muiesan et al.[57] reported that those without reduction in LV mass indexed for body surface area (g/m^2) were at a greater risk for nonfatal cardiovascular events than those with regression of LV hypertrophy (RR = 3.52 vs RR = 1.38, $P < .0001$).

Echocardiographic measures of LV systolic and diastolic function and cardiovascular risk

Other measures obtained from M-mode and two-dimensional echocardiography, such as decreased LV ejection fraction (LVEF) and abnormal segmental wall motion, are also associated with a higher incidence of cardiovascular morbidity and mortality.[58,59] Echocardiographic measures such as left atrial dimension and the presence of mitral annular calcification have been reported to be related to the risk of stroke.[60,61]

Only recently have population studies, including the CHS and CARDIA study, begun to evaluate the distribution and risk factor correlates of LV systolic and diastolic function measures.[62–64] In elderly participants of the CHS, decreased LVEF and LV segmental wall motion abnormalities were more prevalent in men than in women.[62] In the CHS, an abnormal LVEF was one of several risk and subclinical disease factors found to be associated with an increased risk of mortality over 5 years.[63] Decreased LVEF has recently been associated with prevalent CHD in this cohort (RR = 1.9, 95% CI = 1.1–3.3).[64] However, approximately three fourths of those with clinical CHF have systolic function that is intact, but mortality remains high, regardless of whether systolic function is impaired (RR = 6.3, 95% CI = 4.3–9.3) or intact (RR = 3.2, 95% CI = 2.5–4.2) in those with CHF as compared with those with intact LVEF and no CHF.[65]

Among young adults 23 to 35 years of age, male gender, history of hypertension, and current smoking were each independently associated with about a 1% lower LVEF.[66] The prognostic significance of lower levels of LVEF among young adults in the CARDIA study will not be known unless and until a sufficient number of CVD events have occurred.

Various measures of LV diastolic dysfunction obtained from Doppler echocardiography, for example, early diastolic deceleration time, have been related in clinical studies to an increased risk of cardiovascular events.[52,53] Recently, measures of LV diastolic function and their relation to risk factors and events have been assessed in population-based studies. Among 3008 American Indians, aged 45–74 years, participating in the Strong Heart Study, the ratio of peak early to late diastolic filling velocity (E/A) was related to clinical correlates and endpoints.[67] Participants were categorized as having abnormally low (<0.6) or high (>1.5) E/A, with E/A values between 0.6 and 1.5 characterized as normal. Those with low E/A were more likely than those with normal E/A to be female, to be older, and to have lower BMI but elevated systolic blood pressure, pulse pressure, and heart rate. They also had a significantly higher prevalence of hypertension (60%), diabetes (69%), baseline CHD (9%), and aortic regurgitation (16%) compared with controls (43, 52, 4, and 9%, respectively, all P's < .001).

On the other hand, in the Strong Heart Study, those with high E/A were more likely than those with normal E/A to be younger and to have lower BMI, lower diastolic blood pressure, and elevated pulse pressure.[67] Baseline CHD (16%), CHF (16%), and mitral regurgitation (64%) were also more prevalent among those with high E/A than controls (4, 2, and 25%, respectively, all P < .001). All-cause mortality, cardiac death, and incident CHF rates were higher in those with abnormal E/A (either high or low) than in those with normal E/A.

Among 3492 African-American and Caucasian young adults aged 23–35 years in the CARDIA study, women had higher early and late peak flow velocities than men (both P's < .001).[68] Late velocity was positively associated with age, heart rate, systolic blood pressure, LV percentage fractional shortening, and body weight among both men and women (analyzed separately, all P's < .001). Early velocity was inversely related to age, heart rate, and forced expiratory lung capacity in 1 second (all P's < .001).

In the elderly (≥65 years old) participants of the CHS, early diastolic LV Doppler (transmitral) peak filling velocity decreased with age, whereas peak late diastolic (atrial) peak filling velocity increased.[69] Both early and late velocities were higher in women compared with men, even after adjustment for body surface area. Heart rate and blood pressure were also significantly correlated with these diastolic function measures. Both early and late diastolic peak filling velocities were also higher with increased duration of diabetes mellitus.[70] Glucose level, insulin use, oral hypoglycemic agent use, and prevalent diabetes at baseline were all independent predictors of late peak flow velocity (and its integrated flow–velocity

curve), but not of early peak flow velocity or the E/A ratio.

Redfield and colleagues have reported, in a population-based study, on categories of LV diastolic dysfunction, defined as "normal," "mild dysfunction" (impaired LV relaxation without increased atrial filling pressure), "moderate dysfunction" (impaired LV relaxation with moderately elevated atrial filling pressure or "pseudonormal" filling), and "severe dysfunction" (ventricular reduction in LV compliance or reversible or fixed restrictive atrial filling).[71] Their data from Olmsted County, Minnesota, showed that 20.8% of community-dwelling residents aged 45 years and older had mild, 6.6% had moderate, and 0.7% had severe LV diastolic dysfunction (Fig. 3-4).[71] One-hundred subjects (5.6%, 95% CI = 4.5–6.7%) had normal systolic function with moderate or severe diastolic dysfunction. Diastolic dysfunction was associated with increasing age, prevalent CVD, diabetes, and systolic dysfunction, but was equally common among men and women. All-cause mortality also increased as diastolic dysfunction worsened, such that the hazard ratio was 8.31 (95% CI = 3.0–23.1) for those with mild dysfunction versus normal diastolic function and 10.17 (95% CI = 3.28–31.0) for those with moderate to severe dysfunction versus normal diastolic function, independent of age, sex, and LVEF.

Also of recent interest is the occurrence of heart failure with preserved systolic function (LV diastolic heart failure) in community-dwelling populations. Data from Olmsted County also showed that among 45 persons with at least one validated previous diagnosis of CHF, 20 (44%) had preserved systolic function (LVEF >50%).[71] Only one of these persons had normal diastolic function; 21 had abnormal diastolic function (the remainder were indeterminate).

In the CHS, among 272 persons with prevalent CHF and adequate two-dimensional ECGs, 55% had normal LV systolic function, and 80% had either normal or slightly reduced systolic function.[72] Sixty-seven percent of women with CHF had normal systolic function compared with 42% of men (P < .001). Among those who developed CHF over approximately 5.2 years of follow-up, 57% had normal or borderline LVEF at hospitalization.[73]

Among 95 patients with heart failure in the Strong Heart Study, 50 had normal systolic function (LVEF >54%).[74] Compared to those without CHF, those with CHF and normal LVEF were more likely to be smokers and to have lower ankle–arm indexes, lower diastolic blood pressure, and higher serum creatinine levels. Those with CHF and a normal LVEF had a significantly greater BMI than those with CHF and a severely decreased (≤40%) LVEF (33.1 ± 10.9 kg/m² vs 27.7 ± 3.6 kg/m², P < .01).

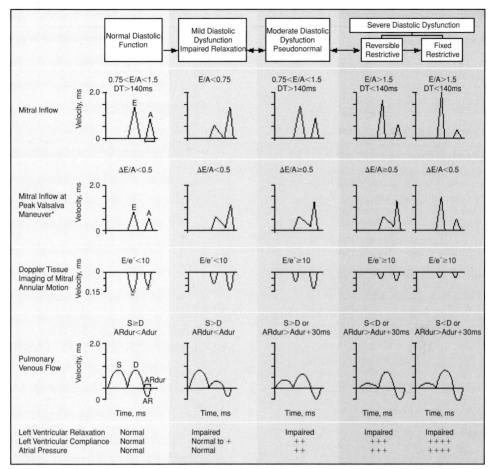

Participants with atrial fibrillation with DT>140ms, other arrhythmia, fusion of E and A, or in whom diastolic parameters were not obtained, who had only 1 criterion suggesting moderate or severe diastolic dysfunction, or in whom diastolic parameters were borderline and suggestive of but not diagnostic of abnormality were classified as having indeterminate diastolic function. E, peak early filling velocity; A, velocity at atrial contraction; DT, deceleration time; Adur, A duration; ARdur, AR duration; S, systolic forward flow; D, diastolic forward flow; AR, pulmonary venous atrial reversal flow; e′, velocity of mitral annulus early diastolic motion; a′, velocity of mitral annulus motion with atrial systolic; DT, mitral E velocity deceleration time.

Corrected for E/A fusion.[80]

FIGURE 3-4 Doppler criteria for classification of diastolic function. (Reproduced, with permission, from Redfield et al.[71])

Clinical recommendations regarding echocardiography in cardiovascular risk assessment

Although selected echocardiographic measures, such as increased LV mass and decreased LVEF, undoubtedly relate to an increased risk of CVD events, there are presently no standardized guidelines for routine echocardiographic assessment in general population groups. A writing group of the American Society of Echocardiography is currently addressing this deficiency. Echocardiographic assessment is part of the standard evaluation of patients with known or suspected cardiac disease, but high-risk asymptomatic patient groups do not routinely undergo such testing. However, some select patient groups, such as those with hypertension, have been recommended as candidates for low-cost, limited, and focused (e.g., on the left ventricle and left atrium) echocardiographic screening.[75] The usefulness of this approach has been demonstrated by studies that have compared the distribution of risk among hypertensive patients according to World Health Organization/International Society of Hypertension (WHO/ISH)

TABLE 3-2 Criteria for Clinical and Subclinical Disease in the Cardiovascular Health Study

Clinical disease criteria	Subclinical disease criteria
Atrial fibrillation or pacemaker	Ankle–arm index of ≤0.9
History of intermittent claudication or peripheral vascular surgery	Internal or common carotid wall thickness >80th percentile
History of congestive heart failure	Carotid diameter stenosis >25%
History of stroke, transient ischemic attack, or carotid surgery	Major electrocardiogram abnormalities* or abnormal ejection fraction
History of coronary artery bypass graft or percutaneous transluminal coronary angioplasty	Abnormal LV wall motion on echocardiogram
History of angina or use of nitroglycerin	
Positive Rose questionnaire for claudication or angina pectoris	
History of myocardial infarction	

*According to the Minnesota Code, ventricular conduction defects (7-1, 7-2, 7-4), major Q/QS abnormalities (1-1, 1-2), left ventricular hypertrophy (high-amplitude R waves with major or minor ST-T abnormalities) (3-1, 3-3, and 4-1 to 4-3 or 5-1 to 5-3), and isolated major ST/T wave abnormalities (4-1, 4-2, 5-1, 5-2).

SOURCE: Adapted, with permission, from Kuller et al.[2]

guidelines.[76–78] In one of these studies, those at low and medium risk (of receiving delayed treatment) represented 17 and 43%, respectively, of the hypertensive population. However, echocardiography demonstrated the prevalence of LV hypertrophy to be 21 and 32%, respectively, in these groups, resulting in modification of the risk classification in 29% of subjects and identifying an immediate need for their drug treatment.[77] Another study that used both echocardiography and carotid ultrasonography revealed an increase in the proportion of patients identified as high-risk from 22 to 45%.[78] Also, the issue has been raised whether individuals taking certain medications (such as weight-reducing drugs) should have echocardiograms to screen for possible subclinical heart valve disease, pulmonary hypertension, or other problems.[79–81]

COMBINED MEASURES FOR SUBCLINICAL DISEASE ASSESSMENT

Considering that atherosclerosis is systemic rather than limited to a single vascular bed, measurements made from several vascular beds combined with other markers of subclinical CVD may provide better prediction of CHD risk than do single measures. A combined subclinical disease index, consisting of measures of ankle–brachial blood pressure, carotid artery stenosis and wall thickness, electrocardiographic and echocardiographic abnormalities, and a positive response to the Rose Angina and Claudication Questionnaire, has been applied to the large elderly population-based CHS to address this question[2] (Table 3-2). Independent of other coronary risk factors, the presence of subclinical disease was

TABLE 3-3 Multivariate Assessment of Group Differences in Incident Clinical Cardiovascular Diseases: Subclinical Disease Compared with No Subclinical Disease Group*

Incident Disease	Men and women		Men only		Women only	
	OR[†]	95% CI	OR	95% CI	OR	95% CI
Total CHD	1.99	1.33–3.00	1.84	1.09–3.09	2.41	1.26–4.62
Total MI	1.32	0.75–2.32	0.93	0.47–1.84	2.54	0.87–7.43
Total mortality	1.82	1.08–3.08	2.52	1.18–5.37	1.21	0.57–2.57

*Included in model: age, systolic blood pressure, LDL cholesterol level, HDL cholesterol level, triglyceride level, diabetes, hypertension, weight, and current smoking status.
[†]OR, odds ratio; CI, confidence interval; CHD, coronary heart disease; MI, myocardial infarction.

SOURCE: Adapted, with permission, from Kuller et al.[2]

TABLE 3-4 Noninvasive Imaging Modalities for Assessing Subclinical Cardiovascular Disease

Parameter	Modality	Advantages	Disadvantages
LV mass/ LV hypertrophy	ECG	Low cost Widespread availability	Poor sensitivity Confounders (thin body habitus, LBBB, etc)
	ECHO	Good sensitivity and specificity Moderate cost Portability Other information, eg, valve regurgitation	Suboptimal image quality, eg, in some COPD, obese, or elderly patients
	MRI	Good sensitivity and specificity Good image resolution	Relatively high cost Nonportability
LV regional wall motion	ECG	Low cost	Poor sensitivity and specificity
	ECHO	Good sensitivity and specificity Moderate cost Portability Other information, eg, valve regurgitation	Suboptimal image quality, eg, in some COPD, obese or elderly patients
	MRI	Good sensitivity and specificity Good image resolution	Relatively high cost Nonportability
	Nuclear	Good sensitivity and specificity Fairly good image resolution	Relatively high cost Low portability
LV regional perfusion	ECHO with contrast	Promising contrast application Moderate cost Portability	Still experimental, especially in terms of quantitation
	Nuclear	Good sensitivity and specificity Fairly good image resolution	Diagnostic challenges include balanced perfusion decreases* Relatively high cost Low portability
	MRI	Good sensitivity and specificity Good image resolution	Relatively high cost Nonportability
Carotid plaque (intimal–media thickness, plaque morphology)	Ultrasound	Good sensitivity and specificity Excellent image resolution Moderate cost Portability	Modest inter examination variability Technician dependent and difficult to standardize
	MRI	Good sensitivity and specificity Very good image resolution	Relatively high cost Nonportability
Flow-mediated dilatation (FMD)	Brachial artery reactivity testing (BART)	Noninvasive Generally low cost May detect early effects from risk factor intervention	Technician dependent, difficult to standardize Incremental value over known risk factors not established

*May occur in triple vessel coronary artery disease.

associated with an increased incidence, over a mean 2.4-year follow-up, of total CHD in both sexes and of total mortality in men, but not with MI in either sex or with total mortality in women[2] (Table 3-3). More extensive follow-up data reported from the CHS showed that among 20 characteristics significantly associated with 5-year mortality, several risk factors and measures of subclinical or clinical disease were included, specifically, high brachial (>169 mm Hg) and low tibial (≤127 mm Hg) systolic blood pressure, low forced vital capacity (≤206 mL), aortic stenosis (moderate or severe), abnormal LVEF (by echocardiography), major electrocardiographic abnormality, and stenosis of the internal carotid artery (by ultrasound). Increased LV mass by echocardiography, however, was not a significant predictor of mortality after these other factors were considered.[63]

The findings suggest that subclinical disease assessment using a combined set of measures representing several vascular beds may provide improved risk prediction over and above standard CHD risk factors.[2] At least in older individuals—from whom these data were derived—assessment of subclinical disease may provide an approach to identifying high-risk individuals who may be candidates for more active intervention to prevent clinical disease. Measurements of subclinical disease from these tests can be done by trained technicians under the supervision of physicians. The costs of performing one or more of these tests in the office-based health care setting, which continue to decrease, will help determine the practical application of such tests in risk stratification for the population as a whole. Further follow-up of the cohort in the CHS and other studies incorporating subclinical disease assessment, such as the ongoing National Institutes of Health-sponsored Multiethnic Study of Atherosclerosis (MESA), should help determine the best combination of measures to efficiently identify those at highest risk of clinical disease outcomes.[82] In the interim, Table 3-4 represents the authors' assessment of the relative value of the various noninvasive modalities available for assessing measures of subclinical disease, including LV mass and hypertrophy, LV regional wall motion and perfusion, brachial artery reactivity FMD, and carotid IMT and plaque morphology. Coronary artery calcium, magnetic resonance imaging, and ankle–brachial index are discussed in Chapter 4.

CONCLUSIONS

Over the past decade, evidence from large population-based studies has established the prognostic value for CVD of several noninvasive subclinical disease measures, including carotid artery IMT measured by ultrasound; echocardiographic LV mass and hypertrophy and LV global systolic function (ejection fraction). Although these measures do show predictive value over and above standard risk factor assessment, their utility in screening general or selected population groups has yet to be determined, and limited consensus regarding such screening currently exists.

A major challenge will be to establish consensus on a limited set of indicators or measures of subclinical disease that not only are cost-effective and able to be efficiently implemented in the office-based setting, but also provide information over and above standard CHD risk factor assessment.

REFERENCES

1. Califf RM, Armstrong PW, Carver JR, et al. 27th Bethesda Conference: matching the intensity of risk factor management with the hazard for coronary disease events. Task Force 5. Stratification of patients into high, medium and low risk subgroups for purposes of risk factor management. *J Am Coll Cardiol* 1996;27:1007–1019.

2. Kuller LH, Shemanski L, Psaty BM, et al. Subclinical disease as an independent risk factor for cardiovascular disease. *Circulation* 1995;92:720–726.

3. Celermajer DS. Noninvasive detection of atherosclerosis [editorial]. *N Engl J Med* 1998;339:2014–2015.

4. Gardin JM, Wong ND, Bommer W, et al. Echocardiographic design of a multicenter investigation of free-living elderly subjects: the Cardiovascular Health Study. *J Am Soc Echocardiogr* 1992;5:63–72.

5. O'Leary DH, Polak JF, Kronmal RA, et al, for the Cardiovascular Health Study Collaborative Research Group. Thickening of the carotid wall: a marker of atherosclerosis in the elderly? *Stroke* 1996;27:224–231.

6. Chambless LE, Heiss G, Folson AR, et al. Association of coronary heart disease incidence with carotid arterial wall thickness and major risk factors: the Atherosclerosis Risk in Communities (ARIC) Study, 1987–1993. *Am J Epidemiol* 1997;146:483–494.

7. Polak JF. Carotid ultrasound. *Radiol Clin North Am* 2001;39:569–589.

8. Clarkson P, Celermajer DS, Donald AE, et al. Impaired vascular reactivity in insulin-dependent diabetes mellitus is related to disease duration and low density lipoprotein cholesterol levels. *J Am Coll Cardiol* 1996;28:573–579.

9. Celermajer DS, Sorensen KE, Bull C, et al. Endothelium-dependent dilatation in the systemic arteries of asymptomatic subjects relates to coronary risk factors and their interaction. *J Am Coll Cardiol* 1994;24:1468–1474.

10. Mercuri M. Noninvasive imaging protocols to detect and monitor carotid atherosclerosis progression. *Am J Hypertens* 1994;7(Pt 2):23S–29S.

11. Salonen JT, Salonen R. Ultrasonographically assessed carotid morphology and the risk of coronary heart disease. *Arterioscler Thromb* 1991;11:1245–1249.

12. Bots ML, Hoes AW, Koudstaal PJ, et al. Common carotid intima–media thickness and risk of stroke and myocardial infarction: the Rotterdam Study. *Circulation* 1997;96:1432–1437.

13. Sharrett AR, Patsch W, Sorlie PD, et al. Associations of lipoprotein cholesterols, apolipoproteins A1 and B, and triglycerides with carotid atherosclerosis and coronary heart disease: the Atherosclerosis Risk in Communities (ARIC) Study. *Arterioscler Thromb* 1994;14:1098–1104.

14. Krisnan P, Balamurugan A, Urbina E, et al. Cardiovascular risk profile of asymptomatic healthy young adults with increased carotid artery intima–media thickness: the Bogalusa Heart Study. *J La State Med Soc* 2003;155:165–169.

15. O'Leary DH, Polak JF, Kronmal RA, et al, for the Cardiovascular Health Study Collaborative Research Group. Carotid-artery intima and media thickness as a risk factor for myocardial infarction and stroke in older adults. *N Engl J Med* 1999;340:14–22.

16. Khoury Z, Schwartz R, Gottlieb S, et al. Relation of coronary artery disease to atherosclerotic disease in the aorta, carotid, and femoral arteries evaluated by ultrasound. *Am J Cardiol* 1997;80:1429–1433.

17. Nagai Y, Metter J, Earley CJ, et al. Increased carotid artery intima–media thickness in asymptomatic older subjects with exercise-induced myocardial ischemia. *Circulation* 1998;98:1504–1509.

18. Gnasso A, Irace C, Mattioli PL, Pujia A. Carotid intima–media thickness and coronary heart disease risk factors. *Atherosclerosis* 1996;119:7–15.

19. Visona A, Pesavento R, Lusiani L, et al. Intima medial thickening of common carotid artery as indicator of coronary artery disease. *Angiology* 1996;47:61–66.

20. Adams MR, Nakagomi A, Keech A, et al. Carotid intima–media thickness is only weakly correlated with the extent and severity of coronary artery disease. *Circulation* 1995;92:2127–2134.

21. Hodis HN, Mack WJ, LaBree L, et al. The role of carotid arterial intima–media thickness in predicting clinical coronary events. *Ann Intern Med* 1998;128:262–269.

22. Furberg CD, Adams HP, Applegate WB, et al, for the Asymptomatic Carotid Artery Progression Study (ACAPS) Research Group. Effect of lovastatin on early carotid atherosclerosis and cardiovascular events. *Circulation* 1994;90:1679–1687.

23. Salonen R, Nyyssonen K, Porkkala E, et al. Kuopio Atherosclerosis Prevention Study (KAPS): a population-based primary prevention trial of the effect of LDL-lowering on atherosclerotic progression in carotid and femoral arteries. *Circulation* 1995;92:1758–1764.

24. Jonas HA, Kronmal RA, Psaty BM, et al, for the CHS Collaborative Research Group. Current estrogen–progestin and estrogen replacement therapy in elderly women: association with carotid atherosclerosis: Cardiovascular Health Study. *Ann Epidemiol* 1996;6:314–324.

25. Greenland P, Abrams J, Aurigemma GO, et al, for Write Group III. Prevention Conference V: beyond secondary prevention: identifying the high-risk patient for primary prevention: noninvasive tests of atherosclerotic burden. *Circulation* 2000;86:615–618.

26. Whitty CJ, Sudlow CL, Warlow CP. Investigating individual subjects and screening populations for asymptomatic carotid stenosis can be harmful. *J Neurol Neurosurg Psychiatry* 1998;64:619–623.

27. Crouse JR III. Predictive value of carotid two-dimensional ultrasound. *Am J Cardiol* 2001;88:27E–30E.

28. Wilson PWF, Smith SC, Blumenthal RS, Burke GL, Wong ND. 34th Bethesda Conference: Can atherosclerosis imaging improve the detection of patients at risk for ischemic heart disease? Task Force 4—how do we select patients for atherosclerosis imaging? *J Am Coll Cardiol* 2003;1898–1906.

29. Healy B. Endothelial cell dysfunction: an emerging endocrinopathy linked to coronary disease. *J Am Coll Cardiol* 1990;16:357–358.

30. Ross R: The pathogenesis of atherosclerosis: an update. *N Engl J Med* 1986;8:488–500.

31. Furchgott R, Zawadzki D. The obligatory role of endothelial cells in the relaxation of arterial of smooth muscle by acetylcholine. *Nature* 1980;288:373–376.

32. Ludmer PL, Selwyn AP, Shook TL, et al. Paradoxical vasoconstriction induced by acetylcholine in atherosclerotic coronary arteries. *N Engl J Med* 1986;315:1046–1051.

33. Celermajer DS, Sorensen KE, Gooch VM, et al. Non-invasive detection of endothelial dysfunction in children and adults at risk of atherosclerosis. *Lancet* 1992;340:1111–1115.

34. Laurent S, Lacolley P, Brunel P, et al. Flow-dependent vasodilatation of brachial artery in essential hypertension. *Am J Physiol* 1990;258:H1004–H1011.

35. Rubanyi RM, Romero C, Vanhouette TM. Flow-induced release of endothelium-derived relaxing factor. *Am J Physiol* 1986;250:1115–1119.

36. Pohl U, Holtz J, Busse R, Bassenge E. Crucial role of endothelium in the vasodilator response to increased flow in vivo. *Hypertension* 1986;8:37–44.

37. Nabel EL, Selwyn AP, Ganz P. Large coronary arteries in humans are responsive to changing blood flow: an endothelium-dependent mechanism that fails in patients with atherosclerosis. *J Am Coll Cardiol* 1990;16:349–356.

38. Celermajer DS, Sorensen KE, Spiegelhalter DJ, et al. Aging is associated with endothelial dysfunction in healthy men years before the age-related decline in women. *J Am Coll Cardiol* 1994;24:471–476.

39. Weidinger F, Frick M, Alber HF, et al. Association of wall thickness of the brachial artery measured with high-resolution ultrasound with risk factors and coronary artery disease. *Am J Cardiol* 2002;89:1025–1029.

40. Corretti MC, Anderson TJ, Benjamin EJ, et al. Guidelines for the ultrasound assessment of endothelial dependent flow-mediated vasodilation of the brachial artery: a report of the International Brachial Artery Reactivity Task Force. *J Am Coll Cardiol* 2002;39:257–265.

41. Burke GL, Arcilla RA, Culpepper WS, et al. Blood pressure and echocardiographic measures in children: the Bogalusa Heart Study. *Circulation* 1987;75:106–114.

42. Mahoney LT, Schieken RM, Clarke WR, Lauer RM. Left ventricular mass and exercise responses predict future blood pressure: the Muscatine Study. *Hypertension* 1988;12:206–213.

43. Levy D, Garrison RJ, Savage DD, et al. Prognostic implications of echocardiographically determined left ventricular mass in the Framingham Heart Study. *N Engl J Med* 1990;322:1561–1566.

44. Levy D, Garrison RJ, Savage DD, et al. Left ventricular mass and incidence of coronary heart disease in an elderly cohort: the Framingham Heart Study. *Ann Intern Med* 1989;110:101–107.

45. Levy D, Savage DD, Garrison RJ, et al. Echocardiographic criteria for left ventricular hypertrophy: the Framingham Heart Study. *Am J Cardiol* 1987;59:956–960.

46. Gardin JM, Wagenknecht LE, Anton-Culver H, et al. Relationship of cardiovascular risk factors to echocardiographic left ventricular mass in healthy young black and white adult men and women: the CARDIA Study. *Circulation* 1995;92:380–387.

47. Devereux RB, Roman MJ, de Simone G, et al. Relations of left ventricular mass to demographic and hemodynamic variables in American Indians: the Strong Heart Study. *Circulation* 1997;96:1416–1423.

48. Sahn DJ, DeMaria A, Kisslo J, et al, for the Committee on M-mode Standardization of the American Society of Echocardiography. Recommendations regarding quantitation in M-mode echocardiography: results of a survey of echocardiographic methods. *Circulation* 1978;58:1072–1083.

49. Devereux RB, Alonso DR, Lutas EM, et al. Echocardiographic assessment of left ventricular hypertrophy: comparisons with necropsy findings. *Am J Cardiol* 1986; 57:450–458.

50. Xie X, Gidding SS, Gardin JM, et al. Left ventricular diastolic function in young adults: the Coronary Artery Risk Development in Young Adults Study. *J Am Soc Echocardiogr* 1995;8:771–779.

51. Benjamin EJ, Levy D, Anderson KM, et al. Determinants of Doppler indices of left ventricular diastolic function in normal subjects: the Framingham Heart Study. *Am J Cardiol* 1992;70:508–515.

52. Oh JK, Ding JB, Gersh BJ, et al. Restrictive left ventricular diastolic filling identifies patients with heart failure after acute myocardial infarction. *J Am Soc Echocardiogr* 1992;5:497–503.

53. Ortiz J, Matsumoto AY, Ghefter CGM, et al. Prognosis in dilated myocardial disease: influence of diastolic dysfunction and anatomical changes. *Echocardiography* 1993;10:247–253.

54. Kronmal RA, Smith VE, OLeary DH, et al. Carotid artery measures are strongly associated with left ventricular mass in older adults (a report from the Cardiovascular Health Study). *Am J Cardiol* 1996;77:628–633.

55. Gardin JM, Arnold A, Gottdiener JS, et al. Left ventricular mass in the elderly: the Cardiovascular Health Study. *Hypertension* 1997;29:1095–1103.

56. Gardin JM, McClelland R, Kitzman D, et al. M-mode echocardiographic predictors of six-to-seven year incidence of coronary heart disease, stroke, congestive heart failure, and mortality of an elderly cohort: the Cardiovascular Health Study. *Am J Cardiol* 2001;87:1051–1057.

57. Muiesan ML, Salvetti M, Rizzoni D, et al. Persistence of left ventricular hypertrophy is a stronger indicator of cardiovascular events than baseline left ventricular mass or systolic performance: 10-years of follow-up. *J Hypertens* 1996;14(suppl):S43–S49.

58. Taylor GJ, Humphries JO, Mellits ED, et al. Predictors of clinical course, coronary anatomy, and left ventricular function after recovery from acute myocardial infarction. *Circulation* 1980;62:960–970.

59. Ong L, Green S, Reiser P, Morrison J. Early prediction of mortality in patients with acute myocardial infarction: a prospective study of clinical and radionuclide risk factors. *Am J Cardiol* 1986;57:33–38.

60. Benjamin E, Levy D, Plehn J, et al. Left atrial size and the risk of stroke and death: the Framingham Heart Study. *Circulation* 1995;92:835–841.

61. Aronow WS, Koenigsberg M, Kronzon I, Gutstein H. Association of mitral annular calcium with new thromboembolic stroke and cardiac events at 39-month follow-up in elderly patients. *Am J Cardiol* 1990;65:1511–1512.

62. Gardin JM, Siscovick D, Anton-Culver H, et al. Sex, age, and disease affect echocardiographic left ventricular mass and systolic function in the free-living elderly: the Cardiovascular Health Study. *Circulation* 1995;91:1739–1748.

63. Fried LP, Kronmal RA, Newman AB, et al. Risk factors for 5-year mortality in older adults: the Cardiovascular Health Study. *JAMA* 1998;279:585–592.

64. Gottdiener JS, Arnold AM, Marshall RJ, et al. LV function and congestive heart failure in the elderly: relevance to therapeutic trials: the Cardiovascular Health Study [abstract]. *Circulation* 1998; 98:I–718.

65. Gottdiener JS, McClelland RL, Marshall R, et al. Outcome of congestive heart failure in elderly persons: influence of left ventricular systolic function: the Cardiovascular Health Study. *Ann Intern Med* 2002;137:631–639.

66. Wong ND, Gardin JM, Kurosaki T, et al. Echocardiographic left ventricular systolic function and volumes in young adults: distribution and factors influencing variability. *Am Heart J* 1995;129:571–577.

67. Bella JN, Palmieri V, Roman MJ, et al. Mitral ratio of peak early to late diastolic filling velocity as a predictor of mortality in middle-aged and elderly adults: the Strong Heart Study. *Circulation* 2002;105:1928–1933.

68. Xie X, Gidding SS, Gardin JM, et al. Left ventricular diastolic function in young adults: the Coronary Artery Risk Development in Young Adults study. *J Am Soc Echocardiogr* 1995;8:771–779.

69. Gardin JM, Arnold AM, Bild DE, et al. Left ventricular diastolic filling in the elderly: the Cardiovascular Health Study. *Am J Cardiol* 1998;82:345–351.

70. Lee M, Gardin JM, Lynch JC, et al. Diabetes mellitus and echocardiographic left ventricular function in free-living elderly men and women: the Cardiovascular Health Study. *Am Heart J* 1997;133:36–43.

71. Redfield MM, Jacobsen SJ, Burnett JC Jr, et al. Burden of systolic and diastolic ventricular dysfunction in the community: appreciating the scope of the heart failure epidemic. *JAMA* 2003;289:194–202.

72. Kitzman DW, Gardin JM, Gottdiener JS, et al. Importance of heart failure with preserved systolic function in patients ≥65 years of age. *Am J Cardiol* 2001;87:413–419.

73. Aurigemma GP, Gottdiener JS, Shemanski L, et al. Predictive value of systolic and diastolic function for incident congestive heart failure in the elderly: the Cardiovascular Health Study. *J Am Coll Cardiol* 2001;37:1042–1048.

74. Devereux RB, Roman MJ, Liu JE, et al. Congestive heart failure despite normal left ventricular systolic function in a population-based sample: the Strong Heart Study. *Am J Cardiol* 2000;86:1090–1096.

75. Black HR, Weltin G, Jaffe CC. The limited echocardiogram: a modification of standard echocardiography for use in the routine evaluation of patients with systemic hypertension. *Am J Cardiol* 1991;67:1027–1030.

76. Cuspidi C, Michev L, Severgnini B, et al. Change in cardiovascular risk profile by echocardiography in medium-risk elderly hypertensives. *J Hum Hypertens* 2003;17:101–106.

77. Schillaci G, DeSimone G, Revoldi G, et al. Change in cardiovascular risk profile by echocardiography in low- or medium-risk hypertension. *J Hypertens* 2002;20:1519–1525.

78. Cuspidi C, Lonati L, Macca G, et al. Cardiovascular risk stratification in hypertensive patients: impact of echocardiography and carotid ultrasonography. *J Hypertens* 2001;19:375–380.

79. Gardin JM, Schumacher D, Constantine G, et al. Valvular abnormalities and cardiovascular status following exposure to dexfenfluramine or phentermine/fenfluramine. *JAMA* 2000;283:1703–1709.

80. Gardin JM, Weissman NJ, Leung C, et al. Clinical and echocardiographic follow-up of patients previously treated with dexfenfluramine or phentermine/fenfluramine. *JAMA* 2001;286:2011–2014.

81. Bonow RO, Carabello B, de Leon AC Jr, et al. ACC/AHA guidelines for the management of patients with valvular heart disease: a report of the American College of Cardiology/American Heart Association Task Force on Practice Guidelines (Committee on Management of Patients with Valvular Heart Disease). *J Am Coll Cardiol* 1998;32:1486–1588.

82. Bild DE, Bluemke DA, Burke GL, et al. The multi-ethnic study of atherosclerosis: objectives and design. *Am J Epidemiol* 2002;156:871–881.

Surrogate measures of atherosclerosis

4

Nathan D. Wong
Michael H. Criqui

KEY POINTS

- *Noninvasive methods of measuring atherosclerosis, including computed tomography, magnetic resonance imaging, ankle–brachial index, and pulse wave analysis provide an opportunity to measure the effect of primary prevention efforts, as well as the progress of treatment.*

- *Coronary calcium burden has a variable relationship to overall atherosclerosis quantity, is directly associated with future risk of cardiovascular events, and may provide incremental value over standard risk factor assessment.*

- *Noninvasive identification of the vulnerable plaque (eg, using magnetic resonance imaging) and estimation of atherosclerotic burden (eg, using computed tomography techniques) may help identify those at highest risk. The quantitative accuracy and prognostic value of magnetic resonance imaging-assessed atherosclerotic plaque remains to be established.*

- *Ankle–brachial index is independently and directly associated with the risk of future cardiovascular events and mortality. Its measurement is office-based and provides a high degree of sensitivity and specificity for detecting peripheral arterial disease. However, it is of limited value in patients under the age of 50 years.*

- *Persons at intermediate risk of coronary heart disease based on Framingham risk scoring (eg, 6–20% 10-year risk of a coronary heart disease event) can be considered possible candidates for noninvasive atherosclerosis screening, and those with significant findings (eg, calcium scores ≥75th percentile for age or gender or ≥400, or carotid intima–media thickness in highest quintile) may be suitable for more intensive risk factor intervention and further diagnostic evaluation. This represents up to 40% of US adults.*

RATIONALE FOR USING SURROGATE MEASURES OF ATHEROSCLEROSIS

Coronary heart disease (CHD) events often occur among those with no clinical history of CHD, and who not infrequently have blood pressure or cholesterol levels considered to be in the normal range and not warranting treatment. Studies show a third or more of CHD events occur in persons without a previous history of chest pain.[1] More importantly, less than one sixth of clinical events occur in lesions of 70% or greater diameter stenosis, with most events occurring in sites of "hemodynamically insignificant" lesions,[2] often undetectable by traditional methods (eg, exercise test, angiogram). This indicates a need for identifying subclinical atherosclerotic burden long before it has become physiologically significant if we are to institute therapies known to be effective in retarding or reversing coronary atherosclerosis.

57

This chapter reviews the role and methodology of computed tomography, magnetic resonance imaging, and ankle–brachial index in assessing subclinical cardiovascular disease, their relationship to clinical cardiovascular events, and how they may be able to be used in cardiovascular risk stratification. Finally, pulse wave analysis for assessing arterial stiffness is described.

FEATURES OF USING SURROGATE MEASURES OF ATHEROSCLEROSIS

Among the most common reasons for conducting studies involving surrogate endpoints is consideration of these as "intermediate endpoints" that can be realized within a much shorter time frame than can hard endpoints (eg, myocardial infarction, stroke, death). Such endpoints are also used principally for their ability to designate earlier, subclinical disease, and to track this subclinical disease burden, as well as the effects of therapies aimed at retarding or even reversing its progression. Compared with clinical event studies, studies of surrogate endpoints are lower in cost, and require fewer subjects and less treatment or follow-up time. The suitability of classifying surrogate measures as continuous nature variables, as opposed to hard endpoints that must be defined as binary outcomes, provides significant advantages with respect to statistical power.

CORONARY AND AORTIC CALCIUM EVALUATION: ELECTRON BEAM TOMOGRAPHY AND MULTIDETECTOR SCANNERS

Coronary artery calcium (CAC) scanning is widely touted as the "mammogram of the heart" and has over recent years become widely commercialized. Initially performed exclusively with electron beam tomography (EBT) computed tomography (CT) scanners, but now widely performed with multidetector CT scanners, CAC scanning is noninvasive, of moderate cost, and convenient to many segments of the population. CT scanning detects location and quantity (score, mass, volume) of CAC, estimating the "burden of atherosclerosis," and is highly sensitive to angiographic disease, but variably specific, depending on the standard used (eg, any vs significant angiographic disease). There is, however, significant variability in the relationship between amount of calcium burden and overall amount of atherosclerosis, as shown by comparison studies with histology.

MEASUREMENT OF CORONARY CALCIUM

EBT scanners use an electron sweep of stationary tungsten target rings to generate x-ray images that can reveal small amounts of calcium, whereas multidetector scanners use a continuously rotating x-ray source. A sequence of 50- to 100-millisecond-speed, 3- to 6-mm-thick slices are usually obtained within 40 seconds from an EBT scan, whereas multidetector scanners have somewhat slower scan times, but take multiple slices simultaneously, especially with the advent of newer 16- and 32-slice scanners. The entire test takes about 15 minutes to complete, and involves a moderate radiation dose.[3] The presence of coronary calcium is normally defined as at least four contiguous calcified pixels that exceed a radiographic density of 130 Hounsfield units (HU); the calcium score for a given lesion is based on the product of the area of the calcified focus and a multiplier based on the peak density in HU (1 = 131–199, 2 = 200–299, 3 = 300–399, 4 = 400 or higher). The sum of the scores for the lesions in a given artery is the artery-specific score, and adding

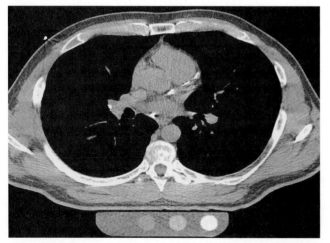

FIGURE 4-1 Example of electron beam tomography (EBT) slice showing significant coronary artery calcium.

the scores for the four coronary arteries (left main, left anterior descending, left circumflex, and right) yields a total calcium score. A coronary calcium score of 400 or greater and/or seventy-fifth percentile or greater for age and gender has been widely described as clinically significant and warranting more intensive risk factor intervention and further diagnostic follow-up[4] (Fig. 4-1). Although interscan concordance in calcium absence/presence is very high (often ≥95%), there is wide interscan variability in quantitative calcium scores, with absolute variability (absolute difference in score) directly proportional, and relative variability (percentage difference in scores) inversely proportional, to the absolute extent of coronary calcium. Given this, reporting results occurring within a category of scores, in addition to the age- and gender-

specific percentile level, has been recommended by some investigators.

PREVALENCE AND PROGNOSIS OF CORONARY CALCIUM

Coronary calcium quantity and prevalence increase with age and are related to major cardiovascular risk factors (self-reported and measured), including diabetes, hypertension, hypercholesterolemia, and cigarette smoking.[5–8] Figure 4-2 shows the prevalence of coronary calcium by age group based on one recently published study of a screened cohort.[6] In men, prevalence is roughly equivalent to age in years, and in women, about 10 to 15 points below age.[4] In addition, the greater the number of risk

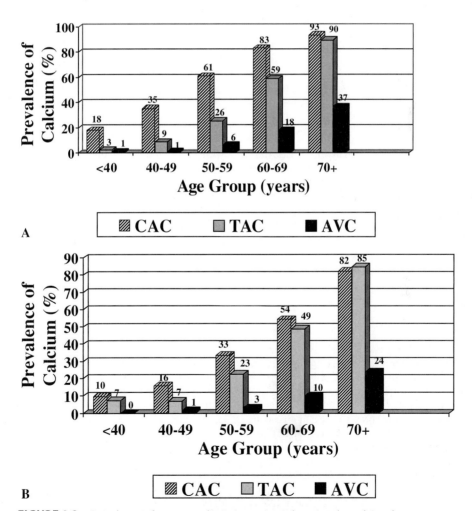

FIGURE 4-2 Prevalence of coronary, thoracic aortic, and aortic valve calcium by age group in men (a) and women (b). CAC, coronary artery calcium; TAC, thoracic aortic calcium; AVC, aortic valve calcium. (Reproduced, with permission, from Wong et al.[6])

TABLE 4-1 Selected Prospective Studies Relating Coronary Calcium to Clinical Events

Author	Sample studied and follow-up	Endpoint and results
Detrano et al.[9]; Yang et al. [10]	1196 asymptomatic intermediate/high risk subjects followed for 3.4 years	RR = 2.2 for CHD events above vs. below median score; 3.1 for more with vs. without calcium after adjustment for risk factors.
Wong et al., 2000[13]	926 asymptomatic, intermediate-risk subjects followed for average of 3.1 y	RR = 4.5 for CHD events above vs. below median score of 4, or RR = 8.8 for scores ≥75th percentile of positive scores, after adjustment for other risk factors.
Arad et al., 2000[14]	1172 asymptomatic subjects followed for average of 3.6 y	RR = 14.3 for all CHD events, and RR = 20.2 for nonfatal MIs and deaths for calcium scores ≥160 after adjustment for other risk factors.
Kondos et al., 2003[15]	5635 asymptomatic subjects followed for 37 mo	RR = 10.5 (P <.001) for men, and RR = 2.6 (P = .04) for women for predicting CHD events in those with vs without calcium. Calcium provided incremental information over risk factors.
Shaw et al., 2003[16]	10,377 asymptomatic individuals followed for 5 y	RR = 1.64, 1.74, 2.54, and 4.03 for total mortality for calcium scores 11–100, 101–400, 401–1000, and >1000, respectively, compared with <10, all P < .001. Calcium provided incremental information over risk factors.

factors present, the higher the calcium score.[5,8] A recent report demonstrated that in 30,908 asymptomatic individuals 30 to 90 years old, major conventional risk factors were significantly associated with any calcium in both men and women, with odds ratios similar to those reported for the development of clinical coronary disease.[8]

The amount of coronary calcium has also been examined in relation to the risk of cardiovascular events from numerous, selected cohort studies[9–17] (Table 4-1). The South Bay Heartwatch reported, for 1196 asymptomatic high-risk individuals, relative risks for hard coronary events of 2.2 for those above versus below the median calcium score[9] and 3.1 for those with versus. without calcium[10]; however, receiver operator curve analyses did not show a significant incremental value of coronary calcium for predicting events over Framingham and derived risk scores.[9] More recent reports from the South Bay Heartwatch cohort have shown CHD events to relate to extent of CAC among those without, but not with, diabetes at baseline,[11] as well as to provide incremental value over C-reactive protein levels in predicting CHD events in nondiabetic individuals.[12] Wong and associates showed in 926 subjects that, compared with those subjects with nonzero calcium scores, those in the fourth versus first quartile of positive scores were at an 8.8-fold greater risk of events, and those in the third versus first quartile were at a 4.5-fold greater risk of events.[13] Arad and colleagues, in the St. Francis Heart Study, reported particularly high relative risks (RRs) of 14.3 and 20.2 for predicting all CHD events and non-

fatal myocardial infarction or death, respectively, in those with scores 160 and higher.[14] Kondos and co-workers showed that persons with versus without calcium were at an increased risk of CHD events that was higher in men (RR = 10.5, P < .001) than in women (RR = 2.6, P = .04).[15] Most recently, Shaw and colleagues reported significantly increased risks of mortality in a graded fashion with increasing calcium scores, with significant improvement in the concordance index from the receiver operator curve from 0.72 for cardiac risk factors alone to 0.78 (P < .001) when the calcium score was added to the model. One published meta-analysis of several studies noted an unadjusted odds ratio of 4.2 (95% confidence interval [CI] = 1.6–11.3) for a myocardial infarction or death for those above versus below the median calcium score.[17]

One potentially important benefit of coronary calcium screening (as well as detection of other types of subclinical disease) is its effect on motivating patients to undertake beneficial lifestyle behaviors. In one cohort of 703 men and women without prior coronary disease who received CAC screening and were subsequently told their scores, after adjusting for baseline risk factors, the extent of CAC was significantly associated with the likelihood of new aspirin usage, taking new cholesterol medication, consulting with a physician, losing weight, and decreasing dietary fat, but also with new coronary revascularization and hospitalization and increased worry.[18] The question of whether receiving coronary calcium results truly motivates changes in lifestyle or treatment sufficient to lower risk of CHD was recently tested in a clinical trial among 450 asymptomatic active-duty US army personnel. Possibly because the prevalence of CAC was low (15%), those receiving their results did not show a significant reduction in change in Framingham risk score after 1 year, but those receiving intensive case management for risk factor modification did show significant reductions in risk score.[19] Further study of populations at higher risk may provide further insight into this question of "whether a picture is worth a thousand words."

PROGRESSION OF CORONARY CALCIUM

Studies of serial EBT scanning in selected patient groups have reported annual increases in CAC of 22 to 52% per year[20] (Fig. 4-3). While this translates to a doubling of CAC every 2 to 4.5 years, particularly among persons with preexisting CAC (the annual incidence of new positive scans for those negative at baseline is lower), observational studies incorporating serial scanning, such as the Multiethnic Study of Atherosclerosis, are needed to confirm CAC progression rates. One recently published observational study of 149 patients with hypercholesterolemia showed calcium volume to progress by 52% over 1 year in those not treated, whereas CAC regressed 7% among those treated aggressively to a low-density lipoprotein cholesterol (LDL-C) below 120 mg/dL, and progressed moderately (25%) in those treated less aggressively (LDL-C <120 mg/dL).[21] Other observational studies also relate cholesterol-lowering or other therapy to a reduced rate of progression (up to

50% in some cases). In addition, with respect to progression of coronary calcium and risk of cardiovascular events, among 269 asymptomatic patients observed for 2.5 years, 20 of 22 events occurred in those whose CAC scores increased.[22] Others, however, do not relate aggressiveness of lipid treatment to progression of CAC,[23] and while a recent follow-up of 761 subjects scanned twice over seven years did show higher high-density lipoprotein cholesterol (HDL-C) levels to relate to less progression of CAC, better LDL-C cholesterol control did not have less progression of CAC.[24]

Differences in CAC assessed among two scans in the same individual, whether done at the same time or across time, can be highly variable. In the Multiethnic Study of Atherosclerosis, among more than 6000 persons scanned twice, relative percentage interscan variability was reported to be approximately 20%, was greatest at lower calcium scores, but did not significantly differ by type of scanner (EBT vs multidetector CT); large interscan differences were most likely to be the result of misregistration of image slices or cardiac motion artifact.[25] Given the variable extent of interscan reproducibility that has been reported and the fact that the clinical significance of progression of CAC has not been confirmed by large-scale prospective studies, serial testing to follow progression of coronary calcium is not currently recommended.[4]

AORTIC AND AORTIC VALVE CALCIUM

There is also increasing interest in the measurement of aortic calcium and aortic valve calcium as surrogate markers of atherosclerosis. As with coronary calcium,

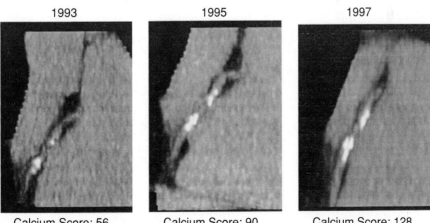

1993	1995	1997
Calcium Score: 56	Calcium Score: 90	Calcium Score: 128
Volume Score: 45	Volume Score: 78	Volume Score: 113

FIGURE 4-3 Example of serial electron beam tomography (EBT) slices demonstrating progression of coronary calcium.

the prevalence of both thoracic aortic calcium and aortic valve calcium increases dramatically with age in both men and women[6] (Figs. 4-2a and 4-2b). Calcification of the aortic arch measured on a chest radiograph is related to greater risk of CHD and, in women, increased risk of ischemic stroke.[26] Aortic valve calcium (AVC) also predicts stroke in the elderly.[27] Extent of aortic calcium in either the ascending or descending aorta has also been shown to be closely associated with AVC,[28] as well as with advanced CAC,[29] suggesting a common underlying systemic vascular atherosclerotic process. Although AVC is usually not considered part of the atherosclerotic process, recent reports suggest a common mechanism for AVC and vascular calcification.[30,31] Several major coronary risk factors have been shown to be common to coronary, thoracic aortic, and aortic valve calcium. LDL-C was consistently related to calcium in all three areas. But while diastolic blood pressure was predictive of CAC, increased systolic blood pressure, but reduced diastolic blood pressure, predicted the likelihood of thoracic aortic calcium[6] (Table 4-2). The prevalence and clinical significance of overall aortic calcium, particularly that in the descending aorta and abdominal aorta where most aortic calcium is present, are being examined in relation to the prevalence and clinical significance of coronary calcium in the prediction of future cardiovascular events in the ongoing Multiethnic Study of Atherosclerosis.[32] Some important features of abdominal aortic calcium are that it is (1) easier to measure (less motion) than CAC; (2) occurs earlier and in larger amounts than CAC, making it a potentially better predictor of overall cardiovascular events (although this requires confirmation from prospective comparison studies); (3) appears to be related to iliac calcium and peripheral arterial disease; and (4) on plain abdominal radiographs in the Framingham Heart Study, was a strong predictor of subsequent cardiovascular events.

GUIDELINES FOR CORONARY CALCIUM ASSESSMENT

Although some investigators have proposed clinical guidelines regarding the interpretation and recommended clinical action based on coronary calcium score

TABLE 4-2 Association of Coronary Risk Factors with Presence of Coronary, Thoracic Aortic, and Aortic Valve Calcium from Multiple Logistic Regression*

Risk factor (increment)	Odds of CAC (95% CI)	P value	Odds of TAC (95% CI)	P value	Odds of AVC (95% CI)	P value
Age (10 y)	3.15 (2.81–3.54)	<.0001	4.35 (3.78–5.01)	<.0001	3.13 (2.57–3.81)	<.001
Sex (F vs M)	.35 (0.28–0.44)	<.0001	0.75 (0.58–0.97)	.03	0.41 (0.27–0.63)	<.001
LDL-C (10 mg/dL)	1.03 (1.01–1.06)	.007	1.05 (1.02–1.08)	.001	1.06 (1.01–1.11)	.01
HDL-C (10 mg/dL)	0.99 (0.92–1.06)	.71	0.98 (0.91–1.05)	.55	1.06 (0.94–1.19)	.38
Triglycerides (10 mg/dL)	1.01 (0.99–1.02)	.51	0.99 (0.98–1.01)	.46	1.00 (0.98–1.03)	.80
BMI (kg/m²)	1.01 (0.99–1.03)	.26	1.03 (1.00–1.05)	.04	1.05 (1.01–1.09)	.006
Systolic BP (10 mm Hg)	1.00 (0.94–1.07)	.95	1.15 (1.07–1.24)	.0002	1.11 (0.997–1.23)	.06
Diastolic BP (10 mm Hg)	1.16 (1.04–1.30)	.009	0.82 (0.73–0.94)	.003	0.76 (0.62–0.92)	.006
Smoking (% current)	1.16 (0.86–1.55)	.34	1.58 (1.13–2.21)	.007	0.88 (0.49–1.60)	.68
Diabetes (yes vs no)	1.51 (1.06–2.15)	.02	1.02 (0.71–1.47)	.91	1.40 (0.86–2.28)	.17

*Sample size = 2647 with complete risk factor data available. CI, confidence interval; BMI, body mass index; CAC, coronary artery calcium; TAC, thoracic aortic calcium; AVC, aortic valve calcium. (Reproduced, with permission, from Wong et al.[6])

or quantity,[33,34] the American College of Cardiology/American Heart Association, in their initial scientific advisory statement, did not recommend populationwide screening of CAC.[35] While this panel does not recommend unselected screening of the asymptomatic population, the recent American Heart Association Prevention V Conference indicated that persons of intermediate cardiovascular risk (eg, 6–20% 10-year risk of CHD as calculated by Framingham algorithms) may be appropriate candidates for coronary calcium screening.[36] More recently, the 34th Bethesda Conference suggested that persons at intermediate risk of CHD events (eg, 6–20% 10-year risk of CHD as calculated by Framingham algorithms) may be suitable for screening for coronary calcium, and that those found to have increased levels of coronary calcium (≥75th percentile for age and gender or score >400) are suggested for more intensive clinical evaluation and/or risk factor modification.[4] This statement also recommended against the screening of persons either at low risk or at very high risk (eg, CHD risk equivalents, including persons with diabetes) of CHD. Ongoing large-scale prospective studies such as the Multiethnic Study of Atherosclerosis will provide further verification of the value of coronary calcium and its progression for predicting cardiovascular events.[32]

AORTIC AND CAROTID MAGNETIC RESONANCE IMAGING

Magnetic resonance imaging (MRI) of the aorta or carotid artery offers direct visualization of the atherosclerotic plaque, allowing identification of plaque components such as the fibrous cap, lipid core, calcium, hemorrhage, and thrombosis (vunerable plaques have thin fibrous cap and large lipid core).[37] MRI differentiates plaque components on the basis of biophysical and biochemical parameters such as chemical composition and concentration, water consent, physical state, molecular motion, or diffusion.[38] The technique is non-invasive and free of ionizing radiation. Computerized morphometric analysis involves following the edge of significant contrast, providing measures of total vascular and lumen area, the difference being the vessel wall area (Image Pro-Plus, Media Cybernetics). A recent report from the Framingham Heart Study offspring cohort found that plaques detected by MRI were two to three times more common in the abdominal than in the thoracic aorta, and, similar to coronary CT and carotid IMT, the extent of plaque was directly related to age.[39] Challenges include obtaining sufficient sensitivity for sub-mm imaging and exclusion of artifacts from respiratory motion and blood flow. Multicontrast approaches include performing T1-, PD-, and T2-weighted images with high resolution "black blood" spin used to visualize the adjacent vessel wall. Matched MRI and transesophageal echocardiographic cross-sectional aortic images show strong correlation for plaque composition and maximum plaque thickness.

Challenges of MRI scanning include obtaining sufficient sensitivity for sub-mm imaging essential for evaluating the coronary arteries and exclusion of artifacts from respiratory motion and blood flow. For imaging of coronary artery plaque, the ultimate goal of MRI atherosclerotic imaging, preliminary studies in a pig model have shown difficulties to include cardiac and respiratory motion, nonlinear course of coronary arteries, and small size and location of coronary arteries. Wall thickness in human coronaries can be differentiated between normal and >40% stenosis; breathholding can minimize respiratory motion.[37,40,41]

Studies involving lipid-lowering and other interventions to demonstrate effects on MRI vessel wall area have just begun to emerge. An image-specific error of 2.6% for aortic and 3.5% for carotid plaques allows accurate measurement of changes in plaque size of >5.2% for aortic lesions and >7% for carotid lesions.[42] In one study report, 18 asymptomatic hypercholesterolemic patients were studied, with a total of 35 aortic and 25 carotid plaques measured. Serial black-blood MRI of aorta and carotid artery was performed at baseline, 6, and 12 months. After 12 months (but not 6 months) of simvastatin therapy, significant reductions in vessel wall thickness and area (8% reduction in aorta and 15% reduction in carotid artery vessel wall area), without lumen area changes, were observed[42] (Figure 4-4). These beneficial effects as assessed by MRI continued even after two years of follow-up.[43]

It has been noted, however, that the optimal vascular bed and method for quantifying extent of atherosclerosis measured by noninvasive MRI remains to be established, as does the prognostic significance of quantitative (e.g., plaque thickness or cross-sectional area) versus qualitative (e.g., presence of "thin" fibrous cap) atherosclerosis measures.[3] Moreover, ongoing studies such as the Multiethnic Study of Atherosclerosis[32] are conducting measures of left ventricular size geometry and function, as well as aortic plaque; the significance of these measures in predicting risk of future cardiovascular events in relation to other measures of subclinical disease will be determined.

ANKLE–BRACHIAL INDEX

While the "gold standard" for the diagnosis of peripheral arterial disease (PAD) is arteriography, the ease and convenience of the office-based ankle-brachial index (ABI)—the ratio of the ankle systolic blood pressure (SBP) to the brachial SBP—has established this technique as an important clinical and research tool. The ABI is associated with major cardiovascular risk factors, including cigarette smoking, SBP, and diastolic blood pressure,[44] and has been demonstrated to be a significant

Baseline   **6 Months**   **12 Months**

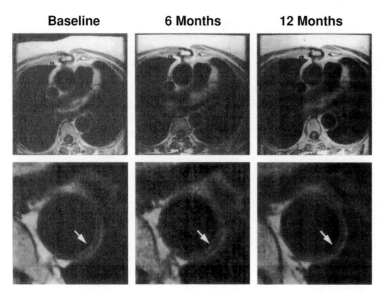

FIGURE 4-4 MRI serial T2-weighted images during simvastatin treatment: coronary vessels (top) and descending aorta (bottom). (Reproduced, with permission, from Corti et al.[42])

risk factor for cardiovascular events and mortality.[45] It is based on the principle of a peripheral artery stenosis reaching a critical level and causing a decrease in perfusion pressure distal to the stenosis that is roughly proportional to the severity of the disease. The test is inexpensive to perform.[3]

The higher of the SBP measures taken in each arm using a handheld Doppler is used as the denominator for the ABI calculation for each leg. A 12 cm cuff is normally used for the ankle. The higher of the two pressures in each ankle (from posterior tibial and dorsalis pedis arteries using the handheld Doppler) forms the numerator for the left and right ABI, respectively. A value of less than or equal to 0.90 is generally defined as an abnormal ABI, which has a sensitivity of about 90% and specificity of about 98% for moderate or greater obstructive peripheral arterial disease on angiography. It has modest test-retest reliability (as good as ± 10% when the mean of four measures is taken), and while suitable for cross-sectional population screening, is not ideally suited for serial testing.[3]

More recently, the Third Adult Treatment Panel for the Detection, Evaluation, and Treatment of High Blood Cholesterol has defined a low ABI diagnostic of PAD to be a "coronary heart disease equivalent," providing justification for treating persons with low ABI as candidates for aggressive lipid-lowering to an LDL-cholesterol level of under 100 mg/dl, the same as for persons with established CHD.[46] The Prevention V conference[36] recently indicated that persons aged >50 years, or those at intermediate or higher risk of CHD, could be suitable for screening for ABI. Some clinical trials have provided

evidence that the progression of PAD and extent of ABI can be altered by lipid-lowering or other therapy. The CLAS trial[47] showed less progression and more regression in femoral arteries in patients treated with niacin and colestipol. The Scandinavian Simvastatin Survival Study showed a lower incidence of new claudication in those on simvastatin.[48] Therapy with atorvastatin[49] and simvastatin[50] appear to benefit.

SCREENING FOR PERIPHERAL ARTERY DISEASE IN CARDIOVASCULAR RISK ASSESSMENT

In screening higher-risk patients for atherosclerotic cardiovascular disease (CVD), an often overlooked area is screening for peripheral arterial disease (PAD). In a recently published cross-sectional evaluation in 350 primary care practices throughout the United States comprising 6,979 patients aged 50 or greater with a history of cigarette smoking or diabetes, or 70 years or older irrespective of risk factors, PAD based on an ABI of 0.90 or less was detected in 29% of patients: 44% of these patients had PAD without other known cardiovascular disease. Moreover, of those patients with PAD, only 49% of their physicians were aware of this diagnosis.[51]

Historically as well as currently, the "gold standard" for PAD diagnosis is arteriography. However, this procedure is inappropriate not only for asymptomatic persons but also for symptomatic persons as well, unless an interventional procedure is contemplated. Current technology allows rather sophisticated noninvasive

TABLE 4-3 Measurement of Ankle–Brachial Index and Toe–Brachial Index

Measurement of ABI*
1. Patients should be studied in the supine position at rest.
2. When the ABI is measured alone, an appropriate-sized blood pressure cuff is used in the arm, and a 12-cm cuff is nearly always the correct size at the ankel.
3. Six SBPs are recorded: left arm pressure, right arm pressure, two right ankle pressures, two left ankle pressures. Each is recorded using a handheld Doppler over the brachial artery at the antecubital fossa in the arm and over the posterior tibial and dorsalis pedis arteries at the ankle. If neither ankle pulse can be located with the Doppler, the patient can be considered to have peripheral arterial disease.
4. The higher arm SBP is used as the denominator for both the left and right ABI (because of the possibility of subclavian stenosis in the arm with the lower pressure).
5. The right ankle SBP is the higher of the two right ankle SBPs, and the left ankle SBP, similarly, is the higher of the two left ankle SBPs.
6. The most commonly used cutpoint defining an abnormal ABI is <0.90, although cutpoints from 0.95 to 0.80 have been employed in various studies.

Measurement of TBI
1. As the TBI can be influenced by cold, the feet should be covered with a blanket prior to evaluation and minimum room temperature should be 25°C.
2. Measurement of the TBI requires arm and toe cuffs, a PPG sensor at the hands and toes, and a recorder.
3. Using PPG sensors on the middle finger of each hand (to assess brachial SBP) and on each great toe (to assess toe SBP) and with cuffs on both arms and both toes, one can rapidly assess all four SBPs.
4. Toe cuffs (2.5 cm) are employed, and the PPG sensors are applied to both middle fingers and the plantar aspect of the great toes.
5. Because transient vasomotor changes in small vessels can change the TBI, the cutpoint for abnormality is lower; it is normally defined as ≤0.70.

*ABI, ankle–brachial index; TBI, toe–brachial index; SBP, systolic blood pressure; PPG, photoplethysmographic.

assessment of PAD in symptomatic as well as asymptomatic persons. Major categories of evaluation, in descending order of ease and simplicity of assessment, are (1) segmental (e.g., ankle-brachial) blood pressure ratios, (2) flow velocity by Doppler ultrasound, (3) Doppler waveform analysis, and (4) duplex imaging and flow velocity evaluation. For office assessment of CVD risk in persons without leg symptomatology, the last three methods are probably not currently cost-effective, since each requires fairly sophisticated equipment and technical skill. Conversely, segmental blood pressure ratios are conceptually and operationally relatively straightforward, especially for measurement of the ratio of ankle systolic blood pressure (SBP) to SBP in the arm, i.e., or the ankle-brachial index (ABI). In terms of sensitivity, specificity, and positive and negative predictive value for significant PAD determined angiographically, the ABI gives most of the information that would be obtained by, in addition, measuring segment-to-arm SBP ratios at the upper thigh, above the knee, and below the knee.[52] However, measurement of the ratio of SBP at the toe to the arm, or the toe-brachial index (TBI), does provide incremental information and is discussed below.

Procedures for measuring ABI and TBI appear in Table 4-3.

RELATION OF ABIs AND TBIs TO CARDIOVASCULAR RISK

The ABI has been employed in clinical practice for over a half-century.[53] It is fairly simple to measure (Table 4-3) and shows good reproducibility, with the 95 percent confidence interval variability of a single measurement being about ±16 percent.[54,55] The normalized reproducibility of the ABI is actually considerably better than that of many standard clinical, hematologic, and biochemical measurements, such as heart rate, white blood cell count, and blood urea nitrogen.[56] The ABI correlates highly with angiographically determined PAD.[57] Extensive data document the association of the ABI with traditional CVD risk factors, such as cigarette smoking, SBP and diastolic blood pressure (DBP), and dyslipidemia, particularly low HDL-C and high triglycerides.[58–61] Other studies have shown ABI correlations with lipoprotein(a)[62,63] homocysteine[64] and fibrinogen and blood viscosity.[65]

Cross-sectionally, PAD shows considerable overlap with CHD and cerebrovascular disease.[66] In the lower extremities, it has been shown that PAD, diagnosed by both segmental blood pressure and flow velocities, increased the risk of total mortality threefold and the risk of CVD mortality sixfold in both men and women.[67] Again, nearly all the segmental blood pressure information for prognosis was carried in the ABI alone.[52] In addition, CVD morbidity was also sharply increased in subjects with PAD.[68] Several other investigators have reported similar results for morbidity and mortality.[69,70] Also demonstrated is a clear dose-response relationship between the severity of PAD and CVD mortality[67] (Figure 4-5), with severe cases being more likely to be symptomatic. Nonetheless, only one in five cases of PAD had typical symptoms of claudication,[71] and even among completely asymptomatic PAD patients (i.e., true subclinical PAD), the relative risk (RR) for CVD mortality was fivefold and highly statistically significant. This study also showed the striking independence of PAD as a predictor of CVD mortality. Relative risks were little changed after exclusion of subjects with clinical CVD at baseline as well as after adjustment for CVD risk factors. An indication of the clinical importance of these findings was the use of these and related data to revise the National Cholesterol Education Program Adult Treatment Guidelines to treat patients with PAD, even if asymptomatic, as secondary prevention.[72]

Two other follow-up studies using the ABI alone to diagnose PAD have reported quite similar results.[73,74] In both these studies, the ABI predicted CVD mortality independent of both CVD diagnosed at baseline and CVD risk factors, and in a graded dose-response fashion. Another study restricted to 422 patients with abnormal ABIs showed a strong ABI dose-response gradient

for mortality,[75] and similarly, a study of over 2000 PAD patients showed low ABI to independently predict all CVD events and total mortality.[76] ABI abnormalities increase sharply with age, but even in adults aged 40 to 59 years, the ABI is abnormal in 2 to 3 percent of persons,[61,77] which highlights its potential importance in screening higher-risk middle-aged and older persons.

The ABI is noninvasive, simple to measure, highly reproducible, shows a strong correlation with angiographically determined PAD, and is strongly predictive of CVD events in middle-aged and older persons, suggesting its utility as a screening test in these age groups. Measurement of the TBI at present is limited to vascular laboratories. The procedures are presented in Table 4-3. The TBI may add additional information in predicting CVD morbidity and mortality even when the ABI is normal. As is well known in vascular laboratories, some patients, particularly diabetics, may have falsely normal (false negative) ABIs due to rigid, calcified vessels; in these cases, the TBI may demonstrate the true reduced pressure.[78] However, only some abnormal TBIs fit into this category. In a recent natural history study of vascular laboratory patients, change in limb classification was examined over an average of 5 years of follow-up.[79] In limbs with a normal ABI (≥ 0.9) and a low TBI (<0.7) at baseline, 33.1 percent progressed to an abnormal ABI, 28.2 percent were stable, and 38.7 percent showed a normal TBI and ABI at follow-up. Thus some isolated low-TBI limbs have early large-vessel PAD, while some such limbs appear to reflect temporary vasomotor changes.

The TBI (may detect subclinical or clinical PAD in diabetics or other patients with false-negative ABIs, and thus provide incremental information on appropriate treatment and prognosis.

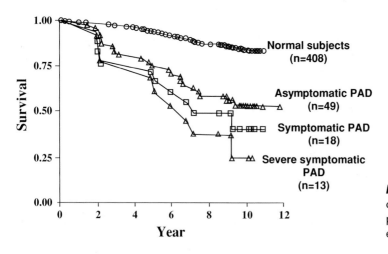

FIGURE 4-5 Relationship of ABI to cardiovascular and total mortality. (Reproduced, with Permission, from Criqui et al.[67])

ARTERIAL STIFFNESS AND PULSE WAVE ANALYSIS

Increased arterial stiffness, assessed noninvasively by pulse wave velocity (PWV), is a potentially important surrogate marker of atherosclerosis, and has been shown to correlate with increased risk and burden of coronary artery disease. One of several methods for measuring PWV involves assessing peripheral pressure waveforms from the radial artery at the wrist, using applanation tonometry with a high fidelity micromanometer (Millar Instruments and AtCor Medical). After acquiring about 20 sequential waveforms, a generalized transfer function is used to generate the corresponding central aortic pressure waveform.[80] A principal feature of increased arterial stiffness is an augmentation of central aortic systolic peak pressure due to an increased pulse wave velocity and rate of wave reflection.

Studies performed in various populations have shown PWV, used as an index of regional arterial stiffness, to be related to cardiovascular risk factors, with aortic PWV shown to be an independent predictor of all-cause mortality in patients with essential hypertension.[81] Recently, investigators have shown levels of inflammation, measured by C-reactive protein, to be independently correlated with augmentation index, a measure of arterial stiffness.[82] Another study also shows those with both diabetes and hypertension to have significantly higher PWV than healthy subjects or those with only one of the conditions.[83]

Regarding associations with other measures of atherosclerosis, in one study of 465 symptomatic men undergoing coronary angiography and arterial stiffness evaluated noninvasively using applanation tonometry of the radial artery, an 7-fold increased likelihood of angiographic coronary artery disease was seen among those in the highest quartile of augmentation index.[80] Among subjects with end-stage renal disease, pulse wave velocity was strongly correlated with coronary calcium, which has been suggested to increase vascular stiffness.[84] Others have shown carotid-radial pulse wave velocity (but not augmentation index) to be significantly associated with coronary artery plaque burden measured by intravascular ultrasound.[85]

Clinical trials have shown effects of long-term treatment certain antihypertensive agents, particularly ACE inhibitors and calcium channel antagonists, on reducing arterial stiffness. Pulse wave changes with these agents include reduced pulse wave velocity, vascular stiffness, wave reflection and central augmentation.[1,86] Among type 2 diabetic patients, treatment with the thiazolidinedione pioglitazone was associated with significant reductions in PWV, independent of changes in glucose metabolism.[87]

Large-scale prospective investigation is required to confirm the prognostic importance of measures of PWV in intermediate risk asymptomatic persons before this tool can be recommended as a possible screening tool for cardiovascular risk stratification. While recent emerging data are promising documenting the significance of PWV measures as surrogate markers of atherosclerosis, and its potential usefulness in selected patient populations such as persons with hypertension, there are currently no recommendations regarding the routine assessment of PWV in populations of intermediate risk asymptomatic patients.

REFERENCES

1. *Heart and Stroke Facts.* American Heart Association; 2000.

2. Little WC, Constantinescu M, Applegate RJ, et al. Can coronary angiography predict the site of a subsequent myocardial infarction in patients with mild-to-moderate coronary artery diameter? *Circulation* 1988;78:1157–1166.

3. Redberg RF, Vogel RA, Criqui MH, et al. Task Force ♯3: What is the spectrum of current and emerging techniques for the noninvasive measurement of atherosclerosis. In: 34th Bethesda Conference: can atherosclerosis imaging techniques improve the detection of patients at risk for ischemic heart disease. *J Am Coll Cardiol* 2003;41:1886–1898.

4. Wilson PWF, Smith SC, Blumenthal RS,et al. Task Force ♯4: How do we select patients for atherosclerosis imaging? In: 34th Bethesda Conference: can atherosclerosis imaging techniques improve the detection of patients at risk for ischemic heart disease. *J Am Coll Cardiol* 2003;41:1898–1906.

5. Wong ND, Kouwabunpat D, Vo AN, et al. Coronary calcium and atherosclerosis by ultrafast computed tomography in asymptomatic men and women: relation to age and risk factors. *Am Heart J* 1994;127:422–430.

6. Wong ND, Sciammarella M, Miranda-Peats R, et al. Relation of thoracic aortic and aortic valve calcium to coronary artery calcium and risk assessment. *Am J Cardiol* 2003;92:951–955.

7. Maher JE, Raz JA, Bielak LF, et al. Potential of quantity of coronary artery calcification to identify new risk factors for asymptomatic atherosclerosis. *Am J Epidemiol* 1996;144:943–953.

8. Hoff JA, Daviglus ML, Chomka EV, et al. Conventinoal coronary artery disease risk factors and coronary artery calcium detected by electron beam tomography in 30,908 healthy individuals. *Ann Epidemiol* 2003;13:163–169.

9. Detrano RC, Wong ND, Doherty TM, et al. Coronary calcium does not accurately predict near-term future coronary events in high-risk adults. *Circulation* 1999;99:2633–2638.

10. Yang T, Doherty TM, Wong ND, Detrano RC. Alcohol consumption, coronary calcium, and coronary heart disease events. *Am J Cardiol* 1999;84:802–806.

11. Qu W, Le TT, Azen SP, et al. Predictive value of CT coronary artery calcium scanning for coronary heart disease in subjects with diabetes mellitus. *Diabetes Care* 2003;26:905–910.

12. Park R, Detrano R, Xiang M, et al. Combined use of computed tomography coronary calcium scores and C-reactive protein levels in predicting cardiovascular events in nondiabetic individuals. *Circulation* 2002;106:2073–2077.

13. Wong ND, Hsu JC, Detrano RC, et al. Coronary artery calcium evaluation by electron beam computed tomography: relation to new cardiovascular events. *Am J Cardiol* 2000;86:495–498.

14. Arad Y, Spadaro LA, Goodman K, et al. Prediction of coronary events with electron beam computed tomography. *J Am Coll Cardiol* 2000;36:1253–1260.

15. Kondos GT, Hoff JA, Sevrukov A, et al. Electron-beam tomography coronary artery calcium and cardiac events: a 37-month follow-up of 5,635 initially asymptomatic low to intermediate-risk adults. *Circulation* 2003;107:2571–2576.

16. Shaw LJ, Raggi P, Schisterman E, et al. Prognostic value of cardiac risk factors and coronary artery calcium for all-cause mortality. *Radiology* 2003;228:826–833.

17. O'Malley PG, Taylor AJ, Jackson JL, et al. Prognostic value of coronary electron-beam computed tomography for coronary heart disease events in asyptomatic populations. *Am J Cardiol* 2000;85:945–948.

18. Wong ND, Detrano RC, Diamond G, et al. Does coronary artery screening by electron beam computed tomography motivate potentially beneficial lifestyle behaviors? *Am J Cardiol* 1996;78:1220–1223.

19. O'Malley PG, Fuerstein IM, Taylor AJ. Impact of electron beam tomography, with or without case management, on motivation, behavioral change, and cardvascular risk profile. *JAMA* 2003;289:2215–2223.

20. Budoff MJ, Raggi P. Coronary artery disease progression assessed by electron beam computed tomography. *Am J Cardiol* 2001;88 (suppl):46E–50E.

21. Callister TQ, Raggi P, Cooil B, et al. Effect of HMG-CoA reductase inhibitors on coronary artery disease as assessed by electron beam computed tomography. *N Engl J Med* 1998;339:1972–1978.

22. Raggi P, Callister TQ, Nicheolas J, et al. Cardiac events in patients with progression of coronary calcification on electron beam computed tomography [abstract]. *Radiology* 1999; 213:351.

23. Hecht HS, Harman SM. Change in calcified plaque burden in relation to aggressiveness of treatment and baseline LDL cholesterol levels. *J Am Coll Cardiol* 2002;39(suppl A):236A.

24. Wong ND, Kawakubo M, LaBree L, et al. Relation of coronary calcium progression and control of lipids according to National Cholesterol Education Program guidelines. *Am J Cardiol* 2004 (in press).

25. Detrano R, Anderson M, Nelson J, et al. Effect of scanner type and calcium measure on the re-scan variability of calcium quantity by computed tomography [abstract]. *Circulation* 2002;106:II–479.

26. Iribarren C, Sidney S, Sternfeld B, Browner WS. Calcification of the aortic arch: risk factors and association with coronary heart disease, stroke, and peripheral vascular disease. *JAMA* 2000;283:2810–2815.

27. Otto CM, Lind BK, Kitzman DW, et al. Association of aortic-valve sclerosis with cardiovascular mortality and morbidity in the elderly. *N Engl J Med* 1999;341:142–147.

28. Adler Y, Motro M, Tenenbaum A, et al. Aortic valve calcium on spiral computed tomography is associated with calcification of the thoracic aorta in hypertensive patients. *Am J Cardiol* 2002;89:632–634.

29. Adler Y, Shemesh J, Tenenbaum A, et al. Aortic valve calcium on spiral computed tomography (dual slice mode) is associated with advanced coronary calcium in hypertensive patients. *Coron Artery Dis* 2002;13:209–213.

30. Olsson M, Thyberg J, Nilsson J. Presence of oxidized low density lipoprotein in nonrheumatic stenotic aortic valves. *Arterioscler Thromb Vasc Biol* 1999;19:1218–1222.

31. Demer LL. Cholesterol in vascular and valvular calcification. *Circulation* 2001; 104:1881–1883.

32. Bild DE, Bluemke DA, Burke GL. Multi-ethnic study of atherosclerosis: objectives and design. *Am J Epidemiol* 2002;156: 871–881.

33. Rumberger JA, Brundage BH, Rader DJ, Kondos G. Electron beam computed tomographic coronary calcium scanning: a review and guidelines for use in asymptomatic persons. *Mayo Clin Proc* 1999;74:243–252.

34. Taylor AJ, O'Malley PG. Detecting coronary calcification with electron beam computed tomography: its role in managing coronary artery disease. *West J Med* 1999;171: 339–341.

35. O'Rourke RA, Brundage BH, Froelicher VF, et al. American College of Cardiology/American Heart Association Expert Consensus Document on Electron-Beam Computed Tomography for the Diagnosis and Prognosis of Coronary Artery Disease. *Circulation* 2000;101:126–140.

36. Greenland P, Abrams J, Aurigemma GP, et al, for Writing Group III. Prevention Conference V: beyond secondary prevention: identifying the high-risk patient for primary prevention: tests for silent and inducible ischemia. *Circulation* 2000;101 E16–E22.

37. Fayad ZA, Fuster V. The human high-risk plaque and its detection by magnetic resonance imaging. *Am J Cardiol* 2000; 88(suppl):42E–45E.

38. Wood ML, Wehrli FW. Principles of magnetic resonance imaging. In: Stark DD, Bradley WG, eds. *Magnetic Resonance Imaging.* 3rd ed. St Louis: Mosby; 1999:1–14.

39. Jaffer FA, O'Donnell CJ, Larson MG, et al. Age and sex distribution of subclinical aortic atherosclerosis: a magnetic resonance imaging examination of the Framingahm Heart Study. *Arterioscler Thromb Vasc Biol* 2002;22:849–854.

40. Worthley SF, Helft G, Fuster V, et al. High resolution ex vivo magnetic resonance imaging of an in situ coronary and aortic atherosclerotic plaque in a porcine model. *Atherosclerosis* 2000;150:321–329.

41. Worthley SF, Helft G, Fuster V, et al. Noninvasive in vivo magnetic resonance imaging of experimental coronary artery lesions in a porcine model. *Circulation* 2000;101:2956–2961.

42. Corti R, Fayad ZA, Fuster V, et al. Effects of lipid-lowering by simvastatin on human atherosclerotic lesions: a longitudinal study by high-resolution, noninvasive magnetic resonance imaging. *Circulation* 2001;104:249–252.

43. Corti R, Fuster V, Fayad ZA, et al. Lipid lowering by simvastatin induces regression of human atherosclerotic lesions: two years' follow-up by high-resolution noninvasive magnetic resonance imaging. *Circulation* 2002;106: 2884–2887.

44. Doherty TM, Detrano RC, Criqui MH, Wong ND. Exercise testing, ankle–brachial index, and coronary calcium screening. In: Wong ND, Black HR, Gardin JM, eds. *Preventive Cardiology.* New York: McGraw–Hill; 2000:49–73.

45. Criqui MH, Langer RD, Fronek A, et al. Mortality over a period of 10 years in patients with peripheral arterial disease. *N Engl J Med* 1992;326:381–386.

46. Expert Panel on Detection, Evaluation, and Treatment of High Blood Cholesterol in Adults. *Third report of the National Cholesterol Education Program (NCEP) expert panel on detection, evaluation, and treatment of high blood cholesterol in adults (Adult Treatment Panel III).* Bethesda, Md: National Heart Lung and Blood Institute, National Institutes of Health; 2001.

47. Blankenhorn DH, Azen SP, Crawford DW, et al. Effects of colestipol-niacin therapy on human femoral atherosclerosis. *Circulation* 1991;83:438–447.

48. Pederson TR, Kjekshus J, Pyorala K, et al. Effect of simvastatin on ischemic signs and symptoms in the Scandinavian simvastatin survival study (4S). *Am J Cardiol* 1998;81:333–335.

49. Aronow WS, Nayak D, Woodworth S, Ahn C. Effect of simvastatin versus placebo on treadmill exercise time until the onset of intermittent claudication in older patients with peripheral arterial disease at six months and at one year after treatment. *Am J Cardiol* 2003;92:711–712.

50. Mondillo S, Ballo P, Barbati R, et al. Effects of simvastatin on walking performance and symptoms of intermittent claudication in hypercholesterolemia patients with peripheral vascular disease. *Am J Med* 2003;114:359–364.

51. Hirsch AT, Criqui MH, Treat-Jacobson D, et al. Peripheral arterial disease detection, awareness, and treatment in primary care. *JAMA* 2001;286:1317–1324.

52. Feigelson HS, Criqui MH, Fronek A, et al. Screening for peripheral arterial disease: the sensitivity, specificity, and predictive value of non-invasive tests in a defined population. *Am J Epidemiol* 1994;140:526–534.

53. Winsor T. Influence of arterial disease on the systolic blood pressure gradients of the extremity. *Am J Med Sci* 1950;220:117–126.

54. Osmundson PJ, O'Fallon WM, Clements IP, et al. Reproducibility of noninvasive tests of peripheral occlusive arterial disease. *J Vasc Surg* 1985;2:678–683.

55. Fowkes FGR, Housley E, Macintyre CCA, et al. Variability of ankle and brachial systolic pressures in the measurement of atherosclerotic peripheral arterial disease. *J Epidemiol Community Health* 1988;42:128–133.

56. Johnston KW, Hosang MY, Andrews DF. Reproducibility of noninvasive vascular laboratory measurements of the peripheral circulation. *J Vasc Surg* 1987;6:147–151.

57. Kiekara O, Riekkinen H, Soimakallio S, Lansimies E. Correlation of angiographically determined reduction of vascular lumen with lower-limb systolic pressures. *Acta Chir Scand* 1985;151:437–440.

58. Criqui MH, Browner D, Fronek A, et al. Peripheral arterial disease in large vessels is epidemiologically distinct from small vessel disease: an analysis of risk factors. *Am J Epidemiol* 1989;129:1110–1119.

59. Criqui MH, Langer RD, Fronek A, et al. Large vessel and isolated small vessel disease. In: Fowkes, FGR, ed. *Epidemiology of Peripheral Vascular Disease.* London: Springer-Verlag; 1991.

60. Fowkes FGR, Housley E, Riermersma RA, et al. Smoking, lipids, glucose intolerance, and blood pressure as risk factors for peripheral atherosclerosis compared with ischemic heart disease in the Edinburgh Artery Study. *Am J Epidemiol* 1992;135: 331–340.

61. Hiatt WR, Hoag S, Hamman RF. Effect of diagnostic criteria on the prevalence of peripheral arterial disease. *Circulation* 1995;91:1472–1479.

62. Tyrrell J, Cooke T, Reilly M, et al. Lipoprotein [Lp(a)] and peripheral vascular disease. *J Intern Med* 1992;232:349–352.

63. Valentine RJ, Grayburn PA, Vega Gl, Grundy SM. Lp(a) lipoprotein is an independent, discriminating risk factor for premature peripheral atherosclerosis among white men. *Arch Intern Med* 1994;154:801–806.

64. Malinow MR, Kang SS, Taylor LM, et al. Prevalence of hyperhomocyst(e)inemia in patients with peripheral arterial occlusive disease. *Circulation* 1989;79:1180–1188.

65. Lowe DGO, Fowkes FGR, Dawes J, et al. Blood viscosity, fibrinogen, and activation of coagulation and leukocytes in peripheral arterial disease and the normal population in the Edinburgh Artery Study. *Circulation* 1993;87:1915–1920.

66. Criqui MH, Denenberg JO, Langer RD, et al. The epidemiology of peripheral arterial disease: importance of identifying the population at risk. *Vasc Med* 1997;2:221–226.

67. Criqui MH, Langer RD, Fronek A, et al. Mortality over a period of 10 years in patients with peripheral arterial disease. *N Engl J Med* 1992;326:381–386.

68. Criqui MH, Langer RD, Fronek A, Feigelson HS. Coronary disease and stroke in patients with large vessel peripheral arterial disease. *Drugs* 1991;42(suppl 5):16–21.

69. Ogren M, Hedblad B, Jungquist G, et al: Low ankle–brachial pressure index in 68-year-old men: prevalence, risk factors and prognosis. *Eur J Vasc Surg* 1993;7:500–556.

70. Newman AB, Sutton-Tyrrell K, Vogt MT, Kuller LH. Morbidity and mortality in hypertensive adults with a low ankle/arm blood pressure index. *JAMA* 1993;270:487–498.

71. Criqui MH, Fronek A, Klauber MR, et al. The sensitivity, specificity, and predictive value of traditional clinical evaluation of peripheral arterial disease: results from non-invasive testing in a defined population. *Circulation* 1985;71:516–521.

72. Expert Panel on Detection, Evaluation and Treatment of High Blood Cholesterol in Adults: Summary of the Second Report of the National Cholesterol Education Program (NCEP) Expert Panel on Detection, Evaluation and Treatment of High Blood Cholesterol in Adults (Adult Treatment Panel II). *JAMA* 1993;269:3015–3023.

73. McKenna M, Wolfson S, Kuller L. The ratio of ankle and arm arterial pressure as an independent predictor of mortality. *Atherosclerosis* 1991;87:119–128.

74. Vogt MT, Cauley JA, Newman AB, et al. Decreased ankle/arm blood pressure index and mortality in elderly women. *JAMA* 1993;270:465–469.

75. McDermott MM, Feinglass J, Slavensky R, Pearce WH. The ankle–brachial index as a predictor of survival in patients with peripheral vascular disease. *J Gen Intern Med* 1994;9:445–449.

76. Violi F, Criqui M, Longoni A, Castiglioni C. Relation between risk factors and cardiovascular complications in patients with peripheral vascular disease: results from the ADEP study. *Atherosclerosis* 1996;120:25–35.

77. Criqui MH, Fronek A, Barrett-Connor E, et al. The prevalence of peripheral arterial disease in a defined population. *Circulation* 1985;71:510–515.

78. Fronek A: Arterial system (evaluation of the lower and upper extremities). In: *Noninvasive Diagnostics in Vascular Diseases.* New York: McGraw-Hill; 1989:88–120.

79. Bird CE, Criqui MH, Fronek A, et al. Qualitative and quantitative progression of peripheral arterial disease by non-invasive testing. *Vasc Med* 1999;4:15–21.

80. Weber T, Auer J, O'Rourke MF, et al. Arterial stiffness, wave reflections, and the risk of coronary artery disease. *Circulation* 2004;109:184–189.

81. Asmar R. Effect of antihypertensive agents on artieral stiffness as evaluated by pulse wave velocity: clinical implications. *Am J Cardiovasc Drugs* 2001;1:387–397.

82. Kampus P, Kals J, Ristimae T, et al. High-sensitivity C-reactive protein affects central haemodynamics and augmentation index in apparently healthy persons. *J Hypertens* 2004;22:1133–1139.

83. Tedesco MA, Natale F, Salvo GD. Effects of coexisting hypertension and type II diabetes mellitus on arterial stiffness. *J Hum Hypertens* 2004;Feb 26 Epub.

84. Haydar AA, Covic A, Colhoun H, et al. Coronary artery calcification and aortic pulse wave velocity in chronic kidney disease patients. *Kidney Int* 2004;65:1790–1794.

85. McLeod AL, Uren NG, Wilkinson IB, et al. Non-invasive measures of pulse wave velocity correlate with coronary arterial plaque load in humans. *J Hypertens* 2004;22:363–368.

86. Ting C-T, Chen C-H, Chang M-S, et al. Short-and long-term effects of antihyertensive drugs on arterial reflections, compliance, and impedance. *Hypertension* 1995;26:524–530.

87. Satoh N, Ogawa Y, Usui T, et al. Antiatherogenic effect of pioglitazone in type 2 diabetic patients irrespective of the responsiveness to its antidiabetic effect. *Diabetes Care* 2003;26:2493–2499.

PART III

Risk Factors and Intervention

| Tobacco use, passive smoking, and smoking cessation interventions | 5 |

Russell V. Luepker
Harry A. Lando

KEY POINTS

- *The evidence linking tobacco use to the incidence and mortality from CVD is substantial; approximately a half-million deaths annually in the US are attributed to cigarette smoking.*

- *Tobacco use remains an important problem in many segments of the US population as well as in other developed and in developing countries worldwide.*

- *Environmental tobacco smoke is responsible for some 35,000–40,000 deaths from heart disease annually.*

- *Important interventions among youth include school-based prevention programs,*

- *community-based prevention programs, state and federal initiatives, as well as cessation assistance.*

- *For adults, interventions include behavioral treatment, self-help approaches, and pharmacologic therapy. Health care, worksite, and other community programs are invaluable.*

- *Physicians and other healthcare providers need to take greater initiative in reviewing and following up on tobacco use, and in informing patients about appropriate community and healthcare resources for those needing help.*

There are approximately 46 million adult smokers in the United States.[1,2] It is estimated that 440,000 deaths annually are attributable to cigarette smoking (Fig. 5-1).

These deaths are replenished by the estimated 3000 teenagers per day who begin the smoking habit. The economic costs are estimated to be more than $75 billion per

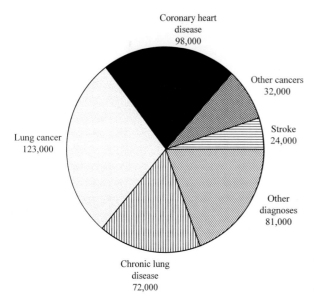

FIGURE 5-1 The number of annual deaths attributable to cigarette smoking in the United States, 1990–1994, was 430,000. SOURCE: Centers for Disease Control. *MMWR* 1997;46:448–451.

year in direct medical expenses and $50 billion in indirect costs. The costs in lost health and in human suffering are incalculable.

The causal links between cigarette smoking and human disease are incontrovertible. Cigarette smoking is linked to many cancers and is the prime factor in lung cancer. Cigarette smoking is also linked to acute and chronic pulmonary diseases, including emphysema. Finally, tobacco smoking is among the three major risk factors for cardiovascular disease. It is linked to sudden death, myocardial infarction, and stroke.[3] There is growing evidence that environmental tobacco smoke, which results in exposure of nonsmokers, poses health risks to that group. Lung cancer and respiratory tract infection among those exposed to environmental tobacco smoke is well recognized. More recent evidence suggests that environmental tobacco smoke increases the risk of coronary heart disease. These observations and others have resulted in the widespread call for prevention of tobacco intake by teens, cessation among smoking adults, and restriction in the environment. In this chapter, the epidemiologic evidence relating active and passive tobacco use to cardiovascular risk and the benefits of quitting are presented. Also described are the trends in cigarette use. Finally, individual and population intervention strategies among youth and adults are discussed.

EFFECTS OF CIGARETTE SMOKING ON CARDIOVASCULAR DISEASE

Over the past five decades, a wealth of evidence linking cigarette smoking to major cardiovascular disease (CVD),

including myocardial infarction, sudden death, stroke, and peripheral vascular disease, has accumulated.[3,4] These associations are observed across all age, gender, and ethnic groups.

The relationship of coronary heart disease (CHD) mortality to smoking status reported in the 1959–1965 Cancer Prevention Study is shown in Fig. 5-2. Death from CHD increases with age for both men and women, with women having lower rates at all ages, and ever smokers having significantly higher death rates than never smokers. These differences are greatest in the younger age groups, in which the relative risk of smoking (vs. non-smoking) approaches 8. However, the differences remain into the older years, when relative risks are less, but absolute risk is significantly greater. Smoking cessation among adults significantly reduces the risk of CHD and all CVD as shown in many populations.[5,6]

More recent data from the Multiple Risk Factor Screening Study of 316,099 white men also support a graded relationship between number of cigarettes and death from CHD.[7] The relative risk associated with smoking 1 to 25 cigarettes per day is 2.1, and rises to 2.9 for smoking more than 25 cigarettes per day. Similarly, the Multiple Risk Factor Intervention Trial (MRFIT) Research Group found that quitting smoking reduces mortality from CVD.[8]

In addition to age and gender effects, it is apparent that smoking-related disease also affects all of the major ethnic and racial groups in the United States.[3] The ill effects of smoking cut across national boundaries, as demonstrated in the Seven Countries Study of Keys and colleagues.[9]

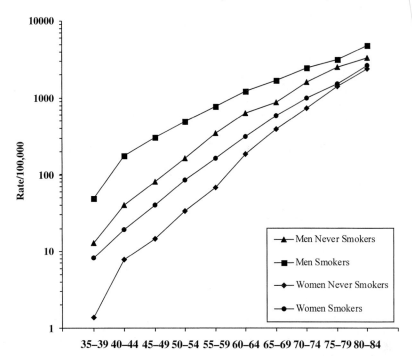

FIGURE 5-2 Coronary heart disease mortality. SOURCE: from *Changes in Cigarette-Related Disease Risks and Their Implication for Prevention and Control.* Monograph 8. Rockville, Md: US Department of Health and Human Services; 1997.

One of the most disturbing aspects of cigarette smoking is its strong association with sudden, unexpected death, particularly among younger individuals. Although sudden death is common among those with known CVD, Escobedo and Caspersen found that smoking alone predicted sudden death in those thought to be disease free.[10] Similarly, in both men and women, acute myocardial infarction in younger individuals (<50 years) is strongly associated with cigarette smoking.[11,12] The interaction of cigarette smoking with other known risk factors is well studied. Some suggest that the effect is additive; others find a multiplicative effect. Cigarette smoking adds to the risk associated with lipids, obesity, diabetes mellitus, hypertension, oral contraceptive use, and electrocardiogram (ECG) abnormalities.[13–17] Even without additional risk factors, however, smoking can increase the risk of CVD.[4] Smokers who continue in the habit after an acute myocardial infarction have significantly higher rates of recurrent events and death.[18,19] Individuals who quit smoking reduce that risk of a subsequent event.[18]

The mechanisms by which cigarette smoking and the constituents of tobacco smoke affect CVD have been studied in both animal models and humans. Both acute and chronic mechanisms are postulated, and it is likely both contribute. There is accumulating evidence that smoking plays an important role in the basic atherosclerotic process. This was elegantly confirmed by the Pathobiological Determinants of Atherosclerosis in Youth (PDAY) Research Group.[20] In that study, autopsies were performed on 1443 men and women aged 15 to 34 who died of external causes such as violence and auto accidents. Smoking was associated with an excess of fatty streaks and raised lesions in the abdominal aorta in these otherwise healthy individuals.[20] Injury of the arterial endothelium is suggested by some as the mechanism for the atherosclerotic lesions.[21] Other mechanisms are also postulated.[22] Acute effects of smoking are supported by the known short-term vascular effects of nicotine and the rapid improvement in prognosis with smoking cessation. Postulated mechanisms for acute effects include alterations in clotting, increased platelet adhesion, and acute coronary vasoconstriction with nicotine.[23,24] In any event, there are significant data indicating an association of cigarette use with acute and chronic CVD effects.

ENVIRONMENTAL TOBACCO SMOKE

Recently, increased emphasis has been placed on exposure of nonsmokers to environmental tobacco smoke (ETS) in the home, workplace, and public settings. ETS is more hotly debated than individual smoking because it affects others who may not have a choice about being exposed to tobacco smoke. In the 1986 Surgeon General's Report, *The Health Consequences of Involuntary Smoking*, CVD was barely mentioned.[25] The report focused principally on the cancer and respiratory disease effects of ETS. Recent increased research on ETS and CVD suggests a much larger problem.[26,27]

A number of prospective epidemiologic studies have evaluated the role of ETS in CVD (Table 5-1). They are hampered by the difficulty of ascertaining the level of ETS exposure and the potential for confounding by unmeasured or poorly measured risk factors for CVD. Some authors have suggested that cause and effect does not exist.[28,29] However, two recent meta-analyses determined that the vast majority of studies report similar increased relative risks for both fatal and nonfatal CHD from ETS.[26,27] A follow-up of the American Cancer Society Cancer Prevention Study cohort from 1982 to 1989 found that male nonsmokers with smoking wives had a 1.22 relative risk, which was significant. Women living with smoking husbands had a relative risk of 1.1, which was not significant. There was no increase in risk for spouses of former smokers. This study was able to control for other CVD risk factors. Ten-year follow-up data on 32,046 women aged 36 to 61 who had never smoked indicated that those exposed to ETS had relative risks (adjusted for other cardiovascular risk factors) of 1.58 (95% confidence interval = 0.93–2.68) in those with occasional exposure and 1.91 (95% confidence interval = 1.11–3.78) in those reporting regular exposure at work or home.[30] The recently published analysis of

the National Health and Nutrition Examination Survey (NHANES) attempted to answer the questions about confounders by comparing other risk measures, including classic risk factors and diet, in that large population sample. They found few differences in CVD risk factors between nonsmokers living in nonsmoking households and nonsmokers living in households with a smoker.[31] They stated that confounding by unmeasured CVD risk factors was unlikely.

Recently, a meta-analysis incorporating more home-based studies along with workplace studies (total of 1699 cases) showed an overall increased risk associated with passive smoking (relative risk = 1.49, 95% confidence interval = 1.29–1.72) and suggested similar relative risks for heart disease from work- versus home-based exposure.[32]

The mechanism by which ETS affects individuals is still debated, but considerable data are available. It is clear that mainstream smoke, that inhaled by the smoker, differs from sidestream smoke, which is released immediately into the environment.[33] Sidestream smoke may be more toxic. It is apparent that nonsmokers who are exposed regularly to cigarette smoke develop a number of physiologic changes. Some studies find that nonsmokers are more sensitive to these changes than those smokers regularly exposed.[34] These include the chronic effects of cigarette smoke such as lower high-density lipoprotein cholesterol (HDL-C), increased fibrinogen, and platelet abnormalities.[32–34] It is also apparent that exposed nonsmokers have acute effects, including endothelial dysfunction and lower exercise tolerance.[34–36]

These observations are all compatible with pathologic cardiovascular effects in nonsmokers exposed to ETS.

TABLE 5-1   Cohort Studies of Environmental Tobacco Smoke and CHD

Source	Year	Location	Cases/Population	Adjusted RR (CI)*
Hirayama[130]	1984	Japan	494/91,540	1.15 (0.93–1.42)
Garland et al[131]	1985	USA	19/695	2.7 (0.7–10.5)
Svendsen et al[132]	1987	USA	88/1245	2.2 (0.72–6.92)
Helsing et al[133]	1988	USA	1358/19,035	M 1.31 (1.05–1.64) F 1.24 (1.10–1.40)
Hole et al[134]	1989	UK	53/7987	2.01 (1.2–3.4)
Layard[135]	1995	USA	1389/2916	M 0.97 (0.73–1.28) F 0.99 (0.84–1.16)
Tunstall-Pedoe et al[136]	1995	UK	70/2278	2.7 (1.3–5.6)
Steenland et al[27]	1996	USA	3819/309,599	M 1.22 (1.07–1.40) F 1.10 (0.96–1.27)
Kawachi et al[30]	1997	US	152/32,046	F 1.91 (1.11–3.28)

* RR, relative risk; CI, confidence interval.

Recent estimates suggest that 35,000 to 40,000 deaths per year from acute myocardial infarction are associated with ETS. This effect is much larger than observed for lung cancer and suggests that attempts to reduce exposure of nonsmokers to tobacco smoke should be a high priority.[37]

PREVALENCE AND TRENDS IN CIGARETTE SMOKING AMONG YOUTH

Youth smoking issues are well described in the 1994 Surgeon General's Report.[38] Most smokers begin this habit in their teenage years. It begins with social pressure from friends, siblings, and parents who smoke. Youth feel that smoking makes one look more adult and is associated with social success. It is related to independence and rebelliousness, common themes in the teenage years. The environment provides important support through advertising that reinforces the "coolness" of smoking. The highly effective Joe Camel ads were clearly aimed at, and successful with, new-onset smokers.[39] The most vulnerable period is the sixth to eighth grades (ages 12–14), when most smokers start.

Early surveys of national trends showed a steady rise in cigarette smoking from 1968 to 1974.[40] During that time, smoking by female teenagers began to exceed that by male teenagers. From 1975 to 1990, a national sample of high school seniors noted a steady fall in smoking rates among this group. Importantly, the category "never smoked" was increasing. Smoking by females exceeded that by males, but recently those differences have disappeared. There were also socioeconomic status differences, with college-bound seniors much less likely to smoke than seniors who did not plan to attend college.[41]

The prevalence of cigarette smoking nationwide among high school students increased during the 1990s.[42] To determine the prevalence of cigarette, smokeless tobacco (ie, chewing tobacco and snuff), cigar, and pipe use among middle school and high school students nationwide, the American Legacy Foundation, in collaboration with the CDC Foundation, conducted the National Youth Tobacco Survey (NYTS) during the fall of 1999. Table 5-2 summarizes the prevalence of various types of tobacco use among middle and high school students by gender and race/ethnicity. The overall reported tobacco use (used tobacco on one or more of the 30 days preceding the survey) was 12.8% for middle school students and 34.8% for high school students.

To examine changes in cigarette smoking among US high school students during 1991–2001, the Centers for Disease Prevention and Control (CDC) analyzed data from the national Youth Risk Behavior Survey (YRBS). Results of the analysis indicated that although cigarette smoking rates increased during most of the 1990s, they have declined significantly since 1997. In 1997, current smoking among high school students (defined as smoking cigarettes on at least one of the 30 days preceding the survey) was 36.4%; in 2001, current smoking had declined to 28.5%. For current frequent smoking (defined as having smoked on at least 20 of the 30 days preceding the survey), the figures were 16.7% in 1997 and 13.8% in 2001.

If the long-term health of the nation is to be improved, prevention of cigarette smoking initiation among youth is essential.

PREVALENCE AND TRENDS AMONG ADULTS

Cigarette consumption per capita for individuals aged 18 and older rose steadily from 1900 to the late 1960s. Since that time, it steadily declined, at least until the late 1990s.[4] This pattern was the result of competing trends, including increased levels of smoking cessation and increasing recruitment of women smokers. There have also been early signs of a trend of increasing never smokers. The National Health Interview Survey (NHIS) found that 37.6% of adult men smoked in 1980 and 28.4% in 1990. Among women, the prevalence of current smoking was 29.3% in 1980 and 23.5% in 1990. These national rates confirm a declining number of adult smokers. But although national rates have decreased further since 1990, there still exists significant variation by region of the country.[43] In 1996, the percentage of adults who smoked ranged from a high of 31.7% in Kentucky to 15.8% in Utah, with most states reporting a prevalence under 25% (Table 5-3).

The Minnesota Heart Survey has surveyed random samples of adults aged 25 to 74 in the Minneapolis–St. Paul metropolitan area since 1980. Self-report of cigarette smoking is validated by serum chemical measures. As shown in Table 5-4, the "never smoked" category has been growing for both men and women. This trend combined with the increase in ex-smokers to cause a decrease in the rates of cigarette smoking from 1980 to 2002.

Although cigarette smoking among adults has substantially declined, a sizable proportion of the population is still addicted.[41,44] One of the national health objectives for 2010 is to reduce the prevalence of cigarette smoking among adults to 12% or less. To assess progress toward this objective, CDC analyzed self-reported data from the 2000 NHIS. In 2000, approximately 23.3% of adults were current smokers, compared with 25.0% in 1993. Although this decline is modest, it is statistically significant. Overall, 19.1% of adults reported smoking every day and 4.1% reported smoking some days. Smoking was more prevalent among men (25.7%) than women (21.0%). Prevalence was lowest among Asians (14.4%) and Hispanics (18.6%) and highest among American

TABLE 5-2 Percentage of Students in Middle School (Grades 6–8) and High School (Grades 9–12) Currently* Using Tobacco Products, by Type of Tobacco Product, Sex, Race/Ethnicity—United States, National Youth Tobacco Survey, 1999

| | Sex | | | | Race/Ethnicity | | | | | | | | Total | |
| | Male | | Female | | White | | African-American | | Hispanic | | | | | |
Type of tobacco product	%	95% CI	%	95% CI	%	95% CI	%	95% CI	%	95% CI			%	95% CI
Any use†														
Middle school	14.2	±2.2	11.3	±2.2	11.6	±2.3	14.4	±2.7	15.2	±5.2			12.8	±2.0
High school	38.1	±3.2	31.4	±3.1	39.4	±3.2	24.0	±4.2	30.7	±4.4			34.8	±2.7
Cigarette														
Middle school	9.6	±1.7	8.8	±1.7	8.8	±2.0	9.0	±1.8	11.0	±4.1			9.2	±1.6
High school	28.7	±2.8	28.2	±3.3	32.8	±3.1	15.8	±3.8	25.8	±4.7			28.4	±2.7
Smokeless														
Middle school	4.2	±1.3	1.3	±0.5	3.0	±1.1	1.9	±0.9	2.2	±0.9			2.7	±0.7
High school	11.6	±2.8	1.5	±0.6	8.7	±2.1	2.4	±1.3	3.6	±1.6			6.6	±1.6
Cigar														
Middle school	7.8	±1.3	4.4	±1.3	4.9	±1.0	8.8	±2.3	7.6	±2.9			6.1	±1.1
High school	20.3	±1.9	10.2	±1.6	16.0	±1.6	14.8	±3.5	13.4	±2.9			15.3	±1.4
Pipe														
Middle school	3.5	±0.8	1.4	±0.6	2.0	±0.6	2.0	±0.9	3.8	±1.7			2.4	±0.5
High school	4.2	±0.9	1.4	±0.5	2.6	±0.6	1.8	±0.9	3.8	±1.4			2.8	±0.5
Bidi														
Middle school	3.1	±0.8	1.8	±0.6	1.8	±0.5	2.8	±1.3	3.5	±1.6			2.4	±0.6
High school	6.1	±1.0	3.8	±1.0	4.4	±0.9	5.8	±2.1	5.6	±2.1			5.0	±0.8
Kretek														
Middle school	2.2	±0.6	1.7	±0.7	1.7	±0.7	1.7	±0.8	2.1	±0.6			1.9	±0.5
High school	6.2	±1.1	5.3	±1.5	6.5	±1.5	2.8	±1.5	5.5	±1.9			5.8	±1.2

* Used tobacco on one or more of the 30 days preceeding the survey
† Use of cigarettes, smokeless tobacco, cigars, pipes, bidis, or kreteks.

SOURCE: MMWR 2000;49:49–53.

TABLE 5-3   Percentage of Adults Who Reported Cigarette Smoking* 1996[†]

Rank	State	Percent	Rank	State	Percent
1	Kentucky	31.7	26	Massachusetts	23.7
2	Ohio	29.5	28	New Jersey	23.6
3	Indiana	28.8	28	New York	23.6
4	Nevada	28.1	28	Oregon	23.6
5	Missouri	28.0	28	Washington	23.6
5	Tennessee	28.0	32	Colorado	23.5
7	West Virginia	27.0	33	Mississippi	23.1
8	Arkansas	26.5	33	Rhode Island	23.1
9	Alaska	26.2	35	Nebraska	23.0
10	Maine	26.1	36	Florida	22.9
11	Louisiana	25.8	36	Kansas	22.9
11	Michigan	25.8	38	New Mexico	22.8
13	New Hampshire	25.7	38	Texas	22.8
13	North Carolina	25.7	40	Alabama	22.6
15	Pennsylvania	25.3	41	Connecticut	22.2
16	Wisconsin	25.2	42	Montana	21.7
17	Illinois	25.1	43	South Dakota	21.5
18	Iowa	24.6	44	Idaho	21.3
19	Oklahoma	24.6	45	Minnesota	21.1
20	Virginia	24.6	46	District of Columbia	20.8
21	South Carolina	24.4	46	Maryland	20.8
22	Delaware	24.3	48	Georgia	19.9
22	North Dakota	24.3	49	California	18.7
24	Vermont	24.2	50	Hawaii[‡]	17.5
25	Wyoming	24.0	51	Utah	15.8
26	Arizona	23.7			

* Ever smoked at least 100 cigarettes and now smoke every day or some days.
[†] All data are age adjusted, 1970 total US population.
[‡] Hawaii data are from 1995.
SOURCE: Centers for Disease Control and Prevention. Behavioral Risk Factor Surveillance System (provisional data)

TABLE 5-4   Smoking Status 1980–1992 in the Minnesota Heart Survey

	1980–1982	1985–1987	1990–1992	1995–1997	2000–2002
Men					
Never	30.2%	34.5%	40.6%	45.2%	49.7%
Former	35.6%	35.9%	33.1%	31.0%	28.2%
Current	34.2%	29.6%	26.3%	24.0%	22.5%
Women					
Never	45.7%	46.9%	50.4%	50.5%	54.2%
Former	20.4%	25.3%	24.1%	26.7%	25.5%
Current	33.9%	27.8%	25.5%	23.3%	20.9%

Indians/Alaska Natives (36.0%). Adults who lived below the poverty level were more likely to smoke (31.7%). Persons with graduate or professional degrees were far less likely to smoke (8.4%) than were those with less than a high school education or a general equivalency diploma. Smoking prevalence was far lower in those 65 and older (9.7%) than in the younger age groups.

PREVENTION AND INTERVENTION AMONG YOUTH

School-based prevention programs

Much of the effort in preventing youth smoking has focused on the school setting. School-based prevention programs generally target children in junior high or middle school, where the habit begins. Unfortunately, however, school-based programming alone may have limited impact in the absence of active parental and community involvement.[38] At one time, it was assumed that simply educating youths about the harmful effects of smoking would be sufficient to prevent them from initiating cigarette use.[45] However, it soon became apparent that information alone was not sufficient to deter adolescents from beginning to smoke.

Social influence approaches have identified the social environment as a critical determinant of smoking onset. Rather than focusing on long-term disease risk, these interventions have stressed more immediate consequences of smoking, including negative social consequences. Adolescents are viewed as often lacking in skills needed to resist peer pressure and other influences that promote smoking.[46] As described in the 1994 Surgeon General's Report, the principal messages of skill-based interventions have focused on the negative, short-term social consequences of smoking, on the techniques of tobacco advertising that may be falsely appealing to adolescents, and on the socially salient advantages of being a nonsmoker.

Meta-analyses of school-based smoking prevention programs have indicated that these contemporary programs do have an impact in preventing smoking onset.[47–51] Furthermore, social influence approaches appear to be the most effective type of school-based program. Based on the results of her meta-analysis, Rooney concluded that the best results were obtained by social influence programs that: (1) were delivered to sixth-grade students, (2) included booster sessions, (3) concentrated the program within a short period, and (4) used an untrained peer to present the program.[50]

Glynn listed essential elements of effective smoking prevention programs based on the consensus of a panel of experts.[52] These elements were summarized in the 1994 Report of the Surgeon General as follows:

1. Classroom sessions should be delivered at least five times per year in each of 2 years in the sixth through eighth grades.
2. The program should emphasize the social factors that influence smoking onset, short-term consequences, and refusal skills.
3. The program should be incorporated into the existing school curricula.
4. The program should be introduced during the transition from elementary school to junior high or middle school (sixth or seventh grades).
5. Students should be involved in the presentation and delivery of the program.
6. Parental involvement should be encouraged.
7. Teachers should be adequately trained.
8. The program should be socially and culturally acceptable to each community.

Although some of these points might appear self-evident (eg, adequate training of teachers, social and cultural acceptability of programs), they have often been overlooked in practice. Furthermore, in high-risk populations, including those of low socioeconomic status, many inner city residents, and some ethnic minorities, a considerable number of children will have already begun to smoke by sixth grade. In these populations, it may be advisable to focus prevention efforts on younger children as well.

Peterson and his colleagues reported the results of the Hutchinson Smoking Prevention Project (HSPP), which was conducted from 1984 through 1999.[53] The goal of this project was to assess the long-term impact of a theory-based, social influence approach implemented in grades 3 to 12. Study participants included 8388 children enrolled in two consecutive third grades in 40 Washington state school districts. Participants were followed until 2 years after high school. Prevalence of daily smoking for girls was 24.4% for experimental school districts and 24.7% for control school districts. Prevalence of daily smoking for boys was 26.3 and 26.7% for experimental and control school districts, respectively. This trial is noteworthy for its rigor. The negative findings cast some doubt on the long-term effectiveness of school-based programs.

Community-based prevention programs

A few model prevention programs have actively involved parents and the larger community in addition to schools. One example is a project by Perry and her colleagues in the context of the Minnesota Heart Health Program (MHHP),[54] a research and demonstration project designed to reduce CVD at the community level.[55] Initiated in 1980, MHHP involved the entire population in three participating communities in the north-central

United States. These communities were exposed to a 5-year educational program that encouraged modifications in eating, exercise, and smoking.

Perry and co-workers hypothesized that school-based smoking prevention would be more effective in communities in which multiple complementary school and community programs were established.[54] Students participated in 5 years of school-based health education, including peer-led prevention in a context in which adults were actively involved in community smoking cessation programs and smoking restrictions were being considered both in schools and in the larger community. Results were very encouraging, with smoking prevalence significantly lower among students in the intervention community than among students in the control community. These differences persisted throughout junior and senior high school. At the end of the twelfth grade, smoking was 40% less prevalent among students in the intervention community than among students in the comparison community: 14.6% of students were weekly smokers at the end of high school compared with 24.1% in the reference community.

State and federal prevention initiatives

California, Massachusetts, and Arizona have operated comprehensive anti-tobacco programs funded by cigarette excise taxes. A major emphasis of these programs has been on preventing tobacco use in youth. Each of these initiatives has included aggressive and well-funded anti-tobacco media campaigns. Florida launched an aggressive media campaign that directly targeted the tobacco industry.[56] After 2 years, current cigarette use dropped from 18.5 to 11.1% among middle school students and from 27.4 to 22.6% among high school students.[57] The National Cancer Institute American Stop Smoking Intervention Study for Cancer Prevention (ASSIST) is the largest tobacco-control project undertaken in the United States. ASSIST is based on a coalition model and is intended to demonstrate that a comprehensive, coordinated intervention can significantly reduce tobacco use. A major emphasis of ASSIST as well has been on primary prevention of tobacco use among children, adolescents, and young adults.

Flynn and colleagues found that a combination of media intervention and school-based programming fared better than school-based intervention alone.[58] The media campaign included both radio and television spots, which were broadcast as paid advertisements over local media. Reported smoking in the past week was 35% less among youth in the school-and-media group than in the school-only group (12.8% vs. 19.8%).

Prevention efforts should be considered within a broader context that also addresses policy issues and counteradvertising, in addition to youth-focused prevention and cessation initiatives.[59] According to the most recent Federal Trade Commission report, in 2001 the tobacco industry spent $11.2 billion in the United States on advertising and promotion, with these expenditures heavily targeted toward youth. A comprehensive public policy on tobacco should address tobacco advertising and promotion, access of minors to tobacco products, and tobacco excise taxes, in addition to school-based and other community initiatives.

Restrictions on tobacco advertising targeted at youth, including use of cartoon imagery, may be effective in reducing the appeal of such advertising to youth. Restrictions on smoking in public places, including schools, and on tobacco availability to minors also may reduce smoking prevalence, although findings have been inconsistent.[59,60] All 50 states and the District of Columbia have adopted a minimum age of 18 for the purchase of tobacco, but these laws have not been widely enforced.

Increased taxation also may have an impact on adolescent smoking. Adolescents appear to be at least as price sensitive, if not more so, than adults. The impact of significantly higher prices may be even greater in discouraging initiation than in reducing consumption among existing smokers. Furthermore, not only could a substantial increase in excise taxes be an important tool to discourage adolescent smoking, but revenue from these taxes can be dedicated to comprehensive tobacco control programs that will further reduce youth onset of smoking.

CDC published Best Practices for Comprehensive Tobacco Control Programs (1999). This document provides recommendations to the states for establishing initiatives that include local community programs, chronic disease programs to reduce the burden of tobacco-related diseases, school interventions, enforcement, statewide programs, countermarketing, cessation methods, surveillance and evaluation, and administration and management. Recommended funding levels are given for each of these components. Local community programs can engage young people; school-based interventions can be linked with local community coalitions and statewide counteradvertising; enforcement can reduce access of minors; and statewide initiatives can provide skill, resources, and information for coordinated strategic implementation of community programs. The Best Practices guide notes that funds can be awarded directly to school districts and programs can be supported by statewide technical assistance. Best Practices dictates allocating $500,000 to $750,000 annually for statewide infrastructure and technical assistance to support individual school districts. In addition, $4 to $6 per student in grades K to 12 should be budgeted for annual awards to school districts. Unfortunately, few states have funded comprehensive statewide programs at levels close to those recommended by CDC, and the recent trend has been to cut funding for state tobacco control initiatives.

Cessation

The vast majority of the work done with youth has focused on prevention rather than cessation of smoking. One of the most comprehensive studies was the Project Towards No Tobacco Use.[61] This study was conducted in rural and suburban high schools in two states. The cessation component of this project was a group-based clinic. Students were randomly assigned to a clinic or to a waitlist control. Clinics consisted of five sessions over 1 month, with an additional follow-up session held 3 months after the fifth session. Unfortunately, the clinics suffered high attrition, and results at the 3-month follow-up indicated no benefit from the clinic (6.8% chemically confirmed abstinence) over the waitlist control (7.9% chemically confirmed abstinence). These results are especially discouraging because the investigators had previously undertaken extensive formative work that included 31 focus groups with adolescents.

Hollis and co-workers reported a less intensive, but well-designed intervention in an HMO setting.[62] Adolescents who indicated on a screening questionnaire having smoked in the past week were asked to participate in the study. Participants were randomly assigned to an intervention consisting of a 60-minute office visit with a nurse practitioner or to usual care. Intervention subjects who wished to quit smoking received a follow-up call 1 week later; additional calls were dependent on adolescents' continued interest in quitting. Those who quit smoking were eligible for a lottery with opportunities to win $100. One-year outcome data failed to indicate an intervention effect.

Importantly, many of the interventions that have been demonstrated to be effective in adults have not achieved comparable success in adolescent populations. Thus, although nicotine replacement has consistently led to good outcomes with adult smokers,[63] findings to date with adolescents have been disappointing. In a study by Smith and colleagues, only 1 of 22 adolescent smokers aged 13 to 17 who received nicotine patch therapy was abstinent at 6-month follow-up.[64] In a second unpublished study with 101 adolescent smokers, 6-month abstinence was only 5%.

A more promising preliminary study was recently published by Colby and colleagues.[65] Intervention consisted of brief motivational interviewing of adolescent smokers (without follow-up) in a hospital emergency room. Motivational interviewing has been widely used with adults,[66] but there is very little published work with adolescents. Colby and co-workers randomly assigned 40 adolescents to either motivational interviewing or usual care. Three months after the intervention, 22% of

the intervention group had quit smoking, compared with 10% in the control group. However, with only 40 adolescents, this difference was not significant. Motivational interviewing appears feasible with adolescents, and, indeed, this client-centered method may be especially appropriate for adolescent smokers.

Lando and his colleagues implemented a systems-based approach with adolescents in the context of dental practices within a large HMO.[67] Adolescent smokers aged 14 to 17 years who had scheduled routine dental appointments were randomly assigned either to dental advice only or to dental advice plus face-to-face counseling and follow-up telephone support. The face-to-face counseling session and follow-up support emphasized motivational interviewing. Although the project had been intended as a cessation trial, self-reported smoking among adolescents in this setting was far lower than expected from prior survey data (eg, approximately 13% of respondents reported having smoked within the past 30 days as opposed to more than 30% of comparably aged respondents to a statewide survey conducted in 1996). Eligibility criteria were expanded to include susceptible never smokers, as well as susceptible ever smokers. (Susceptibility was defined by answers to three questions, including: "If your best friend were to give you a cigarette, would you smoke it," and "Do you think you will be smoking a year from now?"). Results failed to indicate an intervention effect at either the 3- or 12-month follow-up.

A recent review examined the literature on smoking cessation in adolescents.[68] The authors evaluated 17 cessation studies. Program content for these studies was derived from a wide range of theoretical perspectives. Most studies were conducted in school settings and reached less than half of the potential population of adolescent smokers. End-of-treatment quit rates reported in 12 of the 17 studies averaged 20.7% (range = 0 − 36%), and abstinence at follow-up declined to 13%. The most successful programs generally included some type of cognitive-behavioral intervention such as instruction in coping skills and a focus on the immediate consequences of quitting.

Grantees funded under special requests for applications for youth tobacco intervention have reported their results at annual meetings sponsored by the National Cancer Institute. The most recent of these meetings took place in June 2003. Results of funded cessation trials reported at these meetings have been almost uniformly negative. It is apparent we know less about how to intervene with youths than we do with adults. Behavioral and pharmacologic methods that have proven effective with adults generally have not been demonstrated to work with adolescents. The vast majority of adolescents are not actively considering quitting. Most adolescents who smoke regularly believe it would be very difficult to

TABLE 5-5 Prevention and Intervention Strategies in Youth

School-based prevention programs
Social influence approaches produce good results
Community-based prevention programs
May also enhance effects of school-based programs
State and federal prevention initiatives
Anti-tobacco media campaigns
May enhance school-based programs
Restrictions on tobacco advertising
Restrictions on tobacco availability to minors
Restrictions on smoking in public places, including schools
Increased taxation
Adolescents may be sensitive to price increases
Limited work in adolescent cessation
School-based cessation approaches
Adolescent cessation in managed care

quit,[69] but adolescents are unlikely either to enroll or to remain in formal cessation programs.[38] Adolescents often have withdrawal symptoms much like adults. Despite these withdrawal symptoms and perceived difficulty in quitting, many adolescents view organized cessation programs as irrelevant largely on the grounds that there is no immediate need for assistance. The importance of effective cessation programs for adolescents is underscored, however, by the fact that more than 80% of those who smoked a half-pack a day or more as high school seniors were smoking five to six years later as young adults; more than half of these smokers were consuming a pack or more a day at follow-up. Programs among youth are summarized in Table 5-5.

INTERVENTIONS AMONG ADULTS

Interventions with adults have focused on cessation rather than prevention for obvious reasons. There is, however, some initiation of smoking even in adulthood. Adult interventions are summarized in Table 5-6. Adult initiation is relatively common in certain settings, such as the military. Thus, Klesges and colleagues reported that 7% of never smokers who entered the Air Force and completed Basic Military Training were regular smokers 1 year later.[70] Ethnic differences also have been observed in smoking initiation: African-Americans tend to initiate later than Euro-Americans.[71] In some other countries, initiation of smoking tends to occur considerably later than in the United States. In China, for example, one cohort study found the mean age for starting smoking to be 22 years.[72] Initiation also has been demonstrated among college students. Until recently, it had been widely

assumed that those who reached the age of 18 without smoking were very unlikely to initiate smoking as adults. However, the tobacco industry has increasingly targeted advertising and promotion efforts at young adults. In contrast to older adults, smoking prevalence has not been declining in the young adult (18- to 24-year-old) population.

The vast majority of the published work with adults has been limited not only to individual smokers, but also to smokers who have sought assistance in quitting. Unfortunately, individual smokers who are ready to quit and who seek help represent a very small proportion of the overall smoking population.[73] Furthermore, even in these smokers, absolute long-term outcomes with formal quit smoking programs have tended to be disappointing. Intensive multisession group clinics generally produce no more than about 25% abstinence at 1 year.[74] Unaided quit attempts fare substantially less well: of the approximately 17 million smokers in the United States who attempt to quit on their own each year, fewer than 10% are successful.

Traditionally, interventions have focused on a single, assisted quit attempt. A more effective approach may be to view smoking as a chronic disease and to support multiple quit attempts if necessary.[67] More recently, larger-scale public health efforts have been undertaken to address smoking cessation at the community level and to target adults who may not present for treatment or who may not be immediately interested in quitting.[75,76] For many years, smoking and other tobacco use were seen as essentially learned behaviors. More recently, however, smoking and use of other tobacco products have been recognized as physically addictive.[77]

Interventions targeted at individuals

There has been far more progress in developing effective smoking cessation interventions with adults than with adolescents. An exhaustive review of the published smoking cessation literature between 1975 and 1994 was undertaken by a panel appointed by the Agency for Health Care Policy and Research.[63] An overall conclusion of the panel was that effective smoking cessation treatments are available for adults. More specific conclusions were that brief cessation treatments improve outcome and that a dose–response relationship exists between the intensity and duration of a program and effectiveness, with more intensive treatments generally producing better long-term abstinence. In addition, the panel recognized three specific treatment elements as effective: nicotine replacement therapy (nicotine patches or gum), social support (clinician-provided encouragement and assistance), and skills training/problem solving (techniques for achieving and maintaining abstinence).

TABLE 5-6 Adult Cessation Strategies

Strategy	Comments on risk
Aversion (rapid smoking, oversmoking)	May pose significant risk, especially for smokers with existing cardiovascular disease
Contingency contracting (rewards for abstinence)	
Social support (support from clinician, group support, support from family and friends)	
Relaxation techniques (progressive relaxation, deep breathing)	
Stimulus control and cue extinction (restricting where and when smoking takes place)	
Coping skills (problem solving, cognitive and behavioral strategies)	
Reduced smoking and nicotine fading (gradual reduction in numbers of cigarettes, switching to lower-tar and nicotine brands)	
Multicomponent treatment programs (combinations of behavioral techniques)	
Hypnosis	
Acupuncture	
Nonprofit and proprietary programs	
Self-help (written materials, videos, tapes, hotlines/helplines)	
Computer-tailored messages	
Pharmacologic intervention	
Nicotine patch	Skin rashes and irritation, usually mild
Nicotone polacrilex (nicotine gum)	Mouth soreness, hiccups, dyspepsia, jaw ache, generally mild and transient, often alleviated by correcting patient's chewing technique
Nicotine nasal spray	Nose and eye irritation is common, but usually disappears within 1 wk
Nicotine inhaler	Few side effects, may cause mouth or throat irritation
Bupropion hydrochloride (Zyban)	Slight risk of seizure; should not be used by patients with eating disorders or seizure disorders, or those taking certain other medications

An updated clinical practice guideline was published in 2000. The accelerating pace of tobacco research that prompted the update is reflected by the fact that 3000 articles were published between 1975 and 1994 and screened as part of the original guideline, and an additional 3000 were published between 1995 and 1999 and contributed to the updated guideline. The updated guideline largely reiterated the recommendations of the earlier guideline. Several additional medications were recognized as effective. These included bupropion SR (Zyban), which is the first nonnicotine medication shown to be effective for smoking cessation and approved by the Food and Drug Administration for that purpose. Bupropion SR is available exclusively as a prescription med-

ication, with both an indication for smoking cessation and an indication for depression (Wellbutrin). Nicotine nasal spray and nicotine inhaler were also shown to reliably increase abstinence rates. Both of these medications require a prescription, and they have had very limited popularity with consumers. One additional medication, a nicotine-containing lozenge, has been approved since publication of the updated guideline.

Behavioral treatments

Despite the addictive properties of nicotine, behavioral aspects of smoking are still seen as critical. The most effective intervention programs have included behavioral treatment components. The clinical practice guidelines report findings for a number of specific behavioral components, including aversive smoking, intratreatment social support, problem solving/skills training, quit day, extratreatment social support, motivation, weight/diet/nutrition, exercise/fitness, contingency contract, relaxation/breathing, and cigarette fading. Most of these specific treatment components have not been proven effective in isolation, but may contribute to an overall multicomponent intervention.

AVERSION

Although the guideline found aversive smoking to be effective (and indeed to achieve the highest absolute abstinence levels), aversive techniques have largely gone out of favor. These techniques have included rapid smoking[78,79] and oversmoking, or satiation.[80,81] Rapid smoking requires smokers to take very frequent puffs, typically every 6 seconds, for as long as they can tolerate. Oversmoking requires subjects to dramatically increase (perhaps double) their usual cigarette consumption for an arbitrary period, typically 1 week. Concerns have been expressed about the safety of rapid smoking and oversmoking.[82] Acceptability of these techniques to smokers has been an additional issue. Another option is reduced aversion techniques,[83,84] including focused smoking (smoking at a regulated but slower rate) and smoke holding (retaining smoke in the mouth and throat while breathing through the nose).

CONTINGENCY CONTRACTING

Several studies have required participants to submit monetary deposits that are refunded contingent on maintained abstinence.[85,86] Contracts may also call for self-administered rewards for progressively longer periods of abstinence. Typically, contingency contracting has been included as part of multicomponent behavioral programs.

SOCIAL SUPPORT

Supportive intervention during direct contact with a clinician or in a group (intratreatment social support) increases smoking cessation rates.[63] However, although social support from friends and family is strongly related to successful outcomes in smoking cessation treatments, efforts to systematically enhance natural social support as part of treatment intervention generally have proven unsuccessful.[87]

RELAXATION TECHNIQUES

Progressive relaxation and deep breathing strategies have been employed for smoking cessation, although rarely in isolation. A major rationale for the use of these procedures is that smoking relapses are very likely to occur during negative emotional states.[88,89] Relaxation training allows an alternative response for coping with negative emotions or stressful situations and with the stress of quitting smoking and nicotine withdrawal effects. However, there is little evidence to support the efficacy of relaxation training as a stand-alone technique.[90]

STIMULUS CONTROL AND CUE EXTINCTION

Stimulus control and cue extinction procedures also have tended to produce weak results. These procedures have been used in an effort to reduce the huge number of environmental cues that have been associated with smoking.[91] In theory, if some of the cues governing smoking can be weakened or extinguished, quitting should be facilitated. One strategy has been to gradually reduce smoking consumption by progressively restricting the types of situations in which smoking is permitted. Another type of stimulus control strategy permits smoking only at set times (eg, every hour on the half-hour), regardless of the individual's desire to smoke.[92]

COPING SKILLS

Favorable results have been obtained with specific training in coping skills. Coping skills include problem solving and methods for managing stress and preventing relapse. Shiffman found that a combination of cognitive (eg, mentally reviewing benefits of quitting) and behavioral (eg, physical activity, leaving a tempting situation) coping responses provided maximum protection against smoking in a potential crisis situation.[89]

REDUCED SMOKING AND NICOTINE FADING

Nicotine fading is a nonaversive preparation technique based on the logical premise that withdrawal discomfort might be ameliorated if nicotine consumption is progressively reduced prior to abstinence. This premise may appear to be in conflict with the results of gradual reduction or cigarette "tapering" procedures. Strategies that have emphasized cutting down the numbers of cigarettes smoked have been almost uniformly unsuccessful.[93] Smokers typically appear to reach a "stuck point," often at 10 to 12 cigarettes per day.[93] For the typical smoker of approximately a pack per day, compensatory changes in puffing can compensate for reduced numbers of cigarettes at this level. Nicotine fading is an alternative in which smokers switch, in a series of progressive steps over several weeks, to cigarettes rated lower in tar and nicotine[94] or use commercially available nicotine reduction filters (95). These procedures have not proven successful in improving smoking cessation outcomes.

MULTICOMPONENT TREATMENT PROGRAMS

The most successful behavioral programs have incorporated multiple treatment components. Emphasis has been placed on both initial preparation for quitting and longer-term maintenance. Reported long-term abstinence rates for these multicomponent treatment programs have approached 50%.[84,96] More recent outcomes have tended to be less successful, however.[97]

Hypnosis and acupuncture

There are numerous approaches to smoking cessation that are not primarily behavioral or pharmacologic. Two commonly advertised methods include hypnosis and acupuncture. Unfortunately, there are few good studies of these methods, and overall results tend to be disappointing. Telling, perhaps, was the fact that only three acceptable studies that examined hypnosis were found in preparation of the AHCPR guidelines, despite the widespread use of this technique. Because the studies were of poor quality and their results were inconsistent, the evidence was insufficient to assess the effectiveness of hypnosis. No additional studies that met inclusion criteria were found in preparing the updated clinical practice guideline. Studies that have compared acupuncture at theoretically correct sites versus "incorrect" or sham sites have generally found no differences in outcome.

Nonprofit and proprietary programs

The oldest of the nonprofit programs are the Five-Day Plans sponsored by the Seventh-Day Adventist Church.[98] An estimated 14 million smokers in more than 150 countries have attended Five-Day Plans. This program considers both physical and psychologic aspects of cigarette dependence, but uses few cognitive-behavioral strategies. Treatment consists of five 90-minute to 2-hour sessions on consecutive days. The Five-Day Plan has been revised and renamed The Breathe-Free Plan to Stop Smoking, which includes eight sessions over a 3-week period.

Both the American Cancer Society and the American Lung Association offer formal group programs. Lando and co-workers compared these two programs.[99] Smokers ($n = 1041$) in three Iowa communities were randomly assigned to American Cancer Society clinics, American Lung Association clinics, or an intensive multicomponent behavioral program derived from laboratory research. Although results initially favored the laboratory program over both nonprofit clinics, by 1-year follow-up, differences between the laboratory program and the American Lung Association program were no longer significant. Sustained abstinence rates at 1 year were 22.2, 19.0, and 12.1% for the laboratory, American Lung Association, and American Cancer Society clinics, respectively. The American Lung Association program (Freedom from Smoking) was more intensive than the American Cancer Society program (FreshStart), with the former program consisting of seven 90-minute to 2-hour group sessions in addition to an initial orientation over

a 7-week period, and the latter consisting of four 1-hour group sessions over either 2 or 4 weeks. Content of the American Cancer Society FreshStart program recently has been revised.

A number of commercial programs are available, usually concentrated in larger metropolitan areas. Most programs tend not to be highly profitable and therefore do not remain active. In evaluating commercial methods, it again appears that the most successful are those that include multicomponent cognitive-behavioral techniques. A number of commercial products (eg, lozenges, filters) have been introduced as aids to smoking cessation. Currently, none of these products, other than nicotine replacement and Zyban, are recognized as effective.

Self-help

Simply handing smokers written self-help materials has not been demonstrated to be effective. There is evidence based on a limited number of studies that smoker-initiated calls to telephone hotlines/helplines for cessation counseling or assistance does improve abstinence rates.[63] Although results have been mixed, several studies have reported good results for proactive telephone support in which calls are initiated by the helpline rather than by the smoker.[100–102]

Computer-tailored messages

Computer-tailored messages or "expert systems" have the potential to individualize cessation content to the individual smoker. These programs use computer-based algorithms to characterize the individual smoker and provide messages most appropriate to their smoking pattern, environment, and needs. Some encouraging preliminary results have been reported with these types of programs.[103–108]

Pharmacologic intervention

Currently, a number of pharmacologic aids are recognized as effective by the Food and Drug Administration. Most of these aids involve some form of nicotine replacement: nicotine patch, nicotine polacrilex (nicotine gum), nicotine nasal spray, nicotine inhaler, and nicotine lozenge. Each of these products has specific advantages and disadvantages. Suggestions for effective clinical use of medications are included in the clinical practice guideline.

The patch is easy to use and needs to be applied only once each day. However, it does not allow very flexible dosing (eg, once the patch is placed on the skin, the delivered dose is not controlled by the patient), and delivery of nicotine is relatively slow. The gum allows more flexible dosing, but is somewhat harder to use correctly. Most gum users underdose with this medication. Nicotine nasal spray also has the advantage of flexible dosing, plus it provides faster delivery of nicotine. However, many users are bothered by initial eye and nose irritation, and frequent use is necessary to obtain adequate nicotine levels. The nicotine inhaler allows flexible dosing and, at least partially, mimics the hand-to-mouth behavior of smoking. The inhaler also has few side effects. A major limitation, however, may be the need to do far more puffing than on a cigarette. For optimal nicotine dosage, many hundreds of puffs may be needed, as opposed to perhaps 200 for a regular pack-per-day smoker. The nicotine lozenge also allows flexible dosing and is easier for many people to use than is nicotine gum.

The only FDA-approved nonnicotine medication is bupropion hydrochloride (trade name Zyban). This product is available in tablet form. Its appears to act on brain chemistry to bring about some of the same effects that nicotine has in people who smoke, although its action is not fully understood. The product is easy to use and can be combined with nicotine replacement. Preliminary evidence suggests that the combination of nicotine patch and Zyban may be more effective than either alone.[109] The main ingredient in Zyban has been available for many years as a treatment for depression under the trade name Wellbutrin. However, Zyban works well in smokers with no symptoms of depression. The major risk of this product is a very slight possibility of seizures.

There is evidence that combinations of medications may be more effective in producing abstinence. A combination of passive dosing (eg, through nicotine patch) and active dosing (eg, ad libitum use such as with nicotine gum) has been demonstrated to be more effective than a single form of dosing in isolation.[110–112]

Community and public health approaches

Fewer than 1% of all smokers have attended formal group or individual treatment programs. Even if half of these smokers achieved permanent abstinence, the overall impact on smoking prevalence would be extremely modest. There is need for a comprehensive public health approach to smoking that includes community and systems changes in addition to treatment programs of varying types and intensities.[73,113] These approaches are summarized in Table 5-7.

HEALTH CARE APPROACHES

Primary care and other clinicians have unique access to the smoking population. At least 70% of smokers see a physician each year.[63] Smokers cite physician advice to quit as an important motivator.[114,115] Unfortunately, however, only about half of current smokers report having ever been asked about their smoking status or urged to quit by physicians, and substantially fewer have re-

TABLE 5-7 Community and Public Health Approaches

Interventions in health systems
    Clinician advice (brief advice significantly increases
        quitting)
    Pharmacologic treatment

Worksite interventions (convenient access to large
    population of smokers, opportunities to capitalize on
    social support)

Community programs
    Overall mixed results
    Quit and Win contests widely disseminated

Policy changes

ceived advice on how to quit smoking successfully. Brief physician advice alone has been associated with a 30% increase in the probability of quitting.[63] Although absolute abstinence rates were modest, universal application of physician or other clinician advice could have major public health impact. Combining brief advice with offers of pharmacologic treatment could further increase the likelihood of success.

A major issue in health system implementation is lack of reimbursement for smoking cessation services. Curry and colleagues found that use of smoking cessation services varies with the extent of coverage.[116] Full coverage of both behavioral intervention and nicotine replacement therapy led to the highest rates of use of smoking cessation services and to the greatest impact on the overall prevalence of smoking.

WORKSITE INTERVENTIONS

Worksites provide convenient access to a large population of smokers, as well as the opportunity to capitalize on social support in this setting. Some very positive results have been reported for worksite interventions, although not all studies have been successful. Jeffery and colleagues reported modest, but significant, reductions in overall worksite smoking prevalence with an intervention that provided structured group programs and incentives (eg, refundable payroll deductions) for quitting.[117] The Working Well Trial conducted in 111 worksites was the largest worksite cancer control trial in the United States.[118] Interventions addressed dietary patterns and smoking. Although reductions in tobacco use were in the predicted direction, differences in tobacco use between intervention and control worksites were not significant.

COMMUNITY PROGRAMS

Several major community smoking interventions were offered as part of multicomponent heart disease prevention studies.[55,119,120] The Stanford Five-City project reported significant smoking reductions in the intervention cohort relative to the control, but changes were not found in cross-sectional samples. The Pawtucket Heart Health Program failed to obtain differences in smoking prevalence between an intervention city and a comparison city. The Minnesota Heart Health Program obtained mixed, but primarily negative results for smoking intervention. The only evidence of a significant intervention effect was for women in cross-sectional survey data.[121]

Although the overall impact of these communitywide trials on smoking prevalence was disappointing, a useful innovation resulting from these programs was the Quit and Win smoking cessation contest. These contests have been successful at the community level in engaging relatively large proportions of the smoking population. Contests also have engaged large numbers of nonsmokers in support of smokers' quit efforts and have increased community awareness around issues of quitting. Community contests have enrolled as many as 7% of all eligible smokers and have involved many more in reported quit attempts during the contest period.[122] The Quit and Win contest model has been applied in communities in a number of countries around the world and also in national smoking cessation contests in the United Kingdom and Finland.

A direct successor to these community trials was the Community Intervention Trial for Smoking Cessation (COMMIT) project, which focused only on smoking.[123,124] In contrast to the earlier studies, COMMIT randomly assigned communities to intervention or control conditions and included sufficient numbers of communities to allow use of the community as the unit of analysis. One community within each of 11 matched community pairs (10 in the United States, 1 in Canada) was randomly assigned to intervention. The initial target of COMMIT was heavy smokers, defined as those who smoked 25 or more cigarettes per day. Intervention channels focused on public education through media and communitywide events; health care providers; worksites and other organizations; and cessation resources.[123]

No differences were found between intervention and comparison communities in quit rates among heavy smokers. There was a significant intervention effect on quitting in light to moderate smokers.[123] Evaluation of overall smoking prevalence failed to indicate significant differences between intervention and comparison communities, however.[124] Results indicated rather modest differences between smokers in intervention and comparison communities in receipt of intervention activities.

More promising results have been reported for the American Stop Smoking Intervention Study (ASSIST). ASSIST is the largest tobacco control project ever undertaken in the United States.[125] In this initiative, 17 US states funded through ASSIST were compared with 32 others (California, which already had extensive tobacco control activities, was omitted). The primary goal of ASSIST was to reduce smoking prevalence and cigarette consumption among adults in ASSIST states. ASSIST was designed as a collaborative effort between the National Cancer Institute and the American Cancer Society. The primary contractors for ASSIST were state health departments. State health departments and American Cancer Society divisions formed coalitions with health organizations, health and social service agencies, and community groups to develop and implement comprehensive smoking control plans.

ASSIST targeted those considered at higher risk for smoking, including youth, ethnic minorities, blue collar workers, unemployed, women, heavy smokers, and smokeless tobacco users. Interventions were delivered to target populations through five channels: community environment, worksites, schools, health care settings, and community groups such as churches and chambers of commerce. Emphasis was placed primarily on policy and media interventions, with less emphasis on programmatic services. Per capita consumption was almost identical in intervention and comparison states before 1993, when full funding for ASSIST interventions began. By 1996, smokers in the intervention states were consuming approximately 7% fewer cigarettes per capita.[126]

POLICY CHANGES

Perhaps one of the largest impacts on society may be from improvements in health that can result from policy changes, such as the passage of anti-tobacco legislation. An excellent example stems from a study of respiratory health before and after recent tobacco prohibition began in bars and taverns in California.[127] In a small study of 53 bartenders in San Francisco, of those with respiratory symptoms at baseline, 59% no longer had symptoms at follow-up; of those with sensory irritations, 78% had resolution of symptoms (both $P < .001$). Further, a significant improvement (increase) in mean forced vital capacity (FVC) (increase of 4.2%) was reported after prohibition, and after cessation, significant improvements in both FVC (6.8% increase) and mean forced expiratory volume in 1 second (FEV1) (4.5% increase) were reported.

SUMMARY

The evidence linking tobacco use to incidence of, and mortality from, CVD is substantial. Approximately a half-million deaths annually are attributed to cigarette smoking, and economic costs total some $100 billion in medical expenses and indirect costs. Environmental tobacco smoke is also an important culprit, responsible for some 35,000 to 40,000 deaths from heart disease annually. Important interventions among youth include school-based prevention programs, community-based prevention programs, state and federal initiatives, as well as cessation assistance. For adults, various behavioral treatments, self-help approaches, and pharmacologic therapy are available. Community and public health approaches, including health care and worksite programs, are invaluable. Physicians and other health care providers need to take greater initiative in reviewing and following up on tobacco use, and in informing patients about appropriate community and health care resources for those needing help.

Reductions in adult smoking will have the most immediate benefit in terms of reduced hospitalizations from myocardial infarction and stroke, as well as saving associated medical costs of more than $3 billion over 7 years for a program reducing smoking prevalence by 1% per year.[128] Nonetheless, the key to making future progress is primary prevention of smoking in children and teenagers. The fact that tobacco use is dangerous, lethal, and disabling when used as directed has resulted in the call by many experts for the Food and Drug Administration to take steps to regulate its sale and use.[129]

REFERENCES

1. US Department of Health and Human Services. *Targeting Tobacco Use: The Nation's Leading Cause of Death, At-A-Glance.* Atlanta, Ga: Centers for Disease Control and Prevention; 1998.

2. Porter S, Jackson K, Trosclari A, et al. Prevalence of current cigarette smoking among adults and changes in prevalence of current and some day smoking, United States, 1996–2001. *MMWR* 2003;52:303–307.

3. US Public Health Service. *The Health Consequences of Smoking: Cardiovascular Disease: A Report of the Surgeon General.* DHHS publication (PHS) 84-50204. Rockville, Md: US Department of Health and Human Services; 1983.

4. US Department of Health and Human Services. *Changes in Cigarette-Related Disease Risks and Their Implication for Prevention and Control.* Monograph 8. NIH publication 97-4213. Rockville, Md: US Department of Health and Human Services, Public Health Services, National Institutes of Health, National Cancer Institute; 1997.

5. Kawachi I, Colditz GA, Stampfer MJ, et al. Smoking cessation and time course of decreased risks of coronary heart disease in middle-aged women. *Arch Intern Med* 1994;154:169–175.

6. Centers for Disease Control. *The Health Benefits of Smoking Cessation: A Report of the Surgeon General.* DHHS publication (CDC) 90-8416. Washington, DC: Public Health Service, Office on Smoking and Health; 1990.

7. Neaton JD, Wentworth D, for the Multiple Risk Factor Intervention Trial Research Group. Serum cholesterol, blood pressure, cigarette smoking, and death from coronary heart disease: overall findings and differences by age for 316,099 white men. *Arch Intern Med* 1992;152:56–64.

8. The Multiple Risk Factor Intervention Trial Research Group. Mortality after 16 years for participants randomized to the Multiple Risk Factor Intervention Trial. *Circulation* 1996;94:946–951.

9. Keys A, Menotti A, Aravanis C, et al. The seven countries study: 2,289 deaths in 15 years. *Prev Med* 1984;13:141–154.

10. Escobedo LG, Caspersen CJ. Risk factors for sudden coronary death in the United States. *Epidemiology* 1997;8:175–180.

11. Rosenberg L, Miller DR, Kaufman DW, et al. Myocardial infarction in women under 50 years of age. *JAMA* 1983;250:2801–2806.

12. Kannel WB, McGee DL, Castelli WP. Latest perspectives on cigarette smoking and cardiovascular disease: the Framingham Study. *J Cardiac Rehabil* 1984;4:267–277.

13. Miettinen TA, Gulling H. Mortality and cholesterol metabolism in familial hypercholesterolemia: long-term follow-up of 96 patients. *Arteriosclerosis* 1988;8:163–167.

14. Pooling Project Research Group. Relationship of blood pressure, serum cholesterol, smoking habit, relative weight, and ECG abnormalities to incidence of major coronary events: final report of the Pooling Project. *J Chronic Dis* 1978;31:201–306.

15. Suarez L, Barrett-Connor E. Interaction between cigarette smoking and diabetes mellitus in the prediction of death attributed to cardiovascular disease. *Am J Epidemiol* 1984;120:670–675.

16. Mishell DR. Use of oral contraceptives in women of older reproductive age. *Am J Obstet Gynecol* 1988;158:1652–1657.

17. Williams RR, Hasstedt SJ, Wilson DE, et al. Evidence that men with familial hypercholesterolemia can avoid early coronary death: an analysis of 77 gene carriers in four Utah pedigrees. *JAMA* 1986;255:219–224.

18. Hermanson B, Omenn GS, Kronmal RA, et al. Beneficial six-year outcome of smoking cessation in older men and women with coronary artery disease: results from the CASS registry. *N Engl J Med* 1988;319:1365–1369.

19. Rosenberg L, Kaufman DW, Helmrich SP, et al. The risk of myocardial infarction after quitting smoking in men under 55 years of age. *N Engl J Med* 1985;313:1511–1514.

20. McGill HC, McMahan CA, Malcom GT, et al, for the PDAY Research Group. Effects of serum lipoproteins and smoking on atherosclerosis in young men and women. *Arterioscler Thromb Vasc Biol* 1997;17:95–106.

21. Zimmerman M, McGeachie J. The effect of nicotine on aortic endothelium: a quantitative ultrastructural study. *Atherosclerosis* 1987;63:33–41.

22. Fried LP, Moore RD, Pearson TA. Long-term effects of cigarette smoking and moderate alcohol consumption on coronary artery diameter: mechanisms of coronary artery disease independent of atherosclerosis or thrombosis? *Am J Med* 1986;80:37–44.

23. Meade TW, Imeson J, Stirling Y. Effects of changes in smoking and other characteristics on clotting factors and the risk of ischaemic heart disease. *Lancet* 1987;2:986–988.

24. Maouad J, Fernandez F, Barrillon A, et al. Diffuse or segmental narrowing (spasm) of coronary arteries during smoking demonstrated on angiography. *Am J Cardiol* 1984;53:354–355.

25. US Department of Health and Human Services. *The Health Consequences of Involuntary Smoking: A Report of the Surgeon General.* Rockville, Md: Office on Smoking and Health;1986.

26. Lam TH, He Y. Passive smoking and coronary heart disease: a brief review. *Clin Exp Pharmacol Physiol* 1997;24:993–996.

27. Steenland K, Thun M, Lally C, et al. Environmental tobacco smoke and coronary heart disease in the American Cancer Society CPS-II cohort. *Circulation* 1996;94:622–628.

28. Gori GB. Environmental tobacco smoke and coronary heart syndromes: absence of an association. *Regul Toxicol Pharmacol* 1995;21:281–295.

29. Enstrom JE, Kabat GC. Environmental tobacco smoke and tobacco related mortality in a prospective study of Californians, 1960–98. *BMJ* 2003;326:1057–1066.

30. Kawachi I, Colditz GA, Speizer FE, et al. A prospective study of passive smoking and coronary heart disease. *Circulation* 1997;95:2374–2379.

31. Steenland K, Sieber K, Etzel RA, et al. Exposure to environmental tobacco smoke and risk factors for heart disease among never smokers in the Third National Health and Nutrition Examination Survey. *Am J Epidemiol* 1998;147:932–939.

32. Wells AH. Heart disease from passive smoking in the workplace. *J Am Coll Cardiol* 1998;31:1–9.

33. Kritz H, Schmid P, Sinzinger H. Passive smoking and cardiovascular risk. *Arch Intern Med* 1995;155:1942–1948.

34. Glantz SA, Parmley WW. Passive smoking and heart disease: mechanisms and risk. *JAMA* 1995;273:1047–1053.

35. Celermajer DS, Adams MR, Clarkson P, et al. Passive smoking and impaired endothelium-dependent arterial dilation in healthy young adults. *N Engl J Med* 1996;334:150–154.

36. Otsuka R, Watanabe H, Hirata K, et al. Acute effects of passive smoking on the coronary circulation in healthy young adults. *JAMA* 2001;286:436–441.

37. Weiss ST. Cardiovascular effects of environmental tobacco smoke. *Circulation* 1996;94:599.

38. U.S. Department of Health and Human Services. *Preventing Tobacco Use Among Young People: A Report of the Surgeon General.* Atlanta, Ga: US Department of Health and Human Services, Public Health Service, Centers for Disease Control and Prevention, National Center for Chronic Disease Prevention and Health Promotion, Office on Smoking and Health; 1994.

39. DiFranza JR, Richards JW, Paulman PM, et al. RJR Nabisco's cartoon camel promotes camel cigarettes to children. *JAMA* 1991;266:3149–3153.

40. Johnston LD, O'Malley PM, Bachman JG. *National Survey Results on Drug Use from the Monitoring the Future Study, 1968–1974,* vol 1: *Secondary School Students.* Rockville, Md: National Institutes on Drug Abuse.

41. Centers for Disease Control. Surveillance for selected tobacco-use behaviors—United States, 1900–1994. *MMWR* 1994;43:143.

42. *MMWR* 1998. Cited by: Centers for Disease Control. Tobacco Use Among Middle and High School Students—United States, 1999. *MMWR* 2000;49:49–53.

43. Centers for Disease Control. *Chronic Diseases and Their Risk Factors,* 1998.

44. Arnett DK, Sprafka JM, McGovern PG, et al. Trends in cigarette smoking: the Minnesota Heart Survey, 1980 through 1992. *Am J Public Health* 1998;88:1230–1233.

45. Thompson EL. Smoking education programs 1960–1976. *Am J Public Health* 1978;68:250–257.

46. Botvin GJ, Wills TA. Personal and social skills training: cognitive-behavioral approaches to substance abuse prevention. In: Bell CS, Battjes R, eds. *Prevention Research: Deterring Drug Abuse Among Children and Adolescents.* Monograph 63. Bethesda, Md: US Department of Health and Human Services, Public Health Service, Alcohol, Drug Abuse, and Mental Health Administration, National Institute on Drug Abuse; 1985. DHHS Publication (ADM) 85-1334.

47. Tobler NS. Meta-analysis of 143 adolescent drug prevention programs: quantitative outcome results of program participants compared to a control or comparison group. *J Drug Issues* 1986;16:537–567.

48. Tobler NS. Drug prevention programs can work: research findings. *J Addict Dis* 1992;11:1–28.

49. Rundall TG, Bruvold WH. A meta-analysis of school-based smoking and alcohol use prevention programs. *Health Educ Q* 1988;15:317–334.

50. Rooney B. *A meta-analysis of smoking-prevention programs after adjustment for study design* [dissertation]. Minneapolis: University of Minnesota; 1992.

51. Bruvold WH. A meta-analysis of adolescent smoking-prevention programs. *Am J Public Health* 1993;83:872–880.

52. Glynn TJ. Essential elements of school-based smoking-prevention programs. *J Sch Health* 1989;59:181–188.

53. Peterson AV, Kealey KA, Mann SL, et al. Hutchinson Smoking Prevention Project: long-term randomized trial in school-based tobacco use prevention. *J Natl Cancer Inst* 2000;92:1979–1991.

54. Perry CL, Kelder SH, Murray DM, et al. Community-wide smoking prevention: long-term outcomes of the Minnesota Heart Health Program and the class of 1989 study. *Am J Public Health* 1992;82:1210–1216.

55. Luepker RV, Murray DM, Jacobs DR, et al. Community education for cardiovascular disease prevention: risk factor changes in the Minnesota Heart Health Program. *Am J Public Health* 1994;84:1383–1393.

56. Sly DF, Heald GR, Ray S. The Florida "truth" anti-tobacco media evaluation: design, first year results, and implications for planning future state media evaluations. *Tobacco Control* 2001;10:9–15.

57. Bauer UE, Johnson TM, Hopkins RS, Brooks RG. Changes in youth cigarette use and intentions following implementation of a tobacco control program: findings from the Florida Youth Tobacco Survey, 1998–2000. *JAMA* 2000;284:723–728.

58. Flynn BS, Worden JK, Secker-Walker RH, et al. Prevention of cigarette smoking through mass media intervention and school programs. *Am J Public Health* 1992;82:827–834.

59. Forster JL, Murray DM, Wolfson M, et al. The effects of community policies to reduce youth access to tobacco. *Am J Public Health* 1998;88:1193–1198.

60. Rigotti NA, DiFranza JR, YuChiao C, et al. The effect of enforcing tobacco-sales laws on adolescents' access to tobacco and smoking behavior. *N Engl J Med* 1997;337:1044–1051.

61. Sussman S, Dent CW, Burton D, et al. *Developing School-Based Tobacco Use Prevention and Cessation Programs.* Thousand Oaks, Calif: Sage; 1995.

62. Hollis JF, Vogt TM, Stevens V, et al. The tobacco reduction and cancer control (TRACC) program: team approaches to counseling in medical and dental settings. In: National Cancer Institute. *Tobacco and the Clinician: Interventions for Medical and Dental Practice, Smoking and Tobacco Control.* Monograph 5. Rockville, Md: US Department of Health and Human Services; 1994. NIH publication 94-3693.

63. Fiore MC, Bailey WC, Cohen SJ, et al. *Smoking Cessation.* Clinical Practice Guideline 18. Rockville, Md: US Department of Health and Human Services, Public Health Service, Agency for Health Care Policy and Research; April 1996. AHCPR publication 96-0692.

64. Smith TA, House RF Jr., Crogham IT, et al. Nicotine patch therapy in adolescent smokers. *Pediatrics* 1996;98:659–667.

65. Colby S, Monti P, Barnett N, et al. Motivational interviewing with teen smokers in a hospital setting: 3-month treatment outcome results. *Ann Behav Med* 1997;19:S049.

66. Miller WR, Rollnick S. *Motivational Interviewing: Preparing People to Change Addictive Behavior.* New York: Guilford Press; 1991.

67. Lando H, Rolnick S, Klevan D, et al. Telephone support as an adjunct to transdermal nicotine. *Am J Public Health* 1997;87: 1670–1674.

68. Sussman S, Lichtman K, Ritt A, et al. Effects of thirty-four adolescent tobacco use cessation and prevention trials on regular users of tobacco products. *Substance Use Misuse* 1999;34:1469–1503.

69. Barker D. Reasons for tobacco use and symptoms of nicotine withdrawal among adolescent and young adult tobacco users—United States. *MMWR* 1993;43:745–750.

70. Klesges R, Haddock K, Lando H, et al. Efficacy of forced smoking cessation and an adjunctive behavioral treatment on long term smoking rates. *J Consult Clin Psychol* 1999;67:952–958.

71. US Department of Health and Human Services. *Tobacco Use Among US Racial/Ethnic Minority Groups—African Americans, American Indians and Alaska Natives, Asian Americans and Pacific Islanders, and Hispanics: A Report of the Surgeon General.* Atlanta, Ga: US Department of Health and Human Services, Centers for Disease Control and Prevention, National Center for Chronic Disease Prevention and Health Promotion, Office on Smoking and Health; 1998.

72. Lam TH, He Y, Li LS, et al. Mortality attributable to cigarette smoking in China. *JAMA* 1997;278:1505–1508.

73. Lichtenstein E, Glasgow RE. Smoking cessation: what have we learned over the past decade? *J Consult Clin Psychol* 1992;60: 518–527.

74. U.S. Department of Health and Human Services. *Treating Tobacco Use and Dependence.* Rockville, Md: Public Health Services; June 2000.

75. Lichtenstein E, Glasgow RE. A pragmatic framework for smoking cessation: implications for clinical and public health programs. *Psychol Addict Behav* 1997;11:142–151.

76. DiClemente C, Prochaska J, Fairhurst S, et al. The process of smoking cessation: an analysis of precontemplation, contemplation, and preparation stages of change. *J Consult Clin Psychol* 1991;59:295–304.

77. US Department of Health and Human Services. *The Health Consequences of Smoking: Nicotine Addiction: A Report of the Surgeon General.* Rockville, Md: US Department of Health and Human Services, Public Health Service, Centers for Disease Control, Center for Health Promotion and Education, Office on Smoking and Health; 1994.

78. Lichenstein E, Harris DE, Birchler GR, et al. Comparison of rapid smoking, warm, smoky air, and attention placebo in the modification of smoking behavior. *J Consult Clin Psychol* 1973;40:92–98.

79. Poole AD, Sanson-Fisher RW, German GA. The rapid-smoking technique: therapeutic effectiveness. *Behav Res Ther* 1981;19: 89–397.

80. Resnick JH. Effects of stimulus satiation on the overlearned maladaptive response of cigarette smoking. *J Consult Clin Psychol* 1968;32:501–505.

81. Lando HA. A comparison of excessive and rapid smoking in the modification of chronic smoking behavior. *J Consult Clin Psychol* 1975;43:350–355.

82. Hauser R. Rapid smoking as a technique of behavior modification: caution in selection of subjects. *J Consult Clin Psychol* 1974;42:625.

83. Powell DR, McCann BS. The effects of a multiple treatment program and maintenance procedures on smoking cessation. *Prev Med* 1981;10:94–104.

84. Tiffany ST, Martin EM, Baker TB. Treatments for cigarette smoking: an evaluation of the contributions of aversion and counseling procedures. *Behav Res Ther* 1986;24:437–452.

85. Elliott R, Tighe T. Breaking the cigarette habit: effects of a technique involving threatened loss of money. *Psychol Record* 1968;18:503–513.

86. Lando HA. Aversive conditioning and contingency management in the treatment of smoking. *J Consult Clin Psychol* 1976; 44:312.

87. Lichenstein E, Glasgow RE, Abrams DB. Social support in smoking cessation: in search of effective interventions. *Behav Res Ther* 1986;17:607–619.

88. Brandon TH, Tiffany ST, Baker TB. The process of smoking relapse. In: Tims FM, Leukefeld CG, eds. *Relapse and Recovery in Drug Abuse.* NIDA Research Monograph 72. Rockville, Md: US Department of Health and Human Services, Public Health Service, Alcohol, Drug Abuse, and Mental Health Administration, National Institute on Drug Abuse; 1986. DHHS Publication (ADM) 86-1473.

89. Shiffman S. Relapse following smoking cessation: a situational analysis. *J Consult Clin Psychol* 1982;50:71–86.

90. Hatsukami DK, Lando H. Smoking cessation. In: Ott PJ, Tartar RE, Ammerman RT, eds. *Sourcebook on Substance Abuse: Etiology, Epidemiology, Assessment, and Treatment.* Needham Heights, Mass: Allyn & Bacon; 1999:399–415.

91. Abrams DB. Roles of psychosocial stress, smoking cues and coping in smoking-relapse prevention. *Health Psychol* 1986; 5(suppl):91–92.

92. Shapiro D, Tursky B, Schwartz GE, et al. Smoking on cue: a behavioral approach to smoking reduction. *J Health Soc Behav* 1971;12:108–113.

93. Flaxman J. Quitting smoking now or later: gradual, abrupt, immediate, and delayed quitting. *Behav Res Ther* 1978;9: 260–270.

94. Foxx RM, Brown RA. A nicotine fading and self-monitoring program to produce cigarette abstinence or controlled smoking. *J Appl Behav Anal* 1979;12:111–125.

95. McGovern PG, Lando HA: Reduced nicotine exposure and abstinence outcome in two nicotine fading methods. *Addict Behav* 1991:1611–1620.

96. Hall SM, Rugg D, Tunstall C, et al. Preventing relapse to cigarette smoking by behavioral skill training. *J Consult Clin Psychol* 1984;52:372–382.

97. Lando H, Sipfle CL, McGovern PG. A statewide public service smoking cessation clinic. *Am J Health Promotion* 1995;10: 9–11.

98. McFarland MI. When five became twenty-five. A silver anniversary of the Five-Day Plan to stop smoking. *Adventist Heritage* 1986;11:57–64.

99. Lando H, McGovern P, Barrios F, et al. Comparative evaluation of American Cancer Society and American Lung Association smoking cessation clinics. *Am J Public Health* 1990;80: 554–559.

100. Lando H, Johnson K, McGovern P, et al. Smoking patterns and interest in quitting in Urban American Indians. *Public Health Rep* 1992;107:340–344.

101. Orleans CT, Schoenbach VJ, Wagner EH, et al. Self-help quit smoking intervention: effects of self-help materials, social support intervention, and telephone counseling. *J Consult Clin Psychol* 1991;59:439–448.

102. Zhu S-H, Stretch V, Balabanis M, et al. Telephone counseling for smoking cessation: effects of single-session and multiple-session interventions. *J Consult Clin Psychol* 1996;64: 202–221.

103. Velicer WF, Prochaska JO, Bellis JM, et al. An expert system intervention for smoking cessation. *Addict Behav* 1993;18:269–290.

104. Strecher VJ, Kreuter M, Den Boer DJ, et al. The effects of computer-tailored smoking cessation messages in family practice settings. *J Fam Pract* 1994;39:262–270.

105. Pallonen UE, Velicer WF, Prochaska JO, et al. Computer-based smoking cessation interventions in adolescents: description, feasibility, and six-month follow-up findings. *Substance Use Misuse* 1998;33:1–31.

106. Dijkstra A, de Vries H, Roijackers J, et al. Tailoring information to enhance quitting in smokers with low motivation to quit: three basic efficacy questions. *Health Psychol* 1998;17: 513–519.

107. Strecher V. Computer-tailored smoking cessation materials: a review and discussion. *Patient Educ Counsel* 1999;36: 107–117.

108. Velicer W, Prochaska JO. An expert system intervention for smoking cessation. *Patient Educ Counsel* 1999;36: 119–129.

109. Hurt RD, Sachs DPL, Glover ED, et al. Comparison of sustained-release buproprion and placebo for smoking cessation. *N Engl J Med* 1997;337:1195–1202.

110. Kornitzer M, Bousten M, Thijs J, et al. Efficiency and safety of combined use of nicotine patches and nicotine gum in smoking cessation: a placebo controlled double-blind trial. *Eur Respir J* 1993;6:630s.

111. Puska P, Korhonen H, Vartiainen E, et al. Combined use of nicotine patch and gum compared with gum alone in smoking cessation: a clinical trial in North Karelia. *Tob Control* 1995;4:231–235.

112. Blondal T, Gudmundsson LJ, Olafsdottir I, et al. Nicotine nasal spray with nicotine patch for smoking cessation: randomized trial with six year follow up. *BMJ* 1999;318: 285–288.

113. Abrams DB, Orleans CT, Niaura RS, et al. Integrating individual and public health perspectives for treatment of tobacco dependence under managed health care: a combined stepped-care and matching model. *Ann Behav Med* 1996;18: 290–304.

114. National Cancer Institute. *Tobacco and the Clinician: Interventions for Medical and Dental Practice. Monogr Natl Cancer Inst* 1994;5:1–22. NIH publication 94-3693.

115. Ockene JK. Smoking intervention: the expanding role of the physician. *Am J Public Health* 1994;77:782–783.

116. Curry SJ, Grothaus LC, McAfee T, et al. Use and cost effectiveness of smoking-cessation services under four insurance plans in a health maintenance organization. *N Engl J Med* 1998;339:673–679.

117. Jeffery RW, Forster JL, French SA, et al. The Healthy Worker Project: a work-site intervention for weight control and smoking cessation. *Am J Public Health* 1993;83:395–401.

118. Sorenson G, Thompson B, Glanz K, et al, for the Working Well Trial. Work site-based cancer prevention: primary results from the Working Well Trial. *Am J Public Health* 1996;86:939–947.

119. Carleton RA, Lasater TM, Assaf AR, et al, and the Pawtucket Heart Health Program Writing Group. The Pawtucket Heart Health Program: community changes in cardiovascular risk factors and projected disease risk. *Am J Public Health* 1995;85:777–785.

120. Farquhar JW, Fortmann SP, Flora JA, et al. Effects of community-wide education on cardiovascular disease risk factors. *JAMA* 1990;264:359–365.

121. Lando H, Pechacek TF, Pirie PL, et al. Changes in adult cigarette smoking in the Minnesota Heart Health Program. *Am J Public Health* 1995;85:201–208.

122. Pechacek TF, Lando HA, Nothwehr F, et al. Quit and Win: a community-wide approach to smoking cessation. *Tobacco Control* 1994;3:236–241.

123. The COMMIT Research Group. Community Intervention Trial for Smoking Cessation (COMMIT): I. Cohort results from a four-year community intervention. *Am J Public Health* 1995;85:183–192.

124. The COMMIT Research Group. Community Intervention Trial for Smoking Cessation (COMMIT): II. Changes in adult cigarette smoking prevalence. *Am J Public Health* 1995;85:193–200.

125. Manley M, Lynn W, Epps RP, et al. The American Stop Smoking Intervention Study for cancer prevention: an overview. *Tobacco Control* 1997;6:S5–S11.

126. Manley MW, Pierce JP, Gilpin EA, et al. Impact of the American Stop Smoking Intervention Study on cigarette consumption. *Tobacco Control* 1997;6:S12–S16.

127. Eisner MD, Smith AK, Blanc PD. Bartenders' respiratory health after establishment of smoke-free bars and taverns. *JAMA* 1998;280:1909–1914.

128. Lightfoot JM, Glantz SA. Short-term economic and health benefits of smoking cessation: myocardial infarction and stroke. *Circulation* 1997;96:1089–1096.

129. Kannel WB. Curbing the tobacco menace. *Circulation* 1997; 96:1070.

130. Hirayama T. Lung cancer in Japan: effects of nutrition and passive smoking. In: Mizell M, Correa P, eds. *Lung Cancer: Causes and Prevention.* New York: Verlag Chemie International; 1984:175–195.

131. Garland C, Barrett-Connor E, Suarez L, et al. Effects of passive smoking on ischemic heart disease mortality of non-smokers. *Am J Epidemiol* 1985;121:645–650.

132. Svendsen KH, Kuller LH, Martin MJ, Ockene JK. Effects of passive smoking in the Multiple Risk Intervention Trial. *Am J Epidemiol* 1987;126:783–795.

133. Helsing KJ, Sandler DP, Comstock GW, Chee E. Heart disease mortality in nonsmokers living with smokers. *Am J Epidemiol* 1988;127:915–922.

134. Hole DJ, Gillis CR, Chopra C, Hawthorne VM. Passive smoking and cardiorespiratory health in a general population in the west of Scotland. *BMJ* 1989;299:423–427.

135. Layard MW. Ischemic heart disease and spousal smoking in the National Mortality Followback Survey. *Regul Toxicol Pharmacol* 1995;21:180–183.

136. Tunstall-Pedoe H, Brown CA, Woodward M, Travendale R. Passive smoking by self-report and serum cotinine and the prevalence of respiratory and coronary heart disease in the Scottish Heart Health Study. *J Epidemiol Community Health* 1995;49:139–143.

Family History and Genetic Factors

6

Paul N. Hopkins
Steven C. Hunt
Lily L. Wu

KEY POINTS

- *Premature coronary heart disease is strongly familial, but in most cases, the underlying cause of the excess risk for a given family cannot be ascertained by genetic or other special testing.*

- *Increased prevalence of standard coronary heart disease risk factors may account for a substantial portion of excess risk in high-risk families. Each of the standard risk factors is strongly heritable.*

- *Targeting of high-risk families for standard coronary heart disease risk factor intervention may be an effective means of preventing premature coronary heart disease.*

- *Much evidence for common variants in a number of candidate genes has been published. As yet, however, none of the evidence is sufficiently validated or convincing to provide strong impetus for genetic testing in the clinical environment.*

- *Familial hypercholesterolemia remains one of the few well-understood, monogenic disorders*

- *that are sufficiently common and severe to contribute importantly to premature coronary heart disease in the general population.*

- *Risks for familial combined hyperlipidemia and familial hypertriglyceridemia are similar, and both may be considered as subsets of the metabolic syndrome.*

- *Identification of the genetic basis for a number of monogenic disorders leading to hypertension and hypotension has underscored the importance of the kidney in long-term blood pressure control. None of these genes, however, contributes importantly to common hypertension.*

- *Gene therapy shows considerable promise in the setting of acute coronary syndromes and severe coronary artery disease using discrete, catheter-based delivery of gene-carrying vectors to specific sites. In contrast, lipid intervention by gene therapy must still overcome a number of technical hurdles before it will be feasible in humans.*

Cardiovascular disease (CVD) accounts for about 40% of all deaths each year in the United States and many Western nations. Recent statistics show that the Ukraine, the Russian Federation, and other Eastern European countries have by far the highest rates of mortality from both coronary heart disease (CHD) (340–398 per 100,000) and cerebrovascular disease in the world.[1] In contrast, Asian countries, particularly Japan (36/100,000) and rural China,[2] report the lowest CHD rates but intermediate rates of cerebrovascular disease.[1] The striking gradient in CHD risk between populations is thought to be due primarily to lifestyle factors, not racial or genetic differences.[3–6] In contrast, genetic factors contribute importantly to individual risk within a population. When heart attacks and strokes occur at a relatively early age, a large fraction can be attributed to inherited or familial predisposition or susceptibility. Knowledge of an individual's family history can help guide preventive efforts. Even if the underlying cause of a positive family history is not entirely understood, a strong positive family history justifies more aggressive intervention for known risk factors.

FAMILY HISTORY AS A CHD RISK FACTOR

The Centers for Disease Control and Prevention have recognized the public health implications and clinical utility of family history, particularly for CHD.[7,8] Premature CHD is a familial disease. A simple family history, if competently obtained, can provide substantial insights and risk estimates comparable in predictive power to virtually any laboratory-measured risk factor. Recall bias appears to have only a small impact on familial estimates of risk.[9] Higher risk is associated with earlier onset of disease and more family members affected.[10–12] At least 10 studies have reported that family history is an independent CHD risk predictor.[11,13–15] Perhaps most impressive was a 26-year follow-up of 21,004 Swedish twins. Among men, when a twin died of CHD before age 55, the relative risk to the remaining twin was 8.1 for monozygous and 3.8 for dizygous twins. For women, relative risks of 15.0 and 2.6, respectively, were reported. The earlier the death of the first twin, the greater the relative risk of the remaining twin. The excess risk persisted after adjustment for standard CHD risk factors.[16]

To obtain a population perspective of the extent of CHD familial aggregation, risk to remaining siblings was studied as a function of CHD experience of older siblings in 15,200 Utah families (Table 6-1).[17] Up to 12-fold increases in risk were seen for surviving siblings when two or more siblings had already experienced early onset of CHD. A more recent examination of 122,155 families, providing a net experience of 16,602 early CHD cases, found that an impressive 35% of all early CHD aggregated in just 3.2% of families with strong positive family histories (quantified by a family history score).[18] A comparison of different methods to calculate family history

scores has been published. Generally, any method that accounts for both the age at onset and the number affected is more predictive than other methods.[12]

The kinds of genetic and environmental risk factors associated with a family history of premature CHD are depicted in figure 6-1. A substantial, but currently unknown proportion of the risk associated with a family history of premature CHD may be explained by standard CHD risk factors, including smoking, hypercholesterolemia, low high-density lipoprotein cholesterol (HDL-C), hypertension, and diabetes.[19,20] Family aggregation of such risk factors was first demonstrated many years ago.[21–23] Prior to onset, only about 10% of individuals developing premature clinical CHD are found without any of these standard risk factors; an even smaller proportion have truly favorable levels.[24] It should not come as a surprise to find that the same was true in a study of sibling pairs with premature CHD.[25] An excess of hypercholesterolemia and hypertension were especially evident in these sibling pairs.[25] Such findings may have been anticipated given the high heritability of most coronary risk factors.

Heritability (h^2) is an estimate of the fraction of the variance of a quantitative trait in the population explained by inheritance and can range from 0 (no evidence of inheritance) to 1.0 (all of the variance explained by inherited factors). In twin studies, the classic estimate of heritability is $2(r_m - r_d)$, where r_m is the correlation coefficient between monozygous twins (eg, the systolic blood pressure in twin 1 vs twin 2), and r_d is the correlation coefficient between dizygous twins. In family studies, $2r_s$ (where r_s is the correlation of the trait between siblings) is another reasonable estimate of heritability. Heritability in twin studies is often higher than in family studies, probably because monozygotic twins are more similar in their behavior and dietary preferences than dizygotic twins, violating one of the assumptions in the calculation. Heritability of a variety of traits related to CHD is summarized in Table 6-2.[26,27] In this table, c^2 is an estimate of the shared household effect or "cultural

TABLE 6-1 Relative Risk for CHD by Family History in 15,200 Utah Families*

CHD FHx definition	Prevalence	Relative risk		
		20–39 y	50–59 y	70+ y
1+ Affected	38%	2.9	1.3	1.3
1+ Age < 55	13%	3.9	1.5	1.1
2+ Affected	8%	5.9	1.8	2.0
2+ Age < 55	2%	12.7	2.9	0.7
FHx score > 1.0	6%	6.9	2.0	3.0
FHx score > 2.0	3%	9.1	2.5	4.2

*Data for 94,292 persons.

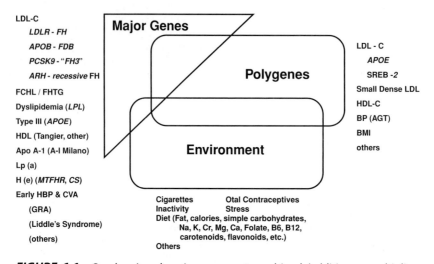

LDL-C
  LDLR - FH
  APOB - FDB
  PCSK9 - "FH3"
  ARH - recessive FH
FCHL / FHTG
Dyslipidemia (*LPL*)
Type III (*APOE*)
HDL (Tangier, other)
Apo A-1 (A-I Milano)
Lp (a)
H (e) (*MTFHR, CS*)
Early HBP & CVA
  (GRA)
  (Liddle's Syndrome)
  (others)

Major Genes

Polygenes

Environment

LDL - C
  APOE
  SREB -2
Small Dense LDL
HDL-C
BP (AGT)
BMI
others

Cigarettes   Otal Contraceptives
Inactivity   Stress
Diet (Fat, calories, simple carbohydrates,
      Na, K, Cr, Mg, Ca, Folate, B6, B12,
      carotenoids, flavonoids, etc.)
Others

FIGURE 6-1 Overlapping domains represent combined (additive or multiplicative) effects of monogenic, polygenic, and environmental factors promoting atherosclerosis.

heritability" for the trait. Most standard cardiovascular risk factors, including low-density lipoprotein (LDL-C) and HDL-C, systolic and diastolic blood pressure, body mass index (BMI), and scapular skinfold, show 40 to 60% heritability in twin studies, with somewhat lower heritabilities in family studies.[26–32] Changes in lipids with age also appear to be heritable.[33] Complex modeling of blood pressure in families suggests inheritance of a gene or genes that lead to a steeper rise in blood pressure with age.[34,35] Both type I diabetes and type II diabetes are highly heritable. High sensitivity C-reactive protein was found to be 40% heritable in the National Heart Lung and Blood Institute (NHLBI) Family Heart Study.[36] Small, dense LDL (as peak particle

diameter) were 50 to 60% heritable in the Quebec Family Study.[37] Lipoprotein(a) levels are at least 90% heritable in most populations.[32,38] Increased risk factor levels in family members or offspring of premature CHD patients have been reported for most of the standard risk factors,[39] as well as for emerging risk factors, including homocysteine,[40] fibrinogen,[39,41,42] fibrin D-dimer,[42] plasminogen activator inhibitor 1 (PAI-1),[43,44] tissue-type plasminogen activator,[42] microalbuminuria,[45] and insulin resistance.[42] The high heritability of most CHD risk factors further justifies a public health approach that focuses attention on high-risk families. Heritability of CHD death in twin registries has been reported to be approximately 40 to 60%.[46,47] In one study, familial risk

TABLE 6-2 Heritability (h^2) of Selected Traits in Twins and Pedigree*

	h^2 twins	h^2 pedigrees	c^2 pedigrees
Standing Height	—	.75	.11
BMI	.54	.24	.00
Scapular Skinfold	—	.32	.03
Sitting Systolic BP	.42	.17	.07
Sitting Diastolic BP	.46	.22	.03
Total Cholesterol	.61	.45	.08
Triglycerides	.81	.37	.06
HDL Cholesterol	.74	.45	.15

*Includes 146 male monozygous twins, 162 male dizygous twins, and 1102 adults in 67 Utah pedigrees.
SOURCE: Reproduced, with permission, from Hunt et al[26] and Williams et al.[27]

appeared to be specific for sudden cardiac death versus myocardial infarction,[48] whereas in most studies these conditions were considered together. Studies considering only parental history of CHD have found lower relative risks than studies that use a more comprehensive family history including all first-degree relatives.[48,49]

Although standard and some emerging risk factors mediate some of the risk associated with a positive family history, they clearly do not explain it all. A number of studies have reported that a positive family history of premature CHD continues to be associated with increased subsequent risk after controlling for risk factors.[13–16,50,51] Carotid intima–media thickness and brachial artery flow-mediated dilation, but not most other risk factors, were significantly worse in 19-year-old offspring of premature CHD cases than in 19-year-old controls.[52] Even among patients with familial hypercholesterolemia (FH), a positive family history of premature CHD is predictive of individual risk.[53–55]

Genomewide scans have successfully identified gene loci for many monogenic disorders. Much less success has been realized for common diseases such as CHD, which are likely to be highly heterogeneous.[56] Nevertheless, reports of significant linkage for atherosclerosis-related endpoints have begun to appear. Most recently, a LOD score of 4.2 at chromosome 15q26 was found in a two-generation family with 10 coronary cases and 9 unaffected members (or too young to provide strong phenotype information). All the affected family members had at least one coronary risk factor and 93 genes were located in the indicted region. Nevertheless, every affected member was found to carry a 21-bp (7-amino-acid) deletion in the myocyte enhancer factor 2 (MEF2A) gene located in that region. MEF2A is a transcription factor strongly expressed in endothelial cells, and the investigators postulated that the deletion may result in defective endothelial defenses against atherosclerosis.[57] This represents the first gene for premature CHD identified through linkage analysis and may open avenues of research into how the mutation leads to disease expression. However, MEF2A mutations may be a relatively rare cause of familial CHD, as no mutations of MEF2A were found in 50 sporadic cases of myocardial infarction (MI).[57] The first genomewide association study for MI identified a variant in the lymphotoxin-α gene (LTA on 6p21) that was modestly (odds ratio 1.78) associated with MI. The variant could increase expression of some adhesion molecules.[58] Other genomewide scans have identified only regions, and none so far correspond to the region of LTA or MEF2A. Regions identified include chromosomes 2q21.1 (153 cM) and Xq23-26 in Finnish families,[59] chromosome 16p13 in Indo-Mauritians (with an additional locus linked to metabolic syndrome and diabetes on 3q27),[60] chromosome 14 (123-130 cM) in Western Europeans,[61] and chromosome 2q36 (255 cM)

in Australian sibling pairs with acute coronary syndrome before age 70.[62] The first genome scan of coronary artery calcium, a sensitive and specific marker of coronary atherosclerosis, identified two different potential loci (6p21.3 with LOD 2.2 and 10q21.3 with LOD 3.2).[63]

PROGRESS ON CANDIDATE GENES FOR PREMATURE CHD

Investigators have had no difficulty in assembling lists of favorite gene targets for association studies. However, replication of findings and reliable estimates of risk has been fraught with difficulty.[64] Initial reports of highly significant odds ratios associated with a particular gene are consistently followed by less significant findings, probably due to a statistical phenomenon termed "winner's curse."[65] Studies aimed at replicating initial reports are often underpowered or use different definitions of phenotype, yielding conflicting results. Nevertheless, a recent meta-analysis of reported genetic association studies with a variety of phenotypes suggests that as many as 25% of reported genetic associations are real, though typically more modest than the initial report.[65] Replication, pooling of results with meta-analysis, and demonstration of biological plausibility by pathophysiologic investigations appear to be key for demonstrating real associations.

A case-in-point is the so-called "heat-labile" methylenetetrahydrofolate reductase (MTHFR) variant (677C > T causing Ala222Val), which increases homocysteine levels primarily in homozygotes with low folate intake. The first report was positive for CHD risk[66]; subsequent reports were less so. In the NHLBI Family Heart Study, low plasma folate (<15.4 nmol/L) had to be present before the heat-labile MTHFR mutation (only for homozygotes) increased plasma homocysteine.[67] In Utah, the heat labile variant of MTHFR was identified and homocysteine measured in 224 cases of premature, familial CHD and in 146 controls. There were significant interactions between case status, folate, and association with homocysteine level.[68] However, no association with CHD risk was observed for the heat-labile variant overall. Nevertheless, among cases and controls with plasma folate below 16 nmol/L, a nonsignificant increase in risk for homozygous carriers of the heat-labile variant was seen (odds ratio = 1.8, 95% CI = 0.6–5.5, P = 0.3, in 46 cases and 47 controls with low folate) (Fig. 6-2).[69] This small series was subsequently included in a very large, international meta-analysis that obtained, from numerous investigators, the individual data on more than 11,000 cases and a comparable number of controls. A small, but statistically significant association with CHD risk was demonstrated for homozygosity of the heat-labile variant (odds ratio = 1.16).[70] Slightly stronger associated risks were reported in another recent meta-analysis.[71] The attendant CHD risk associated with the heat-labile

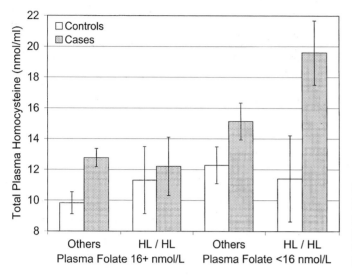

FIGURE 6-2 Plasma homocysteine levels [H(e)] (mean ± SEM) as a function of the presence of heat-labile (HL) *MTHFR* mutation, plasma folate intake levels, and premature CHD case status. Interactions exist for both folate and CHD case status.

MTHFR variant was restricted to studies conducted outside North America, where folate intakes were presumably lower. When the studies that reported folate status were examined separately (including the Utah series), risk associated with the heat-labile variant was observed only among subjects with below-average folate status (odds ratio = 1.44).[70] Thus, the results of this very large meta-analysis essentially confirmed and provided statistical significance for the findings of the small Utah study. The authors concluded that there was no clinical or public health utility in determining MTHFR genotype, but that a plentiful folate intake should be encouraged.

A large Japanese study provides several insights into future testing of candidate genes.[72] The investigators tested a panel of 112 variants in 71 candidates in a large series of MI patients (2003 men and 816 women) and 2242 controls with at least one standard risk factor. The investigators divided their large series into a screening group (about one fifth of the available subjects) and a confirmation group (the remainder). Among the men, 19 variants were identified for further testing, and among the women, 18 variants (mostly different). Of all these variants, just 3 (connexin 37 in men and PAI-1 and stromelysin 1 in women) were considered statistically significant. Only the stromelysin 1 (also called MMP3 for matrix metalloproteinase 3) variant was considered predictive enough by itself to be potentially useful. Additional evidence supporting the MMP3 association has been reported.[73,74] Another recent large Japanese case–control study also found association with variants in the stromelysin 1 and connexin 37 genes, as well as apoE.[75] Yamada and colleagues describe a model study in many ways, including very large size and a planned replication population.[72] The lack of replication for most of the

genes identified in the screening set may have been due in part to the very low *P* value required for the replication set. One could argue that *P* values of .05 should be imposed on all such associations, acknowledging that 5% will be expected to be false positives.[76] Nevertheless, another smaller study also failed to verify previously reported associations in most instances.[77]

Despite the limitations mentioned above, it is nevertheless instructive to consider at least some of the many studies that have examined one or more polymorphisms associated with premature CHD in candidate genes. Some of the more promising candidate genes are listed in Table 6-3. Most of the candidates in this table are unrelated to standard CHD risk factors. They may be considered to be acting by one or more potential atherogenic mechanisms using a scheme proposed more than 20 years ago.[78] In this scheme, factors contributing to atherosclerosis are classified into four categories based on demonstrated or presumed steps or mechanisms of atherogenesis. The steps include *initiation* of endothelial activation, dysfunction, or inflammation; *promotion* of lipoprotein modification and foam cell formation; *potentiation* of thrombosis; and *precipitation* of acute events, particularly through plaque destabilization. Factors, particularly major risk factors, frequently act at more than one step. For example, elevated lipids can contribute to endothelial dysfunction or activation,[79–83] impair nitric oxide synthesis by endothelium or its availability,[84–87] lead to foam cell formation (after a variety of possible modifications),[88–90] increase platelet activation and thrombotic potential,[91] and also lead to reversible plaque destabilization.[92–95] Obviously, factors that increase thrombotic potential may also help precipitate an acute event if they lead to formation of a larger

TABLE 6-3 Candidate Genes for Premature Atherosclerosis, Potentially Independent of Standard Risk Factors*

Name abbreviation location	Variant frequency in control	Relative risks on odds ratio	Comments
Initiation of endothelial activation, dysfunction, or inflammation			
Angiotensin converting enzyme (*ACE*), 17q23	I/D D 55%	1.10	DD associated with greater risk in some studies.[604–607] A meta-analysis found larger studies did not generally find excess risk.[608] OR = 1.10 (95% CI = 1.00–1.21) in the largest study of 4629 myocardial infarction cases and 5934 controls.[609]
Angiotensinogen (*AGT*), 1q42–q43	Met235Thr (complete linkage disequilibrium with −6A > G)	1.8 (*P* = .009)	Higher risk after correction for other risk factors.[610] Others have also found similarly increased risk.[611–615] Interaction with ACE I/D has also been reported.[616–619] Others show no associated risk.[620–622]
CD14 (lipopolysaccharide receptor), 5q31.1	−260C > T 35%	1.8 (*P* = .0005)	178 men with MI prior to age 65 and 135 controls.[623] An OR of 3.8 (*P* = .0001) was reported in a small Japanese study.[624] No association in Physicians' Health Study.[625] Suggestive in female screening group but not confirmed in Yamada et al.[72]
	−159T > C	1.6–3.8	Genotypes in 2228 men who had undergone coronary angiography for diagnostic purposes. Higher risk for CAD in otherwise low-risk patients.[626]
Connexin 37 (gap junction protein, ALPHA-4; *GJA4*), 1p35.1	1019C > T Pro319Ser 1019T 28%	1.4 (*P* <.001)	Risk for MI shown for Japanese men only though screen was suggestive for women.[72] Opposite association (increased risk with C allele) with CAD in Taiwanese men[627] and for carotid plaque in Swedish study.[628] Allele frequency of 1019T is 28% in North Americans, 12% for Japanese and Taiwanese.
C-reactive protein (*CRP*), 1q21–q23	1059G > C C 6.0%	1.01 (*P* = .8)	GC had CRP of 1.05 vs 1.38 mg/L in GG but *no* effect of genotype on risk of MI/stroke with >700 cases and matched controls.[150]
CYP1A1, 15q22–q24	*Msp*I 11%	3.44 (in light smokers only)	Variants of CYP1A1 *Msp*I polymorphism at the 3′-flanking region associated with susceptibility to lung cancer in smokers, especially light smokers. Association in this study among patients referred for angiography was only for triple-vessel disease in light smokers (no association with diagnosis of CAD, prior MI, any CAD, or overall severity).[629]

(Continued)

TABLE 6-3 (Continued)

Name abbreviation location	Manual frequency control	Relative risks on odds ratio	Comments
E-selectin (*SELE*), 1q23–q25	Ser128Arg (561A > C) 9%	1.9 (*P* = .02)	Variant may modify binding to ligands.[97] Severe coronary or peripheral artery disease patients vs controls. Higher relative risks in cases under age 41.[630] Increased risk also seen in another small case–control study.[631] No association seen in the ECTIM study.[632] Suggestive in female screening group, negative overall in Yamada et al.[72]
	Leu554Phe (1839C > T) 2%	3.1 (*P* = .02)	From Wenzel et al.[631]
Endothelial nitric oxide synthase (*NOS3*), 7q36	−786T > C 4%	3.7 *P* <.0001	The frequency of the C allele was significantly higher in the MI group than in the control group (*P* <.001), especially those with minimal disease.[633] This allele also associated with coronary spasm.[634] Lower cerebral blood flow seen in smokers only with CC genotype.[635] The "4a" allele (in intron 4) associated with risk only in smokers.[157] 4a/a homozygotes appeared to be protected from MI or coronary thrombosis but not coronary atherosclerosis in an autopsy study.[636] Near-complete linkage disequilibrium with −786T>C polymorphism and 4 a/b polymorphism. Mildly suggestive in screening sets only in Yamada et al.[72]
	Glu298Asp (894G > T) 10.2%	2.4–4.2	Comparing Asp/Asp homozygotes with others (MI and angiographic CAD)[637–639]
Estrogen receptor 1 (*ESR1*), 6q25.1	*Pvu*II (p/p)	6.2–10.6 (*P* = .007)	Risk shown for coronary thrombosis in autopsy study.[640]
Fractalkine receptor (*CX3CR1*), 3pter-p21	Val249Iso (84635G > A) I/I or V/I 51%	0.54 (*P* = .03)	Fractalkine (CX3CL1), expressed on inflamed endothelial cells, attaches to the CX3CR1 receptor expressed on monocytes, T cells, and natural killer cells and promotes leukocyte adhesion. I249 shown to be associated with fewer binding sites and appears to be protective in this study.[641] Confirmatory results from the Framingham Offspring Study have been published.[642]
Interleukin-1α, interleukin-1β, and receptors, 2q14–q21	—	—	Several generally negative studies.[136]
Interleukin-6 (*IL6*), 7p21	−174G > C 43%	1.54 (*P* = .048)	−572G > C not associated with risk. Greater risk (RR = 2.66, *P* = sig) in smokers.[162] Reported RR = 1.34 m ECTIM.[643] Greater risk associated with this variant in those taking pravastatin in WOSCOPS.[166] −634G > C also negative.

TABLE 6-3   (Continued)

Name abbreviation location	Manual frequency control	Relative risks on odds ratio	Comments
Interleukin-10 (*IL10*). 1q31–q32	−1082G > A −819T > C −592A > C		From Jenkins et al.[644] Mild association for −819T > C and −592A > C in male screening group but overall negative in Yamada et al.[72]
Lewis blood group, (*FUT3*), 19p13.3	a − b-6.3%	2.0	Mechanism unknown. Independent of known cardiovascular risk factors in NHLBI Family Heart Study.[645] Also seen in Copenhagen Male Study. Four common mutations in the fucosyltransferase 3 gene explain most a-b- types and are each mildly associated with CAD and increased CRP.[646]
5-Lipoxygenase (*ALOX5*), 10	Sp1 promoter tandem repeats 6%	Increased IMT	Carriers of either of two common promoter variants had significantly greater IMT.[647]
Mannose-binding lectin (*MBL2*), 10q11.2–q21	"non-A" alleles 11% American Indians 45.7% Whites	3.2 (p = 0.004)	CAD increased in American Indians in Strong Heart Study.[648] Originally, carotid plaque area associated with infection susceptibility "non-A" alleles (associated with lower levels of mannose-binding lectin).[149]
Methylenetetrahydrofolate reductase (*MTHFR*), 1p36.3	Ala222Val (677C > T) 10.7% TT	1.16 (1.05–1.28)	Shown are the pooled odds ratio and 95% CI comparing TT with CC homozygotes (46.4% of controls) from a large meta-analysis.[70] Similar results were found in another meta-analysis.[71] The effect was seen only in persons with low folate status.[69,70]
Monocyte chemoattractant protein 1 (*MCP1*), 17q11.2–q12	−2518A > G GG 6%	2.2 (p = 0.005)	G allele carriers produce more MCP-1 than AA homozygotes.[649]
Platelet activating factor acetyl hydrolase (*PLA2G7*); 6p21.2–p12	Ala379Val 24%	0.46 (0.22–0.93)	Also called lipoprotein-associated phospholipase A2. Shown is risk for MI in ValVal homozygotes after adjustment for other risk factors including CRP.[650]
Platelet–endothelium cell adhesion molecule 1 (*PECAM-1*, also referred to as CD31), 17q23	53G > A 1–2%	–	The 53A allele disrupts a putative sheer stress response element with decreased production of endothelial PECAM-1 during sheer stress. Decreased progression of atherosclerosis seen in carriers.[651]
	Leu125Val 51%	1.8 (*P* = .006)	Variant known to alter immunologic properties of PECAM-1. *P* value based on allele frequencies. There were 98 patients with CAD and 103 healthy controls.[652] No association with CAD in another study but increase in 125Val in patients without diabetes or hypertension.[653]
	Ser563Asn (4428G > A) 50%	1.7 (*P* = .012)	Positive association in Wenzel et al. Homozygotes for both 125Val and 563Ser had greater risk.[652]

(Continued)

TABLE 6-3   (Continued)

Name abbreviation location	Manual frequency control	Relative risks on odds ratio	Comments
P-selectin (*SELP*), 1q23–q25	Thr715Pro (76666A > C) Pro715 17.4%	0.67 (*P* = .002)	In the ECTIM study (647 patients with MI and 758 controls), homozygote Pro715 vs homozygotes Thr715 risk was 0.29 (*P* = .02).[632] CAD risk was not significant in the AtheroGene Study though P-selectin variants were associated with different plasma levels of soluble P-selectin.[654]
Toll-like receptor 4 (*TLR4*), 9q32–q33	Asp299Gly 3.1%	0.54 (*P* < .05)	Shown is association with carotid atherosclerosis in an Italian study.[655] Thr399Ile may have had an additive effect. Carriers of the 299Gly variant had lower levels of several soluble inflammatory factors and fibrinogen and possibly more infections. Carotid IMT was less than that of wild type (*P* = .01).
Transforming growth factor β1 (*TGFβ1*) 19q13.1–13.3	−509C > T	—	
	Leu10Pro (869T > C) 29T > C.	3.5 (*P* < .0001 with T in men only)	Variant in signal peptide. In both male MI patients and controls, the serum concentration of TGF-β1 was significantly higher in individuals with the CC genotype than in subjects with the TT or TC genotype.[656] No association in ECTIM.[657] Mild association in male screening group only (not overall) in Yamada et al.[72]
	Arg25Pro (74G > C)		Associated with MI in some but not all populations included in ECTIM.[657] Other negative studies.[658]
Tumor necrosis factor α (*TNFα*), 6p21.1–21.3	−863C > A −850C > T −238G > A	—	Mild association in screening sets of men (−863C > A) and women (−850C > T) but negative in larger sets in Yamada et al.[72] −238G > A not associated with MI in same study.
	−308G > A	—	Modest increase in obesity associated with this variant but no relation to CAD in one study.[659] Several other negative reports.[136] Others suggest some associated CAD risk.[660]
Tumor necrosis factor β (*TNFβ*), 6p21	Asp26Thr	—	Several negative studies reported even though variant is functional. Other variants also show no association.[136]
Werner helicase gene (*RECOL2*), 8p12–p11.2	Cys1367Arg 85% CC	2.78	Cys homozygotes (most common) association with MI. Not associated with NIDDM in this Japanese population.[661] Viability/senescence of endothelial cells thought possibly associated with this gene.

TABLE 6-3   (Continued)

Name abbreviation location	Manual frequency control	Relative risks on odds ratio	Comments
Promotion of lipoprotein oxidation, other modification, and foam cell formation			
ABCA1 transporter (*ABCA1*), 9q22–q31	Arg219Lys. 46% carriers	0.85 (*P* = .02)	219Lys associated with fewer coronary events, less severe atherosclerosis, lower triglycerides, and a tendency to higher HDL. Atherosclerosis progressed less in 219Lys carriers.[662]
	−477C>T		Inconsistent increased risk associated with T allele.[663]
	−191G>C 22%	3.96 (*P* = .003)	Relative risk for incident CAD events for CC homozygotes vs others in REGRESS study. Risk appeared to be independent of plasma lipids. Also associated with positive family history and risk in a group of FH patients.[274]
	−17C > G 32%	0.67 (*P* = .04)	Relative risk for CAD events in REGRESS.[274] No association with plasma lipids.
ABCC6 transporter, 16p13.1	Arg1141X 0.8%	4.2 (*P* = .001)	R1141X is the most common mutation leading to pseudoxanthoma elasticum.[664] No association of carrier status in this study to serum lipids. In another study, ABCC6 mutations were associated with elevated triglycerides and low HDL but the mechanism of association with CAD is not known.[665]
Alcohol dehydrogenase type 3 (*ADH3*), 4q22	γ_2 17% $\gamma_2\gamma_2$	0.65 (*P* = .04, entire study) 0.14 (*P* < .001 for those consuming 1+ drink/day)	Interaction with alcohol intake and CAD risk in historical prospective analysis of Physician's Health Study. Two amino acid differences at positions 271 and 349 between γ_1 and γ_2 alleles. 2.5-fold difference in maximal velocity of ethanol oxidation by homodimeric γ_1 (faster) vs homodimeric γ_2 enzymes. Higher HDL associated with men and women with γ_2 allele.[666]
Aldosterone synthase (*CYP11B2*), 8q21	−344C > T		OR associated with smoking increased from 1.1 in TT (ns) to 4.7 in CC homozygotes. Similar interaction with low HDL.[158]
Apolipoprotein AIV (*APOA4*), 11q23	Thr347Ser 19.5% carry Ser	2.0 (*P* < .05)	Increased MI risk in Northwick Park II study. Also associated with lower ApoA-IV.[667]
Apolipoprotein CIII (*APOC3*), 11q23	−482C > T	—	Mild association with MI male and female screening sets. Not associated in larger set in Yamada et al.[72]
	−455T > C 9.2% homozygous	2.5 (*P* < .001)	Associated with both higher triglycerides and higher ApoC-III. 549 angiographic cases, 251 controls.[668]
Cholesterol ester transfer protein (*CETP*), 16q21	Ala373Pro Arg451Gln (1200G > A) 5%	0.64	All carriers of the 451Gln allele also carried the 373Pro allele. Lower HDL associated with 373P or 451Q but paradoxical decreased CAD risk when adjusting for HDL levels.[281]

(Continued)

TABLE 6-3 (Continued)

Name abbreviation location	Manual frequency control	Relative risks on odds ratio	Comments
	Ile405Val (1061A > G) 30%	2.1	Additive risk (homozygous women given here). Nonsignificant in men. Complex risk pattern dependent on variant, remnants, and HDL levels. Some common variants raise HDL but still associated with increased CHD risk.[669] Recently reviewed.[670]
	Asp442Gly (1163A > G)	—	
Haptoglobin (*HP*), 16q22.1, starch-gel electrophoresis polymorphism	Hb2 vs Hb1 Hb2 60%	3.3 (*P* = .01)	Shown is risk of MI age <45 in Hp2-2 CABG candidates compared with controls. Also, Hp2 was associated with younger CABG and shorter graft survival.[671] LDL in Hp2-2 person were more susceptible to copper-induced oxidation.[672] Monocytes from Hp2-2 subjects took up Hp–Hb complexes much more avidly and acquired more iron.[673] Hp2 but not Hp1 inhibits *streptococcus pyogenes* growth in human serum.[674] Other associations with infarct size,[675] and peripheral vascular disease reported.[676]
Hemochromatosis-associated gene (*HFE*), 6p21.3	Cys282Tyr (845G > A) 0.25%	2.3	Significant for men in Kuopio Heart Study.[677] Not significant in two case–control studies.[678,679]
Hepatic lipase (*LIPC* or *IIL*), 15q21–q23	−514C > T	—	Greater CAD extent reported in those with T allele. T allele associated with lower postheparin HL activity and promoter activity.[146] Other studies with mixed findings cited. The −514C > T is in complete linkage disequilibrium with the −480C > T allele.[680]
	−480C > T 14%	2.90 (*P* < .05)	OR shown is for presence of CAC in type 1 diabetics. The proportion with CAC was 44% in LIPC −480CC subjects, 71% in heterozygotes, and 83% in LIPC −480TT subjects (*P* <.01).[143] Higher activity genotype (CC) associated with greater coronary flow reserve.[144]
	−250G > A	—	
Insulin receptor substrate 1 (*IRS1*), 2q36	Gly972Arg (3494G > A) 6.8%	2.93	Relative odds 6.97 in obese, 27.3 in those with multiple features of the insulin resistance syndrome.[681] Borderline association in female screening group, negative in larger groups in Yamada et al.[72]

TABLE 6-3   (Continued)

Name abbreviation location	Manual frequency control	Relative risks on odds ratio	Comments
Lamin A (*LMNA*), 1q21.2	Arg482Gln R482W	5.9 (*P* = .033 for CAD at any age; more significant for premature CAD)	The *LMNA* mutations listed here dominantly transmit Dunnigan-type familial partial lipodystrophy with loss of fat from extremities and glutcal region and central accumulation of fat. It may be a rare monogenic model of multiple metabolic syndrome as affected patients develop hypertension, dyslipidemia (high TG, low HDL, normal LDL), type II diabetes, and premature CHD.
Lipoprotein lipase (*LPL LIPD*), 8p22	Asp9Agn (280G > A) 1.4%	5.36	Linked to −93T > G. Risk given for 762 Dutch males with angiographically diagnosed CAD and 296 healthy normolipidemic Dutch male controls.[682] Mean HDL levels lower in carriers but OR independent of HDL. Meta-analysis suggested positive association with CAD risk.[234]
	Gly188Glu rare	5.25 (*P* <.05)	From a meta-analysis.[234]
	Asn291Ser (1127A > G) 2.5%	1.98 F 1.02 M	Female heterozygous probands had increased plasma triglycerides and risk, whereas HDL-C was reduced in both female and male carriers.[683]
	Ser447X 17%	0.4	Lower risk in 447X carriers. They have higher HDL, lower TG, and higher LPL activity.[684] Less striking OR of 0.8 in a recent meta-analysis.[234] 60% lower risk of CAD in parents of children with X447.[685] Similar risks reported by our group for *Hind*III polymorphism.[686] Association may be due to strong linkage disequilibrium with S447X.[235]
Myeloperoxidase (*MPO*), 17q23.1	−463G > A 30%	0.14 (*P* <.0009)	OR shown for AA homozygotes vs all others.[151] The A allele has less myeloperoxidase activity. Substantial protection from in AA and GA also seen in renal dialysis patients.[152]
NAD(P)H oxidase p22*phox* gene (*CYBA*), 16q24	His72Lys (242C > T)	0.49	The 72Y (242T) variant appeared protective.[687] Presence of the 242T allele was associated with significantly reduced vascular NAD(P)H oxidase activity.[688] Inconsistent results for CAD.[689–691] Significant, mild association (OR = 1.8) for stroke.[692] Associated with OR of 0.7 (*P* = .007) for MI in men, not women, in Yamada et al.[72]
	640A > G	0.74 (*P* = .038)	2205 males with coronary angiography. OR is for CAD present vs not present.[691]

(Continued)

TABLE 6-3 (Continued)

Name abbreviation location	Manual frequency control	Relative risks on odds ratio	Comments
Paraoxonase 1 (*PON1*), 7q21.3	−107 T > C	—	
	Met54Leu (172A > T) 30%	1.9–3.4	Carotid therosclerosis associated with LI (OR = 1.9).[693] No association with Gln191 Arg variant in that study. Up to 3.4-fold risk in a small case–control study.[694]
	Gln191Arg (584G > A) 26–59%	1.4–3.0	Some investigators refer to this variant as 192. Much higher prevalence in Japanese, in whom it was a risk factor.[695] Lower risk reported in Costa Rica. Risk seen only in nonsmokers.[159] Associated with MI in female screening group, not larger groups, in Yamada et al.[72]
Paraoxonase 2 (*PON2*), 7q21.3	Cys311Ser 61%	2.5	Variants in *PON2* possibly associated with CAD.[696]
Peroxisome proliferator-activated receptor α (*PPARA*), 22q12–q13.1	Leu 62Val (696C > G) 2.8–6.3% Intron 7 G > C (13.4–17.4%)	2.61	OR of 2.61 (*P* = .009) associated with intron 7 CC only in those with 162 LL genotype in Northwick Park Heart Study (162Val appeared to be protective). Also, association with CAD progression in LOCAT study.[697] No clear differences in gene expression studied except that V162 has higher transcriptional activation in vitro. The two polymorphisms are in linkage disequilibrium.
Peroxisome proliferator-activated receptor γ (*PPARG*), 3p25	Cys161Thr 16.3%	0.46	T allele associated with less coronary disease but not with obesity.[698]
Potentiation of thrombosis			
Coagulation factor V (*F5*), 1q23	Arg507Gln (1691G > A) (Leiden) 2–3%	1.4—men 2.4—young women	1.4 increased risk in men was not significant. Greater risk if other risk factors present.[699] Other studies negative.[699–701] Higher risk in young women, particularly smokers.[702]
Coagulation factor VII (*F7*), 13q34	Arg353Glu (11496G > A) 20%	0.47	Lower risk of MI in those with CAD, no association with CAD.[703] Supported in prior study reporting lower FVII with 353Glu and other variants.[704] No association with CVD in another study.[705] Twofold greater activation after fatty meal in RR homozygotes.[706]
Coagulation factor XIIIA subunit (*F13A1*), 6p25–p24	Va134Leu (163G > T) 50%	0.47 (*P* = .005)	Prevalence of 34Leu lower in patients with MI than in controls (32% of 398 vs 48% of 196), *P* = .005 in one study.[707] Another case–control study also suggested decreased risk.[708] Greater effect of aspirin in 34Leu carriers.[709] No protection or association with CAD or risk factors in prospective ARIC study.[710]

TABLE 6-3   (Continued)

Name abbreviation location	Manual frequency control	Relative risks on odds ratio	Comments
Factor VII-activating protease (*FSAP*)	Gly511Glu 4.4% carriers	6.6 (*P* = .01)	Marburg 1 mutation of *FSAP* associated with incident or progressive carotid atherosclerosis in Bruneck Study (shown here).[711] Marburg 1 showed much lower activity in conversion of pro-urokinase to urokinase.
Plasminogen activator inhibitor type 1 (*PAI1*), 7q21.3–q22	−668 4G > 5G 67%	1.6 (*P* <.001)	Shown is OR for women only in Yamada et al.[72] Other studies do not support association in US men[712] or Dutch women.[713] Dutch women with 4G/4G had significantly lower cerebrovascular mortality (OR = 0.4).
Platelet glycoprotein Ia (GP Ia), 5q23–q31	807C > T	0.44 (*P* = .0045)	Association shown here was for CC homozygotes in low-risk subjects (those with high ApoA-1/ApoB)[714] Prior study suggested risk for MI only, not extent of CAD.[715]
	1648A > G	0.44 (*P* = .0003)	Association shown was with angiographic CAD in 2163 males only in low-risk subjects (shown here for nonsmokers and those with high ApoA-1/ApoB)[714]
Platelet glycoprotein IIIa (*GP3A*), 17q21.32	Leu33Pro (1565T > C)	—	
	PI(A1/A2) A2 15%	1.4–2.5	PI(A2) allele associated with nonsignificant trends toward increased risk in one study. Risk diminished with adjustment for standard risk factors.[716] Higher OR reported in sudden death in men under 50, particularly with proven thrombosis.[717] Not associated with premature familial CAD in author's study (unpublished observations).
Thrombomodulin (*THBD*), 20p11.2	−9/−10 GG > AT, −33G > A, −133C > A 1% (any of the 3)	5.2	Any of the three promoter mutations found in 5% of CAD patients in one study.[718] −33G > A associated with CAD in another study.[77,719]
	Ala455Val (2135C > T) VA or V V 7% in blacks, 33% in whites	6.1 in blacks 1.1 in whites	Significant risk in blacks only (*P* = .016). Genotype had no effect on soluble thrombomodulin levels.[720] Borderline association in male screening group, but not larger groups, in Yamada et al.[72]
Thrombospondin I (*THBS1*), 15q15	Asn700Ser (2210A > G) 0.3%	11.9 (*P* = .041)	Thrombospondin is important activator of transforming growth factor β1 with a potential link between platelet thrombosis and atherosclerosis. OR is from study of premature familial CAD cases and general population controls.[77]
Thrombospondin 2 (*THBS2*), 6q27	5755T > G	0.31 (*P* = .0018)	From Topol et al.[77]

(Continued)

TABLE 6-3   (Continued)

Name abbreviation location	Manual frequency control	Relative risks on odds ratio	Comments
Thrombospondin 4 (*THBS4*)	Ala387Pro (1186G > C)	1.9 (*P* = .002)	387Pro associated with increased risk in Topol et al.[77] Significant association in male screening group, but not larger groups, in Yamada et al.[72]
Precipitation of acute events, plaque destabilization			
Adenosine monophosphate deaminase 1 (*AMPD1*), 1p21–p13	Cys34Thr 13%	0.37 (*P* = .046)	Shown is RR for total CVD mortality.[721] C34T results in enzymatic inactivity and has been associated with prolonged survival in heart failure. The dysfunctional AMPD1(−) allele may lead to increased cardiac adenosine and increased cardioprotection during ischemic events.
Gelatinase B (*MMP9*), 20q11.2–q13.1	−1562C > T 14%		T allele had higher promoter activity than C allele. 584 male patients with MI, 645 controls. Allele frequencies did not significantly differ between cases and control subjects. However, in 374 patients with available angiographic data, 26% of those carrying one or two copies of the T allele had >50% stenosis in three coronary arteries, whereas only 15% of C/C homozygotes had triple-vessel disease.[722]
Matrix Gla protein (*MGP*), 12p13.1–p12.3	Thr83Ala 37%	3.8 (*P* < .002)	Increased risk of MI in Ala/Ala homozygotes only in low-risk subjects. Other variants associated with femoral plaque calcification.[723]
Microsomal triglyceride transport protein (*MTP*), 4q22–q24	−493G > T 25%	5.1 (*P* < .005)	The −493G > T is in complete linkage disequilibrium with −164T > C and Ileu128Thr. Despite modestly lower total and LDL cholesterol levels,[724] TT homozygotes had increased CHD event rates in the Uppsala Longitudinal Study (shown here) and in WOSCOPS (OR = 4, *P* < .0001).[725] No association with prevalent CHD in Framingham offspring.[726]
Stromelysin 1 (*MMP3*), 11q23	−1171 5A > 6A 6A— 55%	4.9 (*P* < .001)	More rapid progression of CAD in homozygotes for the 6A allele, who represent 25–30% of population.[73] OR estimate for females only in a Japanese population.[72]

*Loci are alphabetically arranged within categories (initiation, promotion, potentiation, precipitation). OR, odds ratio; CI, confidence interval. CAD, coronary artery disease; IMT, intima–media thickness; CRP, C-reactive protein; CABG, coronary artery bypass graft; CAC, coronary artery calcium.

thrombus on a ruptured plaque. Factors that initiate inflammation also likely lead to an unstable plaque.[96]

Demonstrating biologic plausibility for a gene or gene product provides substantial impetus for continued investigation. An elegant model is the demonstration of effects on disease development in atherosclerosis-prone mice using knockout and transgenic techniques. ApoE-deficient and LDL receptor-deficient mice are the usual models. Substantially less atherosclerosis was seen in these animals lacking a number of genes involved in the initiation of endothelial dysfunction or inflammation.[97–111] Manipulation of genes related to lipoprotein oxidation and foam cell formation have also been reported.[112–124] Severe, fulminant atherosclerosis, including coronary lesions with appearance similar to human disease, develops in apoE-deficient mice lacking the SR-B1 receptor, which is involved in reverse cholesterol transport.[125] Examples of manipulating genes that affect thrombosis and plaque stability have also been published.[126–135] These studies offer exciting insights into the intricacies of atherogenesis. Nevertheless, demonstrating that a gene participates in atherogenesis in an animal model does not constitute evidence that human variants of that gene will affect CHD risk.[136]

Novel mechanisms operating at various stages of atherogenesis will likely be found through genetic research. For example, some strains of inbred mice (such as BL/6) are susceptible to atherosclerosis, whereas others (such as C3H) are not. Endothelial cells isolated from BL/6 mice exhibited dramatic induction of the pro-inflammatory cytokines MCP-1 and M-CSF when incubated with certain oxidized phospholipids, whereas endothelial cells from C3H mice did not.[137] Further, endothelial cell responses to minimally modified or mildly oxidized LDL (MM-LDL) cosegregated with aortic lesion size in inbred strains derived from BL/6 and C3H parental strains. Endothelial cell response to MM-LDL or oxidized phospholipids appeared to be mediated by peroxisome proliferator-activated receptor α (PPARα) and was inhibited by troglitazone (a PPARγ).[138]

Hepatic lipase provides an example of interaction and complexity in humans. Four common variants in complete linkage disequilibrium and forming a single haplotype in the promoter region of the hepatic lipase gene have been found to affect hepatic lipase activity. Although most investigators did not find a direct association with coronary artery disease,[72,139,140] differences in response to treatment in one study appeared to be striking. Thus, the $-514C > T$ polymorphism, which accounted for 20 to 30% of the variability of hepatic lipase activity, was strongly predictive of both change in angiographic outcome and change in small, dense LDL and HDL in response to aggressive treatment of lipids in the Familial Atherosclerosis Treatment Study.[141,142] The more common $-514C$ allele was associated with

higher hepatic lipase activity and higher levels of small, dense LDL and HDL particles. All but one of the 25 aggressively treated subjects with CC genotype experienced regression of CHD during the trial. In contrast, about half of the subjects with CT genotype showed regression, and all of the 4 patients with TT genotype experienced progression ($P < 0.001$ for gene effect). Another study reported greater coronary artery calcium associated with the less common allele of the $-480C > T$ polymorphism.[143] Greater coronary flow reserve was associated with the higher CC genotype of the $-480C > T$ polymorphism.[144] The C allele of an unlinked hepatic lipase variant, $-586T > C$, was paradoxically associated with higher HDL-C and lower hepatic lipase promoter activity, yet greater risk for CHD, in a Chinese cohort.[145] Other investigators reported increased CHD risk in persons with lower hepatic lipase activity associated with common variants despite higher HDL.[146,147] Increased risk for premature CHD has been reported in hepatic lipase deficiency.[148] These studies suggest a paradoxical finding of greater risk of CHD generally for lower-activity hepatic lipase variants, but improved response to aggressive lipid lowering for CHD patients who happen to have the higher-activity variants.

Included in Table 6-3 are several reports of novel associations that may open new avenues of inquiry. For example, an increased risk of carotid atherosclerosis was reported in carriers of "non-A" alleles of mannose-binding lectin, a variant associated with increased susceptibility to a variety of common infections.[149] Interestingly, a common variant for C-reactive protein that affects levels of this risk factor was not associated with CHD in a recent study.[150] A common variant ($-463G > A$) in myeloperoxidase resulting in lower transcription activity was associated with apparent protection from CHD in two studies.[151,152] Deficiency of myeloperoxidase was also suggestively associated with protection in another study.[153] It is possible that there are many interactions between variants listed in Table 6-3, as well as interactions with unknown variants, unmeasured genetic background, and various environmental factors. Further, there may be an additive effect for many of the variants, with a resultant "genetic burden" that could potentially be calculated as a simple score.[154] or likelihood ratio.[155] Evaluation of these effects will require very large samples, comprehensive gene testing, and possibly sophisticated statistical methods. Nevertheless, such avenues of research may yield information useful to the clinician in the future.

INTERACTION BETWEEN GENES AND ENVIRONMENT

Environmental risk factors can have an exaggerated adverse effect in patients with genetic susceptibility, as noted

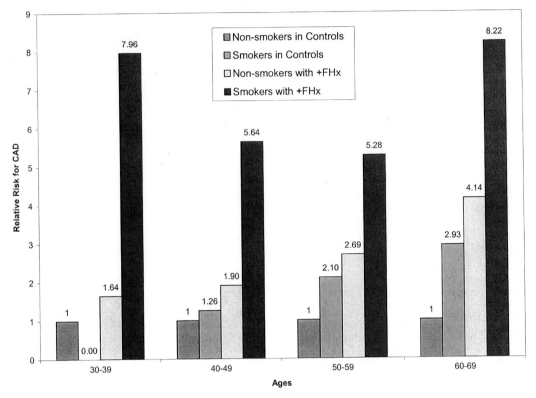

FIGURE 6-3 Relative risks for incident CHD by family history and smoking status illustrate a significant interaction, especially in the younger two age groups. (Adapted, with permission, from Hopkins et al. *West J Med* 1984;141:196.)

above for the folic acid intake and the heat-labile variant of MTHFR. Another example is cigarette smoking. Among younger persons, a positive family history greatly increases the risk of early CHD associated with cigarette smoking, as illustrated in Fig. 6-3.[10] Others have also noted a strong interaction between cigarette smoking and a positive family history of premature CHD.[156] Variants of at least eight different loci have been suggested to interact specifically with smoking, providing a plausible molecular explanation for prior epidemiologic observations.[157–164] Other classic risk factors such as HDL-C also showed evidence of interaction with a positive family history of premature CHD.[158] Such a history should therefore be used to strongly motivate against smoking and to target intervention efforts for known risk factors. Gene variants may also influence the beneficial effects of medications, such as the statins.[165–168] Optimum control of environmental risks is particularly important for all persons with a positive family history of CHD, especially if the molecular or metabolic basis of the risk is unknown.

LIPID DISORDERS

Familial hypercholesterolemia

Familial hypercholesterolemia (FH) has come to be understood as a severe, autosomal codominant hypercholesterolemia caused by mutations of the LDL receptor on chromosome 19. FH is one of the most common and best studied of all genetic diseases, with one of the more than 900 LDL receptor mutations (www.ucl.ac.uk/fh) affecting at least one heterozygote in 500 persons in most populations.[169,170] A substantial number of additional, previously unrecognized FH-causing mutations may exist in unsuspected intronic regions.[171] How the several mutations affect LDL receptor function is illustrated in Fig. 6-4. The dominant transmission and very early penetrance (essentially at birth) of severely elevated plasma LDL-C make pedigree tracing relatively easy (see Fig. 6-5). Because about two thirds of LDL is normally removed by way of the LDL receptor pathway, and because LDL receptors affect the fraction of very low density lipoprotein (VLDL) converted to LDL (and possibly

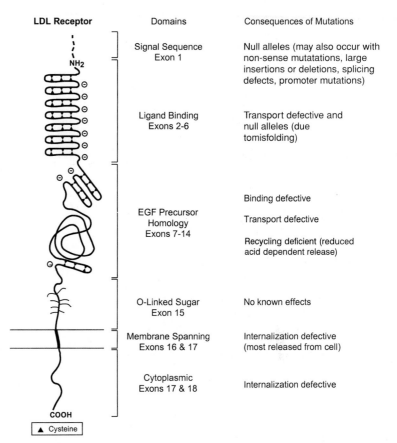

FIGURE 6-4 Structure of the LDL receptor and consequences of defined mutations. Five functional classes of LDL receptor mutations have been identified. Null alleles produce no protein product. Transport-defective alleles (due mostly to abnormal protein folding) display impaired movement of protein product from endoplasmic reticulum to Golgi. Binding-defective alleles bind reduced amounts of LDL (some bind normally to β-VLDL). Recycling deficient alleles do not release LDL normally in endosomes in the presence of acid pH. Internalization-defective alleles do not group normally in clathrin-coated pits and do not internalize LDL. (Adapted, with permission, from Hobbs et al. *Annu Rev Genet* 1990;24:133.)

net VLDL production), a 50% reduction in activity due to one nonfunctional allele results in an approximately twofold elevation of LDL-C. Thus, in untreated adults, total cholesterol is generally above 300 mg/dL (LDL-C > 220 mg/dL).

In patients with FH, standard risk factors increase CHD risk as does small, dense LDL.[172,173] Additional risk associated with elevated lipoprotein(a) appears to be less than initially thought.[172,173] Significant correlation for age at coronary death between sibling pairs with FH from different families has been reported,[174] and a positive family history is a significant risk factor in FH patients.[54,55,175] Less severe atherosclerosis was evident in FH homozygotes with LDL receptor mutations having some residual activity, compared with those with no activity.[176,177]

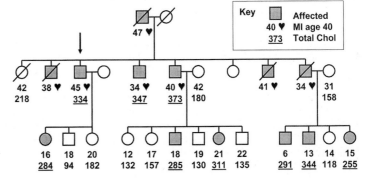

FIGURE 6-5 Familial hypercholesterolemia pedigree.

TABLE 6-4 Total Cholesterol (and LDL-C) Criteria for Diagnosis of Heterozygous Familial Hypercholesterolemia

Age group	Degree of relatedness to closest FH relative			General population	"100%" probability
	First	Second	Third		
<20	220 (155)	230 (165)	240 (170)	270 (200)	(240)
20–29	240 (170)	250 (180)	260 (185)	290 (220)	(260)
30–39	270 (190)	280 (200)	290 (210)	340 (240)	(280)
40+	290 (205)	300 (215)	310 (225)	360 (260)	(300)

FH is a clinically important cause of very early CHD death and disability, but is consistently under-diagnosed.[178,179] A reasonably secure diagnosis of het-erozygous FH can be made (without resorting to special testing such as DNA or fibroblast studies) if the lipid criteria in Table 6-4 are met, together with a clear bi-modal pattern of LDL levels in the family and the pres-ence of affected children or one or more patients with tendon xanthoma in the pedigree.[180] The 10- to 20-fold relative risks for CHD that accompany FH are well documented[181,182] and constitute a major threat to sur-vival in these patients. Although only 1 in 500 in the gen-eral population are affected by FH, about 4% of CHD under age 60, and just over 16% of CHD under age 45, is attributable to FH.[19,20,183,184] FH has been recognized as a significant public health threat, and approaches to screening have been assessed for cost-effectiveness in pre-venting death and disability. Generally, family tracing is most cost-effective, but considering the opportunity for finding nearly all cases and long-term preventive efforts, screening the entire population at high school age is al-most equally cost-effective.[185]

FH is an excellent model of clinical hypercholes-terolemia because of its diversity of presentation, severity, and responsiveness to treatment with regression of coronary atherosclerosis.[186,187] More aggressive LDL lowering has been shown to prevent CHD events[188] and progression of carotid atherosclerosis.[189] The approach to lowering LDL in FH may be considered as a paradigm for other patients with elevated LDL. An effective statin is the drug of first choice. If LDL levels remain above goal, ezetimibe is probably the most convenient and well-tolerated second drug. Bile acid sequestrants (primarily colesevelam) are an alternative. Niacin may be added as a third agent if needed, or may be used as a second choice if triglycerides are elevated and HDL-C is low. LDL apheresis is reserved for the most severe heterozygotes and homozygotes.[190] The FDA requirement for beginning LDL apheresis is an LDL-C level of at least 200 mg/dL with CHD, or 300 mg/dL without CHD, after max-imally tolerated drug therapy. Several recent reviews on diagnosis and management of FH are available.[191–194]

Several other less common forms of dominantly trans-mitted hypercholesterolemia have been described, in-cluding familial defective apoB-100 (most commonly found in northern Europeans)[195–198] and persons with a mutation in the *PCSK9* gene, which encodes neural apoptosis-regulated convertase (NARC-1).[199–202] These patients appear to respond to various treatments similarly to FH patients.[203–205] Two rare forms of autosomal re-cessive hypercholesterolemia have been described.[206–209]

Sitosterolemia

Sitosterolemia is a rare recessive disorder characterized by elevated plasma and tissue sterols, tendon xanthomata, and premature CHD. Sitosterolemia was recently shown to be caused by mutations in either ABCG5 or ABCG8 (both on chromosome 2p21).[210] Serum cholesterol is variably elevated, but hypercholesterolemia can be se-vere and can be accompanied by extremely premature CHD, exemplified by the recently reported MI death of a 5-year-old girl.[211] Common variants in these genes may contribute to net cholesterol absorption, which, in turn, has been related to responsiveness to statin drugs.[212]

Abetalipoproteinemia

This rare recessive disorder is of interest primarily because of the identification of its cause: deficiency of microso-mal transfer protein (MTP), with resultant inability to assemble triglyceride-rich, ApoB-containing lipoproteins in the endoplasmic reticulum.[213] Only about 100 pa-tients have been identified and 18 mutations (mostly truncations) are known.[214] A mild phenotype associated with a less severe missense mutation has been reported.[215]

The potential for lipid lowering using MTP in-hibitors was recognized early. Use of one of these agents in Watanabe heritable hyperlipidemic rabbits (with homozygous genetic deficiency of the LDL receptor and severe hypercholesterolemia) resulted in normalization of lipid levels.[216] Unfortunately, however, these agents have demonstrated a narrow margin of safety, primarily due to the development of fatty liver. Fatty intestine and fat malabsorption, which may also occur, can be avoided if the drug is not given with meals. Nevertheless, there is apparently continued interest in development of these agents because of their marked triglyceride-lowering capacity.[217] Interestingly, naringenin, the chief flavonoid of grapefruit, also possesses MTP inhibitory activity.[218]

Hypobetalipoproteinemia

More than 40 defects in ApoB gene structure (on chromosome 2p24), mostly truncations, have been found to result in diminished serum levels of ApoB-containing lipoproteins due to reduced synthesis.[219] However, these apparently do not account for the majority of families with very low LDL-C.[220] A range in plasma total cholesterol levels among heterozygotes has been reported (40–180 mg/dL), but, on average, plasma LDL and VLDL lipid concentrations are 50% lower than those in unaffected first-degree relatives. Generally, heterozygotes are asymptomatic and appear to be protected from premature CHD, though many appear to harbor nonalcoholic fatty liver.[221] Nevertheless, the lack of adverse clinical effects for most patients with hypobetalipoproteinemia has frequently been cited as evidence that low LDL-C levels per se (achievable with lipid-lowering agents such as statin drugs) would be unlikely to have significant adverse consequences.

Chylomicronemia and lipoprotein lipase deficiency

Chylomicrons are usually present in plasma when fasting triglyceride levels are above 800 mg/dL (9.0 mmol/L), and are almost always present when levels rise above 1200 mg/dL (13.5 mmol/L).[222] Acute pancreatitis is the major clinical concern above these levels, and risk is particularly elevated when plasma triglycerides exceed 2000 mg/dL. Approximately 20% of cases of acute pancreatitis can be attributed to severe hypertriglyceridemia.[223] Eruptive xanthomas can occur when chylomicrons or VLDL is engulfed by skin macrophages.

CHD risk is generally considered to be low with chylomicronemia, whereas pancreatitis risk is high.[224,225] Indeed, severe hypertriglyceridemia actually *protected* diabetic, cholesterol-fed rabbits from arterial atherosclerotic changes owing to the large size of accumulating particles, which were unable to penetrate the artery wall.[226] Nevertheless, premature atherosclerosis can occur in persons with a total deficiency of lipoprotein lipase (LPL) activity (usually with other risk factors present), as elegantly demonstrated in a series of four patients.[227] The progression of atherosclerosis in such patients may be due to accumulation of triglyceride-rich remnants, which are highly atherogenic but poorly detected when chylomicrons are present in plasma.

Nearly 100 functional mutations of the LPL gene on chromosome 8p22 have been described that affect the production of end product, active site, conformation, and ability to self-dimerize, with a wide range of severity of associated phenotype.[123,228] Heterozygotes have moderately elevated triglycerides (that increase with age and higher BMI) and lower HDL,[229] increased postprandial lipemia,[230,231] and small, dense LDL.[232] Interestingly, even LPL lacking enzymatic activity can facilitate uptake of triglyceride-rich remnants into the liver.[233] A meta-analysis of studies examining CHD risk in heterozygous LDL deficiency found a significant 2.03-fold increase in risk associated with the common D9N variant, a 5.25-fold risk for the relatively rare G188E mutation, a marginally increased risk for the common N291S variant, and a significantly decreased risk (odds ratio = 0.81) associated with the S447X variant.[234] The S447X actually shows increased activity, lower triglycerides, and higher HDL-C.[235] It was also associated with lower familial risk of CHD.[236] The N9 allele is associated with increased binding of LDL.[237] The increased risk associated with the D9N variant is consistent with findings of substantial penetrance of low HDL in a family identified by premature CHD and examined for genetic linkage to possible loci associated with low HDL-C.[238]

Type III hyperlipidemia or familial dysbetalipoproteinemia

Type III hyperlipidemia is characterized by the presence of significant concentrations of abnormal chylomicrons and VLDL remnants, often called β-VLDL. Persons with type III hyperlipidemia have long been noted to be at severely increased risk for premature CHD.[239,240] The most objective estimates of the prevalence of type III hyperlipidemia (0.4% in men, 0.2% in women) come from the Lipid Research Clinics Prevalence Study.[241] Type III hyperlipidemia (defined as measured VLDL-C/total triglycerides ≥ 0.30) accounts for as much as 5% of early CHD.[19,183,242,243] Later investigators suggested that more than 90% of patients with type III hyperlipidemia also have an ApoE-2-2 genotype, though this may apply primarily to patients with severe lipid elevations.[244] Patients with less severe type III hyperlipidemia that still meets the Fredrickson measured VLDL/triglyceride criteria frequently do not have the ApoE-2-2 genotype.[243] A quantitative estimate of β-VLDL can be derived from the composition of normal VLDL and reported composition of β-VLDL, with estimated β-VLDL = [VLDL-C− 0.17 (total triglycerides)]/0.521.[245] Estimated β-VLDL-C levels above 40 to 60 mg/dL are abnormal and highly suggestive of type III hyperlipidemia.[245] A newly developed immunosorption assay for remnant particles supports the validity of this estimate.[243,246]

Clinical features of type III hyperlipidemia may include tuberous xanthomas (specific but insensitive), palmar striae, and xanthelasma (nonspecific and insensitive). Cholesterol and triglycerides are elevated together (both usually >250 mg/dL untreated). Remarkable reductions in serum lipids may be seen with treatment. Often, weight loss alone results in a 50% or greater reduction in both cholesterol and triglycerides. These patients are often responsive to niacin, fibrates, or (as second-line agents) statins.[247,248] Note that this disorder cannot be diagnosed with a simple lipid panel in which LDL-C and VLDL-C levels are calculated. A typical case of type III hyperlipidemia is presented in Table 6-5.

Hepatic lipase deficiency

Only a few individuals with hepatic lipase deficiency have been described.[249–252] Some of the affected individuals had premature coronary disease. Serum lipids of affected individuals range from 260 to 1495 mg/dL for total cholesterol and 350 to 8200 mg/dL for triglycerides. Such individuals can respond to a strict metabolic diet restrictive in calories, saturated fat, and cholesterol. The presence of abnormal VLDL remnants and markedly reduced conversion of VLDL to LDL in hepatic lipase deficiency support a role for hepatic lipase in remnant clearance.[253] This role in remnant clearance may be mediated largely by a tethering function (regardless of lipase activity).[252] Heterozygosity for hepatic lipase deficiency has tentatively been associated with CHD.[254] Other studies suggest increased risk for CHD in association with lower-activity variants as noted above.

Severe low-HDL syndromes

Several rare recessive, severe HDL deficiency syndromes have been described.[255] These syndromes account for

TABLE 6-5   A Case of Type III Hyperlipidemia

A 43-year-old male was first seen in our lipid clinic after his cardiologist noted abnormal lipids with total cholesterol of 223 mg/dL, triglycerides of 333 mg/dL, HDL-C of 32 mg/dL, and calculated LDL-C of 124 mg/dL. He was taking 20 mg of lovastatin twice daily at the time of the blood draw. He had experienced his first myocardial infarction at age 31 with recurrent infarcts at ages 38 and 40. After angiography disclosed diffuse coronary disease, he underwent coronary bypass grafting at age 40 but was being evaluated for worsening angina. A call to his primary care physician provided some important insights. The following information was obtained:

Age	Serum Total Cholesterol	Serum Triglycerides	Comments
31	215	328	Lipids at time of first MI
40	461	688	No treatment
40.5	377	395	Low-fat, low-cholesterol diet
41	371	503	Started lovastatin
41.5	306	410	On lovastatin 20 mg bid
42	256	418	On lovastatin 20 mg bid

HDL-C levels were consistently between 30 and 39 mg/dL. The parallel and marked changes in total cholesterol and triglycerides suggested type III hyperlipidemia. After the initial consultation at our lipid clinic, the patient stopped (but then restarted) lovastatin and began a strict weight loss diet. After a 13-pound weight loss and while taking lovastatin 20 mg daily, his lipids were analyzed with ultracentrifugation and ApoE phenotype was determined. Total cholesterol had fallen to 176 mg/dL, triglycerides were 209 mg/dL, HDL-C was 35 mg/dL, measured LDL-C was 45 mg/dL, and measured VLDL-C was 93 mg/dL. Virtually 100% of this VLDL was estimated to be β-VLDL, a highly atherogenic lipoprotein characteristic of type III hyperlipidemia. He was found to have an ApoE phenotype of 2–2, confirming the diagnosis of type III hyperlipidemia. Adding niacin to his regimen (increasing gradually to 1000 mg bid) resulted in a dramatic reduction of his lipids. Subsequent total cholesterol levels have remained under 144 mg/dL and triglycerides remained consistently below 120 mg/dL.

This is an example of typical type III hyperlipidemia. However, this patient never had xanthomas, and a diagnosis of type III hyperlipidemia would not have been possible at the time of initial consultation without making use of ultracentrifugation and ApoE phenotyping. The historical lipids certainly pointed to the diagnosis, but many physicians do not take the time to obtain a complete record. Focusing only on calculated LDL-C levels (which in this case were entirely misleading) had contributed to the inappropriate treatment (gemfibrozil or niacin would have been more appropriate as single initial agents). The marked reduction in lipids when niacin was added to the regimen is typical of type III hyperlipidemia.

only a tiny proportion of the cases of low HDL-C associated with early-onset CHD. Surprisingly, some severe deficiencies of HDL are associated with premature coronary disease, whereas others are not. It has been suggested that low HDL-C due to decreased production is associated with early CHD (especially if production of small HDL is impaired), and syndromes resulting in increased catabolism are not necessarily atherogenic.[256] Thus, ApoA–I(Milano)[257] and ApoA-1(Paris),[258] associated with increased ApoA–I removal but normal production, result in low HDL-C, yet little or no increased risk for CHD, possibly even decreased risk. In contrast, among families or cases with deficient A-I production (such as absent A-I/C-III), early CHD risk is high. A defective ApoA-I with apparent dominant transmission of low HDL and increased CHD risk has been reported.[259] Theoretically, if sufficient HDL is present to promote reverse cholesterol transport, then increased catabolism will not be atherogenic. In fact, increased catabolism may contribute to cholesterol transport by way of the prematurely removed HDL. Recent evidence of rapid removal of atherosclerotic plaque cholesterol by infusion of ApoA-1 (Milano) in both animals[260,261] and humans[262] bolsters this view.

Tangier disease is characterized by severely depressed HDL-C levels accompanied by large orange tonsils, followed by gradual development of peripheral neuropathy, hepatomegaly, and splenomegaly. Tangier disease is caused by a homozygous (or compound heterozygous) defect in the ABCA1 transmembrane cholesterol and phospholipid transporter, resulting in hypercatabolism of ApoA-I.[263] The ABCA1 transporter shuttles cholesterol and phospholipid from inner to outer cell membranes and from there to nascent HDL.[264,265] At least 52 mutations in the ABCA1 gene have been shown to result in either Tangier disease (homozygous or compound heterozygous state) or familial hypoalphalipoproteinemia (heterozygous state).[266] Heterozygotes have low HDL-C (usually below 30 mg/dL, but often as low as 10–15 mg/dL),[267,268] but usually normal triglycerides. A relatively small percentage (about 16%) of persons with HDL in the lowest fifth percentile appear to have an ABCA1 defect.[268] Initially, premature coronary disease was not thought to be a prominent feature of homozygous Tangier disease; more recent estimates suggest up to a sixfold increase in CHD risk.[269] The heterozygous state is associated with an approximately threefold greater risk of CHD (as compared with unaffected pedigree members).[267] Further, the ABCA1 transporter appears to be particularly instrumental in transporting cholesterol out of lipid-laden macrophages in atherosclerotic plaques.[270,271] Nevertheless, ABCA1 deficiency does not appear to be a major contributor to low HDL associated with premature coronary artery disease.[272,273] Several relatively common variants of *ABCA1* may be associated with an increased or decreased incidence of CHD independent of effects on HDL or other lipids.[274]

Deficiency of cholesterol ester transfer protein

It appears that cholesterol ester is acquired by VLDL and other triglyceride-rich particles during their sojourn through the plasma. Cholesterol ester is transferred to VLDL from HDL by way of the cholesterol ester transfer protein (CETP) reaction. In kinetic studies in humans, up to 50 mg/kg per day is transferred from HDL to VLDL by this reaction,[275] similar to estimates for the total rate of esterification of free cholesterol by lecithin-cholesterol acyltransferase (LCAT).[276] Animals such as rats, which lack CETP, have high HDL-C and low LDL-C and are resistant to atherosclerosis. In contrast, rabbits with abundant CETP have much lower plasma HDL-C levels and are more susceptible to atherosclerosis. In humans, mutations of the CETP gene, particularly common in Japan, result in substantial elevations in HDL-C (164 mg/dL in homozygotes, 66 mg/dL in heterozygotes). LDL-C tends to be low, with a relative increase in LDL triglyceride content.[277,278] Surprisingly, however, higher CHD rates may be seen with CETP deficiency despite generally higher HDL, particularly if HDL levels are not above 80 mg/dL.[279–281] Although this issue remains controversial, with some studies showing decreased CHD with CETP variants that have lower activity,[282–288] it raises the possibility that decreased CETP activity may interfere with reverse cholesterol transport and promote atherosclerosis, despite the increased levels of HDL-C. Accordingly, inhibition of CETP with drugs[289] must be tested with atherosclerosis-related endpoints, not simply effects on plasma HDL levels.

Elevated lipoprotein(a)

Lipoprotein(a) (Lp(a)) particles are formed by the covalent disulfide linkage of the glycoprotein apoprotein(a) to apoprotein B of LDL. Nearly all the population variance of plasma Lp(a) can be explained by genetic variability at the apoprotein(a) locus.[38] Renal disease can result in substantial elevations, whereas estrogen lowers Lp(a).[290,291] Plasma concentrations of Lp(a) above 30 to 40 mg/dL (approximately the ninetieth percentile) have generally been associated with modestly increased risk for premature CHD (relative odds = 2–4) in numerous retrospective case–control and angiographic studies among white subjects and in most prospective studies.[290,292,293] Although elevated Lp(a) is difficult or impractical to modify directly, several studies have identified a significant interaction of elevated Lp(a) with other lipids. Risk associated with an elevated Lp(a) imparted little excess risk unless total cholesterol or HDL-C was unfavorable, whereas in those with a modestly elevated total/HDL-C ratio, elevated Lp(a) was associated with a strikingly elevated risk.[294–297][292,293] Persons with total/HDL-C ratio above 5.8 (a modest elevation) may particularly benefit from measurement of Lp(a) and aggressive management of lipids if Lp(a) is elevated.

Polygenic hypercholesterolemia

The most common cause of type IIa hyperlipidemia (elevation of LDL-C only) with serum total cholesterol between 240 and 350 mg/dL is probably polygenic predisposition, often aggravated by a poor diet, increased adiposity with age, and other poorly defined factors. Mechanisms for such elevations probably include both increased production and, to a lesser extent, decreased removal of LDL-C.[298–300] Figure 6-6 depicts a sibship with polygenic hypercholesterolemia.

Genes contributing to polygenic hypercholesterolemia are largely unknown. A prototype, however, is ApoE. About 7 to 14% of population variance has been attributed to the combined effects of ApoE-2, -E-3, and –E-4.[160,301] Persons with the ApoE-3-2 genotype have approximately 10% lower total cholesterol and LDL-C compared with persons having the ApoE-3-3 genotype. The presence of an Apo-E-4 allele raises total and LDL-C approximately 7%. About 2 to 3% of CHD events can be attributed to these lipid effects with an approximate 40% increase in risk, particularly with ApoE-4.[160,302] In the 4S study, ApoE-4 carriers experienced a 1.8-fold increased CHD risk, but also experienced the greatest reduction in risk from simvastatin treatment.[303] It has been suggested that the lesser affinity of ApoE-2 for the LDL receptor results in reduced deposition of cholesterol ester–rich particles in the liver, with subsequently less downregulation of LDL receptors. The converse may

occur with ApoE-4.[304,305] Recently, a common variant (−595A > G) in one of the cholesterol regulatory genes, *SREB-2*, was found to be another significant, modest contributor to plasma cholesterol variation, particularly among hypercholesterolemic subjects.[306]

Familial combined hyperlipidemia, familial hypertriglyceridemia, and small, dense LDL

Familial combined hyperlipidemia (FCHL) is characterized by the presence of hypercholesterolemia (type IIa), hypertriglyceridemia (type IV), or both (type IIb), with two or more of these patterns present among first-degree relatives. Small, dense LDL and increased plasma ApoB are reported to be the most consistent lipid findings in patients with FCHL.[307,308] Typically, the hyperlipidemia is in the ninetieth to ninety-fifth percentile range and, thus, is not nearly as striking as in familial hypercholesterolemia. Age dependency of expression is a prominent feature. Affected persons are generally not recognizable until the third decade, though in some families affected children can be identified by reference to age-specific percentiles.[309] Estimates of FCHL prevalence in the general population range from 0.5 to 5% or higher, depending on cut points used. The genetics of FCHL remain unclear, though a locus on chromosome 1q appears to be the most consistently identified linkage region to date.[310,311] Traditionally, FCHL was considered distinct from familial hypertriglyceridemia (FHTG). Also, FCHL was thought to carry higher CHD risk than FHTG. FHTG shares the same definition with FCHL with respect to the hypertriglyceridemia phenotype (type IV), but type II and type IIb phenotypes are not seen in FHTG first-degree relatives by definition. This may be an artificial distinction, as recent results from the NHLBI Family Heart Study suggest the two entities are indistinguishable with respect to CHD risk (both diagnoses carry an approximate twofold increased risk) and with respect to clinical correlates such as low HDL, hypertension, and diabetes. Indeed, both may be considered variant manifestations of metabolic syndrome (see below).[312] Further, both syndromes probably share the kinetic hallmark of VLDL overproduction,[313–315] though impaired removal of both VLDL and LDL can occur in some FCHL families.[316]

Both FCHL and FHTG are also associated with small, dense LDL and an increase in ApoB. Hyperapobetalipoproteinemia, defined as elevated LDL ApoB with relatively normal LDL-C, is essentially the same entity.[317,318] A pattern of predominantly small, dense LDL appears to be dominantly transmitted and has been linked to several loci, including the LDL receptor, CETP, manganese superoxide dismutase, and the AI–CIII–AIV

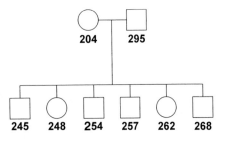

FIGURE 6-6 Sibship illustrating common polygenic hypercholesterolemia.

gene cluster.[310] Small, dense LDL has been reported as a risk factor for premature CHD by several investigators, usually with modest odds ratios of 2 to 3.[319–325] Some have found the associated risk independent of HDL-C and triglycerides[321,324–326]; others have not.[322,323] Accelerated atherosclerosis progression is also associated with small, dense LDL.[327,328] Plausible mechanisms for accelerated atherosclerosis associated with small, dense LDL are increased susceptibility to oxidation,[329,330] greater penetration of the smaller particles into the subintima,[331] and increased interaction with proteoglycans.[332] Expression of small, dense LDL is strongly dependent on plasma triglycerides; most persons will have pattern B when triglycerides are above 200 mg/dL (2.26 mmol/L). Although some support its clinical utility,[333] most lipid specialists consider determination of LDL particle size a research tool at present, owing to technical difficulties or expense.

METABOLIC SYNDROME

Metabolic syndrome has been variously designated as visceral fat syndrome, insulin resistance syndrome, multiple metabolic syndrome, pleurimetabolic syndrome, cardiovascular dysmetabolic syndrome, syndrome X, Reaven's syndrome, and dyslipidemic hypertension. The simplified term, *metabolic syndrome*, has become almost universally accepted after being adopted by the ATP-III panel.[334] In 1988, a syndrome descriptively named *familial dyslipidemic hypertension* (FDH) was described.[335] After the first 131 participants in a Utah study of familial hypertension selected *only* on the basis of early hypertension present in two or more siblings were screened, a very high prevalence of lipid abnormalities (65% of individuals, concordant in 48% of sibships) was noted, with high triglycerides (30%) and low HDL-C (39%) being most common. High LDL-C (19%) was also more prevalent than the 10% expected for each abnormality. Further studies demonstrated a pattern of FCHL in approximately half of those with FDH, while the other half had elevated triglycerides and/or low HDL-C, without elevated LDL-C. Both FDH groups had elevated fasting plasma insulin concentrations.[336] Follow-up in more than 300 participants in this study confirmed and strengthened these initial findings and clearly placed FDH in the same realm as metabolic syndrome.[337]

The combination of insulin resistance, hypertriglyceridemia, central obesity, and hypertension has been termed "the deadly quartet."[338] Very possibly, central or visceral obesity, rather than insulin resistance, is the central causative feature of this syndrome.[337,339] This model would be consistent with detailed genetic analysis of the metabolic syndrome in a group of 289 Swedish twins[340] and a recent linkage study from the NHLBI Family Heart Study.[341] In a study of twins by NHLBI, exaggerated risks of CHD were evident when hypertension and dyslipidemia were present jointly (Fig. 6-7). Furthermore, the combination of hypertension and dyslipidemia did appear to be genetically determined.[342] Approximately 12% of early familial CHD is associated with dyslipidemic hypertension.[343] Several practical implications are derived from these observations. First, in persons with hypertension, lipid profiles including total cholesterol, triglycerides, and HDL-C should be measured to assess risk more fully. Second, antihypertensive medications that do not adversely affect lipids should be used in persons with dyslipidemic hypertension. Third, weight loss and exercise should be central features of intervention.

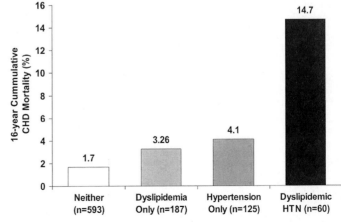

FIGURE 6-7 Prospective study demonstrating risk associated with dyslipidemia and hypertension separately and combined. (Adapted from Selby et al. *JAMA* 1991; 265:2079.)

Fourth, other family members of persons with dyslipidemic hypertension should be screened for both hypertension and dyslipidemia and treated accordingly.

Genetic evidence for the common inheritance of lipid abnormalities (particularly FCHL),[311,344,345] diabetes,[346] and blood pressure[347–349] comes from linkage in various genome scans to 1q21–q23 (near 170–180 cM). Similar loci on chromosomes 4p[350] and 7q[351] may exist. Several candidate gene variants appear to interact with BMI to increase the risk for metabolic syndrome.[352–357]

HYPERTENSION

Rare monogenic hypertension syndromes

The brilliant work by Guyton and co-workers, identifying the kidney as the dominant, long-term regulator of blood pressure,[358–361] illustrates the need for an appreciation of pathophysiology when considering genetic factors potentially contributing to hypertension. Recent identification of the genetic basis of most rare, monogenic forms of hypertension and hypotension reiterates the central role of the kidney in long-term control of blood pressure (Table 6-6).[362] Virtually all the monogenic hypertension syndromes identified to date are caused by defects resulting in renal salt retention, whereas all the low blood pressure syndromes share a common mechanism of excess renal sodium loss. These findings should direct researchers to carefully consider the effects on renal salt handling of proposed hypertension gene variants.

Common essential hypertension

Essential hypertension may be considered the result of interactions between genes and environment. The environmental effects are powerful and probably explain most or all of the substantial blood pressure differences between different populations. Genetic effects explain much of blood pressure distribution in populations with homogeneous nutrient intakes. One of the most powerful influences is body weight or obesity (itself largely genetically determined). Central or upper-body obesity is the major contributor in this relationship. An impressive 80% of all new-onset hypertension could be explained by subscapular skinfolds above the lowest quintile in the Framingham study.[363] Salt has a lesser but probably important effect.[364–366] Alcohol, physical activity, potassium intake (especially in fruits and vegetables), and possibly psychosocial stress are other potentially important environmental factors.[367] The mechanism of interaction probably involves how effectively the kidneys modulate changes in salt intake. Indeed, the hypertension in virtually every genetically hypertensive animal model can

be reversed by transplantation of the kidneys of a normotensive animal.[368]

Formal estimates of heritability of blood pressure usually range between 50 and 70% for systolic and diastolic blood pressure in twin studies. Lower estimates (around 20–25%) are typically reported for family studies.[26,27,369] Complex segregation analysis continues to show evidence for hypertension-related "major" genes.[370,371] Linkage analysis has identified potential blood pressure or hypertension loci on virtually every chromosome.[372]

Susceptibility to hypertension-related end-organ damage

In addition to heritability of blood pressure, predisposition to end-organ damage may be inherited separately from blood pressure. For example, there are "stroke-prone" and "stroke-resistant" spontaneously hypertensive rats (SHRs). Cross-breeding the two strains demonstrated independent segregation of the stroke-prone trait.[373] These investigators further identified a variant in the atrial natriuretic peptide gene associated with a twofold increased risk of stroke in the large, prospective, Physician's Health Study.[374] There are relatively rare mendelian forms of stroke, both hemorrhagic[375] and lacunar (cerebral autosomal dominant arteriopathy with subcortical infarcts and leukoencephalopathy, or CADASIL),[376] that are unrelated to hypertension. CADASIL has a prevalence of at least 1 per 100,000 and accounts for about 2% of lacunar strokes under age 65.[377] Leukoaraiosis[378] is a diffuse lesion of white matter resulting in hyperintensity on MRI scans, and was found to be 71% heritable in World War II veteran twins.[379]

Family history appears to influence more common types of end-organ damage, even after adjustment for blood pressure. Family history of atherothrombotic stroke increased risk up to threefold for this most common form of stroke.[380–382] A strong linkage to chromosome 5q12 has been reported, independent of known risk factors.[383] Family history of intracerebral hemorrhage was associated with sixfold increased risk of having this form of stroke, independent of blood pressure.[384] For subarachnoid hemorrhage, risk was increased fourfold by a definite positive family history.[385] Left ventricular mass[386] and other measures of left ventricular size and function[387] are heritable. Pulse pressure, a measure of arterial stiffness or distensibility, was strongly heritable and related to telomere length (which was also highly heritable).[388,389] Carotid intima–media thickness (IMT) has been reported to be up to 30 to 64% heritable.[390–393] Presence of carotid plaque was 23% heritable after correction for hypertension.[394] A possible candidate gene variant was associated with increased carotid IMT at high

TABLE 6-6   Monogenic Syndromes Resulting in Early-Onset, Severe Hypertension or Marked Low Blood Pressure*

Syndrome, transmission, defect (abbreviation, gene location)	Pathophysiology, comments
High blood pressure syndromes	
Glucocorticoid remedial hyperaldosteronism (GRA) Autosomal dominant Unequal fusion (chimera) of two, similar and adjacent genes, aldosterone synthase (*CYP11B2*) and 11β-hydroxylase (*CYP11B1*) due to an unequal crossing over event (8p21)	Aldosterone synthase activity is ectopically expressed in the adrenal zona fasciculata due to the chimeric promoter region of 11β-hydroxylase (under control of ACTH). Results in elevated aldosterone despite low plasma renin, increased ENaC expression, and increased Na$^+$ resorption in connecting tubule and collecting duct. Excess aldosterone secretion suppressed by glucocorticoid administration (suppresses ACTH). Hypokalemia and metabolic alkalosis (due to increased secretion of K$^+$ and H$^+$) are variably expressed. Hypertension responsive to spironolactone, suppressed by prednisone. May be diagnosed by the presence of abnormal urinary metabolites (18-hydroxy- and 18-oxocortisol steroids).
Apparent mineralocorticoid excess Autosomal recessive Deficiency of 11β-hydroxysteroid dehydrogenase-2 (*HSD11B2*, *AME1*, 16q22)	Cortisol, which activates the MR, as well as aldosterone, is not converted normally to cortisone (no MR activity). Low renin, absence of circulating aldosterone, hypokalemia, metabolic alkalosis. A mouse model also shows hypertension.
Steroid 11β-hydroxylase deficiency (congenital adrenal hyperplasia IV) Autosomal recessive (*CYP11B1*, 8q21)	11β-Hydroxylase is required for cortisol synthesis. Deficiency results in increased ACTH and increased production of both deoxycorticosterone and corticosterone, which can activate MR. Aldosterone is suppressed, hypokalemic alkalosis present.
Steroid 17α-hydroxylase deficiency (congenital adrenal hyperplasia V) Autosomal recessive (*CYP17*, 10q24.3)	Similar to steroid 11β-hydroxylase deficiency.
Hypertension with severe exacerbation in pregnancy Autosomal dominant MR Ser810Leu (*NR3C2*, *MR*, 4q31.1)	Carriers have hypertension onset before age 20 with severe worsening in pregnancy. Low renin phenotype. 801 Leu variant results in modification of MR, causing promiscuous activation by a variety of compounds (eg, progesterone, spironolactone) that normally bind without activating MR. Normally, MR has specificity for 21-hydroxylated steroids.
Liddle syndrome Autosomal dominant Deletions of cytoplasmic tail and some missense mutations of ENaC (*SCNN1B*, 16p13–p12)	Defect or loss of PPPXY sequence in the cytoplasmic C terminus of either the β or γ subunits o ENaC results in loss of affinity for clathrin (and loss of normal removal into clathrin-coated pits) and reduced clearance of ENaC from luminal brush border. Nedd4–1 and Nedd4–2, proteins that recognize the PPPXY domain and ubiquitinate ENaC, marking it for degradation, may also be involved.
Pseudohypoaldosteronism, type II (Gordon's syndrome) Autosomal dominant (*WNK1*, 12p13) (*WNK4*, 17q21–q22) (also linkage to 1q31–q42)	Clinical features of Gordon's syndrome include hypertension, hyperkalemia, hyperchloremia, metabolic acidosis, salt (and chloride) sensitivity, and responsiveness to low-dose thiazide diuretics. WNK1 mutations causing Gordon's syndrome are gain-in-function mutations. WNK1 appears to increase activity of thiazide-sensitive Na–Cl cotransporter (NCCT), causing increased NaCl transport. WNK4 normally suppresses NCCT, with the mutant form leading to impaired WNK4 activity and increased NCCT activity.

(Continued)

TABLE 6-6   (Continued)

Syndrome, transmission, defect (abbreviation, gene location)	Pathophysiology, comments
Hypertension with brachydactyly mapped to 12p12.2–11.2	Not salt sensitive or associated with abnormalities of the renin–angiotensin system. Unknown mechanism.
Bardet–Biedl syndrome (*BBS2*, 16q21) (*BBS4*, 15q22.3–q23)	Mechanism of disease unknown.
Autosomal dominant polycystic kidney disease (*PKD1*, 16p 13.3) (*PKD2*, 4q21–q23)	Common (1/500 to 1/1000). May be considered genetic cause of secondary hypertension (due to activation of renin–angiotensin system secondary to compressive effects of cysts). 75% of patients have hypertension, frequently severe.
Low blood pressure syndromes	
Aldosterone synthase deficiency Autosomal recessive (*CYP11B2*, 8p21)	Impaired aldosterone synthesis leads to impaired distal sodium resorption, hypovolemia, hypotension, and shock. Impaired K^+ and H^+ exertion with hyperkalemia and metabolic acidosis also seen.
Congenital adrenal hyperplasia 1 Steroid 21-hydroxylase deficiency Autosomal recessive (*CYP21A2*, 6p21.3)	Similar to aldosterone synthase deficiency. Other endocrine abnormalities.
Dominant pseudohypoaldosteronism, type I Autosomal dominant Mineralocorticoid receptor loss of function (various mutations seen) (*MR*, 4q31.1)	Neonatal hypotension, severe salt wasting, marked hyperkalemia, and metabolic acidosis despite elevated aldosterone. Normally, ENaC, under control of aldosterone, establishes the luminal electronegative potential that allows normal K^+ and H^+ excretion. Once a typical salt-rich diet is established, the phenotype reverts to normal with no manifestations of disease in the adult.
Recessive pseudohypoaldosteronism, type I Autosomal recessive (*SCNN1A*, 12p13) (*SCNN1B*, 16p13–p12) (*SCNN1G*, 16p13–p12)	Loss of ENaC function leads to salt wasting, hypovolemia, hyperkalemia, metabolic acidosis (due to impaired K^+ and H^+ excretion) in neonatal period despite high serum aldosterone. Unlike dominant form, recessive does not correct with age.
Gitelman syndrome Autosomal recessive Sodium chloride cotransporter (*SLC12A3*, 16q13)	Impaired function of thiazide-sensitive Na–Cl cotransporter (*SLC12A3*) of distal convoluted tubule results in salt wasting. Compensatory increase in the renin–angiotensin–aldosterone system minimizes salt loss, but increase in distal ENaC leads to increased K^+ and H^+ excretion. A decrease in urinary calcium is seen together with excess magnesium excretion. Heterozygotes frequently maintain normal blood pressure by increased salt intake.
Bartter syndrome Autosomal recessive Type 1 (*SLC12A1*, 15q15–q21) Type 2 (*ROMK or KCNJ1*, 11q24) Type 3 (*CLCNKB*, 1q36)	Loss of function of apical, furosemide-sensitive, Na–K–2Cl contransporter (*SLC12A1*) in thick ascending loop of Henle results in marked salt wasting, activation of renin–angiotensin–aldosterone system, hypokalemia, and metabolic alkalosis. Deficiency of ROMK (ATP-sensitive K^+ channel) leads to a similar phenotype. ROMK is required in the TAL because K^+ is low in the TAL tubular fluid and must be excreted back into the tubular lumen to facilitate further NaCl reabsorption. CLCNKB is a chloride channel in the basolateral membrane of TAL epithelial cells. Na^+ entering via Na–K–2CL contransporter exits by way of the basolateral Na^+ K^+-ATPase. Cl^- must leave by way of CLCNKB. All forms have increased urinary calcium and less magnesium wasting as compared with Gitelman syndrome.

*MR, mineralocorticoid receptor; ENaC, epithelial sodium channel; TAL, thick ascending loop of Henle.

alcohol intakes.[395] A substantial number of gene variants have been associated with carotid IMT; some were also associated with CHD.[396]

Candidate genes for hypertension

The first candidate gene to show linkage with human essential or primary hypertension was angiotensinogen (*AGT*).[397] In addition to linkage to the *AGT* locus (ie, cosegregation within families of hypertension with genetic markers of the *AGT* gene), hypertension and plasma angiotensinogen levels were both found to be *associated* with the 235T and 174M variants of *AGT* (ie, more hypertension was found associated with these particular gene variants in the entire population).[397] Numerous studies followed with mixed, but mostly positive results. A meta-analysis of 69 association studies with 27,906 subjects concluded that the *AGT* 235TT genotype conferred a 31% greater risk for hypertension ($P = 0.001$), whereas those with the MT genotype had 11% greater risk ($P = 0.03$).[398] Subsequent studies have continue to find a mixed, but generally positive association.[399–405] The *AGT* 235T polymorphism, although without any apparent functional significance itself, is in almost complete linkage disequilibrium with the -6A variant in the promoter region of *AGT*, which, in in vitro studies, resulted in greater expression of a marker gene product compared with the -6G allele.[406] Exposure of tissues to increased angiotensinogen, and thereby angiotensin II, likely mediates the increase blood pressure associated with this variant.[372,407,408] Other phenotypes besides blood pressure may be affected by the *AGT* genotype. These include left ventricular mass index,[409–412] stroke,[413] renal disease,[414–417] and long-term response to reductions of salt intake[418,419] or increased fruit and vegetable intake.[420] There is less evidence demonstrating significant effects on relationship to hypertension for other genes of the renin–angiotensin system, though evidence exists for angiotensin-converting enzyme (*ACE*) (primarily in interaction with other genes), angiotensin type 1 (AT1) receptor, 11β-hydroxysteroid dehydrogenase (particularly with salt sensitivity), and aldosterone synthase (*CYP11B2*).[372]

The α-adducin gene (*ADD1*) is another gene for which there is substantial evidence of a modest role in human hypertension. Recognition of a potential role of *ADD1* in hypertension began with the Milan hypertensive rat, a salt-sensitive strain with mild hypertension with modestly increased proximal tubular sodium reabsorption. Further detailed studies led to identification of variants in both the α and β subunits of adducin that accounted for 50% of the difference in systolic blood pressure between Milan hypertensive rats and normotensive strains. Adducin is a cytoskeletal protein that interacts with Na,K-ATPase. Adducin variants associated with both rat and human hypertension show greater affinity for Na,K-ATPase, resulting in increased membrane expression and activity of Na,K-ATPase.[421,422] Initial positive association studies in humans[423] were followed by significant linkage studies in hypertensive siblings[424] and identification of a common variant associated with hypertension. Mechanistic studies suggest increased salt retention in carriers of a common variant (460Trp) associated with hypertension.[424–428] As with *AGT*, subsequent studies were mixed but generally positive, particularly in Caucasian populations.[355,429] Further, adducin appears to interact with other genes (particularly *ACE*).[425,430] and affect other phenotypes, including CHD[431,432] and left ventricular hypertrophy.[433] Variants in other genes affecting ion transport have also been reported, including the endothelial sodium channel,[434–438] a G-protein-coupled receptor kinase 4 (*GRK4γ*) affecting activity of the dopamine receptor,[439–441] and possibly variants in the D_1 and D_2 receptor genes.[442,443]

Several genes of the adrenergic system may contribute to hypertension. Evidence has been presented for the 825C>T variant in G-protein β3 subunit (*GNB3*) (also associated with overweight and insulin resistance), the $β_2$-adrenergic receptor, the $β_1$- and $β_3$-adrenergic receptors, and the G_s-protein α subunit (*GNAS1*). Other genes for which evidence of an effect on hypertension in human populations exists include endothelial nitric oxide synthase (*NOS3*), atrial natriuretic peptide receptor, endothelin-1 (in the context of overweight), and prostacyclin synthase.[372] Currently, none of these gene variants are readily available to the clinician, and none can be endorsed as a means of directing antihypertensive therapy or predicting hypertension risk in an individual. Treatment of hypertension remains largely empirical. Treatment choices, however, may be influenced by the experience of other family members, such as a good response to a particular agent in a close relative. The field of pharmacogenomics promises considerable contributions to the treatment of hypertension in the future, but no clear examples of clinical utility are available yet.[444–446] Possibly, large panels of gene variants assessed simultaneously will yield useful information someday.[447]

TYPE 2 DIABETES

Diabetes is a major risk factor for CHD, resulting in three- to fivefold elevations in risk of new-onset CHD in numerous studies.[448] Elevated fasting glucose, especially clinically diagnosed diabetes, is also a strong predictor of subsequent mortality in persons undergoing percutaneous coronary interventions.[449] Both type 1 and type 2 diabetes are associated with increased risk, but the excess prevalence of lipid abnormalities and hypertension, or metabolic syndrome, accompanying and preceding type 2 diabetes may help explain the strong cardiovascular risk associated with this disorder.[450–453] Even after adjusting for these risk factors, however, persons destined to develop type 2 diabetes were at increased risk of MI before their diagnosis of diabetes.[454] CHD risk in diabetes may be restricted those who also display features of metabolic syndrome.[455]

The genetics of type 1 diabetes is considerably better understood than that of type 2 diabetes. The sibling of a type 1 diabetic is at 15 times the risk of for type 1 diabetes than the general population. Most cases of type 1 diabetes probably involve a genetic predisposition to autoimmune destruction of the pancreatic beta cells.[456] Even so, at least 20 genomic regions have been identified in genomewide scans, though the strongest LOD scores are found on 6p21, the human histocompatibility locus.[457] Particular combinations of HLA type II are particularly associated with type 1 diabetes, with up to 30% of the disease being associated with HLA DQ2/DQ8 heterozygotes and up to 50% attributable to variation at the human histocompatibility locus generally.[458] The insulin gene has also been implicated.[457,458] Type 1 diabetes is not discussed further here.

A strong genetic component for type 2 diabetes has also long been recognized. Lifetime concordance in monozygous twins may approach 100%, compared with about 25 to 38% in dizygous twins, consistent with very high heritability.[459,460] But like hypertension, type 2 diabetes is a complex quantitative disease with varying degrees of genetic and environmental contributions, making the identification and confirmation of contributing genes difficult. Environmental effects are well illustrated by the Pima Indians. Pima Indians in Mexico living a traditional lifestyle in a remote mountainous area are lean

(mean BMI = 24.9) and physically active; they have about the same prevalence of diabetes as the general US population (about 6).[461,462] In contrast, Pima Indians in southern Arizona are, on average, 26 kg heavier (mean BMI = 33.4) and have an exceedingly high frequency of diabetes: approximately 37% in women and 54% in men.[461] The interaction of overweight and genetic predisposition is perhaps best illustrated in Fig. 6-8 by the strongly increasing gradient of risk associated with higher BMI among offspring of one and, especially, two diabetic parents. Higher BMI only modestly increased risk if family history of diabetes was negative.[463] A clear interaction was also seen in a large English population; those with a positive family history of diabetes had much greater risk of diabetes associated with both obesity and low level of exercise.[464] Related risk factors predicting development of type 2 diabetes include a number of features of the metabolic syndrome and C-reactive protein.[453] These findings provide one of the most clinically useful messages for prevention of diabetes: if you have a family history of type 2 diabetes, get lean and stay lean. Exercise is a particularly important element of this approach, as benefit independent of BMI has been documented.[465–467] The utility of weight loss and exercise has been powerfully demonstrated, in recent intervention studies, to prevent progression from glucose intolerance to frank diabetes.[468,469]

The emergence of diabetes among Pima Indians and several other populations, after changing from a spartan traditional lifestyle to one in which food is more abundant, has been attributed to a "thrifty genotype": a gene or set of genes favoring efficient storage of body fat, thereby increasing survival in times of famine.[470] In times of

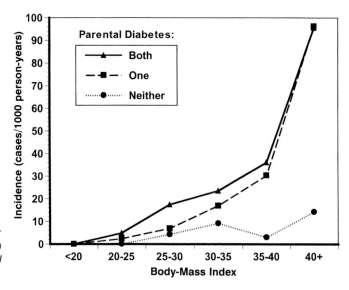

FIGURE 6-8   Interaction between family history of type 2 diabetes mellitus and BMI in Pima Indians. (Adapted from Knowler et al. *Am J Epidemiol* 1981;113:144.)

relative abundance, however, the deposition of excess fat, particularly visceral fat, promotes insulin resistance.[337] It may well be that the inability of peripheral fat cells to proliferate adequately in the face of overabundance, with resultant "overfilling" of fat cells and inappropriate deposition of fat into muscle, liver, and pancreatic beta cells, is the underlying feature of most type 2 diabetes.[471,472] This is consistent with the finding that lipodystrophic mice that lack white adipose tissue have severe insulin resistance, which is largely reversed by white adipose tissue transplantation.[473] These findings help explain the cause of the insulin resistance that is probably the precursor of much, if not most, diabetes.[474,475] Overt diabetes later emerges if insulin resistance is superimposed on a primarily genetic failure of the beta cell to compensate adequately.[451,476,477]

A recent, particularly enlightening study compared glucose-tolerant, lean offspring of diabetics to age-, height-, and weight-matched controls. All were relatively sedentary. BMI was 21 to 23. The offspring of the diabetics were also selected to be insulin resistant but glucose tolerant, whereas controls were selected to be insulin sensitive. A euglycemic insulin clamp confirmed the insulin resistance as due to a marked reduction in insulin-stimulated whole-body glucose uptake and a decrease in nonoxidative glucose metabolism. The factor most strongly correlated with insulin resistance was intramyocellular fat content measured by magnetic resonance spectroscopy of the soleus muscle. There were no differences between the two groups with respect to intrahepatic fat content, nor were there differences in whole-body lipolysis or plasma levels of adiponectin, tumor necrosis factor α, interleukin-6, or resistin. Further, there was a significant decrease in muscle mitochondrial phosphorylation in the offspring of diabetics.[478] These findings are consistent with other investigators who found an increase in type IIb muscle fibers (mitochondria poor) in offspring of diabetics.[479] Variants of the peroxisome proliferator-activated receptor-γ coactivator-1 gene (*PGC-1*), which helps to control PPARγ and several genes of fatty acid oxidative metabolism, have been found to be associated with type 2 diabetes in at least two populations.[480,481] Gene expression studies are also consistent, showing a decrease in *PGC-1*-related gene expression in those with diabetes or a positive family history with insulin resistance.[482,483]

These findings suggest that for many future diabetics, impaired metabolism of fatty acids in muscle may be a primary lesion leading to insulin resistance and, later, to type 2 diabetes. Later in life, in the face of caloric excess and more generalized fat accumulation, both glucotoxicity and lipotoxicity could also be involved with promoting beta cell dysfunction and failure.[484–487] Saturated fatty acids particularly aggravate glucolipotoxicity.[488] Complications in diabetes may also be tied to excess

availability of energy substrates in general, particularly in vascular endothelial cells.[489] These insights suggest that many genes of intermediate metabolism of energy substrates could be considered as potential candidate genes for type 2 diabetes. Recognition that adipocytes are complex endocrine organs, not merely passive fat storage cells, further increases the panoply of candidate genes for diabetes. Thus, besides free fatty acids, adipocytes release tumor necrosis factor α (TNF-α), interleukins, prostaglandins, plasminogen activator inhibitor type 1, angiotensinogen, adipsin, interleukin-6, leptin, adiponectin, and resistin.[490] Of particular recent interest has been the most abundant of these proteins, adiponectin. Higher levels of adiponectin are anti-inflammatory and protect against diabetes, obesity, and, probably, atherosclerosis.[491–494] Adipocytes secrete less adiponectin as weight increases. Two adiponectin receptors, one expressed in muscle, the other in liver, mediate the fatty acid-oxidizing and insulin-sensitizing effects of adiponectin through increased activities of AMP kinase and PPARα.[495] At least three genomewide scans have identified a type 2 diabetes susceptibility locus at chromosome 3q27, the location of adiponectin.[496–498] Several variants in the adiponectin gene seem to affect adiponectin and diabetes or obesity risk.[499–504] Nevertheless, other, as yet unknown genes appear to have major effects on adiponectin levels.[505,506]

Several other gene loci have been suggested to be involved with development of both diabetes and obesity, including the β_3-adrenergic receptor,[507–509] the β_2-adrenergic receptor,[510] glycogen synthase (also associated with hypertension, possibly aggravated by a high-fat diet),[511–513] the sulfonylurea receptor,[514] and a human uncoupling protein (UCP2).[515] Subsequent studies have not confirmed the association with UCP2.[516–519] The findings with UCP2 illustrate the general difficulty in replicating associations for candidate genes.[520,521]

Less than one third of the 10-fold variation seen in insulin sensitivity among young, healthy individuals can be explained by obesity and other known environmental factors.[522] Much of the remainder is likely to involve genetic variation. Several examples have begun to be identified, particularly involving the insulin signaling cascade, including mutations or variants of insulin receptor substrate 1 (IRS-1), the p85 subunit of the phosphatidylinositol 3 (PI3)-kinase, and the regulatory subunit of glycogen-associated protein phosphate 1 (PP1G).[522] Additional support has been reported for a role for the Gly972Arg variant of IRS-1, resulting primarily in defective insulin release from pancreatic beta cells.[523] Another group could not identify mutations in several genes involved in control of intracellular glucose and glycogen homeostasis.[524] Several rare, severe, inherited forms of insulin resistance have been explained by mutations of the insulin receptor.[525,526] In one study,

3 of 51 Japanese patients with ordinary type 2 diabetes had insulin receptor mutations that may have explained their disease.[527]

The genetic bases of several other relatively rare syndromes that cause severe or early-onset type 2 diabetes have been described. One group of these disorders has been called maturity-onset diabetes of the young (MODY). Features include an autosomal dominant inheritance, age of onset below 25, and nonketotic diabetes without insulin dependence. Five molecular etiologies of MODY have been described. These include mutations in hepatocyte nuclear factor 4α (HNF-4α, MODY1), glucokinase (GCK, MODY2), hepatocyte nuclear factor 1α (HNF-1α, MODY3), insulin-promoter factor-1 (IPF-1, MODY4), hepatocyte nuclear factor-1β (HNF-1β, MODY5), and the NeuroD1 gene (MODY6). Of these, MODY2 and MODY3 are the most common; at least 130 mutations of the glucokinase gene causing MODY2 have been described. The common pathophysiologic feature of MODY syndromes is dysfunction of beta cell insulin secretion.[528,529] Maternally inherited diabetes and deafness (MIDD), caused by a mutation in mitochondrial DNA (also leading to impaired insulin secretion), has also been described.[459] An additional form of rare autosomal dominant diabetes with features of both types 1 and 2 has been identified as a mutation in the sulfonylurea receptor 1, which causes congenital hyperinsulinism in infancy but later results in reduced insulin secretion, possibly because of increased calcium levels in beta cells as a result of constant stimulation from the defective ATP-sensitive potassium channel.[530] Mutations and variants in the PPARγ gene have provided new insights into the complex role of this intracellular regulator of adipocyte differentiation. Gene variants with supraphysiologic activity lead to proliferation of subcutaneous fat depots and severe obesity, but with lower insulin resistance than expected for the excess adiposity, whereas reduced activity leads to a form of peripheral lipodystrophy but severe insulin resistance.[531] These results are consistent with studies in animals and with thiazolidinediones.[532,533]

The first example of a clear difference in response to treatment based on genetic background in type 2 diabetes was recently reported. Persons with the relatively common MODY3 genotype responded much better to a sulfonylurea than persons with common type 2 diabetes. The MODY3 patients also had much greater insulin responses to intravenous tolbutamide and were not insulin resistant, even after matching for BMI.[534] Insights into the pathophysiology of the rare causes of monogenic diabetes have not translated into success in finding genetic causes of common type 2 diabetes. Thus, no evidence of linkage to older-onset diabetes has been demonstrated for the glucokinase gene.[535] In fact, efforts to identify linkage or association with more than 250 candidate genes

have largely been unsuccessful,[459,460,536–539] despite evidence for segregation of a major gene for type 2 diabetes in Pima Indians[540] and segregation of fasting insulin levels in Utah type 2 diabetes families.[541] Indeed, lack of replication has brought into question nearly all suggested candidate genes.[459]

Another approach to finding genes, or at least genetic regions containing genes, is genomewide scans. A number of such scans have been performed and the results reviewed.[459,542] Although initial review of the results have been disappointing to some, there are some regions for which reasonable replication is beginning to emerge. One such region contains the adiponectin gene as noted above. Other regions include 1q21–1q24, 2q, and 12q.[542] A composite factor representing the metabolic syndrome was also recently linked to the same region on chromosome 2q, as reported for diabetes linkage studies.[341] No strong candidate genes are known under these peaks, but efforts are underway to identify responsible genes, particularly for the 1q21–q24 which has also been linked to FCHL and obesity. Models that include interaction between genes are just beginning to be considered, and interaction with environmental factors is particularly problematic. The complexity of type 2 diabetes mellitus will continue to challenge geneticists. Nevertheless, this should not deter efforts directed at prevention through achieving and maintaining a lean body habitus through diet and exercise, particularly in persons with apparent familial predisposition.[543]

OBESITY

Obesity is a major determinant of hypertriglyceridemia, low HDL-C, small, dense LDL-C, hypertension, and diabetes. Coupled with genetic predisposition to these problems, excess body fat can have far more severe consequences for the individual than might be suggested by general population surveys. Substantial progress has been made in finding causal genes for rare, monogenic causes of obesity. As of October 2002, 91 persons whose monogenic obesity could be clearly attributed to a specific mutation in one of just six known genes have been identified in the world literature. These genes include leptin (*LEP*), the leptin receptor (*LEPR*), proopiomelanocortin (*POMC*), proprotein convertase subtilisin/kexin type 1 (*PCSK1*), single-minded (Drosophila) homolog 1 (*SIM1*), and the melanocortin 4 receptor (*MC4R*). Variants for these same gene loci, however, have generally not been found to be associated with common obesity.[544] For instance, just six patients have been identified with obesity due to leptin mutations. Melanocortin 4 receptor deficiency is the most common of these monogenic obesity syndromes, accounting for approximately 6% of severe, childhood obesity; homozygosity and null mutations have greater effects than mutations leaving partial activity.[545] Bardet–Biedl syndrome (progressive retinal dystrophy, central obesity, polydactyly, renal dysplasia, reproductive tract anomalies, and mental retardation, all variably expressed) displays complex inheritance patterns involving at least eight loci, the most common being *BBS1*. Some patients may need to be homozygous only at *BBS1*, whereas in others, interaction with one of the other loci appears to be required to express the phenotype. It may be one of the few examples of a truly oligogenic trait.[546,547]

Obesity is a highly heritable trait, suggesting multiple genes contribute to common obesity.[548–550] In Utah twins, heritability was estimated to be 54% for BMI (Table 6-2). Others have reported heritabilities up to 90%t.[550] Interestingly, segregation analysis shows stronger major gene effects for younger persons, whereas multifactorial factors predominated in older individuals.[551] Perhaps this explains the extraordinarily high heritability of 80% for BMI in a large series of Finnish twins aged 16 to 17 years.[552] One of the most persuasive arguments for the strong heritability of body mass is the finding that the BMI of twins reared apart resembled that of their biologic parents much more closely than that of their adoptive parents.[550,553] Also of great interest is the finding of a wide range of weight gains between monozygous twin pairs fed excess calories, with a high correlation of weight gain within the twin pairs.[554]

Fat patterning is also highly heritable in humans.[555,556] Accumulation of visceral fat was one of the most heritable changes in body composition observed in studies of overfeeding among monozygous twins.[548,554] Evidence of a major recessive gene causing increased accumulation of truncal fat has been presented.[557] Increased sharing of alleles on chromosome 1 was seen in sibling pairs with more similar BMI and waist/hip ratios in a study from Muscatine, Iowa.[558] Increased waist/hip ratios are also associated with a polymorphism of the angiotensinogen gene on chromosome 1 among Hutterites.[559] The authors suggested that another gene near the angiotensinogen locus on chromosome 1 may be related to control of abdominal obesity in humans. In the pig, a locus corresponding to chromosome 1 in humans has been described that does control abdominal and back fatness.[560] The β_3-adrenergic receptor gene is an important candidate for central obesity and ensuing features of the multiple metabolic syndrome.[561] Besides these loci, there is increasing, though often conflicting, evidence of contributions to central fat accumulation from common variants in the β_2-adrenergic receptor, leptin receptor, glucocorticoid receptor, PPARγ, and tumor necrosis factor genes. Evidence of a number of other variants in various genes has also been presented, but in no case is the evidence strong enough to consider an association with central obesity confirmed.[562] Similar conclusions can be reached regarding most of the 71 or more genes with variants reported to be associated with general obesity-related phenotypes.[544]

Linkage studies have identified at least 68 potential regions related to adiposity. The locus showing the strongest linkage (LOD = 9.2 at chromosome 4p15 or 49.5 cM) was found for the female-only phenotype (males treated as unknown) in 37 pedigrees having three or more female relatives with BMIs of 40 or higher. Different, much less significant, regions were identified for male-only phenotypes and for non-gender-specific phenotypes. These pedigrees were identified from a resource of 435 families with two or more relatives with BMIs of at least 35.[563] Others have also identified this region as an obesity locus.[564] Another notable region is 20q13, found in a series of 92 nuclear families,[565] and verified (LOD = 4.2) in 103 extended Utah families including 1711 individuals.[544,566] The incentive to find genes for obesity remains strong, with the hope of identifying metabolic pathways that could be amenable to pharmacologic treatment.

HYPERHOMOCYSTEINEMIA

Original observations of atherosclerotic changes in the arteries of young persons dying of severe recessive forms of homocystinuria can be attributed to McCully.[567] Subsequently, other investigations, including studies in Utah,[68,568] found modest elevations in plasma homocysteine to be an important independent risk factor for premature CHD[71,569,570] and continued increased risk in patients with CHD.[571] In the Utah series, 10 to 14% of early-onset, familial CHD could be attributed to elevated total homocysteine.[568] Modest doses of B vitamins, primarily folate, can significantly lower plasma homocysteine[572] and lead to improved endothelial function in CHD patients[573] and fewer subsequent coronary events in initial trials.[574,575]

Severe elevations of plasma homocysteine are associated with recessive defects in enzymes of homocysteine, folate, and vitamin B_{12} metabolism. Nevertheless, genetic contributions to more common hyperhomocysteinemia are poorly understood. A common mutation of the methylenetetrahydrofolate reductase gene is associated with greater sensitivity to low folate,[576,577] but appears to be associated with premature CHD only where folate intakes are low, as noted above.[70] The cystathionine β-synthase gene is another important candidate and has been related to moderately to severely elevated homocysteine in a number of studies.[578,579] Hyperhomocysteinemia has also been associated with a variant of the endothelial nitric oxide synthase gene.[580] It is currently unknown whether these loci sufficiently explain the excess familial aggregation of homocysteine, which is seen particularly in close relatives of patients with premature vascular disease.[581]

MEDPED: A GENETICALLY ORIENTED PUBLIC HEALTH APPROACH FOR HIGH-RISK PEDIGREES

Make Early Diagnoses to Prevent Early Deaths in Medical Pedigrees (MEDPED) is a nonprofit humanitarian project organized in 38 collaborating countries to collect all known index cases with FH or FDB (Familial Defective Apo B). Investigators contact relatives for screening and treatment in both close and distant medical pedigrees. From one index case, 5 to 15 new FH cases can often be found among "close relatives" (siblings, parents, offspring, aunt, uncles, nieces, nephews, first cousins, and their offspring) applying the lipid criteria in Table 6-4. In some families, hundreds of FH cases have been found by extending screening to "distant relatives" (second, third, and fourth cousins and their offspring).[582] This family screening approach has been shown to be the most cost-effective way to find new FH cases.[185] This program can be considered an effective public health measure as the cost-effectiveness of drug therapy for FH has been rigorously documented.[180,583]

At present, the MEDPED collaborators are setting an example of case detection through relative screening. Assistance for patients suspected or known to have FH is available by phone at 1-888-2Hi-CHOL or on the web at *www.medped.org*. MEDPED collaborators in 38 countries have collectively identified well more than 40,000 patients with FH, in part by contacting relatives of known FH cases. By educating patients and their personal physicians and by helping them get additional help from referral specialists, the MEDPED effort has made it possible for many FH patients to experience dramatic (40–50%) reductions in LDL-C levels. The World Health Organization has convened two meetings devoted to FH and the MEDPED concept and has published a report with practical recommendations for this approach.[191] This same approach could work for similar diseases as long as they meet these criteria:

1. A single dominant gene causes preventable serious illness.
2. Validated diagnostic tests are available (gene test or clinical test).
3. Some form of treatment or prevention is available and has been shown to be effective.

Although some social scientists have raised concerns that projects like MEDPED might cause psychologic stress by contacting relatives to talk about their family history, MEDPED collaborators in several countries report a large preponderance of positive reactions from relatives in FH families. In a recent study of patient attitudes regarding diagnosis of FH, patients diagnosed with FH reported modest anxiety about high serum cholesterol, use of cholesterol-lowering drugs, and risk of heart disease. But nearly 90% believed that their family should be screened and that people should be told of disease risks and what they can do to reduce risk.[584]

INCORPORATING FAMILY HISTORY AND GENETICS INTO CLINICAL PRACTICE

Although gene testing in the clinical setting is currently impractical and unproven, family history remains a powerful predictor of subsequent cardiovascular risk. The clinical workup of any new patient, particularly one with CVD (including hypertension), diabetes, or overweight, should include a careful family history, including *age at onset* of coronary artery disease (MI, coronary artery bypass graft, percutaneous transluminal coronary angioplasty, sudden death), hypertension, stroke, and diabetes, as well as some indication of body weight, smoking and diabetic status, and plasma lipids for all first-degree relatives. Similar information on second-degree relatives can be useful as well. Such a family history is conveniently obtained by providing the patient with a form that can be filled out in consultation with other family members prior to the clinic visit (Appendix 1). Knowledge obtained from such a family history should empower the clinician and patient to be more vigilant with preventive measures—not only in the patient, but among his or her close relatives. Among the most important of these measures are: firm advice to stop smoking or never start, aggressive lipid lowering when indicated, careful blood pressure and blood sugar monitoring and management, attainment or maintenance of an ideal body weight, and encouragement of a healthy diet and exercise program.

GENE THERAPY

Gene therapy is often heralded as the logical and definitive approach to treating genetic disorders. However, technical difficulties and shortcomings still limit the utility of this promising modality. To date, the only example of replacing a defective gene to prevent atherosclerosis in humans is that of the LDL receptor in homozygous FH in a small pilot study.[585,586] Five patients with homozygous FH underwent gene therapy, which required removal of a portion of liver, ex vivo transfection of the cultured hepatocytes using a retroviral vector, and infusion of the transfected hepatocytes into the liver through a portal vein catheter placed during the first procedure. Reductions in LDL-C levels were 6 to 25% and prolonged in only three of the five patients; two patients had no reduction in LDL-C.[586] The study provided proof-of-concept, but the benefits did not justify the risks or costs of the procedures. Animal studies are proceeding in an effort to find safer and more efficient vectors and gene transfer, and even different genes to lower LDL. Short-term success in gene therapy of LDL receptor-deficient mice and rabbits continues.[587–590] However, the development of humoral and cellular immune responses to the vector and to the LDL receptor eliminated expression of the transgene within a few weeks in most of these studies.[587–589] One approach circumventing this problem is use of an alternative strategy of ectopic expression of the VLDL receptor in the liver of mice.[591–593] Examples of long-term expression in animals include the VLDL receptor using adeno-associated virus[592] or helper-dependent adenovirus,[593] and apoE in apoE-deficient mice using helper-dependent adenovirus.[594] A more complete genomic transcript may have an advantage over the usual cDNA transfected.[595] Nonviral vectors have been more actively pursued after death, due to hypersensitivity to adenovirus, which occurred in a human study.[596]

Other approaches to gene therapy include increasing expression of protective genes and promoting angiogenesis in the face of marked stenosis. Promising results have been reported for upregulating nitric oxide production in endothelium,[597] decreasing cholesterol levels in ApoE-deficient mice,[598] efficient gene transfer to the liver using ApoE-3 peptides,[599] and stable transfer of apoA-I into LDL receptor-deficient mice.[600] Promotion of reverse cholesterol transport with ApoA–I (Milano) infusion might be considered a form of gene therapy, as recombinant protein was used.[260,262,601] Gene therapy for hypertension has progressed in various animal models and has involved primarily antisense oligonucleotides (including against angiotensinogen and other genes of the renin–angiotensin system).[602] Promotion of angiogenesis (as with VEGF and FGF) and other treatment for acute ischemia is beyond the scope of this chapter, but has been reviewed recently.[603]

REFERENCES

1. Levi F, Lucchini F, Negri E, La Vecchia C. Trends in mortality from cardiovascular and cerebrovascular diseases in Europe and other areas of the world. *Heart* 2002;88:119–124.

2. Campbell TC, Parpia B, Chen J. Diet, lifestyle, and the etiology of coronary artery disease: the Cornell China study. *Am J Cardiol* 1998;82:18T–21T.

3. Robertson TL, Kato H, Rhoads GG, et al. Epidemiologic studies of coronary heart disease and stroke in Japanese men living in Japan, Hawaii and California: incidence of myocardial infarction and death from coronary heart disease. *Am J Cardiol* 1977;39:239–243.

4. Robertson TL, Kato H, Gordon T, et al. Epidemiologic studies of coronary heart disease and stroke in Japanese men living in Japan, Hawaii and California: coronary heart disease risk factors in Japan and Hawaii. *Am J Cardiol* 1977;39:244–249.

5. Keys A, Menotti A, Aravanis C, et al. The Seven Countries Study: 2,289 deaths in 15 years. *Prev Med* 1984;13:141–154.

6. Keys A, Menotti A, Karvonen MJ, et al. The diet and 15-year death rate in the Seven Countries Study. *Am J Epidemiol* 1986;124:903–915.

7. Yoon PW, Scheuner MT, Khoury MJ. Research priorities for evaluating family history in the prevention of common chronic diseases. *Am J Prev Med* 2003;24:128–135.

8. Kardia SL, Modell SM, Peyser PA. Family-centered approaches to understanding and preventing coronary heart disease. *Am J Prev Med* 2003;24:143–151.

9. Kee F, Tiret L, Robo JY, et al. Reliability of reported family history of myocardial infarction. *BMJ* 1993;307:1528–1530.

10. Hopkins PN, Williams RR, Hunt SC. Magnified risks from cigarette smoking for coronary prone families in Utah. *West J Med* 1984;141:196–202.

11. Hopkins PN, Williams RR, Kuida H, et al. Family history as an independent risk factor for incident coronary artery disease in a high-risk cohort in Utah. *Am J Cardiol* 1988;62:703–707.

12. Silberberg J, Fryer J, Wlodarczyk J, et al. Comparison of family history measures used to identify high risk of coronary heart disease. *Genet Epidemiol* 1999;16:344–355.

13. Hopkins PN, Williams RR. Human genetics and coronary heart disease: a public health perspective. *Annu Rev Nutr* 1989;9:303–345.

14. Ciruzzi M, Schargrodsky H, Rozlosnik J, et al. Frequency of family history of acute myocardial infarction in patients with acute myocardial infarction. *Am J Cardiol* 1997;80:122–127.

15. Friedlander Y, Siscovick DS, Weinmann S, et al. Family history as a risk factor for primary cardiac arrest. *Circulation* 1998;97:155–160.

16. Marenberg ME, Risch N, Berkman LF, et al. Genetic susceptibility to death from coronary heart disease in a study of twins. *N Engl J Med* 1994;330:1041–1046.

17. Hunt SC, Williams RR, Barlow GK. A comparison of positive family history definitions for defining risk of future disease. *J Chron Dis* 1986;39:809–821.

18. Williams RR, Hunt SC, Heiss G, et al. Usefulness of cardiovascular family history data for population-based preventive medicine and medical research (The Health Family Tree Study and the NHLBI Family Heart Study). *Am J Cardiol* 2001;87:129–135.

19. Williams RR, Hopkins PN, Hunt SC, et al. Population-based frequency of dyslipidemia syndromes in coronary prone families in Utah. *Arch Intern Med* 1990;150:582–588.

20. Genest JJ, Martin-Munley SS, McNamara JR, et al. Familial lipoprotein disorders in patients with premature coronary artery disease. *Circulation* 1992;85:2025–2033.

21. Deutscher S, Epstein FH, Kjelsberg MO. Familial aggregation of factors associated with coronary heart disease. *Circulation* 1966;33:911–924.

22. Deutscher S, Epstein F, Keller J. Relationships between familial aggregation of CHD and risk factors in the general population. *Am J Epidemiol* 1969;89:510–520.

23. Deutscher S, Ostrander L, Epstein F. Familial factors in premature coronary heart disease: a preliminary report from the Tecumseh Community Health Study. *Am J Epidemiol* 1970;91:233–237.

24. Greenland P, Knoll MD, Stamler J, et al. Major risk factors as antecedents of fatal and nonfatal coronary heart disease events. *JAMA* 2003;290:891–897.

25. Jomini V, Oppliger-Pasquali S, Wietlisbach V, et al, for the GENECARD Project. Contribution of major cardiovascular risk factors to familial premature coronary artery disease. *J Am Coll Cardiol* 2002;40:676.

26. Hunt SC, Hasstedt SJ, Kuida H, et al. Genetic heritability and common environmental components of resting and stressed blood pressures, lipids, and body mass index in Utah pedigrees and twins. *Am J Epidemiol* 1989;129:625–638.

27. Williams RR, Hasstedt SJ, Hunt SC, et al. Genetic traits related to hypertension and electrolyte metabolism. *Hypertension* 1991;17(suppl I):I-69–I-73.

28. Heller DA, Faire UD, Pedersen NL, et al. Genetic and environmental influences on serum lipid levels in twins. *N Engl J Med* 1993;328:1150–1156.

29. Mitchell BD, Kammerer CM, Blangero J, et al. Genetic and environmental contributions to cardiovascular risk factors in Mexican Americans: the San Antonio Family Heart Study. *Circulation* 1996; 94:2159–2170.

30. Snieder H, van Doornen LJ, Boomsma DI. Dissecting the genetic architecture of lipids, lipoproteins, and apolipoproteins: lessons from twin studies. *Arterioscler Thromb Vasc Biol* 1999;19:2826–2834.

31. Higgins M. Epidemiology and prevention of coronary heart disease in families. *Am J Med* 2000;108:387–395.

32. Lichtenstein P, De Faire U, Floderus B, et al. The Swedish Twin Registry: a unique resource for clinical, epidemiological and genetic studies. *J Intern Med* 2002;252:184–205.

33. Friedlander Y, Austin MA, Newman B, et al. Heritability of longitudinal changes in coronary-heart-disease risk factors in women twins. *Am J Hum Genet* 1997;60:1502–1512.

34. Perusse L, Moll PP, Sing CF. Evidence that a single gene with gender- and age-dependent effects influences systolic blood pressure determination in a population-based sample. *Am J Hum Genet* 1991;49:94–105.

35. Cheng LS-C, Carmelli D, Hunt SC, Williams RR. Evidence for a major gene influencing 7-year increases in diastolic blood pressure with age. *Am J Hum Genet* 1995;57:1169–1177.

36. Pankow JS, Folsom AR, Cushman M, et al. Familial and genetic determinants of systemic markers of inflammation: the NHLBI Family Heart Study. *Atherosclerosis* 2001;154:681–689.

37. Bosse Y, Vohl MC, Despres JP, et al. Heritability of LDL peak particle diameter in the Quebec Family Study. *Genet Epidemiol* 2003;25:375–381.

38. Boerwinkle E, Leffert CC, Lin J, et al. Apolipoprotein(a) gene accounts for greater than 90% of the variation in plasma lipoprotein(a) concentrations. *J Clin Invest* 1992;90:52–60.

39. Kelishadi R, Zadegan S, Naderi G, et al. Atherosclerosis risk factors in children and adolescents with or without family history of premature coronary artery disease. *Med Sci Monit* 2002;8:CR425–429.

40. Greenlund KJ, Srinivasan SR, Xu JH, et al. Plasma homocysteine distribution and its association with parental history of coronary artery disease in black and white children: the Bogalusa Heart Study. *Circulation* 1999; 99:2144–2149.

41. Bara L, Nicaud V, Tiret L, et al, for the European Atherosclerosis Research Study Group. Expression of a paternal history of premature myocardial infarction on fibrinogen, factor VIIC and PAI-1 in European offspring: the EARS study. *Thromb Haemost* 1994;71:434–440.

42. Mills JD, Mansfield MW, Grant PJ. Tissue plasminogen activator, fibrin d-dimer, and insulin resistance in the relatives of patients with premature coronary artery disease. *Arterioscler Thromb Vasc Biol* 2002;22:704–709.

43. Margaglione M, Cappucci G, Colaizzo D, et al. The PAI-1 gene locus 4G/5G polymorphism is associated with a family history of coronary artery disease. *Arterioscler Thromb Vasc Biol* 1998;18:152–156.

44. Rallidis LS, Megalou AA, Papageorgakis NH, et al. Plasminogen activator inhibitor 1 is elevated in the children of men with premature myocardial infarction. *Thromb Haemost* 1996;76:417–421.

45. Freedman BI, Beck SR, Rich SS, et al. A genome-wide scan for urinary albumin excretion in hypertensive families. *Hypertension* 2003;42:291–296.

46. Zdravkovic S, Wienke A, Pedersen NL, et al. Heritability of death from coronary heart disease: a 36-year follow-up of 20 966 Swedish twins. *J Intern Med* 2002;252:247–254.

47. Wienke A, Holm NV, Skythe A, Yashin AI. The heritability of mortality due to heart diseases: a correlated frailty model applied to Danish twins. *Twin Res* 2001;4:266–274.

48. Friedlander Y, Siscovick DS, Arbogast P, et al. Sudden death and myocardial infarction in first degree relatives as predictors of primary cardiac arrest. *Atherosclerosis* 2002;162:211–216.

49. Sesso HD, Lee IM, Gaziano JM, et al. Maternal and paternal history of myocardial infarction and risk of cardiovascular disease in men and women. *Circulation* 2001;104:393–398.

50. Bensen JT, Li R, Hutchinson RG, et al. Family history of coronary heart disease and pre-clinical carotid artery atherosclerosis in African-Americans and whites: the ARIC study: Atherosclerosis Risk in Communities. *Genet Epidemiol* 1999;16:165–178.

51. Hawe E, Talmud PJ, Miller GJ, Humphries SE. Family history is a coronary heart disease risk factor in the Second Northwick Park Heart Study. *Ann Hum Genet* 2003;67:97–106.

52. Gaeta G, De Michele M, Cuomo S, et al. Arterial abnormalities in the offspring of patients with premature myocardial infarction. *N Engl J Med* 2000;343:840–846.

53. Sijbrands EJ, Westendorp RG, Paola Lombardi M, et al. Additional risk factors influence excess mortality in heterozygous familial hypercholesterolaemia. *Atherosclerosis* 2000;149:421–425.

54. Taira K, Bujo H, Kobayashi J, et al. Positive family history for coronary heart disease and 'midband lipoproteins' are potential risk factors of carotid atherosclerosis in familial hypercholesterolemia. *Atherosclerosis* 2002;160:391–397.

55. de Jongh S, Lilien MR, Bakker HD, et al. Family history of cardiovascular events and endothelial dysfunction in children with

familial hypercholesterolemia. *Atherosclerosis* 2002;163:193–197.

56. Altmuller J, Palmer LJ, Fischer G, et al. Genomewide scans of complex human diseases: true linkage is hard to find. *Am J Hum Genet* 2001;69:936–950.

57. Wang L, Fan C, Topol SE, et al. Mutation of MEF2A in an inherited disorder with features of coronary artery disease. *Science* 2003;302:1578–1581.

58. Ozaki K, Ohnishi Y, Iida A, et al. Functional SNPs in the lymphotoxin-alpha gene that are associated with susceptibility to myocardial infarction. *Nat Genet* 2002;32:650–654.

59. Pajukanta P, Cargill M, Viitanen L, et al. Two loci on chromosomes 2 and X for premature coronary heart disease identified in early- and late-settlement populations of Finland. *Am J Hum Genet* 2000;67:1481–1493.

60. Francke S, Manraj M, Lacquemant C, et al. A genome-wide scan for coronary heart disease suggests in Indo-Mauritians a susceptibility locus on chromosome 16p13 and replicates linkage with the metabolic syndrome on 3q27. *Hum Mol Genet* 2001;10:2751–2765.

61. Broeckel U, Hengstenberg C, Mayer B, et al. A comprehensive linkage analysis for myocardial infarction and its related risk factors. *Nat Genet* 2002;30:210–214.

62. Harrap SB, Zammit KS, Wong ZY, et al. Genome-wide linkage analysis of the acute coronary syndrome suggests a locus on chromosome 2. *Arterioscler Thromb Vasc Biol* 2002;22:874–878.

63. Lange LA, Lange EM, Bielak LF, et al. Autosomal genome-wide scan for coronary artery calcification loci in sibships at high risk for hypertension. *Arterioscler Thromb Vasc Biol* 2002;22:418–423.

64. Ioannidis JP, Ntzani EE, Trikalinos TA, Contopoulos-Ioannidis DG. Replication validity of genetic association studies. *Nat Genet* 2001;29:306–309.

65. Lohmueller KE, Pearce CL, Pike M, et al. Meta-analysis of genetic association studies supports a contribution of common variants to susceptibility to common disease. *Nat Genet* 2003;33:177–182.

66. Kang S-S, Wong PWK, Bock H-GO, et al. Intermediate hyperhomocysteinemia resulting from compound heterozygosity of methylenetetrahydrofolate reductase mutations. *Am J Hum Genet* 1991;48:546–551.

67. Jacques PF, Bostom AG, Williams RR, et al. Relation between folate status, a common mutation in methylenetetrahydrofolate reductase, and plasma homocysteine concentrations. *Circulation* 1996;93:7–9.

68. Hopkins PN, Wu LL, Wu J, et al. Higher plasma homocyst(e)ine and increased susceptibility to adverse effects of low folate in early familial coronary artery disease. *Arterioscler Thromb Vasc Biol* 1995;15:1314–1329.

69. Hopkins PN, Rozen R, Hunt SC. Is the heat labile variant of methylene tetrahydrofolate reductase (MTHFR-HL) associated with elevated plasma total homocysteine (tHcy) and premature coronary artery disease (CAD) [abstract]? *Circulation* 2001;103:1354.

70. Klerk M, Verhoef P, Clarke R, et al. MTHFR 677C?T polymorphism and risk of coronary heart disease: a meta-analysis. *JAMA* 2002;288:2023–2031.

71. Wald DS, Law M, Morris JK. Homocysteine and cardiovascular disease: evidence on causality from a meta-analysis. *BMJ* 2002;325:1202–1209.

72. Yamada Y, Izawa H, Ichihara S, et al. Prediction of the risk of myocardial infarction from polymorphisms in candidate genes. *N Engl J Med* 2002;347:1916–1923.

73. Humphries SE, Luong LA, Talmud PJ, et al. The 5A/6A polymorphism in the promoter of the stromelysin-1 (MMP-3) gene predicts progression of angiographically determined coronary artery disease in men in the LOCAT gemfibrozil study. *Atherosclerosis* 1998;139:49–56.

74. Pollanen PJ, Lehtimaki T, Ilveskoski E, et al. Coronary artery calcification is related to functional polymorphism of matrix metalloproteinase 3: the Helsinki Sudden Death Study. *Atherosclerosis* 2002;164:329–335.

75. Hirashiki A, Yamada Y, Murase Y, et al. Association of gene polymorphisms with coronary artery disease in low- or high-risk subjects defined by conventional risk factors. *J Am Coll Cardiol* 2003;42:1429–1437.

76. Rothman KJ. No adjustments are needed for multiple comparisons. *Epidemiology* 1990;1:43–46.

77. Topol EJ, McCarthy J, Gabriel S, et al. Single nucleotide polymorphisms in multiple novel thrombospondin genes may be associated with familial premature myocardial infarction. *Circulation* 2001;104:2641–2644.

78. Hopkins PN, Williams RR. A survey of 246 suggested coronary risk factors. *Atherosclerosis* 1981;40:1–2.

79. Watson AD, Subbanagounder G, Welsbie DS, et al. Structural identification of a novel pro-inflammatory epoxyisoprostane phospholipid in mildly oxidized low density lipoprotein. *J Biol Chem* 1999; 274:24787–24798.

80. Subbanagounder G, Leitinger N, Schwenke DC, et al. Determinants of bioactivity of oxidized phospholipids: specific oxidized fatty acyl groups at the sn-2 position. *Arterioscler Thromb Vasc Biol* 2000;20:2248–2254.

81. Suriyaphol P, Fenske D, Zahringer U, et al. Enzymatically modified nonoxidized low-density lipoprotein induces interleukin-8 in human endothelial cells: role of free fatty acids. *Circulation* 2002;106:2581–2587.

82. Zhu Y, Lin JH-C, Liao H-L, et al. LDL induces transcription factor activator protein-1 in human endothelial cells. *Arterioscler Thromb Vasc Biol* 1998;18:473–480.

83. Doi H, Kugiyama K, Oka H, et al. Remnant lipoproteins induce proatherothrombogenic molecules in endothelial cells through a redox-sensitive mechanism. *Circulation* 2000;102:670–676.

84. Leung W-H, Lau C-P, Wong C-K. Beneficial effect of cholesterol-lowering therapy on coronary endothelium-dependent relaxation in hypercholesterolaemic patients. *Lancet* 1993;341:1496–1500.

85. Tamai O, Matsuoka H, Itabe H, et al. Single LDL apheresis improves endothelium-dependent vasodilation in hypercholesterolemic humans. *Circulation* 1997;95:76–82.

86. Plotnick GD, Corretti MC, Vogel RA. Effect of antioxidant vitamins on the transient impairment of endothelium-dependent brachial artery vasoactivity following a single high-fat meal. *JAMA* 1997;278:1682–1686.

87. Aikawa M, Sugiyama S, Hill CC, et al. Lipid lowering reduces oxidative stress and endothelial cell activation in rabbit atheroma. *Circulation* 2002; 106:1390–1396.

88. Aviram M. Modified forms of low density lipoprotein and Atherosclerosis. *Atherosclerosis* 1993;98:1–9.

89. Tabas I. Nonoxidative modifications of lipoproteins in atherogenesis. *Annu Rev Nutr* 1999;19:123–139.

90. Steinberg D, Witztum JL. Is the oxidative modification hypothesis relevant to human Atherosclerosis? Do the antioxidant trials conducted to date refute the hypothesis? *Circulation* 2002;105:2107–2111.

91. Nofer J-R, Tepel M, Kehrel B, et al. Low-density lipoproteins inhibit the Na+/H+ antiport in human platelets: a novel mechanism enhancing platelet activity in hypercholesterolemia. *Circulation* 1997;95:1370–1377.

92. Geng YJ, Libby P. Progression of atheroma: a struggle between death and procreation. *Arterioscler Thromb Vasc Biol* 2002;22:1370–1380.

93. Felton CV, Crook D, Davies MJ, Oliver MF. Relation of plaque lipid composition and morphology to the stability of human aortic plaques. *Arterioscler Thromb Vasc Biol* 1997;17:1337–1345.

94. Kockx MM, De Meyer GR, Buyssens N, et al. Cell composition, replication, and apoptosis in atherosclerotic plaques after 6 months of cholesterol withdrawal. *Circ Res* 1998;83:378–387.

95. Crisby M, Nordin-Fredriksson G, Shah PK, et al. Pravastatin treatment increases collagen content and decreases lipid content, inflammation, metalloproteinases, and cell death in human carotid plaques: implications for plaque stabilization. *Circulation* 2001;103:926–933.

96. Libby P. Inflammation in Atherosclerosis. *Nature* 2002;420:868–874.

97. Cybulsky MI, Iiyama K, Li H, et al. A major role for VCAM-1, but not ICAM-1, in early atherosclerosis. *J Clin Invest* 2001;107:1255–1262.

98. Johnson RC, Chapman SM, Dong ZM, et al. Absence of P-selectin delays fatty streak formation in mice. *J Clin Invest* 1997; 99:1037–1043.

99. Dong ZM, Chapman SM, Brown AA, Frenette PS, Hynes RO, Wagner DD. The combined role of P- and E-selectins in atherosclerosis. *J Clin Invest* 1998;102:145–152.

100. Gu L, Okada Y, Clinton SK, et al. Absence of monocyte chemoattractant protein-1 reduces atherosclerosis in low density lipoprotein receptor-deficient mice. *Mol Cell* 1998;2:275–281.

101. Boring L, Gosling J, Cleary M, Charo IF. Decreased lesion formation in CCR2−/− mice reveals a role for chemokines in the initiation of atherosclerosis. *Nature* 1998;394:894–897.

102. Guo J, Van Eck M, Twisk J, et al. Transplantation of monocyte CC-chemokine receptor 2-deficient bone marrow into ApoE3-Leiden mice inhibits atherogenesis. *Arterioscler Thromb Vasc Biol* 2003;23:447–453.

103. Lutgens E, Gorelik L, Daemen MJ, et al. Requirement for CD154 in the progression of atherosclerosis. *Nat Med* 1999;5:1313–1316.

104. Combadiere C, Potteaux S, Gao JL, et al. Decreased atherosclerotic lesion formation in CX3CR1/apolipoprotein E double knockout mice. *Circulation* 2003;107:1009–1016.

105. Kwak BR, Veillard N, Pelli G, et al. Reduced connexin43 expression inhibits atherosclerotic lesion formation in low-density lipoprotein receptor-deficient mice. *Circulation* 2003;107:1033–1039.

106. Nagano H, Libby P, Taylor MK, et al. Coronary arteriosclerosis after T-cell-mediated injury in transplanted mouse hearts: role of interferon-gamma. *Am J Pathol* 1998;152:1187–1197.

107. Boisvert WA, Santiago R, Curtiss LK, Terkeltaub RA. A leukocyte homologue of the IL-8 receptor CXCR-2 mediates the accumulation of macrophages in atherosclerotic lesions of LDL receptor-deficient mice. *J Clin Invest* 1998;101:353–363.

108. Elhage R, Jawien J, Rudling M, et al. Reduced atherosclerosis in interleukin-18 deficient apolipoprotein E-knockout mice. *Cardiovasc Res* 2003;59:234–240.

109. Qiao JH, Tripathi J, Mishra NK, et al. Role of macrophage colony-stimulating factor in atherosclerosis: studies of osteopetrotic mice. *Am J Pathol* 1997;150:1687–1699.

110. Zhou X, Nicoletti A, Elhage R, Hansson GK. Transfer of CD4(+) T cells aggravates atherosclerosis in immunodeficient apolipoprotein E knockout mice. *Circulation* 2000;102:2919–2922.

111. Robertson AK, Rudling M, Zhou X, et al. Disruption of TGF-β signaling in T cells accelerates atherosclerosis. *J Clin Invest* 2003;112:1342–1350.

112. Mehrabian M, Allayee H, Wong J, et al. Identification of 5-lipoxygenase as a major gene contributing to atherosclerosis susceptibility in mice. *Circ Res* 2002;91:120–126.

113. Cyrus T, Witztum JL, Rader DJ, et al. Disruption of the 12/15-lipoxygenase gene diminishes atherosclerosis in apo E-deficient mice. *J Clin Invest* 1999;103:1597–1604.

114. Barry-Lane PA, Patterson C, van der Merwe M, et al. p47phox is required for atherosclerotic lesion progression in ApoE(−/−) mice. *J Clin Invest* 2001;108:1513–1522.

115. Blanc J, Alves-Guerra MC, Esposito B, et al. Protective role of uncoupling protein 2 in atherosclerosis. *Circulation* 2003;107:388–390.

116. Shih DM, Gu L, Xia YR, et al. Mice lacking serum paraoxonase are susceptible to organophosphate toxicity and atherosclerosis. *Nature* 1998;394:284–287.

117. Brennan ML, Anderson MM, Shih DM, et al. Increased atherosclerosis in myeloperoxidase-deficient mice. *J Clin Invest* 2001;107:419–430.

118. Sakaguchi H, Takeya M, Suzuki H, et al. Role of macrophage scavenger receptors in diet-induced atherosclerosis in mice. *Lab Invest* 1998;78:423–434.

119. Febbraio M, Podrez EA, Smith JD, et al. Targeted disruption of the class B scavenger receptor CD36 protects against atherosclerotic lesion development in mice. *J Clin Invest* 2000;105:1049–1056.

120. Fazio S, Major AS, Swift LL, et al. Increased atherosclerosis in LDL receptor-null mice lacking ACAT1 in macrophages. *J Clin Invest* 2001;107:163–171.

121. Tabas I. Phospholipid metabolism in cholesterol-loaded macrophages. *Curr Opin Lipidol* 1997;8:263–267.

122. Pentikainen MO, Oksjoki R, Oorni K, Kovanen PT. Lipoprotein lipase in the arterial wall: linking LDL to the arterial extracellular matrix and much more. *Arterioscler Thromb Vasc Biol* 2002;22:211–217.

123. Merkel M, Eckel RH, Goldberg IJ. Lipoprotein lipase: genetics, lipid uptake, and regulation. *J Lipid Res* 2002;43:1997–2006.

124. Skalen K, Gustafsson M, Rydberg EK, et al. Subendothelial retention of atherogenic lipoproteins in early atherosclerosis. *Nature* 2002;417:750–754.

125. Braun A, Trigatti BL, Post MJ, et al. Loss of SR-BI expression leads to the early onset of occlusive atherosclerotic coronary artery disease, spontaneous myocardial infarctions, severe cardiac dysfunction, and premature death in apolipoprotein E-deficient mice. *Circ Res* 2002;90:270–276.

126. Methia N, Andre P, Denis CV, et al. Localized reduction of atherosclerosis in von Willebrand factor-deficient mice. *Blood* 2001;98:1424–1428.

127. Xiao Q, Danton MJ, Witte DP, et al. Fibrinogen deficiency is compatible with the development of atherosclerosis in mice. *J Clin Invest* 1998;101:1184–1194.

128. Lou XJ, Boonmark NW, Horrigan FT, et al. Fibrinogen deficiency reduces vascular accumulation of apolipoprotein(a) and development of atherosclerosis in apolipoprotein(a) transgenic mice. *Proc Natl Acad Sci USA* 1998;95:12591–12595.

129. Silence J, Lupu F, Collen D, Lijnen HR. Persistence of atherosclerotic plaque but reduced aneurysm formation in mice with stromelysin-1 (MMP-3) gene inactivation. *Arterioscler Thromb Vasc Biol* 2001;21:1440–1445.

130. Silence J, Collen D, Lijnen HR. Reduced atherosclerotic plaque but enhanced aneurysm formation in mice with inactivation of the tissue inhibitor of metalloproteinase-1 (TIMP-1) gene. *Circ Res* 2002;90:897–903.

131. Lemaitre V, O'Byrne TK, Borczuk AC, et al. ApoE knockout mice expressing human matrix metalloproteinase-1 in macrophages have less advanced atherosclerosis. *J Clin Invest* 2001;107:1227–1234.

132. von der Thusen JH, van Vlijmen BJ, Hoeben RC, et al. Induction of atherosclerotic plaque rupture in apolipoprotein E−/− mice after adenovirus-mediated transfer of p53. *Circulation* 2002;105:2064–2070.

133. Mallat Z, Gojova A, Marchiol-Fournigault C, et al. Inhibition of transforming growth factor-beta signaling accelerates atherosclerosis and induces an unstable plaque phenotype in mice. *Circ Res* 2001;89:930–934.

134. Lutgens E, Gijbels M, Smook M, et al. Transforming growth factor-beta mediates balance between inflammation and fibrosis during plaque progression. *Arterioscler Thromb Vasc Biol* 2002;22:975–982.

135. Pyo R, Lee JK, Shipley JM, et al. Targeted gene disruption of matrix metalloproteinase-9 (gelatinase B) suppresses development of experimental abdominal aortic aneurysms. *J Clin Invest* 2000;105:1641–1649.

136. Andreotti F, Porto I, Crea F, Maseri A. Inflammatory gene polymorphisms and ischaemic heart disease: review of population association studies. *Heart* 2002;87:107–112.

137. Shi W, Haberland ME, Jien ML, et al. Endothelial responses to oxidized lipoproteins determine genetic susceptibility to atherosclerosis in mice. *Circulation* 2000;102:75–81.

138. Lee H, Shi W, Tontonoz P, et al. Role for peroxisome proliferator-activated receptor alpha in oxidized phospholipid-induced synthesis of monocyte chemotactic protein-1 and interleukin-8 by endothelial cells. *Circ Res* 2000;87:516–521.

139. Shohet RV, Vega GL, Anwar A, et al. Hepatic lipase (LIPC) promoter polymorphism in men with coronary artery disease: allele frequency and effects on hepatic lipase activity and plasma HDL-C concentrations. *Arterioscler Thromb Vasc Biol* 1999;19:1975–1978.

140. Hong SH, Song J, Kim JQ. Genetic variations of the hepatic lipase gene in Korean patients with coronary artery disease. *Clin Biochem* 2000;33:291–296.

141. Zambon A, Hokanson JE, Brown BG, Brunzell JD. Evidence for a new pathophysiological mechanism for coronary artery disease regression: hepatic lipase-mediated changes in LDL density. *Circulation* 1999;99:1959–1964.

142. Zambon A, Deeb SS, Brown BG, et al. Common hepatic lipase gene promoter variant determines clinical response to intensive lipid-lowering treatment. *Circulation* 2001;103:792–798.

143. Hokanson JE, Cheng S, Snell-Bergeon JK, et al. A common promoter polymorphism in the hepatic lipase gene (LIPC-480C > T) is associated with an increase in coronary calcification in type 1 diabetes. *Diabetes* 2002;1:1208–1213.

144. Fan Y, Laaksonen R, Janatuinen T, et al. Hepatic lipase gene variation is related to coronary reactivity in healthy young men. *Eur J Clin Invest* 2001;31:574–580.

145. Su Z, Zhang S, Nebert DW, et al. A novel allele in the promoter of the hepatic lipase is associated with increased concentration of HDL-C and decreased promoter activity. *J Lipid Res* 2002;43:1595–1601.

146. Dugi KA, Brandauer K, Schmidt N, et al. Low hepatic lipase activity is a novel risk factor for coronary artery disease. *Circulation* 2001;104:3057–3062.

147. Andersen RV, Wittrup HH, Tybjaerg-Hansen A, et al. Hepatic lipase mutations, elevated high-density lipoprotein cholesterol, and increased risk of ischemic heart disease: the Copenhagen City Heart Study. *J Am Coll Cardiol* 2003;41:1972–1982.

148. Connelly PW, Hegele RA. Hepatic lipase deficiency. *Crit Rev Clin Lab Sci* 1998;35:547–572.

149. Hegele RA, Ban MR, Anderson CM, Spence JD. Infection-susceptibility alleles of mannose-binding lectin are associated with increased carotid plaque area. *J Invest Med* 2000;48:198–202.

150. Zee RY, Ridker PM. Polymorphism in the human C-reactive protein (CRP) gene, plasma concentrations of CRP, and the risk of future arterial thrombosis. *Atherosclerosis* 2002;162:217–219.

151. Nikpoor B, Turecki G, Fournier C, et al. A functional myeloperoxidase polymorphic variant is associated with coronary artery disease in French-Canadians. *Am Heart J* 2001;142:336–339.

152. Pecoits-Filho R, Stenvinkel P, Marchlewska A, et al. A functional variant of the myeloperoxidase gene is associated with cardiovascular disease in end-stage renal disease patients. *Kidney Int Suppl* 2003;63(suppl 84):S172–S176.

153. Kutter D, Devaquet P, Vanderstocken G, et al. Consequences of total and subtotal myeloperoxidase deficiency: risk or benefit? *Acta Haematol* 2000;104:10–15.

154. Horne BD, Anderson JL, Muhlestein JB, et al. Genetic burden of polymorphisms related to lipid metabolism increases the risk of angiographic coronary artery disease. *Circulation* 2002;106(suppl II):II-3583.

155. Yang Q, Khoury MJ, Botto L, et al. Improving the prediction of complex diseases by testing for multiple disease-susceptibility genes. *Am J Hum Genet* 2003;72:636–649.

156. Khaw KT, Barrett-Connor E, Khoury MJ, et al. Family history of heart attack: a modifiable risk factor? *Circulation* 1986;74:239–244.

157. Wang XL, Sim AS, Badenhop RF, et al. A smoking-dependent risk of coronary artery disease associated with a polymorphism of the endothelial nitric oxide synthase gene. *Nat Med* 1996;2:41–45.

158. Hautanen A, Toivanen P, Manttari M, et al. Joint effects of an aldosterone synthase (CYP11B2) gene polymorphism and classic risk factors on risk of myocardial infarction. *Circulation* 1999;100:2213–2218.

159. Sen-Banerjee S, Siles X, Campos H. Tobacco smoking modifies association between Gln-Arg192 polymorphism of human paraoxonase gene and risk of myocardial infarction. *Arterioscler Thromb Vasc Biol* 2000;20:2120–2126.

160. Humphries SE, Talmud PJ, Hawe E, et al. Apolipoprotein E4 and coronary heart disease in middle-aged men who smoke: a prospective study. *Lancet* 2001;358:115–119.

161. Fisher RM, Humphries SE, Talmud PJ. Common variation in the lipoprotein lipase gene: effects on plasma lipids and risk of Atherosclerosis. *Atherosclerosis* 1997;135:145–159.

162. Humphries SE, Luong LA, Ogg MS, et al. The interleukin-6 −174 G/C promoter polymorphism is associated with risk of coronary heart disease and systolic Blood pressure in healthy men. *Eur Heart J* 2001;22:2243–2252.

163. Risley P, Jerrard-Dunne P, Sitzer M, et al. Promoter polymorphism in the endotoxin receptor (CD14) is associated with increased carotid atherosclerosis only in smokers: the Carotid Atherosclerosis Progression Study (CAPS). *Stroke* 2003;34:600–604.

164. Dahl M, Tybjaerg-Hansen A, Sillesen H et al. Blood pressure, risk of ischemic cerebrovascular and ischemic heart disease, and longevity in alpha(1)-antitrypsin deficiency: the Copenhagen City Heart Study. *Circulation* 2003;107:747–752.

165. de Maat MP, Jukema JW, Ye S, et al. Effect of the stromelysin-1 promoter on efficacy of pravastatin in coronary atherosclerosis and restenosis. *Am J Cardiol* 1999;83:852–856.

166. Basso F, Lowe GD, Rumley A, et al. Interleukin-6 -174G > C polymorphism and risk of coronary heart disease in West of Scotland coronary prevention study (WOSCOPS). *Arterioscler Thromb Vasc Biol* 2002;22:599–604.

167. Zito F, Lowe GD, Rumley A, et al. Association of the factor XII 46C>T polymorphism with risk of coronary heart disease (CHD) in the WOSCOPS study. *Atherosclerosis* 2002;165:153–158.

168. Boekholdt SM, Agema WR, Peters RJ, et al. Variants of toll-like receptor 4 modify the efficacy of statin therapy and the risk of cardiovascular events. *Circulation* 2003;107:2416–2421.

169. Hobbs HH, Russel DW, Brown MS, Goldstein JL. The LDL receptor locus in familial hypercholesterolemia: mutational analysis of a membrane protein. *Annu Rev Genet* 1990;24:133–170.

170. Goldstein JL, Hobbs HH, Brown MS. Familial hypercholesterolemia. In: Scriver CR, Beaudet AL, Sly WS, Valle D, eds. *The Metabolic and Molecular Bases of Inherited Disease.* New York: McGraw–Hill; 1995:1981–2030.

171. Amsellem S, Briffaut D, Carrie A, et al. Intronic mutations outside of Alu-repeat-rich domains of the LDL receptor gene are a cause of familial hypercholesterolemia. *Hum Genet* 2002;111:501–510.

172. Hopkins PN, Stephenson S, Wu LL, et al. Evaluation of coronary risk factors in patients with heterozygous familial hypercholesterolemia. *Am J Cardiol* 2001;87:547–553.

173. Jansen AC, van Wissen S, Defesche JC, Kastelein JJ. Phenotypic variability in familial hypercholesterolaemia: an update. *Curr Opin Lipidol* 2002;13:165–171.

174. Heiberg A, Slack J. Family similarities in the age at coronary death in familial hypercholesterolaemia. *BMJ* 1977;2:493–495.

175. Wiegman A, Rodenburg J, de Jongh S, et al. Family history and cardiovascular risk in familial hypercholesterolemia: data in more than 1000 children. *Circulation* 2003;107:1473–1478.

176. Goldstein JL, Hobbs HH, Brown MS. Familial hypercholesterolemia. In: Scriver CR, Beaudet AL, Sly WS, Valle D, eds. *The Metabolic and Molecular Bases of Inherited Disease.* New York: McGraw–Hill; 2001:2863–2913.

177. Umans-Eckenhausen MA, Sijbrands EJ, Kastelein JJ, Defesche JC. Low-density lipoprotein receptor gene mutations and cardiovascular risk in a large genetic cascade screening population. *Circulation* 2002;106:3031–3036.

178. Williams RR, Schumacher MC, Barlow GK, et al. Documented need for more effective diagnosis and treatment of familial hypercholesterolemia according to data from 502 heterozygotes in Utah. *Am J Cardiol* 1993;72:18D–24D.

179. Neil HA, Hammond T, Huxley R, et al. Extent of underdiagnosis of familial hypercholesterolaemia in routine practice: prospective registry study. *BMJ* 2000;321:148.

180. World Health Organization Familial Hypercholesterolemia Consultation Group. Familial Hypercholesterolemia: report of a WHO Consultation. Paris: World Health Organization; October 3, 1997. Report WHO/HGN/FH/CONS/98.7.

181. Stone N, Levy R, Fredrickson D, Verter J. Coronary artery disease in 116 kindred with familial type II hyperlipoproteinemia. *Circulation* 1974;49:476–488.

182. Mabuchi H, Miyamoto S, Ueda K, et al. Causes of death in patients with familial hypercholesterolemia. *Atherosclerosis* 1986;61:1–6.

183. Goldstein J, Schrott H, Hazzard W. Hyperlipidemia in coronary heart disease: II. Genetic analysis of lipid levels in 176 families and delineation of a new inherited disorder, combined hyperlipidemia. *J Clin Invest* 1973;52:1544–1568.

184. Gaudet D, Vohl MC, Julien P, et al. Relative contribution of low-density lipoprotein receptor and lipoprotein lipase gene mutations to angiographically assessed coronary artery disease among French Canadians. *Am J Cardiol* 1998;82:299–305.

185. Marks D, Wonderling D, Thorogood M, et al. Cost effectiveness analysis of different approaches of screening for familial hypercholesterolemia. *BMJ* 2002;324:1303.

186. Kane JP, Malloy MJ, Ports TA, et al. Regression of coronary atherosclerosis during treatment of familial hypercholesterolemia with combined drug regimens. *JAMA* 1990;264:3007–3012.

187. Thompson GR, Maher VMG, Matthews S, et al. Familial Hypercholesterolaemia Regression Study: a randomised trial of low-density-lipoprotein apheresis. *Lancet* 1995;345:811–816.

188. Mabuchi H, Koizumi J, Shimizu M, et al, for the Hokuriku-FH-LDL- Apheresis Study Group. Long-term efficacy of low-density lipoprotein apheresis on coronary heart disease in familial hypercholesterolemia. *Am J Cardiol* 1998;82:1489–1495.

189. Smilde TJ, van Wissen S, Wollersheim H, et al. Effect of aggressive versus conventional lipid lowering on atherosclerosis progression in familial hypercholesterolaemia (ASAP): a prospective, randomised, double-blind trial. *Lancet* 2001;357:577–581.

190. Thompson GR. LDL apheresis. *Atherosclerosis* 2003;167:1–13.

191. WHO Familial Hypercholesterolemia Consultation Group.

Familial Hypercholesterolemia: report of a WHO Consultation. Paris: World Health Organization; October 3, 1997. Report WHO/HGN/FH/CONS/98.7.

192. Marks D, Thorogood M, Neil HA, Humphries SE. A review on the diagnosis, natural history, and treatment of familial hypercholesterolaemia. *Atherosclerosis* 2003;168:1–14.

193. Hopkins PN. Familial hypercholesterolemia: improving treatment and meeting guidelines. *Int J Cardiol* 2003;89:13–23.

194. Rader DJ, Cohen J, Hobbs HH. Monogenic hypercholesterolemia: new insights in pathogenesis and treatment. *J Clin Invest* 2003;111:1795–1803.

195. Innerarity TL, Weisgraber KH, Arnold KS, et al. Familial defective apolipoprotein B-100: low density lipoproteins with abnormal receptor binding. *Proc Natl Acad Sci USA* 1987;84:6919–6923.

196. Innerarity TL, Mahley RW, Weisgraber KH, et al. Familial defective apolipoprotein B-100: a mutation of apolipoprotein B that causes hypercholesterolemia. *J Lipid Res* 1990;31:1337–1349.

197. Ludwig EH, Hopkins PN, Allen A, et al. Association of genetic variations in apolipoprotein B with hypercholesterolemia, coronary artery disease, and receptor binding of low density lipoproteins. *J Lipid Res* 1997;38:1361–1373.

198. Boren J, Ekstrom U, Agren B, et al. The molecular mechanism for the genetic disorder familial defective apolipoprotein B100. *J Biol Chem* 2001;276:9214–9218.

199. Haddad L, Day INM, Hunt S, et al. Evidence for a third genetic locus causing familial hypercholesterolaemia: a non-LDLR, non-apoB kindred. *J Lipid Res* 1999;40:1113–1122.

200. Varret M, Rabes JP, Saint-Jore B, et al. A third major locus for autosomal dominant hypercholesterolemia maps to 1p34–p32. *Am J Hum Genet* 1999;64:1378–1387.

201. Abifadel M, Varret M, Rabes JP, et al. Mutations in PCSK9 cause autosomal dominant hypercholesterolemia. *Nat Genet* 2003;34:154–156.

202. Timms KM, Wagner S, Samuels ME, et al. A mutation in PCSK9 causing autosomal-dominant hypercholesterolemia in a Utah pedigree. *Hum Genet* 2004;114:349–353.

203. Schmidt EB, Illingworth DR, Bacon S, et al. Hypocholesterolemic effects of cholestyramine and colestipol in patients with familial defective apolipoprotein B-100. *Atherosclerosis* 1993;98:213–217.

204. Hansen PS, Meinertz H, Gerdes LU, et al. Treatment of patients with familial defective apolipoprotein B-100 with pravastatin and gemfibrozil: a two-period cross-over study. *Clin Invest* 1994;72:1065–1070.

205. Raal FJ, Pilcher G, Rubinsztein DC, et al. Statin therapy in a kindred with both apolipoprotein B and low density lipoprotein receptor gene defects. *Atherosclerosis* 1997;129:97–102.

206. Norman D, Sun XM, Bourbon M, et al. Characterization of a novel cellular defect in patients with phenotypic homozygous familial hypercholesterolemia. *J Clin Invest* 1999;104:619–628.

207. Garcia CK, Wilund K, Arca M, et al. Autosomal recessive hypercholesterolemia caused by mutations in a putative LDL receptor adaptor protein. *Science* 2001;292:1394–1398.

208. Cohen JC, Kimmel M, Polanski A, Hobbs HH. Molecular mechanisms of autosomal recessive hypercholesterolemia. *Curr Opin Lipidol* 2003;14:121–127.

209. Pullinger CR, Eng C, Salen G, et al. Human cholesterol 7alpha-hydroxylase (CYP7A1) deficiency has a hypercholesterolemic phenotype. *J Clin Invest* 2002;110:109–117.

210. Berge KE, Tian H, Graf GA, et al. Accumulation of dietary cholesterol in sitosterolemia caused by mutations in adjacent ABC transporters. *Science* 2000;290:1771–1775.

211. Mymin D, Wang J, Frohlich J, Hegele RA. Image in cardiovascular medicine: aortic xanthomatosis with coronary ostial occlusion in a child homozygous for a nonsense mutation in ABCG8. *Circulation* 2003;107:791.

212. Berge KE, von Bergmann K, Lutjohann D, et al. Heritability of plasma noncholesterol sterols and relationship to DNA sequence polymorphism in ABCG5 and ABCG8. *J Lipid Res* 2002;43:486–494.

213. Wetterau JR, Aggerbeck LP, Bouma M-E, et al. Absence of microsomal triglyceride transfer protein in individuals with abetalipoporteinemia. *Science* 1992;258:999–1001.

214. Berriot-Varoqueaux N, Aggerbeck LP, Samson-Bouma M, Wetterau JR. The role of the microsomal triglygeride transfer protein in abetalipoproteinemia. *Annu Rev Nutr* 2000;20:663–697.

215. Al-Shali K, Wang J, Rosen F, Hegele RA. Ileal adenocarcinoma in a mild phenotype of abetalipoproteinemia. *Clin Genet* 2003;63:135–138.

216. Wetterau JR, Gregg RE, Harrity TW, et al. An MTP inhibitor that normalizes atherogenic lipoprotein levels in WHHL rabbits. *Science* 1998;282:751–754.

217. Chandler CE, Wilder DE, Pettini JL, et al. CP-346086: an MTP inhibitor that lowers plasma cholesterol and triglycerides in experimental animals and in humans. *J Lipid Res* 2003;44:1887–1901.

218. Borradaile NM, de Dreu LE, Barrett PH, et al. Hepatocyte apoB-containing lipoprotein secretion is decreased by the grapefruit flavonoid, naringenin, via inhibition of MTP-mediated microsomal triglyceride accumulation. *Biochemistry* 2003;42:1283–1291.

219. Schonfeld G. Familial hypobetalipoproteinemia: a review. *J Lipid Res* 2003;44:878-883.

220. Wu J, Kim J, Li Q, et al. Known mutations of apoB account for only a small minority of hypobetalipoproteinemia. *J Lipid Res* 1999;40:955–959.

221. Schonfeld G, Patterson BW, Yablonskiy DA, et al. Fatty liver in familial hypobetalipoproteinemia: triglyceride assembly into VLDL particles is affected by the extent of hepatic steatosis. *J Lipid Res* 2003;44:470–478.

222. Hopkins PN, Wu LL, Williams RR. Dyslipidemias. In: Noe DA, Rock RC, eds. *Laboratory medicine: The selection and interpretation of clinical laboratory studies.* Baltimore: Williams & Wilkins; 1994:476–511.

223. Brunzell JD. Familial lipoprotein lipase deficiency and other causes of chylomicronemia syndrome. In: Scriver CR, Beaudet AL, Sly WS, Valle D, eds. *The metabolic and molecular bases of inherited disease.* 7th ed. New York: McGraw-Hill, Inc.; 1995:1913–1932.

224. Greenberg BH, Blackwelder WC, Levy RI. Primary type V hyperlipoproteinemia. A descriptive study in 32 families. *Ann Intern Med* 1977;87:526–534.

225. Malekzadeh S, Dressler FA, Hoeg JM, et al. Left atrial endocardial lipid deposits and absent to minimal arterial lipid deposits in familial hyperchylomicronemia. *Am J Cardiol* 1991;67:1431–1434.

226. Nordestgaard BG, Zilversmit DB. Large lipoproteins are excluded from the arterial wall in diabetic cholesterol-fed rabbits. *J Lipid Res* 1988;29:1491–1500.

227. Benlian P, De Gennes JL, Foubert L, et al. Premature atherosclerosis in patients with familial chylomicronemia caused by mutations in the lipoprotein lipase gene. *N Engl J Med* 1996;335:848–854.

228. Brunzell JD, Deeb SS. Familial lipoprotein lipase deficiency, apo CII deficiency and hepatic lipase deficiency. In: Scriver CR, Beaudet AL, Sly WS, Valle D, eds. *The Metabolic and Molecular Basis of Inherited Disease.* 8th edition. New York: McGraw-Hill Book Co; 2000:2789–2816.

229. Wilson DE, Emi M, Iverius PH, et al. Phenotypic expression of heterozygous lipoprotein lipase deficiency in the extended pedigree of a proband homozygous for a missense mutation. *J Clin Invest* 1990;86:735–750.

230. Miesenböck G, Hölzl B, Foger B, et al. Heterozygous lipoprotein lipase deficiency due to a missense mutation as the cause of impaired triglyceride tolerance with multiple lipoprotein abnormalities. *J Clin Invest* 1993;91:448–455.

231. Pimstone SN, Clee SM, Gagne SE, et al. A frequently occurring mutation in the lipoprotein lipase gene (Asn291Ser) results in altered postprandial chylomicron triglyceride and retinyl palmitate response in normolipidemic carriers. *J Lipid Res* 1996;37:1675–1684.

232. Hokanson JE, Brunzell JD, Jarvik GP, et al. Linkage of low-density lipoprotein size to the lipoprotein lipase gene in heterozygous lipoprotein lipase deficiency. *Am J Hum Genet* 1999;64:608–618.

233. Heeren J, Niemeier A, Merkel M, Beisiegel U. Endothelial-derived lipoprotein lipase is bound to postprandial triglyceride-rich lipoproteins and mediates their hepatic clearance in vivo. *J Mol Med* 2002;80:576–584.

234. Hokanson JE. Functional variants in the lipoprotein lipase gene and risk cardiovascular disease. *Curr Opin Lipidol* 1999;10:393–399.

235. Ukkola O, Garenc C, Perusse L, et al. Genetic variation at the lipoprotein lipase locus and plasma lipoprotein and insulin levels in the Quebec Family Study. *Atherosclerosis* 2001;158:199–206.

236. Humphries SE, Nicaud V, Margalef J, et al. Lipoprotein lipase gene variation is associated with a paternal history of premature coronary artery disease and fasting and postprandial plasma triglycerides: the European Atherosclerosis Research Study (EARS). *Arterioscler Thromb Vasc Biol* 1998;18:526–534.

237. Fisher RM, Benhizia F, Schreiber R, et al. Enhanced bridging function and augmented monocyte adhesion by lipoprotein lipase N9: insights into increased risk of coronary artery disease in N9 carriers. *Atherosclerosis* 2003;166:243–251.

238. Samuels M, Forbey K, Reid J, et al. Identification of a common variant in the lipoprotein lipase gene in a large Utah kindred ascertained for coronary heart disease: the -93G/D9N variant predisposes to low HDL-C/high triglycerides. *Clin Genet* 2001;59:88–98.

239. Fredrickson DS, Morganroth J, Levy RI. Type III hyperlipoproteinemia: an analysis of two contemporary definitions. *Ann Intern Med* 1975;82:150–157.

240. Morganroth J, Levy RI, Fredrickson DS. The biochemical, clinical, and genetic features of Type III hyperlipoproteinemia. *Ann Intern Med* 1975;82:158–174.

241. LaRosa JC, Chambless LE, Criqui MH, et al. Patterns of dyslipoproteinemia in selected North American populations: the Lipid Research Clinics Program Prevalence Study. *Circulation* 1986;73:1–12.

242. Goldstein J, Hazzard W, Schrott H. Hyperlipidemia in coronary heart disease: I. Lipid levels in 500 survivors of myocardial infarction. *J Clin Invest* 1973;52:1533–1543.

243. Hopkins PN, Wu LL, Williams RR, et al. Type III hyperlipidemia and lipoprotein remnants in early onset familial coronary artery disease. *Circulation* 1998;98 (suppl I):I–791.

244. Mahley RW, Rall SC. Type III hyperlipoproteinemia (dysbetalipoproteinemia): the role of apolipoprotein E in normal and abnormal lipoprotein metabolism. In: Scrover CR, Beaudet AL, Sly WS, Valle D, eds. *The metabolic basis of inherited disease.* 6th ed. New York: McGraw– Hill; 1989:1195–1213.

245. Hopkins PN, Wu LL, Schumacher MC, et al. Type III dyslipoproteinemia in patients heterozygous for familial hypercholesterolemia and apolipoprotein E2: evidence for a gene–gene interaction. *Arterioscler Thromb* 1991;11:1137–1146.

246. Wang T, Nakajima K, Leary ET, et al. Ratio of remnant-like particle-cholesterol to serum total triglycerides is an effective alternative to ultracentrifugal and electrophoretic methods in the diagnosis of familial type III hyperlipoproteinemia. *Clin Chem* 1999;45:1981–1987.

247. Mahley RW, Rall SC. Type III hyperlipoproteinemia (dysbetalipoproteinemia): the role of apolipoprotein E in normal and abnormal lipoprotein metabolism. In: Scriver CR, Beaudet AL, Sly WS, Valle D, eds. *The metabolic and molecular bases of inherited disease.* 7th ed. New York: McGraw–Hill; 1995:1953–1980.

248. Ishigami M, Yamashita S, Sakai N, et al. Atorvastatin markedly improves type III hyperlipoproteinemia in association with reduction of both exogenous and endogenous apolipoprotein B-containing lipoproteins. *Atherosclerosis* 2003;168:359–366.

249. Connelly PW, Maguire GF, Lee M, Little JA. Plasma lipoproteins in familial hepatic lipase deficiency. *Arteriosclerosis* 1990;10:40–48.

250. Carlson LA, Holmquist L, Nilsson-Ehle P. Deficiency of hepatic lipase activity in post-heparin plasma in familial hypertriglyceridemia. *Acta Med Scand* 1986;219:435–447.

251. Auwerx JH, Babirak SP, Hokanson JE, et al. Coexistence of abnormalities of hepatic lipase and lipoprotein lipase in a large family. *Am J Hum Genet* 1990;46:470–477.

252. Zambon A, Deeb SS, Bensadoun A, et al. In vivo evidence of a role for hepatic lipase in human apoB-containing lipoprotein metabolism, independent of its lipolytic activity. *J Lipid Res* 2000;41:2094–2099.

253. Demant T, Carlson LA, Holmquist L, et al. Lipoprotein metabolism in hepatic lipase deficiency: studies on the turnover of apolipoprotein B and on the effect of hepatic lipase on high density lipoprotein. *J Lipid Res* 1988;29:1603–1611.

254. Moennig G, Wiebusch H, Enbergs A, et al. Detection of missense mutations in the genes for lipoprotein lipase and hepatic triglyceride lipase in patients with dyslipidemia undergoing coronary angiography. *Atherosclerosis* 2000;149:395–401.

255. Funke H. Genetic determinants of high density lipoprotein levels. *Curr Opin Lipidol* 1997;8:189–196.

256. Rader DJ, Ikewaki K, Duverger N, et al. Very low high-density lipoproteins without coronary atherosclerosis. *Lancet* 1993;342:1455–1458.

257. Sirtori CR, Calabresi L, Franceschini G, et al. Cardiovascular status of carriers of the apolipoprotein A-I(Milano) mutant: the Limone sul Garda study. *Circulation* 2001;103:1949–1954.

258. Bruckert E, von Eckardstein A, Funke H, et al. The replacement of arginine by cysteine at residue 151 in apolipoprotein A-I produces a phenotype similar to that of apolipoprotein A-IMilano. *Atherosclerosis* 1997;128:121–128.

259. Miller M, Aiello D, Pritchard H, et al. Apolipoprotein A-I(Zavalla) (Leu159?Pro): HDL cholesterol deficiency in a kindred associated with premature coronary artery disease. *Arterioscler Thromb Vasc Biol* 1998;18:1242–1247.

260. Shah PK, Yano J, Reyes O, et al. High-dose recombinant apolipoprotein A-I(Milano) mobilizes tissue cholesterol and rapidly reduces plaque lipid and macrophage content in apolipoprotein E-deficient mice: potential implications for acute plaque stabilization. *Circulation* 2001;103:3047–3050.

261. Chiesa G, Monteggia E, Marchesi M, et al. Recombinant apolipoprotein A-I(Milano) infusion into rabbit carotid artery rapidly removes lipid from fatty streaks. *Circ Res* 2002;90:974–980.

262. Nissen SE, Tsunoda T, Tuzcu EM, et al. Effect of recombinant ApoA-I Milano on coronary atherosclerosis in patients with acute coronary syndromes: a randomized controlled trial. *JAMA* 2003;290:2292–2300.

263. Rust S, Rosier M, Funke H, et al. Tangier disease is caused by mutations in the gene encoding ATP-binding cassette transporter 1. *Nat Genet* 1999;22:352–355.

264. Brewer HB, Santamarina-Fojo S. Clinical significance of high-density lipoproteins and the development of atherosclerosis: focus on the role of the adenosine triphosphate-binding cassette protein A1 transporter. *Am J Cardiol* 2003;92:10–16.

265. Rye KA, Barter PJ. Formation and metabolism of prebeta-migrating, lipid-poor apolipoprotein A-I. *Arterioscler Thromb Vasc Biol* 2004:24:1.

266. Miller M, Rhyne J, Hamlette S, et al. Genetics of HDL regulation in humans. *Curr Opin Lipidol* 2003;14:273–279.

267. Clee SM, Kastelein JJ, van Dam M, et al. Age and residual cholesterol efflux affect HDL cholesterol levels and coronary artery disease in ABCA1 heterozygotes. *J Clin Invest* 2000;106:1263–1270.

268. Marcil M, Bissonnette R, Vincent J, et al. Cellular phospholipid and cholesterol efflux in high-density lipoprotein deficiency. *Circulation* 2003;107:1366–1371.

269. Serfaty-Lacrosniere C, Civeira F, Lanzberg A, et al. Homozygous Tangier disease and cardiovascular disease. *Atherosclerosis* 1994;107:85–98.

270. van Eck M, Bos IS, Kaminski WE, et al. Leukocyte ABCA1 controls susceptibility to atherosclerosis and macrophage recruitment into tissues. *Proc Natl Acad Sci USA* 2002;99:6298–6303.

271. Aiello RJ, Brees D, Bourassa PA, et al. Increased atherosclerosis in hyperlipidemic mice with inactivation of ABCA1 in macrophages. *Arterioscler Thromb Vasc Biol* 2002;22:630–637.

272. Kakko S, Kelloniemi J, von Rohr P, et al. ATP-binding cassette transporter A1 locus is not a major determinant of HDL-C levels in a population at high risk for coronary heart disease. *Atherosclerosis* 2003;166:285–290.

273. Kort EN, Ballinger DG, Ding W, et al. Evidence of linkage of familial hypoalphalipoproteinemia to a novel locus on chromosome 11q23. *Am J Hum Genet* 2000;66:1845–1856.

274. Zwarts KY, Clee SM, Zwinderman AH, et al. ABCA1 regulatory variants influence coronary artery disease independent of effects on plasma lipid levels. *Clin Genet* 2002;61:115–125.

275. Nestel PJ, Poyser A. Changes in cholesterol synthesis and excretion when cholesterol intake is increased. *Atherosclerosis* 1979;34:193–196.

276. Fielding PE, Fielding CJ, Havel RJ. Cholesterol net transport, esterification, and transfer in human hyperlipidemic plasma. *J Clin Invest* 1983;71:449–460.

277. Inazu A, Brown ML, Hesler CB, et al. Increased high-density lipoprotein levels caused by a common cholesteryl-ester transfer protein gene mutation. *N Engl J Med* 1990;323:1234–1238.

278. Inazu A, Jiang XC, Haraki T, et al. Genetic cholesteryl ester transfer protein deficiency caused by two prevalent mutations as a major determinant of increased levels of high density lipoprotein cholesterol. *J Clin Invest* 1994;94:1872–1882.

279. Zhong S, Sharp DS, Grove JS, et al. Increased coronary heart disease in Japanese-American men with mutation in the cholesteryl ester transfer protein gene despite increased HDL levels. *J Clin Invest* 1996;97:2917–2923.

280. Hirano K-i, Yamashita S, Nakajima N, et al. Genetic cholesteryl ester transfer protein deficiency is extremely frequent in the Omagari area of Japan: marked hyperalphalipoproteinemia caused by CETP gene mutation is not associated with longevity. *Arterioscler Thromb Vasc Biol* 1997;17:1053–1059.

281. Agerholm-Larsen B, Tybjaerg-Hansen A, et al. Common cholesteryl ester transfer protein mutations, decreased HDL cholesterol, and possible decreased risk of ischemic heart disease: the Copenhagen City Heart Study. *Circulation* 2000;102:2197–2203.

282. Moriyama Y, Okamura T, Inazu A, et al. A low prevalence of coronary heart disease among subjects with increased high-density lipoprotein cholesterol levels, including those with plasma cholesteryl ester transfer protein deficiency. *Prev Med* 1998;27:659–667.

283. Kuivenhoven JA, Jukema JW, Zwinderman AH, et al, for the Regression Growth Evaluation Statin Study Group. The role of a common variant of the cholesteryl ester transfer protein gene in the progression of coronary atherosclerosis. *N Engl J Med* 1998;338:86–93.

284. Ordovas JM, Cupples LA, Corella D, et al. Association of cholesteryl ester transfer protein-TaqIB polymorphism with variations in lipoprotein subclasses and coronary heart disease risk: the Framingham Study. *Arterioscler Thromb Vasc Biol* 2000;20:1323–1329.

285. Brousseau ME, O'Connor JJ, Jr., Ordovas JM, et al. Cholesteryl ester transfer protein TaqI B2B2 genotype is associated with higher HDL cholesterol levels and lower risk of coronary heart disease end points in men with HDL deficiency: Veterans Affairs HDL Cholesterol Intervention Trial. *Arterioscler Thromb Vasc Biol* 2002;22:1148–1154.

286. Barzilai N, Atzmon G, Schechter C, et al. Unique lipoprotein phenotype and genotype associated with exceptional longevity. *JAMA* 2003;290:2030–2040.

287. Blankenberg S, Rupprecht HJ, Bickel C, et al. Common genetic variation of the cholesteryl ester transfer protein gene strongly predicts future cardiovascular death in patients with coronary artery disease. *J Am Coll Cardiol* 2003;41:1983–1989.

288. Anderson JL, Carlquist JF. Genetic polymorphisms of hepatic lipase and cholesteryl ester transfer protein, intermediate phenotypes, and coronary risk. Do they add up yet? *J Am Coll Cardiol* 2003;41:1990–1993.

289. Barter PJ, Brewer HB, Jr., Chapman MJ, et al. Cholesteryl ester transfer protein: a novel target for raising HDL and inhibiting atherosclerosis. *Arterioscler Thromb Vasc Biol* 2003;23:160–167.

290. Stein JH, Rosenson RS. Lipoprotein Lp(a) excess and coronary heart disease. *Arch Intern Med* 1997;157:1170–1176.

291. Espeland MA, Marcovina SM, Miller V, et al, for the PEPI Investigators. Effect of postmenopausal hormone therapy on lipoprotein(a) concentration. *Circulation* 1998;97:979–986.

292. Hopkins PN, Wu LL, Hunt SC, et al. Lipoprotein(a) interactions with lipid and non-lipid risk factors in early familial coronary artery disease. *Arterioscler Thromb Vasc Biol* 1997;17:2783–2792.

293. Hopkins PN, Hunt SC, Schreiner PJ, et al. Lipoprotein(a) interactions with lipid and non-lipid risk factors in patients with early onset coronary artery disease: results from the NHLBI Family Heart Study. *Atherosclerosis* 1998;141:333–345.

294. Maher MG, Brown BG. Lipoprotein(a) and coronary heart disease. *Curr Opin Lipidol* 1995;6:229–235.

295. Armstrong VW, Cremer P, Eberle E, et al. The association between serum Lp(a) concentrations and angiographically assessed coronary atherosclerosis: dependence on serum LDL levels. *Atherosclerosis* 1986;62:249–257.

296. Cambillau M, Simon A, Amar J, et al. Serum Lp(a) as a discriminant marker of early atherosclerotic plaque at three extracoronary sites in hypercholesterolemic men. The PCVMETRA Group. *Arterioscler Thromb* 1992;12:1346–1352.

297. Solymoss BC, Marcil M, Wesolowska E, et al. Relation of coronary artery disease in women <60 years of age to the combined elevation of serum lipoprotein(a) and total cholesterol to high-density cholesterol ratio. *Am J Cardiol* 1993;72:1215–1219.

298. Kesaniemi YA, Grundy SM. Significance of low density lipoprotein production in the regulation of plasma cholesterol level in man. *J Clin Invest* 1982;70:13–22.

299. Turner PR, Konarska R, Revill J, et al. Metabolic study of variation in plasma cholesterol level in normal men. *Lancet* 1984;2:663–665.

300. Grundy SM, Vega GL, Bilheimer DW. Kinetic mechanisms determining variability in low density lipoprotein levels and rise with age. *Arteriosclerosis* 1985;5:623–630.

301. Davignon J, Gregg RE, Sing CF. Apolipoprotein E polymorphism and atherosclerosis. *Arteriosclerosis* 1988;8:1–21.

302. Wilson PW, Schaefer EJ, Larson MG, Ordovas JM. Apolipoprotein E alleles and risk of coronary disease: a meta-analysis. *Arterioscler Thromb Vasc Biol* 1996;16:1250–1255.

303. Gerdes LU, Gerdes C, Kervinen K, et al. The apolipoprotein epsilon4 allele determines prognosis and the effect on prognosis of simvastatin in survivors of myocardial infarction: a substudy of the Scandinavian Simvastatin Survival Study. *Circulation* 2000;101:1366–1371.

304. Miettinen TA, Gylling H, Vanhanen H, Ollus A. Cholesterol absorption, elimination, and synthesis related to LDL kinetics during varying fat intake in men with different apoprotein E phenotypes. *Arterioscler Thromb* 1992;12:1044–1052.

305. Gylling H, Aalto SK, Kontula K, Miettinen T, A. Serum low density lipoprotein cholesterol level and cholesterol absorp-

tion efficiency are influenced by apolipoprotein B and E polymorphism and by the FH-Helsinki mutation of the low density lipoprotein receptor gene in familial hypercholesterolemia. *Arterioscler Thromb* 1991;11:1368–1375.

306. Miserez AR, Muller PY, Barella L, et al. Sterol-regulatory element-binding protein (SREBP)-2 contributes to polygenic hypercholesterolaemia. *Atherosclerosis* 2002;164:15–26.

307. Veerkamp MJ, de Graaf J, Bredie SJ, et al. Diagnosis of familial combined hyperlipidemia based on lipid phenotype expression in 32 families: results of a 5-year follow-up study. *Arterioscler Thromb Vasc Biol* 2002;22:274–282.

308. Ayyobi AF, McGladdery SH, McNeely MJ, et al. Small, dense LDL and elevated apolipoprotein B are the common characteristics for the three major lipid phenotypes of familial combined hyperlipidemia. *Arterioscler Thromb Vasc Biol* 2003;23:1289–1294.

309. Cortner JA, Coates PM, Liacouras CA, Jarvik GP. Familial combined hyperlipidemia in children: clinical expression, metabolic defects, and management. *J Pediatr* 1993;123:177–184.

310. Aouizerat BE, Allayee H, Bodnar J, et al. Novel genes for familial combined hyperlipidemia. *Curr Opin Lipidol* 1999;10:113–122.

311. Coon H, Myers RH, Borecki IB, et al. Replication of linkage of familial combined hyperlipidemia to chromosome 1q with additional heterogeneous effect of apolipoprotein A- I/C-III/A-IV locus: the NHLBI Family Heart Study. *Arterioscler Thromb Vasc Biol* 2000;20:2275–2280.

312. Hopkins PN, Heiss G, Ellison RC, et al. Coronary artery disease risk in familial combined hyperlipidemia and familial hypertriglyceridemia: a case–control comparison from the National Heart, Lung, and Blood Institute Family Heart Study. *Circulation* 2003;108:519–523.

313. Kane JP, Havel RJ. Disorders of the biogenesis and secretion of lipoproteins containing the B apolipoproteins. In: Scriver CR, Beaudet AL, Sly WS, Valle D, eds. The Metabolic and Molecular Bases of Inherited Disease. *New York: McGraw–Hill*, 2001:2717–2752.

314. Kissebah AH, Alfarsi S, Adams PW. Integrated regulation of very low density lipoprotein triglyceride and apolipoprotein-B kinetics in man: normolipemic subjects, familial hypertriglyceridemia and familial combined hyperlipidemia. *Metabolism* 1981;30:856–868.

315. Sane T, Nikkila EA. Very low density lipoprotein triglyceride metabolism in relatives of hypertriglyceridemic probands. *Arteriosclerosis* 1988;8:217–226.

316. Aguilar-Salinas CA, Hugh P, Barrett R, et al. A familial combined hyperlipidemic kindred with impaired apolipoprotein B catabolism: kinetics of apolipoprotein B during placebo and pravastatin therapy. *Arterioscler Thromb Vasc Biol* 1997;17:72–82.

317. Sniderman A, Teng B, Genest J, et al. Familial aggregation and early expression of hyperapobetalipoproteinemia. *Am J Cardiol* 1985;55:291–295.

318. Sniderman A, Vu H, Cianflone K. Effect of moderate hypertriglyceridemia on the relation of plasma total and LDL apoB levels. *Atherosclerosis* 1991;89:109–116.

319. Austin MA, Breslow JL, Hennekens CH, et al. Low-density lipoprotein subclass patterns and risk of myocardial infarction. *JAMA* 1988;260:1917–1921.

320. Austin MA, King MC, Vranizan KM, Krauss RM. Atherogenic

lipoprotein phenotype: a proposed genetic marker for coronary heart disease risk. *Circulation* 1990;82:495–506.

321. Griffin BA, Freeman DJ, Tait GW, et al. Role of plasma triglyceride in the regulation of plasma low density lipoprotein (LDL) subfractions: relative contribution of small, dense LDL to coronary heart disease risk. *Atherosclerosis* 1994;106:241–253.

322. Gardner CD, Fortmann SP, Krauss RM. Association of small low-density lipoprotein particles with the incidence of coronary artery disease in men and women. *JAMA* 1996;276:875–881.

323. Stampfer MJ, Krauss RM, Ma J, et al. A prospective study of triglyceride level, low-density lipoprotein particle diameter, and risk of myocardial infarction. *JAMA* 1996;276:882–888.

324. Lamarche B, Tchernof A, Moorjani S, et al. Small, dense low-density lipoprotein particles as a predictor of the risk of ischemic heart disease in men: prospective results from the Québec Cardiovascular Study. *Circulation* 1997;95:69–75.

325. Lamarche B, Tchernof A, Mauriege P, et al. Fasting insulin and apolipoprotein B levels and low-density lipoprotein particle size as risk factors for ischemic heart disease. *JAMA* 1998;279:1955–1961.

326. Koba S, Hirano T, Yoshino G, et al. Remarkably high prevalence of small dense low-density lipoprotein in Japanese men with coronary artery disease, irrespective of the presence of diabetes. *Atherosclerosis* 2002;160:249–256.

327. Williams PT, Superko HR, Haskell WL, et al. Smallest LDL particles are most strongly related to coronary disease progression in men. *Arterioscler Thromb Vasc Biol* 2003;23:314–321.

328. Vakkilainen J, Steiner G, Ansquer JC, et al. Relationships between low-density lipoprotein particle size, plasma lipoproteins, and progression of coronary artery disease: the Diabetes Atherosclerosis Intervention Study (DAIS). *Circulation* 2003;107:1733–1737.

329. Tribble DL, van den Berg JJ, Motchnik PA, et al. Oxidative susceptibility of low density lipoprotein subfractions is related to their ubiquinol 10 and alpha tocopherol content. *Proc Natl Acad Sci USA* 1994;91:1183–1187.

330. Tribble DL, Krauss RM, Lansberg MG, et al. Greater oxidative susceptibility of the surface monolayer in small dense LDL may contribute to differences in copper induced oxidation among LDL density subfractions. *J Lipid Res* 1995;36:662–671.

331. Bjornheden T, Babyi A, Bondjers G, Wiklund O. Accumulation of lipoprotein fractions and subfractions in the arterial wall, determined in an in vitro perfusion system. *Atherosclerosis* 1996;123:43–56.

332. Anber V, Griffin BA, McConnell M, et al. Influence of plasma lipid and LDL-subfraction profile on the interaction between low density lipoprotein with human arterial wall proteoglycans. *Atherosclerosis* 1996;124:261–271.

333. Superko HR. What can we learn about dense low density lipoprotein and lipoprotein particles from clinical trials? *Curr Opin Lipidol* 1996;7:363–368.

334. Expert Panel on Detection, Evaluation, and Treatment of High Blood Cholesterol in Adults (Adult Treatment Panel III). Executive Summary of the Third Report of the National Cholesterol Education Program (NCEP) Expert Panel on Detection, Evaluation, and Treatment of High Blood Cholesterol in Adults (Adult Treatment Panel III). *JAMA* 2001;285:2486–2497.

335. Williams RR, Hunt SC, Hopkins PN, et al. Familial dyslipidemic hypertension: evidence from 58 Utah families for a syndrome present in approximately 12% of patients with essential hypertension. *JAMA* 1988;259:3579–3586.

336. Hunt SC, Wu LL, Hopkins PN, Stults BM, et al. Apolipoprotein, low density lipoprotein subfraction, and insulin associations with familial combined hyperlipidemia: study of Utah patients with familial dyslipidemic hypertension. *Arteriosclerosis* 1989;9:335–344.

337. Hopkins PN, Hunt SC, Wu LL, et al. Hypertension, dyslipidemia, and insulin resistance: links in a chain or spokes on a wheel? *Curr Opin Lipidol* 1996;7:241–253.

338. Kaplan NM. The deadly quartet. Upper-body obesity, glucose intolerance, hypertriglyceridemia, and hypertension. *Arch Intern Med* 1989;149:1514–1520.

339. Hall JE, Brands MW, Zappe DH, et al. Insulin resistance, hyperinsulinemia, and hypertension: causes, consequences, or merely correlations? *Proc Soc Exp Biol Med* 1995;208:317–329.

340. Hong Y, Pedersen NL, Brismar K, de Faire U. Genetic and environmental architecture of the features of the insulin-resistance syndrome. *Am J Hum Genet* 1997;60:143–152.

341. Tang W, Miller MB, Rich SS, et al. Linkage analysis of a composite factor for the multiple metabolic syndrome: the National Heart, Lung, and Blood Institute Family Heart Study. *Diabetes* 2003;52:2840–2847.

342. Selby JV, Newman B, Quiroga J, et al. Concordance for dyslipidemic hypertension in male twins. *JAMA* 1991;265:2079–2084.

343. Williams RR, Hunt SC, Wu LL, et al. Dyslipidemic hypertension in families with hypertension, non-insulin-dependent diabetes mellitus, and coronary heart disease. *Atheroscler Rev* 1991;22:107–111.

344. Pajukanta P, Terwilliger JD, Perola M, et al. Genomewide scan for familial combined hyperlipidemia genes in Finnish families, suggesting multiple susceptibility loci influencing triglyceride, cholesterol, and apolipoprotein B levels. *Am J Hum Genet* 1999;64:1453–1463.

345. Pei W, Baron H, Muller-Myhsok B, et al. Support for linkage of familial combined hyperlipidemia to chromosome 1q21–q23 in Chinese and German families. *Clin Genet* 2000;57:29–34.

346. Elbein SC, Hoffman MD, Teng K, et al. A genome-wide search for type 2 diabetes susceptibility genes in Utah Caucasians. *Diabetes* 1999;48:1175–1182.

347. Krushkal J, Ferrell R, Mockrin SC, et al. Genome-wide linkage analyses of systolic blood pressure using highly discordant siblings. *Circulation* 1999;99:1407–1410.

348. Levy D, DeStefano AL, Larson MG, et al. Evidence for a gene influencing blood pressure on chromosome 17: genome scan linkage results for longitudinal blood pressure phenotypes in subjects from the Framingham Heart Study. *Hypertension* 2000;36:477–483.

349. Hunt SC, Ellison RC, Atwood LD, et al. Genome scans for blood pressure and hypertension: the National Heart, Lung, and Blood Institute Family Heart Study. *Hypertension* 2002;40:1–6.

350. Allayee H, de Bruin TW, Michelle Dominguez K, et al. Genome scan for blood pressure in Dutch dyslipidemic families reveals linkage to a locus on chromosome 4p. *Hypertension* 2001;38:773–778.

351. Cheng LS, Davis RC, Raffel LJ, et al. Coincident linkage of fasting plasma insulin and blood pressure to chromosome 7q

in hypertensive hispanic families. *Circulation* 2001;104:1255–1260.

352. Tiret L, Poirier O, Hallet V, et al. The Lys198Asn polymorphism in the endothelin-1 gene is associated with blood pressure in overweight people. *Hypertension* 1999;33:1169–1174.

353. Asai T, Ohkubo T, Katsuya T, et al. Endothelin-1 gene variant associates with blood pressure in obese Japanese subjects: the Ohasama Study. *Hypertension* 200138:1321–1324.

354. Jin JJ, Nakura J, Wu Z, Yamamoto M, et al. Association of endothelin-1 gene variant with hypertension. *Hypertension* 2003;41:163–167.

355. Province MA, Arnett DK, Hunt SC, et al. Association between the alpha-adducin gene and hypertension in the HyperGEN Study. Am J Hypertens 2000;13:710–718.

356. Iwai N, Katsuya T, Mannami T, et al. Association Between SAH, an acyl-CoA synthetase gene, and hypertriglyceridemia, obesity, and Hypertension. *Circulation* 2002;105:41–47.

357. Ringel J, Kreutz R, Distler A, Sharma AM. The Trp64Arg polymorphism of the beta3-adrenergic receptor gene is associated with hypertension in men with type 2 diabetes mellitus. *Am J Hypertens* 2000;13:1027–1031.

358. Guyton AC, Coleman TG. Quantitative analysis of the pathophysiology of hypertension. *Circ Res* 1969;24:1–19.

359. Guyton A, Coleman T, Cowley A. Arterial pressure regulation: overriding dominance of the kidneys in long-term regulation and in hypertension. *Am J Med* 1972;52:584–594.

360. Guyton A, Coleman T, Cowley A. A systems analysis approach to understanding long-range arterial blood pressure control and hypertension. *Circ Res* 1974;35:159–176.

361. Guyton AC. *Circulatory Physiology III: Arterial Pressure and Hypertension.* Philadelphia: WB Saunders; 1980.

362. Lifton RP, Gharavi AG, Geller DS. Molecular mechanisms of human hypertension. *Cell* 2001;104:545–556.

363. Garrison RJ, Kannel WB, Stokes J, Castelli WP. Incidence and precursors of hypertension in young adults: the Framingham Offspring Study. *Prev Med* 1987;16:235–251.

364. He FJ, MacGregor GA. Effect of modest salt reduction on blood pressure: a meta-analysis of randomized trials. Implications for public health. *J Hum Hypertens* 2002;16:761–770.

365. de Wardener HE, MacGregor GA. Sodium and blood pressure. *Curr Opin Cardiol* 2002; 17:360–367.

366. Jurgens G, Graudal NA. Effects of low sodium diet versus high sodium diet on blood pressure, renin, aldosterone, catecholamines, cholesterols, and triglyceride. *Cochrane Database Syst Rev* 2003:CD004022.

367. Chobanian AV, Bakris GL, Black HR, et al. The Seventh Report of the Joint National Committee on Prevention, Detection, Evaluation, and Treatment of High Blood Pressure: the JNC 7 Report. *JAMA* 2003;289:2560–2572.

368. Guyton AC, Hall JE, Coleman TG, et al. The dominant role of the kidney in long-term arterial pressure regulation in normal and hypertensive states. In: Laragh JH, Brenner BM, eds. *Hypertension: Pathophysiology, Diagnosis, and Management.* 2nd ed. New York: Raven Press; 1995:1311–1326.

369. Ward R. Familial aggregation and genetic epidemiology of blood pressure. In: Laragh JH, Brenner BM, eds. *Hypertension: Pathophysiology, Diagnosis, and Management.* 2nd ed. New York: Raven Press; 1995:67–88.

370. Hasstedt SJ, Wu LL, Ash KO, et al. Hypertension and sodium–lithium countertransport in Utah pedigrees: evidence for major-locus inheritance. *Am J Hum Genet* 1988;43:14–22.

371. Chien KL, Yang CY, Lee YT. Major gene effects in systolic and diastolic blood pressure in families receiving a health examination in Taiwan. *J Hypertens* 2003;21:73–79.

372. Hopkins PN, Hunt SC. Genetics of hypertension. *Genet Med* 2003;5:413–429.

373. Rubattu S, Volpe M, Kreutz R, et al. Chromosomal mapping of quantitative trait loci contributing to stroke in a rat model of complex human disease. *Nat Genet* 1996;13:429–434.

374. Rubattu S, Ridker P, Stampfer MJ, et al. The gene encoding atrial natriuretic peptide and the risk of human stroke. *Circulation* 1999;100:1722–1726.

375. Palsdottir A, Abrahamson M, Thorsteinsson L, et al. Mutation in cystatin C gene causes hereditary brain haemorrhage. *Lancet* 1988;2:603–604.

376. Joutel A, Corpechot C, Ducros A, et al. Notch3 mutations in CADASIL, a hereditary adult-onset condition causing stroke and dementia. *Nature* 1996;383:707–710.

377. Dong Y, Hassan A, Zhang Z, et al. Yield of screening for CADASIL mutations in lacunar stroke and leukoaraiosis. *Stroke* 2003;34:203–205.

378. Wardlaw JM, Sandercock PA, Dennis MS, et al. Is breakdown of the blood–brain barrier responsible for lacunar stroke, leukoaraiosis, and dementia? *Stroke* 2003;34:806–812.

379. Carmelli D, DeCarli C, Swan GE, et al. Evidence for genetic variance in white matter hyperintensity volume in normal elderly male twins. *Stroke* 1998;29:1177–1181.

380. de Faire U, Friberg L, Lundman T. Concordance for mortality with special reference to ischaemic heart disease and cerebrovascular disease: a study on the Swedish Twin Registry. *Prev Med* 1975;4:509–517.

381. Welin L, Svardsudd K, Wilhelmsen L, et al. Analysis of risk factors for stroke in a cohort of men born in 1913. *New Engl J Med* 1987;317:521–526.

382. Bak S, Gaist D, Sindrup SH, et al. Genetic liability in stroke: a long-term follow-up study of Danish twins. *Stroke* 2002;33:769–774.

383. Gretarsdottir S, Sveinbjornsdottir S, Jonsson HH, et al. Localization of a susceptibility gene for common forms of stroke to 5q12. *Am J Hum Genet* 2002;70:593–603.

384. Woo D, Sauerbeck LR, Kissela BM, et al. Genetic and environmental risk factors for intracerebral hemorrhage: preliminary results of a population-based study. *Stroke* 2002;33:1190–1195.

385. Okamoto K, Horisawa R, Kawamura T, et al. Family history and risk of subarachnoid hemorrhage: a case–control study in Nagoya, Japan. *Stroke* 2003;34:422–426.

386. Garner C, Lecomte E, Visvikis S, et al. Genetic and environmental influences on left ventricular mass: a family study. *Hypertension* 2000;36:740–746.

387. Tang W, Arnett DK, Devereux RB, et al. Sibling resemblance for left ventricular structure, contractility, and diastolic filling. *Hypertension* 2002;40:233–238.

388. Jeanclos E, Schork NJ, Kyvik KO, et al. Telomere length inversely correlates with pulse pressure and is highly familial. *Hypertension* 2000;36:195–200.

389. Camp NJ, Hopkins PN, Hasstedt SJ, et al. Genome-wide multipoint parametric linkage analysis of pulse pressure in large, extended Utah pedigrees. *Hypertension* 2003;42:322–328.

390. Jartti L, Ronnemaa T, Kaprio J, et al. Population-based twin study of the effects of migration from Finland to Sweden on endothelial function and intima–media thickness. *Arterioscler Thromb Vasc Biol* 2002;22:832–837.

391. Lange LA, Bowden DW, Langefeld CD, et al. Heritability of carotid artery intima–medial thickness in type 2 diabetes. *Stroke* 2002;33:1876–1881.

392. Xiang AH, Azen SP, Buchanan TA, et al. Heritability of sub-clinical atherosclerosis in Latino families ascertained through a hypertensive parent. *Arterioscler Thromb Vasc Biol* 2002;22:843–848.

393. Fox CS, Polak JF, Chazaro I, et al. Genetic and environmental contributions to atherosclerosis phenotypes in men and women: heritability of carotid intima–media thickness in the Framingham Heart Study. *Stroke* 2003;34:397–401.

394. Hunt KJ, Duggirala R, Goring HH, et al. Genetic basis of variation in carotid artery plaque in the San Antonio Family Heart Study. *Stroke* 2002;33:2775–2780.

395. Jerrard-Dunne P, Sitzer M, Risley P, et al. Interleukin-6 promoter polymorphism modulates the effects of heavy alcohol consumption on early carotid artery atherosclerosis: the Carotid Atherosclerosis Progression Study (CAPS). *Stroke* 2003;34:402–407.

396. Zannad F, Benetos A. Genetics of intima–media thickness. *Curr Opin Lipidol* 2003;14:191–200.

397. Jeunemaitre X, Soubrier F, Kotelevtsev YV, et al. Molecular basis of human hypertension: role of angiotensinogen. *Cell* 1992;71:169–180.

398. Staessen JA, Kuznetsova T, Wang JG, et al. M235T angiotensinogen gene polymorphism and cardiovascular renal risk. *J Hypertens* 1999;17:9–17.

399. Province MA, Boerwinkle E, Chakravarti A, et al. Lack of association of the angiotensinogen-6 polymorphism with blood pressure levels in the comprehensive NHLBI Family Blood Pressure Program. National Heart, Lung and Blood Institute. *J Hypertens* 2000;18:867–876.

400. Rankinen T, Gagnon J, Perusse L, et al. Body fat, resting and exercise blood pressure and the angiotensinogen M235T polymorphism: the HERITAGE family study. *Obes Res* 1999;7:423–430.

401. Iso H, Harada S, Shimamoto T, et al. Angiotensinogen T174M and M235T variants, sodium intake and hypertension among non-drinking, lean Japanese men and women. *J Hypertens* 2000;18:1197–1206.

402. Ishikawa K, Baba S, Katsuya T, et al. T+31C polymorphism of angiotensinogen gene and essential hypertension. *Hypertension* 2001;37:281–285.

403. Tiago AD, Samani NJ, Candy GP, et al. Angiotensinogen gene promoter region variant modifies body size–ambulatory blood pressure relations in hypertension. *Circulation* 2002;106:1483–1487.

404. Pereira AC, Mota GF, Cunha RS, et al. Angiotensinogen 235T allele "dosage" is associated with blood pressure phenotypes. *Hypertension* 2003;41:25–30.

405. Tsai CT, Fallin D, Chiang FT, et al. Angiotensinogen gene haplotype and hypertension: interaction with ACE gene I allele. *Hypertension* 2003;41:9–15.

406. Inoue I, Nakajima T, Williams CS, et al. A nucleotide substitution in the promoter of human angiotensinogen is associated with essential hypertension and affects basal transcription in vitro. *J Clin Invest* 1997;99:1786–1797.

407. Lalouel JM, Rohrwasser A, Terreros D, et al. Angiotensinogen in essential hypertension: from genetics to nephrology. *J Am Soc Nephrol* 2001;12:606–615.

408. Hopkins PN, Hunt SC, Jeunemaitre X, et al. Angiotensinogen genotype affects renal and adrenal responses to angiotensin II in essential hypertension. *Circulation* 2002;105:1921–1927.

409. Jeng JR. Left ventricular mass, carotid wall thickness, and angiotensinogen gene polymorphism in patients with hypertension. *Am J Hypertens* 1999;12:443–450.

410. Kurland L, Melhus H, Karlsson J, et al. Polymorphisms in the angiotensinogen and angiotensin II type 1 receptor gene are related to change in left ventricular mass during antihypertensive treatment: results from the Swedish Irbesartan Left Ventricular Hypertrophy Investigation versus Atenolol (SILVHIA) trial. *J Hypertens* 2002;20:657–663.

411. Tang W, Devereux RB, Rao DC, et al. Associations between angiotensinogen gene variants and left ventricular mass and function in the HyperGEN Study. *Am Heart J* 2002;143:854–860.

412. Ortlepp JR, Vosberg HP, Reith S, et al. Genetic polymorphisms in the renin–angiotensin–aldosterone system associated with expression of left ventricular hypertrophy in hypertrophic cardiomyopathy: a study of five polymorphic genes in a family with a disease causing mutation in the myosin binding protein C gene. *Heart* 2002;87:270–275.

413. Schmidt R, Schmidt H, Fazekas F, et al. Angiotensinogen polymorphism M235T, carotid atherosclerosis, and small-vessel disease-related cerebral abnormalities. *Hypertension* 2001;38:110–115.

414. Pei Y, Scholey J, Thai K, et al. Association of angiotensinogen gene T235 variant with progression of immunoglobin A nephropathy in Caucasian patients. *J Clin Invest* 1997;100:814–820.

415. Maruyama K, Yoshida M, Nishio H, et al. Polymorphisms of renin–angiotensin system genes in childhood IgA nephropathy. *Pediatr Nephrol* 2001;16:350–355.

416. Lovati E, Richard A, Frey BM, et al. Genetic polymorphisms of the renin–angiotensin–aldosterone system in end-stage renal disease. *Kidney Int* 2001;60:46–54.

417. Tomino Y, Makita Y, Shike T, et al. Relationship between polymorphism in the angiotensinogen, angiotensin-converting enzyme or angiotensin II receptor and renal progression in Japanese NIDDM patients. *Nephron* 1999;82:139–144.

418. Hunt SC, Cook NR, Oberman A, et al. Angiotensinogen genotype, sodium reduction, weight loss, and prevention of hypertension: Trials of Hypertension Prevention, Phase II. *Hypertension* 1998;32:393–401.

419. Hunt SC, Geleijnse JM, Wu LL, et al. Enhanced blood pressure response to mild sodium reduction in subjects with the 235T variant of the angiotensinogen gene. *Am J Hypertens* 1999;12:460–466.

420. Svetkey LP, Moore TJ, Simons-Morton DG, et al. Angiotensinogen genotype and blood pressure response in the Dietary Approaches to Stop Hypertension (DASH) study. *J Hypertens* 2001;19:1949–1956.

421. Ferrandi M, Salardi S, Tripodi G, et al. Evidence for an interaction between adducin and Na(+)-K(+)-ATPase: relation to genetic hypertension. *Am J Physiol* 1999;277:H1338–1349.

422. Glorioso N, Filigheddu F, Cusi D, et al. Alpha-adducin 460Trp allele is associated with erythrocyte Na transport rate in North Sardinian primary hypertensives. *Hypertension* 2002;39:357–362.

423. Casari G, Barlassina C, Cusi D, et al. Association of the a-adducin locus with essential hypertension. *Hypertension* 1995;25:320–326.

424. Cusi D, Barlassina C, Azzani T, et al. Polymorphisms of alpha-adducin and salt sensitivity in patients with essential hypertension. *Lancet* 1997;349:1353–1357.

425. Barlassina C, Schork NJ, Manunta P, et al. Synergistic effect of alpha-adducin and ACE genes causes blood pressure changes with body sodium and volume expansion. *Kidney Int* 2000;57:1083–1090.

426. Manunta P, Cusi D, Barlassina C, et al. Alpha-adducin polymorphisms and renal sodium handling in essential hypertensive patients. *Kidney Int* 1998;53:1471–1478.

427. Grant FD, Romero JR, Jeunemaitre X, et al. Low-renin hypertension, altered sodium homeostasis, and an alpha-adducin polymorphism. *Hypertension* 2002;39:191–196.

428. Sugimoto K, Hozawa A, Katsuya T, et al. Alpha-adducin Gly460Trp polymorphism is associated with low renin hypertension in younger subjects in the Ohasama study. *J Hypertens* 2002;20:1779–1784.

429. Bianchi G, Cusi D. Association and linkage analysis of alpha-adducin polymorphism: is the glass half full or half empty? *Am J Hypertens* 2000;13:739–743.

430. Staessen JA, Wang JG, Brand E, et al. Effects of three candidate genes on prevalence and incidence of hypertension in a Caucasian population. *J Hypertens* 2001;19:1349–1358.

431. Morrison AC, Bray MS, Folsom AR, Boerwinkle E. ADD1 460W allele associated with cardiovascular disease in hypertensive individuals. *Hypertension* 2002;39:1053–1057.

432. Psaty BM, Smith NL, Heckbert SR, et al. Diuretic therapy, the alpha-adducin gene variant, and the risk of myocardial infarction or stroke in persons with treated hypertension. *JAMA* 2002;287:1680–1689.

433. Winnicki M, Somers VK, Accurso V, et al. Alpha-adducin Gly460Trp polymorphism, left ventricular mass and plasma renin activity. *J Hypertens* 2002;20:1771–1777.

434. Baker EH, Dong YB, Sagnella GA, et al. Association of hypertension with T594M mutation in beta subunit of epithelial sodium channels in black people resident in London. *Lancet* 1998;351:1388–1392.

435. Iwai N, Baba S, Mannami T, et al. Association of a sodium channel alpha subunit promoter variant with blood pressure. *J Am Soc Nephrol* 2002;13:80–85.

436. Wong ZY, Stebbing M, Ellis JA, et al. Genetic linkage of beta and gamma subunits of epithelial sodium channel to systolic blood pressure. *Lancet* 1999;353:1222–1225.

437. Baker EH, Duggal A, Dong Y, et al. Amiloride, a specific drug for hypertension in black people with T594M variant? *Hypertension* 2002;40:13–17.

438. Rayner BL, Owen EP, King JA, et al. A new mutation, R563Q, of the beta subunit of the epithelial sodium channel associated with low-renin, low-aldosterone hypertension. *J Hypertens* 2003;21:921–926.

439. Felder RA, Sanada H, Xu J, et al. G protein-coupled receptor kinase 4 gene variants in human essential hypertension. *Proc Natl Acad Sci USA* 2002;99:3872–3877.

440. Williams SM, Addy JH, Phillips JA 3rd, et al. Combinations of variations in multiple genes are associated with hypertension. *Hypertension* 2000;36:2–6.

441. Jose PA, Eisner GM, Felder RA. Dopamine and the kidney: a role in hypertension? *Curr Opin Nephrol Hypertens* 2003;12:189–194.

442. Sato M, Soma M, Nakayama T, Kanmatsuse K. Dopamine D1 receptor gene polymorphism is associated with essential hypertension. *Hypertension* 2000;36:183–186.

443. Rosmond R, Rankinen T, Chagnon M, et al. Polymorphism in exon 6 of the dopamine D(2) receptor gene (DRD2) is associated with elevated blood pressure and personality disorders in men. *J Hum Hypertens* 2001;15:553–558.

444. Cadman PE, O'Connor DT. Pharmacogenomics of hypertension. *Curr Opin Nephrol Hypertens* 2003;12:61–70.

445. Turner ST, Boerwinkle E. Genetics of blood pressure, hypertensive complications, and antihypertensive drug responses. *Pharmacog J* 2003;4:53–65.

446. Arnett DK, Boerwinkle E, Davis BR, et al. Pharmacogenetic approaches to hypertension therapy: design and rationale for the Genetics of Hypertension Associated Treatment (GenHAT) study. *Pharmacog J* 2002;2:309–317.

447. Liljedahl U, Karlsson J, Melhus H, et al. A microarray minisequencing system for pharmacogenetic profiling of antihypertensive drug response. *Pharmacogenetics* 2003;13:7–17.

448. Hopkins PN, Williams RR. Identification and relative weight of cardiovascular risk factors. *Cardiol Clin* 1986;4:3–31.

449. Muhlestein JB, Anderson JL, Horne BD, et al. Effect of fasting glucose levels on mortality rate in patients with and without diabetes mellitus and coronary artery disease undergoing percutaneous coronary intervention. *Am Heart J* 2003;146:351–358.

450. Haffner SM, Stern MP, Hazuda HP, et al. Cardiovascular risk factors in confirmed prediabetic individuals: does the clock for coronary heart disease start ticking before the onset of clinical diabetes? *JAMA* 1990;263:2893–2898.

451. Haffner SM, Mykkanen L, Festa A, et al. Insulin-resistant prediabetic subjects have more atherogenic risk factors than insulin-sensitive prediabetic subjects: implications for preventing coronary heart disease during the prediabetic state. *Circulation* 2000;101:975–980.

452. Khaw KT, Wareham N, Luben R, et al. Glycated haemoglobin, diabetes, and mortality in men in Norfolk cohort of European Prospective Investigation of Cancer and Nutrition (EPIC-Norfolk). *BMJ* 2001;322:15–18.

453. Sattar N, Gaw A, Scherbakova O, et al. Metabolic syndrome with and without C-reactive protein as a predictor of coronary heart disease and diabetes in the West of Scotland Coronary Prevention Study. *Circulation* 2003;108:414–419.

454. Hu FB, Stampfer MJ, Haffner SM, et al. Elevated risk of cardiovascular disease prior to clinical diagnosis of type 2 diabetes. *Diabetes Care* 2002;25:1129–1134.

455. Alexander CM, Landsman PB, Teutsch SM, Haffner SM. NCEP-defined metabolic syndrome, diabetes, and prevalence of coronary heart disease among NHANES III participants age 50 years and older. *Diabetes* 2003;52:1210–1214.

456. Morwessel NJ. The genetic basis of diabetes mellitus. *AACN Clin Issues* 1998;9:539–554.

457. Pociot F, McDermott MF. Genetics of type 1 diabetes mellitus. *Genes Immun* 2002;3:235–249.

458. Cox NJ, Wapelhorst B, Morrison VA, et al. Seven regions of the genome show evidence of linkage to type 1 diabetes in a consensus analysis of 767 multiplex families. *Am J Hum Genet* 2001;69:820–830.

459. Elbein SC. Perspective: the search for genes for type 2 diabetes in the post-genome era. *Endocrinology* 2002;143:2012–2018.

460. Ghosh S, Schork NJ. Genetic analysis of NIDDM: the study of quantitative traits. *Diabetes* 1996;45:1–14.

461. Ravussin E, Valencia ME, Esparza J, et al. Effects of a traditional lifestyle on obesity in Pima Indians. *Diabetes Care* 1994;17:1067–1074.

462. Pratley RE. Gene–environment interactions in the pathogenesis of type 2 diabetes mellitus: lessons learned from the Pima Indians. *Proc Nutr Soc* 1998;57:175–181.

463. Knowler W, Pettitt D, Savage P, Bennett P. Diabetes incidence of Pima Indians: contributions of obesity and parental diabetes. *Am J Epidemiol* 1981;113:144–156.

464. Sargeant LA, Wareham NJ, Khaw KT. Family history of diabetes identifies a group at increased risk for the metabolic consequences of obesity and physical inactivity in EPIC-Norfolk: a population-based study. The European Prospective Investigation into Cancer. *Int J Obes Relat Metab Disord* 2000;24:1333–1339.

465. Manson JE, Stampfer MJ, Colditz GA, et al. A prospective study of exercise and incidence of myocardial infarction in women. *Circulation* 1993;88:I-220.

466. Hu FB, Sigal RJ, Rich-Edwards JW, et al. Walking compared with vigorous physical activity and risk of type 2 diabetes in women: a prospective study. *JAMA* 1999;282:1433–1439.

467. Hu FB, Li TY, Colditz GA, et al. Television watching and other sedentary behaviors in relation to risk of obesity and type 2 diabetes mellitus in women. *JAMA* 2003;289:1785–1791.

468. Tuomilehto J, Lindstrom J, Eriksson JG, et al. Prevention of type 2 diabetes mellitus by changes in lifestyle among subjects with impaired glucose tolerance. *N Engl J Med* 2001;344:1343–1350.

469. Knowler WC, Barrett-Connor E, Fowler SE, et al. Reduction in the incidence of type 2 diabetes with lifestyle intervention or metformin. *N Engl J Med* 2002;346:393–403.

470. Neel JV. Diabetes mellitus: a "thrifty" genotype rendered detrimental by "progress"? *Am J Hum Genet* 1962;14:353–362.

471. Ravussin E, Smith SR. Increased fat intake, impaired fat oxidation, and failure of fat cell proliferation result in ectopic fat storage, insulin resistance, and type 2 diabetes mellitus. *Ann NY Acad Sci* 2002;967:363-378.

472. Bays H, Mandarino L, DeFronzo RA. Role of the adipocyte, free fatty acids, and ectopic fat in pathogenesis of type 2 diabetes mellitus: peroxisomal proliferator-activated receptor agonists provide a rational therapeutic approach. *J Clin Endocrinol Metab* 2004;89:463–478.

473. Gavrilova O, Marcus-Samuels B, Graham D, et al. Surgical implantation of adipose tissue reverses diabetes in lipoatrophic mice. *J Clin Invest* 2000;105:271–278.

474. Ferrannini E. Insulin resistance versus insulin deficiency in non-insulin-dependent diabetes mellitus: problems and prospects. *Endocr Rev* 1998;19:477–490.

475. DeFronzo RA, Ferrannini E. Insulin resistance: a multifaceted syndrome responsible for NIDDM, obesity, hypertension, dyslipidemia, and atherosclerotic cardiovascular disease. *Diabetes Care* 1991;14:173–194.

476. Pimenta W, Korytkowski M, Mitrakou A, et al. Pancreatic beta cell dysfunction as the primary genetic lesion in NIDDM: evidence from studies in normal glucose tolerant individuals with a first degree NIDDM relative. *JAMA* 1995;273:1855–1861.

477. Polonsky KS, Sturis J, Bell GI. Non-insulin-dependent diabetes mellitus: a genetically programmed failure of the beta cell to compensate for insulin resistance. *N Engl J Med* 1996;334:777–783.

478. Petersen KF, Dufour S, Befroy D, et al. Impaired mitochondrial activity in the insulin-resistant offspring of patients with type 2 diabetes. *N Engl J Med* 2004;350:664–671.

479. Nyholm B, Qu Z, Kaal A, et al. Evidence of an increased number of type IIb muscle fibers in insulin-resistant first-degree relatives of patients with NIDDM. *Diabetes* 1997;46:1822–1828.

480. Ek J, Andersen G, Urhammer SA, Gaede PH, et al. Mutation analysis of peroxisome proliferator-activated receptor-gamma coactivator-1 (PGC-1) and relationships of identified amino acid polymorphisms to type II diabetes mellitus. *Diabetologia* 2001;44:2220–2226.

481. Muller YL, Bogardus C, Pedersen O, Baier L. A Gly482Ser missense mutation in the peroxisome proliferator-activated receptor gamma coactivator-1 is associated with altered lipid oxidation and early insulin secretion in Pima Indians. *Diabetes* 2003;52:895–898.

482. Mootha VK, Lindgren CM, Eriksson KF, et al. PGC-1alpha-responsive genes involved in oxidative phosphorylation are coordinately downregulated in human diabetes. *Nat Genet* 2003;34:267–273.

483. Patti ME, Butte AJ, Crunkhorn S, et al. Coordinated reduction of genes of oxidative metabolism in humans with insulin resistance and diabetes: potential role of PGC1 and NRF1. *Proc Natl Acad Sci USA* 2003;100:8466–8471.

484. Schaffer JE. Lipotoxicity: when tissues overeat. *Curr Opin Lipidol* 2003;14:281–287.

485. Maedler K, Sergeev P, Ris F, et al. Glucose-induced beta cell production of IL-1beta contributes to glucotoxicity in human pancreatic islets. *J Clin Invest* 2002;110:851–860.

486. Prentki M, Joly E, El-Assaad W, Roduit R. Malonyl-CoA signaling, lipid partitioning, and glucolipotoxicity: role in beta-cell adaptation and failure in the etiology of diabetes. *Diabetes* 2002;51(suppl 3):S405–S413.

487. Poitout V, Robertson RP. Minireview: Secondary beta-cell failure in type 2 diabetes: a convergence of glucotoxicity and lipotoxicity. *Endocrinology* 2002;143:339–342.

488. El-Assaad W, Buteau J, Peyot ML, et al. Saturated fatty acids synergize with elevated glucose to cause pancreatic beta-cell death. *Endocrinology* 2003;144:4154–4163.

489. Brownlee M. Biochemistry and molecular cell biology of diabetic complications. *Nature* 2001;414:813–820.

490. Pittas AG, Joseph NA, Greenberg AS. Adipocytokines and insulin resistance. *J Clin Endocrinol Metab* 2004;89:447–452.

491. Lindsay RS, Funahashi T, Hanson RL, et al. Adiponectin and development of type 2 diabetes in the Pima Indian population. *Lancet* 2002;360:57–58.

492. Spranger J, Kroke A, Mohlig M, et al. Adiponectin and protection against type 2 diabetes mellitus. *Lancet* 2003;361:226–228.

493. Diez JJ, Iglesias P. The role of the novel adipocyte-derived hormone adiponectin in human disease. *Eur J Endocrinol* 2003; 148:293-300.

494. Ouchi N, Kihara S, Funahashi T, et al. Obesity, adiponectin and vascular inflammatory disease. *Curr Opin Lipidol* 2003;14:561–566.

495. Yamauchi T, Kamon J, Ito Y, et al. Cloning of adiponectin receptors that mediate antidiabetic metabolic effects. *Nature* 2003;423:762–769.

496. Kissebah AH, Sonnenberg GE, Myklebust J, et al. Quantitative trait loci on chromosomes 3 and 17 influence phenotypes of the metabolic syndrome. *Proc Natl Acad Sci USA* 2000;97:14478–14483.

497. Vionnet N, Hani El H, Dupont S, et al. Genomewide search for type 2 diabetes-susceptibility genes in French whites: evidence for a novel susceptibility locus for early-onset diabetes on chromosome 3q27-qter and independent replication of a type 2-diabetes locus on chromosome 1q21–q24. *Am J Hum Genet* 2000;67:1470–1480.

498. Mori Y, Otabe S, Dina C, et al. Genome-wide search for type 2 diabetes in Japanese affected sib-pairs confirms susceptibility genes on 3q, 15q, and 20q and identifies two new candidate loci on 7p and 11p. *Diabetes* 2002;51:1247–1255.

499. Stumvoll M, Tschritter O, Fritsche A, et al. Association of the T–G polymorphism in adiponectin (exon 2) with obesity and insulin sensitivity: interaction with family history of type 2 diabetes. *Diabetes* 2002;51:37–41.

500. Vasseur F, Helbecque N, Dina C, et al. Single-nucleotide polymorphism haplotypes in the both proximal promoter and exon 3 of the APM1 gene modulate adipocyte-secreted adiponectin hormone levels and contribute to the genetic risk for type 2 diabetes in French Caucasians. *Hum Mol Genet* 2002;11:2607–2614.

501. Menzaghi C, Ercolino T, Di Paola R, et al. A haplotype at the adiponectin locus is associated with obesity and other features of the insulin resistance syndrome. *Diabetes* 2002;51:2306–2312.

502. Hara K, Boutin P, Mori Y, et al. Genetic variation in the gene encoding adiponectin is associated with an increased risk of type 2 diabetes in the Japanese population. *Diabetes* 2002;51: 536–540.

503. Waki H, Yamauchi T, Kamon J, et al. Impaired multimerization of human adiponectin mutants associated with diabetes: molecular structure and multimer formation of adiponectin. *J Biol Chem* 2003;278:40352–40363.

504. Ukkola O, Ravussin E, Jacobson P, et al. Mutations in the adiponectin gene in lean and obese subjects from the Swedish obese subjects cohort. *Metabolism* 2003;52:881–884.

505. Comuzzie AG, Funahashi T, Sonnenberg G, et al. The genetic basis of plasma variation in adiponectin, a global endophenotype for obesity and the metabolic syndrome. *J Clin Endocrinol Metab* 2001;86:4321–4325.

506. Lindsay RS, Funahashi T, Krakoff J, et al. Genome-wide linkage analysis of serum adiponectin in the Pima Indian population. *Diabetes* 2003;52:2419–2425.

507. Walston J, Silver K, Bogardus C, et al. Time of onset of non-insulin-dependent diabetes mellitus and genetic variation in the beta 3-adrenergic-receptor gene. *N Engl J Med* 1995;333:343–347.

508. Sakane N, Yoshida T, Umekawa T, et al. Beta 3-adrenergic-receptor polymorphism: a genetic marker for visceral fat obesity and the insulin resistance syndrome. *Diabetologia* 1997;40:200–204.

509. Sakane N, Yoshida T, Umekawa T, et al. Effects of Trp64Arg mutation in the beta 3-adrenergic receptor gene on weight loss, body fat distribution, glycemic control, and insulin resistance in obese type 2 diabetic patients. *Diabetes Care* 1997;20:1887–1890.

510. Yamada K, Ishiyama-Shigemoto S, Ichikawa F, et al. Polymorphism in the 5′-leader cistron of the beta2-adrenergic receptor gene associated with obesity and type 2 diabetes. *J Clin Endocrinol Metab* 1999;84:1754–1757.

511. Groop LC, Kankuri M, Schalin-Jantti C, et al. Association between polymorphism of the glycogen synthase gene and non-insulin-dependent diabetes mellitus. *N Engl J Med* 1993;328:10–14.

512. Seldin MF, Mott D, Bhat D, et al. Glycogen synthase: a putative locus for diet-induced hyperglycemia. *J Clin Invest* 1994;94:269–276.

513. Schalin-Jantti C, Nikula-Ijas P, Huang X, et al. Polymorphism of the glycogen synthase gene in hypertensive and normotensive subjects. *Hypertension* 1996;27:67–71.

514. Hani EH, Clement K, Velho G, et al. Genetic studies of the sulfonylurea receptor gene locus in NIDDM and in morbid obesity among French Caucasians. *Diabetes* 1997;46:688–694.

515. Fleury C, Neverova M, Collins S, et al. Uncoupling protein-2: a novel gene linked to obesity and hyperinsulinemia. *Nat Genet* 1997;15:269–272.

516. Elbein SC, Leppert M, Hasstedt S. Uncoupling protein 2 region on chromosome 11q13 is not linked to markers of obesity in familial type 2 diabetes. *Diabetes* 1997;46:2105–2107.

517. Urhammer SA, Dalgaard LT, Sorensen TI, et al. Mutational analysis of the coding region of the uncoupling protein 2 gene in obese NIDDM patients: impact of a common amino acid polymorphism on juvenile and maturity onset forms of obesity and insulin resistance. *Diabetologia* 1997;40:1227–1230.

518. Shiinoki T, Suehiro T, Ikeda Y, et al. Screening for variants of the uncoupling protein 2 gene in Japanese patients with non-insulin-dependent diabetes mellitus. *Metabolism* 1999;48:581–584.

519. Cassell PG, Neverova M, Janmohamed S, et al. An uncoupling protein 2 gene variant is associated with a raised body mass index but not type II diabetes. *Diabetologia* 1999;42:688–692.

520. Caramori ML, Mauer M. Diabetes and nephropathy. *Curr Opin Nephrol Hypertens* 2003;12:273–282.

521. Warpeha KM, Chakravarthy U. Molecular genetics of microvascular disease in diabetic retinopathy. *Eye* 2003;17:305–311.

522. Pedersen O. Genetics of insulin resistance. *Exp Clin Endocrinol Diabetes* 1999;107:113–118.

523. Marchetti P, Lupi R, Federici M, et al. Insulin secretory function is impaired in isolated human islets carrying the Gly(972)?Arg IRS-1 polymorphism. *Diabetes* 2002;51:1419–1424.

524. Hansen L, Fjordvang H, Rasmussen SK, et al. Mutational analysis of the coding regions of the genes encoding protein kinase B-alpha and -beta, phosphoinositide-dependent protein kinase-1, phosphatase targeting to glycogen, protein phosphatase inhibitor-1, and glycogenin: lessons from a search for genetic variability of the insulin-stimulated glycogen synthesis

pathway of skeletal muscle in NIDDM patients. *Diabetes* 1999; 48:403–407.

525. Taylor SI, Moller DE. Mutations of the insulin receptor gene. In: Moller DE, ed. *Insulin Resistance.* Chichester: Wiley; 1993:83–121.

526. Kahn CR, Vicent D, Doria A. Genetics of non-insulin-dependent (type-II) diabetes mellitus. *Annu Rev Med* 1996; 47:509–531.

527. Kan M, Kanai F, Iida M, et al. Frequency of mutations of insulin receptor gene in Japanese patients with NIDDM. *Diabetes* 1995;44:1081–1086.

528. Fajans SS, Bell GI, Polonsky KS. Molecular mechanisms and clinical pathophysiology of maturity-onset diabetes of the young. *N Engl J Med* 2001;345:971–980.

529. Winter WE. Newly defined genetic diabetes syndromes: maturity onset diabetes of the young. *Rev Endocr Metab Disord* 2003;4:43–51.

530. Huopio H, Otonkoski T, Vauhkonen I, et al. A new subtype of autosomal dominant diabetes attributable to a mutation in the gene for sulfonylurea receptor 1. *Lancet* 2003;361:301–307.

531. Gurnell M. PPARgamma and metabolism: insights from the study of human genetic variants. *Clin Endocrinol (Oxf)* 2003;59:267–277.

532. Yamauchi T, Waki H, Kamon J, et al. Inhibition of RXR and PPARgamma ameliorates diet-induced obesity and type 2 diabetes. *J Clin Invest* 2001;108:1001–1013.

533. Kadowaki T, Hara K, Yamauchi T, et al. Molecular mechanism of insulin resistance and obesity. *Exp Biol Med (Maywood)* 2003;228:1111–1117.

534. Pearson ER, Starkey BJ, Powell RJ, et al. Genetic cause of hyperglycaemia and response to treatment in diabetes. *Lancet* 2003;362:1275–1281.

535. Zouali H, Vaxillaire M, Lesage S, et al. Linkage analysis and molecular scanning of glucokinase gene in NIDDM families. *Diabetes* 1993;42:1238–1245.

536. Elbein SC, Chiu KC, Hoffman MD, et al. Linkage analysis of 19 candidate regions for insulin resistance in familial NIDDM. *Diabetes* 1995;44:1259–1265.

537. Vionnet N, Hani EH, Lesage S, et al. Genetics of NIDDM in France: studies with 19 candidate genes in affected sib pairs. *Diabetes* 1997;46:1062–1068.

538. Lesage S, Zouali H, Vionnet N, et al. Genetic analyses of glucose transporter genes in French non-insulin- dependent diabetic families. *Diabetes Metab* 1997;23:137–142.

539. Lepretre F, Vionnet N, Budhan S, et al. Genetic studies of polymorphisms in ten non-insulin-dependent diabetes mellitus candidate genes in Tamil Indians from Pondichery. *Diabetes Metab* 1998;24:244–250.

540. Hanson RL, Elston RC, Pettitt DJ, et al. Segregation analysis of non-insulin-dependent diabetes mellitus in Pima Indians: evidence for a major-gene effect. *Am J Hum Genet* 1995;57:160–170.

541. Schumacher MC, Hasstedt SJ, Hunt SC, et al. Major gene effect for insulin levels in familial NIDDM pedigrees. *Diabetes* 1992;41:416–423.

542. Stern MP. The search for type 2 diabetes susceptibility genes using whole-genome scans: an epidemiologist's perspective. *Diabetes Metab Res Rev* 2002;18:106–113.

543. Harrison TA, Hindorff LA, Kim H, et al. Family history of diabetes as a potential public health tool. *Am J Prev Med* 2003;24:152–159.

544. Chagnon YC, Rankinen T, Snyder EE, et al. The human obesity gene map: the 2002 update. *Obes Res* 2003;11:313–367.

545. Farooqi IS, Keogh JM, Yeo GS, et al. Clinical spectrum of obesity and mutations in the melanocortin 4 receptor gene. *N Engl J Med* 2003;348:1085–1095.

546. Beales PL, Badano JL, Ross AJ, et al. Genetic interaction of BBS1 mutations with alleles at other BBS loci can result in non-Mendelian Bardet–Biedl syndrome. *Am J Hum Genet* 2003;72:1187–1199.

547. Ansley SJ, Badano JL, Blacque OE, et al. Basal body dysfunction is a likely cause of pleiotropic Bardet–Biedl syndrome. *Nature* 2003;425:628–633.

548. Bouchard C. Current understanding of the etiology of obesity: genetic and nongenetic factors. *Am J Clin Nutr* 1991;53:1561S–1565S.

549. Barsh GS, Farooqi IS, O'Rahilly S. Genetics of body-weight regulation. *Nature* 2000;404:644–651.

550. Cummings DE, Schwartz MW. Genetics and pathophysiology of human obesity. *Annu Rev Med* 2003;54:453–471.

551. Rice T, Sjostrom CD, Perusse L, et al. Segregation analysis of body mass index in a large sample selected for obesity: the Swedish Obese Subjects study. *Obes Res* 1999;7:246–255.

552. Pietilainen KH, Kaprio J, Rissanen A, et al. Distribution and heritability of BMI in Finnish adolescents aged 16y and 17y: a study of 4884 twins and 2509 singletons. *Int J Obes Relat Metab Disord* 1999;23:107–115.

553. Stunkard AJ, Sorensen TIA, Hanis G, et al. An adoption study of human obesity. *N Engl J Med* 1986;314:193–198.

554. Bouchard C, Tremblay A, Despres JP, et al. The response to long-term overfeeding in identical twins. *N Engl J Med* 1990;322:1477–1482.

555. Hasstedt SJ, Ramirez ME, Hiroshi K, Williams RR. Recessive inheritance of a relative fat pattern. *Am J Hum Genet* 1989;45:917–928.

556. Bouchard C, Perusse L, Leblanc C, et al. Inheritance of the amount and distribution of human body fat. *Int J Obes* 1988;12:205–215.

557. Borecki IB, Rice T, Pérusse L, et al. Major gene influence on the propensity to store fat in trunk versus extremity depots: evidence from the Québec Family Study. *Obes Res* 1995;3:1–8.

558. Burns TL, Donohoue PA, Leibel R. Identification of obesity genes using sib-pair linkage analysis: the Muscatine Study. *Circulation* 1995;91:929.

559. Hegele Ra, Brunt J, connelly PW. Genetic variation on chromosome 1 associated with variation in body fat distribution in men. *Circulation* 1995;92:1089–1093.

560. Andersson L, Haley CS, Ellegren H, et al. Genetic mapping of quantitative trait loci for growth and fatness in pigs. *Science* 1994;263:1771–1774.

561. Widen E, Lehto M, T, K, Walston J, et al. Association of a polymorphism in the b3-adrenergic-receptor gene with features of the insulin resistance syndrome in Finns. *N Engl J Med* 1995;333:348–351.

562. Rosmond R. Association studies of genetic polymorphisms in central obesity: a critical review. *Int J Obes Relat Metab Disord* 2003;27:1141–1151.

563. Stone S, Abkevich V, Hunt SC, et al. A major predisposition locus for severe obesity, at 4p15–p14. *Am J Hum Genet* 2002;70:1459–1468.

564. Perusse L, Rice T, Chagnon YC, et al. A genome-wide scan for abdominal fat assessed by computed tomography in the Quebec Family Study. *Diabetes* 2001;50:614–621.

565. Lee JH, Reed DR, Li WD, et al. Genome scan for human obesity and linkage to markers in 20q13. *Am J Hum Genet* 1999;64:196–209.

566. Hunt SC, Abkevich V, Hensel CH, et al. Linkage of body mass index to chromosome 20 in Utah pedigrees. *Hum Genet* 2001;109:279–285.

567. McCully KS. Homocysteine and vascular disease. *Nat Med* 1996;2:386–389.

568. Wu LL, Wu J, Hunt SC, James BC, et al. Plasma homocyst(e)ine as a risk factor for early familial coronary artery disease. *Clin Chem* 1994;40:552–561.

569. Graham IM, Daly LE, et al. Plasma homocysteine as a risk factor for vascular disease. the European Concerted Action Project. *JAMA* 1997;277:1775–1781.

570. The Homocysteine Studies Collaboration. Homocysteine and risk of ischemic heart disease and stroke: a meta-analysis. *JAMA* 2002;288:2015–2022.

571. Matetzky S, Freimark D, Ben-Ami S, et al. Association of elevated homocysteine levels with a higher risk of recurrent coronary events and mortality in patients with acute myocardial infarction. *Arch Intern Med* 2003;163:1933–1937.

572. den Heijer M, Brouwer IA, Bos GMJ, et al. Vitamin supplementation reduces blood homocysteine levels: a controlled trial in patients with venous thrombosis and healthy volunteers. *Arterioscler Thromb Vasc Biol* 1998;18:356–361.

573. Willems FF, Aengevaeren WR, Boers GH, et al. Coronary endothelial function in hyperhomocysteinemia: improvement after treatment with folic acid and cobalamin in patients with coronary artery disease. *J Am Coll Cardiol* 2002;40:766–772.

574. Schnyder G, Roffi M, Pin R, et al. Decreased rate of coronary restenosis after lowering of plasma homocysteine levels. *N Engl J Med* 2001;345:1593–1600.

575. Schnyder G, Roffi M, Flammer Y, et al. Effect of homocysteine-lowering therapy with folic acid, vitamin B12, and vitamin B6 on clinical outcome after percutaneous coronary intervention: the Swiss Heart Study: a randomized controlled trial. *JAMA* 2002;288:973–979.

576. Christensen B, Frosst P, Lussier-Cacan S, et al. Correlation of a common mutation in the methylenetetrahydrofolate reductase gene with plasma homocysteine in patients with premature coronary artery disease. *Arterioscler Thromb Vasc Biol* 1997;17:569–573.

577. Gudnason V, Stansbie D, Scott J, et al, for the EARS group. C677T (thermolabile alanine/valine) polymorphism in methylenetetrahydrofolate reductase (MTHFR): its frequency and impact on plasma homocysteine concentration in different European populations. *Atherosclerosis* 1998;136:347–354.

578. Clarke R, Daly L, Robinson K, et al. Hyperhomocysteinemia: an independent risk factor for vascular disease. *N Engl J Med* 1991;324:1149-1155.

579. Kluijtmans LA, Boers GH, Kraus JP, et al. The molecular basis of cystathionine beta-synthase deficiency in Dutch patients with homocystinuria: effect of CBS genotype on biochemical and clinical phenotype and on response to treatment. *Am J Hum Genet* 1999;65:59–67.

580. Brown KS, Kluijtmans LA, Young IS, et al. Genetic evidence that nitric oxide modulates homocysteine: the NOS3 894TT genotype is a risk factor for hyperhomocystenemia. *Arterioscler Thromb Vasc Biol* 2003;23:1014–1020.

581. de Jong SC, Stehouwer CDA, Mackaay AJC, et al. High prevalence of hyperhomocysteinemia and asymptomatic vascular disease in siblings of young patients with vascular disease and hyperhomocysteinemia. *Arterioscler Thromb Vasc Biol* 1997;17:2655–2662.

582. Takada D, Emi M, Ezura Y, et al. Interaction between the LDL-receptor gene bearing a novel mutation and a variant in the apolipoprotein A-II promoter: molecular study in a 1135-member familial hypercholesterolemia kindred. *J Hum Genet* 2002; 7:656–664.

583. Goldman L, Goldman PA, Williams LW, Weinstein MC. Cost effectiveness considerations in the treatment of heterozygous familial hypercholesterolemia with medications. *Am J Cardiol* 1993;72:75D–79D.

584. Andersen LK, Jensen HK, Juul S, Faergeman O. Patients' attitudes toward detection of heterozygous familial hypercholesterolemia. *Arch Intern Med* 1997;157:553–560.

585. Grossman M, Raper SE, Kozarsky K, et al. Successful ex vivo gene therapy directed to liver in a patient with familial hypercholesterolaemia. *Nat Genet* 1994;6:335–341.

586. Grossman M, Rader DJ, Muller DW, et al. A pilot study of ex vivo gene therapy for homozygous familial hypercholesterolaemia. *Nat Med* 1995;1:1148–1154.

587. Ishibashi S, Brown MS, Goldstein JL, et al. Hypercholesterolemia in low density lipoprotein receptor knockout mice and its reversal by adenovirus-mediated gene delivery. *J Clin Invest* 1993;92:883–893.

588. Kozarsky KF, McKinley DR, Austin LL, et al. In vivo correction of low density lipoprotein receptor deficiency in the Watanabe heritable hyperlipidemic rabbit with recombinant adenoviruses. *J Biol Chem* 1994;269:13695–13702.

589. Li J, Fang B, Eisensmith RC, Li XH, et al. In vivo gene therapy for hyperlipidemia: phenotypic correction in Watanabe rabbits by hepatic delivery of the rabbit LDL receptor gene. *J Clin Invest* 1995;95:768–773.

590. Shichiri M, Tanaka A, Hirata Y. Intravenous gene therapy for familial hypercholesterolemia using ligand-facilitated transfer of a liposome:LDL receptor gene complex. *Gene Ther* 2003;10:827–831.

591. Kozarsky KF, Jooss K, Donahee M, et al. Effective treatment of familial hypercholesterolaemia in the mouse model using adenovirus-mediated transfer of the VLDL receptor gene. *Nat Genet* 1996;13:54–62.

592. Chen SJ, Rader DJ, Tazelaar J, et al. Prolonged correction of hyperlipidemia in mice with familial hypercholesterolemia using an adeno-associated viral vector expressing very-low-density lipoprotein receptor. *Mol Ther* 2000;2:25–261.

593. Oka K, Pastore L, Kim IH, et al. Long-term stable correction of low-density lipoprotein receptor-deficient mice with a helper-dependent adenoviral vector expressing the very low-density lipoprotein receptor. *Circulation* 2001;103:1274–1281.

594. Kim IH, Jozkowicz A, Piedra PA, et al. Lifetime correction of genetic deficiency in mice with a single injection of

helper-dependent adenoviral vector. *Proc Natl Acad Sci USA* 2001;98:13282–13287.

595. Wade-Martins R, Saeki Y, Antonio Chiocca E. Infectious delivery of a 135-kb LDLR genomic locus leads to regulated complementation of low-density lipoprotein receptor deficiency in human cells. *Mol Ther* 2003;7:604–612.

596. Ferber D. Gene therapy: safer and virus-free? *Science* 2001; 294:1638–1642.

597. Kullow IJ, Mozes G, Schwartz RS, et al. Adventitial gene transfer of recombinant endothelial nitric oxide synthase to rabbit carotid arteries alters vascular reactivity. *Circulation* 1997;96:2254–2261.

598. Fazio VM, Rinaldi M, Ciafre SA, et al. Functional chronic correction of dyslipidemia in apo E deficient mice by direct intramuscular injection of naked plasmid DNA. In: Abstract Book, 66th Congress of the European Atherosclerosis Society, Florence, Italy. Milan: Giovanni Lorenzini Medical *Foundation*; 1996:28.

599. Gottschalk S, Sparrow JT, Hauer J, et al. A novel DNA–peptide complex for efficient gene transfer and expression in mammalian cells. *Gene Ther* 1996;3:48–57.

600. Belalcazar LM, Merched A, Carr B, et al. Long-term stable expression of human apolipoprotein A-I mediated by helper-dependent adenovirus gene transfer inhibits atherosclerosis progression and remodels atherosclerotic plaques in a mouse model of familial hypercholesterolemia. *Circulation* 2003;107:2726–2732.

601. Chiesa G, Stoltzfus LJ, Michelagnoli S, et al. Elevated triglycerides and low HDL cholesterol in transgenic mice expressing human apolipoprotein A-I(Milano). *Atherosclerosis* 1998;136:139–146.

602. Phillips MI. Gene therapy for hypertension: the preclinical data. *Hypertension* 2001;38:543–548.

603. Freedman SB. Clinical trials of gene therapy for atherosclerotic cardiovascular disease. *Curr Opin Lipidol* 2002;13:653–661.

604. Anderson JL, Carlquist JF, King GJ, et al. Angiotensin-converting enzyme genotypes and risk for myocardial infarction in women. *J Am Coll Cardiol* 1998;31:790–796.

605. Cambien F, Poirier O, Lecerf L, et al. The deletion polymorphism of the angiotensin converting enzyme gene is a potent risk factor for myocardial infarction. *Nature* 1992;359:641–644.

606. Ludwig E, Corneli PS, Anderson JL, et al. Angiotensin-converting enzyme gene polymorphism is associated with myocardial infarction but not with development of coronary stenosis. *Circulation* 1995;91:2120–2124.

607. Olivieri O, Trabetti E, Grazioli S, et al. Genetic polymorphisms of the renin–angiotensin system and atheromatous renal artery stenosis. *Hypertension* 1999;34:1097–1100.

608. Agerholm-Larsen B, Nordestgaard BG, Tybjaerg-Hansen A. ACE gene polymorphism in cardiovascular disease: meta-analyses of small and large studies in whites. *Arterioscler Thromb Vasc Biol* 2000;20:484–4920.

609. Keavney B, McKenzie C, Parish S, et al, for the International Studies of Infarct Survival (ISIS) Collaborators. Large-scale test of hypothesised associations between the angiotensin-converting-enzyme insertion/deletion polymorphism and myocardial infarction in about 5000 cases and 6000 controls. *Lancet* 2000;355:434–442.

610. Katsuya T, Koike G, Yee TW, et al. Association of angiotensinogen gene T235 variant with increased risk of coronary heart disease. *Lancet* 1995;345:1600–1603.

611. Ishigami T, Umemura S, Iwamoto T, et al. Molecular variant of angiotensinogen gene is associated with coronary atherosclerosis. *Circulation* 1995;91:951–954.

612. Winkelmann BR, Russ AP, Nauck M, et al. Angiotensinogen M235T polymorphism is associated with plasma angiotensinogen and cardiovascular disease. *Am Heart J* 1999;137:698–705.

613. Gardemann A, Stricker J, Humme J, et al. Angiotensinogen T174M and M235T gene polymorphisms are associated with the extent of coronary atherosclerosis. *Atherosclerosis* 1999;145:309–314.

614. Fatini C, Abbate R, Pepe G, et al. Searching for a better assessment of the individual coronary risk profile: the role of angiotensin-converting enzyme, angiotensin II type 1 receptor and angiotensinogen gene polymorphisms. *Eur Heart J* 2000;21:633–638.

615. Rodriguez-Perez JC, Rodriguez-Esparragon F, Hernandez-Perera O, et al. Association of angiotensinogen M235T and A(-6)G gene polymorphisms with coronary heart disease with independence of essential hypertension: the PROCAGENE study. Prospective Cardiac Gene. *J Am Coll Cardiol* 2001;37:1536–1542.

616. Kamitani A, Rakugi H, Higaki J, et al. Enhanced predictability of myocardial infarction in Japanese by combined genotype analysis. *Hypertension* 1995;25:950–953.

617. Ludwig EH, Borecki IB, Ellison RC, et al. Associations between candidate loci angiotensin-converting enzyme and angiotensinogen with coronary heart disease and myocardial infarction: the NHLBI Family Heart Study. *Ann Epidemiol* 1997;7:3–12.

618. Fomicheva EV, Gukova SP, Larionova-Vasina VI, et al. Gene-gene interaction in the RAS system in the predisposition to myocardial infarction in elder population of St. Petersburg (Russia). *Mol Genet Metab* 2000;69:76–80.

619. Petrovic D, Zorc M, Kanic V, Peterlin B. Interaction between gene polymorphisms of renin–angiotensin system and metabolic risk factors in premature myocardial infarction. *Angiology* 2001;52:247–252.

620. Jeunemaitre X, Ledru F, Battaglia S, et al. Genetic polymorphisms of the renin–angiotensin system and angiographic extent and severity of coronary artery disease: the CORGENE study. *Hum Genet* 1997;99:66–73.

621. Tiret L, Ricard S, Poirier O, et al. Genetic variation at the angiotensinogen locus in relation to high blood pressure and myocardial infarction: the ECTIM Study. *J Hypertens* 1995;13:311–317.

622. Ko YL, Ko YS, Wang SM, et al. Angiotensinogen and angiotensin-I converting enzyme gene polymorphisms and the risk of coronary artery disease in Chinese. *Hum Genet* 1997;100:210–214.

623. Hubacek JA, Rothe G, Pit'ha J, et al. C(-260)?T polymorphism in the promoter of the CD14 monocyte receptor gene as a risk factor for myocardial infarction. *Circulation* 1999;99:3218–3220.

624. Shimada K, Watanabe Y, Mokuno H, et al. Common polymorphism in the promoter of the CD14 monocyte receptor gene is associated with acute myocardial infarction in Japanese men. *Am J Cardiol* 2000;86:682–684.

625. Zee RY, Lindpaintner K, Struk B, et al. A prospective evaluation of the CD14 C(-260)T gene polymorphism and the risk of myocardial infarction. *Atherosclerosis* 2001;154:699–702.

626. Unkelbach K, Gardemann A, Kostrzewa M, et al. A new promoter polymorphism in the gene of lipopolysaccharide receptor CD14 is associated with expired myocardial infarction in patients with low atherosclerotic risk profile. *Arterioscler Thromb Vasc Biol* 1999;19:932–938.

627. Yeh HI, Chou Y, Liu HF, et al. Connexin37 gene polymorphism and coronary artery disease in Taiwan. *Int J Cardiol* 2001;81:251–255.

628. Boerma M, Forsberg L, Van Zeijl L, et al. A genetic polymorphism in connexin 37 as a prognostic marker for atherosclerotic plaque development. *J Intern Med* 1999;246:211–218.

629. Wang XL, Greco M, Sim AS, et al. Effect of CYP1A1 MspI polymorphism on cigarette smoking related coronary artery disease and diabetes. *Atherosclerosis* 2002;162:391–397.

630. Wenzel K, Felix S, Kleber FX, et al. E-selectin polymorphism and atherosclerosis: an association study. *Hum Mol Genet* 1994;3:1935–1937.

631. Wenzel K, Ernst M, Rohde K, et al. DNA polymorphisms in adhesion molecule genes: a new risk factor for early atherosclerosis. *Hum Genet* 1996;97:15–20.

632. Herrmann SM, Ricard S, Nicaud V, et al. The P-selectin gene is highly polymorphic: reduced frequency of the Pro715 allele carriers in patients with myocardial infarction. *Hum Mol Genet* 1998;7:1277–1284.

633. Nakayama M, Yasue H, Yoshimura M, et al. T(-786)?C mutation in the 5′-flanking region of the endothelial nitric oxide synthase gene is associated with myocardial infarction, especially without coronary organic stenosis. *Am J Cardiol* 2000;86:628–634.

634. Nakayama M, Yasue H, Yoshimura M, et al. T-786 to C mutation in the 5′-flanking region of the endothelial nitric oxide synthase gene is associated with coronary spasm. *Circulation* 1999;99:2864–2870.

635. Nasreen S, Nabika T, Shibata H, et al. T-786C polymorphism in endothelial NO synthase gene affects cerebral Circulation in smokers: possible gene–environmental interaction. *Arterioscler Thromb Vasc Biol* 2002;22:605–610.

636. Kunnas TA, Ilveskoski E, Niskakangas T, et al. Association of the endothelial nitric oxide synthase gene polymorphism with risk of coronary artery disease and myocardial infarction in middle-aged men. *J Mol Med* 2002;80:605–609.

637. Hingorani AD, Liang CF, Fatibene J, et al. A common variant of the endothelial nitric oxide synthase (Glu298?Asp) is a major risk factor for coronary artery disease in the UK. *Circulation* 1999;100:1515–1520.

638. Shimasaki Y, Yasue H, Yoshimura M, et al. Association of the missense Glu298Asp variant of the endothelial nitric oxide synthase gene with myocardial infarction. *J Am Coll Cardiol* 1998;31:1506–1510.

639. Colombo MG, Andreassi MG, Paradossi U, et al. Evidence for association of a common variant of the endothelial nitric oxide synthase gene (Glu(298)?Asp polymorphism) to the presence, extent, and severity of coronary artery disease. *Heart* 2002;87:525–528.

640. Lehtimaki T, Kunnas TA, Mattila KM, et al. Coronary artery wall atherosclerosis in relation to the estrogen receptor 1 gene polymorphism: an autopsy study. *J Mol Med* 2002;80:176–180.

641. McDermott DH, Halcox JP, Schenke WH, et al. Association between polymorphism in the chemokine receptor CX3CR1 and coronary vascular endothelial dysfunction and atherosclerosis. *Circ Res* 2001;89:401–407.

642. McDermott DH, Fong AM, Yang Q, et al. Chemokine receptor mutant CX3CR1-M280 has impaired adhesive function and correlates with protection from cardiovascular disease in humans. *J Clin Invest* 2003;111:1241–1250.

643. Georges JL, Loukaci V, Poirier O, et al. Interleukin-6 gene polymorphisms and susceptibility to myocardial infarction: the ECTIM study. Etude Cas-Temoin de l'Infarctus du Myocarde. *J Mol Med* 2001;79:300–305.

644. Jenkins NP, Brooks NH, Perey C, et al. An interleukin-10 promoter haplotype may protect against coronary artery disease. *J Am Coll Cardiol* 2000;35:259A.

645. Ellison RC, Zhang Y, Myers RH, et al. Lewis blood group phenotype as an independent risk factor for coronary heart disease (the NHLBI Family Heart Study). *Am J Cardiol* 1999;83:345–348.

646. Salomaa V, Pankow J, Heiss G, et al. Genetic background of Lewis negative blood group phenotype and its association with atherosclerotic disease in the NHLBI family heart study. *J Intern Med* 2000;247:689–698.

647. Dwyer JH, Allayee H, Dwyer KM, et al. Arachidonate 5-lipoxygenase promoter genotype, dietary arachidonic acid, and atherosclerosis. *N Engl J Med* 2004;350:29–37.

648. Best LG, Davidson M, North KE, et al. Prospective analysis of mannose-binding lectin genotypes and coronary artery disease in American Indians: the Strong Heart Study. *Circulation* 2004;109:471–475.

649. Szalai C, Duba J, Prohaszka Z, et al. Involvement of polymorphisms in the chemokine system in the susceptibility for coronary artery disease (CAD): coincidence of elevated Lp(a) and MCP-1 -2518 G/G genotype in CAD patients. *Atherosclerosis* 2001;158:233–239.

650. Abuzeid AM, Hawe E, Humphries SE, Talmud PJ. Association between the Ala379Val variant of the lipoprotein associated phospholipase A2 and risk of myocardial infarction in the north and south of Europe. *Atherosclerosis* 2003;168:283–288.

651. Elrayess MA, Webb KE, Flavell DM, et al. A novel functional polymorphism in the PECAM-1 gene (53G>A) is associated with progression of atherosclerosis in the LOCAT and REGRESS studies. *Atherosclerosis* 2003;168:131–138.

652. Wenzel K, Baumann G, Felix SB. The homozygous combination of Leu125Val and Ser563Asn polymorphisms in PECAM1 (CD31) gene is associated with early severe coronary heart disease. *Hum Mutat* 1999;14:545.

653. Gardemann A, Knapp A, Katz N, et al. No evidence for the CD31 C/G gene polymorphism as an independent risk factor of coronary heart disease. *Thromb Haemost* 2000;83:629.

654. Barbaux SC, Blankenberg S, Rupprecht HJ, et al. Association between P-selectin gene polymorphisms and soluble P-selectin levels and their relation to coronary artery disease. *Arterioscler Thromb Vasc Biol* 2001;21:1668–1673.

655. Kiechl S, Lorenz E, Reindl M, et al. Toll-like receptor 4 polymorphisms and atherogenesis. *N Engl J Med* 2002;347:185–192.

656. Yokota M, Ichihara S, Lin TL, et al. Association of a T29–>C polymorphism of the transforming growth factor-beta1 gene with genetic susceptibility to myocardial infarction in Japanese. *Circulation* 2000;101:2783–2787.

657. Cambien F, Ricard S, Troesch A, et al. Polymorphisms of the transforming growth factor-beta 1 gene in relation to myocardial infarction and blood pressure: the Etude Cas-Temoin de l'Infarctus du Myocarde (ECTIM) Study. *Hypertension* 1996;28:881–887.

658. Syrris P, Carter ND, Metcalfe JC, et al. Transforming growth factor-beta1 gene polymorphisms and coronary artery disease. *Clin Sci (Lond)* 1998;95:659–667.

659. Herrmann SM, Ricard S, Nicaud V, et al. Polymorphisms of the tumour necrosis factor-alpha gene, coronary heart disease and obesity. Eur *J Clin Invest* 1998;28:59–66.

660. Wang XL, Oosterhof J. Tumour necrosis factor alpha G-308?A polymorphism and risk for coronary artery disease. *Clin Sci (Colch)* 2000;98:435–437.

661. Ye L, Miki T, Nakura J, et al. Association of a polymorphic variant of the Werner helicase gene with myocardial infarction in a Japanese population. *Am J Med Genet* 1997;68:494–498.

662. Clee SM, Zwinderman AH, Engert JC, et al. Common genetic variation in ABCA1 is associated with altered lipoprotein levels and a modified risk for coronary artery disease. *Circulation* 2001;103:1198–1205.

663. Lutucuta S, Ballantyne CM, Elghannam H, et al. Novel polymorphisms in promoter region of ATP binding cassette transporter gene and plasma lipids, severity, progression, and regression of coronary atherosclerosis and response to therapy. *Circ Res* 2001;88:969–973.

664. Trip MD, Smulders YM, Wegman JJ, et al. Frequent mutation in the ABCC6 gene (R1141X) is associated with a strong increase in the prevalence of coronary artery disease. *Circulation* 2002;106:773–775.

665. Wang J, Near S, Young K, et al. ABCC6 gene polymorphism associated with variation in plasma lipoproteins. *J Hum Genet* 2001;46:699–705.

666. Hines LM, Stampfer MJ, Ma J, et al. Genetic variation in alcohol dehydrogenase and the beneficial effect of moderate alcohol consumption on myocardial infarction. *N Engl J Med* 2001;344:549–555.

667. Wong WM, Hawe E, Li LK, et al. Apolipoprotein AIV gene variant S347 is associated with increased risk of coronary heart disease and lower plasma apolipoprotein AIV levels. *Circ Res* 2003;92:969–975.

668. Olivieri O, Stranieri C, Bassi A, et al. ApoC-III gene polymorphisms and risk of coronary artery disease. *J Lipid Res* 2002;43:1450–1457.

669. Agerholm-Larsen B, Nordestgaard BG, Steffensen R, et al. Elevated HDL cholesterol is a risk factor for ischemic heart disease in white women when caused by a common mutation in the cholesteryl ester transfer protein gene. *Circulation* 2000;101:1907–1912.

670. Inazu A, Koizumi J, Mabuchi H. Cholesteryl ester transfer protein and atherosclerosis. *Curr Opin Lipidol* 2000;11:389–396.

671. Delanghe J, Cambier B, Langlois M, et al. Haptoglobin polymorphism, a genetic risk factor in coronary artery bypass surgery. *Atherosclerosis* 1997;132:215–219.

672. Bernard D, Christophe A, Delanghe J, et al. The effect of supplementation with an antioxidant preparation on LDL-oxidation is determined by haptoglobin polymorphism. *Redox Rep* 2003;8:41–46.

673. Langlois MR, Martin ME, Boelaert JR, et al. The haptoglobin 2-2 phenotype affects serum markers of iron status in healthy males. *Clin Chem* 2000;46:1619–1625.

674. Delanghe J, Langlois M, Ouyang J, et al. Effect of haptoglobin phenotypes on growth of Streptococcus pyogenes. *Clin Chem Lab Med* 1998;36:691–696.

675. Chapelle JP, Albert A, Smeets JP, et al. Effect of the haptoglobin phenotype on the size of a myocardial infarct. *N Engl J Med* 1982;307:457–463.

676. Delanghe J, Langlois M, Duprez D, et al. Haptoglobin polymorphism and peripheral arterial occlusive disease. *Atherosclerosis* 1999;145:287–292.

677. Tuomainen TP, Kontula K, Nyyssonen K, et al. Increased risk of acute myocardial infarction in carriers of the hemochromatosis gene Cys282Tyr mutation: a prospective cohort study in men in eastern Finland. *Circulation* 1999;100:1274–1279.

678. Nassar BA, Zayed EM, Title LM, et al. Relation of HFE gene mutations, high iron stores and early onset coronary artery disease. *Can J Cardiol* 1998;14:215–220.

679. Battiloro E, Ombres D, Pascale E, et al. Haemochromatosis gene mutations and risk of coronary artery disease. *Eur J Hum Genet* 2000;8:389–392.

680. Guerra R, Wang J, Grundy SM, Cohen JC. A hepatic lipase (LIPC) allele associated with high plasma concentrations of high density lipoprotein cholesterol. *Proc Natl Acad Sci USA* 1997;94:4532–4537.

681. Baroni MG, D'Andrea MP, Montali A, et al. A common mutation of the insulin receptor substrate-1 gene is a risk factor for coronary artery disease. *Arterioscler Thromb Vasc Biol* 1999;19:2975–2980.

682. Kastelein JJ, Groenemeyer BE, Hallman DM, et al, for the REGRESS Study Group. The Asn9 variant of lipoprotein lipase is associated with the -93G promoter mutation and an increased risk of coronary artery disease. *Clin Genet* 1998;53:27–33.

683. Wittrup HH, Tybjaerg-Hansen A, Abildgaard S, et al. A common substitution (Asn291Ser) in lipoprotein lipase is associated with increased risk of ischemic heart disease. *J Clin Invest* 1997;99:1606–1613.

684. Gagne SE, Larson MG, Pimstone SN, et al. A common truncation variant of lipoprotein lipase (Ser447X) confers protection against coronary heart disease: the Framingham Offspring Study. *Clin Genet* 1999;55:450–454.

685. Chen W, Srinivasan SR, Hallman DM, et al. Influence of lipoprotein lipase serine 447 stop polymorphism on tracking of triglycerides and HDL cholesterol from childhood to adulthood and familial risk of coronary artery disease: the Bogalusa Heart Study [abstract]. *Circulation* 2000; 102(suppl II):II-31.

686. Anderson JL, King GJ, Bair TL, et al. Association of lipoprotein lipase gene polymorphisms with coronary artery disease. *J Am Coll Cardiol* 1999;33:1013–1020.

687. Inoue N, Kawashima S, Kanazawa K, et al. Polymorphism of the NADH/NADPH oxidase p22phox gene in patients with coronary artery disease. *Circulation* 1998;97:135–137.

688. Guzik TJ, West NE, Black E, et al. Functional effect of the C242T polymorphism in the NAD(P)H oxidase p22phox gene

on vascular superoxide production in atherosclerosis. *Circulation* 2000;102:1744–1747.

689. Lee WH, Hwang TH, Oh GT, et al. Genetic factors associated with endothelial dysfunction affect the early onset of coronary artery disease in Korean males. *Vasc Med* 2001;6:103–108.

690. Stanger O, Renner W, Khoschsorur G, et al. NADH/NADPH oxidase p22phox C242T polymorphism and lipid peroxidation in coronary artery disease. *Clin Physiol* 2001;21:718–722.

691. Gardemann A, Mages P, Katz N, et al. The p22phox A640G gene polymorphism but not the C242T gene variation is associated with coronary heart disease in younger individuals. *Atherosclerosis* 1999;145:315–323.

692. Ito D, Murata M, Watanabe K, et al Y. C242T polymorphism of NADPH oxidase p22 PHOX gene and ischemic cerebrovascular disease in the Japanese population. *Stroke* 2000;31:936–939.

693. Schmidt H, Schmidt R, Niederkorn K, et al. Paraoxonase PON1 polymorphism leu-Met54 is associated with carotid atherosclerosis: results of the Austrian Stroke Prevention Study. *Stroke* 1998;29:2043–2048.

694. Salonen JT, Malin R, Tuomainen TP, et al. Polymorphism in high density lipoprotein paraoxonase gene and risk of acute myocardial infarction in men: prospective nested case–control study. *BMJ* 1999; 19:487–489; discussion 490.

695. Zama T, Murata M, Matsubara Y, et al. A 192Arg variant of the human paraoxonase (HUMPONA) gene polymorphism is associated with an increased risk for coronary artery disease in the Japanese. *Arterioscler Thromb Vasc Biol* 1997;17:3565–3569.

696. Sanghera DK, Aston CE, Saha N, Kamboh MI. DNA polymorphisms in two paraoxonase genes (PON1 and PON2) are associated with the risk of coronary heart disease. *Am J Hum Genet* 1998;62:36–44.

697. Flavell DM, Jamshidi Y, Hawe E, et al. Peroxisome proliferator-activated receptor alpha gene variants influence progression of coronary atherosclerosis and risk of coronary artery disease. *Circulation* 2002;105:1440–1445.

698. Wang XL, Oosterhof J, Duarte N. Peroxisome proliferator-activated receptor gamma C161?T polymorphism and coronary artery disease. *Cardiovasc Res* 1999;44:588–594.

699. Doggen CJ, Cats VM, Bertina RM, Rosendaal FR. Interaction of coagulation defects and cardiovascular risk factors: increased risk of myocardial infarction associated with factor V Leiden or prothrombin 20210A. *Circulation* 1998;97:1037–1041.

700. Ridker PM, Hennekens CH, Lindpaintner K, et al. Mutation in the gene coding for coagulation factor V and the risk of myocardial infarction, stroke, and venous thrombosis in apparently healthy men. *N Engl J Med* 1995;332:912–917.

701. Garg UC, Arnett DK, Evans G, Eckfeldt JH. No association between factor V Leiden mutation and coronary heart disease or carotid intima media thickness: the NHLBI Family Heart Study. *Thromb Res* 1998;89:289–293.

702. Rosendaal FR, Siscovick DS, Schwartz SM, et al. Factor V Leiden (resistance to activated protein C) increases the risk of myocardial infarction in young women. *Blood* 1997;89:2817–2821.

703. Girelli D, Russo C, Ferraresi P, et al. Polymorphisms in the factor VII gene and the risk of myocardial infarction in patients with coronary artery disease. *N Engl J Med* 2000;343:774–780.

704. Iacoviello L, Di Castelnuovo A, De Knijff P, et al. Polymor-

phisms in the coagulation factor VII gene and the risk of myocardial infarction. *N Engl J Med* 1998;338:79–85.

705. Feng D, Tofler GH, Larson MG, et al. Factor VII gene polymorphism, factor VII levels, and prevalent cardiovascular disease: the Framingham Heart Study. *Arterioscler Thromb Vasc Biol* 2000;20:593–600.

706. Mennen LI, de Maat MP, Meijer G, et al. Postprandial response of activated factor VII in elderly women depends on the R353Q polymorphism. *Am J Clin Nutr* 1999;70:435–438.

707. Kohler HP, Stickland MH, Ossei-Gerning N, et al. Association of a common polymorphism in the factor XIII gene with myocardial infarction. *Thromb Haemost* 1998;79:8–13.

708. Wartiovaara U, Perola M, Mikkola H, et al. Association of FXIII Val34Leu with decreased risk of myocardial infarction in Finnish males. *Atherosclerosis* 1999;142:295–300.

709. Undas A, Sydor WJ, Brummel K, et al. Aspirin alters the cardioprotective effects of the factor XIII Val34Leu polymorphism. *Circulation* 2003;107:17–20.

710. Aleksic N, Ahn C, Wang YW, et al. Factor XIIIA Val34Leu polymorphism does not predict risk of coronary heart disease: the Atherosclerosis Risk in Communities (ARIC) Study. *Arterioscler Thromb Vasc Biol* 2002;22:348–352.

711. Willeit J, Kiechl S, Weimer T, et al. Marburg I polymorphism of factor VII-activating protease: a prominent risk predictor of carotid stenosis. *Circulation* 2003;107:667–670.

712. Ridker PM, Hennekens CH, Lindpaintner K, et al. Arterial and venous thrombosis is not associated with the 4G/5G polymorphism in the promoter of the plasminogen activator inhibitor gene in a large cohort of US men. *Circulation* 1997;95:59–62.

713. Roest M, van der Schouw YT, Banga JD, et al. Plasminogen activator inhibitor 4G polymorphism is associated with decreased risk of cerebrovascular mortality in older women. *Circulation* 2000;101:67–70.

714. Kroll H, Gardemann A, Fechter A, et al. The impact of the glycoprotein Ia collagen receptor subunit A1648G gene polymorphism on coronary artery disease and acute myocardial infarction. *Thromb Haemost* 2000;83:392–396.

715. Santoso S, Kunicki TJ, Kroll H, et al. Association of the platelet glycoprotein Ia C807T gene polymorphism with nonfatal myocardial infarction in younger patients. *Blood* 1999;93:2449–2453.

716. Anderson JL, King GJ, Bair TL, et al. Associations between a polymorphism in the gene encoding glycoprotein IIIa and myocardial infarction or coronary artery disease. *J Am Coll Cardiol* 1999;33:727–733.

717. Mikkelsson J, Perola M, Laippala P, et al. Glycoprotein IIIa PI(A1/A2) polymorphism and sudden cardiac death. *J Am Coll Cardiol* 2000;36:1317–1323.

718. Ireland H, Kunz G, Kyriakoulis K, et al. Thrombomodulin gene mutations associated with myocardial infarction. *Circulation* 1997;96:15–18.

719. Li Y-H, Chen J-H, Wu H-L, et al. G-33A mutation in the promoter region of thrombomodulin gene and its association with coronary artery disease and plasma soluble thrombomodulin levels. *Am J Cardiol* 2000;85:8–12.

720. Wu KK, Aleksic N, Ahn C, et al. Thrombomodulin Ala455Val polymorphism and risk of coronary heart disease. *Circulation* 2001;103:1386–1389.

721. Anderson JL, Habashi J, Carlquist JF, et al. A common

variant of the AMPD1 gene predicts improved cardiovascular survival in patients with coronary artery disease. *J Am Coll Cardiol* 2000;36:1248–1252.

722. Zhang B, Ye S, Herrmann SM, et al. Functional polymorphism in the regulatory region of gelatinase B gene in relation to severity of coronary atherosclerosis. *Circulation* 1999;99:1788–1794.

723. Herrmann SM, Whatling C, Brand E, et al. Polymorphisms of the human matrix gla protein (MGP) gene, vascular calcification, and myocardial infarction. *Arterioscler Thromb Vasc Biol* 2000;20:2386–2393.

724. Ledmyr H, Karpe F, Lundahl B, et al. Variants of the microsomal triglyceride transfer protein gene are associated with plasma cholesterol levels and body mass index. *J Lipid Res* 2002;43:51–58.

725. Ledmyr H, McMahon AD, Ehrenborg E, et al. The microsomal triglyceride transfer protein -493T allele confers increased risk of coronary heart disease. *Circulation* 2002;106(suppl II):II–746.

726. Couture P, Otvos JD, Cupples LA, et al. Absence of association between genetic variation in the promoter of the microsomal triglyceride transfer protein gene and plasma lipoproteins in the Framingham Offspring Study. *Atherosclerosis* 2000;148:337–343.

APPENDIX 6–1   A QUESTIONNAIRE FOR OBTAINING A DETAILED LIPID FAMILY HISTORY[*]

Medical Family History   *This section is important. Please complete it as accurately as possible*

RELATIONSHIP	First Name	Living (L) or Dead (D)	Age (now or at death)	CAUSE OF DEATH IF DECEASED	HEART ATTACK	CORONARY BYPASS SURGERY	CORONARY ANGIOPLASTY (PTCA)	STROKE	HIGH BLOOD PRESSURE (treated)	DIABETES	CIGARETTES (C)urrent (F)ormer (N)ever	WEIGHT (A)verage (O)verweight 50+ lbs	Total Cholesterol	Triglycerides	HDL Cholesterol
Example	John	D	70	Heart Attack	50	52			40		C	A	255	140	35
You															
Father															
Mother															
Bro / Sis															
Bro / Sis															
Bro / Sis															
Bro / Sis															
Bro / Sis															
Spouse															
Son / Dau															
Son / Dau															
Son / Dau															
Son / Dau															
Pat GF															
Pat GM															
Pat A / U															
Pat A / U															
Pat A / U															
Pat A / U															
Pat A / U															
Mat GF															
Mat GM															
Mat A / U															
Mat A / U															
Mat A / U															
Mat A / U															
Mat A / U															

Header instructions (left block): List all relatives, not just those with problems. Please make an effort to obtain as much information as possible. **Give approximate age for first occurrence or diagnosis for each disease or problem listed.** See the example provided. **You may need to call your relatives for missing information. Circle either Bro / Sis, Son / Dau, A / U for gender.**

AGE OF FIRST OCCURRENCE

BLOOD LEVELS: List the worst levels known - highest serum cholesterol, triglycerides. Approximate levels may be listed. Phone calls may be necessary to verify.

[*]It may often take about 6 months of writing letters and making phone calls to collect all of this information from the relatives listed. Once collected, this information usually leads to a specific diagnosis and also identifies affected relatives needing treatment.

Key: Pat = paternal, Mat = maternal, GF = grandfather, GM = grandmother, A = aunt, U = uncle.

Source: Reproduced with permission from Cardiovascular Genetics Research, University of Utah, Salt Lake City, UT.

Hypertension

7

William J. Elliott
Henry R. Black

KEY POINTS

- *Blood pressure, especially systolic blood pressure, has a strong, positive, and continuous relationship with the risk of future coronary heart disease and stroke. High blood pressure (or "hypertension") is currently diagnosed if the systolic blood pressure is 140 mm Hg or higher, if the diastolic blood pressure is 90 mm Hg or higher, or if the person is taking antihypertensive medications.*

- *Although hypertension is but one of several major risk factors for cardiovascular disease, its importance as a global public health problem is expected to increase in the near future; currently about half of all heart attacks and two thirds of strokes worldwide are attributed to high blood pressure.*

- *Clinical trials have demonstrated that lowering blood pressure significantly reduces the risk of cardiovascular events and end-stage renal disease. In head-to-head comparisons, the most*

- *effective initial treatment has been a low-dose diuretic, although usually more than one drug is required to achieve the blood pressure goal.*

- *Most patients with newly diagnosed hypertension do not need an extensive evaluation before starting therapy, usually with a low-dose diuretic.*

- *The recommended blood pressure targets during therapy are less than 140/90 mm Hg for uncomplicated hypertensive patients and less than 130/80 mm Hg for diabetics and patients with worse than stage 2 chronic kidney disease.*

- *Achieving and maintaining controlled blood pressure is a chronic clinical challenge that requires cooperation of the patient, health care provider, pharmacy, and health plan. Currently, only 34% of Americans have controlled hypertension, although some managed care organizations and specialty clinics have reported better results.*

High blood pressure (BP), or "hypertension," is responsible for more deaths than any other risk factor for cardiovascular disease (CVD), which is already the leading cause of death and disability in the developed world, and is expected to become the leading cause of death and disability worldwide by the year 2020.[1–3] Compared with other risk factors for stroke, acute myocardial infarction, and heart failure, hypertension is among the simplest to diagnose, has the widest range of therapies, and (particularly in high-risk individuals) lends itself to the most cost-effective preventive strategy.[4] Because of its high prevalence (eg, 28.7% of adults) in the United States,[4] hypertension ranks first among the chronic conditions for which Americans visit a health care provider.[5] Among the major reasons for the impressive reduction in age-adjusted stroke mortality (~62%) and coronary heart disease mortality (~45%) in the United States since 1972 is the widespread acceptance of the need to treat hypertension and our increased ability to reduce BP effectively.

DEFINITION AND CLASSIFICATION OF HYPERTENSION

From 1974 to 1993, hypertension in the United States was defined using only a criterion of diastolic BP ≥ 90 mm Hg, and was classified as "mild, moderate, or severe." Since then, burgeoning evidence from both epidemiologic studies[6] and clinical trials[7] has demonstrated that systolic BP is a better predictor of future CVD and renal events than are diastolic or pulse pressure. Since the Fifth Report of the Joint National Committee on Detection, Evaluation, and Treatment of High Blood Pressure in 1993 (JNC-V), the classification scheme used in the United States has included both systolic and diastolic BP (Table 7-1). JNC-V, -VI and now -7 indicate that hypertension should be diagnosed if *either* the systolic BP is 140 mm Hg or higher or the diastolic BP is 90 mm Hg or higher. In addition, these reports have abandoned the descriptive classifications ("mild," "moderate," and "severe") in favor of a staging system, similar to that used in oncology. Many authorities felt that the term *mild hypertension* was especially inappropriate, as stage 1 hypertension describes about 70% of those diagnosed with hypertension, and accounts (on a population basis) for well more than half the deaths and disability attributed to hypertension. The "cut points" for the stages of hypertension were chosen to reflect roughly equal future CVD or renal risk. A diastolic reading of 100 mm Hg carries about the same prognostic importance as a systolic reading of 160 mm Hg. When the systolic and diastolic readings for a given patient fall into different stages, the BP is classified based on the higher stage. For instance, both 162/94 mm Hg and 142/104 mm Hg should now be properly placed in stage 2 (see Table 7-1), the former because of the systolic reading, and the latter because of the diastolic elevation. Although hypertension is more common in older women (Fig. 7-1), the current classification of hypertension is not modified by either age or gender. In large populations, systolic BP increases with age, but the diastolic pressure tends to decrease after the sixth decade.

JNC-7 has made two major changes to the system for classification of hypertension.[4] In the current scheme (Table 7-1), there are only two stages of hypertension (stage 1 and stage 2), with the latter defined at or above the cut points of 160 mm Hg for systolic or 100 mm Hg for diastolic. This was done because the prevalence of higher levels is very small in the general population, and because prognosis depends more on the BP achieved during treatment than the BP before treatment.[7] The second major change was introduction of the term *prehypertension* to characterize those with what was formerly called either "borderline hypertension," "high-normal blood pressure," or "normal blood pressure." The primary reason for this was the finding that, in the Framingham Heart Study (Fig. 7-2), individuals with BPs greater than 120/80 mm Hg had a graded increase in CVD risk, compared with those with what was formerly called "optimal blood pressure" (<120/80 mm Hg).[8] The other reason for choosing the new term *prehypertension* was the finding that, in Framingham, approximately 90% of people aged 55 to 65 with BPs of 120/80 mm Hg or higher develop hypertension (≥140/90 mm Hg) if they live 25 years.[9]

In recent years, pulse pressure (systolic minus diastolic pressure) has also been associated with higher risk of CVD and renal events, especially in older people. In the absence of aortic insufficiency, an arteriovenous fistula, and other uncommon conditions, a wide pulse pressure is often a marker for noncompliant, and often atherosclerotic, large arteries. In several studies, pulse pressure was a better predictor of heart failure, mortality, heart attack, stroke, and all CVD events than either mean arterial or systolic pressure alone.[10–12] However, the largest meta-analysis (which included 61 epidemiologic studies and more than a million persons) showed no significant additional prognostic value of pulse pressure over systolic BP.[6]

MEASUREMENT OF BLOOD PRESSURE

Currently, terminology first introduced by Nicolai Korotkoff in 1905 is used: systolic BP is recognized when clear and repetitive tapping sounds are heard; diastolic BP is recorded when the sounds disappear. Only when audible sounds are heard down to 0 mm Hg is the "muffling" of sound (Korotkoff phase IV) recorded, between the systolic reading and zero (eg, 178/72/0).

Techniques of measuring blood pressure

The proper technique of accurate BP measurement is typically taught very early during medical training, but seldom followed thereafter. Many expert panels have made recommendations regarding methodology of BP measurement,[13] and these frequently do not agree in all details, but they share several general principles:

TABLE 7-1 JNC-7 Classification of Blood Pressures

Category	Systolic (mm Hg)		Diastolic (mm Hg)
Normal	<120	and	<80
Prehypertension	120–139	or	80–89
Stage 1 hypertension	140–159	or	90–99
Stage 2 hypertension	≥160	or	≥100

SOURCE: Modified from JNC-7.[4]

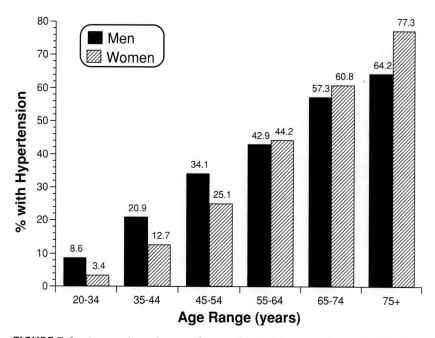

FIGURE 7-1 Age- and gender-specific prevalence of hypertension in the Third National Health and Nutrition Examination Survey (Part 1, 1988–1991). In this large epidemiologic study, nearly 9901 Americans had a blood pressure measurement taken at their homes by specially trained nurses; hypertension was defined as blood pressure ≥ 140/90 mm Hg or taking antihypertensive medication. (Modified from Burt VL, et al. Prevalence of hypertension in the U.S. adult population: results from the Third National Health and Nutritional Examination Survey, 1988–91. *Hypertension* 1995;25:305–313.)

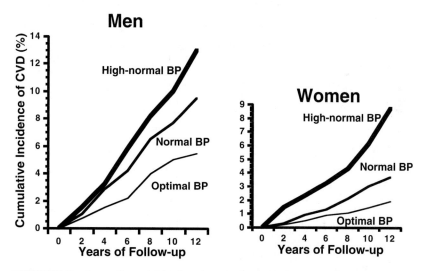

FIGURE 7-2 Age-adjusted risk of cardiovascular disease (CVD) events for men (left) and women (right) with various levels of initial blood pressures in the Framingham Heart Study. The terminology used is that of JNC-VI (high-normal BP: 130–139/85–89 mm Hg; normal BP: 120–129/80–84 mm Hg; optimal BP: <120/80 mm Hg). The elevated CVD risk for those with "high-normal BP and normal BP," as compared with "optimal BP" was one of the major reasons for the new term *prehypertension* in JNC-7. (Modified from Vasan et al.[8])

- The cuff size appropriate for the patient's arm circumference should be used. The deflation rate of the column of mercury should be 2 to 3 mm Hg/s.
- Multiple measurements should be made on different occasions to decide if a person should have his or her BP lowered. In research, the average of the second and third readings is typically used for treatment decisions.

BP measurements are intrinsically quite variable. Several steps can be taken to minimize this, including:

- Taking multiple measurements, especially when the pulse is irregular. Quality assurance auditors typically transcribe only the lowest recorded BP reading at a given visit, irrespective of position or arm.
- Centering the bladder of the cuff over the brachial artery, with its lower edge within 2.5 cm of the antecubital fossa. Have the subject rest silently and comfortably (with back support if seated) for at least 5 minutes before a measurement.
- Having the patient abstain from drinking caffeine or alcohol-containing beverages or using tobacco within 30 minutes prior to a BP measurement.
- Measuring BP when the rectum and bladder are not full. The arm is supported at the level of the heart.
- Listening over the brachial artery using the bell of the stethoscope with minimal pressure exerted on the skin. The cuff is inflated 20 mm Hg higher than the pressure at which the palpable pulse at the radial artery disappears. A properly calibrated sphygmomanometer should be used.
- Attempting to avoid "terminal digit preference" (more than 20% of measurements end with a specific even digit).
- Measuring BP in both arms initially and in the arm with the higher BP thereafter if the difference is greater than 10/5 mm Hg.

Home blood pressure measurements

Technology for accurate and reproducible BP measurements outside the traditional medical environment has improved greatly over the last 35 years.[14] Many convenient, inexpensive, and relatively accurate machines are now available. Some authorities feel such devices should be provided to every person with elevated BP, but others are concerned about their widespread use, as clinical trials have seldom based their decision making solely on this method of measuring BP.

Home BP readings are typically lower than measurements taken in the traditional medical environment (by about 12/7 mm Hg on average[14]), even in normotensive subjects. Home readings are better correlated with both the extent of target-organ damage and the risk of future mortality, than are readings taken in the health care provider's office. Home readings can also be helpful in evaluating symptoms suggestive of hypotension, especially if intermittent or infrequent. During treatment, reliable home readings can lower costs by substituting for multiple visits to health care providers.

Home BP readings should be interpreted cautiously, carefully, and conservatively. Many of the factors that contribute to BP variability (discussed above) are more difficult to control in the home environment, including intrinsic circadian variation, food and alcohol ingestion, exercise, and stress. If home readings are taken, the instrument should be calibrated against a standard sphygmomanometer using a Y-tube, and the technique of the measurer must be checked. Several reports claim benefit to supplementing office BP measurements with home readings.[15,16] Prognosis is better predicted by home readings compared with one or two "casual" office BP measurements. Several long-term studies have shown that people with much lower home BP readings (compared with those at the physician's office) suffer fewer major CVD events than people who have elevated readings both in the office and at home.[17-19]

Ambulatory blood pressure monitoring

Extensive research has better defined the role of automatic recorders that measure BP frequently over a 24-hour period during a person's usual daily activities (including sleep).[20] The clinical use of these devices in the United States was extremely limited until April 1, 2002, when the Center for Medicare and Medicaid Services authorized reimbursement at the federal level (approximately $40–55 per session) for ambulatory BP monitoring, only when performed for the evaluation of "white coat hypertension."[21] Despite the low level of reimbursement, this decision may remove one of the barriers to more widespread use of this important diagnostic modality. As a research tool, the advantages and disadvantages of ambulatory blood pressure monitoring (ABPM) have been well documented (Table 7-2), normal values have been defined (Table 7-3),[22,23] and publications correlating abnormal results of ABPM with adverse outcomes have appeared.[24-26] Several expert panels have defined the special situations in which ABPM is particularly useful (Table 7-4).[27,28]

Several varieties of ABPM devices are currently available. In the United States, those that measure BP indirectly (ie, without arterial cannulation) use either an auscultatory or an oscillometric technique. In the former type a microphone is placed over the artery to detect Korotkoff sounds in the traditional fashion. The latter technique is used to measure biophysical oscillations of the brachial artery, which are compared (using a standardized algorithm) with those measured with a mercury sphygmomanometer: systolic BP is determined directly

TABLE 7-2 Advantages and Disadvantages of Ambulatory Blood Pressure Monitoring

Advantages
Measures blood pressure (BP) frequently during 24-h period
Measures diurnal variation (including BPs during sleep).
Measures BP during daily activities
Can identify and diagnose "white-coat hypertension"
No "alerting response"
Little, if any, placebo effect
Better correlation with target-organ damage than other methods of BP measurement
Disadvantages
Cost
Limited availability of equipment
Disruption of daily activities due to noise or discomfort (eg, sleep quality, need to keep arm flaccid during measurement)
Lack of evidence-based guidelines for treatment
Few long-term prospective studies demonstrating utility compared with traditional (and much less expensive) methods of BP measurement

SOURCE: Modified from Elliott WJ, Black HR. Special situations in the management of hypertension. In: Hollenberg NK, ed. *Atlas of Hypertension*. 4th ed. Philadelphia: Current Medicine; 2003: 257–281.

TABLE 7-3 American Society of Hypertension Thresholds for Home and Ambulatory Blood Pressure Monitoring

BP measure	Probably normal	Borderline	Probably abnormal
Systolic Average (mm Hg)			
Awake	<135	135–140	>140
Asleep	<120	120–125	>125
24 h	<130	130–135	>135
Diastolic Average (mm Hg)			
Awake or asleep	<85	85–89	>90
24 h	<80	80–85	>85
Systolic load* (%)			
Awake or asleep	<15	15–30	>30
Diastolic load† (%)			
Awake	<15	15–30	>30
Asleep	<15	15–30	>30

*Percentage of systolic BP measurements above 140 mm Hg.
†Percentage of diastolic BP measurements above 90 mm Hg.

SOURCE: Modified from Pickering T. Recommendations for the use of home (self) and ambulatory blood pressure monitoring. *Am J Hypertens* 1995;9:1–11.

TABLE 7-4 Uses of Ambulatory Blood Pressure Monitoring

Diagnosis and prognosis
Evaluation of suspected "white-coat" hypertension
Evaluation of refractory or resistant hypertension
Evaluation of circadian pattern of blood pressure
Symptoms
Evaluation of dizziness, presyncope, and syncope
Evaluation of relationship of blood pressure to clinical symptoms
Evaluation of antihypertensive agents (research-based)
Evaluation of trough:peak ratios
Evaluation of antihypertensive efficacy
Evaluation of effects of timing of dosing of antihypertensive agents

SOURCE: Modified from Elliott WJ, Black HR. Diagnosis and management of patients with hypertension. In: Goldman L, Braunwald E, eds. *Cardiology for the Primary Care Physician.* 2nd ed. New York: WB Saunders, 2003:277–304.

from the threshold oscillation, mean arterial pressure is estimated, and diastolic BP is calculated. Both types of monitors are lightweight (<450 g), simple to apply and use, accurate, relatively quiet and tolerable, and powered by two to four small batteries. Data from 80 to 120 measurements of BP and pulse typically are stored in a small microprocessor and then downloaded into a desktop computer, which then edits the readings and prints the report.

ABPM makes it possible to measure BP routinely during sleep and has reawakened interest in the circadian variation of heart rate and BP. Most normotensive and perhaps 80% of hypertensive persons have at least a 10% drop in BP during sleep compared with the daytime average. Although there may be some important demographic confounders (blacks and the elderly have less prominent "dips"[29]), several prospective studies have shown an increased risk of cardiovascular events (and proteinuria in type 1 diabetics[30]) among those with a nocturnal "nondipping" BP or pulse pattern.[24,31–33] Several Japanese studies have raised concern that elderly persons with more than a 20% difference between nighttime and daytime average BPs ("excessive dippers") may suffer unrecognized ischemia in "watershed areas" (of the brain and other organs) during sleep if their BP declines below the autoregulatory threshold.[25,34,35]

Compared with other methods of measuring BP, ABPM readings are most strongly associated with the prevalence and extent of target-organ damage (TOD) in hypertensive individuals. Compared with "casual" BP measurements (obtained in the health care provider's office), ABPM measurements are a better predictor of left ventricular hypertrophy, cardiac function, and overall scores summing optic, carotid, cardiac, renal, and peripheral vascular damage resulting from hypertension. Ambulatory BP monitoring is probably also the only way to identify "white coat normotensives." This term describes a small minority of patients who have normal BP readings in the physician's office but elevated ABPM readings with left ventricular hypertrophy and carotid wall thickening similar to that usually seen in sustained hypertensives.[36] Perhaps the most important data demonstrating the value of ABPM come from studies of CVD events (eg, death, myocardial infarction, stroke). In the initial Italian study, ABPM was the best predictor of CVD events; "nondipper hypertensives" had approximately three times the risk of hypertensives whose BP was at least 10% lower at night compared with daytime ("dippers"). A population-based study of ABPM versus casual and home BPs in 1572 Japanese showed, after an average of approximately 5 years of follow-up, no significant relationship between one casual BP measurement and future CVD mortality. However, there was a highly significantly increased risk of CVD death in the quintile with the highest ABPM, and the lowest risk was found in those in the lowest quintile of ABPM.[37] The value of ABPM in refractory hypertension was demonstrated in another study of 86 hypertensive people taking an average of three antihypertensive medications daily.[38] Approximately 4 years after the ABPM, the patients having average BPs in the lowest tertile had significantly lower rates of CVD complications: 2.2 versus 9.5 versus 13.5 events per 100 patient-years. These data suggest that ABPM may be helpful in sorting out which patients with elevated office BP measurements who already are taking multiple antihypertensive medications ought to have intensified treatment and which ones can be spared the additional expense and risk. In the placebo-treated group of 808 patients in the Systolic Hypertension in Europe (Syst-EUR) trial who had ABPM in addition to the usual clinic BP measurements, ABPM was clearly a better predictor of future CV events than was the office BP measurement.[24]

White coat hypertension

According to several ABPM studies, approximately 10 to 20% of hypertensive Americans have substantially lower BP measurements outside the health care provider's office than in it (so-called "white coat hypertension"). The "white coat" itself is unlikely to be the only factor that increases BP. Careful studies originally done in Italy (and now corroborated elsewhere) show that BP rises in response to an approaching physician who is not previously known to the subject. The acute elevation in BP apparently is less marked if the subject is approached by a nurse, even if he or she is wearing a white coat. The pathophysiologic and psychologic "reasons" for this exaggerated BP response are uncertain.[39]

The clinical consequences and prognostic significance of white coat hypertension are controversial. One point of view suggests that if a person has an acute rise in BP due to "stress" from an approaching physician, similar elevations in BP are likely whenever any stressful stimulus is encountered. In several convenience samples and population-based studies, people with white coat hypertension had a greater prevalence of subclinical CVD risk factors, including: left ventricular hypertrophy, family history of hypertension and heart disease, hypertriglyceridemia, elevated fasting insulin levels, and lower high-density lipoprotein (HDL-C) levels.[40–44]

A minority view, based on more conservative definitions of the "white coat effect," proposes that some individuals consistently show a similar and marked elevation in BP in response to the health care environment. Several long-term observational studies have shown a greatly reduced risk of either TOD or major CVD among people with lower BPs measured either at home or by 24-hour

BP monitoring, as compared with measurements taken in the same person in the physician's office.[17,45] An intermediate viewpoint is that white coat hypertension is merely regression to the mean among the subset of patients with high BP variability.

The best treatment for white coat hypertension is still unclear. Individuals with white coat hypertension should benefit from lifestyle modifications, which presumably would reduce the probability of progression to sustained hypertension. Complete abstention from antihypertensive medication by white coat hypertensives appears unwise.[46] In the largest series of patients studied over the long term, the risk of future CVD events did not differ between white coat and sustained hypertensives, assuming both were treated with antihypertensive medications.[19]

BLOOD PRESSURE AND CARDIOVASCULAR RISK

Several large, representative surveys of the noninstitutionalized civilian US population indicate that BP is nearly normally distributed (Fig. 7-3). Very few individuals have BPs in excess of 210/120 mm Hg. As a result,

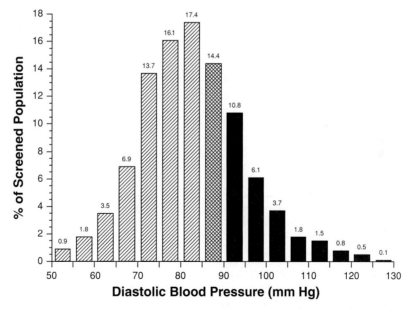

FIGURE 7-3   Distribution of diastolic blood pressures (measured in the home) of a representative sample of about 157,000 untreated, noninstitutionalized, civilian citizens of the United States in the First National Health and Nutritional Evaluation Survey (NHANES-I). In 1974–1977, hypertension was diagnosed in those with diastolic blood pressures ≥ 90 mm Hg (dark bars, 25.3% of the population); high-normal blood pressure was diagnosed in those with diastolic pressures between 85 and 89 mm Hg (cross-hatched bar, 14.4% of the population). (Modified from *Circ Res* 1977;40(suppl 1):1106–1109.)

"stage 4 hypertension" of JNC-V was removed in JNC-VI and incorporated into stage 3; a similar rationale was followed to combine stages 2 and 3 of JNC-VI into stage 2 hypertension of JNC-7.

The first estimates of how much hypertension predisposes to heart attack, heart failure, stroke, and other CVD events were derived from prospective epidemiologic surveys. Perhaps the most well known of these in the United States is the Framingham Heart Study, involving 5209 healthy men and women who were extensively evaluated initially, and then followed over time. After a sufficient number had events, a quantitative estimate could be made of the importance of hypertension in the development of these events, even after adjusting statistically for the presence of other risk factors (eg, elevated plasma lipid levels, smoking). Data have now been pooled from this and 60 other observational and epidemiologic databases, and have firmly established *a strong, positive, and continuous relationship* (Fig. 7-4) between initial BP and future risk of death from ischemic heart disease.[6] Within each decade of life, for each BP increase of 20/10 mm Hg, beginning at 115/75 mm Hg, the risk of ischemic heart disease-related death *doubles*.[6] Similar graphs exist showing a similar direct, positive, and continuous relationship between initial BP and future risk of fatal stroke or other vascular death.[6]

Perhaps more important than epidemiologic and observational studies of large numbers of people that correlate risk of death from heart disease with BP levels many years earlier are the results of randomized clinical trials that show, separately and in aggregate, that antihypertensive drug therapy reduces the risk of CVD events over a 4- to 6-year time frame. Most impressive are the results of early studies comparing placebo or no treatment with antihypertensive drugs (typically diuretics and/or beta blockers in older studies, although a few studies with angiotensin-converting enzyme (ACE) inhibitors or calcium antagonists exist). Figure 7-5 shows the results of

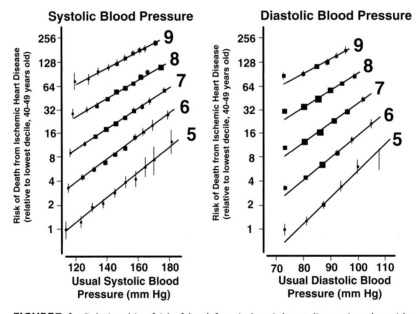

FIGURE 7-4 Relationship of risk of death from ischemic heart disease (on a logarithmic scale) and the initial blood pressures (systolic at left, diastolic at right) measured at the beginning of each decade of life (given at the top left of each line, from 40 to 89 years) in nearly 1 million participants in 61 epidemiologic studies. Larger boxes indicate estimates with smaller 95% confidence intervals, which are indicated for smaller boxes by the vertical lines. The total number of fatal ischemic cardiac deaths was 30,143. The best-fit regression line for each decade of life ignores the point corresponding to the lowest blood pressure (<115/70 mm Hg), which includes some individuals with *very* low blood pressures. These age-specific regression lines demonstrate the *strong, positive, and continuous* relationship between blood pressure and risk of death from ischemic heart disease. (Modified from the Prospective Studies Collaborative.[6])

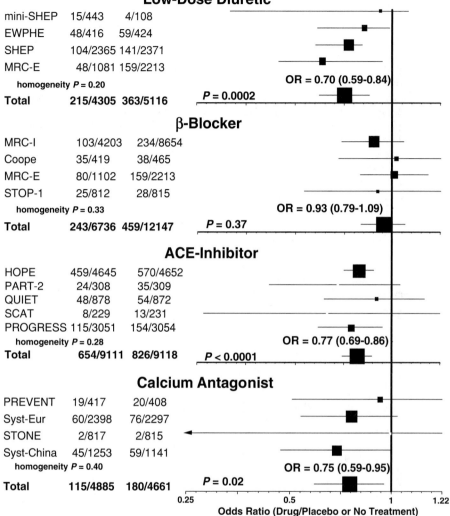

Low-Dose Diuretic

mini-SHEP	15/443	4/108
EWPHE	48/416	59/424
SHEP	104/2365	141/2371
MRC-E	48/1081	159/2213
homogeneity P = 0.20		OR = 0.70 (0.59-0.84)
Total	215/4305	363/5116	P = 0.0002

β-Blocker

MRC-I	103/4203	234/8654
Coope	35/419	38/465
MRC-E	80/1102	159/2213
STOP-1	25/812	28/815
homogeneity P = 0.33		OR = 0.93 (0.79-1.09)
Total	243/6736	459/12147	P = 0.37

ACE-Inhibitor

HOPE	459/4645	570/4652
PART-2	24/308	35/309
QUIET	48/878	54/872
SCAT	8/229	13/231
PROGRESS	115/3051	154/3054
homogeneity P = 0.28		OR = 0.77 (0.69-0.86)
Total	654/9111	826/9118	P < 0.0001

Calcium Antagonist

PREVENT	19/417	20/408
Syst-Eur	60/2398	76/2297
STONE	2/817	2/815
Syst-China	45/1253	59/1141
homogeneity P = 0.40		OR = 0.75 (0.59-0.95)
Total	115/4885	180/4661	P = 0.02

0.25   0.5   1   1.22
Odds Ratio (Drug/Placebo or No Treatment)

FIGURE 7-5   Results of a meta-analysis of clinical trials involving placebo or no treatment, compared with an initial low-dose diuretic, beta blocker, ACE inhibitor, or calcium antagonist, in the prevention of coronary heart disease. (Updated from Elliott WJ. Cardiovascular events during long-term antihypertensive drug treatment: Meta-analysis of four major drug classes vs. placebo or no treatment [abstract]. *Am J Hypertension*, 2003;16:113A.) The four studies that used a low-dose diuretic (LD diuretic) were: mini-SHEP (feasibility study for the Systolic Hypertension in the Elderly Program, *Stroke* 1989;20:4–13); SHEP (Systolic Hypertension in the Elderly Program, *JAMA* 1991;265:3255–3264); MRC-E (Medical Research Council Trial in the Elderly, *BMJ* 1992;304:405–412); and EWPHE (European Working Party on Hypertension in the Elderly, *Lancet* 1985;1:1349–1354). The four studies that used a beta blocker were: MRC-1 (Medical Research Council Trial of Treatment of Mild Hypertension, *BMJ (Clin Res)* 1985;291:97–104); Coope and Warrender (*BMJ* 1986;293:1145–1151); STOP-Hypertension (Swedish Trial of Older Persons with Hypertension, *Lancet* 1991;338:1281–1285); and MRC-E (Medical Research Council Trial in the Elderly, *BMJ* 1992;304:405–412). The five studies that used an ACE inhibitor were: HOPE (*N Engl J Med* 2000;342:145–153); (Contd.)

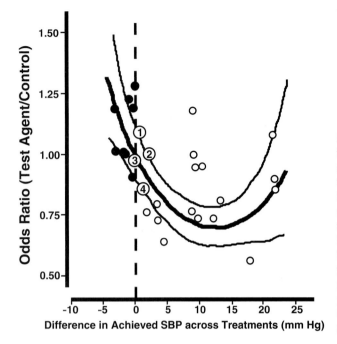

FIGURE 7-6 Relationship of the odds ratio for fatal or nonfatal myocardial infarction (y axis, test agent/control) to the achieved difference in systolic blood pressure between randomized groups (control vs test agent) in 27 clinical trials (placebo control represented by open circles, active control by filled circles) and 4 recently reported studies (numbered circles). The regression line (and its 95% confidence intervals) are plotted for data from the 27 older clinical trials. The recently reported studies are: (1) LIFE, (2) ALLHAT (lisinopril vs chlorthalidone), (3) ALLHAT (amlodipine vs chlorthalidone), (4) CONVINCE. Updated from Staessen et al.[7]

a meta-analysis of clinical trials that compared placebo or no treatment with low-dose diuretics, beta blockers, calcium antagonists, and ACE inhibitors in the prevention of coronary heart disease events (primarily fatal and nonfatal myocardial infarction). With the possible exception of beta blockers (largely because of an inhomogeneity due to the Medical Research Council Trial in the Elderly), antihypertensive drug therapy was associated with a significantly reduced risk of coronary heart disease events.

The most persuasive evidence in favor of the link between BP and coronary heart disease events in clinical trials was gathered from a meta-regression analysis of 27 clinical trials involving more than 136,124 patients.[7] The differences in myocardial infarction rates across randomized treatment groups in these trials was not at all explained by the initial BPs of the participants in each trial

$(r^2 = .02, P = .37)$, but was instead highly significantly correlated with differences across groups in achieved systolic BPs $(r^2 = .53, P = .0005)$ (Fig. 7-6).[7] It is likely that when the more recently completed clinical trials (LIFE, ALLHAT, CONVINCE, INVEST, discussed below) are included in a similar regression analysis, this conclusion will become even stronger.

These data (both epidemiologic and those derived from clinical trials) have several important consequences for the treatment of BP in individual patients. First, BP is only a "risk factor," strongly affecting the probability that a given person will develop CVD, but *not* a central *cause* of this problem. The sensitivity and specificity of BP are low: not everyone with a high reading will eventually have an event, just as, regrettably, not every person with a "normal" BP will be spared. Any strategy that attempts to fix a value above which everyone

←

FIGURE 7-5 (Contd.) PART-2 (Prevention of Atherosclerosis with Ramipril Trial 2, *J Am Coll Cardiol* 2000;36:438–443); QUIET (Quinapril Ischemic Events Trial, *Am J Cardiol* 2001;87:1058–1063); SCAT (Simvastatin/Enalapril Coronary Atherosclerosis Trial, *Circulation* 2000;102:1748–1754); PROGRESS (Perindopril Protection Against Recurrent Stroke Study, *Lancet* 2001;358:1033–1041). The four studies that used a calcium antagonist were: Syst-EUR (Systolic Hypertension in Europe, *Lancet* 1997;360:757–764); Syst-China (Systolic Hypertension in China, *J Hypertens* 1998;16:1823–1829); PREVENT (Prospective Randomized Evaluation of the Vascular Events of Norvasc Trial, *Circulation* 2000;102:1503–1510); STONE (Shanghai Trial of Nifedipine in the Elderly, *Hypertension* 1996;14:1237–1245).

should receive treatment is unlikely to be successful and cost-effective. The strategy recommended below is based on estimates of absolute risk, which can now be easily calculated for an individual, and requires (eg, for the Framingham Risk Equation recommended by the National Cholesterol Education Program[47]) only the age, gender, systolic BP, tobacco habit, and total cholesterol and HDL-C levels. People with only modest BP and no other risk factors are at such low risk that preventing even one event with therapy would require many thousands to be treated. Such treatment "wastes" the time and effort of the vast majority, and puts them at risk for side events related to it. Conversely, hypertensive diabetics are at such high risk of CVD that treatment can be justified even if the initial BP is the only risk factor that is elevated.

BRIEF REVIEW OF OUTCOME-BASED CLINICAL TRIALS

Because so much information about hypertension and its treatment has been derived from clinical trials, many excellent, evidence-based recommendations can now be made about its diagnosis and management.[4] Although details of many of the older studies are available in an excellent monograph,[48] the results of most of these trials have been combined and summarized in other forms (eg, meta-analyses[49,50]).

In the early 1990s, the most frequently cited meta-analysis involving antihypertensive drug therapy compared the observed results of lowering BP in clinical trials with those expected from epidemiologic studies. Although stroke reduction in clinical trials (by about $42 \pm 6\%$) was nearly exactly what would have been expected, prevention of myocardial infarction was substantially less (about $14 \pm 5\%$, compared with the expected 25–28%).[51] This led some to believe that the drugs used in the early trials (nearly exclusively diuretics and/or beta blockers) might be somewhat less effective in preventing heart disease than stroke.

Just prior to publication of the Sixth Report of the Joint National Committee on Prevention, Detection, Evaluation and Treatment of High Blood Pressure, Psaty and co-workers compared the results of 18 clinical trials pitting placebo against either high- or low-dose diuretics or beta blockers. They concluded that beta blockers and high-dose diuretics prevented stroke and heart failure, but low-dose diuretics additionally provided significant protection against coronary disease events and all-cause mortality.[52] They called attention to the lack of long-term outcome data with newer classes of drugs, and suggested that short-acting dihydropyridine calcium antagonists might have been harmful. These conclusions were cited by JNC-VI as central to the recommendation to use low-dose diuretics (and perhaps beta blockers) for uncomplicated hypertension.

During the nearly 5 years between JNC-V and JNC-VI (1993–1997), five major clinical trials in hypertension were published or presented. During the 5.5 years between JNC-VI and JNC-7, there were at least 17 major trials involving antihypertensive drugs; most included one or more of the newer classes of drug therapy about which few data had been available through 1997.

ACE inhibitors

Three of these major trials demonstrated impressive benefits for ACE inhibitors. The first, and most important in terms of impact on prescribing, was the Heart Outcomes Prevention Evaluation (HOPE) study.[53] This international study enrolled 9297 subjects, aged 55 and older, with either current evidence of vascular disease or diabetes and one other CVD risk factor, but without either heart failure or a subnormal ejection fraction. Two randomized treatments (either ramipril, an ACE inhibitor [up to 10 mg/d], or placebo; or vitamin E 400 IU/d or placebo) were provided, in addition to any other appropriate drug therapy (including antihypertensive agents) thought to be indicated by the treating physician. The Data Safety and Monitoring Board halted the study prematurely, because subjects given ramipril had a significant 22% lower risk of the composite primary endpoint (myocardial infarction, stroke, or CVD death). Vitamin E had no beneficial effect. The benefits were alleged to be independent of BP reduction, but this view is not universally shared. The authors claimed that the 3/2 mm Hg average difference in BP between randomized groups during nearly 5 years of treatment could account for perhaps 40% of the observed reduction in stroke and a quarter of the reduction in myocardial infarction. The 3577 diabetics in HOPE were the subject of a separate publication, which showed benefits in CVD event reduction even greater than those of the entire cohort (eg, myocardial infarction, −22%; stroke, −33%; CVD death, −37%).[54]

The second study showing major benefits of an initial ACE inhibitor was the Perindopril Protection Against Recurrent Stroke Study (PROGRESS).[55] This clinical trial was done largely in Australasia and Europe, and involved 6105 patients who had had a stroke or transient ischemic attack in the preceding 5 years. They were randomized to perindopril, an ACE inhibitor (with or without indapamide, a diuretic) or matching placebo(s); the diuretic was recommended as part of the initial treatment strategy, but could be withheld at the discretion of the investigator. The mean BP across groups over 4 years was lower in the group receiving active antihypertensive drugs by 9/4 mm Hg, and was accompanied by a 28% reduction in the risk of recurrent stroke and a 26% reduction in major CVD events. The benefit in secondary stroke prevention was seen across all levels of both systolic and diastolic BPs.

The African American Study of Kidney Diseases and Hypertension (AASK) trial also supported the use of an ACE inhibitor over (first) a dihydropyridine calcium antagonist and (later) a beta blocker.[56,57] In AASK, 1094 nondiabetic African Americans with hypertensive nephrosclerosis were randomized to ramipril, amlodipine, or metoprolol succinate, to which could be added any other antihypertensive agent except an ACE inhibitor, angiotensin receptor blocker (ARB), calcium antagonist, or beta blocker. Although the primary endpoint was decline in glomerular filtration rate (GFR, measured directly by iothalamate clearance), the amlodipine arm was stopped prematurely because of major differences in clinical events (reduction in GFR, end-stage renal disease, or death).[56] Similar, but not quite as striking, conclusions were later provided for comparison of the ACE inhibitor with the beta blocker.[57] These data provided strong support for use of an ACE inhibitor (along with appropriate diuretics) to prevent progressive renal deterioration in African Americans with chronic kidney disease, despite the greater risk of cough and angioedema in this racial/ethnic group.

Calcium antagonists

Since 1995, several epidemiologic and cohort studies have implicated calcium antagonists as being associated with higher rates of myocardial infarction and other adverse outcomes. However, nearly all clinical trials reported thereafter did not verify these allegations, with the exception of heart failure. Syst-China, like Syst-Eur, compared an initial dihydropyridine calcium antagonist (nitrendipine, followed by captopril and hydrochlorothiazide, if needed) with placebo, but (unlike Syst-Eur) was not randomized. It nonetheless showed results very similar to the results of Syst-Eur, with a significant 38% reduction in stroke (as opposed to 42% in Syst-Eur). The conclusions of Syst-China were very strongly supportive of a beneficial role for calcium antagonists in the treatment of hypertension.

Although not a comparative trial of calcium antagonists against another class of drugs, the Hypertension Optimal Treatment (HOT) Study was important, because it compared long-term outcomes in hypertensive patients treated to three different target diastolic BPs.[58] The most intensively treated group had better outcomes in the diabetics, and overall did as well as those treated to the "minimally acceptable level of diastolic BP." One interpretation of these data is that those who received higher doses of the calcium antagonist did NOT have more major CVD events. The alternative argument is that those treated more intensively also received other antihypertensive drugs that may have protected them from the adverse effects of the high-dose calcium antagonist. In any case, the HOT study enrolled the greatest number of patients who received calcium antagonists in a long-term study; most of them appeared to benefit, and there was little evidence of harm.

Three large, actively controlled clinical trials between 1999 and 2000 directly compared the outcome for a calcium antagonist with the outcome of initial therapy with either a diuretic or a beta blocker. The first of these was the Swedish Trial in Older Patients with Hypertension 2 (STOP-Hypertension-2).[59] In this prospective, randomized, open-label, blinded-endpoint (PROBE) study, 6614 hypertensive patients, 70 to 84 years old, were randomized to "conventional therapy" (atenolol 50 mg/d, metoprolol 100 mg/d, pindolol 5 mg/d, or hydrochlorothiazide 25 mg + amiloride 5 mg/d), or a calcium antagonist (felodipine 2.5 or isradipine 2.5 mg/d), or an ACE inhibitor (enalapril 10 or lisinopril 10 mg/d). BP was controlled similarly in all groups by adding either a diuretic (if the initial therapy was either an ACE inhibitor or a beta blocker) or a beta blocker (if the initial therapy was either a diuretic or calcium antagonist). After an average follow-up of 5 years, there was no significant difference between newer and older drugs with respect to any endpoint, leading the authors to conclude that calcium antagonists and ACE inhibitors have similar effects in preventing major CVD events in older hypertensive patients. On further post hoc analysis, there was a 23% lower risk of acute myocardial infarction and a 22% lower risk of heart failure among patients randomized to ACE inhibitors, as compared with those randomized to calcium antagonists.

The International Nifedipine GITS Study: Intervention as a Goal in Hypertension Treatment (INSIGHT) study compared a calcium antagonist and a diuretic.[60] In this study, 6321 hypertensive patients from Europe and Israel with an additional CVD risk factor were randomized to 30 mg of nifedipine GITS or co-amilozide (hydrochlorothiazide 25 mg + amiloride 2.5 mg) once daily. Doses were doubled, if necessary, and atenolol 25 to 50 mg or enalapril 5 to 10 mg could be added to achieve goal BP. Despite nearly identical BP control, the primary outcome (CVD death, myocardial infarction, stroke, or heart failure) was observed in 200 patients in the nifedipine group and 182 in the co-amilozide group (relative risk [RR] = 1.10, 95% confidence interval (CI) = 0.91–1.34, $P = .35$). There were similarly no significant differences between randomized groups with respect to all-cause mortality, nonfatal endpoints, combined primary and secondary endpoints or in stratified analyses according to baseline risk factors (eg, diabetes). Peripheral edema was significantly more common with nifedipine (725 patients vs 518 patients, $P < .0001$), but significantly more serious adverse events occurred in the co-amilozide group (880 vs 796, $P = .02$). The authors suggested that, as the primary results were so similar, the side effects of the drugs may be more important than their effects on CVD morbidity and mortality.

The results of the Nordic Diltiazem (NORDIL) study were published immediately following the INSIGHT results.[61] In this clinical trial with PROBE design, 10,881 previously untreated hypertensive patients, aged 50 to 74 years, with a diastolic BP of 100 mm Hg or higher were randomized to 180 mg/d diltiazem or the physician's choice of a diuretic or beta blocker. An ACE inhibitor was added if either diltiazem at 360 mg/d or both a diuretic and beta blocker did not achieve a diastolic BP less than 90 mm Hg. During a mean follow-up of 4.5 years, a primary event (stroke, myocardial infarction, or CVD-related death) occurred in 403 patients initially given diltiazem and 400 patients given the diuretic or beta blocker (RR = 1.00, 95% CI = 0.87–1.15, $P = .97$). Diltiazem was associated with about 3 mm Hg higher systolic BP throughout follow-up ($P < .001$). Interestingly, myocardial infarction was slightly (but not significantly) more common with diltiazem (183 vs 157, $P = .17$) than with the diuretic/beta blocker, and stroke was less common (159 vs 196, respectively, $P = .04$). Many patients required more than monotherapy (50% for diltiazem, 55% for the diuretic/beta blocker), but more patients abandoned diltiazem (23%) than the diuretic/beta blocker (7%) during the study.

These and some earlier data were then combined in several meta-analyses. One that compared outcomes for patients randomized to calcium antagonists with outcomes for patients randomized to *any* other initial therapy concluded that an initial calcium antagonist was associated with a significant 25% increased risk of myocardial infarction and a 26% increased risk of heart failure.[62] Little media attention was given to the next pages of *The Lancet*, which summarized all the prospectively gathered individual-patient-level data from these clinical trials, and concluded that both ACE inhibitors and calcium antagonists were more effective than placebo in reducing CVD events, and that the few substantive differences noted would be overwhelmed in the next few years when the results of ongoing trials were revealed.[63]

Angiotensin II receptor blockers

Five outcome-based clinical trials involving angiotensin II receptor blockers in hypertension were published between 2001 and 2003. All involved specific, high-risk patient groups; none were conducted in a broad range of hypertensive patients (like most studies discussed above and below).

The Irbesartan Diabetic Nephropathy Trial (IDNT)[64] and The Reduction of Endpoints in Non-Insulin Dependent Diabetes Mellitus with the Angiotensin II Antagonist Losartan (RENAAL) study[65]

used the same primary endpoint (doubling of serum creatinine, end-stage renal disease, or death), and compared an angiotensin II receptor blocker with placebo (or amlodipine) in type 2 hypertensive diabetics with nephropathy. Although neither study showed significant differences across randomized arms in major CVD events,[66] the US Food and Drug Administration (FDA) approved both losartan and irbesartan to retard the progression of type 2 diabetic nephropathy, based on the results of these trials. The Irbesartan Microalbuminuria (IRMA-2) trial showed a significant benefit for only high-dose irbesartan in preventing the progression of microalbuminuria to proteinuria,[67] which had already been seen with ramipril in the HOPE trial.[54]

Two early clinical trials directly comparing captopril with low-dose losartan in heart failure did not show significant differences in long-term prognosis.[68,69] Two other clinical trials compared outcomes with ARB or placebo in heart failure patients who were already receiving an ACE inhibitor. Both the Valsartan in Heart Failure (Val-HeFT) and the Candesartan Heart Failure Assessment of Reduction in Morbidity and Mortality (CHARM-Added) trials showed a significant benefit for the combination of ACE inhibitor and ARB.[70,71] Either ARB (in Val-HeFT or CHARM-Alternative) was superior to placebo in patients who could not take an ACE inhibitor[72]; this has resulted in FDA approval for valsartan for this special situation. Although patients who received "triple therapy" (ACE inhibitor, beta blocker, and ARB) in Val-HeFT had significantly increased mortality in a post hoc analysis, this was not observed in CHARM. The largely unstudied group of heart failure patients with preserved left ventricular function did not significantly benefit from candesartan in CHARM-Preserved[73]; other studies using different ARBs are in progress.

The most positive long-term trial involving CVD endpoints in hypertensive patients treated with ARBs was the Losartan Intervention For Endpoint reduction (LIFE) trial.[74] Because of the important role of left ventricular hypertrophy (LVH) as a risk factor for CVD events in hypertensive patients, 9193 patients fulfilling very strict electrocardiographic criteria for LVH were enrolled and randomized initially to losartan or atenolol (50 mg/d). Doses could be doubled and hydrochlorothiazide and then other drugs (excluding beta blockers, ARBs, or ACE inhibitors) added, if needed, to control BP. The primary endpoint was a composite of myocardial infarction, stroke, and CVD death. After 4.8 years (on average), BPs were reduced slightly better (1.3/0.4 mm Hg) in the losartan group. Even after adjustment for baseline degree of LVH and Framingham risk score, the losartan group had a significantly lower risk of the primary endpoint (by 13%, $P = .021$), which was largely driven by a 25% reduction in stroke ($P < .001$). Although the losartan group had a higher risk of myocardial infarction (7%,

$P = .49$), there was also an improvement in LVH ($P < .0001$) and a lower risk of new diabetes (26%, $P < .001$) and adverse events ($P < .0001$). Subgroup analyses have also shown the benefits of losartan among diabetics[75] and individuals with "isolated systolic hypertension."[76] These data were the basis on which the US FDA approved losartan for stroke prevention in hypertensive patients with LVH.

More recent trials

The largest and most important comparative trial of initial antihypertensive drug therapy was the Antihypertensive and Lipid Lowering Treatment to prevent Heart Attack Trial (ALLHAT).[77] It had been designed and funded by the US National Institutes of Health to see if the newer antihypertensive agents were better than chlorthalidone (the best-studied thiazide-like diuretic) in preventing fatal and nonfatal myocardial infarction. In January 2000, two independent bodies recommended early termination of the doxazosin arm of ALLHAT. Two major reasons were cited: the futility of finding it superior to chlorthalidone, and its association with an increased incidence of all CVD events (most of which was due to a highly significant 2.04 times higher risk of heart failure).[78] In the other three arms, the primary endpoint of coronary heart disease was nearly identical for chlorthalidone, amlodipine (the calcium antagonist), and lisinopril (the ACE inhibitor); systolic BP control was better with chlorthalidone than with either of the other drugs. In addition, combined CVD events were higher with lisinopril than chlorthalidone, and heart failure (which was not a prespecified, independent, or even tertiary endpoint) was significantly better prevented with chlorthalidone than with either of the other drugs. These results and their implications have been hotly debated, but they are the primary reason why JNC-7 indicated that "a thiazide-type diuretic should be first-line drug therapy for most hypertensive patients." Some ALLHAT investigators have recommended that all hypertensive patients should receive thazide-like diuretics as initial therapy unless contraindicated, and that clinicians should consider switching patients who are taking other regimens to thiazide-like diuretics. Although we do not generally recommend that effective treatment be stopped, ALLHAT was a "switch study," and that approach to hypertension management is worthy of consideration if the benefits are felt to outweigh the risks.

Several months after release of the ALLHAT data, the results of the Second Australian National Blood Pressure Trial were published.[79] In this clinical trial with PROBE design used in the offices of 1594 Australian general practitioners, 6083 older hypertensive patients (between 65 and 85 years of age) were taken off their usual antihypertensive drugs and randomized to hydrochlorothiazide or enalapril, although the agent and dose were left to the physician. Beta blockers, calcium antagonists, and alpha blockers could be added sequentially, if needed. The change in BP was nearly exactly equal across randomized groups (a decrease of 26/12 mm Hg). After a median of 4.1 years, there were 695 total CVD events or deaths among those assigned to the ACE inhibitor, as compared with 736 such events for the diuretic. Although this achieved putative statistical significance ($P = .05$), the traditional time to first event was not significant ($P = .06$). In subgroup analyses, the ACE inhibitor appeared to be better in men and in prevention of nonfatal CVD events and myocardial infarctions.

A completely different study objective was planned in the Controlled Onset Verapamil Investigation of Cardiovascular Endpoints (CONVINCE) trial.[80] This head-to-head comparison of the physician's choice of hydrochlorothiazide or atenolol versus controlled-onset extended-release verapamil was intended as an "equivalence trial" from the very beginning. As such, 2024 primary events (stroke, myocardial infarction, or CVD death) were originally required to establish "equivalence," which was expected to take 5 years to accrue. Despite enrolling 16,602 hypertensive subjects with at least one additional risk factor (including obesity) for CVD events, the study was stopped prematurely by the sponsor "for business reasons." Nonetheless, 729 primary events were observed, and they were split between the two randomized treatment regimens in a nearly equal proportion. Unfortunately, CONVINCE failed to meet its objective of showing "equivalence" of the two treatments. Heart failure and bleeding were both significantly more common in the group randomized to verapamil.

The International Verapamil SR/Trandolapril Study was performed in 22,576 subjects with *both hypertension and coronary artery disease*, and compared a regimen starting with verapamil SR (followed by trandolapril) to a more traditional regimen starting with atenolol (followed by hydrochlorothiazide). More than 17,000 eligible individuals were recruited from the United States, with the majority of the remainder coming from other countries in North America. After an average of 2.7 years of open-label treatment, BPs were equally well controlled in both randomized groups (despite discontinuation of study medication in about 43% in both groups), and the primary endpoint (nonfatal myocardial infarction, nonfatal stroke, or all-cause mortality) was also not significantly different ($P = .62$). The results were homogeneous across a wide variety of baseline parameters (eg, age, gender, race/ethnicity), but a post hoc analysis showed a significant decrease in new-onset diabetes in the verapamil/trandolapril group.[81]

Meta-analyses

The results of most outcome-based studies in hypertension have been combined in meta-analyses. The results and value of these meta-analyses are controversial, as they sometimes reach different conclusions. Psaty and colleagues combined data from 42 clinical trials that included 192,478 patients randomized to seven major treatment strategies (including placebo).[49] Using a complex statistical scheme that allows internal comparisons, interpolations, extrapolations, and indirect calculations of relative risks for treatments, their "network meta-analysis" method allows estimates to be made for comparisons that are not based on head-to-head studies. The results of this meta-analysis closely parallel the results of ALLHAT. Low-dose diuretics were significantly better than placebo for any CVD outcome, and no other initial therapy was superior to a low-dose diuretic for any outcome. Low-dose diuretics were superior to calcium antagonists, ACE inhibitors, and alpha blockers in the prevention of heart failure. They were also superior to calcium antagonists, ACE inhibitors, beta blockers, and alpha blockers in the prevention of CVD events. The authors therefore concluded that low-dose diuretics are the most effective first-line treatment for preventing CVD morbidity and mortality, and that a low-dose diuretic should hereinafter serve alone as the "gold standard" initial therapy in all future clinical trials of antihypertensive drugs.

We have performed a set of more traditional meta-analyses to compare the prevention of CVD endpoints in clinical trials that directly compared either an initial diuretic or beta blocker with an initial calcium antagonist or an initial ACE inhibitor.[82] The results are shown in Fig. 7-7. We attempted to standardize all definitions of events across trials; for example, "major CVD events" included only myocardial infarction, stroke, and CVD death. This required estimation of the numbers of events in each arm of several trials (eg, INSIGHT, ALLHAT, INVEST), as each of these included other endpoints in their definitions of "major CVD events." The results of our meta-analyses indicate that heart failure events are significantly more common with calcium antagonists or ACE inhibitors than with diuretics or beta blockers. The effect of a calcium antagonist on stroke is just barely significantly better than that of an initial diuretic or beta blocker, whereas an ACE inhibitor is just slightly worse ($P = .04$ in each case). These estimates may change after ongoing trials are completed and reported. Before the results of many recent studies were reported, the Blood Pressure Lowering Treatment Trialists'

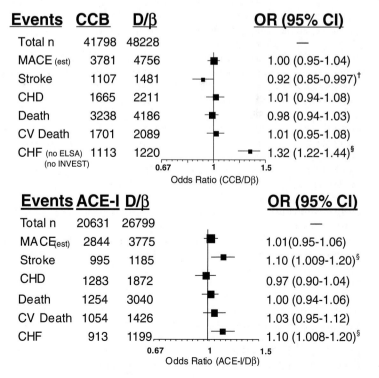

FIGURE 7-7 Results of meta-analyses comparing an initial diuretic or beta blocker with an initial calcium antagonist (top) or ACE inhibitor (bottom I). (Updated from Elliott WJ. Cardiovascular events during initial antihypertensive therapy with either a calcium antagonist or a diuretic/beta-blocker: meta-analysis of 7 clinical trials [abstract]. *Am J Hypertens* 2003;16:9A–10A.[†]$P = .03$;[§]$P < .0001$; CCB, calcium channel blocker; D/β, diuretic or beta blocker; OR, odds ratio; CL, confidence interval; Total *n*, total number of patients; MACE(est), estimated number of major adverse cardiovascular events; CHD, coronary heart disease; CV death, cardiovascular death; CHF, congestive heart failure (excluding CHF data from the European Lacidipine Study of Atherosclerosis, which have not yet been reported); ACE-I, angiotensin-converting enzyme inhibitor.

Events	CCB	D/β		OR (95% CI)
Total n	41798	48228		—
MACE (est)	3781	4756		1.00 (0.95-1.04)
Stroke	1107	1481		0.92 (0.85-0.997)[†]
CHD	1665	2211		1.01 (0.94-1.08)
Death	3238	4186		0.98 (0.94-1.03)
CV Death	1701	2089		1.01 (0.95-1.08)
CHF (no ELSA) (no INVEST)	1113	1220		1.32 (1.22-1.44)[§]

Odds Ratio (CCB/Dβ)

Events	ACE-I	D/β		OR (95% CI)
Total n	20631	26799		—
MACE(est)	2844	3775		1.01(0.95-1.06)
Stroke	995	1185		1.10 (1.009-1.20)[§]
CHD	1283	1872		0.97 (0.90-1.04)
Death	1254	3040		1.00 (0.94-1.06)
CV Death	1054	1426		1.03 (0.95-1.12)
CHF	913	1199		1.10 (1.008-1.20)[§]

Odds Ratio (ACE-I/Dβ)

Collaboration gathered data from 29 trials involving 162,341 patients for a prospective meta-analysis.[50] They found no significant difference in major CVD events between regimens that began with either an ACE inhibitor, calcium antagonist, or diuretic/beta blocker. With the exception of heart failure, any difference in outcomes was directly related to the difference in achieved BP between randomized groups. This meta-analysis suggests that it may matter more that BP is reduced than which agent is chosen initially to lower it.

Combination therapy

A few trials have been designed to explore the potential benefits of combination therapy, that is, drugs from different pharmacologic classes. The majority of patients with hypertension will eventually require more than one drug.[4] Even in ALLHAT, which denied enrollment to those with initial BPs greater than 180/110 mm Hg, by the end of the trial, the average number of drugs used per patient was 2.0.[83] The potential benefits of combination therapy are perhaps best illustrated with PROGRESS: the ACE inhibitor alone lowered BP by 4.9/2.8 mm Hg, whereas the combination (ACE inhibitor + diuretic) reduced BP by 12.3/5.0 mm Hg. Compared with placebo, monotherapy reduced stroke by only 5% (95% CI = −19 to 23%), but the combination therapy reduced stroke by 43% (95% CI = 30–54%). Similarly, CVD events were reduced by only 4% (95% CI = −15 to 20%) with monotherapy, but by 40% (95% CI = 29–49%) with the combination.

The potential benefits of combining an ACE inhibitor with an ARB have been explored in two populations of chronic kidney disease patients. Half-maximal doses of each were used in 199 type 2 diabetics in the Candesartan and Lisinopril Microalbuminuria (CALM) trial.[84] The combination was associated with significantly lower BPs than either the ACE inhibitor or ARB. The combination also showed a further, nearly significant improvement in proteinuria compared with either drug alone. In 263 Japanese with nondiabetic renal disease, therapy with full-dose ACE inhibitor + ARB was compared with therapy with either drug alone. Although the group receiving the combination had nearly identical BPs to the other groups, this group had the lowest amount of proteinuria and the lowest risk of doubling serum creatinine or end-stage renal disease.[85] Further studies will clarify the role of combined ACE inhibitor + ARB therapy in patients with renal disease.

Summary of current evidence from clinical trials

There is little doubt, based on the clinical trial evidence gathered to date and summarized above, that BP reduc-

tion is a powerful means of achieving decreases in CVD events. One of the bigger challenges has been to identify any benefit of antihypertensive drug therapy *over and above* the confounding issue of differential BP lowering that occurred during the trial with the regimens used. Multiple economic analyses also indicate that, in addition to being effective in preventing CVD events, antihypertensive drug therapy is also relatively cost-effective, compared with other commonly employed treatment strategies used in medicine today.[86]

EVALUATION OF THE HYPERTENSIVE PATIENT

Four key issues must be addressed during the initial evaluation of a person with elevated BP readings:

1. Documenting an accurate diagnosis of hypertension (see above).
2. Stratifying the person's risk for CVD, which involves: (i) defining the presence or absence of existing CVD or renal disease, or "target-organ damage" related to hypertension; and (ii) screening for other CVD risk factors that often accompany hypertension.
3. Assessing whether the person is likely to have an identifiable cause for their hypertension (secondary hypertension), and should have further diagnostic testing for it.
4. Obtaining information that may be helpful in choosing appropriate therapy.

Although extensive and expensive laboratory studies are rarely necessary in the evaluation of the hypertensive patient, the physician must be able to recognize when additional studies or consultation with a specialist is appropriate and warranted. Delaying discovery of a potentially curable form of hypertension places the patient at unnecessary risk, and delays implementing specific treatment. Failing to properly assess whether end-organ damage or comorbidity is present may lead to inappropriate therapeutic choices or delay proper therapy.

Documenting the diagnosis

BP should be measured under relaxed and controlled conditions after appropriate rest (typically 5 minutes), and taken by someone whose ability to perform the measurement accurately has been certified. Approximately 10 to 15% of Americans cannot properly hear Korotkoff sounds; it is unlikely that measurements reported by every observer are accurate. Excellent programs are available that can train, validate, and recertify the competency of the person performing BP measurements. Careful attention should be given to proper, standardized technique, as discussed above.

Before the diagnosis of hypertension is made, an individual usually should have elevated BP measurements documented at least twice, at visits separated by a week or longer. Each measurement should be an average of two or three readings differing by less than 5 mm Hg from each other, taken a few minutes apart in the seated or supine position. Patients who exhibit wide fluctuations in BP, or who are hypertensive at some evaluations, but normotensive at others, may need additional measurements, either in the office, at home, or by use of ABPM, to confirm that they are indeed hypertensive. Treatment should generally NOT be instituted until the diagnosis is clearly proven. In some circumstances, such as when end-organ damage is present, treatment may need to be started after a single set of measurements.

Stratifying risk for cardiovascular disease

Before beginning a treatment program directed at lowering BP, a thorough assessment of the person's risk for developing CVD is warranted. Little guidance is provided about this in JNC-7,[4] but many other schemes are available to assist the physician.[87–89] Some of these (including the National Cholesterol Education Program's Adult Treatment Panel III[47]) are semiquantitative, and allow a reasonable estimate of the patient's 10-year risk of CVD to be calculated. JNC-VI stratified people with elevated BP into three risk categories (A, B, or C). Risk group C included patients with existing CVD, TOD, or diabetes, and constituted about 19.2% of the hypertensive population in NHANES-I.[90] Risk group A included only patients with no other CVD risk factors (including male gender) and, therefore, was the least common risk group (9% of the hypertensives in NHANES-I). Risk group B therefore included more than 71% of the hypertensive population, and did not distinguish very well between those at relatively high and those at low CVD risk.[89] This may have been one of the reasons why JNC-7 did not include the previously recommended and simple, but somewhat imprecise, method of stratifying CVD risk in hypertensive patients.

Many of the currently available CVD risk calculators are based on the approach taken by the Framingham Heart Study. The European Society of Cardiology has published an estimator of coronary heart disease (CHD) risk for European patients, which uses a modification of the Framingham risk equations, and weighted coefficients for each traditional risk factor that are based on epidemiologic data from European populations (especially Northern Europe).[91,92] This risk estimator includes serum total cholesterol (rather than the National Cholesterol Education Program-recommended LDL-C), and assumes a constant HDL-C of 1.0 mmol/L (39 mg/dL). This model provides overall estimates that are quite similar to those provided by the Framingham risk equa-

tion, with perhaps slightly less specificity in American patients.[93] The Joint British Societies (Cardiac, Hyperlipidaemia, Hypertension, and Diabetes) agreed in 1998 on recommendations for prevention of coronary disease, which includes a different risk estimator that is based on the Framingham risk equations, but weights the risk factors according to British national statistics.[94]

Investigators from Sheffield, England, have actively promoted a different series of tables, the simplest of which is based on the Framingham equations, supplemented by data from the 1995 Scottish Health Survey.[87] Their reasonably well validated new tables (one for men, another for women) use age and total/HDL-C ratio (with 22 choices for men, 18 for women), and simply dichotomize hypertension (defined as ≥140/90 mm Hg or taking treatment), smoking, and diabetes. Surprisingly, their data indicate that hypertension (whether treated or untreated) affects overall risk of CHD only slightly: when other risk factors are incorporated into the risk equation, the absolute level of BP (especially at diagnosis) is nearly irrelevant.

Despite the availability of reasonably precise and quantitative risk estimators, several important principles about CVD risk remain unchanged since JNC-V. Individuals with the highest short-term risk of a stroke or heart attack are those who already have concomitant CVD or renal disease, for instance, or a history of a recent transient ischemic attack or previous myocardial infarction. These individuals' BP should be treated promptly, intensively, and to a lower BP goal than uncomplicated hypertensive people. The search for evidence of concomitant CVD or renal disease need not be extensive or expensive, however. Typically a complete medical history, directed physical examination, and a few routine laboratory tests (including an electrocardiogram, urinalysis, and serum chemistry panel) are sufficient.

Hypertensive people with TOD are also at substantial risk for CVD events. TOD encompasses many subclinical features of the physical examination or laboratory tests that indicate there has already been an alteration of structure or function in the eyes, heart, kidneys, or blood vessels related to hypertension. Although these people may not have as yet suffered an irreversible hypertension-related event (eg, stroke), some are at substantial risk for these sequelae (eg, those with chronic kidney disease), and the presence of TOD usually indicates that hypertension has been present for some time. These people also should receive prompt and intensive efforts to lower BP to a lower than usual goal.

Data from both epidemiologic studies and clinical trials have shown that hypertensive diabetics have about twice the risk of CVD events as hypertensive persons without diabetes, essentially equivalent to the presence of existing CVD disease in a nondiabetic. JNC-VI recognized this by categorizing all diabetics as Risk Category C;

a similar approach was taken by the National Cholesterol Education Program, in which the presence of diabetes was considered a "coronary heart disease equivalent."[47] JNC-7 recommended that a diabetic person with a BP of 130/80 mm Hg or higher should receive antihypertensive drug therapy, even though the diagnosis of hypertension may NOT be confirmed. This is perhaps the most striking example of how JNC-VI and JNC-7 embraced the concept of treating individual patients according to their absolute risk for CVD events, and *not* by BP levels alone.

Other CVD risk factors (tobacco use, family history of premature CVD) are often found in hypertensive people, and central obesity, dyslipidemia, diabetes, and hypertension tend to cluster. Because other risk factors tend to be additive (if not multiplicative) in increasing the probability of CVD events, it is important to screen a newly diagnosed hypertensive person for these other risk factors to more accurately estimate CVD and renal risk (see below for specific recommendations about screening tests).

Even though age is the most important (nonmodifiable) predictor of CVD risk (see Fig. 7-4), the treatment scheme and BP goals recommended in JNC-7 are independent of the patient's age.[4] There are now good data, and a large meta-analysis, showing that older people, even those older than 80, benefit greatly by lowering their BPs.[95]

Considerations for secondary hypertension

For more than 95% of Americans with hypertension the specific cause of their elevated BPs is not known (ie, idiopathic or primary hypertension). There are three reasons to consider the possibility that hypertension in a newly diagnosed patient might have a specific cause. First, BP control is often difficult to achieve in those with secondary causes of hypertension; early diagnosis is likely to result in more rapid attainment of the BP goal. Second, and particularly important in younger people, diagnosing and treating secondary hypertension with specific modalities with the potential to cure the underlying problem will reduce the future burden of treatment (with respect to medication and follow-up, adverse effects of therapy, and quality of life). Last, routine consideration of secondary causes when the diagnosis of hypertension is made will ensure that the potential diagnoses are entertained, and the pros and cons of further testing critically evaluated.

Guiding therapy

The more than 100 antihypertensive agents and fixed-dose combinations currently available in the United States differ in BP-lowering efficacy in various situations. It is often helpful to discuss these potential confounders of treatment with the patient, in an effort to "individualize" treatment according to the patient's specific dietary, medical, and personal considerations. For example, diuretics and calcium antagonists are more effective than ACE inhibitors and angiotensin II receptor antagonists when dietary sodium is excessive. JNC-VI and JNC-7 both recommended treating hypertension and a concomitant illness/condition with a specific antihypertensive drug when that drug has been shown in clinical trials to improve CVD morbidity and mortality (so-called "compelling indication" for a specific class of antihypertensive drug). Therefore, even though ACE inhibitors were not routinely recommended as initial therapy for an uncomplicated hypertensive patient, if the patient has heart failure of the systolic type, an ACE inhibitor could be prescribed. It would be expected not only to lower the BP, but also to provide the impressive benefits seen in many long-term studies in every stage of heart failure. Lastly, some patients are particularly fearful of specific potential adverse effects of certain antihypertensive drugs, for example, erectile dysfunction. If this information is known to the physician, efforts may be taken to avoid medications associated with a high incidence of this particular problem.

Medical history

In addition to assessment of the risk of CVD and renal disease, a careful drug, environmental, and nutritional history should be obtained during initial evaluation of a hypertensive patient and intermittently during subsequent management. It is particularly important to ascertain whether the patient is taking any drug (prescription or over-the-counter) or other substance that might elevate BP (Table 7-5). Of particular concern are the nonsteroidal anti-inflammatory drugs (NSAIDs), which are widely used and available over-the-counter, and are sometimes not recognized as "drugs" by many patients. Sympathomimetic amines (once commonly found in weight loss, cold, and allergy preparations) have been associated with both increased BP and risk of intracerebral hemorrhage and stroke. Hypertensive people should avoid both NSAIDs and sympathomimetic amines, and attempt to obtain relief of pain with acetaminophen and relief of the symptoms of nasal congestion with antihistamines, if possible. When these modalities are ineffective, short-term use of the usually prescribed drugs may be condoned, but with the recognition that BP control is likely to be suboptimal during and immediately after their consumption.

Oral contraceptive pills containing estrogens and progestins may raise BP in some women, although this is much less of a problem with the lower doses in common use today. If a newly diagnosed hypertensive woman uses

TABLE 7-5 Substances That Can Raise Blood Pressure (Partial List)

Nonsteroidal anti-inflammatory drugs (including the newer COX-2* inhibitors, celecoxib, roficoxib, valdecoxib)
Corticosteroids
Sympathomimetic amines
Oral contraceptive hormones
Methylxanthines (including theophylline and caffeine[†])
Cyclosporine
Erythropoeitin
Cocaine
Nicotine[‡]
Phencyclidine (PCP)

*COX-2, cyclooxgygenase 2; PCP, phenylcyclohexyl piperidine ("angel dust").
[†]Short duration (minutes to hours).
[‡]Very short duration (seconds to minutes).

these pills, discontinuation for 6 months and observation of the BP may allow a decision to be made about whether the pills are the cause of hypertension. Conjugated estrogens (with or without progesterone), typically given for postmenopausal hormone replacement therapy, do not raise BP, although they have been associated with a wide variety of other problems, including increased rates of CVD events.[96]

Other prescription drugs can either elevate BP or interfere with certain antihypertensive agents. Of the former, cyclosporine, erythropoeitin, corticosteroids, cocaine, and theophylline are perhaps the most widely recognized. Of the latter, monoamine oxidase inhibitors, NSAIDs, and tricyclic antidepressants are the most common. It is important to ascertain whether a hypertensive patient has taken any of these agents, as well as several other illicit drugs (eg, phencyclidine). Some chemical elements, particularly lead[97] and chromium, may elevate BP long after exposure; questioning about these and other environmental toxins may sometimes be helpful.

A focused dietary history is very important, as the most effective lifestyle modifications involve limiting calories or sodium, or both.[98] Dietary salt and saturated fat intake can both be estimated from an informal survey of dietary habits and preferences. Many processed foods, "fast foods," "diet foods," condiments, and snack items are very concentrated, often-unrecognized sources of salt. Now that most of these items bear labels attesting to their high salt content, many patients are more easily able to choose healthier foods. A sensible target (now validated in several clinical trials, including DASH-Sodium[99] and

PREMIER[100]) is 100 mEq (2.4 g or 2400 mg) of sodium per day; this usually can be achieved if the high-salt items mentioned above are avoided, and the patient does not add salt, either at the table or in cooking. Occasionally it is useful (and relatively inexpensive, compared with formal dietary counseling) to have the patient collect a 24-hour urine for sodium, particularly when the patient claims to be avoiding salt, but the physician is suspicious. Although not all hypertensive patients will experience a reduction in BP on a low-salt diet or an increase in BP on a high-salt diet, individuals who are "salt-sensitive" will benefit from reducing dietary sodium. In general, African American, elderly, obese, and diabetic patients are more likely to be "salt-sensitive," with BPs that are more responsive to dietary salt restriction.

The nutritional history should also include questions about saturated fat consumption, dairy product intake, and use of mineral or vitamin supplements. As obesity is a major problem for many hypertensive patients, the caloric intake, eating pattern, and changes in weight should be included. Weight loss remains the most successful of all the lifestyle modifications for hypertension, and should be a part of the therapeutic plan in all overweight, hypertensive persons from the outset.[98]

Social history

Although alcohol in moderation (one or two usual-sized drinks—less than 24 oz of beer, 8 oz of wine, or 3 oz of distilled spirits) protects against coronary heart disease, excessive alcohol intake ($\geq$4 drinks/day) raises both BP and all-cause mortality. In some patients, reducing or stopping alcohol ingestion can have very salutary effects on BP. A clinical trial in veterans who consumed approximately six drinks per day when enrolled was unsuccessful in demonstrating a significant reduction in BP in those enrolled in a cognitive-behavioral alcohol reduction program, despite their consuming significantly fewer drinks per day (1.3 fewer, on average) than the control group, who were in a much less intensive educational program.[101] Nonetheless, a meta-analysis suggests there is a place for alcohol restriction in nonpharmacologic therapy for hypertension.[102]

Large populations of smokers have, on average, lower BPs than nonsmokers, probably because smokers tend to be less obese than nonsmokers. Consuming tobacco has both acute and chronic adverse effects on BP and hypertensive patients. Smoking a single cigarette raises BP and heart rate acutely (within seconds to minutes), due to nicotine's stimulation of catecholamine secretion. This effect disappears in about 15 minutes, so BP should be measured at least 15 to 30 minutes after the most recent cigarette is extinguished. Chronic tobacco abuse roughly doubles the long-term risk of coronary disease, and has an even larger effect on peripheral arterial disease (including renovascular hypertension). Inquiry about tobacco abuse and advice to discontinue it (if present) should be a part of every encounter with a health care professional.

Hypertensive patients should also be questioned about a sedentary lifestyle and whether there is willingness and/or ability to engage in regular physical activity. Even limited aerobic exercise, including brisk walking for 30 minutes on most days, can reduce BP and all-cause and CVD mortality. Snoring, daytime sleepiness, and other clinical features of sleep apnea, especially in obese, hypertensive persons, should lead to consideration of a formal evaluation for this underappreciated and underdiagnosed form of secondary hypertension.[103,104]

Physical examination

The "directed" physical examination of the hypertensive patient should pay special attention to weight, TOD, and features consistent with secondary hypertension. It should focus on items that were suggested by the medical history.

- The pattern of fat distribution should be noted. Android obesity (waist-to-hip ratio > 0.95) is associated with increased CVD risk, whereas gynecoid obesity (waist-to-hip ratio < 0.85) is not. Men whose waists are 100 cm (40 in.) or larger and women whose waists are 88 cm (34 in.) or larger are at increased risk.
- The skin should be carefully examined for café-au-lait spots (suggesting neurofibromatosis and possible pheochromocytoma), acanthosis nigricans (suggesting insulin resistance), xanthomata at tendons, and xanthelasma (indicating dyslipidemia). Other skin signs suggesting pheochromocytoma (axillary freckles, ashleaf patches, port-wine stains in the trigeminal distribution, and adenoma sebaceum) are uncommon.
- Common physical signs associated with other secondary causes should be sought, particularly if suggested by the medical history. The signs of Cushing's syndrome (purple striae, moon facies, dorsocervical fat pad, atrophic skin changes) or thyroid disease (abnormal Achilles reflexes, hair quality, eye signs) are typically difficult to ignore.
- The funduscopic examination is important in assessing the duration and severity of hypertension. The presence of hypertensive retinopathy (grade 1: arterial tortuosity, silver wiring; grade 2: arteriovenous crossing changes ["nicking"]; grade 3: hemorrhages or exudates; grade 4: papilledema) provides definitive evidence of TOD.
- The neck should be examined for an enlarged thyroid gland, abnormalities of the venous circulation (eg, jugular venous distention, abnormal or "canon" a-waves), and carotid bruits.
- The chest should be auscultated for evidence of heart failure or bronchospasm; the latter would make beta blockers relatively contraindicated.
- The heart should be examined carefully for cardiomegaly, murmurs, and extra sounds.
- The abdominal examination is one of the most important parts of the "directed" physical examination, because the finding of an abdominal bruit is one of the most cost-effective ways of screening for renovascular hypertension. All four abdominal quadrants and the back should be auscultated, typically using the pulse at the wrist as the synchronizing stimulus. Diastolic or continuous bruits are common in renovascular hypertension, but systolic bruits in young and especially thin hypertensive subjects may not be indicative of renal artery stenosis. Abdominal masses can sometimes be palpated in patients with pheochromocytoma or polycystic kidney disease.
- The groin and legs should be examined for evidence of peripheral arterial disease, which often manifests as bruits, absent or decreased pulses, and abnormal hair growth patterns. Edema can be a sign of heart failure or renal disease, and can be exacerbated by high doses of dihydropyridine calcium antagonists.
- The neurologic examination need not be extensive in a hypertensive patient with no history of cerebrovascular disease, but it should be complete if a history of stroke or transient ischemic attack is present.

Laboratory testing

In most hypertensive patients, only a few inexpensive and simple laboratory tests are needed as part of the initial evaluation. In selected patients, however, more extensive testing is not only appropriate, but also necessary to diagnose secondary hypertension and avoid delaying proper treatment. The laboratory tests that are recommended for all hypertensive persons are listed in Table 7-6, and can be divided into those that are done to assess risk, to establish etiology, to screen for important common diseases, and, finally, to guide the choice of initial therapy.

For uncomplicated hypertensive patients whose history and physical examination do not suggest a secondary cause, the simple battery of tests in Table 7-6 is all that is needed. A lipid profile and fasting glucose are indicated because of the high prevalence of the metabolic syndrome in hypertensive patients. The presence of diabetes or additional risk factors not only requires institution of therapy for these conditions, but also indicates substantially increased CVD risk, thus requiring more intensive therapy for hypertension, a lower goal BP, and closer follow-up.

TABLE 7-6 Laboratory Tests Appropriate for All Newly Diagnosed Hypertensive Patients

Assessing risk
Lipid profile (including total cholesterol, HDL-C, and triglycerides)
Serum glucose (preferably fasting)
Serum creatinine
Urinalysis (both dipstick and microscopic)
12-Lead electrocardiogram
Establishing cause
Serum potassium
Serum creatinine
Urinalysis (both dipstick and microscopic)
?Thyroid-stimulating hormone
Screening for common asymptomatic diseases
Complete blood count
Serum calcium
Guiding therapy
Lipid profile (including total cholesterol, HDL-C, and triglycerides)
Serum glucose (preferably fasting)
Serum creatinine

Routine measurement of serum creatinine and a full urinalysis are recommended for three reasons. First, the urinalysis is useful to assess risk, as hypertensive patients with microalbuminuria, proteinuria, and chronic kidney disease have a distinctly worse prognosis. Second, the urinalysis may identify hypertension secondary to chronic renal disease, characterized by an elevated serum creatinine, often proteinuria, and typically an active sediment. Chronic kidney disease (manifesting as an elevated serum creatinine) with a normal urinary sediment may be a valuable clue suggesting ischemic nephropathy perhaps due to renal artery stenosis. Third, knowledge of the serum creatinine level frequently guides therapy, as loop diuretics are routinely needed and are more effective than thiazide or thiazide-like diuretics when the creatinine clearance is less than 30 to 50 mL/min.

An electrocardiogram may provide important, but limited information in most hypertensive patients. Although it may identify an occasionally important dysrhythmia or even an unsuspected old myocardial infarction, its biggest role is in screening for left ventricular hypertrophy (LVH), which is an objective measure of both the severity and the duration of elevated BP. Despite a sensitivity of only 10 to 50% (depending on which criteria are used in its interpretation) in the

Framingham Heart Study, electrocardiographic evidence of LVH was associated with an approximately threefold increase in incidence of CVD events. LVH detected by an echocardiogram appears to be an even better predictor of future events.[105] Echocardiography is not recommended for routine evaluation because of its high cost and the high intrinsic variability of a single echocardiogram (~10–15%). A "limited echo" has been recommended as one way around this problem, but is not widely used in the United States for this indication.

Because hypothyroidism is a cause of remediable hypertension that is subtle, especially in the elderly, a thyroid-stimulating hormone assay may be helpful. Serum calcium is useful in evaluating hyperparathyroidism, and is often included in automated chemistry panels. It is not necessary to measure plasma renin activity to screen for secondary causes of hypertension, to determine prognosis, or to guide therapy. However, this test is useful in the diagnosis of mineralocorticoid excess states, such as primary hyperaldosteronism.

SECONDARY HYPERTENSION

Important clues to the presence of secondary hypertension are often provided by a carefully obtained medical history (see above). Many patients with primary hypertension report an isolated elevated BP reading or two sometime in their twenties and thirties that was not reproducible or sustained until at least a decade or more later. The level of BP gradually rises until it reaches a threshold level, and then hypertension is diagnosed.

In contrast, patients with an identifiable secondary cause of hypertension usually present with a very different history. Instead of the gradual onset of elevated BPs, they usually have a relatively abrupt onset of hypertension, typically presenting at a higher stage and with considerable TOD. The sudden onset of elevated BPs below 30 or above 50 years of age should alert the clinician to the possibility that the patient may have secondary hypertension. Thus, the history of the patient's presentation with hypertension should be carefully documented. At what age were the BP readings first elevated? How high were the readings? Were all prior readings within the normal range? Was it discovered during a routine office visit, or did the patient have clinical problems related to BP elevation or related TOD?

As patients with secondary hypertension typically do not respond as well to antihypertensive drug therapy as patients with primary hypertension, the history of the patient's response to treatment must be ascertained. What drugs were used and at which doses? Did the patient's BP respond initially, and then become resistant? A positive answer to this question is frequently elicited from patients with primary hypertension who later develop secondary hypertension, particularly atherosclerotic renovascular disease.

Laboratory testing for secondary hypertension

All types of secondary hypertension are uncommon in the general hypertensive population. In interpretation of test results in a given patient, Bayesian analysis (which incorporates the pretest probability of finding disease) is therefore more important than the sensitivity of the test (ie, the percentage of people with disease who have a positive test). Medical history, physical examination, and routine laboratory studies can be used to identify the hypertensive patients with a higher likelihood of having a particular kind of secondary hypertension. Those tests that are commonly used in evaluating patients for secondary hypertension in our Center are listed in Table 7-7.

MANAGEMENT

Successful management of hypertension requires a major commitment from the patient, the health care provider, and the health care system. The patient must continue to take what could be a costly medication with potential side effects and see a physician frequently, for an asymptomatic condition, in the belief that this will reduce the risk of a major complication, or even death. The physician must help the patient achieve goal BP and maintain surveillance on this and other CVD risk factors, without being sure that such treatment will prevent an event that would have occurred without it.

Lifestyle modifications

Nearly all hypertension guidelines (including JNC-7) (Fig. 7-8) recommend nutritional-hygienic measures to control BP, despite the absence of clinical trial data demonstrating that these modalities significantly reduce CVD morbidity and mortality. There is, however, a good public health rationale for advocating weight loss, dietary salt restriction, and other lifestyle modifications as preventive, adjunctive, and (occasionally) definitive treatment for hypertension. In multicenter clinical trials involving overweight subjects, weight loss is the most effective single modality that reduces BP in the short term. Dietary salt restriction to about 90 to 100 mmol (2000–2400 mg) of sodium per day is also effective in lowering BP. Recidivism can be a problem for both weight loss and sodium restriction, however, and long-term adherence to such programs is uncommon in many clinics. Also recommended (if appropriate for the individual) are: alcohol restriction to one to two drinks per day (two to three in the British Hypertension Society guidelines), tobacco avoidance, major exercise (30 minutes most days of the week), reduction of caffeine (if excessive), and supplements of potassium, calcium, and/or magnesium (only if a deficiency state is present).

In the Treatment of Mild Hypertension Study (TOMHS), a vigorous program of lifestyle modifications, executed by experts with very motivated participants, was inferior to antihypertensive drug therapy *plus* lifestyle modifications in both reducing BP and preventing overall CVD events.[106] Because of the difficulties in sustaining initial efforts using lifestyle modifications alone, many patients and most clinicians prefer a strategy that adds effective antihypertensive drug therapy even earlier than the 6 to 12 months that JNC-VI recommended, particularly when initial efforts at weight

TABLE 7-7   Screening and Other Tests for Common Forms of Secondary Hypertension

Diagnosis	Preferred screening test(s)	Other tests
Renovascular hypertension	Captopril scintigraphy	Doppler ultrasound of renal arteries, magnetic resonance angiography, renal angiogram
Mineralocorticoid excess states	24-h urinary aldosterone during salt loading, plasma aldosterone/renin ratio	Computed tomographic scan of adrenals
Pheochromocytoma	24-h urine for vanillylmandelic acid (VMA) and metanephrines	Plasma metanephrines, plasma catecholamines, T_2-weighted magnetic resonance imaging
Sleep apnea	Formal sleep study	
Cushing's syndrome	8 AM plasma cortisol	Dexamethasone suppression test(s)
Hypothyroidism	Thyroid-stimulating hormone (TSH)	Serum thyroxine, triiodothyronine levels

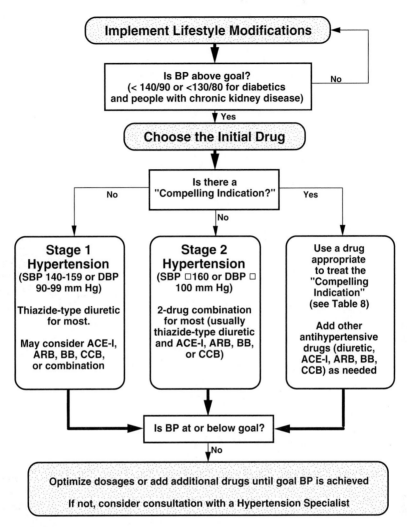

FIGURE 7-8 Authors' algorithm for choosing antihypertensive drug therapy, modified slightly from JNC-7.[4] If the initial BP is more than 20/10 mm Hg above goal, two drugs are recommended, one of which should be a diuretic in most people. JNC-7 recommended an angiotensin II receptor blocker as a co-equal choice with an ACE inhibitor; some would use these newer and more expensive drugs only when an ACE inhibitor is contraindicated or not tolerated.

loss and sodium restriction are unsuccessful or troublesome.

Choice of initial drug therapy

INITIAL ANTIHYPERTENSIVE DRUG THERAPY FOR "COMPLICATED PATIENTS"

Both JNC-VI and JNC-7 formally recognized that many hypertensive people begin treatment too late, after they have already developed CVD or other medical condi-

tions that may be positively affected by specific antihypertensive drug therapies.[4,27] JNC-VI divided these situations into "compelling conditions" and "clinical conditions." In the former, a specific class of antihypertensive drug should be prescribed if clinical trials showed that class of drug reduces morbidity and/or mortality for that condition.[4] Thus, for a hypertensive person with systolic heart failure, an ACE inhibitor will be likely not only to lower BP, but also to reduce clinical events and hospitalizations. Table 7-8 lists antihypertensive drugs that

TABLE 7-8 Compelling Conditions for Which Specific Antihypertensive Drug Therapy Has Reduced Morbidity and/or Mortality in Clinical Trials

"Compelling indication"	Treatment prevents/delays	Recommended in 1997	Recommended in 2003
Heart Failure (Systolic Type)	CV events	ACE-I*(CONSENSUS,[†] SAVE, etc)	Beta blockers (MERIT-HF, etc); spironolactone (RALES); ARB (Val-HeFT, CHARM)
After recent MI	Recurrent infarction or death	Beta blocker (ISIS, etc)	
Diminished LV function after recent MI	Recurrent infarction, CHF hospitalization	ACE-I (SAVE, TRACE)	Eplerenone (EPHESUS)
Known CVD	CV events		ACE-I (HOPE)
Type 1 diabetes mellitus	Deterioration in renal function	ACE-I (CCSG)	
Type 2 diabetes	CV events		ACE-I (MICRO-HOPE)
Type 2 diabetic nephropathy	Deterioration in renal function		ARBs (IDNT, RENAAL)
Type 2 diabetes	Progression of micro-albuminuria		ACE-I (MICRO-HOPE); ARB (IRMA-2)
Older hypertensive persons	CV events	Diuretic (SHEP); DHP-CA (Syst-Eur)	ACE-I or DHP-CA (STOP-2); DHP-CA (Syst-China); ARB (SCOPE, second-line); ARB (LIFE)
Nondiabetic chronic kidney disease	Deterioration in renal function		ACE-I (REIN, AIPRI, AASK)
Prior Stroke/TIA	Stroke and CV events		ACE-I (PROGRESS)
LVH (using strict criteria)	CV events (perhaps limited to stroke?)		ARB (LIFE)

*ACE-I, angiotensin-converting enzyme inhibitor; ARB, angiotensin receptor blocker, DHP-CA, dihydropyridine calcium antagonist.

[†]CONSENSUS = Cooperative North Scandinavian Enalapril Survival Study (*N Engl J Med* 1987; 316:1429–1435); SAVE = Survival and Ventricular Enlargement Study (*N Engl J Med* 1992;327:669–677); CCSG = Captopril Cooperative Study Group (*N Engl J Med* 1993; 323:1456–1462); SHEP = Systolic Hypertension in the Elderly Program (*JAMA* 1991;265:3255–3264); Syst-Eur = Systolic Hypertension in Europe Trial (*Lancet* 1997;360:757–764); MERIT-HF = Metoprolol Randomized Intervention Trial in Congestive Heart Failure (*JAMA* 2000;283:1295–1302); RALES = Randomized Aldactone Evaluation Study (*N Engl J Med* 1999;341:709–717); Val-HeFT = Valsartan Heart Failure Trial (*N Engl J Med* 2001;345:1667–1675); CHARM = Candesartan Heart Failure Assessment of Reduction in Morbidity and Mortality (*Lancet* 2003;362:759–781); ISIS = International Study of Infarct Survival (*Lancet* 1986;2:57–66); TRACE = Trandolapril Cardiac Evaluation (*N Engl J Med* 1995;333:1670–1676); EPHESUS = Eplerenone Post-Myocardial Infarction Heart Failure Efficacy and Survival Study (*N Engl J Med* 2003;348:1309–1321); HOPE = Heart Outcomes Prevention Evaluation (*N Engl J Med* 2000;342:145–153); MICRO-HOPE = Microalbuminuria, Cardiovascular and Renal Outcomes Substudy of the Heart Outcomes Prevention Evaluation (*Lancet* 2000;355:253–259); IDNT = Irbesartan Diabetic Nephropathy Trial (*N Engl J Med* 2001;345:841–860); RENAAL = Reduction of Endpoints in Non-Insulin-Dependent Diabetes Mellitus with the Angiotensin II Antagonist Losartan (*N Engl J Med* 2001;345:861–869); IRMA-2 = Irbesartan Microalbuminuria Study 2 (*N Engl J Med* 2001;345:870–878); STOP-2 = Swedish Trial in Old Patients with Hypertension 2 (*Lancet* 1999;354:1751–1756); Syst-China = Systolic Hypertension in China Trial (*J Hypertens* 1998;16:1823–1829); SCOPE = Study on Cognition and Prognosis in the Elderly (*J Hypertens* 2003;21:875–886); LIFE = Losartan Intervention for Endpoint Reduction (*Lancet* 2002;359:995–1003); REIN = Ramipril Evaluation in Nephropathy Trial (*Lancet* 1998;352:1252–1256); AIPRI = Angiotensin-Converting Enzyme Inhibition in Progressive Renal Insufficiency (*Kidney Int* 1997;suppl. 63:S63–S67); AASK = African American Study of Kidney Disease and Hypertension (*JAMA* 2002;288:2421–2431); PROGRESS = Perindopril Protection Against Recurrent Stroke Study (*Lancet* 2001;358:1033–1041).

TABLE 7-9 Contraindications for Specific Antihypertensive Drug Classes

Antihypertensive Drug Class	Contraindication
Thiazide diuretic	Allergy
Beta blocker	Asthma
ACE inhibitor	Angioedema due to ACE inhibitor, pregnancy
Calcium antagonist	Allergy
Angiotensin II receptor blocker	Pregnancy, renal artery stenosis
Alpha blocker	Orthostatic hypotension with frequent falls
α_2-Agonist (centrally acting drug)	Allergy

improve prognosis in conditions commonly seen in hypertensive persons. There are also some absolute and relative contraindications for specific antihypertensive drugs that limit their use as initial therapy in all hypertensive persons (Table 7-9).

INITIAL ANTIHYPERTENSIVE DRUG THERAPY FOR "UNCOMPLICATED HYPERTENSIVES"

Since ALLHAT, the "default choice" for initial antihypertensive drug therapy for most patients is a low-dose thiazide-type diuretic. Those who strictly adhere to "evidence-based medicine" insist on chlorthalidone, but some are willing to accept hydrochlorothiazide. However, data from MRFIT suggested that hydrochlorothiazide was associated with a higher risk of cardiac events than chlorthalidone.[107] Perhaps because a 12.5-mg dose of chlorthalidone is not commercially available, JNC-7 did not distinguish between these two diuretics, but did recommend a thiazide-type diuretic "for most patients."

ADD-ON DRUG THERAPY

Perhaps because there are few clinical trials that directly compared second-step antihypertensive drugs (following an initial diuretic), JNC-7 recommended an ACE inhibitor, ARB, beta blocker, or calcium antagonist, but gave little further guidance. Some would add to the list an alpha blocker, which was inferior to chlorthalidone as *initial* therapy in ALLHAT.[78] Others would routinely favor an ACE inhibitor or an ARB because of the potential synergy on serum potassium when combined with a thiazide or thiazide-like diuretic. Beta blockers have the largest clinical trial experience as a second-line agent to be used after a diuretic. Calcium antagonists have never been tested in clinical trials as a second-line agent after a diuretic, although one combination of a diuretic and calcium antagonist was used successfully in the first factorial design study of antihypertensive agents,[108] and this was the combination used in many volunteers in CONVINCE.[80]

Target blood pressures

Unlike its predecessor, JNC-7 now recommends only one of two BP targets. For uncomplicated hypertensive patients, the BP should be lowered to below 140/90 mm Hg. For diabetic patients or those with chronic kidney disease, the BP should be less than 130/80 mm Hg. The Hypertension Optimal Treatment (HOT) study showed (in 18,790 hypertensive patients) the benefit of reducing the BP to 138.5/82.6 mm Hg, which was the achieved BP associated with "optimal reduction in CVD risk." Risk was not significantly increased by reducing BP to a diastolic target of 80 mm Hg or lower, but there was no further benefit, either.[58] Because the probability of drug-related side effects often increases as dose is increased, it is likely that the target BP of less than 140/90 mm Hg for uncomplicated hypertensive patients will be defensible for some time to come.

JNC-7 recommended that diabetic patients, and those with chronic kidney disease, should have a BP target less than 130/80 mm Hg. It is easier to justify this for diabetics than for patients with chronic kidney disease. The first clinical trial to demonstrate the benefit of a lower BP target for diabetics was the United Kingdom Prospective Diabetes Study (UKPDS) 38.[109] Over 8.4 years of follow-up, among 1148 type 2 diabetics randomized to two different BP goals (<150/85 or <180/105 mm Hg), those treated to the lower goal did much better. Interestingly, the difference in achieved BPs between groups was 10/5 mm Hg (154/87 mm Hg vs 144/82 mm Hg), which, when subtracted from the usual current BP goal for nondiabetic patients (140/90 mm Hg), gives a target for diabetics *identical* to that recommended by JNC-VI: 130/85 mm Hg! In the 1501 diabetics in the HOT study, the lowest risk of stroke, heart attack, or CVD death in the intent-to-treat analysis was seen in those randomized to a diastolic BP of 80 mm Hg or lower.[58] Thus, the target BP of less than 130/80 mm Hg has now been recommended by nearly all authorities for diabetics, including JNC-7.[4]

There were concerns that the lower BP goal recommended for diabetics would be expensive, as it requires more antihypertensive medication and more visits to health care providers. A cost analysis of the UKPDS clinical trial, however, did not support this: despite higher drug and provider costs, the strategy of the lower BP goal saved lives, strokes, limbs, and *money*. The cost-effectiveness ratio for the lower BP goal was -£720 per year of life saved, and an even more impressive -£1049 per year of life without diabetic complications.[110] A similar conclusion was derived from an economic analysis of US epidemiologic and clinical trial data for older (≥60 years) diabetics treated to a goal of less than 130/85 mm Hg (recommended initially by JNC-VI), compared with leaving the target BP at less than 140/90 mm Hg.[111] Because the lower BP goal impressively reduces the risk of expensive CVD events, including stroke, heart attack, heart failure, and renal replacement therapy, the incremental cost-effectiveness ratio for the lower BP goal is negative (meaning more intensive treatment saves money!), just as in UKPDS.

JNC-7 recommended the BP target of less than 130/80 mm Hg for patients with chronic kidney disease, but there are fewer clinical trial data on this topic. In the African American Study of Kidney (AASK) Diseases, there was no benefit to reducing BP to less than 125/75 mm Hg (compared with <140/90 mm Hg). JNC-7 therefore backed away from the <125/75 mm Hg target, and simply suggested a target identical to that for diabetics.

Constructing a regimen

Because most hypertensive patients require more than a single drug to achieve the more intensive treatment goals recommended currently, one probably needs to worry less about the initial choice of therapy than the appropriate combinations of drugs necessary to achieve the goal BP. Even in ALLHAT, which restricted enrollment to those with a high chance of being controlled on single-drug therapy (untreated BP <180/110 mm Hg or BP <160/100 on one or two drugs), an average of two medications per patient were required at the end of the study.[83]

The ideal drug regimen would have many characteristics. In addition to lowering the BP to goal, the regimen should be able to be administered once daily, without regard to meals, be relatively inexpensive, cause few adverse effects (and perhaps even result in fewer side effects than single-drug therapy), and be widely available in all pharmacies and benefit plans. Several of the newer fixed-dose combination products have several of these attributes; those combining a dihydropyridine calcium antagonist and an ACE inhibitor, for instance, cause less pedal edema than the calcium channel blocker alone,

even at the same doses. It is unfortunate that only one triple-drug combination, containing a diuretic, reserpine, and low-dose hydralazine, is available in the United States.

Management in special circumstances

Aside from patients who have a "special indication" for a particular antihypertensive drug (see Table 7-8), hypertensive patients at increased risk for CVD require more attention. Those falling into this category include hypertensive patients of older age, those with diabetes, those who are pregnant, those awaiting surgery, those with refractory hypertension or chronic kidney disease, and those in hypertensive crisis.

OLDER PATIENTS WITH HYPERTENSION

There is now no question that older patients derive major benefit from antihypertensive drug therapy (Fig. 7-9). In fact, the "number needed to treat" to prevent a single CVD event is far lower for older (compared with younger) patients, simply because their age places them at a higher absolute risk. A meta-analysis that included all 1870 patients over age 80 enrolled in eight clinical trials showed that substantial and significant reductions in stroke, CVD events, and heart failure accrue in people over age 80 who are given antihypertensive medications (Fig. 7-10).[95]

DIABETIC PATIENTS WITH HYPERTENSION

The regimen used to treat diabetics to a BP goal of less than 130/80 mm Hg should include either an ACE inhibitor or an ARB (see Table 7-8).[112] An ARB can be justified if the patient is intolerant of an ACE inhibitor, or if the patient has type 2 diabetes, chronic kidney disease, and major proteinuria (eg, patients in IDNT and RENAAL). An ACE inhibitor exhibited renoprotective effects in type 1 diabetics. Both an ACE inhibitor and an ARB have been shown to reduce the progression of microalbuminuria to overt proteinuria (in MICRO-HOPE and IRMA-2). The CVD benefits of an ACE inhibitor in type 2 diabetics have been seen in MICRO-HOPE. Further studies are needed to determine whether both an ACE inhibitor and an ARB (as in COOPERATE) will be useful in diabetics. The challenge for most diabetics is to achieve the BP goal. Most surveys of BP control in large groups of patients have shown much worse control of BP in diabetic subjects, as compared with nondiabetics, even when equivalent target BPs (<140/90 mm Hg) are used.

PREGNANT PATIENTS WITH HYPERTENSION

Many antihypertensive drugs are either contraindicated or a potential threat to the mother or fetus.[113] Diuretics, the preferred first-line therapy for nonpregnant hypertensive individuals, are generally avoided during pregnancy

FIGURE 7-9   Results of a meta-analysis of 14 controlled treatment trials of antihypertensive drug therapy in ~23,996 older adults. The number of each type of endpoint is given in the left column. The dark vertical bars indicate the point estimate of the risk reduction with antihypertensive drug therapy; shaded boxes indicate the 95% confidence intervals. In this meta-analysis, because the odds ratios for all cardiovascular events are significantly different from 1.00, antihypertensive drug therapy was associated with a statistically significant reduction in all endpoints, including all-cause mortality. (Modified from Elliott WJ. Treatment of hypertension in the elderly: an updated meta-analysis [abstract]. *Am J Hypertens* 2001;14:145A.)

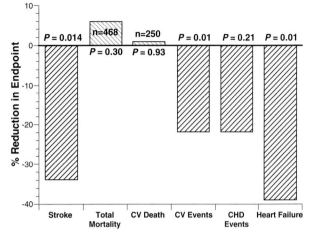

due to the risk of oligohydramnios. ACE inhibitors and ARBs are contraindicated due to the risk of renal and other fetal malformations. Nitroprusside is transformed to cyanide, which is very toxic to the fetus. As a result, time-tested and traditional antihypertensive drug therapy is usually used, including, in order, methyldopa, hydralazine, a beta blocker (typically labetalol), and then perhaps a calcium antagonist.

HYPERTENSIVE PATIENTS AWAITING SURGERY

Most hypertensive patients receive closer scrutiny when elective surgery is planned; occasionally the procedure must be postponed, especially if the BP is higher than 160/95 mm Hg. For individuals who show no evidence of major coronary disease, short-term treatment with a beta blocker is often recommended.[114,115] This is an excellent example of how CVD risk can be reduced by treatment that is given for only a few days.

PATIENTS WITH REFRACTORY HYPERTENSION

The more common causes of refractory hypertension are listed in Table 7-10; the most common may be nonadherence to prescribed antihypertensive therapy. Close behind are other drugs the patient may be taking, especially NSAIDs. The most common successful pharmacologic intervention for patients with resistant hypertension in our clinic is modification of the drug regimen. Adding or switching to an appropriate diuretic (a thiazide if GFR = 50 mL/min, or loop diuretic if GFR is < 50 mL/min) and adding an alpha blocker are the most frequent successful changes.

HYPERTENSIVE PATIENTS WITH CHRONIC KIDNEY DISEASE

People with hypertension and chronic kidney disease should have their dose (or, less commonly, frequency of administration) of renally excreted antihypertensive drugs reduced and should be treated to a lower target

FIGURE 7-10   Results of a meta-analysis of all 1870 patients over age 80 years in eight clinical trials of antihypertensive drug therapy. Results are expressed as percentage reduction in each endpoint seen in those given antihypertensive drug therapy, as compared with those given placebo or no treatment. (Modified from Gueyffier F, et al. Antihypertensive drugs in very old people: a subgroup meta-analysis of randomised clinical trials. *Lancet* 1999;353:793–796.)

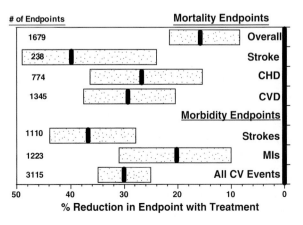

TABLE 7-10   Common Causes of "Resistant Hypertension"

Pseudo-resistant hypertension
"White-coat" hypertension" (clinic responder)
Nonadherence to Antihypertensive Therapy
Dietary indiscretion to salt, ethanol, or other dietary stimulus

Poor adherence to drug treatment, due to:
    Side effects of antihypertensive agents
    Excessive cost of medication(s)
    Inconvenient or inappropriate dosing schedules
    Organic brain syndrome (eg, impairment of memory, forgetfulness)

Poor understanding of the importance of taking pills as directed
    Inadequate patient education
    Instructions not understood
    Lack of continuing, consistent primary source of medical care

Drug-Related Causes
Inadequate doses of antihypertensive drugs
Inappropriate combinations of antihypertensive drugs (eg, clonidine + methyldopa)
Rapid metabolism (eg, rapid acetylators of hydralazine)

Drug–drug interactions
    Nonsteroidal anti-inflammatory drugs
    Sympathomimetic agents (eg, nasal decongestants, appetite suppressants, cocaine, caffeine)
    Oral contraceptive pills (more of a problem with older, high-dose agents)
    Corticosteroids
    Licorice (and similarly flavored chewing tobacco)
    Cyclosporine/tacrolimus
    Erythropoeitin
    Cholestyramine (or other resin-binding agents, taken simultaneously with antihypertensive drugs)
    Antidepressants (monoamine oxidase inhibitors, some tricylics [Venlafaxine])

Rebound hypertension after abrupt discontinuation of centrally acting drugs, beta blockers, or, occasionally, calcium antagonists
Associated Medical Conditions
Tobacco use (especially cigarette smoking during the 15 min before BP measurement) Increasing weight (and obesity)
Chronic pain
Intense, acute vasoconstriction (eg, Raynaud's phenomenon)
Insulin resistance/hyperinsulinemia
Anxiety-induced hypertension, hyperventilation, and/or panic attacks
Secondary Hypertension
Renovascular hypertension
Chronic kidney disease
Sleep apnea
Pheochromocytoma
Mineralocorticoid excess states
Volume Overload
Excessive sodium intake
Progressive renal damage and impairment (eg, hypertensive nephrosclerosis)
Fluid retention due to direct (or indirect) vasodilators (eg, minoxidil)
Inadequate or inappropriate diuretic therapy

SOURCE: Modified from the Sixth Report of the Joint National Committee on Prevention, Detection, Evaluation, and Treatment of High Blood Pressure (JNC VI). *Arch Intern Med* 1997;157:2414–2446.

(currently <130/80 mm Hg).[116] An ACE inhibitor or ARB is highly recommended, after which a modest acute rise in serum creatinine and usually clinically nonsignificant increase in serum potassium should be expected.[117] An ARB was useful in preventing the progression of renal disease in type 2 diabetics in both IDNT and RENAAL; an ACE inhibitor was more effective than the calcium antagonist or beta blocker in AASK. An ACE inhibitor can be recommended for nondiabetic chronic kidney disease.[118]

PATIENTS IN HYPERTENSIVE CRISIS

Hypertensive emergencies are best treated in hospital (typically in the ICU) with a short-acting, rapidly reversible, intravenously administered antihypertensive drug (typically nitroprusside).[119] Hypertensive urgencies may be routinely treated in the outpatient setting with any one of a number of oral antihypertensive agents, including captopril, labetalol, and clonidine. Nifedipine capsules, which had been widely used in this setting for nearly 20 years, are now to be used "with great caution, if at all," according to an FDA advisory, because of their propensity to cause quick and excessive hypotension. Perhaps the most important aspect of the treatment of hypertensive crisis is to arrange quick follow-up for the patient where chronic, better management of BP can be ensured.

Organizing for successful management

The goal of hypertension management is to prevent the morbidity and mortality associated with it and to do so in the "least intrusive" manner (both physiologically and fiscally). As hypertension is not a disease, but a condition that increases the risk of developing CVD and renal disease, its long-term control is a continuing challenge. For many years, it was thought that most patients with hypertension have no noticeable symptoms. Studies using antihypertensive drugs without appreciable side effects have demonstrated a significant decrease in headache when hypertensive patients are successfully treated. The quality of life among treated hypertensive patients was greatest in the group that achieved the lowest BPs in both HOT and TOMHS, suggesting that there may be subtle symptoms that can be attributed to an elevated BP that improve when BP is lowered. It is nonetheless often difficult to convince a person with hypertension that taking a pill or changing his or her lifestyle will result in tangible benefits, especially in the short term. It is also unfortunately true that treating hypertension (even successfully) does not reduce CVD risk to the level of a normotensive person. This provides strong impetus for initiating lifestyle modifications early, even before the levels of BP we call hypertension are present.

It is therefore not surprising that it is difficult in the long term to motivate patients to sustain their lifestyle modifications and adhere to the prescribed medications. National survey data indicate that only 34% of America's hypertensive people have their BPs lower than 140/90 mm Hg[4]; in other parts of the world, the results are even worse. There have been many official reports about, and efforts to improve, adherence to pill taking. Nonadherence results in unnecessary hospitalizations, preventable strokes and myocardial infarctions, and a large portion of the admissions to nursing homes (where drug taking can be more carefully and efficiently supervised).

Many suggestions have been made to increase adherence to pill taking; some have been proven successful in clinical trials. Several clinical trials in conditions besides hypertension (eg, after myocardial infarction or in heart failure) have shown that patients who do not take the pills as directed typically suffer more hard endpoints than those who are adherent. Education of the patient (and family) is the cornerstone of improving adherence; patients with educational or cognitive deficits about hypertension and its treatment are unlikely to follow instructions for very long. Some clinics have improved their hypertension control rates after adding a health educator to the hypertension treatment team. Behavioral suggestions are often useful: integrating pill taking into the activities of daily living (eg, taking pills when caring for teeth), or using a pill organizer (typically to organize pills according to days of the week they are to be consumed). Increasing social support appears to be a beneficial strategy, especially for older individuals. The family member or caretaker can remind the patient of the need to take pills and keep office visits, as well as actually measure BP with a home device.

Missing one's appointments for follow-up care and monitoring of hypertension treatment has been associated with poorer outcomes. Several routine procedures can help to minimize this problem. Appointment reminders (either by telephone or by mail) increase return visit rates. Scheduling a specific time and date with a known health care provider, at the end of the office visit, is more successful than "calling in for a future appointment." Decreased waiting times, convenient office hours, and a solicitous, caring office staff are also helpful. Several characteristics of physicians impact on patients' adherence to taking medications and willingness to keep appointments. The Medical Outcomes Study showed that physicians who are willing to involve the patient (when appropriate) in medical decision making are more successful in controlling BP.[120] A common example is asking whether the patient would prefer to take a less expensive pill more often or a more expensive pill just once a day. Physicians who are perceived as having effective communication skills, who encourage questions from the patient and appropriate family members, and who provide feedback about the patient's progress also achieved better results.

Much of the underachievement of BP control nationwide has been attributed to patients' unwillingness to take pills and appear for follow-up visits, but some of the blame has been attributed to physicians and other components of the health care system.[121] Most systems have accepted the treatment of hypertension as a worthwhile endeavor, one that is actually cost-saving in high-risk patients and relatively cost-effective in others (compared with many other common medical interventions). Efforts to restrict pharmacy benefits, limit the range and doses of drugs on an accepted formulary, and reduce accessibility to health care services have led to increased costs. Systemwide efforts (often called "disease management programs") to encourage acceptance of generic drugs, increase the threshold for beginning antihypertensive drug therapy in low-risk patients, use one drug to treat both hypertension and a concomitant medical condition, and to encourage adherence to medication taking have been more successful. The workload of the health care provider involved in these efforts can be increased by some of these procedures, but is sometimes offset by case managers and other allied health professionals who perform some of these important tasks.

Hypertension control is an important public health goal that requires a long-term commitment from the patient, the physician, and the health care system. When all work together, the benefits of hypertension therapy in clinical trials can be easily and effectively translated into practice. This will eventually reduce the burden of CVD and renal disease that was formerly associated with untreated or undertreated elevated BP.

REFERENCES

1. Wolf-Maier K, Cooper RS, Banegas JR, et al. Hypertension prevalence and blood pressure levels in 6 European countries, Canada, and the United States. *JAMA* 2003;289:2363–2369.

2. Ezzati M, Lopez AD, Rodgers A, et al, and the Comparative Risk Assessment Collaborating Group. Selected major risk factors and global and regional burden of disease. *Lancet* 2002;360:1347–1360.

3. Murray CJ, Lopez AD. Alternative projections of mortality and disability by cause 1990–2020: Global Burden of Disease Study. *Lancet* 1997;349:1498–1504.

4. Chobanian AV, Bakris GL, Black HR, et al. The seventh report of the Joint National Committee on Prevention, Detection, Evaluation, and Treatment of High Blood Pressure: the JNC 7 Report. *JAMA* 2003;289:2560–2572.

5. Cherry DK, Woodwell DA. National Ambulatory Care Survey: 2000 summary. *Advance Data* 2002;328:1–32.

6. Prospective Studies Collaborative. Age-specific relevance of usual blood pressure to vascular mortality: a meta-analysis of individual data for one million adults in 61 prospective studies. *Lancet* 2002;360:1903–1913.

7. Staessen JA, Wang JG, Thijs L. Cardiovascular protection and blood pressure reduction: a meta-analysis. *Lancet* 2001;358:1305–1315.

8. Vasan RS, Larson MG, Leip EP, et al. Impact of high-normal blood pressure on the risk of cardiovascular disease. *N Engl J Med* 2001;345:1291–1297.

9. Vasan RS, Beiser A, Seshadri S, et al. Residual lifetime risk for developing hypertension in middle-aged women and men: the Framingham Heart Study. *JAMA*. 2002;287:1003–1010.

10. Franklin SS, Khan SA, Wong ND, et al. Is pulse pressure useful in predicting risk for coronary heart disease? The Framingham Heart Study. *Circulation* 1999;100:354–360.

11. Blacher J, Staessen JA, Girerd X, et al. Pulse pressure, not mean pressure, determines cardiovasular risk in older hypertensive patients. *Arch Intern Med* 2000;160:1085–1089.

12. Glynn RJ, Chae CU, Guralnik JM, et al. Pulse pressure and mortality in older people. *Arch Intern Med* 2000;160:2765–2772.

13. Perloff D, Grim C, Flack J, et al. Special report: human blood pressure determination by sphygomanometry [AHA Medical/Scientific Statement]. *Circulation* 1993;88:2460–2470.

14. Yarows SA, Julius S, Pickering TG. Home blood pressure monitoring. *Arch Intern Med* 2000;160:1251–1257.

15. Kjeldsen SE, Hedner J, Jamerson K, et al. Hypertension Optimal Treatment (HOT) study: home blood pressure in treated hypertensive subjects. *Hypertension* 1998;31:1014–1020.

16. Broege PA, James GD, Pickering TG. Management of hypertension in the elderly using home blood pressures. *Blood Press Monit* 2001;6:139–144.

17. Perloff D, Sokolow M, Cowan RM, Juster RP. Prognostic value of ambulatory blood pressure measurements: further analyses. *J Hypertens* 1989;7(suppl 3):S3–S10.

18. Verdecchia P, Porcellati C, Schillaci G, et al. Ambulatory blood pressure: an independent predictor of prognosis in essential hypertension. *Hypertension* 1994;24:793–801.

19. Verdecchia P, Schillaci G, Borgioni C, et al. Prognostic significance of the white coat effect. *Hypertension* 1997;29:1218–1224.

20. O'Brien E, Beevers G, Lip GYH. ABC of hypertension: blood pressure measurement: Part III. Automated sphygmomanometry: ambulatory blood pressure measurement. *BMJ* 2001;322:1110–1114.

21. Tunis S, Kendall P, Londner M, Whyte J. Medicare Coverage Policy ~ Decisions: Ambulatory Blood Pressure Monitoring (CAG-00067N): Decision Memorandum. Washington, DC: Health Care Financing Administration; October 17, 2001. Found on the Internet at: www.hcfa.gov/coverage/8b3-ff2.htm; accessed 01 APR 02 at 18:32 CST.

22. Staessen JA, Bieniaszewski L, O'Brien ET, Fagard R. What is normal blood pressure in ambulatory monitoring? *Nephrol Dial Transplant* 1996;11:241–245.

23. Rasmussen SL, Torp-Pedersen C, Borch-Johnsen K, Ibsen H. Normal values for ambulatory blood pressure and differences between casual blood pressure and ambulatory blood pressure: results from a Danish population survey. *J Hypertens* 1998;16:1415–1424.

24. Staessen JA, Thijs L, Fagard R, et al. Predicting cardiovascular risk using conventional vs. ambulatory blood pressure

in older patients with systolic hypertension. *JAMA* 1999;282:589–596.

25. Kario K, Pickering TG, Matsuo T, et al. Stroke prognosis and abnormal nocturnal blood pressure falls in older hypertensives. *Hypertension* 2001;38:852–857.

26. Bur A, Herkner H, Vlcek M, et al. Classification of blood pressure levels by ambulatory blood pressure in hypertension. *Hypertension* 2002;40:817–822.

27. The sixth report of the Joint National Committee on Prevention, Detection, Evaluation, and Treatment of High Blood Pressure (JNC VI). *Arch Intern Med* 1997;157:2413–2446.

28. O'Brien E, Coats A, Owens P, et al. Use and interpretation of ambulatory blood pressure monitoring: recommendations of the British Hypertension Society. *BMJ* 2000;320:1128–1134.

29. Staessen JA, Bieniaszewski L, O'Brien E, et al. Nocturnal blood pressure fall on ambulatory monitoring in a large international database. *Hypertension* 1997;29:30–39.

30. Lurbe E, Redon J, Kesani A, et al. Increase in nocturnal blood pressure and progression to microalbuminuria in type 1 diabetes. *N Engl J Med* 2002;347:797–805.

31. Verdecchia P, Schillaci G, Borgioni C, et al. Adverse prognostic value of a blunted circadian rhythm of heart rate in essential hypertension. *J Hypertens* 1998;16:1335–1343.

32. Verdecchia P, Schillaci G, Reboldi G, et al. Different prognostic impact of 24–hour mean blood pressure and pulse pressure on stroke and coronary artery disease in essential hypertension. *Circulation* 2001;103:2579–2584.

33. Verdecchia P, Reboldi G, Porcellati C, et al. Risk of cardiovascular disease in relation to achieved office and ambulatory blood pressure control in treated hypertensive subjects. *J Am Coll Cardiol* 2002;39:878–885.

34. Elliott WJ. Circadian variation in blood pressure: implications for elderly patients. *Am J Hypertension* 1999;12:43S–49S.

35. Kario K, Eguchi K, Hoshide S, et al. U-Curve relationship between orthostatic blood pressure change and silent cerebrovascular disease in elderly hypertensives: orthostatic hypertension as a new cardiovascular risk factor. *J Am Coll Cardiol* 2002;40:133–141.

36. Liu JE, Roman MJ, Pini R, et al. Cardiac and arterial target organ damage in adults with elevated ambulatory and normal office blood pressure. *Ann Intern Med* 1999;131:564–572.

37. Ohkubo T, Imai Y, Tsuji I, et al. Prediction of mortality by ambulatory blood pressure monitoring versus screening blood pressure measurements: a pilot study in Ohasama. *J Hypertens* 1997;15:357–364.

38. Redon J, Campos C, Narciso ML, et al. Prognostic value of ambulatory blood pressure monitoring in refractory hypertension: a prospective study. *Hypertension* 1998;31:712–718.

39. Pierdomenico SD, Bucci A, Constantini F, et al. Twenty-four hour autonomic nervous function in sustained and "white coat" hypertension. *Am Heart J* 2000;140:672–677.

40. Muscholl MW, Hense HW, Brockel U, et al. Changes in left ventricular structure and function in patients with white coat hypertension: cross sectional survey. *BMJ* 1998;317:565–570.

41. Owens PE, Lyons SP, Rodriguez SA, O'Brien ET. Is elevation of clinic blood pressure in patients with white coat hypertension who have normal ambulatory blood pressure associated with target organ changes? *J Hum Hypertens* 1998;12:743–748.

42. Palatini P, Mormini P, Santonastaso M, et al, for the HARVEST Study Investigators. Target organ damage in stage 1 hypertensive subjects with white coat and sustained hypertension: results from the HARVEST Study. *Hypertension* 1998;31:57–63.

43. Grandi AM, Broggi R, Colombo S, et al. Left ventricular changes in isolated office hypertension: a blood pressure-matched comparison with normotension and sustained hypertension. *Arch Intern Med* 2001;161:2677–2681.

44. Sega R, Trocino G, Lanzarotti A, et al. Alterations of cardiac structure in patients with isolated office, ambulatory, or home hypertension: data from the general population (Pressione Arteriose Monitorate E Loro Associazioni [PAMELA] Study). *Circulation* 2001;104:1385–1392.

45. Verdecchia P, Schillaci G, Borgioni C, et al. White-coat hypertension: not guilty when correctly defined. *Blood Press Monit* 1998;3:147–152.

46. Moser M. White-coat hypertension: to treat or not to treat: a clinical dilemma [editorial]. *Arch Intern Med* 2001;161:2655–2656.

47. Executive Summary of the Third Report of the National Cholesterol Education Program (NCEP) Expert Panel on Detection, Evaluation, and Treatment of High Blood Cholesterol in Adults (Adult Treatment Panel III). *JAMA* 2001;285:2486–2497.

48. Black HR. *Clinical Trials in Hypertension.* New York: Marcel Dekker, Inc; 2001.

49. Psaty BM, Lumley T, Furberg CD, et al. Health outcomes associated with various antihypertensive therapies used as first-line agents: a network meta-analysis. *JAMA* 2003;289:2534–2544.

50. Turnbull F. Blood Pressure Lowering Treatment Trialists' Collaboration: effects of different blood-pressure-lowering regimens on major cardiovascular events: results of prospectively-designed overviews of randomised trials. *Lancet* 2003;362:1527–1535.

51. Collins R, Peto R, MacMahon S, et al. Blood pressure, stroke, and coronary heart disease: Part 2, Short-term reductions in blood pressure: overview of randomised drug trials in their epidemiological context. *Lancet* 1990;335:827–838.

52. Psaty BM, Smith NL, Siscovick DS, et al. Health outcomes associated with antihypertensive therapies used as first-line agents: a systematic review and meta-analysis. *JAMA* 1997;277:739–745.

53. The Heart Outcomes Prevention Evaluation (HOPE) Study Investigators. Effects of an angiotensin-converting-enzyme inhibitor, ramipril, on death from cardiovascular causes, myocardial infarction, and stroke in high-risk patients. *N Engl J Med* 2000;342:145–153.

54. Heart Outcomes Prevention Evaluation (HOPE) Study Investigators. Effects of ramipril on cardiovascular and microvascular outcomes in people with diabetes mellitus: The HOPE study and MICRO-HOPE substudy. *Lancet* 2000;355:253–259.

55. PROGRESS Collaborative Group. Randomised trial of a perindopril-based blood-pressure-lowering regimen among 6105 individuals with previous stroke or transient ischaemic attack. *Lancet* 2001;358:1033–1041.

56. Agodoa LY, Appel L, Bakris GL, et al, for the African American Study of Kidney Disease and Hypertension (AASK) Study

Group. Effect of ramipril vs. amlodipine on renal outcomes in hypertensive nephrosclerosis: a randomized controlled trial. *JAMA* 2001;285:2719–2728.

57. Wright JT Jr, Bakris GL, Greene T, et al. Effect of blood pressure lowering and antihypertensive drug class on progression of hypertensive kidney disease: results from the AASK Trial. *JAMA* 2002;288:2421–2431.

58. Hansson L, Zandretti A, Carruthers SG, et al, for the HOT Study Group. Effects of intensive blood pressure lowering and low-dose aspirin in patients with hypertension: principal results of the Hypertension Optimal Treatment (HOT) randomised trial. *Lancet* 1998;351:1755–1762.

59. Hansson L, Lindholm LH, Ekbom T, et al, for the Swedish Trial in Old Patients with Hypertension-2 Study. Randomised trial of old and new antihypertensive drugs in elderly patients: cardiovascular mortality and morbidity. *Lancet* 1999;354:1751–1756.

60. Brown MJ, Palmer CR, Castaigne A, et al. Morbidity and mortality in patients randomised to double-blind treatment with a long-acting calcium-channel blocker or diuretic in the International Nifedipine GITS Study: Intervention as a Goal in Hypertension Treatment (INSIGHT). *Lancet* 2000;356:366–372.

61. Hansson L, Hedner T, Lund-Johansen P, et al, for the NORDIL Study Group. Randomised trial of effects of calcium antagonists compared with diuretics and beta-blockers on cardiovascular morbidity and mortality in hypertension: the Nordic Diltiazem (NORDIL) Study. *Lancet* 2000;356:359–365.

62. Pahor M, Psaty BM, Alderman MH, et al. Health outcomes associated with calcium antagonists compared with other first-line antihypertensive therapies: a meta-analysis of randomised controlled trials. *Lancet* 2000;356:1949–1951.

63. Blood Pressure Lowering Treatment Trialists' Collaborative. Effects of ACE-inhibitors, calcium antagonists, and other blood-pressure-lowering drugs: Results of prospectively designed overviews of randomised trials. *Lancet* 2000;356:1955–1964.

64. Lewis EJ, Hunsicker LG, Clarke WR, et al, for the Collaborative Study Group. Renoprotective effect of the angiotensin-receptor antagonist irbesartan in patients with nephropathy due to type 2 diabetes. *N Engl J Med* 2001;345:841–860.

65. Brenner BM, Cooper ME, de Zeeuw D, et al, for the Reduction of Endpoints in Non-Insulin Dependent Diabetes Mellitus with the Angiotensin II Antagonist Losartan (RENAAL) Study Group. Effects of losartan on renal and cardiovascular outcomes in patients with type 2 diabetes and nephropathy. *N Engl J Med* 2001;345:861–869.

66. Berl T, Hunsicker LG, Lewis JB, et al, for the Irbesartan Diabetic Nephropathy Trial Collaborative Study Group. Cardiovascular outcomes in the Irbesartan Diabetic Nephropathy Trial of patients with type 2 diabetes and overt nephropathy. *Ann Intern Med* 2003;138:542–549.

67. Parving H-H, Lehnert H, Brochner-Mortensen J, et al, for the The Irbesartan in Patients with Type 2 Diabetes and Microalbuminuria Study Group. The effect of irbesartan on the development of diabetic nephropathy in patients with type 2 diabetes. *N Engl J Med* 2001;345:870–878.

68. Pitt B, Segal R, Martinez FA, et al, for the ELITE Investigators. Results of the Evaluation of Losartan In The Elderly (ELITE) Trial. *Lancet* 1997;349:757–762.

69. Pitt B, Poole-Wilson PA, Segal R, et al. Effect of losartan compared with captopril on mortality in patients with symptomatic heart failure: randomised trial. The Losartan Heart Failure Survival Study ELITE II. *Lancet* 2000;355:1582–1587.

70. Cohn JN, Tognoni G, for the Val-HeFT Investigators. A randomized trial of the angiotensin-receptor blocker valsartan in chronic heart failure. *N Engl J Med* 2001;345:1667–1675.

71. McMurray JJV, Östergren J, Swedberg K, et al, for the CHARM Investigators and Committees. Effects of candesartan in patients with chronic heart failure and reduced left-ventricular systolic function taking angiotensin-converting-enzyme inhibitors: the CHARM-Added trial. *Lancet* 2003;362:767–771.

72. Granger CB, McMurray JJV, Yusuf S, et al, for the CHARM Investigators and Committees. Effects of candesartan in patients with chronic heart failure and reduced left-ventricular function intolerant to angiotensin-converting-enzyme inhibitors: the CHARM-Alternative trial. *Lancet* 2003;362:772–776.

73. Yusuf S, Pfeffer MA, Swedberg K, et al, for the CHARM Investigators and Committees. Effects of candesartan in patients with chronic heart failure and preserved left-ventricular ejection fraction: the CHARM-Preserved trial. *Lancet* 2003;362:777–781.

74. Dahlöf B, Devereux RB, Kjeldsen SE, et al, for the LIFE Study Group. Cardiovascular morbidity and mortality in the Losartan Intervention For Endpoint Reduction in Hypertension Study (LIFE): a randomised trial against atenolol. *Lancet* 2002;359:995–1003.

75. Lindholm L, Ibsen H, Dahlöf B, et al, for the LIFE Gtudy Group. Cardiovascular morbidity and mortality in patients with diabetes in the Losartan Intervention For Endpoint Reduction in Hypertension Study (LIFE): a randomised trial against atenolol. *Lancet* 2002;359:1004–1010.

76. Kjeldsen SE, Dahlöf B, Devereux RB, et al, for the LIFE (Losartan Intervention for Endpoint Reduction) Study Group. Effects of losartan on cardiovascular morbidity and mortality in patients with isolated systolic hypertension and left ventricular hypertrophy: a Losartan Intervention for Endpoint Reduction (LIFE) Substudy. *JAMA* 2002;288:1491–1498.

77. The ALLHAT Officers and Coordinators for the ALLHAT Collaborative Research Group. Major outcomes in high-risk hypertensive patients randomized to angiotensin-converting enzyme inhibitor or calcium channel blocker vs. diuretic: the Antihypertensive and Lipid Lowering Treatment to Prevent Heart Attack Trial (ALLHAT). *JAMA* 2002;288:2981–2997.

78. The ALLHAT Collaborative Research Group. Major cardiovascular events in hypertensive patients randomized to doxazosin vs. chlorthalidone: the Antihypertensive and Lipid-Lowering Treatment to Prevent Heart Attack Trial (ALLHAT). *JAMA* 2000;283:1967–1975.

79. Wing LMH, Reid CM, Ryan P, et al, for the Second Australian National Blood Pressure Study Group. A comparison of outcomes with angiotensin-converting-enzyme inhibitors and diuretics for hypertension in the elderly. *N Engl J Med* 2003;348:583–592.

80. Black HR, Elliott WJ, Grandits G, et al., for the CONVINCE Research Group. Principal results of the Controlled ONset Verapamil INvestigation of Cardiovascular Endpoints (CONVINCE) Trial. *JAMA* 2003;289:2073–2082.

81. Pepine CJ, Handberg EM, Cooper-DeHoff RM, et al, for the INVEST Investigators. A calcium antagonist vs. a non-calcium

antagonist hypertension treatment strategy for patients with coronary artery disease: the International Verapamil-Trandolapril Study (INVEST): a randomized controlled trial. *JAMA* 2003;290:2805–2816.

82. Elliott WJ. Cardiovascular events during initial antihypertensive therapy with either a calcium antagonist or a diuretic/beta-blocker: meta-analysis of 7 clinical trials [abstract]. *Am J Hypertens* 2003;16:9A–10A.

83. Cushman WC, Ford CE, Cutler JA, et al. Success and predictors of blood pressure control in diverse North American settings: the Antihypertensive and Lipid-Lowering Treatment to Prevent Heart Attack Trial (ALLHAT). *J Clin Hypertension* 2002;4:393–404.

84. Mogensen CE, Neldam S, Tikkanen I, et al. Randomised controlled trial of dual blockade of rennin–angiotensin system in patients with hypertension, microalbuminuria, and non-insulin dependent diabetes: the Candesartan and Lisinopril Microalbuminuria (CALM) Study. *BMJ* 2000;321:1440–1444.

85. Nakao N, Yoshimura A, Morita H, et al. Combination treatment of angiotensin-II receptor blocker and angiotensin-converting-enzyme inhibitor in non-diabetic renal disease (COOPERATE): a randomised controlled trial. *Lancet* 2003;361:117–124.

86. Elliott WJ. Economic considerations in the management of hypertension. In: Izzo JL, Black HR, eds. *Hypertension Primer*. 3rd ed. Baltimore, Md: Lippincott, Williams & Wilkins; 2003:317–319.

87. Wallis EJ, Ramsay LE, Haq IU, et al. Coronary and cardiovascular risk estimation for primary prevention: validation of a new Sheffield table in the 1995 Scottish Health Survey population. *BMJ* 2000;320:671–676.

88. Pocock S, McCormack V, Gueyffier F, et al, for the INDANA Project Steering Committee. A score for predicting risk of death from cardiovascular disease in adults with raised blood pressure, based on individual patient data from randomised controlled trials. *BMJ* 2001;323:75–81.

89. Wallis EJ, Ramsay LE, Jackson PR. Cardiovascular and coronary risk estimation in hypertension management. *Heart.* 2002;88:306–312.

90. Ogden LG, He J, Lydick E, Whelton PK. Long-term absolute benefit of lowering blood pressure in hypertensive patients according to the JNC VI Risk Stratification. *Hypertension* 2000;34:539–543.

91. Prevention of coronary heart disease in clinical practice: recommendations of the Second Joint Task Force of European and Other Societies on Coronary Prevention. *Eur Heart J* 1998;19:1434–1503.

92. De Backer G, Ambrosioni E, Borch-Johnsen K, et al. Executive summary: European guidelines on cardiovascular disease prevention in clinical practice. *Eur Heart J* 2003;24:1601–1610.

93. Orford JL, Sesso HD, Stedman M, et al. A comparison of the Framingham and European Society of Cardiology coronary heart disease risk prediction models in the normative aging study. *Am Heart J* 2002;144:95–100.

94. Wood D, Durrington P, Poulter N, et al, for the British Cardiac Society, British Hyperlipidaemia Association, British Hypertension Society and endorsed by the British Diabetic Association. Joint British recommendations on prevention of coronary

heart disease in clinical practice. *Heart* 1998;80(suppl 2):S1–S29.

95. Gueyffier F, Bulpitt C, Boissel J-P, et al, for the INDANA Group. Antihypertensive drugs in very old people: a subgroup meta-analysis of randomised controlled trials. *Lancet* 1999;353:793–796.

96. Writing Group for the Women's Health Initiative Investigators. Risks and benefits of estrogen plus progestin in healthy postmenopausal women. *JAMA* 2002;288:321–333.

97. Nash D, Magder L, Lustberg M, et al. Blood lead, blood pressure, and hypertension in perimenopausal and postmenopausal women. *JAMA* 2003;289:1523–1532.

98. Whelton PK, He J, Appel LJ, et al. Primary prevention of hypertension: clinical and public health advisory from the National High Blood Pressure Education Program. *JAMA* 2002;288:1882–1888.

99. Sacks FM, Svetkey LP, Vollmer WM, et al. Effects on blood pressure of reduced dietary sodium and the Dietary Approaches to Stop Hypertension (DASH) diet. *N Engl J Med* 2001;344:3–9.

100. Writing Group of the PREMIER Collaborative Research Group. Effects of comprehensive lifestyle modification on blood pressure control: main results of the PREMIER clinical trial. *JAMA* 2003;289:2083–2093.

101. Cushman WC, Cutler JA, Hanna E, et al, for the PATHS Group. The Prevention and Treatment of Hypertension Study (PATHS): effects of an alcohol treatment program on blood pressure. *Arch Intern Med* 1998;152:1197–1207.

102. Xin X, He J, Frontini MG, et al. Effects of alcohol reduction on blood pressure: a meta-analysis of randomized controlled trials. *Hypertension* 2001;38:1112–1117.

103. Nieto FJ, Young TB, Lind BK, et al. Association of sleep-disordered breathing, sleep apnea, and hypertension in a large community-based study. *JAMA* 2000;283:1829–1836.

104. Dart RA, Gregoire JR, Gutterman DD, Woolf SH. The association of hypertension and secondary cardiovascular disease with sleep-disordered breathing. *Chest* 2003;123:244–260.

105. Levy D, Garrison RJ, Savage DD, et al. Prognostic implications of echocardiographically determined left ventricular mass in the Framingham Heart Study. *N Engl J Med* 1990;322:1561–1566.

106. Neaton JD, Grimm RH, Prineas RJ, et al. Treatment of mild hypertension study: final results. *JAMA.* 1993;270:713–724.

107. Mortality after 10 1/2 years for hypertensive participants in the Multiple Risk Factor Intervention Trial. *Circulation* 1990;82:1616–1628.

108. Burris J, Weir M, Oparil S, et al. An assessment of diltiazem and hydrochlorothiazide in hypertension. *JAMA* 1990;263:1507–1512.

109. Turner R, Holman R, Stratton I, et al, for the United Kingdom Prospective Diabetes Study Group. Tight blood pressure control and risk of macrovascular and microvascular complications in type 2 diabetes: UKPDS 38. *BMJ* 1998;317:707–713.

110. Raikou M, Gray A, Briggs A, et al. Cost-effectiveness analysis of improved blood pressure control in hypertensive patients with type 2 diabetes: UKPDS 40. U.K. Prospective Diabetes Study Group. *BMJ* 1998;317:720–726.

111. Elliott WJ, Weir DR, Black HR. Cost-effectiveness of lowering treatment goal of JNC VI for diabetic hypertensives. *Arch Intern Med* 2000;160:1277–1283.

112. American Diabetes Association. Treatment of hypertension in adults with diabetes. *Diabetes Care* 2003;26(suppl 1):S80–S83.

113. Report of the National High Blood Pressure Education Program Working Group on High Blood Pressure in Pregnancy. *Am J Obstet Gynecol* 2000;183:S1–S22.

114. Mangano DT, Layug EL, Wallace AR, et al. Effect of atenolol on mortality and cardiovascular morbidity after non-cardiac surgery. *N Engl J Med* 1996;335:1713–1720.

115. Poldermans D, Boersma E, Bax JJ, et al. The effect of bisoprolol on perioperative mortality and myocardial infarction in high-risk patients undergoing vascular surgery. *N Engl J Med* 1999;341:1789–1794.

116. Bakris GL, Williams M, Dworkin L, et al, for the National Kidney Foundation Hypertension and Diabetes Executive Committee Working Group. Preserving renal function in adults with hypertension and diabetes: a consensus approach. *Am J Kidney Dis* 2000;35:646–661.

117. Bakris GL, Weir MR. ACE inhibitor associated elevations in serum creatinine: is this a cause for concern? *Arch Intern Med* 2000;160:685–693.

118. Jafar TH, Schmid CH, Landa M, et al. Angiotensin-converting enzyme inhibitors and progression of nondiabetic renal disease: a meta-analysis of patient-level data. *Ann Intern Med* 2001;135:73–87.

119. Elliott WJ. Hypertensive emergencies. *Crit Care Clin* 2001;17:435–451.

120. DiMatteo MR, Sherbourne CD, Hays RD, et al. Physicians' characteristics influence patients' adherence to medical treatment: results from the Medical Outcomes Study. *Health Psychol* 1993;12:93–102.

121. Berlowitz DR, Ash AS, Hickey C, et al. Inadequate management of blood pressure in a hypertensive population. *N Engl J Med* 1998;339:1967–1963.

Dyslipidemia

Nathan D. Wong
Shaista Malik
Moti L. Kashyap

8

KEY POINTS

- Epidemiologic studies have demonstrated a consistent relation of elevated total and low-density lipoprotein cholesterol and reduced high-density lipoprotein cholesterol with the risk of coronary heart disease.

- Several studies have also shown increased lipoprotein(a) levels, levels of small, dense low-density lipoprotein cholesterol particles, and other lipid abnormalities to be associated with the risk of coronary heart disease.

- Primary and secondary prevention studies have shown the efficacy of lowering levels of low-density lipoprotein cholesterol in reducing the risk of cardiovascular events. Benefit appears similar regardless of gender, age group, baseline levels of low-density lipoprotein cholesterol, and presence of hypertension, diabetes, or other risk factors.

- Secondary prevention trials show a consistent effect of lowering levels of low-density lipoprotein cholesterol on reducing risk of stroke.

- The National Cholesterol Education Program (NCEP) Third Adult Treatment Panel recommends initial assessment with a full fasting lipid profile and recommends, in the population, low-density lipoprotein cholesterol levels less than 100 mg/dL, high-density lipoprotein cholesterol

levels greater than 60 mg/dL, and triglyceride levels less than 150 mg/dL as optimal. Persons with a prior history of coronary heart disease, other vascular disease, or 10-year estimated risk of coronary heart disease greater than 20% are classified as coronary heart disease risk equivalents with a goal level of low-density lipoprotein cholesterol set at less than 100 mg/dL (and less than 70 mg/dL if at very high risk).

- Therapeutic lifestyle approaches, including a diet emphasizing increased intake of high-fiber foods, use of monounsaturated fats while minimizing other sources of fat, and physical activity most days of the week, are the initial recommended treatment for persons with dyslipidemia.

- Treatment with hydroxymethylglutaryl coenzyme A reductase inhibitors (statins) remains the primary pharmacologic approach for lowering levels of low-density lipoprotein cholesterol; however, combination therapy with niacin (especially in those with low levels of high-density lipoprotein cholesterol or elevated triglycerides), bile acid sequestrants, and the newer cholesterol absorption inhibitors are also options for control of dyslipidemia. Fibric acid derivatives are most useful for hypertriglyceridemia and/or low high-density lipoprotein cholesterol.

The importance of elevated total and low-density lipoprotein cholesterol (LDL-C) in the etiology of coronary heart disease (CHD) and the value of their reduction in the primary and secondary prevention of CHD are well recognized.[1,2] In addition, high-density lipoproteins have been linked to protection for CHD.[3,4] Evidence indicates that high-density lipoprotein cholesterol (HDL-C) participates in the process of reverse cholesterol transport, whereby excess cholesterol is removed from tissues,[5] and may also inhibit atherogenesis.[6,7] The raising of HDL-C levels has also been shown to protect against initial coronary events[8] and has been documented to be of benefit in the secondary prevention of CHD.[9] Despite lower rates of CHD events and mortality among those receiving lipid-regulating therapy, many individuals still remain inadequately treated, and many of those who receive effective treatment still suffer events.

Important challenges we face include: (1) adequate identification of the many individuals in need of treatment, among those both with and without coronary artery disease; (2) more effective treatment of the many persons with preexisting coronary artery disease who are either not on lipid-regulating treatment or are inadequately treated; and (3) adequate treatment of other high-risk patient populations, such as diabetics, hypertensives, and the elderly, who would clearly benefit from lipid management.

EPIDEMIOLOGIC PERSPECTIVE

Total cholesterol and LDL-C

A direct relation between levels of total cholesterol or LDL-C and the risk of CHD has been demonstrated by numerous studies, both across and within populations. The Seven Countries Study showed that, among populations with higher mean levels of total cholesterol, rates of CHD were also higher (Fig. 8-1).[10] Migration studies in Japanese showed mean total cholesterol levels and corresponding rates of CHD to be lowest in their native country (181 mg/dL and 25.4/1000, respectively), intermediate among those living in Hawaii (218 mg/dL and 34.7/1000, respectively), and highest among Japanese living in San Francisco (228 mg/dL and 44.6/1000, respectively).[11] Within a large sample of middle-aged men, a curvilinear relation of total cholesterol to CHD risk was demonstrated by the Multiple Risk Factor Intervention Trial (MRFIT) (Fig. 8-2)[12] and in both men and women by the Framingham Heart Study.[3] Similar relationships are also seen among those with elevated levels of LDL-C.[13] In contrast, the US Pooling Project showed the lowest rate of coronary events to be in the second, rather than the first, quintile of cholesterol levels.[14] In addition, the relation of total cholesterol to CHD risk is amplified as a function of the number of other risk factors present, as demonstrated by the Framingham Heart Study (Fig. 8-3).[15] Among persons with a prior history of myocardial infarction, an elevated total cholesterol following recovery remains a significant independent risk factor for reinfarction, death from CHD, and total mortality.[16]

Falling cholesterol levels are associated with future total mortality, possibly being a consequence of certain diseases, such as cancers, predisposing to death.[17] In the Honolulu Heart Study,[18] men with low total cholesterol levels were more likely to have had preexisting adverse health characteristics, such as a higher prevalence of current smoking, heavy drinking, and certain

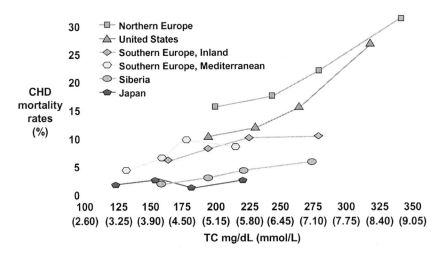

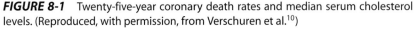

FIGURE 8-1 Twenty-five-year coronary death rates and median serum cholesterol levels. (Reproduced, with permission, from Verschuren et al.[10])

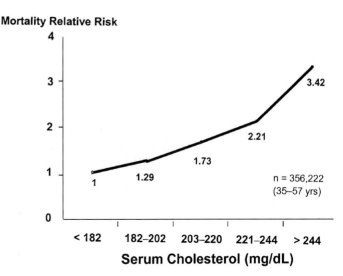

Mortality Relative Risk

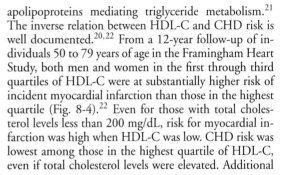

FIGURE 8-2 Total cholesterol and coronary heart disease incidence among MRFIT screenees. (Reproduced, with permission, from Stamler et al.[12])

gastrointestinal conditions, and those with the lowest levels of total cholesterol were at a significantly higher risk for hemorrhagic stroke, cancer, and all-cause mortality. Falling levels of total cholesterol over a 6-year period were also associated with a subsequent increase in the risk of all-cause mortality.[19,20]

HDL-C

HDL-C plays a role in reverse cholesterol transport, protecting against CHD. HDL-C also has antioxidant and profibrinolytic properties and transports important

apolipoproteins mediating triglyceride metabolism.[21] The inverse relation between HDL-C and CHD risk is well documented.[20,22] From a 12-year follow-up of individuals 50 to 79 years of age in the Framingham Heart Study, both men and women in the first through third quartiles of HDL-C were at substantially higher risk of incident myocardial infarction than those in the highest quartile (Fig. 8-4).[22] Even for those with total cholesterol levels less than 200 mg/dL, risk for myocardial infarction was high when HDL-C was low. CHD risk was lowest among those in the highest quartile of HDL-C, even if total cholesterol levels were elevated. Additional

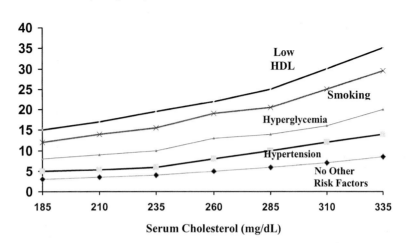

FIGURE 8-3 Impact of multiple risk factors on relation of total cholesterol to coronary heart disease risk: Framingham Heart Study. (Reproduced, with permission, from Kannel.[15])

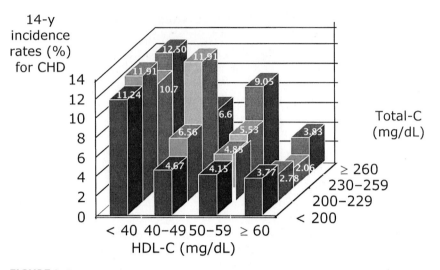

FIGURE 8-4 Fourteen-year incidence of CHD by total and HDL-C levels: Framingham cohort, men. (Adapted, with permission, from Castelli et al.[22])

evidence from the placebo group of the Helsinki Heart Study showed the LDL-C/HDL-C ratio to be the single best predictor of cardiac events.[8] When this ratio exceeded 5.0 in combination with a triglyceride level of 200 mg/dL or higher, the risk of new coronary events was nearly fourfold higher compared with the risk for individuals with lower LDL-C/HDL-C ratios and triglyceride levels. A recent study also showed HDL-C and LDL-C to be the most important independent predictors of incident CHD in diabetic American Indians.[23]

Population levels of total cholesterol, LDL-C, and HDL-Cl

The National Health and Nutrition Examination Survey 1999–2000 and other sources provide data on the distribution (prevalence of high-risk levels) by gender and ethnicity of total cholesterol, LDL-C, and HDL-C levels among large population samples of male and female individuals.[24] These data are summarized in Table 8-1.

Triglycerides

The relation of triglyceride levels to risk for CHD has been controversial. Although triglycerides were associated with an increased risk of CHD among women aged 50 to 69 in the Framingham Heart Study and among men aged 53 to 74 in the Copenhagen Male Study,[25,26] the Lipid Research Clinics Follow-up Study showed no independent relation of triglycerides with CHD mortality, except among subjects with lower HDL-C and higher LDL-C and younger subjects.[27] Further, a large meta-

analysis of population-based prospective studies showed a direct relation of triglycerides (per mmol/L or 88.5 mg/dL) and CHD incidence (relative risk [RR] = 1.14, 95% confidence interval [CI] = 1.05–1.28 for men; RR = 1.37, 95% CI = 1.13–1.66 for women), independent of HDL-C and other risk factors.[28]

Apolipoproteins and lipoprotein(a)

There exist limited prospective data relating apolipoproteins AI and B to CHD risk. The Quebec Cardiovascular Study reported, among 2155 men aged 45 to 76, a direct relation of plasma apolipoprotein B (Apo-B) concentrations with onset of ischemic heart disease over the next 5 years (RR = 1.4, 95% CI = 1.2–1.7), independent of other risk factors. A weaker, inverse association of Apo-AI with ischemic heart disease (RR = 0.85, 95% CI = 0.7–1.0) did not persist after adjustment for risk factors.[29]

Lipoprotein(a) (Lp(a)) excess has been identified as a powerful risk factor for development of CHD (Table 8-2) and is also elevated in those with premature CHD.[30] Lp(a) can contribute to atherosclerosis by impairing fibrinolysis, increasing lipid deposition in the arterial wall, and increasing oxidation of LDL-C.

Elevated Lp(a) is associated with a higher risk for cerebrovascular disease, peripheral arterial disease, myocardial infarction, restenosis after angioplasty, and failure of coronary artery bypass grafts.[31] In Swedish middle-aged asymptomatic men, elevated Lp(a) was also associated with subsequent myocardial infarction,[32] and the Lipid Research Clinics reported a relationship between Lp(a) and CHD.[33] Further, the Framingham Heart Study has

TABLE 8-1   Prevalence of High Blood Cholesterol and Other Lipids by Ethnicity and Gender, 2001

Population group	Prevalence of total cholesterol ≥200 mg/dL, 2001	Prevalence of total cholesterol ≥240 mg/dL, 2001	Prevalence of LDL-C ≥130 mg/dL, 2001	Prevalence of HDL-C <40 mg/dL, 2001
Total population*	104,700,000 (50.7%)	37,000,000 (18.3%)	93,000,000 (45.8%)	53,600,000 (26.4%)
Total males*	49,200,000 (50.4%)	16,500,000 (17.2%)	47,300,000 (48.5%)	38,000,000 (39.0%)
Total females*	55,500,000 (50.9%)	20,500,000 (19.1%)	45,700,000 (43.3%)	15,700,000 (14.9%)
White males[†]	51.0%	17.8%	49.6%	40.5%
White females[†]	53.6%	19.9%	43.7%	14.5%
Black males[†]	37.3%	10.6%	46.3%	24.3%
Black females[†]	46.4%	17.7%	41.6%	13.0%
Mexican males	54.3%	17.8%	43.6%	40.1%
Mexican females	44.7%	13.9%	41.6%	18.4%
Total Hispanics[‡]	—	25.6%	—	—
Total Asian/Pacific Islanders[a]	—	27.3%	—	—
Total American Indians/ Alaska Natives, Alaska[‡]	—	26.0%	—	—
Total American Indians/ Alaska Natives, Oklahoma[‡]	—	28.6%	—	—
Total American Indians/ Alaska Natives, Washington[‡]	—	26.5%	—	—

NOTE: mg/dL = milligrams per deciliter of blood. "Prevalence of Total Cholesterol ≥200 mg/dL" includes people with total cholesterol of ≥240 mg/dL. In adults, levels of 200–239 mg/dL are considered borderline high risk. Levels of ≥240 mg/dL are considered high risk. — data not available.
*Total population data for total cholesterol are for Americans aged 20 and older. Data for LDL-C, HDL-C, and all racial/ethnic groups are age-adjusted for age 20 and older.
[†]Data for 240 mg/dL for whites are white only, and those for blacks are black or African-American only. Source for total cholesterol ≥200 mg/dL. NHANES-IV (1999–2000). *Circulation* 2003:107:2185–2189, ≥240 mg/dl. *Health United States, 2003*, CDC/NCHS; LDL- and HDL-C: NHANES-III (1988–94), CDC/NCHS.
[‡]BRFSS (1977), *MMWR*, Vol. 49, No. SS-2, March 24, 2000, CDC/NCHS: data are for Americans aged 18 and older.
SOURCE: Reproduced, with permission, from the American Heart Association.[24]

reported for both men[34] and women [35] that an elevated Lp(a) is related to an increased risk of future coronary and/or cardiovascular events. Although neither the Helsinki Heart Study[36] nor the Physician's Health Study[37] showed Lp(a) to be a significant risk factor, it was reported in a community-based cohort of 9936 men and women followed for 14 years, that an increased level of Lp(a) was associated with a 1.9-fold increased risk of CHD events in women and a 1.6-fold increased risk in men, but had no consistent relationship to cerebrovascular events.[38]

Most recently, the Scandinavian Simvastatin Survival Study demonstrated Lp(a) levels to be significantly higher in those sustaining major coronary events than in subjects who had not experienced such events. This study also showed a significant relation of Lp(a) levels to total mortality.[39] In patients undergoing coronary angiography, Lp(a) levels are also higher in patients with higher numbers of blocked coronary vessels as well as greater degrees and extents of blockage.[40] Finally, in the Quebec Cardiovascular Study, Lp(a) was not an independent risk factor for ischemic heart disease but, instead, amplified the risks associated with elevated total cholesterol, LDL-C, and ApoB and retarded the protective effect associated with elevated HDL-C.[41]

TABLE 8-2 Observational Studies of the Relation of Lipoprotein(a) to Coronary Heart Disease

Reference	Study population	Result
Rosengren et al, 1990[32]	135 men aged 50, nested case–control, 6-year follow-up	RR* = 3.3, P = .02, unadjusted; P = .01, risk factor-adjusted
Ridker et al, 1993[37]	592 male physicians, nested case–control, 5-year follow-up	RR = 1.07, fifth quintile vs first quintile; P = trend = 0.93
Schaefer et al, 1994[33]	623 men aged 35–39, nested case–control, 7- to 10-year follow-up	RR = 2.08 (1.19–3.63), fifth quintile vs first quintile; age- and risk factor-adjusted
Bostom et al, 1994[35]	3101 women, prospective, 12-year follow-up	MI: RR = 2.37 (1.48–3.81) CAD: RR = 1.61 (1.13–2.29) CVD: RR = 1.44 (1.09–1.91) Age- and risk factor-adjusted
Bostom et al, 1996[34]	2191 men aged 20–54, prospective, CAD age < 55, 15-year follow-up	RR = 1.9 (1.2–2.9), age- and risk factor-adjusted
Nguyen et al, 1997[38]	9936 men and women, 14-year follow-up	CAD: RR = 1.9 (1.3–2.9) (women) RR = 1.6 (1.0–2.5) (men)
Cantin et al, 1998[41]	2156 men aged 47–76, 5-year follow-up	CAD: RR = 1.16 (0.83–1.85) Lp(a) > 33 mg/dL vs < 11 mg/dL

*RR, relative risk, with 95% confidence interval in parentheses; CAD, coronary artery disease; MI, myocardial infarction; CVD, cardiovascular disease.

TABLE 8-3 Studies of the Relation of the Atherogenic Lipoprotein Phenotype (Small, Dense LDL-C) to Heart Disease

Reference	Study population	Result
Austin et al[43]	109 cases and 121 controls; MI hospital admissions	OR* = 3.0 (1.7–5.3) (adjusted for age, sex, BMI) OR = 1.5 (0.7–3.3) (adjusted for age, sex, BMI, other lipids)
Krauss et al[44]	Physicians' Health Survey	Threefold CAD risk associated with pattern B, independent of total cholesterol, HDL-C, and ApoB
Gardner et al[45]	248 individuals, nested case–control within Stanford Five Cities Study	LDL-C size significantly smaller in cases, independent of other factors; also graded odds of CAD with LDL-C size
Phillips et al[46]	335 men and women with CAD; angiographic follow-up	Triglyceride-rich lipoproteins directly related to lesion progression
Zambon et al[47]	Nested case–control within Familial Atherosclerosis Treatment Study (FATS)	LDL-C size most important indicator of CAD progression; explained 48% of variance in model including other lipids
Lamarche et al[48]	Nested case–control within Quebec Cardiovascular Study; 114 cases, 5-year follow-up	RR = 3.6 (1.5–8.8), first tertile vs third tertile of LDL particle diameter

*MI, myocardial infarction; CAD, coronary artery disease; OR, odds ratio; HDL-C, high-density lipoprotein cholesterol; ApoB, apolipoprotein B; LDL-C, low-density lipoprotein cholesterol; RR, relative risk, with 95% confidence interval in parentheses; BMI, body mass index.

Atherogenic lipoprotein phenotype and other inherited lipid disorders

Of increasing interest is the possible relation of small LDL-C particle size, also referred to as the atherogenic lipoprotein phenotype (ALP), to increased risk of CHD. ALP consists of a major peak of small, dense LDL-C particles (denoted phenotype B), distinct from predominantly large, buoyant LDL-C particles (denoted phenotype A). The LDL pattern B trait is associated with a tendency toward elevated levels of triglycerides, very low density lipoprotein (VLDL), and intermediate-density lipoprotein and reduced levels of HDL-C; however, it can occur even when levels of these lipoproteins are normal.[42]

Several observational studies have described a relationship between small, dense LDL-C and risk for CHD (Table 8-3). Austin and colleagues showed small, dense LDL-C to be associated with a threefold greater odds of myocardial infarction (MI) in a case–control study; however, risk was attenuated after adjustment for other lipid fractions.[43] The Physicians' Health Survey also confirmed this threefold increased risk for CHD associated with pattern B individuals,[44] which persisted after adjustment for total cholesterol, HDL-C, and ApoB. In addition, the Stanford Five Cities Project showed, among 248 individuals, LDL size to be significantly smaller among CHD cases compared with controls, independent of HDL-C, non-HDL-C, triglycerides, body mass index, and smoking. Small LDL-C was found in about 50% of cases, and there was a graded relation between LDL-C size and odds of CHD.[45] Although triglycerides, LDL-C, and/or ApoB were associated with progression of angiographic disease in 335 men and women enrolled in a quantitative angiographic follow-up study, triglyceride-rich lipoproteins, which included cholesterol in intermediate-density lipoproteins, were directly related to lesion progression.[46] Moreover, the Familial Atherosclerosis Treatment Study (FATS)[47] demonstrated LDL-C density to be the most important predictor of atherosclerosis regression, followed (in decreasing order of contribution) by LDL-C, hepatic lipase, and Lp(a). Finally, in 2103 men in the Quebec Cardiovascular Study followed for 5 years, those in the first tertile of LDL peak particle diameter had a 3.6-fold increased risk (95% CI = 1.5–8.8) of ischemic heart disease.[48]

ApoE is the most common gene affecting LDL-C levels and includes, as its major isoforms, E2, E3, and E4. LDL-C catabolism is greater in those with the less common E2 isoform than in those with the most common E3 isoform. The E4 isoform is associated with reduced catabolism of LDL and suppression of LDL-C receptors. There is also evidence of an association of increased risk of MI with the E4 allele.[49]

CLINICAL TRIAL EVIDENCE FOR LIPID INTERVENTION

Primary prevention studies

Numerous primary prevention studies document the importance of cholesterol lowering in patients without previous CHD (Table 8-4).[50] The Lipid Research Clinics Coronary Primary Prevention Trial (LRC-CPPT) randomized approximately 3800 men to cholestyramine versus placebo, and after 7 years of follow-up, there was a 20% reduction in LDL-C and a corresponding 19% reduction in coronary events, but no significant reduction in coronary or total mortality.[51] In the Helsinki Heart Study, more than 4000 middle-aged men without prior evidence of CHD were randomized to gemfibrozil (as compared with placebo); there was a highly significant reduction of 34% in the incidence of coronary events.[52] A subanalysis showed that elevation in HDL-C was independently associated with reduction in risk.[8] More recently, the West of Scotland Coronary Prevention Study reported results on 6595 men aged 45 to 64 years with hypercholesterolemia assigned to pravastatin or placebo, with a mean follow-up of 4.9 years.[53] Nonfatal MI or CHD death, the primary endpoint, was reduced significantly by 31% in the pravastatin-treated group. Total mortality was also reduced by 22% ($P = .05$). This mortality advantage widened to a 26% reduction ($P = .01$) by 6 months after completion of the study, but narrowed to 17% (n.s.) after 1 year, suggesting the importance of continuing therapy.[54] A more recent trial (PROSPER) involving pravastatin in elderly patients revealed a significant reduction in CHD events, but not in total mortality, among those randomized to pravastatin versus placebo. This trial, however, showed an unexplained increase in breast cancer risk in those taking pravastatin.[55] A safety analysis done among three major pravastatin studies representing more than 112,000 person-years of exposure comparing placebo and pravastatin 40 mg once daily demonstrated a slight, but nonsignificant ($P = .08$) increased incidence of breast cancer (0.2% in pravastatin-treated vs 0.1% in those on placebo).[56] The Air Force/Texas Coronary Atherosclerosis Prevention Study (AFCAPS/ TexCAPS) provided further evidence for the role of lipid lowering in primary prevention among men and women with average cholesterol levels similar in distribution to those of the national population based on NHANES-III data.[57] In this study, 5608 men and 997 women with "average" total cholesterol and LDL-C levels (means = 221 and 150 mg/dL, respectively) and below-average HDL-C levels (means = 36 mg/dL in men and 40 mg/dL in women) were enrolled and randomized to lovastatin or placebo. After a mean follow-up of 5.2 years, there was a 37% reduction

TABLE 8-4 Primary Prevention Studies of Lipid Modification

	Study/Treatment		LDL-C reduction		Risk reduction (%)	
Trial	Therapy	n	Change (%)	Achieved (mg/dL)	CAD events	Total mortality
WHO	Clofibrate	10,627	−9 (TC)*	224[†]	20	−30
LRC-CPPT[51]	Cholestyramine	3,806	−20	175	19	7
Helsinki[52]	Gemfibrozil	4,081	−10[‡]	174	34	−6
WOSCOPS[53]	Pravastatin	6,595	−26	142	31[¶]	22[§]
AFCAPS/TexCAPS[56]	Lovastatin	6,605	−25	115	37[¶]	−4
ALLHAT-LLT[57]	Pravastatin	10,305	−17	104	9	1
PROSPER[55]	Pravastatin	5,804	−34	97	19[ǁ]	3
ASCOT-LLA[58]	Atorvastatin	19,342 with hypertension	−35	89	36[¶]	13

*Total cholesterol.
[†]Estimated based on baseline of 249 mg/dL.
[‡]Also accompanied by a 43% reduction in triglycerides and a 10% increase in HDL-C.
[§]$P = .05$.
[ǁ]$P < .01$.
[¶]$P < .001$.

in major coronary events (fatal or nonfatal MI, unstable angina, or sudden cardiac death), a 33% reduction in new revascularization, and a 25% reduction in total cardiovascular events.

Two recent clinical trials of lipid lowering involving patients with hypertension are noteworthy to review briefly. The Antihypertensive Lipid Lowering to Prevent Heart Attack Trial (ALLHAT) included a lipid-lowering trial (LLT)[58] component consisting of 10,355 patients assigned to pravastatin 40 mg or usual care. There were no significant benefits in terms of all-cause mortality or coronary and stroke events between treatment groups, which was considered to be a reflection of the limited difference (17%) in on-treatment LDL-C levels between treatment groups, a result of a large number of usual care group participants being placed on treatment. More recently published are the results of the Anglo-Scandinavian Cardiac Outcomes Trial—Lipid Lowering Arm (ASCOT-LLA) involving 10,305 hypertensive patients aged 40 to 79 years with at least three other cardiovascular risk factors who were randomly assigned to atorvastatin 10 mg or placebo.[59] Although an average follow-up of 5 years was planned, treatment was stopped after a median follow-up of 3.3 years. Those assigned to atorvastatin had a 36% lower rates of nonfatal MI and CHD death. There were also significant reductions in stroke (27%), total cardiovascular events (21%), and coronary events (29%), and a nonsignificant 13% reduction in total deaths. On-treatment LDL-C in ASCOT-LLA remained 29 to 35% lower in the treatment group than in the placebo group, a

likely explanation for the difference in outcomes between the ASCOT-LLA and ALLHAT trials.

Secondary prevention studies

A number of clinical trials in persons with preexisting CHD demonstrate the efficacy of lipid intervention in reducing subsequent coronary events and total mortality (Table 8-5, Fig. 8-5). The Coronary Drug Project, originally published in 1975, showed that in men aged 30 to 64 with a history of MI, treatment with niacin for 5 years was associated with a 27% reduction in the incidence of definite nonfatal MI, but little effect on total mortality.[60] A 15-year follow-up of this cohort,[61] however, yielded a significant 11% lower total mortality rate in those originally randomized to niacin. The Program on the Surgical Control of the Hyperlipidemias (POSCH) showed that regression of atherosclerosis and significant reductions in morbidity and mortality from CHD, as well as total mortality, could be obtained from total cholesterol and LDL-C reduction effected by partial ileal bypass in patients with significant hypercholesterolemia.[62]

The Scandinavian Simvastatin Survival Study (4S) demonstrated that lipid lowering in patients with preexisting CHD not only prevented subsequent coronary events, but also reduced total mortality and stroke.[63] In the 4444 men and women aged 35 to 70 with a history of MI or angina pectoris randomized to simvastatin or placebo for a mean follow-up of 5.4 years, the primary endpoint of total mortality was reduced (significantly)

TABLE 8-5   Secondary Prevention Studies of Lipid Modification

	Study/Treatment			LDL-C* reduction		Risk reduction (%)‖	
Trial	Therapy	n	Change (%)	Achieved (mg/dL)	CHD events	Total mortality
CDP[60]†	Niacin	3,908	−10 (TC)	—	27	11¶
	Clofibrate	3,892	− 5 (TC)	—	4.7	− 1
	Dextrothyroxine	3,872	−10 (TC)	—	−13	−22
POSCH[62]	Partial ileal bypass	838	−38	103	35§	22
4S[63]	Simvastatin	4,444	−34	121	42¶	30¶
CARE[2]	Pravastatin	4,159	−28	100	24§	9
LIPID[65]	Pravastatin	9,014	−25	113	24¶	22¶
HIT[9]	Gemfibrozil	2,531	3.6‡	115	22§	10
HPS[67]	Simvastatin	20,536	−37	89	27¶	13

*LDL-C, low-density lipoprotein cholesterol; CHD, coronary heart disease; TC, total cholesterol. Sign indicates increase in risk.
†Lipid changes available only for total cholesterol; CHD events based on 5-year follow-up, total mortality on 15-year follow-up.
‡Accompanied by a 7.5% increase in HDL-C and a 24.5% decrease in triglycerides.
‖$P < .05$.
§$P < .01$.
¶$P < .001$.

by 30% in the treatment group versus those on placebo. Benefit was similar regardless of age group and gender. A later report included published data in the subgroup of 202 diabetic patients; coronary events were reduced significantly by 55% in these individuals, and there was a nonsignificant (RR = 0.57, $P = .09$) reduction in total mortality.[64]

The Cholesterol and Recurrent Events (CARE) study reported data from 5 years of treatment with pravastatin or placebo in 4159 men and women who had sustained a previous MI, but who had a total cholesterol less than 6.2 mmol/L (240 mg/dL) and mean LDL-C averaging

3.6 mmol/L (139 mg/dL).[2] The incidence of fatal coronary events or nonfatal MI was reduced significantly by 24%. There were also significant reductions in coronary bypass surgery (26%), coronary angioplasty (23%), and stroke (31%). No significant difference in total mortality was observed between the treatment and placebo groups (9% reduction, $P = .37$); however, there was an unexpected increased risk of breast cancer in the treatment group.

The Long-Term Intervention with Pravastatin in Ischemic Disease (LIPID) study[65] also investigated whether cholesterol reduction with pravastatin reduces

FIGURE 8-5   Relation of LDL-C achieved to CHD risk reduction from primary and secondary prevention studies involving statins. 4S, Scandinavian Simvastatin Survival Study; AFCAPS, Air Force/Texas Coronary Atherosclerosis Prevention Study; CARE, Cholesterol and Recurrent Events Trial; LIPID, Long-Term Intervention with Pravastatin in Ischaemic Disease Study; WOSCOPS, West of Scotland Coronary Prevention Study. HPS, Heart Protection Study. (Reproduced, with permission, from Ballantyne et al.[88])

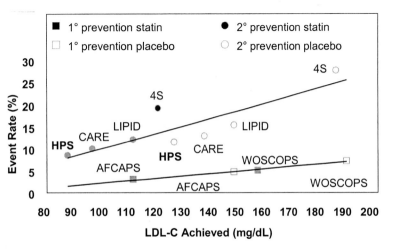

CHD mortality in patients with a previous MI or unstable angina who had cholesterol levels between 155 and 271 mg/dL. Among the 9014 patients aged 31 to 75 years randomized to pravastatin 40 mg daily or placebo, and followed for an average of 6 years, the primary endpoint of CHD mortality was reduced by 24%; there was also a 23% reduction in total mortality and a significant 20% reduction in the risk of stroke.

The efficacy of increasing HDL-C on reducing recurrent coronary events was recently examined in the HDL Intervention Trial (HIT). Subjects also had "normal" LDL-C (≤140 mg/dL) but low HDL-C (≤40 mg/dL) and were randomized to gemfibrozil or placebo.[66] After a median follow-up of 5.1 years, the risk of CHD death or nonfatal MI was reduced by 22% among those treated versus those on placebo.

The largest single lipid-lowering trial to date, the Heart Protection Study,[67] examined the efficacy of simvastatin 40 mg or placebo in 20,536 patients in the United Kingdom aged 40 to 80 with coronary disease, other arterial disease, or diabetes, followed for a 5-year period. All-cause mortality was significantly reduced by 12.9%, with an 18% reduction in coronary deaths. Nonfatal MIs, as well as nonfatal and fatal strokes, were also reduced significantly by about one-fourth. Risk reduction was similar regardless of gender, age, or baseline LDL-C; those with a baseline LDL-C less than 100 mg/dL had a reduction in CHD events similar to that of persons with higher baseline LDL-C levels. Noteworthy was the large sample of nearly 6000 persons with diabetes (but no history of CHD), for whom a consistent reduction in cardiovascular events was observed.[68] This trial is important in documenting the importance of statin treatment in persons with preexisting vascular disease or type 2 diabetes, regardless of baseline LDL-C. Because of this observation, the Heart Protection Study investigators have suggested that all diabetics and individuals at high risk should initially be given statin therapy.[67]

Atherosclerosis regression studies

Coronary angiographic follow-up studies have also demonstrated the importance of lipid intervention on retarding progression and/or stimulating regression of coronary atherosclerosis (Table 8-6). A number of these studies show that, despite fairly modest angiographic changes, event rates are reduced substantially.[69] In the Cholesterol Lowering Atherosclerosis Study,[70] patients with coronary artery bypass surgery were treated for 2 years with a combination of colestipol and niacin, and the results compared with those of a placebo group. Of the treated patients, 16% showed regression of atherosclerosis, compared with only 2% in the placebo group.

The Familial Atherosclerosis Treatment Study (FATS)[71] involved two different treatment arms, one with combined niacin and colestipol treatment and a second with combined lovastatin and colestipol treatment; each was compared with a conventionally treated diet arm. More than one third of treated patients exhibited regression of atherosclerosis, compared with about one tenth of control group patients. Moreover, the incidence of new coronary events was about 70% less in those on treatment than in the control group. The same investigators recently published the results of a second clinical trial showing combination simvastatin–niacin treatment to be related to retarded progression of atherosclerosis (regression of 0.4%, compared with progression of stenosis of 3.9% with placebo, $P < .0001$), but this beneficial effect was blunted with the addition of antioxidants. The incidence of new cardiovascular events in those on the simvastatin–niacin combination was 80 to 90% lower than in the placebo arms of the study.[72] This important trial gives preliminary evidence that combination therapy not only provides additional efficacy in treating the lipid profile, but also may result in an additive reduction in risk.

The Lifestyle Heart Trial[73] involved a lifestyle regimen that included a vegetarian low-fat diet (<10% of calories in fat) and a daily cholesterol intake less than 5 mg, along with smoking cessation, stress management, and increased physical activity. Of note, 81% of patients in the treated group demonstrated regression of atherosclerosis (and there was a 91% reduction in the frequency of angina). A recent follow-up report from this study showed continued improvements among the intervention group as determined in those completing the 5-year follow-up angiogram who maintained comprehensive lifestyle changes.[74]

Other studies have also demonstrated that hydroxymethylglutaryl coenzyme A (HMG-CoA) reductase monotherapy with lovastatin,[75,76] pravastatin,[77,78] or simvastatin[79] retards the angiographic progression of atherosclerosis, as evidenced by less reduction in minimum lumen diameter in the intervention versus the control group. Another study demonstrated regression of atherosclerosis among those with lower total cholesterol and LDL-C levels achieved by therapy with a fibric acid derivative.[80] The Stanford Coronary Risk Intervention Project (SCRIP) used a diet and exercise regimen, as well as lipid-lowering medications, to effectively modify lipid levels in many patients during the course of the study. They demonstrated less progression of atherosclerosis (small reduction in minimum lumen diameter) and fewer cardiac events in the risk reduction group.[81] Another study with multiple drug therapies did not induce regression or reduce progression of atherosclerosis in individuals with normal cholesterol levels.[82] A review of many angiographic trials of lipid lowering showed regression to be more common in trials where baseline mean LDL-C exceeded 170 mg/dL, as compared with those in which

TABLE 8-6 Arteriographic "Regression" Studies of Lipid Modification

Study/Treatment		n*	LDL-C reduction		Percentage of patients*	
Trial	Therapy		Change (%)	Achieved (mg/dL)	Progression	Regression
NHLBI[68]	Cholestyramine	59/57	−26	178	32/49	7/7
CLAS[69]	Colestipol + niacin	80/82	−38	105	9/61	16/2
FATS[70]	Colestipol + niacin	36/46	−32	129	25/46	39/11
	Lovastatin + colestipol	38/46	−46	107	21/46	32/11
Hahmann et al.[80]	Fenofibrate	21/21	−20	—	10/—	11/—
SCOR[68]	Colestipol, niacin,	40/32	−28	172	20/41	33/13
SCRIP[81]	Colestipol, niacin,	119/127	−23	121	50/50	20/10
STARS[68]	Cholestyramine	24/24	−33	136	4/38	21/4
STARS[68]	Diet	26/24	−16	164	15/38	31/4
MARS[76]	Lovastatin	114/106	−45	86	29/40	23/13
CCAIT[79]	Lovastatin	165/166	−30	120	33/50	10/7
MAAS[78]	Simvastatin	178/167	−31	117	23/32	19/12
REGRESS[76]	Pravastatin	314/327	−25	125	45/55	17/9
HARP[81]	Multiple agents	40/39	−39	85	35/38	10/13
POSCH[62]	Partial ileal bypass	333/301	−42	104	38/65	13/5
Post-CABG[84]	Multiple agents	628/628	−38	93–97	27/39	5/4
Lifestyle[73,74]	Diet, other	22/19	−36	95	14/32	41/32
Heidelberg[68]	Diet, exercise	40/52	−9	149	20/42	30/4
LOCAT[84]	Gemfibrozil	395	−12	131	4 (2%)	23 (14%)
HATS[72]†	Simvastatin, Niacin	160 (total)	−43	75	3.9% placebo	0.4% treatment
REVERSAL[83]	Atorvastatin vs Pravastatin	654 total	−46 (atorvastatin vs −25 pravastatin)	79 (TC atorvastatin vs 110 mg/dL TC pravastatin)	Atheroma volume change (−0.4% atorvastatin vs 2.7% pravastatin), ($p = 0.02$)	

*Data presented according to treatment/control group status.
†Data presented according to mean percentage stenosis progression for placebo and regression for treatment with simvastatin and niacin.

SOURCE: Modified, with permission, from Rossouw.[69]

baseline LDL-C was 170 mg/dL or lower.[69] Most recently, the Reversal of Atherosclerosis with Aggressive Lipid Lowering (REVERSAL) study examined, in 654 patients with known CHD, the efficacy of 80 mg atorvastatin compared with 40 mg pravastatin in retarding changes in atheroma volume as measured by intravascular ultrasound. Progression of atheroma volume after 18 months on treatment was significantly less in those on atorvastatin (−0.4%) than in those on pravastatin (2.7%) ($P = .02$).[83]

Atherosclerosis can also be retarded by interventions other than those designed to reduce LDL-C. The Lopid Coronary Angiography Trial (LOCAT) involved 372 patients who had low HDL-C as their principal lipid abnormality and were randomized to gemfibrozil or placebo. These patients underwent two angiograms separated by an average of 32 months. Progression of native coronary atherosclerosis was significantly retarded in the treatment group (−0.04 mm) as compared with the placebo group (−0.09 mm); new lesions in the graft vessels were more common in the placebo group (14%) than in the gemfibrozil group (2%)[84] The results of this trial provide some support for the use of fibrates to treat CHD patients who have normal cholesterol levels, but low HDL-C.[85]

Finally, of promising interest is a study examining the effect of infusing recombinant ApoA-I (Milano)/phospholipid complexes (ETC-216) on atheroma burden among 57 patients with acute coronary syndromes randomly assigned to five weekly infusions of ETC-216 or placebo. ApoA-I(Milano) is a variant of ApoA-I identified in individuals in rural Italy who have very low levels of HDL-C. Those randomized to the ETC-216 group showed significant reductions in atheroma volume from baseline ($P = .02$) as measured by intravascular ultrasound, whereas there were no changes in the placebo group, suggesting infusion of ETC-216 in five doses at weekly intervals produced significant regression of atherosclerosis.[86]

The issue of how low an LDL-C is required to retard progression of angiographic disease was studied in 1351 individuals who had undergone coronary artery bypass surgery; those who received aggressive treatment with lovastatin (and cholestyramine, if needed) to maintain an LDL-C between 93 and 97 mg/dL were less likely to show progression of atherosclerosis (27% of grafts) than those who achieved only moderate lowering of LDL-C, to 132 to 136 mg/dL (39%).[87] Data from most of the recent atherosclerosis regression trials involving measurement of minimum lumen diameter demonstrate less progression of atherosclerosis, the lower the LDL-C achieved (Fig. 8-5).[88]

In many clinical trials, the reduction in cardiovascular disease (CVD) events appears to be beyond what would be expected based on changes in arterial lumen diameter from angiographic trials. An effect of lipid-lowering therapy on plaque stabilization is hypothesized as one mechanism for the prevention of clinical events. Other agents recommended for secondary prevention, for example, antiplatelet agents (such as aspirin) and beta blockers, might explain the magnitude of risk reductions achievable with the addition of cholesterol-lowering agents.[89]

Lipid-lowering in acute coronary syndromes

Given the fact that the risk of complications remains high in the first few months following an acute coronary event, the role of lipid-lowering therapy, particular statins, has been studied and has been shown to reduce angina, rehospitalization, and mortality. Possible mechanisms for this reduced risk may be mediated through beneficial effects on plaque stabilization, endothelial function, inflammation, and thrombus formation.[90] Despite these important findings, statin therapy following a coronary event remains underutilized. In-hospitalization initiation of statin therapy has been shown to result in a markedly increased treatment rate, improved long-term patient compliance, and higher proportion of patients reaching LDL-C goals of <100 mg/dl.[91–95]

Several recently published clinical trials have documented the importance of in-hospitalization initiation of lipid-lowering medication usage in coronary patients. The value of such therapy early in the posthospitalization phase was demonstrated by the Atorvastatin versus Revascularization Treatment (AVERT) study, which showed among 341 patients with stable coronary artery disease, randomization to atorvastatin for 18 months to result in a 36% lower ischemic event rate compared to those assigned to angioplasty, although this reduction in events was due primarily to a smaller number of revascularizations and hospitalizations for worsening angina.[93] The MIRACL study involved treatment with atorvastatin (vs. placebo) initiated 24 to 96 hours after an acute coronary syndrome in 3086 adults and showed after 16 weeks the primary endpoint of death, nonfatal acute myocardial infarction, cardiac arrest with resuscitation, or recurrent symptomatic myocardial ischemia requiring rehospitalization to be 16% lower among those in the atorvastatin group, due mostly to reduced recurrent rehospitalization. There were no significant differences in risk of death, nonfatal myocardial infarction, or cardiac arrest between the groups.[94] The Platelet Receptor Inhibition in Ischemic Syndrome Management (PRISM) study also showed among 1616 patients with coronary disease and chest pain in the previous 24 hours that those continuing statin therapy had a 51% lower 30-day event rate (death and nonfatal myocardial infarction) compared to those not on statins and that those who had their statin therapy withdrawn had nearly a 3-fold greater risk of events compared to those who continued their statin use.[92] More recently, the PROVE-IT study involving 4162 patients hospitalized with an acute coronary syndrome in the past 10 days who were randomized to 80 mg of atorvastatin (intensive therapy) compared to 40 mg of pravastatin (standard therapy) showed median on-treatment LDL-C levels of 62 mg/dl and 95 mg/dl, respectively. A highly significant 16% reduction in the primary endpoint of death, myocardial infarction, unstable angina requiring hospitalization, revascularization within 30 days, and stroke was observed among those in the atorvastatin arm.[95] While many patients in the pravastatin arm did not reach the goal of LDL-C <100 mg/dl, these data are suggestive of a greater benefit from more aggressive lipid goals in acute coronary syndrome patients. Furthermore, recent data suggest the efficacy of statin use on improving survival in heart failure patients.[96]

Recent guidelines from the American College of Cardiology and American Heart Association now recommend statin therapy at discharge among patients with unstable angina and non-ST-segment elevation myocardial infarction and several in-hospitalization programs to implement these and other treatment guidelines for acute coronary syndromes have been initiated[97,98] and are discussed further in Chapter 26. Moreover, patients with acute coronary syndromes are considered *very high risk* where an optional goal of lowering the LDL-C to <70 mg/dL has recently been recommended by the National Cholesterol Education Program.[99]

RELATION OF BASELINE LDL-C AND EXTENT OF LDL-C REDUCTION TO CORONARY EVENT RISK

Coronary event reduction may also depend on the level of baseline LDL-C. In primary prevention, the AFCAPS/TexCAPS study[56] showed event risk to be similar regardless of baseline LDL-C tertile; those in the lowest tertile (91–142 mg/dL) sustained a 34% risk reduction as compared with a reduction of 41% in the highest tertile (157–236 mg/dL). The West of Scotland Coronary Primary Prevention Study (WOSCOPS)[51] had much higher baseline LDL-C levels and also showed greater efficacy among those with LDL-C levels below 189 mg/dL (37% risk reduction) as compared with 189 mg/dL or greater (27% risk reduction).

Although there is generally an incremental value in achieving low LDL-C levels on treatment in both primary and secondary prevention (Fig. 8-5),[100] among participants in the CARE study,[2] there was no benefit of treatment for those with baseline LDL-C levels below 125 mg/dL The LIPID study[64] corroborated these findings with a nonsignificant 16% risk reduction noted for those with LDL-C levels below 135 mg/dL, versus sig-

nificantly greater reductions in risk for those with higher baseline LDL-C levels. But the recently published Heart Protection Study (HPS), with a much larger sample of subjects with lower baseline LDL-C levels, reported the percentage risk reduction to be similar for those with baseline LDL-C levels of less than 100 mg/dL, 100 to 129 mg/dL, and 130 mg/dL or higher.[67]

MECHANISMS OF EVENT REDUCTION

Ongoing investigations have tried to determine the potential mechanisms of action behind the clinical benefit of lipid lowering. The first hypothesis is based on the theory that it is the small, rather than large plaques that result in rupture and thrombosis, leading to the acute, serious, and eventually fatal complications of atherosclerosis. The second theory is that lipid reduction restores the abnormal endothelial function that is often observed in patients with CHD.[101] Possible beneficial, nonlipid effects on endothelial function, inflammatory responses, plaque stability, and thrombus formation have been proposed, and experimental studies have suggested that stability may be achieved through a reduction in macrophages and cholesterol ester content and an increase in volume of collagen and smooth muscle cells. Also, inhibition of platelet aggregation and maintenance of a favorable balance between prothrombotic and fibrinolytic mechanisms may be involved.[102]

SCREENING AND EVALUATION OF DYSLIPIDEMIA

Although there have been substantial increases in awareness of elevated cholesterol, as well as increased treatment compliance during the past two decades, recent national surveys suggest substantial improvement is still needed.[103] A recent study showed that less than half of the patients who met NCEP criteria for initiation of therapy actually received it, and among those given medications, only one third achieved acceptable LDL-C reductions within a year.[104] In a large sample of postmenopausal women with heart disease, only 47% were taking lipid-lowering medication and 91% did not meet the NCEP goal level for an LDL-C less than 100 mg/dL.[105]

Not surprisingly, the blame must be shared by both the health care provider and the patient. A recent retrospective chart review[106] of patients admitted to a coronary care unit showed that physicians followed NCEP guidelines for obtaining a lipid profile only 50% of the time. Moreover, a lipid profile was obtained (at best) in 74% of patients with known CHD, but only in 56% of patients with a known family history of CHD and in 37% of those with diabetes.

CURRENT SCREENING AND MANAGEMENT RECOMMENDATIONS IN ADULTS

The Third Adult Treatment Panel (ATP-III) of the NCEP[1] recommends an initial fasting lipid profile (and, if not possible, at least total cholesterol and HDL-C) in all adults aged 20 and older as an initial screening for primary prevention. If a nonfasting test shows a total cholesterol of 200 mg/dL or higher, or an HDL-C less than 40 mg/dL, a follow-up lipid profile is recommended. New classifications define an optimal LDL-C as less than 100 mg/dL, optimal triglycerides as less than 150 mg/dL, and low HDL-C as less than 40 mg/dL (Table 8-7). If these lipids are normal, a repeat screening is recommended every 5 years.

A major new feature of the ATP-III guidelines is a broader definition of those defined as CHD risk equivalents. Besides those with established CHD, these include persons with diabetes, those with noncoronary atherosclerosis (symptomatic carotid artery disease, abdominal aortic aneurysm, and peripheral arterial disease), and those who are at a 10-year absolute risk of CHD greater than 20%, based on a global risk assessment (eg, Framingham Heart Study algorithms for hard CHD events, as described in Chapter 1). Although few persons with fewer than two CHD risk factors will be at increased risk of CHD, some exceptions do apply and should be considered at the physician's judgment, such as those with familial hypercholesterolemia, those with a strong

TABLE 8-7 ATP III Classification of LDL, Total, and HDL-Cholesterol and Triglycerides

LDL-C: primary target of therapy	
<100 mg/dL	Optimal
100–129 mg/dL	Near optimal/above optimal
130–159 mg/dL	Borderline high
160–189 mg/dL	High
≥190 mg/dL	Very high
Total cholesterol	
<200 mg/dL	Desirable
200–239 mg/dL	Borderline high
≥240 mg/dL	High
HDL-C	
<40 mg/dL	Low
≥60 mg/dL	High
Triglycerides	
<150 mg/dL	Normal
150–199 mg/dL	Borderline high
200–499 mg/dL	High
≥500 mg/dL	Very high

SOURCE: Adapted, with permission, from the National Cholesterol Education Program.[1]

premature family history of CHD, and those with extreme elevations in other risk factors. Moreover, when two or more risk factors are present, a global risk assessment is recommended to identify the subset of individuals in this group at greater than 20% 10-year CHD risk, now defined as a CHD risk equivalent. Finally, special consideration is given to multiple risk factor modification in persons with the metabolic syndrome, which is defined as the presence of three or more of the following: (1) abdominal obesity, defined as a waist circumference greater than 40 in. in men and greater than 35 in. in women; (2) triglyceride levels of 150 mg/dL or greater; (3) HDL-C less than 40 mg/dL in men or less than 50 mg/dL in women; (4) blood pressure of 130/85 mm Hg or higher, or on treatment; (5) fasting glucose of 110 mg/dL or higher. Because these factors increase risk at any level of LDL-C, intensified efforts in weight reduction and physical activity are recommended as initial treatment. More details on treatment of the metabolic syndrome are provided in Chapter 9.

As is the case with persons who have established CHD, those with other CHD risk equivalents also have a recommended goal LDL-C of less than 100 mg/dL. In a recently released update[99] to these guidelines, an LDL-C goal of <70 mg/dL is favored in those who are at *very high risk* (eg, CHD plus multiple major risk factors, metabolic syndrome risk factors, or with severe and poorly controlled risk factors). Those with two or more risk factors who do not exceed 20% risk have a goal LDL-C of less than 130 mg/dL but an optional goal of <100 mg/dL, and those with fewer than two risk factors have a goal LDL-C of less than 160 mg/dL (Table 8-8). Although LDL-C levels exceeding these cut points dictate initiation of therapeutic lifestyle changes, LDL-C levels for initiating drug therapy are 100, 160, and 190 mg/dL or higher for persons in each of these three risk groups, respectively. However, in the case of two or more CHD risk factors, when calculated 10-year risk of CHD is 10 to 20%, pharmacologic treatment should begin at an LDL-C of 130 mg/dL or higher, and is optional at an LDL-C of 100–129 mg/dL. Drug therapy is optional for those with CHD and CHD risk equivalents, if the LDL-C is less than 100 mg/dL, and for persons with one or fewer risk factors whose LDL-C is 160 to 189 mg/dL, where factors such as a severe elevation of a single risk factor (eg, premature family history, hypertension, or very low HDL-C) may indicate treatment at the judgment of the physician.

For persons with fasting triglyceride levels that are 200 mg/dL greater, calculation of non-HDL-C (total cholesterol minus HDL-C) is recommended, in part due to the possible underestimation of calculated LDL-C in persons with elevated (>400 mg/dL) triglycerides. For these individuals, treatment goals are based not on LDL-C goals, but on non-HDL-C goals, which are

TABLE 8-8 LDL-C Goals and Cut Points for Therapeutic Lifestyle Changes and Drug Therapy in Different Risk Categories

Risk category	LDL goal (mg/dL)	LDL level at which to initiate therapeutic lifestyle changes (mg/dL)	LDL level at which to consider drug therapy (mg/dL)
CHD or CHD risk equivalents (10-year risk >20%)	<100 (optional goal <70)*	≥100	≥100 (<100: drug optional)*
2+ risk factors (10-year risk ≤20%)	<130 (optional goal <100)	≥130	10-year risk 10%–20%: ≥130 (100–129 optional) 10-year risk <10%: ≥160
0–1 risk factor†	<160	≥160	≥190 (160–189: LDL-lowering drug optional)

*Optional LDL-C goal of <70 mg/dL for very high risk patients; for those with elevated triglycerides, non–HDL-C <100 mg/dL.
†Almost all people with 0–1 risk factor have a 10-year risk <10%; thus, 10-year risk assessment in people with 0–1 risk factor is not necessary.
SOURCE: Modified from Expert Panel on Detection, Evaluation and Treatment of High Blood Cholesterol in Adults,[1] and adapted from Grundy, et al.[99]

30 mg/dL higher than those specified for LDL-C (<130, <160, and <190 mg/dL for those who are CHD risk equivalents, those with two or more risk factors and 20% 10-year CHD risk or less, or those with fewer than two risk factors, respectively).

Consistent with the revised American Heart Association guidelines for patients with vascular disease,[107] the ATP-III guidelines indicate that lipid-lowering drug treatment for persons with established CHD may begin concurrently while in the hospital, as data show compliance is more likely if such treatment is begun while in the hospital. In fact, many experts believe starting such treatment prior to hospital discharge, even if the LDL-C level is unknown, is more appropriate than waiting for an accurate level. Although studies have shown that fasting lipoprotein measurements made immediately on admission for an acute coronary event reasonably estimate baseline levels, total cholesterol and LDL-C can subsequently fall below baseline after a cardiac event, requiring a wait of several weeks or longer to obtain accurate baseline measures.[108] In the primary prevention setting, however, obtaining the average of two fasting measures on separate occasions a few weeks apart may be the most prudent approach to obtaining an accurate baseline on which to justify initiating lipid-lowering therapy.[109]

DIETARY MANAGEMENT OF DYSLIPIDEMIA

The initial treatment for hypercholesterolemia involves therapeutic lifestyle changes, in particular, diet and other nonpharmacologic measures, including physical activity (Fig. 8-6). These interventions are considered in greater depth in other chapters of this book dealing specifically with nutrition (Chapter 11), physical activity (Chapter 12), and behavioral management (Chapter 14). Basic nutritional principles are based on the previously known "Step II" diet of the American Heart Association and NCEP, now referred to as a single "Therapeutic Lifestyle Change" (TLC) diet, which is somewhat more liberal than the previously known Step II diet in total calories from fat permitted (25–35%); however, a larger proportion of this should be in the form of monounsaturated fat (and up to 20% of total calories), while limiting saturated fat to less than 7% of total calories. Additionally, the use of high-fiber foods (20–30 g/d) and consideration of stanol ester margarines are recommended. After an initial 6 weeks on such a TLC regimen, blood lipids should be retested, and if not at goal, TLC approaches should be intensified for another 6 weeks. Pharmacologic therapy is considered if, after this period, LDL-C goal levels are not reached.[1]

PHARMACOLOGIC MANAGEMENT OF DYSLIPIDEMIA

Table 8-9 lists the preparations currently available in the United States and their efficacy and major toxicity.[110] The drugs that are available for lipid lowering are the bile acid sequestrants, nicotinic acid (niacin), fibric acid derivatives, HMG-CoA reductase inhibitors, and cholesterol absorption inhibitors. Selection of the appropriate agent depends on the lipid disorder, including the extent

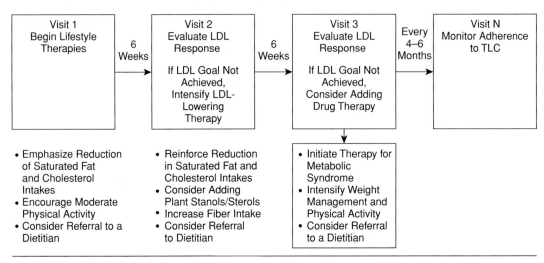

LDL indicates low-density lipoprotein.

FIGURE 8-6 Model of steps in Therapeutic Lifestyle Changes (TLC). (Reproduced, with permission, from the Expert Panel on Detection, Evaluation and Treatment of High Blood Cholesterol in Adults.[1])

of LDL-C elevation, whether triglycerides are elevated or HDL-C is decreased, the presence of other known risk factors,[1] known tolerability to previously used agents, and medical history. Figure 8-7 displays suggested guidelines for the pharmacologic management of dyslipidemia based on the four major phenotypes of dyslipidemia.

Bile acid sequestrants

Bile acid-binding resins, which include cholestyramine and colestipol, primarily lower LDL-C (up to 30% reduction with maximal dosages of 25–30 g/d), do not affect HDL-C significantly, but may increase triglycerides, especially in insulin-resistant patients. Once a mainstay of lipid therapy, these agents now act as adjuncts in combination therapies with statins or other agents. These agents are resins that prevent reabsorption of bile salts. This results in increased conversion of hepatocellular cholesterol to bile acids. Decreased hepatocellular cholesterol content results in upregulation of LDL-C receptors and increased clearance of circulating LDL-C particles.

Gastrointestinal discomfort, including constipation, bloating, and heartburn, is the most common side effect.[110,111] To minimize the likelihood of side effects, the intiation dosage should be small. This dosage is gradually increased over several weeks, and a stool softener or psyllium may be included. One suggested regimen is to start with one dose (4 g of cholestyramine or 5 g of colestipol) at mealtime for 2 weeks and to increase this by a dose every 2 weeks (given subsequently

twice daily) until a dosage of 16 g of cholestyramine or 20 g of colestipol, respectively, is reached. To prevent constipation, it is preferable to precede resin administration with 1 to 2 teaspoons of psyllium powder given for 3 to 5 days. Psyllium itself is a mild bile acid-binding agent and may lower LDL-C by approximately 5%.[112] Higher doses may result in more adverse events and should be reserved for the few patients who fail to reach goal (despite combination therapy).

A relatively recently approved agent, colesevelam, provides an alternative to cholestyramine and colestipol while offering the potential for fewer adverse effects and better compliance. Its efficacy is lower than that of cholestyramine and colestipol. It is approved for use alone or in combination with statins. In clinical trials, colesevelam demonstrated efficacy either alone or in combination with HMG-CoA reductase inhibitors in the treatment of primary hypercholesterolemia. Combination therapy appeared to be more effective than monotherapy. The constipation that typically hinders compliance with traditional bile acid sequestrants is minimal with colesevelam, with one study reporting compliance of 93%.[113]

Cholesterol absorption inhibitors

This is a new class of agents, and currently ezetimibe is the only drug in this class available in the US market. Ezetimibe localizes and appears to act at the brush border of the small intestine to inhibit cholesterol absorption

TABLE 8-9 Pharmacologic Effects of Lipid-Regulating Drugs

Drug	Usual dose	Mode of action	Adverse effects	Efficacy*
HMG-CoA Reductase Inhibitors				
Atorvastatin (Lipitor, Pfizer)	10–80 mg once daily (any time of the day)	↑LDL receptors due to ↓ cholesterol synthesis from inhibition of HMG-CoA reductase	Most common: myalgia, abdominal distress, constipation, diarrhea	↓TC 25–45% ↓LDL 26–60% ↑HDL 5–13% ↓TG 17–53%
Fluvastatin (Lescol, Novartis) Fluvastatin XL	20–80 mg/d as single dose in evening or divided twice daily		If serum transaminase levels rise to three times upper limits of normal, or if patient develops signs/ symptoms of myopathy, should discontinue use	↓TC 16–27% ↓LDL 22–36% ↑HDL 3–11% ↓TG 12–25%
Lovastatin (Mevacor, Merck) (Generic) Lovastatin ES (Altacor, Andrx)	10–80 mg as single dose in evening or divided twice daily			↓TC 16–34% ↓LDL 21–42% ↑HDL 2–10% ↓TG 6–27%
Simvastatin (Zocor, Merck)	5–80 mg/d as single dose in evening or divided twice daily		Interactions with azole antifungals, cyclosporine, diltiazem, verapamil, grapefruit juice, macrolide antibiotics, nefazodone can increase myopathy risk	↓TC 19–36% ↓LDL 26–47% ↑HDL 8–16% ↓TG 12–34%
Pravastatin (Pravachol, Bristol–Myers Squibb)	10–80 mg/d as a single dose at bedtime			↓TC 16–25% ↓LDL 22–34% ↑HDL 2–12% ↓TG 15–24%
Rosuvastatin (Crestor, Astra–Zeneca)	5–40 mg/d as single dose			↓TC 24–46% ↓LDL 28–63% ↑HDL 3–22% ↓TG 10–43%
Bile Acid Sequestrants				
Cholestyramine (Questran, Bristol–Meyers Squibb; Prevalite, Upsher–Smith)	4–24 g/d in two or more divided doses	Bind bile acids in intestine, interrupting enterohepatic recycling of bile acids	Not systemically absorbed	↓TC 10–25% ↓LDL 15–30% ↑HDL 3–5% or no change ↑TG 3–10% or no change
Colesevelam (WelChol, Sankyo Pharma)	3750–4375 mg/d as single dose or divided twice daily with meals	↑Bile acid synthesis from cholesterol, decreased hepatic cholesterol ↑ LDL receptors	Main side effects are nausea, constipation, bloating, and flatulence: some of these may be less with colesevelam	↓TC 8–18% ↓LDL 8–20% ↑HDL 3–5% ↑TG 9–10% or no change
Colestipol (Colestid, Pharmacia)	5–30 g/d as single dose or divided			↓TC 10–25% ↓LDL 15–30% ↑HDL 3–5% or no change ↑TG 3–10% or no change
Fibrates				
Fenofibrate (Tricor, Abbott)	160 mg/d	↑ Lipoprotein lipase activity ↑TG hydrolysis	Common side effects: nausea, diarrhea, and abdominal pain	↓TC 9–22% ↓LDL 31% or ↑45%

(continued)

TABLE 8-9 Continued

Drug	Usual dose	Mode of action	Adverse effects	Efficacy*
HMG-CoA Reductase Inhibitors				
		Inhibit diacylglycerol acyl transferase, thereby decreasing TG synthesis and decreasing ApoB production		↑HDL 9–23% ↓TG 23–54%
Gemfibrozil (Lopid, Pfizer) (Generic)	1200 mg/d in two doses, 30 min before meals		Rarely risk of myositis/ rhabdomyolysis when fibric acids are given with HMG-CoA reducatase inhibitors (risk increased with CRI)	↓TC 2–16% ↓ or ↑LDL up to 30% ↑HDL 10–30% ↓TG 20–60%
Cholesterol Absorption Inhibitors				
Ezetimibe (Zetia, Merck)	10 mg once daily	Acts at brush border of intestine and inhibits absorption of chole- sterol, leading to decrease in delivery of intestinal cholesterol to the liver ↓Hepatic cholesterol stores ↑Clearance of cholesterol from blood	Side effects similar to placebo	↓TC 12–13% ↓LDL 18–20% ↑HDL 1–5% ↓TG 5–9%
Niacin Preparations				
Niacin (nicotinic acid) Extended release (ER) (Niaspan, Kos)	1000–3000 mg once daily at bedtime	Raises HDL-C and ApoA-I by decreasing hepatic catabolism of ApoA-I	Side effects include flushing, itching, gastric distress, headache, hepatotoxicity, hyperglycemia, hyperuricemia	↓TC 3–12% ↓LDL 3–18% ↑HDL 14–26% ↓TG 11–38%
Niacin immediate release (IR) (Generic)	2–6 g/d in three or more divided doses	Reduces plasma triglycerides (TG) by directly inhibiting diacylglycerol transferase 2 (DGAT 2)	Flushing is reduced by giving aspirin, taking with low-fat snack	↓TC 3–25% ↓LDL 5–25% ↑HDL 15–35% ↓TG 20–60%
Niacin time-release preparations (Generic)	Variable, two to three times daily		Flushing and hepatotoxicity may be less with ER niacin than other time-release preparations and high-dose niacin IR	
Combination Products				
Niacin ER with lovastatin (Advicor)	500 mg/20 mg to 2000 mg/40 mg daily at bedtime	See above	See above	↓TC 30% ↓LDL 30–42% ↑HDL 20–41% ↓TG 32–44%

Malik and Kashyap 2003.[100]

*Physicians' Desk Reference, 2003, 57th edition, and product package inserts.

SOURCE: Adapted, with permission, from Malik and Kashyap.[101]

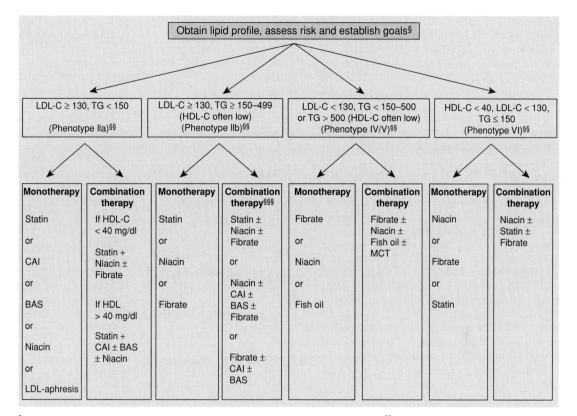

§Rule out secondary causes, eg Type 2 diabetes melitus, hypothyroidism, nephrotic syndrome, etc. §§Phenotype is defined by current guidelines and risk (see text). §§Use fibrate or niacin for predominantly TG problem or low HDL-C problem respectively.
BAS: Bile acid sequestrant; CAI: Cholesterol absorption inhibitor; HDL-C: High-density lipoprotein cholesterol; LDL-C Low-density lipoprotein cholesterol; MCT: Medium-chain triglyceride; TG: Triglyceride.

FIGURE 8-7 Suggested guidelines for pharmacologic management of dyslipidemia. (Reproduced, with permission, from Malik and Kashyap.[101])

without affecting the absorption of triglycerides or fat-soluble vitamins. It has a 24-hour half-life, which allows for once-a-day dosing.[114] This results in a decrease in the delivery of intestinal cholesterol to the liver, a reduction in hepatic cholesterol stores, and an increase in clearance of cholesterol from the blood.

Administered as monotherapy, ezetimibe results in an approximately 20% LDL-C reduction; when added to a statin, studies generally show an additional 15% LDL-C reduction, similar to the additional reduction in LDL-C obtained from a starting to maximum dosage of a statin. Modest additional benefits in lowering triglycerides are also noted from the addition of ezetimibe to a statin.[115] Ezetimibe has been shown to be well tolerated, and does not differ from placebo with respect to laboratory or clinical safety parameters or gastrointestinal, liver, or muscle side effects.

Niacin

Among lipid-regulating agents, niacin is unique in that it is the only agent that favorably affects all major lipoprotein subfractions, resulting in a 15 to 25% reduction in LDL-C, 15 to 30% increases in HDL-C, and even greater reductions in triglycerides (20–50%). It also lowers Lp(a) by as much as 30 to 40%, and may convert individuals from the "small, dense" LDL-C pattern B to a larger, more buoyant pattern A.[49] Recent studies indicate that niacin also increases lipoprotein A-I (LpA-I), a subfraction of HDL that is considered to be antiatherogenic, versus lipoprotein A-II, which is not.[21] Older studies indicated that niacin decreases free fatty acid mobilization by inhibition of adipose tissue lipolysis[116]; however, more recent research indicates that it raises HDL-C and ApoA-I by decreasing the hepatic catabolism of ApoA-I. It decreases hepatic uptake of ApoA-I without affecting cholesterol uptake from the HDL-C. Thus, the half-life of HDL-C is prolonged, but its ability to deliver cholesterol to the liver remains intact, augmenting reverse cholesterol transport.[117] In addition, new information indicates that niacin reduces plasma triglycerides (TGs) and VLDL-C by inhibiting VLDL TG synthetic rate through the inhibition of both fatty acid synthesis and fatty acid esterification to form TGs.[118] A very recent report indicates that niacin noncompetitively, directly, and selectively inhibits diacylglycerol acyltransferase (DGAT2 but not DGAT1), thereby defining a specific target of this agent.[119] DGAT2 is the specific key enzyme involved in VLDL TG synthesis, whereas DGAT1 is involved in nonlipoprotein TG synthesis. Both these enzymes are distinct in their structure and have recently been cloned.[120] Decreased TG synthesis results in poorer lipidation of hepatocellular ApoB, which renders it more susceptible to degradation by proteases. This results in lower secretion of ApoB and smaller TG-poor VLDL-C particles by the liver. Because the larger VLDL-C particles are a precursor of small, dense LDL-C particles, the reduction in VLDL-C size caused by niacin has been proposed as the mechanism by which small, dense LDL-C particles are reduced in concentration and rendered larger (and more buoyant). Decreased VLDL-C concentrations lead to decreased LDL-C concentrations, as VLDL-C is converted into intermediate-density lipoprotein (IDL) cholesterol and then to LDL-C.[121]

In the past, niacin preparations were difficult to tolerate. With the immediate-release niacin preparation, multiple-dosing regimens and intolerable flushing frequently led to noncompliance. A newer formulation, extended-release (ER) niacin,[122] minimizes flushing and hepatotoxicity without eliminating its effectiveness in modifying the lipid levels, and also provides a convenient once-daily regimen. It should be distinguished from other over-the-counter time-release preparations (designated as "sustained-release," "controlled-release"), which have variable efficacy and toxicity. Other side effects include dry skin, itching, gastritis, hepatitis, increased uric acid levels, and hyperglycemia. Tips for improving tolerability include starting at a low dosage and gradually increasing the dosage over several weeks to a maximum in the range of 1 to 3 g per day, as necessary and tolerated. Enteric-coated aspirin minimizes flushing and can be given one-half to one hour before administration. Liver enzyme elevations may accompany use of higher dosages. Enzyme levels should be monitored and niacin dosage reduced or withdrawn if they exceed three times the upper limit of normal.

Niacin is contraindicated in patients with a history of gout or active peptic ulcer disease and hepatic dysfunction. It has been traditionally taught that niacin is also a relative contraindication for patients with diabetes.

However, recent studies have shown that niacin does not significantly worsen hyperglycemia in patients with impaired glucose tolerance/glycemic control.[123,124] The ADMIT study, which looked at the effects of niacin in diabetic patients, concluded that immediate-release niacin was equally effective in modifying lipid and lipoprotein levels in people with or without diabetes.[123] The study showed that plasma glucose levels were increased in people with and without diabetes, but the effects after 60 weeks of follow-up did not significantly increase niacin discontinuation rates or change glycemic therapy.

In addition to ADMIT, Grundy and co-workers examined the use of niacin in diabetics and showed that extended-release niacin had a significant effect on triglyceride as well as HDL-C levels (ADVENT).[124] The changes in HbA1C levels were small in all treatment groups. Increases in fasting blood glucose occurred between weeks 4 and 8 in the niacin-treated groups; levels returned to baseline by week 16. ADVENT demonstrated that extended-release niacin at the doses tested was effective and well tolerated in diabetics. The recommendation is that high niacin doses (>1500–2000 mg/d) not be used.

Fibric acid derivatives

The fibric acid derivatives, or "fibrates" (gemfibrozil and fenofibrate are available in the United States), lower triglycerides by 30% or more and raise HDL-C by as much as 15%, with greater changes for both lipids in patients with severe hypertriglyceridemia. They also lower LDL-C modestly, usually about 10% with gemfibrozil, somewhat more for fenofibrate. In hypertriglyceridemic patients, however, LDL-C levels may increase. By inhibiting diacylglycerol acyltransferase, a key enzyme for triglyceride synthesis, fibrates decrease triglyceride levels.[125] In addition, fibrates activate peroxisome proliferator-activated receptor α (PPAR-α), a nuclear transcription protein that produces several metabolic actions that stimulate reverse cholesterol transport.[126] These actions include increased cholesterol removal from cholesterol-loaded macrophages to HDL-C by the transporter ABC-A1 and the receptor SRB-1 and increased cholesterol uptake from HDL-C to the liver, also by SRB-1. Fibrates also raise HDL-C by increasing synthesis of ApoA-I and ApoA-II by the liver, again by activating PPAR-α.

Gallstone disease, dyspepsia, abdominal pain, and rashes are the most common side effects. Hepatoxicity may occur, but the incidence is low. Myotoxicity is also a rare side effect. The drug should be withdrawn if this occurs. This class of drugs needs to be used with caution in patients with renal insufficiency, liver disease, or gall bladder disease. The dose of gemfibrozil is 600 mg given twice a day orally, half an hour before meals. Fenofibrate comes in tablets of 54 and 160 mg. The usual initial dose is 160 mg/d. Lower starting doses should be used in patients with renal insufficiency and in elderly patients.

HMG-CoA reductase inhibitors

HMG-CoA reductase inhibitors ("statins") have come into wide use in the United States only within the last fifteen years, during which seven such agents have been marketed, each varying in cost and effectiveness in lowering LDL-C. The six currently available ones include lovastatin, pravastatin, simvastatin, fluvastatin, atorvastatin, and rosuvastatin. The statins inhibit HMG-CoA, a key enzyme in cholesterol biosynthesis. In the liver, statins lower free cholesterol concentration, which results in upregulation of LDL-C receptors. LDL-C particles are cleared more rapidly, resulting in lower LDL-C concentrations. Hepatotoxicity, myopathy, and teratogenicity are the adverse events of greatest concern, but they generally affect a small (<1–2%) number of patients and are dose-related; dyspepsia and abdominal discomfort are more common and may occur in up to 5% of patients. Drug interactions can be significant with fibrates and, to a much lesser extent, with niacin, azole antifungals, cyclosporine, diltiazem, verapamil, grapefruit juice, macrolide antibiotics, and nefazodone. These drugs may increase the risk of rhabdomyolysis with HMG-CoA reductase inhibitors by inhibiting their metabolism by cytochrome P450 3A4.[127] Patients should be monitored closely for this side effect if these combinations are used. Cerivastatin was withdrawn from the market due to a higher than expected number of cases of fatal rhabdomyolisis.

At higher dosages of atorvastatin,[128] simvastatin,[129] and rosuvastatin,[130] a 40 to 60% reduction in LDL-C can be expected, with rosuvastatin having the greatest effect on LDL-C lowering compared with equivalent dosages of other statins. Also, statins decrease the concentration of all species of LDL-C, but do not modify the size of LDL-C as powerfully as fibrates or niacin.[131] There is generally a 10 to 35% reduction in triglycerides and less than a 10% increase in HDL-C associated with use of the HMG-CoA reductase inhibitors at lower dosages, although higher recommended dosages of rosuvastatin and atorvastatin have resulted in reductions in triglycerides of as much as 30% or greater. Moreover, increases in HDL-C of up to 10% or more have been noted from use of higher dosages of rosuvastatin.[130] Comparative efficacy data show that at a given dosage of each, rosuvastatin results in successively greater reductions in LDL-C, as well as attainment of LDL-C target goal by a greater proportion of patients than starting dosages of atorvastatin,[132] simvastatin, or pravastatin.[133] The quantity and strength of the research evidence supporting the efficacy of each statin in primary and/or secondary prevention studies

vary dramatically from one drug to the other. Most published clinical trial data have involved lovastatin, pravastatin, simvastatin, and atorvastatin, as noted earlier in this chapter. Hepatic transaminases or creatinine phosphokinase levels elevated to a clinically significant degree occur in less than 1% of persons taking any of the marketed statins, and although rare, rhabdomyolysis can and has occurred with the use of any of the marketed statins. Dipstick positive tubular proteinuria, while shown to be reversible on dosage reduction or withdrawal, also occurs in less than 1% of persons on marketed dosages of any of the statins, although to a slightly higher degree at the higher doses of rosuvastatin. Although the HMG-CoA reductase inhibitors generally provide the greatest LDL-C reduction with the best tolerability, it should be realized that maximal CHD risk reduction may not necessarily require LDL-C reduction beyond that provided by modest dosages of most formulations.[55] However, this question remains open for investigation, as the lowest LDL-C level beyond which no further benefit is achieved is unclear. Clinical trials are underway to address this question.

Estrogen replacement therapy

Estrogen replacement therapy can be used in postmenopausal women and generally results in lowering of LDL-C and raising of HDL-C by approximately 10% each. The use of progestin in combination with estrogen for women with an intact uterus often blunts some of the beneficial lipid effects obtained from estrogens alone.[134] Plasma turnover and in vitro studies indicate that estrogens raise plasma levels of HDL-C and ApoA-I largely by increasing rates of production of ApoA-I-containing particles without altering the fractional catabolic rate.[135–137] Although they also lower plasma LDL-C levels, estrogens increase production of VLDL-C and, therefore, increase plasma triglyceride levels in some women.

Observational studies have shown significant reductions in CHD risk associated both with estrogen used alone[138,139] and estrogens in combination with progestin.[139,140] However, current guidelines do not recommend estrogen replacement therapy for either primary or secondary prevention of CHD.[141] The Heart and Estrogen/Progestin Replacement Study (HERS) in postmenopausal women with known coronary artery disease reported no overall benefit on preventing future cardiovascular outcomes over a 4-year follow-up.[142] The Women's Health Initiative clinical trial arm involving combined estrogen and progestin therapy showed a 29% increased risk of CHD events, 41% increased risk of stroke, a 2.1-fold increased risk of venous thrombotic events, and a 26% increase in the risk of breast cancer in those on the estrogen–progestin combination, compared with placebo.[143] Most recently, a higher risk of stroke was noted in the estrogen-only group which has also now been discontinued.[144] Other recently published trials involving coronary angiographic endpoints have also not shown a benefit.[145,146] In many of these trials, the intervention was given long after menopause; hence, the benefit, if any, of hormone replacement therapy given only in the perimenopausal period remains unclear.

Fish oils

Fish oils contain omega-3 fatty acids, which also lower triglycerides. In total dosages of 3 to 6 g per day, triglyceride lowering can be achieved, but HDL-C levels are largely unaffected. Several fish oil preparations are sold over the counter and are useful (in addition to a very low fat diet) in treating severe hypertriglyceridemia where pancreatitis is a potential risk.

Medium-chain triglycerides

Medium-chain triglycerides (MCTs) are fats that contain 6,8,10, or 12 carbons. The number of carbons distinguishes them from long-chain ($\geq$14 carbons) or short-chain (2 or 4 carbons) fats. The length of the carbon chain affects its metabolism. MCTs are absorbed rapidly and burned for immediate energy, whereas other long-chain fatty acids are absorbed and form chylomicrons, which are metabolized more slowly. Supplements are sold as MCT oil, either fruit-flavored or unflavored. Because the length of the carbon chain affects absorption, and medium-chain triglycerides are rapidly absorbed, they are transported directly to the liver and are quickly oxidized without chylomicron formation, which increases the risk of pancreatitis. Their rapid transport and oxidation make them more similar to carbohydrates than to other fats, and MCTs have less of a tendency to be stored as body fat.

We use MCTs as a substitute for cooking oil in dosages of 1 to 2 tablespoons per day for patients with high triglycerides. The initial dose should be small (ie, one-half tablespoon per day) to make sure there are no gastrointestinal side effects. One tablespoon of MCT oil contains 14 g; ingestion of 85 g has been shown to cause cramping and diarrhea in some individuals. MCT oil should not be used for frying, as the high temperature negatively affects the taste. More research is needed on this agent's effect on lipid metabolism.

CLINICAL APPROACH AND PRINCIPLES OF DRUG SELECTION

The selection of these agents should be highly individualized, although general guidelines can be formulated. Once the decision to initiate drug therapy is made, the choice of agent depends on two major considerations: first, the nature of the lipid disorder, and second, the assessment of risk (for atherosclerotic CVD and pancreatitis). These must be considered and the lipid goal established using NCEP recommendations as a guide. In the vast majority of patients, the lipid disorder falls into one of four patterns as shown in Fig. 8-7. Patients can also be categorized into three broad categories, based on the older Frederickson and Lee classification in adults and a fourth, newer phenotype (VI) proposed recently.[147] The determination of phenotype is defined using cutoff lipid levels based on NCEP ATP-III recommendations described above. In addition to categorizing the patient's lipid phenotype, risk assessment is done to determine therapeutic goal.

The four categories are:

1. Phenotype IIa (hyperbetalipoproteinemia), in which elevated LDL-C is the sole abnormality. Low HDL-C may be present.

2. Phenotype IIb (mixed dyslipidemia, synonymous with combined dyslipidemia), in which LDL-C and triglycerides are elevated and most often HDL-C is low.

3. Phenotype IV/V, in which LDL-C is normal, but triglycerides are elevated (type V characterized by fasting chylomicronemia) and most commonly HDL-C is low.

4. Phenotype VI (not in the Frederickson and Lee classification), in which only HDL-C is low and LDL-C and triglycerides are normal.

If the patient is medication naive, monotherapy may first be used (Fig. 8-8), and in many patients, it may achieve treatment targets. However, results of the Heart Protection Study show that lowering LDL-C in high-risk patients results in further event reduction regardless of baseline LDL-C. Trials are underway that may change LDL-C goals in the future, in which case monotherapy would get even fewer patients to target. The Heart Protection Study also suggests that assessment of risk may be more important than baseline LDL-C levels. Based on this massive study, it could be proposed that a statin should be first-line therapy for most high-risk patients.

Even though monotherapy may result in target goals for some patients, in terms of cardiovascular event reduction, combination therapy should be considered as another effective strategy. Although the HATS trial[72] showed data on only 160 patients, it is the first trial to demonstrate that combination therapy with simvastatin and niacin produces a 70 to 90% reduction in events. The rationale for using combination therapy includes achieving target goals where monotherapy has failed. Using combination therapy results in a lower frequency and

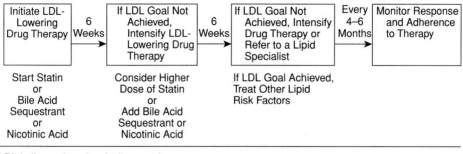

LDL indicates low-density lipoprotein.

FIGURE 8-8   (Reproduced, with permission, from the Expert Panel on Detection, Evaluation and Treatment of High Blood Cholesterol in Adults.[1])

severity of adverse events. Monotherapy usually has dose-dependent side effects, whereas combination therapy allows the use of low doses of two or three agents, thus minimizing side effects from each agent. However, some adverse effects may be increased, for example, myopathy. More research is needed using nonstatin drug combinations, for example, ezetimibe, niacin, fibrate, and other agents.

Prior to initiation of therapy, secondary causes of hyperlipidemia, such as hypothyroidism, nephrotic syndrome, renal failure, diabetes, obstructive liver disease, hyperparathyroidism, and alcoholism, need to be excluded, by appropriate testing. Also, hyperlipidemia can occur as a consequence of such medications as beta blockers, diuretics, estrogens/progestins, glucocorticoids, antiretroviral agents, isotretinoin, tamoxifen, cyclosporine, etretinate, and antipsychotics. In patients with phenotype IIa, in which the only lipoprotein abnormality is an isolated, increased LDL-C, if the goal is not achieved with a statin alone, then combination with niacin, bile acid sequestrant, or cholesterol absorption inhibitor would be desirable. The use of colesevelam, a bile acid sequestrant, and, recently, ezetimibe with 10 mg of atorvastatin was recently shown to produce a reduction in LDL-C similar to that produced by the maximum 80-mg atorvastatin dose. By use of such combinations, the probability of an adverse event due to dose-related side effects is decreased. In patients with combined dyslipidemia (with elevated LDL-C, elevated triglycerides, and, most often, low HDL-C), we prefer, again, to start with a statin to lower the LDL-C and, then, as the next step, to add either a fibrate or niacin. We use a fibrate or niacin if the predominant problem is hypertriglyceridemia or a low HDL-C problem, respectively. A new formulation combining ER niacin and lovastatin was studied in a recent open-labeled multicenter trial.[148] Mean HDL-C was raised by 41% ($P < .001$). Plasma levels of C-reactive

protein and Lp(a) were also reduced in a dose-dependent manner. The most common adverse event was flushing, which led to withdrawal from treatment by 10% of patients. This once-daily fixed-dose ER niacin–lovastatin combination exhibits substantial effects on multiple lipid risk factors and represents a new treatment option in the management of dyslipidemia.

Given recent concerns about increased myotoxicity and rhabdomyolysis, if a fibrate is used at all in combination, it should be used initially with the lowest statin dosage. Fibrate addition does not consistently provide additional LDL-C lowering; however, there is a modest increase in HDL-C. Occasionally, we use more than two agents to get patients to goal. These agents include statins, niacin, and fibrates concurrently; or niacin, cholesterol absorption inhibitor, and bile acid sequestrant, or cholesterol absorption inhibitor and bile acid sequestrant in combination. The use of a cholesterol absorption inhibitor and a fibrate may, in theory, increase gallstones, as both drugs increase biliary cholesterol; however, more research into the combination of these agents is needed.

In patients with phenotype IV/V, in whom triglycerides are elevated with frequently a low HDL-C, we use a fibrate, niacin, fish oil, or their combination and medium-chain triglycerides in patients with persistent fasting chylomicronemia. As niacin and fibrates work by different mechanisms, a combination of these two agents can decrease triglycerides and raise HDL-C better than either alone. If triglycerides are severely elevated, then adding fish oil and/or medium-chain triglycerides can be effective, especially to prevent pancreatitis. With this phenotype, we seldom use statins because of their relatively modest effect in lowering triglycerides in these patients.

Finally, in patients with isolated low HDL-C (phenotype VI); we use a fibrate, niacin, or statin, or their combination. The use of pharmacologic agents in patients with isolated low HDL-C has been controversial; however, current evidence indicates that low HDL-C independently carries an excess risk for ASCVD similar to that of high total cholesterol or LDL-C. If single-drug therapy does not achieve satisfactory results, combinations of a statin and niacin or a fibrate and niacin should be considered. We use statins in this category because they do increase HDL-C synergistically, especially with niacin. More research is needed in this group of patients.

Figure 8-8 illustrates the approach recommended by ATP-III for the progression of drug therapy in primary prevention patients.

OTHER CONSIDERATIONS

The above approach is usually successful in achieving lipid goals in the vast majority of patients. Patients with rare dyslipidemias (eg, type I hypertriglyceridemia) and those with severe lipid level elevations despite maximal drug therapy should be referred to a specialized lipid center. In some high-risk patients (eg, with CHD and LDL-C levels >200 mg/dL despite drug treatment), LDL apheresis must be considered. The Food and Drug Administration has recently approved the use of this procedure, in which the patient's blood plasma is processed through a column that specifically removes ApoB-containing lipoproteins. This procedure is performed twice a month and requires trained personnel.

COST-EFFECTIVENESS OF LIPID-LOWERING

The cost-effectiveness of lipid-lowering therapy depends not only on the actual cost of the medication used for a given patient or in a given institution, but also the risk status of the patient. The cost to produce health benefits (increased longevity and improved quality of life) is generally lowest in groups with the highest near-term risk for CHD, such as those with preexisting CHD.[1] Next in cost effectiveness are those with multiple risk factors or severely elevated cholesterol levels who have a fairly high risk of developing clinical events. Therapy is least cost-effective in those who have only moderate elevations of blood cholesterol without other risk factors.

In the 4S study, among high-risk men and women with preexisting CHD, the cost per year of life gained depended on age, gender, and baseline lipid levels; it ranged from $3800 for 70-year-old men with a mean cholesterol of 309 mg/dL to $27,400 for 35-year-old women with a mean cholesterol of 213 mg/dL.[149] Other models creating estimates for primary prevention of CHD have estimated costs per year of life saved in the range $19,000 to $56,000, depending on dosage and formulation of medication (HMG-CoA reductase inhibitor in all cases).

The cost per life-year saved was about three times greater among women than men at age 40, twice as great at age 60, and 1.3 times as great at age 70 as compared with age 40.[150,151] A recent survey found that although cardiologists tended to recommend pharmacologic treatment in situations where published studies suggested it to be more cost-effective, treatment in the primary prevention setting tended to be more aggressive than would be recommended on the basis of cost-effectiveness analyses.[152] Others have calculated cost-effectiveness based on populationwide approaches to reduce cholesterol levels in the US adult population, estimating cost per year of life saved ($3200) to be similar to that of many medical interventions.[153]

REFERENCES

1. Expert Panel on Detection, Evaluation, and Treatment of High Blood Cholesterol in Adults. Executive Summary of the Third Report of the National Cholesterol Education Program (NCEP) Expert Panel on Detection, Evaluation, and Treatment of High Blood Cholesterol in Adults (Adult Treatment Panel III). *JAMA* 2001;285:2486–2497.

2. Sacks FM, Pfeffer MA, Moye LA, et al. The effect of pravastatin on coronary events after myocardial infarction in patients with average cholesterol levels. *N Engl J Med* 1996;335:1001–1009.

3. Kannel WB, Castelli WP, Gordon T. Cholesterol in the prediction of atherosclerotic disease: new perspective based on the Framingham Heart Study. *Ann Intern Med* 1979;90:85–91.

4. Gordon T, Castelli WP, Hjortland MC, et al. High density lipoprotein as a protective factor against heart disease: the Framingham Heart Study. *Am J Med* 1977;62:707–714.

5. Kashyap ML. Basic considerations in the reversal of atherosclerosis: significance of high-density lipoproteins in stimulating reverse cholesterol transport. *Am J Cardiol* 1989;63:56H–59H.

6. Rubin EM, Krauss RM, Spangler EA, et al. Inhibition of early atherogenesis in transgenic mice by human apolipo-protein AI. *Nature* 1991;353:265–267.

7. Badimon JJ, Badimon L, Fuster V. Regression of atherosclerotic lesions by high-density lipoprotein fraction in the cholesterol-fed rabbit. *J Clin Invest* 1990;85:1234–1241.

8. Manninen V, Tenkanen L, Koskinen P, et al. Joint effects of serum triglyceride and LDL-cholesterol and HDL-cholesterol concentrations on coronary heart disease risk in the Helsinki Heart Study: implications for treatment. *Circulation* 1992;85:37–45.

9. Bloomfield-Rubins H, Robins SJ, Collins D, for the Department of Veterans Affairs HIT Study Group. Gemfibrozil for the secondary prevention of coronary heart disease in men with low levels of high-density lipoprotein cholesterol. *N Engl J Med* 1999;341:410–418.

10. Verschuren WM, Jacobs DR, Bloemberg DP, et al. Serum total cholesterol and long-term coronary heart disease mortality in different cultures: twenty-five-year follow-up of the Seven Countries Study. *JAMA* 1995;274:131–136.

11. Robertson TL, Kato H, Rhoads GG, et al. Epidemiologic studies of coronary heart disease and stroke in Japanese men living in Japan, Hawaii and California: incidence of myocardial

infarction and death from coronary heart disease. *Am J Cardiol* 1977;39:239–243.

12. Stamler J, Wentworth D, Neaton JD. Is the relationship between serum cholesterol and risk of premature death from coronary heart disease continuous and graded? Findings in 356,333 primary screenees of the Multiple Risk Factor Intervention Trial (MRFIT). *JAMA* 1986;256:2823–2828.

13. Kannel WB, Castelli WP, Gordon T, McNamara PM. Serum cholesterol, lipoproteins, and the risk of coronary heart disease: the Framingham study. *Ann Intern Med* 1971;74:1–12.

14. The Pooling Project Research Group. Relationship of blood pressure, serum cholesterol, smoking habit, relative weight and ECG abnormalities to incidence of major coronary events: final report of the Pooling Project. *J Chron Dis* 1978;31:201–306.

15. Kannel WB. High-density lipoproteins: epidemiologic profile and risks of coronary artery disease. *Am J Cardiol* 1983;52:9B–12B.

16. Wong ND, Wilson PWF, Kannel WB. Serum cholesterol as a prognostic factor after myocardial infarction: the Framingham study. *Ann Intern Med* 1991;115:687–693.

17. Anderson KM, Castelli WP, Levy D. Cholesterol and mortality: 30 years of follow-up from the Framingham study. *JAMA* 1987;257:2176–2180.

18. Iribarren C, Reed DM, Chen R, et al. Low serum cholesterol and mortality: which is the cause and which is the effect? *Circulation* 1995;92:2396–2403.

19. Iribarren C, Reed DM, Burchfiel CM, Dwyer JH. Serum total cholesterol and mortality: confounding factors and risk modification in Japanese-American men. *JAMA* 1995;273:1926–1932.

20. Abbott RD, Yano K, Hakim AA, et al. Changes in total and high-density lipoprotein cholesterol over 10- and 20-year periods (the Honolulu Heart Program). *Am J Cardiol* 1998;82:172–178.

21. Kashyap ML. Mechanistic studies of high-density lipoproteins. *Am J Cardiol* 1998;82:42U–48U.

22. Castelli WP, Garrison RJ, Wilson PW, et al. Incidence of coronary heart disease and lipoprotein cholesterol levels: the Framingham Study. *JAMA* 1986;256:2835–2838.

23. Hu D, Jablonski KA, Sparling YH, et al. Accuracy of lipoprotein lipids and apoproteins in predicting coronary heart disease in diabetic American Indians: the Strong Heart Study. *Ann Epidemiol* 2002;12:79–85.

24. Heart Disease and Stroke Statistics, 2004 Update. Dallas, Tex: American Heart Association.

25. Gotto AM. Triglyceride as a risk factor for coronary artery disease. *Am J Cardiol* 1998;82(suppl 9A):22Q–25Q.

26. Jeppesen J, Hein HO, Suadicani P, Gyntelberg F. Triglyceride concentration and ischemic heart disease: an eight-year follow-up in the Copenhagen Male Study. *Circulation* 1998;97:1029–1036.

27. Criqui MH, Heiss G, Cohn R, et al. Plasma triglyceride level and mortality from coronary heart disease. *N Engl J Med* 1993;328:1220–1225.

28. Hokanson JE, Austin MA. Plasma triglyceride level is a risk factor in cardiovascular disease independent of high-density lipoprotein cholesterol level: a meta-analysis of population-based prospective studies. *J Cardiovasc Risk* 1996;3:213–219.

29. Lamarche B, Moorjani S, Lupien PJ, et a. Apolipoprotein AI and B levels and the risk of ischemic heart disease during a five-year follow-up of men in the Quebec Cardiovascular Study. *Circulation* 1996;94:273–278.

30. Stein JH, Rosenson RS. Lipoprotein lp(a) excess and coronary heart disease. *Arch Intern Med* 1997;157:1170–1176.

31. Seed M: Lipoprotein (a): its role in cardiovascular disease. In: Betteridge DJ (ed): *Lipids: Current Perspectives, vol 1: Lipids and Lipoproteins.* London: Martin Dunitz; 1996.

32. Rosengren A, Wilhelmsen L, Eriksson E, et al. Lipoprotein(a) and coronary heart disease risk: a prospective case–control study in a general population sample of middle-aged men. *BMJ* 1990;301:1248–1251.

33. Schaefer EJ, Lamon-Fava S, Janner J, et al. Lipoprotein(a) levels and risk of coronary heart disease in men: the Lipid Research Clinics Primary Prevention Trial. *JAMA* 1994;271:999–1003.

34. Bostom AG, Cupples LA, Jenner JL, et al. Elevated plasma lipoprotein(a) and coronary heart disease in men aged 55 years and younger: a prospective study. *JAMA* 1996;276:544–548.

35. Bostom AG, Gagnon DR, Cupples LA, et al. A prospective investigation of elevated lp(a) detected by electrophoresis and cardiovascular disease in women: the Framingham Heart Study. *Circulation* 1994;90:1688–1695.

36. Jauhiainen M, Koskinen P, Ehnholm C, et al. Lipoprotein(a) and coronary heart disease risk: a nested case–control study of the Helsinki Heart Study participants. *Atherosclerosis* 1991;89:59–67.

37. Ridker PM, Hennekens CH, Stampfer MJ. A prospective study of lipoprotein(a) and risk of myocardial infarction. *JAMA* 1993;270:2195–2199.

38. Nguyen TT, Ellefson RD, Hodge DO, et al. Predictive value of electrophoretically detected lipoprotein(a) for coronary heart disease and cerebrovascular disease in a community-based cohort of 9,936 men and women. *Circulation* 1997;96:1390–1397.

39. Berg K, Dahlen G, Christophersen B, et al. Lp(a) lipoprotein level predicts survival and major coronary events in the Scandinavian Simvastatin Survival Study. *Clin Genet* 1997;52:254–561.

40. Budde T, Fechtrup C, Bosenberg E, et a. Plasma lp(a) levels correlate with the number, severity, and length-extension of coronary lesions in male patients undergoing coronary arteriography for clinically suspected coronary atherosclerosis. *Arterioscler Thromb* 1994;14:1730–1736.

41. Cantin B, Gagnon F, Moorjani S, et al. Lipoprotein(a) is an independent risk factor for ischemic heart disease in man? The Quebec Cardiovascular Study. *J Am Coll Cardiol* 1998;31:519–525.

42. Krauss RM. Heterogeneity of plasma low-density lipoproteins and atherosclerosis risk. *Curr Opin Lipidol* 1994;5:339–349.

43. Austin MA, Breslow JL, Hennekens CH, et al. Low-density lipoprotein subclass patterns and risk of myocardial infarction. *JAMA* 1988;260:1917–1921.

44. Krauss RM, Stampfer MJ, Blanche PJ, et al. Particle diameter and risk of myocardial infarction. *Circulation* 1994;90:I-460.

45. Gardner CD, Fortmann SP, Krauss RM. Small low-density lipoprotein particles are associated with the incidence of coronary artery disease in men and women. *JAMA* 1996;276:875–881.

46. Phillips NR, Waters D, Havel RJ. Plasma lipoproteins and progression of coronary artery disease evaluated by angiography and clinical events. *Circulation* 1993;88:2762–2770.

47. Zambon A, Brown BG, Hokansen JE, Brunzell JD. Hepatic lipase changes predict coronary artery disease regression progression in the Familial Atherosclerosis Treatment Study [abstract]. *Circulation* 1996;94:I–539.

48. Lamarche B, Tchernof A, Moorjani S, et al. Small, dense low-density lipoprotein particles as a predictor of the risk of ischemic heart disease in men: prospective results from the Quebec Cardiovascular Study. *Circulation* 1997;95:69–75.

49. Superko HR. New aspects of risk factors for the development of atherosclerosis, including small low-density lipoprotein, homocysteine, and lipoprotein(a). *Curr Opin Cardiol* 1995;10:347–354.

50. Holme I. Cholesterol reduction and its impact on coronary artery disease and total mortality. *Am J Cardiol* 1995;76:10C–17C.

51. Lipid Research Clinics Program. The Lipid Research Clinics Coronary Primary Prevention Trial results: I. Reduction in incidence of coronary heart disease. *JAMA* 1984;251:351–364.

52. Frick MH, Elo O, Kaapa K, et al. Helsinki Heart Study: primary-prevention trial with gemfibrozil in middle-aged men with dyslipidemia: safety of treatment, changes in risk factors, and incidence of coronary heart disease. *N Engl J Med* 1987;317:1237–1245.

53. Shepherd J, Cobbe SM, Ford I, et al, for the West of Scotland Coronary Prevention Study Group. Prevention of coronary heart disease with pravastatin in men with hypercholesterolemia. *N Engl J Med* 1995;333:1301–1307.

54. Ford I, for the WOSCOPS Study Group. A follow-up report on mortality in the West of Scotland Coronary Prevention Study (WOSCOPS). Paper presented at: 11th International Symposium on Atherosclerosis, Paris, October 1997. Abstract P-145.

55. Prosper Study Group. Pravastatin in elderly individuals at risk of vascular disease (PROSPER): a randomized controlled trial. *Lancet* 2002;360:1623–1630.

56. Pfeffer MA, Keech A, Sacks FM, et al. Safety and tolerability of pravastatin in long-term clinical trials. *Circulation* 2002;105:2341–2346.

57. Downs JR, Clearfield M, Weis S, et al, for the AFCAPS/TexCAPS Research Group. Primary prevention of acute coronary events with lovastatin in men and women with average cholesterol levels. *JAMA* 1998;279:1615–1622.

58. The ALLHAT Officers and Coordinators for the ALLHAT Collaborative Research Group. Major outcomes in moderately hypercholesterolemic, hypertensive patients randomized to pravastatin vs. usual care. *JAMA* 2002;288:2998–3007.

59. Sever PS, Dahlof B, Poulter NR, et al, for the ASCOT Investigators. Prevention of coronary and stroke events with atorvastatin in hypertensive patients who have average or lower-than-average cholesterol concentrations, in the Anglo-Scandinavian Cardiac Outcomes Trial—Lipid Lowering Arm (ASCOT-LLA): a multicenter randomized controlled trial. *Lancet* 2003;361:1149–1158.

60. The Coronary Drug Project Research Group. Clofibrate and niacin in coronary heart disease. *JAMA* 1975;231:360–381.

61. Canner PL, Berge KG, Wenger NK, et al. Fifteen-year mortality in Coronary Drug Project patients: long-term benefit with niacin. *J Am Coll Cardiol* 1986;8:1245–1255.

62. Buchwald H, Varco RL, Matts JP, et al, and the POSCH group. Report of the Program on the Surgical Control of the Hyperlipidemias (POSCH): effect of partial ileal bypass surgery on mortality and morbidity from coronary heart disease in patients with hypercholesterolemia. *N Engl J Med* 1990;323:946–955.

63. Scandinavian Simvastatin Survival Study Group. Randomized trial of cholesterol lowering in 4444 patients with coronary heart disease: the Scandinavian Simvastatin Survival Study (4S). *Lancet* 1994;344:1383–1389.

64. Pyorala K, Pedersen TR, Kjekshus J, et al. Cholesterol lowering with simvastatin improves prognosis of diabetic patients with coronary heart disease: a subgroup analysis of the Scandinavian Simvastatin Survival Study (4S). *Diabetes Care* 1997;20:614–620.

65. The Long-Term Intervention with Pravastatin in Ischaemic Disease (LIPID) Study Group. Prevention of cardiovascular events and death with pravastatin in patients with coronary heart disease and a broad range of initial cholesterol levels. *N Engl J Med* 1998;339:1349–1357.

66. Bloomfield-Rubins H, Robins SJ, Iwane MK, et al, for the Department of Veterans Affairs HIT Study Group. Rationale and design of the Department of Veterans Affairs High-Density Lipoprotein Cholesterol Intervention Trial (HIT) for secondary prevention of coronary artery disease in men with low high-density lipoprotein cholesterol and desirable low-density lipoprotein cholesterol. *Am J Cardiol* 1993;71:45–52.

67. Heart Protection Study Collaborative Group. MRC/BHF Heart Protection Study of cholesterol lowering with simvastatin in 20,536 high-risk individuals: a randomized placebo-controlled trial. *Lancet* 2002;360:7–22.

68. Heart Protection Study Collaborative Group. MRC/BHF Heart Protection Study of cholesterol lowering with simvastatin in 5,963 people with diabetes: a randomized placebo-controlled trial. *Lancet* 2003;361:2005–2006.

69. Rossouw JE. Lipid-lowering interventions in angiographic trials. *Am J Cardiol* 1995;76:86C–92C.

70. Blankenhorn DH, Nessim SA, Johnson RL, et al. Beneficial effects of combined colestipol–niacin therapy on coronary atherosclerosis and coronary venous bypass grafts. *JAMA* 1987;257:3233–3240.

71. Brown BG, Albers JJ, Fisher LD. Regression of coronary artery disease as a result of intensive lipid-lowering therapy in men with high levels of apolipoprotein B. *N Engl J Med* 1990;323:1289–1298.

72. Brown BG, Zhao ZQ, Chait A, et al. Simvastatin and niacin, antioxidant vitamins, or the combination for the prevention of coronary disease. *N Engl J Med* 2001;345:1583–1592.

73. Ornish D, Brown SE, Scherwitz LW, et al. Can lifestyle changes reverse coronary heart disease? The Lifestyle Heart Trial. *Lancet* 1990;336:129–133.

74. Ornish D, Scherwitz LW, Billings JH, et al. Intensive lifestyle changes for reversal of coronary heart disease. *JAMA* 1998;280:2001–2007.

75. Blankenhorn DH, Azen SP, Kramsch DM, et al. The Monitored Atherosclerosis Regression Study (MARS): coronary angiographic changes with lovastatin therapy. *Ann Intern Med* 1993;119:969–976.

76. Jukema JW, Bruschke AVG, Van Boven AJ, et al. Effects of lipid lowering by pravastatin on progression and regression

of coronary artery disease in symptomatic men with normal to moderately elevated serum cholesterol levels: the Regression Growth Evaluation Statin Study (REGRESS). *Circulation* 1995;91:2528–2540.

77. Pitt B, Mancini GBJ, Ellis SG, et al, for the PLAC I Investigators. Pravastatin Limitation of Atherosclerosis in the Coronary Arteries (PLAC I): reduction in atherosclerosis progression and clinical events. *J Am Coll Cardiol* 1995;26:1133–1139.

78. MAAS Investigators. Effect of simvastatin on coronary atheroma in the multicentre anti-atheroma study (MAAS). *Lancet* 1994;344:633–638.

79. Waters D, Hinninson L, Gladstone P, et al. Effects of cholesterol-lowering on the progression of coronary atherosclerosis in women: a Canadian Coronary Atherosclerosis Intervention Trial (CCAIT) substudy. *Circulation* 1995;92:2404–2410.

80. Hahmann HW, Bunte T, Hellwig N, et al. Progression and regression of mild coronary arterial narrowings by quantitative angiography after fenofibrate therapy. *Am J Cardiol* 1991;67:957–961.

81. Haskell WL, Alderman EL, Fair JM, et al. Effects of intensive multiple risk factor reduction on coronary atherosclerosis and clinical cardiac events in men and women with coronary artery disease: the Stanford Coronary Risk Intervention Project (SCRIP). *Circulation* 1994;89:975–990.

82. Sacks FM, Pasternak RC, Gibson CM, et al. Effect on coronary atherosclerosis of decrease in plasma cholesterol concentrations in normocholesterolaemic patients. *Lancet* 1994;344:1182–1186.

83. Nissen SE, Tuzcu EM, Schoenhagen P, et al. Effect of intensive compared with moderate lipid lowering therapy on progression of coronary atherosclerosis: a randomized controlled trial. *JAMA* 2004;291:1076–1080.

84. Frick MH, Syvanne M, Nieminen MS, et al, for the Lopid Coronary Angiography Trial (LOCAT) Study Group. Prevention of the angiographic progression of coronary and vein-graft atherosclerosis by gemfibrozil after coronary bypass surgery in men with low levels of HDL-cholesterol. *Circulation* 1997;96:2137–2143.

85. Havel RJ. Benefits of fibrate drugs in coronary heart disease patients with normal cholesterol levels. *Circulation* 1997;96:2113–2114.

86. Nissen SE, Tsunoda T, Tuzcu EM, et al. Effect of recombinant ApoA-I Milano on coronary atherosclerosis in patients with acute coronary syndromes: a randomized controlled trial. *JAMA* 2003;290:2292–2300.

87. The Post Coronary Artery Bypass Graft Trial Investigators. The effect of aggressive lowering of low-density lipoprotein cholesterol levels and low-dose anticoagulation on obstructive changes in saphenous vein coronary-artery bypass grafts. *JAMA* 1997;336:153–161.

88. Ballantyne CM, Herd JA, Dunn JK, et al. Effects of lipid lowering therapy on progression of coronary and carotid artery disease. *Curr Opin Lipidol* 1997;8:354–361.

89. Yusuf S, Lessem J, Jha P, Lonn E. Primary and secondary prevention of myocardial infarction and strokes: an update of randomly allocated controlled trials. *J Hypertens* 1993;11(suppl 4): S61–S73.

90. Mosca L, Biviano A. Lipid-lowering therapies in the management of acute coronary syndromes. *Curr Cardiol Rep* 2002;4: 320–326.

91. Fonarow GC. In-hospitalization initiation of statin therapy in patients with acute coronary events. *Curr Athero Rep* 2003;5: 394–402.

92. Heeschen C, Hamm CW, Laufs U, et al. Withdrawal of statins increases event rates in patients with acute coronary syndromes. *Circulation* 2002;105:1446–1452.

93. Pitt B, Waters D, Brown WV, et al. Aggressive lipid-lowering therapy compared with angioplasty in stable coronary artery disease. Atorvastatin versus Revascularization Treatment Investigators. *N Engl J Med* 1999;341:70–76.

94. Schwartz GC, Olsson AG, Ezekowitz MD, et al. Effects of atorvastatin on early recurrent ischemic events in acute coronary syndromes: the MIRACL study: a randomized controlled trial. *JAMA* 2001;285:1711–1718.

95. Cannon CP, Braunwald E, McCabe CH, et al. Intensive versus moderate lipid lowering with statins after acute coronary syndromes. *N Engl J Med* 2004;350:1495–1504.

96. Horwich TB, MacLellan WR, Fonarow GC. Statin therapy is associated with improved survival in ischemic and non-ischemic heart failure. *J Am Coll Cardiol* 2004;43:642–648.

97. Braunwald E, Antman EM, Beasley JW, et al. ACC/AHA guideline update for the managmeent of patients with unstable angina and non-ST-segment elevation myocardial infarction—2002: summary article. *Circulation* 2002;106:1893–1900.

98. Pepine CJ. Optimizing lipid management in patients with acute coronary syndromes. *Am J Cardiol* 2003;91:30B–35B.

99. Grundy SM, Cleeman JI, Merz CN, et al. Implications of recent clinical trials for the National Cholesterol Education Program Adult Treatment Panel III Guidelines. *Circulation* 2004;110:227–239.

100. Ballantyne CM. Low-density lipoproteins and risk for coronary artery disease. *Am J Cardiol* 1998;82(suppl 9A):3Q–12Q.

101. Pearson TA, Marx HJ. The rapid reduction in cardiac events with lipid-lowering therapy: mechanisms and implications. *Am J Cardiol* 1993;72:1072–1073.

102. Rosenson RS, Tangney CC. Antiatherothrombotic properties of statins: implications for cardiovascular event reduction. *JAMA* 1998;279:1643–1650.

103. Stafford RS, Blumenthal D, Pasternak RC. Variations in cholesterol management practices by U.S. physicians. *J Am Coll Cardiol* 1997;29:139–146.

104. Danias PG, O'Mahony S, Radford M, et al. Serum cholesterol levels are underevaluated and undertreated. *Am J Cardiol* 1998;81:1353–1355.

105. Schrott HG, Bittner V, Vittinghoff E, et al. Adherence to National Cholesterol Education Program treatment goals in postmenopausal women with heart disease: the Heart and Estrogen/Progestin Replacement Study (HERS). *JAMA* 1997;277:1281–1286.

106. Frolkis JP, Zyzanski SJ, Schwartz JM, Suhan PS. Physician noncompliance with the 1993 National Cholesterol Education Program (NCEP-ATPII) guidelines. *Circulation* 1998;98:851–855.

107. Smith SC, Blair SN, Bonow RO, et al. AHA/ACC Guidelines for Preventing Heart Attach and Death in Patients With Atherslerotic Cardiovascular Disease: 2001 update. A statement for healthcare professionals from the American Heart Association and the American College of Cardiology. *J Am Coll Cardiol* 2001;38:1581–1583.

108. Grundy SM, Balady GJ, Criqui MH, et al. When to start cholesterol-lowering therapy in patients with coronary heart disease: a statement for healthcare professionals from the American Heart Association Task Force on Risk Reduction. *Circulation* 1997;95:1683–1685.

109. Grundy SM, Balady GJ, Criqui MH, et al. AHA Science Advisory: guide to primary prevention of cardiovascular diseases. *Circulation* 1997;95:2329–2331.

110. Malik S, Kashyap ML. Dyslipidemia treatment: current considerations and unmet needs. *Expert Rev Cardiovasc Ther* 2003;1:121–134.

111. Wong ND, Kashyap ML. Dyslipidemia in the elderly: prevalence and implications for clinical management in the prevention of coronary artery disease. *Cardiol Elderly* 1994;2:348–354.

112. Sprecher DL, Harris BV, Goldberg AC, et al. Efficacy of psyllium in reducing serum cholesterol levels in hypercholesterolemic patients on high- or low-fat diets. *Ann Intern Med* 1993;119(7, pt 1):545–554.

113. Davidson MH, Disklin MR, Maki KC, Kleinpell RM. Colesevelam hydrochloride: a non-absorbed, polymeric cholesterol-lowering agent. *Expert Opin Investig Drugs* 2000;9(11):2663–2671.

114. Sudhop T, Lutjohann D, Kodal A, et al. Inhibition of intestinal cholesterol absorption by ezetimibe in humans. *Circulation* 2002;106:1943–1948.

115. Davidson MH, McGarry T, Bettis R, et al. Ezetimibe coadministered with simvastatin in patients with primary hypercholesterolemia. *J Am Coll Cardiol* 2002;40:2125–2134.

116. Carlson LA. Studies on the effect of nicotinic acid on catecholamide stimulated lipolysis in adipose tissue in vitro. *Acta Med Scand* 1963;173:719–722.

117. Jin FY, Kamanna VS, Kashyap ML. Niacin decreases removal of high density lipoprotein apolipoprotein A-I but not cholesterol ester by Hep G2 cells: implications for reverse cholesterol transport. *Arterioscler Thromb Vasc Biol* 1997;17:2020–2028.

118. Jin FY, Kamanna VS, Kashyap ML. Niacin accelerates intracellular apoB degradation by inhibiting triacylglycerol synthesis in human hepatoblastoma (Hep G2) cells. *Arterioscler Thromb Vasc Biol* 1999;19:1051–1059.

119. Gangi SH, Tavintharan S, Zhu D, Kamanna VS, Kashyap ML. Niacin non-competitively inhibits hepatocyte diacylglycerol acyltransferase, a key enzyme for triglyceride synthesis [abstract]. *Arterioscler Thromb Vasc Biol* 2002;22:878A.

120. Cases S, Stones SJ, et al. Cloning of DGAT2, a second mammalian diacylglycerolacyl transferase, and related family members. *J Biol Chem* 276:38870–38876.

121. Kamanna VS, Kashyap ML. Mechanism of action of niacin on lipoprotein metabolism. *Curr Atheroscler Rep* 2000;2:36–46.

122. Morgan JM, Capuzzi DM, Guyton JR. A new extended-release niacin (Niaspan): efficacy, tolerability, and safety in hypercholesterolemic patients. *Am J Cardiol* 1998;82(12A):29V–34V.

123. Elam MB, Hunninghake DB, Davis KB, et al. Effect of niacin on lipid and lipoprotein levels and glycemic control in patients with diabetes and peripheral vascular disease. The ADMIT study: a randomized trial. *JAMA* 2000;284:1263–1270.

124. Grundy SM, Vega GL, McGovern ME et al. Efficacy, safety, and tolerability of once-daily niacin for the treatment of dyslipidemia associated with type 2 diabetes: results of the assessment of diabetes control and evaluation of the efficacy of the niaspan trial. *Arch Intern Med* 2002;162:1568–1576.

125. Zhu D, Ganji SH, Kamanna VS, Kashyap ML. Effect of gemfibrozil on apolipoprotein B secretion and diacylglycerol acyltransferase activity in human hepatoblastoma (HepG2) cells. *Atherosclerosis* 2002;164:221–228.

126. Fruchart J-C. Peroxisome proliferators-activated receptor-activated receptor-alpha activation and high density lipoprotein metabolism. *Am J Cardiol* 2001;88:12A: 9N–24N.

127. Pasternack RC, Smith SC Jr, Bairey-Merz CN, et al. ACC/AHA, NHLBI Clinical Advisory on the Use and Safety of Statins. *Stroke* 2002;33:2337–2341.

128. Nawrocki JW, Weiss SR, Davidson MH, et al. Reduction in LDL cholesterol of 25% to 60% in patients with primary hypercholesterolemia by atorvastatin, a new HMG-CoA reductase inhibitor. *Arterioscl Thromb Vasc Biol* 1995;15:678–682.

129. Stein EA, Davidson MH, Dobs AS, et al. Efficacy and safety of simvastatin 90 mg/day in hypercholesterolemic patients. *Am J Cardiol* 1998; 82:311–316.

130. Schneck DW, Knopp RH, Ballantyne CM, et al. Comparative effects of rosuvastatin and atorvastatin across their dose ranges in patients with hypercholesterolemia and without active arterial disease. *Am J Cardiol* 2003;91:33–41.

131. Marais AD. Therapeutic modulation of low-density lipoprotein size. *Curr Opin Lipid* 2000;11:597–602.

132. Olsson AG, Istad H, Luurila O, et al. Effects of rosuvastatin and atorvastatin compared over 52 weeks of treatment in patients with hypercholesterolemia. *Am Heart J* 2002;144:1044–1051.

133. Brown WV, Bays HE, Hassman DR, et al. Efficacy and safety of rosuvastatin compared with pravastatin and simvastatin in patients with hypercholesterolemia: a randomized, double-blind, 52-week trial. *Am Heart J* 2002;144:1036–1043.

134. Effects of estrogen or estrogen/progestin regimens on heart disease risk factors in postmenopausal women: the Postmenopausal Estrogen/Progestin Interventions (PEPI) Trial. *JAMA* 1995;273:199–208.

135. Schaefer EJ, Foster DM, Zech LA, et al. The effects of estrogen administration on plasma lipoprotein metabolism in postmenopausal females. *J Clin Endocrin Metab* 1983;57:262–267.

136. Brinton EA. Oral estrogen replacement therapy in postmenopausal women selectively raises levels and production rates of lipoprotein A-1 and lowers hepatic lipase activity without lowering the fractional catabolic rate. *Arterioscler Thromb Vasc Biol* 1996;16:431–440.

137. Jin FY, Kamanna VS, Kashyap ML. Estradiol stimulates apolipoprotein A-I but not A-II containing particle synthesis and secretion by stimulating mRNA transcription rate in Hep G2 cells. *Arterioscler Thromb Vasc Biol* 1998;18:999–1006.

138. Bush TL, Barrett-Connor E, Cowan LD, et al. Cardiovascular mortality and noncontraceptive use of estrogen in women: results of the Lipid Research Clinics Program Follow-up Study. *Circulation* 1987;75:1102–1109.

139. Grodstein F, Stampfer MH, Manson JE, et al. Postmenopausal estrogen and progestin use and the risk of cardiovascular disease. *N Engl J Med* 1996; 335:453–461.

140. The Women's Health Initiative Study Group. Design of the Women's Health Initiative clinical trial and observational study. *Control Clin Trials* 1998;19:61–109.

141. Mosca L, Collins P, Herrington DM, et al. Hormone replacement therapy and cardiovascular disease: a statement for healthcare professionals from the American Heart Association. *Circulation* 2001;104:499.

142. Hulley S, Grady D, Bush T, et al. Randomized trial of estrogen plus progestin for secondary prevention of coronary heart disease in postmenopausal women. *JAMA* 1998:280:605–613.

143. Writing Group for the Women's Health Initiative Investigators. Risks and benefits of estrogen plus progestin in healthy postmenopausal women: principal results from the Women's Health Initiative randomized controlled trial. *JAMA* 2002;288:321–333.

144. Anderson GL, Limacher M, Assaf AR, et al. Effects of conjugated equine estrogen in postmenopausal women with hysterectomy: the Women's Health Initiative randomized controlled trial. *JAMA* 2004;291:1701–1712.

145. Herrington DM, Reboussin DM, Brosnihan KB, et al. Effects of estrogen replacement on the progression of coronary artery atherosclerosis. *N Engl J Med* 2000;343:522–529.

146. Hodis HN, Mack WJ, Azen SP, et al. Hormone therapy and the progression of coronary-artery atherosclerosis in postmenopausal women. *N Engl J Med* 2003;349(6):535–545.

147. Kashyap ML, Tavintharan S, Kamanna VS. Optimal therapy of low levels of high density lipoprotein-cholesterol. *Am J Cardiovasc Drugs* 2003;3:53–65.

148. Kashyap ML, McGovern ME, Berra K, et al. Long-term safety and efficacy of a once-daily niacin/lovastatin formulation for patients with dyslipidemia. *Am J Cardiol* 2002;89:672–678.

149. Johannesson M, Jonsson B, Kjekshus J, et al. Cost-effectiveness of simvastatin treatment to lower cholesterol levels in patients with coronary heart disease. *N Engl J Med* 1997;336:332–336.

150. Martens LL, Guibert R. Cost-effectiveness analysis of lipid-modifying therapy in Canada: comparison of HMG-CoA reductase inhibitors in the primary prevention of coronary heart disease. *Clin Therapeut* 1994;16:1052–1062.

151. Thorvik E, Aursnes I, Kristiansen IS, Waller HT. Cost-effectiveness of cholesterol-lowering drugs: a review of the evidence. *Wiener Klin Wochensch* 1996;108:234–243.

152. Gaspoz JM, Kennedy JW, Orav EJ, Goldman L. Cost-effectiveness of prescription recommendations for cholesterol-lowering drugs: a survey of a representative sample of cardiologists. *J Am Coll Cardiol* 1996;27:1232–1237.

153. Tosteson ANA, Weinstein MC, Hunink MGM. Cost-effectiveness of populationwide educational approaches to reduce serum cholesterol levels. *Circulation* 1997;95:24–30.

Diabetes and the Metabolic Syndrome

9

Jennifer Kaseta
James R. Sowers

KEY POINTS

- *Cardiovascular disease, including myocardial infarction and stroke, are leading causes of morbidity and mortality in persons with diabetes.*

- *A substantial increase in the prevalence of diabetes has been noted in recent decades, with more than 17 million (8.4%) of US adults currently estimated to have diabetes.*

- *Twenty-four percent of the US adult population has the metabolic syndrome, characterized by abdominal obesity, atherogenic dyslipidemia, elevated blood pressure, and insulin resistance. Persons with the metabolic syndrome have been demonstrated to be at increased risk of cardiovascular disease.*

- *Lifestyle modifications, including maintenance of optimal weight through therapeutic lifestyle dietary changes, as well as physical activity, are integral in the prevention and treatment of metabolic syndrome and diabetes.*

- *Diabetic dyslipidemia is characterized, in particular, by low high-density lipoprotein cholesterol and elevated triglycerides. A primary treatment target for low-density lipoprotein cholesterol is less than 100 mg/dL (70 mg/dL if accompanied by cardiovascular disease), with secondary goals to reduce triglycerides and increase high-density lipoprotein cholesterol. Treatment with statins has been shown to significantly reduce cardiovascular events in persons with diabetes.*

- *Blood pressure should be kept to below 130 mm Hg/80 mm Hg in persons with diabetes. Treatment with angiotensin-converting enzyme inhibitors or angiotensin receptor blockers as part of required hypertensive therapy (which frequently requires two or more drugs to achieve goal) is recommended.*

- *Glycemic control to more stringent goals (eg, normal hemoglobin A_{1c}, now designated as <6%) is recommended in individual patients.*

Diabetes mellitus is known to be a risk factor for cardiovascular disease (CVD). It causes both macrovascular and microvascular disease, leading to cardiovascular complications. The macrovascular complications include coronary heart disease (CHD), stroke, and peripheral vascular disease, whereas the microvascular complications present as diabetic nephropathy, retinopathy, and cardiomyopathy.[1] CVD, including myocardial in-farction and stroke, is the cause of death among three fourths or more of diabetic persons.[1,2] Several studies have shown that diabetes mellitus is an independent risk factor for CVD.[3-5] In recent years, diabetes has been designated as a CHD risk equivalent,[6] given that the prognosis in those with diabetes without prior myocardial infarction has been shown to be similar to the diagnosis in those without diabetes but with prior myocardial infarction.[7] This has helped to motivate efforts to more aggressively control CHD risk factors in those with diabetes.

EPIDEMIOLOGY

An estimated 17 million have diabetes in the United States, of whom approximately 95% have type 2 diabetes, and an estimated one third of all cases of type 2 diabetes (5–6 million) are undiagnosed and untreated. A dramatic increase in the prevalence of diabetes has been noted over the past several decades. Between 1960 and 1990, the prevalence of diabetes increased from approximately 2.6 to 7.0%.[8] The most recent estimates from 2001 indicate that approximately 5.5% of the US adult population have physician-diagnosed diabetes, with another 2.9% undiagnosed, for a total of 8.4%. Moreover, an additional 7.1% of the population are considered to be prediabetic, based on fasting blood glucose levels of 110 to 125 mg/dL. The prevalence of physician-diagnosed diabetes ranges from approximately 4.6% in Asian/Pacific Islanders to 9.5% in female African-Americans and 11.4% in female Mexican-Americans (Table 9-1).[9] Population- and occupation-based cohort studies generally show type 2 diabetes mellitus to confer about a twofold greater risk for CHD in men, but a threefold greater risk in women. Reported national incidence rates (per 1000 person-years) for CHD range from 4.1 in nondiabetic versus 10.5 in diabetic women aged 40 to 77 years, to 10.2 in nondiabetic versus 28.4 in diabetic men.[5] Multiple studies have also described important risk factors for CVD in diabetics, including hypertension, hyperlipidemia, hyperinsulinemia, advancing age, cigarette smoking, obesity, physical inactivity, and microalbuminuria.[2–12] An overview of cardiovascular risk factors and their degree of evidence in persons with diabetes is given in (Table 9-2).

In the Framingham study,[3] the presence of diabetes doubled the age-adjusted risk of CVD in men and tripled it in women. Myocardial infarction, angina, and sudden death were two times higher in the diabetic as compared with the nondiabetic. Subjects with diabetes in all age groups had a significantly higher rate of cardiac failure as compared with nondiabetic subjects. This difference was more pronounced in the oldest age groups (65–75 years). Diabetes continues to be a major independent cardiovascular risk factor even when all other risk factors for CVD are adjusted for.

Within the Multiple Risk Factor Intervention Trial (MRFIT),[4] more than 5000 diabetics were followed for 12 years and compared with more than 350,000 nondiabetics. The risk of cardiovascular death at the 12-year follow-up was approximately three times higher in male diabetics as compared with their nondiabetic controls, regardless of age, ethnic group, serum cholesterol, systolic blood pressure, or tobacco use. For patients who had optimal control of systolic blood pressure (<120 mm Hg) and serum cholesterol (<200 mg/dL), and were non-smokers, the relative risk (RR) of cardiovascular death was 5.1 times higher in the diabetic than in the nondiabetic. The MRFIT study confirmed that diabetes is a strong independent risk factor for cardiovascular mortality, above the risk incurred from hypercholesterolemia, systolic hypertension, and cigarette use. It also confirmed that hypercholesterolemia, systolic blood pressure, and cigarette smoking were significant independent predictors of mortality in men with and without diabetes. The presence of one or more of these risk factors had a greater impact on increasing CVD risk in diabetics than in nondiabetics (Fig. 9-1).

Although Framingham Heart Study risk algorithms that incorporate diabetes can be used to estimate 10-year global risk of CHD,[13] a recent analysis of 4540 patients from the United Kingdom Prospective Diabetes Study (UKPDS) followed for approximately 10 years was used to construct a risk algorithm for estimating CHD risk. In addition to age, gender, smoking status, systolic blood pressure, and total to high-density lipoprotein cholesterol (HDL-C) ratio, this model additionally incorporates age at diagnosis of diabetes as well as hemoglobin (Hgb) A1c levels. In this model, significant risk ratios were observed for age at diagnosis of diabetes (1.06/year), female gender (0.53), Afro-Carribean ethnicity (0.39), smoking (1.35), Hgb A1c (1.18/1% increase), systolic blood pressure (1.09/10 mm Hg increase), total/HDL-C ratio (3.85/1-unit increase), and duration of diagnosed diabetes (1.08/increase).[14]

Among more than 115,000 female nurses aged 30 to 55 years at baseline, those with onset of diabetes prior to age 30 had an age-adjusted RR for CHD of 12.2, compared with 6.7 for those with diabetes onset at age 30 or older. After adjustment for other risk factors, this risk remained significant but was attenuated (RR = 3.1).[11]

Diabetes mellitus and hypertension often coexist. Hypertension in type 2 diabetics is associated with an increased risk of macrovascular as well as microvascular complications.[15,16] The United Kingdom Prospective Diabetes Study (UKPDS) Group documented an increased risk of stroke over an 8-year observational period in diabetic persons with associated hypertension or elevated levels of systolic blood pressure.[17] They also demonstrated that blood pressure lowering reduced the incidence of macrovascular and microvascular complications in type 2 diabetics.[18] Tight control of blood pressure with either an angiotensin-converting enzyme (ACE) inhibitor or a beta blocker resulted in a reduced risk of both macrovascular and microvascular complications in hypertensive patients with type 2 diabetes.[17–19] The risk of any diabetes-related endpoints

TABLE 9-1 Prevalence of Diabetes Mellitus in the US Population, 2001

Population group	Prevalence of physician-diagnosed diabetes, 2001	Prevalence of undiagnosed diabetes, 2001	Prevalence of prediabetes, 2001	Incidence (type 2 diabetes)	Mortality (diabetes), 2001	Hospital discharges, 2001
Total population	11,100,000 (5.5%)	5,900,000 (2.9%)	14,500,000 (7.1%)	798,000	71,372	562,000
Total males	5,100,000 (5.5%)	3,100,000 (3.3%)	8,800,000 (9.3%)	—	32,841 (46.0%)*	271,000
Total females	6,000,000 (5.5%)	2,800,000 (2.5%)	5,800,000 (5.3%)	—	38,531 (54.0%)*	291,000
White males	5.4%	3.0%	9.4%	—	26,917	—
White females	4.7%	2.1%	4.8%	—	30,263	—
Black males	7.6%	2.8%	8.0%	—	5,049	—
Black females	9.5%	4.7%	6.8%	—	7,256	—
Mexican-American males	8.1%	5.8%	12.1%	—	—	—
Mexican-American females	11.4%	3.9%	6.7%	—	—	—
Total Hispanics[†]	5.5%	—	—	—	—	—
Total Asian/Pacific Islanders[†]	4.6%	—	—	—	—	—
Total American Indians/Alaska Natives[†]	7.6%	—	—	—	—	—

NOTE: Undiagnosed diabetes is a fasting blood glucose of 126 mg/dL or more. Prediabetes is a fasting blood glucose of 110 to less than 126 mg/dL (impaired fasting glucose). Prediabetes also includes impaired glucose tolerance. (—) Data not available.
*These percentages represent the portion of total mortality that is males versus females.
[†]BRFSS (1997). CDC/NCHS, data are for Americans aged 18 and older.

SOURCE: *Prevalence:* NHANESHI [1988–1994]. CDC/NCHS: data for white and black males and females and females are for non-Hispanics: percentages for racial/ethnic groups are age-adjusted for Americans aged 20 and older. *Incidence:* NINDS estimates. *Mortality:* CDC/NCHS. data for white and black males and females include Hispanics. *Hospital discharges:* CDC/NCHS; data include people both living and dead. Reproduced, with permission, from the American Heart Association.[9]

TABLE 9-2   Summary of CVD Risk Factors in Patients With Diabetes

Factor	Longitudinal evidence	Clinical trial evidence
Classic risk factors		
Cholesterol (LDL)*	Conclusive; may be stronger than in ND	+(Subgroup analyses)
Blood pressure	Conclusive	+
Smoking	Conclusive	NA
Sex	Conclusive; weaker than in ND	NA
Additional risk factors		
Glucose	Almost conclusive	+
Insulin	Inconclusive	+ (Insulin Rx—less CVD)
Insulin resistance syndrome	Conclusive	NA
Lipoprotein(a)	Little available	NA
Albuminuria	Conclusive	+ (ACE inhibitors)
Inflammatory markers	None available	NA
Fibrinogen	Suggestive	NA
Subclinical atherosclerosis†	Suggestive	NA
Physical inactivity	Incomplete	NA
Diet	None available	NA

*LDL indicates low-density lipoprotein; ND, nondiabetics; NA, not applicable; Rx, treatment; and ACE, angiotensin converting enzyme.

†Some prefer the term "risk predictor" rather than "risk factor" for subclinical atherosclerosis.

SOURCE: Reproduced, with permission, from Howard et al.[8]

was reduced by 24%, strokes were reduced by 44%, and microvascular endpoints by 37%.[12] The Hypertension Optimal Treatment Trial provides additional support for aggressive treatment of hypertension in diabetics.[20] The most aggressively treated subjects had a 30% reduction in stroke, as compared with the least aggressively treated group, although this difference was not statistically significant, probably due to the small cohort of diabetics and short duration of follow-up.

Type 2 diabetes mellitus is characterized by insulin resistance and decreased insulin production by pancreatic beta cells. Both obesity and physical inactivity predispose individuals to type 2 diabetes mellitus, and both contribute to insulin resistance.[21] Insulin resistance is associated with other cardiovascular risk factors—dyslipidemia, hypertension, and prothrombotic factors.[21] This association underscores the importance of metabolic abnormalities in CVD among diabetics.

FIGURE 9-1 Age adjusted CVD death rates by presence of number of risk factors for men screened for MR-FIT, with and without diabetes at baseline. Risk factors include serum cholesterol ≥200 mg/dL, cigarette smoking (any), and systolic blood pressure ≥120 mmHg. (Adapted from Stamler et al.[4])

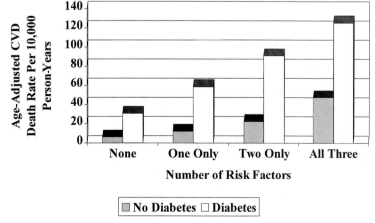

DIAGNOSTIC CRITERIA FOR DIABETES

The most recent American Diabetes Association criteria for the diagnosis of diabetes mellitus[22] are based on having one of the following:

1. Symptoms of diabetes plus casual plasma glucose concentration of 200 mg/dL or greater (where *casual* is defined as any time of the day without respect to time since last meal). Symptoms include polyuria, polydipsia, and unexplained weight loss.
2. Fasting plasma glucose of 126 mg/dL or greater (fasting is defined as no caloric intake for at least 8 hours).
3. Two-hour postload glucose of 200 mg/dL or greater during an oral glucose tolerance test, performed using a glucose load containing the equivalent of 75 g of anhydrous glucose dissolved in water.

Impaired fasting glucose is defined as a fasting plasma glucose of 100 to 125 mg/dL and impaired glucose tolerance is defined as a 2-hour postload glucose of 140–199 mg/dL; these levels are now referred to as "prediabetes" and are associated with the metabolic syndrome, the criteria for which are defined below under Insulin Resistance and the Metabolic Syndrome. Levels above these ranges indicate a provisional diagnosis for diabetes; however, these levels require confirmation.

PATHOPHYSIOLOGY

Many factors contribute to the increased incidence of CVD among diabetics. These include microalbuminuria, lipoprotein and coagulation abnormalities, hypertension, hyperinsulinemia, endothelial dysfunction, increased oxidative stress,[23] and abnormalities of platelet function and coagulation[24] (Tables 9-3 to 9-5). A pathophysiologic model has been proposed that relates the development of predisposing factors to early metabolic abnormalities, measured risk factors, vascular disease, and clinical events (Fig. 9-2).

Microalbuminuria

Microalbuminuria, indicated by an albumin excretion rate of 0.03 to 0.3 g/dL, has been shown to be a risk factor for cardiovascular mortality in type 2 diabetes mellitus. It has also been associated with adverse cardiovascular events in type 1 diabetics.[25–27] The exact mechanism is unknown. It is thought that albuminuria may be the result of generalized endothelial dysfunction that enhances the penetration of atherogenic lipoproteins in the arterial wall.[26] Microalbuminuria has been associated with several cardiovascular risk factors including hyperinsulinemia, insulin resistance, central

TABLE 9-3   Abnormalities of Platelet Function in Diabetes

Increased platelet adhesiveness
Increased platelet aggregation
Decreased platelet survival
Increased platelet generation of vasoconstrictor prostanoids
Reduced platelet generation of prostacyclin and other vasodilator prostanoids
Altered platelet divalent cation homeostasis, ie, decreased $[Mg^{2+}]_i$ and increased $[Ca^{2+}]_i$
Increased nonenzymatic glycosylation of platelet proteins
Decreased platelet polyphosphoinositide content
Decreased platelet production of nitric oxide
Increased platelet myosin light chain phosphorylation
Increased platelet adhesion to endothelium

obesity, and dyslipidemia.[21] Nondiabetic first-degree relatives of patients with type 2 diabetes often have microalbuminuria associated with insulin resistance. This suggests that microalbuminuria in nondiabetic individuals may foreshadow the onset of type 2 diabetes mellitus.[5]

TABLE 9-4   Lipids, Coagulation, and Fibrinolytic Abnormalities in Diabetes

Elevated plasma levels of VLDL*, LDL, and Lp(a)
Decreased plasma HDL-C
Increased small dense LDL-C products
Decreased lipoprotein lipase activity
Elevated plasma levels of factors VII and VIII
Increased levels of fibrinogen and PAI-1
Elevated thrombin–antithrombin complexes
Decreased levels of antithrombin II, protein C, and protein S
Decreased plasminogen activators and fibrinolytic activity
Increased endothelial expression of adhesion molecules
Increased adhesion of platelets and leukocytes to the endothelium

*VLDL, very low density lipoprotein; LDL, low-density lipoprotein; Lp(a), lipoprotein(a); HDL, high-density lipoprotein; C, cholesterol; PAI-1, plasminogen activator inhibitor 1.

TABLE 9-5   Alterations in Vascular Endothelium Associated with Diabetes

Elevated plasma levels of von Willebrand factor
Elevated expression, synthesis, and plasma levels of endothelin-1
Diminished prostacyclin release
Decreased release of endothelium-derived relaxing factor, ie, nitric oxide (NO) and reduced responsiveness to NO
Impaired fibrinolytic activity
Increased endothelial cell surface thrombomodulin
Increased endothelial cell procoagulant activity
Impaired plasmin degradation of glycosylated fibrin
Increased levels of advanced glycosylated end products
Increased superoxide anion generation and NO destruction
Increased expression of adhesion molecules

Lipoprotein abnormalities

Although many diabetics do have elevated levels of total and low-density lipoprotein cholesterol (LDL-C), hypertriglyceridemia and/or low levels of HDL-C are the most commonly occurring lipid abnormalities in diabetics. For any lipoprotein level, diabetics have a greater coronary risk than do nondiabetics. Among the 5163 men in the MRFIT study who reported taking medication for diabetes, those with a total cholesterol of 260 mg/dL and higher were at more than twice the risk of cardiovascular death over 12 years than were those with levels under 180 mg/dL. In contrast, triglycerides, but not total cholesterol, were associated with the pres-ence of ischemic heart disease.[4] The few data regarding the predictive value of lipoprotein levels in diabetics derive from a registry study of 1059 Finnish diabetics receiving drug reimbursement who were followed for 7 years for CHD events.[28] Compared with those with HDL-C of 35 mg/dL or higher, those with HDL-C below 35 mg/dL were at a twofold greater risk of coronary events as were those with triglycerides of 400 mg/dL or greater versus less than 200 mg/dL. Those with LDL-C levels of 160 mg/dL or greater also were at greater risk.

The characteristics of lipoproteins may also differ be-tween diabetics and nondiabetics. Oxidation of lipopro-teins is enhanced in the presence of hyperglycemia and hypertriglyceridemia.[27] Triglycerides are elevated in the diabetic secondary to a decrease in lipoprotein lipase activity.[24] Oxidized lipoproteins are cytotoxic to vascu-lar endothelial and smooth muscle cells and probably contribute to atherogenesis.[23] There is increased glyca-tion of apolipoprotein B (ApoB) in the hyperglycemic state.[20] This results in impaired recognition of LDL by hepatocyte receptors and an increase in LDL half-life. The glycation of HDL increases the clearance of HDL and decreases its half-life. The net result is an increase in plasma very low density lipoprotein (VLDL), LDL, and lipoprotein(a) and a decrease in plasma HDL.[29] Lipopro-tein(a) is a modified form of LDL that can bind to en-dothelium and components of the extracellular matrix.[30] This results in localized cholesterol accumulation. In sev-eral large prospective studies, lipoprotein(a) has been shown to be a powerful predictor of premature atheroscle-rotic vascular disease.[31–33] Its structure is similar to that of plasminogen; it interferes with fibrinolysis and ac-centuates thrombosis by competing with plasminogen for binding sites. Several other mechanisms have been

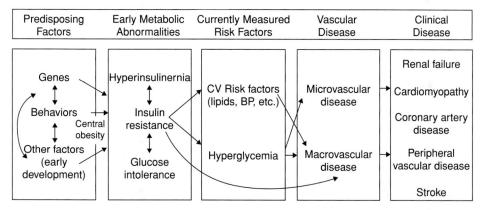

FIGURE 9-2   Pathophysiologic model of development of diabetes and vascular disease. (Reprinted with permission from Howard et al.[8])

elucidated in the diabetic milieu that skew the coagulation cascade in favor of thrombosis. Finally, small, dense LDL (phenotype B) appears to be an important risk factor for the development of type 2 diabetes, possibly mediated through its association with insulin resistance.[34]

Coagulation abnormalities

Diabetic individuals are prone to thrombosis, in part through disruptions in platelet function (Table 9-3) and the vascular endothelium (Table 9-4).[35] Diabetics have higher levels of plasminogen activator inhibitor 1 (PAI-1)[36] than nondiabetics. Elevated levels of PAI-1, which inhibit fibrinolysis, have been associated with hyperinsulinemia and hypertriglyceridemia[37]; they are also found in diabetic survivors of myocardial infarction.[38] This increase in PAI-1 may predispose individuals to recurrent myocardial infarction or abrupt closure of a lesion previously opened by angioplasty.[20] Fibrinolytic activity is also decreased. There are decreased levels of antithrombin III, protein C, and protein S,[29] which predispose these patients to thrombosis. The procoagulant state associated with diabetes can also be attributed to higher-than-normal levels of coagulation factors. Plasma levels of von Willebrand factor are elevated, especially in association with endothelial cell injury, microvascular and macrovascular damage, and poor diabetic control. High concentrations of factor VIII with hyperglycemia accelerate the rate of thrombin formation, which may contribute to occlusive vascular disease. Levels of fibrinogen, factor VII, and thrombin–antithrombin complexes have been noted to be higher in diabetics. This prolongs the survival of provisional clots on injured endothelium. Increased concentrations of thrombin–antithrombin complexes result in increased clot generation.

Platelet adhesion and aggregation are enhanced in diabetics, further contributing to a procoagulant milieu.[39] Studies have suggested that release of the contents of the alpha granules (thromboglobulin and platelet factor 4) is increased in platelets of diabetic individuals.[40] Platelets of diabetics also appear to have decreased levels of platelet-derived growth factor (PDGF) and serotonin, suggesting increased release. Nitric oxide (NO) is produced by platelets[41] as well as by other tissues and inhibits platelet aggregation and adhesion to endothelial cells.[21,38,39,41] In diabetes mellitus, there is reduced production and increased destruction of NO.[1,42] This results in increased platelet aggregation. Other platelet abnormalities in diabetics include decreased platelet survival, increased platelet generation of vasoconstrictor prostanoids, reduced platelet generation of prostacyclin and other vasodilator prostanoids, and increased glycosylation of platelet proteins.[1,39]

Endothelial cell dysfunction

Abnormalities in the vascular endothelium are also associated with diabetes mellitus[1,42] (Table 9-5). Endothelial cell lipoprotein lipase activity is decreased. This impairs conversion of VLDL to LDL, which, in turn, is injurious to the endothelial cells. Hyperglycemia alters endothelial matrix production, which is thought to lead to basement membrane thickening. It also increases endothelial cell collagen and fibronectin synthesis while delaying endothelial cell replication and cell death by enhancing both oxidation and glycation. Hypercholesterolemia, frequently a disease of the diabetic, impairs endothelium-dependent relaxation. There is decreased release of endothelium-derived relaxing factor nitric oxide (NO)[42,43] and reduced responsiveness to NO, as previously discussed with respect to platelets. In addition, there is impaired degradation of glycosylated fibrin, increased concentrations of glycated end products, and elevated expression, synthesis, and plasma concentrations of endothelin-1.

Insulin resistance and the metabolic syndrome

Hyperinsulinemia, or insulin resistance, has traditionally been considered to be an important risk factor for diabetes, as well as for CVD, in diabetics.[10] Hyperinsulinemia is frequently associated with dyslipidemia and central obesity, as well as hypertension.[44,45] In fact, among Framingham offspring subjects (mean age = 54 years), approximately one fourth—now middle-aged adults—were found to have this "central metabolic syndrome" characterized by hyperinsulinemia, dyslipidemia, and obesity.[38] More recent studies in adults with type 2 diabetes or impaired glucose tolerance do not consistently show a relation of endogenous insulin to heart disease.[46] However, among those without diabetes at baseline, a recent meta-analysis involving data from 12 population-based or nested case–control studies showed an overall weak positive association between nonfasting insulin levels and incidence of cardiovascular disease (RR = 1.18, 95% confidence interval [CI] = 1.08–1.29).[47] A recent 22-year follow-up from a study of Helsinki policemen showed a significant positive association for a major coronary event in the highest quintile versus the lower four quintiles of insulin response to an oral glucose tolerance test (area under the curve), with relative risks ranging from 1.32 (22-year follow-up) to 2.36 (5-year follow-up) after adjustment for other risk factors.[48] Hyperinsulinemia may increase cardiovascular risk through its promotion of hypertension, possibly a result of chronic enhancement of sympathetic nervous system activity, thus increasing renal tubular sodium reabsorption, modulating cation transport, or inducing vascular smooth muscle cell hypertrophy.[44] Low HDL-C, also a risk factor for CHD, is promoted by insulin resistance through diminished activity of lipoprotein lipase, which may result in excessive transfer of triglycerides from chylomicrons and VLDL particles from cholesterol esters from HDL particles, thus reducing HDL-C levels.[49]

More recently, the Third Adult Treatment Panel (ATP-III) of the National Cholesterol Education Program (NCEP) came up with a clinically relevant definition for the metabolic syndrome (MetS), based on the presence of three or more of the following: abdominal obesity, elevated triglycerides, low HDL-C, elevated blood pressure, and impaired fasting glucose as defined in (Table 9-6a).[6] An alternative definition, requiring the presence of insulin resistance, has been proposed by the World Health Organization (Table 9-6b).[50] A recent conference convened by the American Heart Association, National Heart Lung and Blood Institute, and American Diabetes Association declared cardiovascular disease as a major clinical outcome of MetS and identified six major components of the syndrome: abdominal obesity, atherogenic dyslipidemia, elevated blood pressure, insulin resistance with or without glucose intolerance, a pro-inflammatory state, and a prothrombotic state.[51] Data from the Third National Health and Nutrition Examination Survey reveal that the vast majority of persons with the metabolic syndrome (but who do not have diabetes) have abdominal obesity, elevated blood pressure, low HDL-C, and elevated triglycerides. Moreover, approximately 60% of such persons have LDL-C levels of 130 mg/dL or higher (Fig. 9-3).[52]

Recent estimates suggest that 24% of the US adult population has the metabolic syndrome based

TABLE 9.6a   NCEP Definition of the Metabolic Syndrome

Risk factor	Defining level
Abdominal obesity, given as waist circumference*†	
Men	>102 cm (>40 in.)
Women	>88 cm (>35 in.)
Triglycerides	≥150 mg/dL
HDL cholesterol	
Men	<40 mg/dL
Women	<50 mg/dL
Blood pressure	≥130/>85 mm Hg
Fasting glucose	≥110 mg/dL‡

*Overweight and obesity are associated with Insulin resistance and the metabolic syndrome. However, the presence of abdominal obesity is more highly correlated with the metabolic risk factors than is an elevated BMI. Therefore, the simple measure of waist circumference is recommended to identify the body weight component of the metabolic syndrome.

†Some male patients can develop multiple metabolic risk factors when the waist circumference is only marginally increased, eg, 94 to 102 cm (37 to 39 in). Such patients may have a strong genetic contribution to insulin resistance. They should benefit from changes in life habits, similarly to men with categorical increases in waist circumference.

‡The American Diabetes Association has recently established a cut point of ≥100 mg/dL, above which persons have either prediabetes (impaired fasting glucose) or diabetes.[14] This new cut point should be applicable for identifying the lower boundary to define an elevated glucose as one criterion for the metabolic syndrome.

TABLE 9.6b   WHO Criteria for the Definition of the Metabolic Syndrome

Insulin resistance, identified by one of the following:
    Type 2 diabetes
    Impaired fasting glucose
    Impaired glucose tolerance
    Or for those with normal fasting glucose levels (<110 mg/dL), glucose uptake below the lowest
        quartile for background population under investigation under hyperinsulinemic, euglycemic
        conditions

Plus any two of the following:
    Antihypertensive medication and/or high blood pressure (≥140 mm Hg systolic or ≥90 mm Hg
        diastolic)
    Plasma triglycerides ≥150 mg/dL (≥1.7 mmol/L)
    HDL-C <35 mg/dL (<0.9 mmol/L) in men or <39 mg/dL (1.0 mmol/L) in women
    BMI >30 kg/m² and/or waist:hip ratio >0.9 in men, >0.85 in women
    Urinary albumin excretion rate ≥20 μg/min or albumin:creatinine ratio ≥30 mg/g

SOURCE: Reprinted with permission, from Grundy et al.[51]

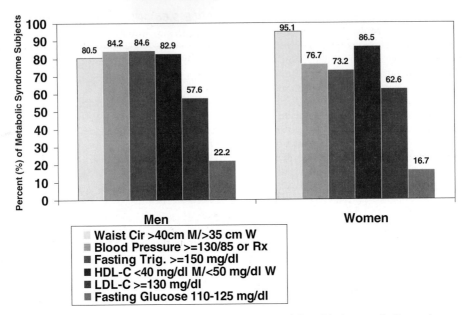

FIGURE 9-3 Prevalence of selected risk factors in US adults with the metabolic syndrome (without diabetes). (Reprinted with permission from Wong et al.[52]) M, men; W, women; Cir, circumference.

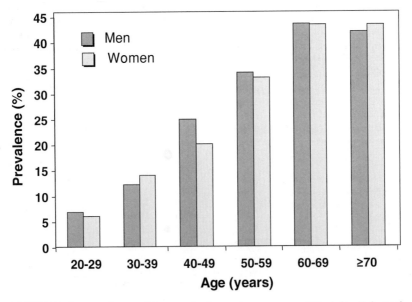

FIGURE 9-4 Prevalence of the metabolic syndrome among US adults. (Adapted from Ford et al.[53])

on the NCEP definition, with greater prevalence in Mexican-Americans and African-Americans than in whites, and with the prevalence rising to approximately 40% by the seventh decade of life (Fig. 9-4) .[53] Several studies have reported on the relationship of MetS to risk of CVD.[54–60] Using the NCEP definition, Lakka and co-workers showed MetS to be associated with a 4.2-fold increased risk of CHD death, a 2.5-fold increased risk of CVD death, and a 2.0-fold increased risk of total mortality in middle-aged men in Finland.[57] Isomaa and co-workers reported CVD and overall mortality to be higher in 35- to 70-year-old persons in Finland and Sweden with a family history of type 2 diabetes who had MetS.[58] Ninomiya and colleagues showed in 10,357 NHANES-III subjects an approximately 2-fold greater odds of preexisting myocardial infarction or stroke in both men and women with versus without MetS.[59] Most recently, Malik et al. showed, in the NHANES-II follow-up study of 6255 subjects representing 64 million US adults, significant risk factor-adjusted hazard ratios of 2.04 for CHD mortality, 1.84 for CVD mortality, and 1.42 for overall mortality in those with versus without MetS, with significant risks also demonstrated among those with MetS who did not have diabetes.[60]

PREVENTION AND MANAGEMENT

The underlying factors that contribute to diabetes also contribute to the development of MetS and include overweight and obesity, physical inactivity, and an atherogenic diet. All current guidelines appropriately emphasize lifestyle modification (weight loss and physical activity) as first-line therapy for the prevention and treatment of MetS and diabetes.[61]

Lifestyle modification

Obesity and physical inactivity can predispose one to type 2 diabetes mellitus and CVD.[62,63] The incidence of type 2 diabetes mellitus increases when obesity is severe. The National Institutes of Health Obesity Education Intiative[64] defines overweight as a body mass index (BMI) of 25 to 29.9 kg/m^2 and obesity as a BMI of greater than 30 kg/m^2. Upper-body obesity (central, android) is usually an indicator of insulin resistance. The waist-to-hip ratio and the waist circumference can be used to assess upper-body obesity. A waist-to-hip ratio greater than 0.9 in men or 0.8 in women indicates upper-body obesity and represents predominant upper-body fat distribution.[45,46] A waist circumference greater than 40 in. (102 cm) in men or 35 in. (88 cm) in women is indicative of abdominal obesity and is one of the components that defines the metabolic syndrome. Approximately 50% of adult Americans are overweight, with nearly half of these classified as obese.[64]

Obesity contributes to hyperlipidemia, low HDL-C, hypertension, insulin resistance, and a prothrombotic state. Obesity acts as a risk factor for both diabetes and CVD by enhancing the metabolic milieu created by the other risk factors of diabetes mellitus and CVD. Regular exercise reduces insulin resistance and a sedentary lifestyle increases it. As with obesity, physical inactivity contributes to the metabolic abnormalities that precede the onset of hyperglycemia and subsequent CVD. There is indirect evidence indicating that decreased physical activity results in an increased risk for type 2 diabetes mellitus, and less active population groups have an increased prevalence of type 2 diabetes. This prevalence increases as physical activity decreases. Physical activity increases insulin sensitivity. Endurance exercise causes weight loss and improves glucose tolerance.

Given the above information, lifestyle modifications are recommended as initial therapy for the prevention and management of diabetes mellitus. These include weight loss if the individual's body weight exceeds the recommendations of the National Institutes of Health Obesity Education Initiative,[64] adherence to American Diabetes Association (ADA) recommendations on medical nutrition therapy,[65] increase in physical activity, and smoking cessation.

The focus of medical nutrition therapy in type 2 diabetes should be on achieving glucose, lipid, and blood pressure goals. Therapy should be individualized, giving consideration to usual eating habits and other lifestyle factors. Weight loss, when needed, as well as hypocaloric diets, can improve glycemic control and may have the potential for long-term metabolic control. The recommended proportion of calories from fat depends on desired glucose, lipid, and weight goals. For those with normal lipid levels at desirable weight, the general goal of 30% or less calories from total fat, less than 10% calories from saturated fat, and less than 300 mg/d dietary cholesterol can be implemented. Less saturated fat and cholesterol, as from the NCEP Therapeutic Lifestyle Changes (TLC) diet (similar to the previously known AHA step 2 diet, eg, <7% of calories from saturated fat and <200 mg of dietary cholesterol), can be recommended for those with elevated LDL-C levels. In general, 10 to 20% of calories should come from protein, which would leave the remaining 50 to 60% from carbohydrates, given the goal of 30% or less calories from fat. Although a commonly held belief has been that simple sugars should be avoided and complex carbohydrates emphasized, there is limited scientific evidence to support this view. There is no reason to avoid consumption of fruits and vegetables, in which fructose occurs naturally. Intake of 20 to 35 g/d dietary fiber is also recommended, as is reduction of sodium intake to no more than 2400 mg/d and less than 2000 mg/d in those with hypertension and nephropathy. Recommendations regarding alcohol use are generally the same for diabetics as for the general public, but reduction or abstention may be advisable in those diabetics with other problems, such as pancreatitis, dyslipidemia, and neuropathy, as well as in those being treated with insulin or sulfonylureas.[65]

Some type of regular exercise is likely to be beneficial in most diabetics. For those patients older than 35 and those who have had diabetes 10 years or longer, a complete physical exam and exercise stress test should be performed prior to the onset of an exercise program. It is well established that sudden exercise in sedentary individuals, including nondiabetics, can precipitate myocardial infarction.[66,67] Patients will be more compliant with activities that they enjoy, and regular encouragement and suggestions should be offered.[68,69] A reasonable initial exercise program should include 10 minutes of warmup and stretching, followed by 20 minutes of aerobic activity (walking, biking, swimming, etc). This should be done undertaken at regular intervals (at least three times a week). The duration and intensity of the exercise program should be increased gradually. Although aerobic exercise is preferred, this may be limited by existing microvascular complications. Patients with proliferative retinopathy should avoid intense isometric exercise (weight lifting), as it can cause an increase in blood pressure and, in turn, intraocular bleeding. Patients with significant neuropathy should avoid traumatic weight-bearing activities (long-distance running, prolonged downhill skiing). These have the potential to precipitate stress fractures in the foot and ankle and to cause pressure ulcers on the feet.

The efficacy of diet and exercise in prevention of diabetes has recently been demonstrated by several trials, including the Diabetes Prevention Program, Finnish Diabetes Prevention Study Group, and DA Qing Impaired Glucose Tolerance and Diabetes Study which each showed a 58% reduction in the risk of new diabetes as a result of such a regimen.[70–72] Nonpharmacologic therapy in diabetic hypertensive patients may be beneficial for hypertension and may be used in combination with pharmacologic therapy to attain adequate blood pressure control, although at blood pressure levels of 140 mm Hg systolic or 90 mm Hg diastolic or higher, concurrent pharmacologic therapy is definitely indicated. The American Diabetes Association (ADA) diet has been reported to lower blood pressure in diabetic patients. Moderate salt restriction can reduce systolic blood pressure. Weight reduction reduces blood pressure. For every 10 lb in weight reduction, systolic and diastolic blood pressures can be expected to decrease by 10 and 5 mm Hg, respectively.[73,74]

Cigarette smoking is an independent risk factor for all-cause mortality, largely due to CVD. Smoking is associated with increased plasma total cholesterol and VLDL, a reduction in HDL, and a greater degree of insulin resistance.[75] In addition, smokers have worse glycemic control than do nonsmokers.[76,77] In type 1 diabetics, smoking is independently associated with an increase in urinary albumin excretion and nonproliferative retinopathy.[78] The degree of albuminuria approaches that of the nonsmoking diabetic when smoking is discontinued.[77,78] A meta-analysis of several cardiovascular risk reduction trials has shown that smoking cessation has a much greater benefit on survival than most other nonpharmacologic interventions.[79] Smoking cessation is one of the most important lifestyle modifications one can make that will decrease cardiovascular morbidity and mortality.[74,80]

Risk assessment and clinical management of the metabolic syndrome

Although therapeutic lifestyle modifications are the initial step for treatment of the metabolic syndrome and its associated risk factors, drug therapy may be recommended to achieve recommended goals.[61] An initial step to deciding on appropriate treatment goals is risk assessment using currently recommended global risk algorithms such as those recommended by the NCEP[6] (see also Chapter 1). Investigators from Framingham have shown that the standard Framingham risk equations, which include cigarette smoking, blood pressure, total cholesterol, HDL-C, and age, capture most of the risk for CVD in those with MetS. Whether the addition of other parameters that may contribute to MetS, such as C-reactive protein, fibrinogen, and LDL particle size, may enhance risk assessment is unknown, although there is preliminary evidence that C-reactive protein levels may help stratify risk in those with MetS and diabetes.[81] Although most persons with MetS are at intermediate calculated risk of CHD (eg, 6 -20% over 10 years),[52] it has recently been shown that approximately 40% of such individuals may be considered CHD risk equivalents based on either a greater than 20% calculated risk of CHD or the presence of significant evidence of subclinical disease from coronary calcium scanning.[82]

Beyond lifestyle modifications, drug treatment could be considered if needed to achieve goals to correct atherogenic dyslipidemia, elevated blood pressure, and hyperglycemia, as well as prothrombotic and proinflammatory states, if present.[61] Goals for LDL-C should be based on risk levels as determined by global risk assessment as recommended above. As in the general population and those with diabetes, efforts should be made to achieve HDL-C levels greater than 40 mg/dL and triglycerides less than 150 mg/dL.

With blood pressure cut points for defining the metabolic syndrome of 130/85 mm Hg or higher, efforts should be made to keep blood pressure levels below this point. As JNC-7 has defined prehypertension as blood pressures of 120 to 139 mm Hg systolic and 80 to 89 mm Hg diastolic,[83] efforts should ideally be made to achieve levels below these points. No particular antihypertensive agents have been identified as being preferable for hypertensive patients who also have the metabolic syndrome, although diuretics and beta blockers in higher doses can worsen insulin resistance and atherogenic dyslipidemia.

With respect to glycemic control, there is growing interest that drugs that reduce insulin resistance may delay the onset of type 2 diabetes. Although some evidence such as that from the Diabetes Prevention Program[70] has shown that metformin therapy can prevent or delay the development of diabetes, neither metformin nor any of the thiazolidinediones currently available have been shown as yet to reduce the risk of CVD in those with MetS, prediabetes, or diabetes.

In patients with the MetS who may be in a prothrombotic state, as evidenced by elevations of fibrinogen, PAI-1, or other factors, aspirin prophylaxis may be appropriate, particularly when their 10-year risk of CHD is 10% or greater. In persons at intermediate risk of CHD, C-reactive protein testing may be appropriate, as recommended by the American Heart Association and Centers for Disease Control, and if it is found to be elevated (≥3 mg/L), may warrant stratification to the next higher risk level for more intensive risk factor intervention.[61,84]

Clinical management of diabetes

A concerted effort to control all major cardiovascular risk factors as well as hyperglycemia maximizes the ability to prevent cardiovascular events in persons with diabetes. Table 9-7 summarizes goals for risk factor management in persons with diabetes.

MANAGEMENT OF HYPERTENSION

The goal in treatment of hypertension in individuals with diabetes mellitus is a blood pressure less than 130/80 mm Hg.[83,85] This is lower than the recommendation for those without diabetes (<140/90 mm Hg) because of the increased risk of CVD in diabetics The UKPDS has previously demonstrated[18,83] that for each 10 mm Hg decrease in mean systolic blood pressure, there is a reduction in risk of 12% for any diabetic complication, 15% for death related to diabetes, 11% for myocardial infarction, and 13% for microvascular complications, with no lower threshold for reduction of risk. In the Hypertension Optimal Treatment (HOT) trial,[20] optimal outcomes were achieved in the group with a target diastolic blood pressure of 80 mm Hg, supporting the benefit of bringing diastolic blood pressure below 80 mm Hg.

At blood pressures of 130 to 139 mm Hg systolic or 80 to 89 diastolic, lifestyle measures, including diet, physical activity, and behavioral therapy, are recommended for a

TABLE 9-7   Goals for Risk Factor Management in Persons with Diabetes

Risk factor	Goal of therapy	Recommending body*
Cigarette smoking	Complete cessation	ADA
Blood pressure	<130/85 mm Hg <130/80 mm Hg	JNC VI (NHLBI) ADA
LDL cholesterol	<100 mg/dL (<70 mg/dL if CVD also present)	ATP-III (NHLBI), ADA
Triglycerides 200–499 mg/dL	Non-HDL cholesterol <130 mg/dL	ATP-III (NHLBI)
HDL cholesterol <40 mg/dL	Raise HDL (no set goal)	ATP-III (NHLBI)
Prothrombotic state	Low-dose aspirin therapy (patients with CHD and other high-risk patients)	ADA
Glucose	Hemoglobin A_{1c} <7%	ADA
Overweight and obesity (BMI >25 kg/m^2)	Lose 10% of body weight in 1 y	OEI (NHLBI)
Physical inactivity	Exercise prescription dependent on patient status	ADA
Adverse nutrition	See text	ADA, AHA, and NHLBI's ATP-III, OEI, and JNC VI

* JNC VI indicates 6th report of the Joint National Committee on Prevention, Evaluation, and Treatment of High Blood Pressure; NHLBI, National Heart, Lung, and Blood Institute; ATP-III, National Cholesterol Education Program Adult Treatment Panel III; HDL, high-density lipoprotein; CVD, Cardiovascular disease; and OEI, Obesity Education Initiative Expert Panel on Identification, Evaluation, and Treatment of Overweight and Obesity in Adults.

SOURCE: Modified, with permission, from Grundy et al. Prevention Conference VI: Diabetes and cardiovascular disease. Writing Group IV: lifestyle and medical management of risk factors. *Circulation* 2002;105:e153–e158.

maximum of 3 months, after which pharmacologic treatment should be considered; at 140 mm Hg or higher systolic or 90 mHg or higher diastolic, concurrent behavioral and pharmacologic therapy (with agents that block the renin–angiotensin system) is recommended. Combinations of two or more drugs are normally needed to achieve the target goal of less than 130/80 mm Hg.[83] Angiotensin-converting enzyme (ACE) inhibitors, angiotensin receptor blockers (ARBs), beta blockers, diuretics, and calcium channel blockers can be used alone or in combination with lifestyle modification for those with blood pressure exceeding 140/90 mm Hg. All patients with type 2 diabetes and hypertension should be treated with an ARB if possible (given the convincing protective effect of ARBs in those with type 2 diabetes), with a thiazide diuretic added if needed to achieve the target blood pressure. Reduction in blood pressure is the goal of antihypertensive therapy and is more important than the antihypertensive agent chosen. The UKPDS[17–19] and other studies have shown benefit with therapy using different classes of antihypertensives, including diuretics, ACE inhibitors, beta blockers, and calcium channel blockers.

ACE inhibitors or ARBs are recommended as an integral part of hypertensive therapy in the diabetic patient[83.86] regardless of the presence or absence of proteinuria. They have no adverse effects on lipid levels or glycemic control[85] and have been shown to slow the progression of diabetic nephropathy.[86–88] Adverse effects of ACE inhibitors include acceleration of renal insufficiency in patients with bilateral renal artery stenosis, angioedema, and cough. When diabetics are intolerant of ACE inhibitors, angiotensin II receptor blockers may be considered, as these have also been shown to favorably affect the progression of diabetic nephropathy.[89,90] In patients with type 2 diabetes, hypertension, macroalbuminuria (>300 mg/d) or proteinuria, and renal insufficiency, an ARB should be strongly considered.[84]

Thiazide diuretics have been shown to reduce cardiovascular morbidity and mortality in large population-based trials. The diabetic hypertensive patient is generally volume-expanded; thus, diuretics are often needed for adequate blood pressure control. Disadvantages of thiazides include short-term dyslipidemia, altered carbohydrate metabolism, hypokalemia, hypomagnesemia, and hyperuricemia. These side effects are minimal if the patient receives a low dose (ie, $\leq$25 mg of hydrochlorothiazide or chlorthalidone). When used in combination with ACE inhibitors, diuretics often have a synergistic effect in blood pressure lowering and the metabolic adverse effects of diuretics are minimized.[85–92]

Calcium channel blockers, alpha blockers, and beta blockers are not recommended as first-line therapy in the treatment of the hypertensive diabetic individual. Calcium channel blockers, however, may be beneficial in the treatment of microalbuminuria. Of note is the fact that nondihydropyridine calcium channel blockers reduce microalbuminuria, but dihydropyridine calcium channel blockers do not. Beta blockers may have adverse effects on glucose and lipid metabolism. They can blunt the catecholamine-mediated symptoms of hypoglycemia and prolong the recovery from hypoglycemia. Beta blockers can also decrease peripheral blood flow and worsen claudication and vasospasm in patients with an already compromised peripheral vasculature. Alpha blockers may have slightly beneficial effects on lipids.

MANAGEMENT OF DYSLIPIDEMIA

The most common pattern of dyslipidemia in patients with type 2 diabetes patients is elevated triglycerides and decreased HDL-C levels, and mean LDL-C levels are not substantially different from those of nondiabetics. Those with diabetes do tend to have a higher proportion of smaller, denser LDL particles, which may be associated with greater risk of CVD events. Given the lipid abnormalities associated with diabetes mellitus, optimal lipid levels in diabetics correspond to an LDL-C of 100 mg/dL or lower, an HDL-C greater than 40 mg/dL, and triglycerides below 150 mg/dL (Table 9-8).[93] Consideration should be given to obtaining a fasting lipid profile annually in adult patients and beginning at age 2 in children with diabetes.

In adults, the primary goal of a reduction of LDL-C to less than 100 mg/dL can usually be achieved with a combination of a low-fat diet, achievement of ideal body weight, and pharmacologic therapy. Medical nutrition therapy normally reduces LDL-C by approximately 10 to 15%. If the baseline LDL-C is 100 mg/dL or lower, cholesterol-lowering agents are not required; if the baseline LDL exceeds 100 mg/dL, dietary therapy is initially recommended, although in patients with both diabetes and preexisting CVD, pharmacologic therapy should be initiated simultaneously with dietary therapy (Table 9-9).[93] A goal to reduce LDL-C below 100 mg/dL is recommended given the status of diabetes as a CHD risk equivalent. However, when diabetes is accompanied by pre-existing cardiovascular disease, now considered criteria for *very high risk* status, a therapeutic option to reduce the LDL-C to below 70 mg/dL has been recently recommended.[94] The favored drugs for treatment of hyperlipidemia in diabetics are the hydroxymethylglutaryl coenzyme A (HMG-CoA) reductase inhibitors ("statins"), recommended in part because of clinical trial data from the Scandinavian Simvastatin Survival Study documenting their efficacy in reducing coronary heart disease events, as shown in subgroup analysis in diabetics.[95] More recently, the Heart Protection Study, the largest lipid-lowering trial to date, demonstrated, in the subset of 5963 patients with diabetes, a 22% reduction in major CVD events, with a similar risk reduction regardless of pretreatment

TABLE 9-8 Treatment Initiation and Goal Levels for Lipoprotein Therapy

	Treatment initiation level (mg/dL)	Target goal (mg/dL)
LDL-C		
Without prior CVD	$\geq$100	<100
With prior CVD	$\geq$100[†]	<70
HDL-C	[‡]	>40
Triglycerides	<400[§]	<150

*LDL-C, low-density lipoprotein, cholesterol; HDL-C high-density lipoprotein cholesterol.
[†]Initiation of pharmacologic therapy concurrently with lifestyle intervention.
[‡]No definite initiation levels for treatment of low HDL-C levels are given; however, treatment may be considered at HDL-C levels <40 mg/dL where LDL-C is not controlled to goal levels.
[§]The decision to start pharmacologic therapy is dependent on the clinician's judgment between triglyceride levels of 200 and 400 mg/dL.

SOURCE: Adapted, with permission, from the American Diabetes Association,[93] and Grundy, et al.[94]

LDL-C levels.[96] Bile acid sequestrants (resins) and nicotinic acid are also effective, but they are less potent and are not as well tolerated. In addition, bile acid sequestrants may raise triglyceride levels, and niacin can exacerbate hyperinsulinemia and hyperglycemia. Cholesterol absorption inhibitors, fenofibrate, and niacin are also options for LDL-C lowering (see Table 9-9).

Secondary goals of lipid therapy in diabetics are to reduce serum triglycerides and raise HDL-C.[93] First-line therapy to attain these goals is attainment of desired body weight and increased physical activity. Smoking cessation also aids in lowering triglycerides and raising HDL-C. The goal for triglycerides is less than 150 mg/dL. While glucose-lowering agents do lower triglyceride levels, a fi-

brate may be added if elevated triglycerides persist and hypertriglyceridemia is the principal lipid abnormality. In cases where elevated LDL-C is the principal problem and a statin was prescribed as the initial agent, a fibrate may be added to provide additional triglyceride lowering beyond the modest reductions in triglycerides possible from high dosages of statins. The down side to this approach is that fibrates and statins in combination place the patient at increased risk for myopathy. Nicotinic acid can be used as an alternative to fibrates, but, unfortunately, nicotinic acid increases insulin resistance and enhances hyperglycemia and has normally been contraindicated in diabetic patients. In some well-controlled diabetics, however, nicotinic acid may be a suitable

TABLE 9-9 Order of Priorities for Treatment of Diabetic Dyslipidemia in Adults

I.	LDL-C lowering
	a. Lifestyle interventions
	b. Preferred therapy: HMGCoA reductase inhibitors (statins)
	c. Other therapy: bile acid-binding resin (resin), cholesterol absorption inhibitor, fenofibrate, or niacin
II.	HDL-C raising
	a. Lifestyle interventions
	b. Niacin or fibrates
III.	Triglyceride lowering
	a. Lifestyle interventions
	b. Glycemic control
	c. Fibric acid derivative (gemfibrozil, fenofibrate)
	d. Niacin
	e. High-dose statins (in those who also have high LDL-C)
IV.	Combined hyperlipidemia
	a. First choice: improved glycemic control plus high-dose statin
	b. Second choice: improved glycemic control plus statin plus fibric acid derivative
	c. Third choice: improved glycemic control plus statin, plus niacin

SOURCE: Adapted, with permission, from the American Diabetes Association.[93]

choice, especially if hypertriglyceridemia and/or low HDL-C are the principal lipid abnormalities. The order of priority for raising HDL-C, lowering triglycerides, and for treating combined dyslipidiemia is given in Table 9-9. Thiazolidinediones may increase HDL-C levels, but may also increase LDL-C levels, and the long-term effects of such therapies on lipids are not known.[93]

ASPIRIN THERAPY

Diabetic individuals have enhanced platelet aggregation and adhesion.[97] Thromboxane, a potent vasoconstrictor and platelet-aggregating agent, is increased in patients with type 2 diabetes and CVD.[97,98] Aspirin inhibits thromboxane synthesis by acetylating platelet cyclooxygenase. It has been used as both a primary and a secondary intervention in nondiabetic and diabetic individuals to prevent CVD.[99–101] The current guidelines for aspirin use provided by the ADA[102,103] include both primary and secondary prevention. Aspirin therapy is recommended as a secondary prevention strategy in diabetic individuals with large-vessel disease, including individuals with a history of myocardial infarction, vascular bypass procedures, stroke or transient ischemic attacks, peripheral vascular disease, claudication, and/or angina. The ADA also recommends the consideration of aspirin therapy as a primary preventive strategy in high-risk individuals with type 1 or type 2 diabetes. This includes those with type 1 or type 2 diabetes who either are older than 40 or have one or more of the following characteristics: family history of CVD, hypertension, smoking, dyslipidemia, and albuminuria. The great majority of diabetics have at least one of these conditions that would warrant aspirin therapy. Aspirin therapy is not recommended in those individuals with an aspirin allergy, bleeding tendencies, anticoagulant therapy, recent gastrointestinal bleeding, and/or clinically active hepatic disease, or in those younger than 21 because of the increased risk of Reye's syndrome in this population. The recommended dose is 75 to 162 mg of enteric-coated aspirin, given the lower risk of adverse effects and the fact that trials have demonstrated similar efficacy in risk reduction with lower dosages of 75 mg/d as compared with higher dosages.[103] Regular use of nonsteroidal anti-inflammatory drugs may increase the risk for developing chronic renal disease and impair blood pressure control in hypertensive patients. Low-dose aspirin is a weak inhibitor of prostaglandin synthesis and has no clinically significant effect on renal function or blood pressure control. Aspirin therapy is not associated with an increased risk or benefit in the progression of diabetic retinopathy and maculopathy.[103]

PHARMACOLOGIC AGENTS FOR GLYCEMIC CONTROL IN TYPE 2 DIABETES MELLITUS

The Diabetes Control and Complications Trial (DCCT)[104] demonstrated a relationship between hy-

perglycemia and the development of microvascular disease and peripheral neuropathy. In patients with type 1 diabetes mellitus, improved glycemic control reduced both microvascular complications and peripheral neuropathy. There is evidence to support the same relationship between glycemic control and microvascular complications and peripheral neuropathy in type 2 diabetics.[105] Although no similar well-controlled prospective trial has been completed in type 2 diabetics, these results have been extrapolated to individuals with type 2 diabetes. The relationship between glycemic control and cardiovascular complications was not statistically significant in the DCCT. It is not known to what degree, if any, glycemic control will affect the progression of macrovascular disease in type 1 and type 2 diabetes. At least there does appear to be a strong relation of glycemic control to risk in nondiabetics, based on a recent report among more than 17,000 working nondiabetic men from three European cohorts. Over 20 years, those in the upper 2.5% of fasting glucose distributions (compared with the lower 80%) were at significantly greater risk of all-cause mortality (age-adjusted hazard ratio = 2.0, 95% CI = 1.6–2.6) and cardiovascular death (hazard ratio = 2.7, 95% CI = 1.7–4.4).[106]

Based on the results of the DCCT and other similar studies, the ADA has recommended treatment goals for individuals with diabetes that emphasize glycemic control.[104] The initial treatment aimed at glycemic control in people with type 2 diabetes is a diet and exercise program. If substantial progress toward glycemic control goals has not been achieved within a 3-month period, pharmacologic therapy is recommended after a diet and exercise program has been initiated.[105] Recent recommendations by the ADA include consideration of more stringent goals for glycemic control (ie, a normal Hgb A1c of < 6%) in individual patients.[107] Some patients may require initial therapy with medications at the time of diagnosis of diabetes. These include individuals with symptoms of hyperglycemia, patients undergoing surgery, and those with ketosis.

Sulfonylureas are recommended as initial pharmacologic intervention in patients with type 2 diabetes because most of these patients are relatively insulin-deficient. An increase in endogenous insulin production is usually observed in patients taking sulfonylureas. After several years of sulfonylurea therapy, endogenous insulin secretion usually decreases and it is difficult to maintain near-normal glycemia.

Biguanides (eg, metformin) have been used alone and in combination with sulfonylureas.[108] As with the sulfonureas, the effectiveness of therapy with biguanides slowly declines with time and other therapeutic interventions become necessary. In the Diabetes Prevention Program,[70] metformin therapy resulted in a 31% reduction in the risk of diabetes in persons with impaired glucose tolerance (compared with a 58% reduction in risk from combined diet and exercise).

The thiazolidinediones (eg, rosiglitazone, pioglitazone) decrease hepatic gluconeogenesis and increase insulin-dependent glucose uptake in skeletal muscle. They require the presence of insulin for their action and can be used as monotherapy or in combination. α-glucosidase inhibitors delay the hydrolysis of complex carbohydrates and thus slow absorption. These agents are useful in patients with postprandial hyperglycemia. As compared with sulfonylureas and biguanides, with which there is usually a reduction in Hgb A1c of 1.5 to 2.0%,[109,110] in α-glucosidase therapy Hgb A1c usually decreases by 0.5 to 1.0%.[110] As the effectiveness of oral agents decreases, insulin therapy is usually required to maintain glycemic control. The insulin regimen should be individualized to the patient.

Adverse events from sulfonylureas include hypoglycemia and weight gain. Biguanides are associated with lactic acidosis, especially in patients with renal disease and congestive heart failure, and are contraindicated in patients with renal insufficiency. The incidence of lactic acidosis with metformin is 0.03 per 1000 patient-years of use. Less concerning than lactic acidosis is gastrointestinal distress, most commonly diarrhea. α-glucosidase inhibitors almost exclusively cause gastrointestinal side effects, most commonly flatulence and abdominal discomfort. This can be avoided by taking the medication with meals and by decreasing the amount of starch in the diet. Thiazolidinediones, also known as PPARs, have been associated with elevated serum transaminase levels as well as hepatic failure in patients taking this class of drug. Although troglitazone has been withdrawn from the market, other drugs in this class are available (rosiglitazone, pioglitazone) and are currently under development. Prescribing thiazolidinediones to patients with serum transaminase levels 2.5 times the upper limit of normal is currently not recommended. Serum transaminase levels should be obtained at the initiation of therapy, then monthly for 8 months, and then every 2 months for the remainder of the first year of therapy.

All of the thiazolidinediones cause weight gain. The weight gain is caused by both proliferation of new adipocytes and redistribution of fat stores. Thiazolidinediones also cause fluid retention and may, in rare cases, precipitate heart failure. This effect is more pronounced in patients on both insulin and thiazolidinediones. Patients who are currently taking rosiglitazone or pioglitazone in addition to insulin therapy should be carefully followed for signs and symptoms of heart failure. The medication should be discontinued if any deterioration in cardiac status occurs. Thiazolidinediones are not recommended in patients with New York Heart Association (NYHA) class III and IV cardiac status.

Both pioglitazone and rosiglitazone affect lipids. In clinically controlled trials, patients treated with pioglitazone had significant decreases in triglycerides and increases in HDL-C, but no consistent mean changes in LDL-C and total cholesterol. Patients treated with rosiglitazone as monotherapy had increases in total cholesterol, LDL-C, and HDL-C and decreases in free fatty acids.[111] In another study, serum total cholesterol and LDL-C concentrations decreased with pioglitazone but not with rosiglitazone.[112] Commonly used pharmacologic agents for glycemic control, including mode of action, duration, dosage, and side effects, are listed in Table 9-10.[113]

SUMMARY

Macrovascular disease is the major cause of mortality in persons with type 2 diabetes mellitus. Many factors contribute to the high prevalence of macrovascular disease in persons with diabetes mellitus. Hypertension and dyslipidemia are two such factors highly prevalent in those with daibetes. The vast majority of diabetes-related cardiovascular complications may be attributed to hypertension and/or dyslipidemia.[114] These observations have contributed to recommendations of more aggressive lowering of blood pressure (ie, to <130/80 mm Hg) and lipids in persons with coexistent diabetes and hypertension and/or dyslipidemia.

Diabetes is often accompanied by other metabolic abnormalities, including insulin resistance. These metabolic abnormalities of the coagulation-fibrinolytic system predispose to a procoagulant state. The nexus for all of these abnormalities may be central (visceral) obesity. The dyslipidemia accompanying hypertension frequently consists of low HDL-C, elevated triglyceride levels, and an abnormal, more atherogenic (small, dense) LDL-C particle. Dyslipidemia interacts with associated hemodynamic (ie, hypertension) and metabolic (ie, increased platelet aggregation and PAI-1 levels) factors in a multiplicative manner, potentiating cardiovascular and renal disease. Accordingly, lipid therapy should be aggressive to attenuate these medical complications. The wide variety of lipid medications currently available, including many that are well tolerated and efficacious, leaves little excuse for not achieving adequate control of dyslipidemia in many persons with diabetes.

Despite the current recommendations regarding the goal of antihypertensive therapy in patients with diabetes mellitus, in many clinical settings, 15% or fewer such persons are adequately controlled at blood pressures less than 130/80 mm Hg. Strategies for better control include combination therapy using several antihypertensive agents at relatively low doses that would result in synergism of their antihypertensive properties. It is also

TABLE 9-10 Commonly Used Pharmacologic Agents for Glycemic Control

Drug class, oral agent	Mode of action	Duration of action	Approved daily dosage range effective dosage	Clearance	Side effects	Efficacy
Sulfonylureas, first generation	Insulin secretagogue				Hypoglycemia, weight gain	60–70 mg/dL decrease in FPG, 0.8–2% decrease in HbA$_{1c}$
(a) Acetohexamide		(a) 12–13 h	(a) 250–1500 mg/ 500–750 mg qd	(a) Renal		
(b) Chlorpropamide		(b) 48 h	(b) 100–500 mg/ 250–500 mg qd	(b) Hepatic/renal		
(c) Tolazamide		(c) 12–24 h	(c)100–1000 mg/ 250–500 mg qd	(c) Hepatic		
(d) Tolbutamide		(d) 6–12 h	(d) 250–3000 mg/ 500–1000 mg bid	(d) Renal		
Sulfonylureas, second generation	Insulin secretagogue				Hypoglycemic, weight gain	60–70 mg/dL decrease in FPG, 0.8–2% decrease in HbA$_{1c}$
(a) Glyburide		(a) 12–24 h	0.75–20 mg/3–5 mg bid	(a) Hepatic, renal		
(b) Glipizide		(b) 12–24 h	2.5–40 mg/5–10 mg qd	(b) Hepatic		
(c) Glimepiride		(c) 24 h	1–8 mg/1–4 mg qd	(c) Hepatic, renal		
Meglitinides	Insulin secretagogue			Hepatic	Hypoglycemia, weight gain	65–75 mg/dL decrease in FPG, 0.5–2% decrease in HbA$_{1c}$
(a) Nateglinide		(a) 2–4 h	(a) 180–360 mg/120 mg tid			
(b) Rapaglinide		(b) 2–6 h	(b) 1.5–16 mg/1–2 mg tid			
Biguanides Metformin	Insulin sensitizer	>3–4 wk	850–2550 mg (500–2000 for XR)/1000 mg bid	Renal	Gastrointestinal	50–70 mg/dL FPG reduction, 1.5–2% HbA$_{1c}$ reduction
Thiazolidinediones	Insulin sensitizer	>3–4 wk		Hepatic	Edema, weight gain, increased LDL-C, potential hepatoxicity	25–50 mg/dL FPG reduction; 0.1–1.5% HbA$_{1c}$ reduction
(a) Pioglitazone			(a) 15–45 mg; 45 mg q.d			
(b) Rosiglitazone			(b) 4–8 mg; 4 mg b.i.d			
α-Glucosidase inhibitors	Delay carbohydrate absorption	<4 h	75–300 mg; 50 mg tid	Renal	Gastrointestinal	35–40 mg/dL FPG reduction; 0.7–1% HbA$_{1c}$ reduction
(a) acarbose						
(b) miglitol						

Adapted from Hsueh et al.[78c] FPG, fasting plasma glucose; XR, extended release.

SOURCE: Adapted, with permission, from Hsueh et al.[112]

likely that less than a minority of diabetic persons lower their LDL-C level to less than 100 mg/dL, which is the goal for most of these patients.

Efforts aimed at preventing diabetes on a population level, however, are essential if we are to reduce the population burden from this disease. Many risk factors for type 2 diabetes, such as obesity, physical inactivity, insulin resistance, and a high-fat diet, can largely be controlled. There exists the tantalizing hypothesis that at least in some people, diabetes can be delayed if not prevented. Although results of some behavioral and drug interventions are promising, further investigation is needed to determine the best approaches to preventing diabetes.[114]

REFERENCES

1. Sowers JR. Diabetes mellitus and cardiovascular disease in women. *Arch Intern Med* 1998;158:617–621.

2. Muggeo M, Verlato G, Bonora E, et al. The Verona Diabetes Study: a population based survey on known diabetes mellitus prevalence and 5-year all cause mortality. *Diabetologia* 1995;38: 318–325.

3. Kannel WB, McGee DL. Diabetes and cardiovascular disease: the Framingham study. *JAMA* 1979;241:2035–2038.

4. Stamler J, Vaccaro O, Neaton JD, Wentworth D, and the Multiple Risk Factor Intervention Trail Group. Diabetes, other risk factors and 12 year cardiovascular mortality for men screened in the Multiple Risk Factor Intervention Trial. *Diabetes Care* 1993; 16:434–444.

5. Wingard DL, Barrett-Conner E. Heart disease and diabetes. In: *Diabetes in America.* 2nd ed. Bethesda, Md: National Institutes of Health; 1995. NIDDK, NIH publication 95–1468.

6. Expert Panel on Detection, Evaluation, and Treatment of High Blood Cholesterol in Adults. Third report of the National Cholesterol Education Program (NCEP) Expert Panel on Detection, Evaluation, and Treatment of High Blood Cholesterol in Adults (Adult Treatment Panel III): final report. *Circulation* 2002;106:3143–3421.

7. Haffner SM, Lehto S, Ronnemaa T, et al. Mortality from coronary heart disease in subjects with type 2 diabetes and in nondiabetic subjects with and without prior myocardial infarction. *N Engl J Med* 1998; 339:229–234.

8. Howard BV, Rodriguez BL, Bennett PH, et al. Prevention Conference VI. Diabetes and Cardiovascular Disease Writing Group I: epidemiology. *Circulation* 2002;105:e132–e137.

9. *2004 Heart and Stoke Facts.* Dallas, Tex: American Heart Association; 2004.

10. Stout RW: Insulin and atheroma: 20-year perspective. *Diabetes Care* 1990;13:631–654.

11. Manson JE, Colditz GA, Stampfer MJ, et al. A prospective study of maturity-onset diabetes mellitus and risk of coronary heart disease and stroke in women. *Arch Intern Med* 1991;151: 1141–1147.

12. Raman M, Nesto RW. Heart disease in diabetes mellitus. *Endocrinol Metab Clin North Am*s 1996;25:425–438.

13. Wilson PWF, D'Agnostino RB, Levy D, et al. Prediction of coronary heart disease using risk factor categories. *Circulation* 1998;97:1837–1847.

14. Stevens RJ, Kothari V, Adler AI, et al. The UKPDS risk engine: a model for the risk of coronary heart disease in Type II diabetes (UKPDS 56). *Clin Sci* 2001;101:671–679.

15. Ali SS, Sowers JR. Update on the management of hypertension; treatment of the elderly and diabetic hypertensives: is the approach to management really different? *Cardiovasc Rev Rep* 1998;6:44–54.

16. The National High Blood Pressure Education Program Working Group. National High Blood Pressure Education Program Working Group report on hypertension in diabetes. *Hypertension* 1994;23:145–158.

17. Davis TM, Millus H, Stratton IM, et al. Risk factors for stroke in type 2 diabetes mellitus: United Kingdom Prospective Diabetes Study (UKPDS) 29. *Arch Intern Med* 1999;159: 1097–1103.

18. UKPDS Group. UK Prospective Diabetes Study 38: tight blood pressure control and risk of macrovascular and microvascular complications in type 2 diabetes. *BMJ* 1998; 317:703–713.

19. UKPDS Group. UK Prospective Diabetes Study 39: efficacy of atenolol and captopril in reducing risk of macrovascular and microvascular complications in type 2 diabetes. *BMJ* 1998;317:713–720.

20. Hansson L, Zanchetti A, Carruthers SG, et al, for the HOT study group. Effects of intensive blood-pressure lowering and low dose aspirin in patients with hypertension: principal results of the Hypertension Optimal Treatment (HOT) randomized trial. *Lancet* 1998;351:1755–1762.

21. Hamaty M, Lamberti M, Sowers JR. Diabetic vascular disease and hypertension. *Curr Opin Cardiol* 1998;13:298–303.

22. American Diabetes Association. Position Statement: diagnosis and classification of diabetes. *Diabetes Care* 2004(suppl 1);S5–S10.

23. Sowers JR, Sowers PS, Peuler JD. Role of insulin resistance and hyperinsulinemia in the development of hypertension and atherosclerosis. *J Lab Clin Med* 1994;123:647–652.

24. Guigliano D, Ceriello A, Paolisso G. Oxidative stress and diabetic complications. *Diabetes Care* 1996;19:257–267.

25. Carmassi F, Morale M, Puccetti R, et al. Coagulation and fibrinolytic system impairment in insulin dependent diabetes mellitus. *Thromb Res* 1992;67:643–654.

26. Kuusisto J, Mykkanen L, Pyorala K, et al. Hyperinsulinemia and microalbuminuria: a new risk indicator for coronary heart disease. *Circulation* 1995;90:831.

27. Dinneen SF, Gerstein HC. The association of microalbuminuria and mortality in non-insulin-dependent diabetes mellitus: a systematic overview of the literature. *Arch Intern Med* 1997;157:1413–1418.

28. Lehto S, Ronnemaa T, Haffner SM, et al. Dyslipidemia and hyperglycemia predict coronary heart disease events in middle-aged patients with NIDDM. *Diabetes* 1997;48: 1354–1359.

29. Lyons T. Lipoprotein glycation and its metabolic consequences. *Diabetes* 1992;41(S2):67.

30. Chisolm G, Irwin K, Penn M: Lipoprotein oxidation and lipoprotein-induced cell injury in diabetes. *Diabetes* 1992; 41(S2):61.

31. Bostom AG, Cupples LA, Jenner JL, et al. Elevated plasma lipoprotein(a) and coronary heart disease in men ages 55 years and younger: a prospective study. *JAMA* 1996;276:544–548.

32. Schaefer EJ, Lamon-Fava S, Jenner JL, et al. Lipoprotein(a) levels and risk of coronary heart disease in men. *JAMA* 1994;271:999–1003.

33. Bostom AG, Gagnon DR, Cupples LA, et al. A prospective investigation of elevated lipoprotein(a) detected by electrophoreseis and cardiovascular disease in women: the Framingham Heart Study. *Circulation* 1994;90:1688–1695.

34. Austin MA, Mykkanen L, Kuusisto, et al. Prospective study of small LDLs as a risk factor for non-insulin dependent diabetes mellitus in elderly men and women. *Circulation* 1995;92:1770–1778.

35. Ford I, Singh TP, Kitchen I, et al. Activation of coagulation in diabetes mellitus in relation to the presence of vascular complications. *Diabetes Med* 1991;8:322–329.

36. Kwaan H. Changes in blood coagulation, platelet function and plasminogen–plasmin system in diabetes. *Diabetes* 1992; 41(S2):31.

37. Landin K, Tengborn L, Smith U. Elevated fibrinogen and plasminogen activator inhibitor (PAI-1) in hypertension is related to metabolic risk factors for cardiovascular disease. *J Intern Med* 1990;227:273–278.

38. Gray R, Patterson D, Yudkin J. Plasminogen activator inhibitor activity in diabetic and nondiabetic survivors of myocardial infarction. *Atherothrombosis* 1993;13:415.

39. Winocour P. Platelet abnormalities in diabetes mellitus. *Diabetes* 1992;41(S2):26.

40. Davi G, Catalano I, Averna M, et al. Thromboxane biosynthesis and platelet function in type 2 diabetes mellitus. *N Eng J Med* 1990;322:1769.

41. Mehta JL, Chen LY, Kone BC, et al. Identification of constitutive and inducible forms of nitric oxide synthase in human platelets. *J Lab Clin Med* 1995;25:370–377.

42. Williams SB, Cusco JA, Roddy MA, et al. Impaired nitric oxide-mediated vasodilation in non-insulin dependent diabetes. *Circulation* 1994;90:1–50.

43. Clarkson P, Celermajer DS, Donald AE, et al. Impaired vascular reactivity in insulin-dependent diabetes mellitus is related to disease duration and low-density lipoprotein cholesterol levels. *J Am Coll Cardiol* 1996;28:573–579.

44. Salone Jt, Lakka TA, Lakka H-M, et al. Hyperinsulinemia is associated with the incidence of hypertension and dyslipidemia in middle-aged men. *Diabetes* 1998;47:270–275.

45. Meigs JB, D'Agostino RB Sr, Wilson PWF, et al. Risk variable clustering in the insulin resistance syndrome. *Diabetes* 1997;46:1594–1600.

46. Wingard DL, Ferrara A, Barrett-Conner EL. Is insulin really a heart disease risk factor? *Diabetes Care* 1995;18:1299–1304.

47. Ruige JB, Assendelft WJJ, Dekker JM, et al. Insulin and risk of cardiovascular disease: a meta-analysis. *Circulation* 1998;97:996–1001.

48. Pyorala M, Miettinen H, Laakso M, Pyorala K. Hyperinsulinemia predicts coronary heart disease risk in healthy middle-aged men: the 22-year follow-up results of the Helsinki Policemen Study. *Circulation* 1998;98:398–404.

49. Garg A. Insulin resistance in the pathogenesis of dyslipidemia. *Diabetes Care* 1996;19:387–389.

50. Alberti KG, Zimmet PZ. Definition, diagnosis and classification of diabetes mellitus and its complications: Part 1. Diagnosis and classification of diabetes mellitus: a provisional report of a WHO consultation. *Diabet Med* 1998;15:539–553.

51. Grundy SM, Brewer HB, Cleeman JI, et al. Definition of metabolic syndrome: report of the National Heart, Lung, and Blood Institute/American Heart Association Conference on Scientific Issues Related to Definition. *Circulation* 2004;109:433–438.

52. Wong ND, Pio J, Franklin SS, et al. Preventing heart disease by nominal and optimal control of blood pressure and lipids in persons with the metabolic syndrome. *Am J Cardiol* 2003;91:1421–1426.

53. Ford ES, Giles WH, Dietz WH. Prevalence of the metabolic syndrome among US adults. *JAMA* 2002;287:356–359.

54. Trevisan M, Liu J, Bahsas FB, Menotti A. Syndrome X and mortality: a population-based study. *Am J Epidemiol* 1998;148:958–966.

55. Burchfiel CM, Sharp DS, Curb DJ, et al. Hyperinsulinemia and cardiovascular disease in elderly men. *Arterioscler Thromb Vasc Biol* 1998;18:450–457.

56. Solymoss BC, Marcil M, Cahour M, et al. Fasting hyperinsulinism, insulin resistance syndrome, and coronary artery disease in men and women. *Am J Cardiol* 1995;76:1152–1156.

57. Lakka HM, Laaksonen DE, Lakka TA, et al. The metabolic syndrome and total and cardiovascular disease mortality in middle-aged men. *JAMA* 2002;288:2709–2716.

58. Isomaa B, Almgren P, Tuomi T, et al. Cardiovascular morbidity and mortality associated with the metabolic syndrome. *Diabetes Care* 2001;24:683–689.

59. Ninomiya JK, L'Italien G, Criqui MH, et al. Association of the metabolic syndrome with history of myocardial infarction and stroke in the Third National Health and Nutrition Examination Survey. *Circulation* 2004;109:42–46.

60. Malik S, Wong ND, Franklin SS, et al. The impact of the metabolic syndrome on mortality from coronary heart disease, cardiovascular disease, and all causes in United States adults. *Circulation* 2004;110:1239–1244.

61. Grundy SM, Hansen B, Smith SC, et al. Clinical management of the metabolic syndrome: report of the American Heart Association/National Heart Lung and Blood Institute/American Diabetes Association Conference on Scientific Issues Related to Management. *Circulation* 2004;109:551–556.

62. Peiris AN, Sothmann MS, Hennes MI, et al. The relative contribution of obesity and body fat distribution to alterations in glucose and insulin homeostasis. *Am J Clin Nutr* 1989;49:758–764.

63. Haffner SM, Stern MP, Hazuda HP, et al. Do upper body and centralized adiposity measure different aspects of regional body fat distribution? Relation to non-insulin-dependent diabetes mellitus, lipids, and lipoproteins. *Diabetes* 1987;36:43–51.

64. *Clinical Guidelines for the Identification, Evaluation, and Treatment of Overweight and Obesity in Adults.* Bethesda, Md: NHBLI, NIH; 1998.

65. American Diabetes Association. Nutrition recommendation and principles for people with diabetes mellitus (position statement). *Diabetes Care* 1998;21:S32–S35.

66. Mittleman MA, Maclure M, Tofler GH, et al. Triggering of acute myocardial infarction by heavy physical exertion: protection against trigger by regular exertion. *N Engl J Med* 1993;329:1677.

67. Curfman, GD. Is exercise beneficial or hazardous to your heart? *N Engl J Med* 1993;329:1730.

68. Calfas KJ, Long BJ, Sallis JF, et al. A controlled trial of physician counseling to promote the adoption of physical activity. *Prev Med* 1996;25:225.

69. Long BJ, Calfas KJ, Wooten W, et al. A multi-site field test of the acceptability of Physical Activity Counseling in primary care: Project PACE. Am J Prev Med 1996;12:73.

70. Knowlet WC, Barrett-Conner E, Fowler SE, et al. Reduction in the incidence of type 2 diabetes with lifestyle intervention or metformin. *N Engl J Med* 2002;346:393–403.

71. Tuomilehto J, Lindstrom J, Eriksson JG, et al. Prevention of type 2 diabetes mellitus by changes in lifestyle among subjects with impaired glucose tolerance. *N Engl J Med* 2001;344:1343–1350.

72. Li G, Hu Y, Yang W, et al. Effects of insulin resistance and insulin secretion on the efficacy of interventions to retard development of type 2 diabetes mellitus: the DA Qing IGT and Diabetes Study. *Diabetes Res Clin Pract* 2002;58:193–200.

73. Sowers JR, Epstein M. Diabetes mellitus and hypertension: an update. *Hypertension* 1995;26:869–879.

74. Sowers JR. Insulin and insulin-like growth factor in normal and pathological cardiovascular physiology. *Hypertension* 1997;29:691–699.

75. Facchini FS, Hollenbeck CB, Jeppesen J, et al. Insulin resistance and cigarette smoking. *Lancet* 1992;339:1128.

76. Lundman B, Asplund K, Norberg A. Smoking and metabolic control in patients with insulin-dependent diabetes mellitus. *J Intern Med* 1990;227:101.

77. Chaturvedi N, Stephenson JM, Fuller JH, et al. The relationship between smoking and microvascular complication in the EURODIAB IDDM Complications Study. *Diabetes Care* 1995;18:785.

78. Chase HP, Garg SK, Marshall G, et al. Cigarette smoking increases the risk of albuminuria among subjects with type 1 diabetes. *JAMA* 1991;265:614.

79. Yudkin JS. How can we best prolong life? Benefits of coronary risk factor reduction in non-diabetic and diabetic subjects. *BMJ* 1993;306:1313.

80. Ford ES, Malarcher AM, Herman WH, et al. Diabetes mellitus and cigarette smoking: findings from the 1989 National Health Interview Survey. *Diabetes Care* 1994;17:688.

81. Malik S, Wong ND, Franklin SS, Pio J, et al. Risk of cardiovascular disease in US persons with metabolic risk factors, diabetes, and elevated C-reactive protein. *J Am Coll Cardiol* 2004;43(suppl A):486A(abstr).

82. Wong ND, Sciammarella M, Miranda-Peats R, et al. The metabolic syndrome, diabetes, and subclinical atherosclerosis assessed by coronary calcium. *J Am Coll Cardiol* 2003;41:1547–1553.

83. Chobanian AV, Bakris GL, Black HR, et al. The seventh report of the Joint National Committee on Prevention, Detection, Evaluation, and Treatment of High Blood Pressure: the JNC 7 Report. *JAMA* 2003;289:2560–2572.

84. Pearson TA, Mensah GA, Alexander RW, et al. Markers of inflammation and cardiovascular disease: application to clinical and public health practice: a statement for healthcare professionals from the Centers for Disease Control and Prevention and the American Heart Association. *Circulation* 2003;107:499–511.

85. American Diabetes Association. Hypertension management in adults with diabetes. *Diabetes Care* 2004; 27(suppl 1):S65–S67.

86. Lebovitz HE, Wiegmann TB, Cnaan A, et al. Renal protective effects of enalapril in hypertensive NIDDM: role of baseline albuminuria. *Kidney Int* 1994;45:S150–S155.

87. Ravid M, Savin H, Jutrin I, et al. Long-term stabilizing effect of angiotensin-converting enzyme inhibition on plasma creatinine and on proteinuria in normotensive type II diabetic patients. *Ann Intern Med* 1993;118:577–581.

88. Lewis EJ, Hunsicker LG, Bain RP, Rohde RD, for the Collaborative Study Group. The effect of angiotensin-converting enzyme inhibition on diabetic nephropathy. *N Engl J Med* 1993;329:1456–1462.

89. Brenner BM, Cooper ME, de Zeeuw D, et al. Effects of losartan on renal and cardiovascular outcomes in patients with type 2 diabetes and nephropathy. *N Engl J Med* 2001;345:861–869.

90. Lewis EJ, Hunsicker LG, Clarke WR, et al. Renoprotective effect of the angiotensin-receptor antagonist irbesartan in patients with nephropathy due to type 2 diabetes. *N Engl J Med* 2001;345:851–860.

91. Sowers JR, Lester MA. Diabetes and cardiovascular disease. *Diabetes Care* 1999;suppl 3:C14–C20.

92. Sowers JR, Epstein M. Diabetes mellitus and associated hypertension, vascular disease, and nephropathy: an update. *Hypertension* 1995;26:869–879.

93. American Diabetes Association. Dyslipidemia management in adults with diabetes. *Diabetes Care* 2004; 27(suppl 1):S68–S71.

94. Grundy SM, Cleeman JI, Merz CN, et al. Implications of recent clinical trials for the National Cholesterol Education Program Adult Treatment Panel III guidelines. *Circulation* 2004;110:227–239.

95. Pyorala K, Pedersen TR, Kjekshus J, et al. Cholesterol lowering with simvastatin improves prognosis of diabetic patients with coronary heart disease. *Diabetes Care* 1997;20:614–620.

96. Heart Protection Study Collaborative Group. MRC/BHF Heart Protection Study of cholesterol lowering with simvastatin in 5,963 people with diabetes: a randomized placebo-controlled trial. *Lancet* 2003;361:2005–2006.

97. Sagel J, Colwell JA, Crook L, Laimins M. Increased platelet aggregation in early diabetes mellitus. *Ann Intern Med* 1975;82:733–738.

98. Halushka PV, Rogers RC, Loadholt CB, et al. Increased platelet thromboxane synthesis in diabetes mellitus. *Ann Intern Med* 1981;97:87–96.

99. Antiplatelet Trialists' Collaboration. Collaborative overview of randomized trials of antiplatelet therapy: I. Prevention of death, myocardial infarction, and stroke by prolonged antiplatelet therapy in various categories of patients. *BMJ* 1994;308:71–72.

100. ETDRS Investigators. Aspirin effects on mortality and morbidity in patients with diabetes mellitus. *JAMA* 1992;268:1292–1300.

101. Steering Committee of the Physicians' Health Study Research Group. Final report on the aspirin components of the ongoing Physicians' Health Study. *N Engl J Med* 1989;321:129–135.

102. Colwell JA. Aspirin therapy in diabetes (technical review). *Diabetes Care* 1997; 20:1767–1771.

103. American Diabetes Association. Aspirin therapy in diabetes. *Diabetes Care* 2004;27(suppl 1):S72–S73.

104. DCCT Research Group. The effect of intensive diabetes treatment on the development and progression of long-term complications in insulin dependent diabetes mellitus. *N Engl J Med* 1983;329:977–986.

105. The Pharmacological Treatment of Hyperglycemia in NIDDM: consensus statement. *Diabetes Care* 1995;18(suppl 7):1413–1418.

106. Balkau B, Shipley M, Jarrett RJ, et al. High blood glucose concentration is a risk factor for mortality middle-aged nondiabetic men. 20-year follow-up in the Whitehall Study, the Paris Prospective Study, and the Helsinki Policemen Study. *Diabetes Care* 1998;21:360–367.

107. American D iabetes Association. Summary of revisions for the 2004 clinical practice recommendations. *Diabetes Care* 2004;27(suppl 1):S3.

108. DeFronzo RA, Goodman AM. The multicenter metformin study group: efficacy of metformin in patients with non-insulin-dependent diabetes mellitus. *N Engl J Med* 1995;333:541–549.

109. Hermann LS, Bitzen PO, Kjellstrom T, et al. Comparative efficacy of metformin and glibenclamide in patients with non-insulin-dependent diabetes mellitus. *Diabetes Metab* 1991;17:201–208.

110. Chiasson JL, Josse RG, Hunt JA, et al. The efficacy of acarbose in treatment of patients with non-insulin-dependent diabetes mellitus. A multi-centered controlled clinical trial. *Ann Intern Med* 1994;121:928–935.

111. *Mosby's Drug Consult,* Copyright 2003.

112. Khan MA, St Peter JV, Xue JL. A prospective, randomized comparison of the metabolic effects of pioglitazone or rosiglitazone in patients with type 2 diabetes who were previously treated with troglitazone. *Diabetes Care* 2002;25:708.

113. Hsueh WA, Moore L, Bryer-Ash M. *Contemporary Diagnosis and Management of Type 2 Diabetes.* Newtown, Penn: Handbooks in Health Care; 2004.

114. Bild D, Teusch SM. The control of hypertension in persons with diabetes: a public health approach. *Public Health Rep* 1987;102:522–529.

115. Knowler WC, Narayan KMV, Hanson RL, et al. Preventing non-insulin-dependent diabetes. *Diabetes* 1995;44:483–488.

Obesity and Weight Control   10

Karen C. McCowen
George L. Blackburn

KEY POINTS

- Obesity rates are increasing dramatically, especially in minorities and children.

- Obesity leads to increased risk of cardiovascular disease, both directly and indirectly, through related comorbidities.

- Relevant obesity comorbidities include diabetes mellitus, obstructive sleep apnea, hypertension, dyslipidemia, hyperviscosity, and systemic inflammation.

- Visceral obesity is more easily correlated with cardiovascular risk factors than is generalized obesity.

- Weight loss diets rarely have sustained effectiveness to maintain reduced body mass index, but in short-term studies, blood pressure, lipids, sleep apnea, and insulin sensitivity can all be improved, and diabetes can be prevented.

- No one particular macronutrient-based diet has been shown to be more effective than others for promotion of weight loss, although fish-based diets may help prevent coronary heart disease (secondary prevention).

- Bariatric surgery is remarkably effective in the morbidly obese patient in leading to long-term weight loss and resolution of hypertension, diabetes, sleep apnea, and dyslipidemia.

INTRODUCTION

In response to mounting evidence relating adiposity to cardiovascular disease (CVD), the American Heart Association has classified obesity as a major, modifiable risk factor. Childhood and minority obesity prevalence continues to increase. Therapy, outside of bariatric surgery, is uniformly abysmal over the long term. It is widely known that obesity promotes the development of hypertension, diabetes mellitus, sleep apnea, and hyperlipidemia, all classic contributors to CVD.[1] Research over the past decade has shown that obesity promotes a state of inflammation. In parallel, coronary heart disease (CHD) has been recognized as resulting from inflammatory processes in atheromatous plaques. Other obesity-associated factors include low levels of plasminogen activator inhibitor 1 (PAI-1) and higher levels of C-reactive protein (CRP), interleukin-6 (IL-6), and tumor necrosis factor α (TNF-α) (Table 10-1). Obesity also causes insulin resistance, with consequent hyperinsulinemia; elevated insulin levels may be linked to atherosclerosis, although this is controversial. Of increasing importance is the role of intraabdominal fat, estimated by waist circumference, which is associated with the insulin resistance syndrome, sleep apnea, and inflammation, three potentially critical players in the obesity–CVD link. We discuss the epidemiologic and pathophysiologic links between obesity and classic and nonclassic CVD risk factors and the impact of weight loss on these risks. The effect of a variety of diets, lifestyle modifications, and anti-obesity medications on sustained weight loss will be contrasted with that of bariatric surgery to modify CVD risk factors.

TABLE 10-1 Risk Factors for Atherosclerosis and Vascular Disease Associated with Obesity

Hypertension
Dyslipidemia
Diabetes mellitus (type 2)
Obstructive sleep apnea
Hyperinsulinemia/insulin resistance
Low levels of plasminogen activator inhibitor 1
Hyperviscosity

OBESITY ASSESSMENT: RISK OF CARDIOVASCULAR DISEASE

Definition and prevalence of obesity

ADULTHOOD

Obesity has traditionally been defined by body mass index (BMI). This is calculated by dividing weight (in kilograms) by the square of the height (in meters). The National Obesity Education Initiative's Clinical Guidelines on the Identification, Evaluation, and Treatment of Overweight and Obesity in Adults has added waist circumference cutpoints to stratify CVD risk at given levels of BMI. Within each of the overweight and obese categories, those with waist circumference >102cm (40 in) if male or >88cm (35 in) if female are noted to be at higher CVD risk than those with lower levels of waist circumference. Table 10-2 documents the range of underweight, normal, overweight, and obese according to standard criteria for BMI, and corresponding CVD risk among normal and increased waist circumference categories.

The National Health and Nutrition Examination Survey (NHANES) has been documenting heights and weights of representative samples of the population for decades (Fig. 10-1). The prevalence of obesity (defined[2] as a BMI equal to or greater than 30 kg/m^2) was stable between 1960 and 1980, but has been increasing since that time.[3] The most recent data published show further significant increases from NHANES-III (published in 1994) to 1999/2000.[4] Currently, the prevalence of obesity is 30.5% in adults, with much of the burden found in black women (50% with obesity, 15% with BMI >40 kg/m^2). Sixty-five percent of adults are overweight (BMI >25 kg/m^2). Clearly, BMI fails to account for body fat distribution; those with central/visceral obesity are at higher cardiovascular risk.

CHILDHOOD

In children as in adults, obesity is associated with a clustering of metabolic risk factors that increase the chance of CVD in later life.[5] Overweight is defined in children as a BMI greater than the 95th percentile for age, whereas risk for overweight is greater than the 85th percentile, the reference ranges having been defined by surveys between 1963 and 1980. NHANES has documented increasing prevalence of overweight, with 10% of 2- through 5-year-olds and 15% of 6- through 19-year-olds in this category (Fig. 10-2).[6-8] One quarter of African-American and Mexican-American adolescents were classified as overweight in the most recent NHANES survey.[8] In a recent Taiwanese study of more than 1300 school-age children, about 70% of obese boys had one cardiovascular risk factor; the prevalence of two or more risk factors was consistently higher among obese than among nonobese children.[9] In European adolescents, BMI above the 95th

TABLE 10-2 Classification of Overweight and Obesity by BMI, Waist Circumference and Associated Disease Risks

	BMI (kg/m³)	Obesity class	Disease risk* relative to normal weight and waist circumference	
			Men ≤102 cm (≤40 in) Women ≤ 88 cm (≤35 in)	>102 cm (>40 in) >88 cm (>35 in)
Underweight	<18.5		—	—
Normal†	18.5–24.9		—	—
Overweight	25.0–29.9		Increased	High
Obesity	30.0–34.9	I	High	Very High
	35.0–39.9	II	Very High	Very High
Extreme Obesity	≥40	III	Extremely High	Extremely High

* Disease risk for type 2 diabetes, hypertension, and CVD.
† Increased waist circumference can also be a marker for increased risk even in persons of normal weight.
From the National Institutes of Health Obesity Education Initiative.

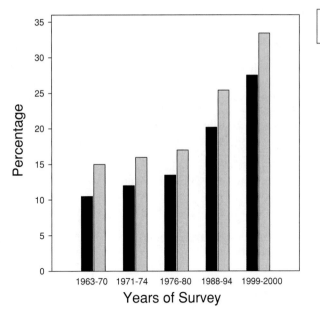

FIGURE 10-1 Increasing prevalence of obesity (BMI > 30 kg/m^2) in U.S. adults. (Adapted, with permission, from Flegal et al.[4])

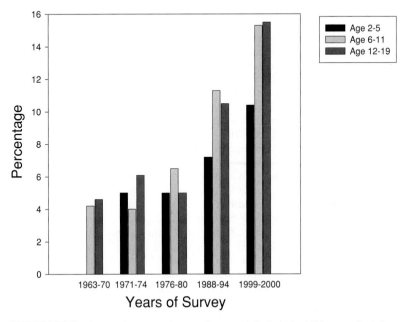

FIGURE 10-2 Increasing prevalence of overweight in U.S. children and adolescents. Overweight was defined here as >95 percentile for a population surveyed in the 1960s for the National Health Education Survey. (Adapted, from Ogden et al.[8])

percentile was associated with higher blood pressure and more atherogenic lipid profiles.[10] Obese children had higher PAI-1 concentrations compared with age- and sex-matched controls, and weight loss was associated with reductions in PAI-1.[11] Left ventricular hypertrophy is related to other risk factors in childhood, including obesity and insulin resistance.[12] Although dietary excess is in part responsible, declining rates of physical activity, especially in minority girls, is an additional culprit.[13] In sum, pediatric obesity is increasing at an alarming rate, and children are developing diabetes and the metabolic syndrome at ever-younger ages, leading to a huge potential pool of obese adult patients with CVD, with major medical burdens on society.

Association of obesity with cardiovascular morbidity and mortality

GENERALIZED OBESITY

Most epidemiologic studies have shown that being overweight or obese is associated with higher overall mortality.[14–17] The Nurses' Health Study showed that in women who were "never smokers" without a recent history of weight loss, a BMI of 27 to 29 kg/m^2 was associated with a relative risk (RR) of death of 1.6, a BMI of 29 to 32 kg/m^2 with a RR of 2.1, and a BMI of 32 kg/m^2 or greater with a RR of 2.2 as compared with the leanest cohort (BMI <19 kg/m^2).[18] Similarly in never-smoking male alumni of Harvard University, a BMI of 26 kg/m^2 or greater was associated with a RR of 1.67, compared with those with a BMI below 22.5 kg/m^2.[19] Mortality was lowest in the leanest participants, without evidence for a J- or U-shaped curve when smokers and those with intercurrent illnesses were excluded. Some of the controversy related to the U-shaped curve is removed when those with low BMI related to low lean body mass are removed from the analysis. In whites, desirable BMI is probably below 25 kg/m^2, based on all-cause mortality, but ideal weight in minorities is not clear.[17]

There are also epidemiologic data to show that CVD risks are directly related to obesity. In the Nurses' Health Study, almost 1300 cases of CHD were ascertained over 14 years.[18–20] After controlling for confounding variables, the risk of CHD rose with increasing BMI above 23 kg/m^2 (Fig. 10-3A). This was striking because it indicated elevated risk even within the "normal" range for BMI. For women with a BMI above 29 kg/m^2, the RR compared with those whose BMI was below 21 kg/m^2 was 3.6. Similarly, a history of weight gain, even in women of normal weight, was strongly associated with the development of CHD (Fig. 10-3B). For stroke, which has been studied less intensively than heart attack, events caused by ischemia are associated with overweight in a variety of studies.[21–23]

NHANES-I reported a relative risk of 1.5 for CVD in later life for a woman with a BMI above 29 kg/m^2 versus the referent population (BMI <21 kg/m^2).[24] Similar findings have been reported for men[25] and many other populations, with the notable exception of the Pima Indian tribe, in which rates of CHD are strangely low, despite obesity and a plethora of other risk factors endemic in this group.[26] In addition, obesity has been associated with myocardial hypertrophy independent of hypertension and with higher rates of heart failure in the Framingham cohort.[27] More than 50% of patients with morbid obesity had moderate diastolic dysfunction, left ventricular hypertrophy, cardiomegaly, and impaired contractility.[28,29]

VISCERAL OBESITY: A BETTER PREDICTOR?

Central adiposity is associated with insulin resistance and hyperinsulinemia, higher blood pressure, and exaggerated dyslipidemia.[30–32] Hemorrheologic factors such as blood viscosity are also elevated in central obesity in comparison with generalized obesity, and may contribute to greater coronary risk.[33,34] Clinical markers of visceral adiposity include increased waist circumference or waist/hip ratio (WHR). Many early studies used WHR to define abdominal obesity; however, waist circumference is a more accurate reflection of abdominal fat and is easier to measure. Studies comparing waist circumference with abdominal fat (measured directly by computed tomography or magnetic resonance imaging) have found the former to be a reasonable substitute for imaging techniques. It must be remembered that WHR and waist circumference measure the magnitude of both visceral fat and subcutaneous fat around the belly and, so, are not pure markers of the most metabolically injurious fat. However, waist circumference greater than 35 in. in women or 40 in. in men has been shown to be associated with increased risk for CHD. Waist circumference above these thresholds should prompt consideration of intervention even if the patient does not fall into the obese category.

Among the largest reviews of the relationship between central obesity and CHD is the Nurses' Health Study, in which a WHR above 0.88 was associated with a RR of 3.25 for CHD compared with a WHR below 0.72. A waist circumference of 38 in. or greater was associated with a RR of 3.[35] The presence of increased abdominal fat is an important predictor of cardiac risk in the absence of obesity.[36] Abdominal obesity as determined by waist circumference, but not BMI, predicted risk of stroke in the Physicians' Health Study.[37]

The pathophysiologic basis for the importance of central obesity may relate to higher rates of lipolysis in visceral adipocytes, which are relatively resistant to insulin-induced suppression of lipolysis following meals; thus, portal vein free fatty acid (FFA) concentrations are

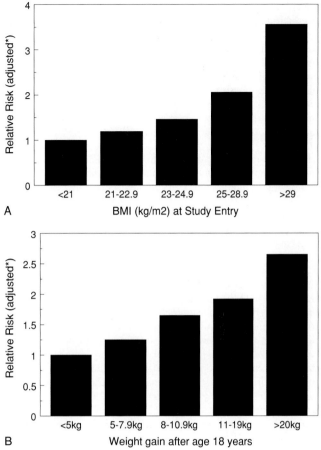

FIGURE 10-3   Relation of obesity to rates of coronary disease. Baseline BMI is correlated with risk over the subsequent 14 years of the development of coronary disease (A), and history of weight gain after the age of 18 years is also associated with increased risk (B). Note that the risk is significantly increased for BMI ≥23 and weight gain ≥5 kg. (Data adapted from reports of the Nurses' Health Study by Manson et al.[18] and Willett et al.[20])

increased in central obesity.[38] Exposing hepatocytes to high rates of FFA delivery increases both gluconeogenesis and very low density lipoprotein (VLDL) secretion. Increased FFA in the peripheral circulation causes decreased rates of insulin-mediated glucose uptake in skeletal muscle. In addition, visceral adipocytes are a rich source of potentially diabetogenic hormones such as resistin and PAI-1, yet are a relatively poor source of insulin-sensitizing factors such as adiponectin.[39–42] The combination of insulin resistance and increased gluconeogenesis can lead to impairment in glucose tolerance and, ultimately, to the development of diabetes.

Epidemiology of cardiovascular disease in obesity

LOW BIRTH WEIGHT

The "Dutch Hunger Winter" occurred at the end of World War II between late November 1944 and early

May 1945. A relatively good food supply was available immediately prior to and following that period; thus, it represents a unique opportunity to study the effect of intrauterine malnutrition. In one study, oral glucose tolerance tests were performed on adult survivors. Postchallenge glycemia was higher in those exposed to famine in utero than in infancy, and was highest in those who were exposed in mid- and late gestation, and especially in those who subsequently became obese.[43] In addition, persons exposed to famine had a more atherogenic lipid profile than controls, although this finding was independent of adult obesity.[44] The prevalence of CVD was significantly higher in those adults exposed to famine early in utero, compared with controls not exposed, especially in those who manifested adulthood obesity.[45] In some studies, small size at birth related to maternal undernutrition predicted increased visceral adiposity in childhood and adulthood.[46] In a British population study of women and men, reduced fetal growth led to insulin resistance and the associated disorders of raised blood pressure and serum triglycerides (TGs) and low high-density lipoprotein cholesterol (HDL-C) concentrations. The highest values of these coronary risk factors occurred in people who were small at birth and became obese.[47] These congruent findings from different continents suggest fetal programming of a thrifty phenotype as an explanation for subsequent obesity and obesity-related cardiovascular risk factors.

Hypertension

Many cross-sectional and longitudinal studies delineate the association between obesity and hypertension. The etiology of the link has not been completely explained.[48] In the Nurses' Health Study, for each 1 kg/m² increment in current BMI, the RR of hypertension increased by 12%.[49] Women with a BMI above 31 had a RR of 6.3 compared with the leanest women. Weight gain after age 18 of 1 kg elevated the risk of hypertension by 5%. The INTERSALT and NHANES cross-sectional studies showed direct correlations between BMI and central obesity and blood pressure.[50,51] The National Heart Foundation of Australia surveyed more than 5500 persons and reported almost identical findings.[52] In addition, they noted that overweight, hypertensive persons were less likely to achieve normal blood pressure control on treatment. The INTERSALT study has shown that an additional 10 kg of body mass is associated with higher systolic (3 mm Hg) and diastolic (2.2 mm Hg) blood pressures.[50] Although there are fewer studies of this topic, central adiposity is a better predictor of hypertension than is BMI.[53,54]

One pathophysiologic explanation for the association between hypertension and obesity may be hyperinsulinemia. Skeletal muscle resistance to the action of insulin is present in obesity, leading to compensatory hyperinsulinemia. Insulin may elevate blood pressure through renal sodium retention and through activation of the sympathetic nervous system. Accordingly, many cross-sectional studies demonstrate that insulin concentrations correlate with blood pressure. Other mediators of the obesity effect on blood pressure include obstructive sleep apnea, which elevates catecholamines, and fetal malnutrition, which can promote the development of both obesity and hypertension as discussed above.

DIABETES MELLITUS

Obesity is a major risk factor for the development of type 2 diabetes, particularly in the presence of low birth weight.[55] Underlying (possibly inherited) insulin resistance is compounded by the fact that obesity worsens insulin sensitivity. Ultimately, beta cell failure results in hyperglycemia and frank diabetes mellitus. Obesity may account for 50% or more of the variance in insulin sen-

sitivity in the general population; abdominal fat bears a particularly strong relation to insulin resistance.

Excessive visceral adiposity and increased intramyocellular fat have been specifically linked to insulin resistance. Rates of lipolysis from omental adipocytes is significantly increased compared with subcutaneous adipocytes as discussed above, leading to insulin resistance in liver and periphery. The presence of fat depots in muscle cells has been similarly associated with reductions in insulin-mediated glucose uptake.[56–58] A potential additional link between obesity and diabetes is obstructive sleep apnea. As with hypertension, sleep apnea-related catecholamine excess can lead to insulin resistance.[59,60]

The association of higher BMI with increased rates of type 2 diabetes has been demonstrated in diverse populations, both those with high[61,62] and those with low[63] rates of diabetes. Studies of the Pima Indian tribe, in which diabetes is rampant, show the importance of this association. The incidence of diabetes was strongly related to preceding obesity, with 0.8 case per 1000 person-years for BMI below 20, in comparison with 72 cases for BMI above 40. Interestingly, diabetes was extremely rare in this tribe in the 1940s, when the diet consisted of complex carbohydrates with very small amounts of fat. Exposure of the Pima Indians to a sedentary lifestyle and change in their diet to a more typical "American" high-energy, high-fat type has led to obesity and a prevalence of diabetes that exceeds 50% in adults.

In the Nurses' Health Study, even among women of average BMI, 23 to 24, the RR of developing diabetes was 3.6 times that of women with BMI below 22.[64] The risk continued to increase in proportion to the BMI (Fig. 10-4). Weight at age 18 bore no relation to future rate of diabetes; instead, weight gain after this age was a major determinant of risk. Thus, even for women of average weight, the relation between BMI and risk of diabetes is continuous. Similarly, in the Health Professionals Study of more than 50,000 male health professionals, BMI was strongly linked to risk of diabetes.[65] From multivariate analysis controlling for confounding variables, BMI above 35 yielded a RR of 42 for the development of diabetes. In another study, truncal obesity and the size of fat cells in the abdomen were highly significantly correlated with insulin and glucose levels following a glucose challenge, whereas thigh and subcutaneous fat were not.[66]

DYSLIPIDEMIA

Obesity and insulin resistance both strongly affect lipoprotein metabolism and classically lead to higher low-density lipoprotein cholesterol (LDL-C) and TGs and lower HDL-C. Weight loss reduces TGs and LDL-C, and increases HDL-C, with HDL-C increases being more pronounced in women and LDL-C changes of greater magnitude in men.[1] Rates of cholesterol

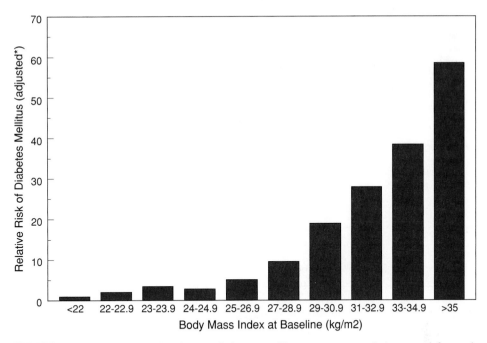

FIGURE 10-4   The risk of developing diabetes mellitus over 8 years is increased for each increment in BMI. Note that the risk was significantly elevated for all BMI ranges ≥22. (Data from Colditz et al.[62])

production correlate with excess body mass, with an approximately 20 mg/dL increase per kilogram rise in body fat.[67,68] The "low-HDL-C, high-TG" phenotype is the most frequently described dyslipidemia among the obese in both longitudinal and cross-sectional studies.[69,70] In the Framingham Offspring Study, increases in BMI are associated with decreases in HDL-C and increases in LDL-C, as seen in Fig. 10-5. A 10 kg/m^2 increment in BMI is associated with a 3.2 mg/dL (in women) to 10 mg/dL (in young men) lower HDL-C level.[71] Cross-sectional data indicate that this magnitude of weight difference may cause a 10 mg/dL rise in LDL-C and is associated with a more atherogenic (small and dense) LDL particle.[72] As with other coronary risk factors, visceral adiposity may impact many of these relationships. In one study, negative correlations between deep abdominal fat mass and HDL-C, or HDL-C/LDL-C ratio, were demonstrated in obese, premenopausal women.[66] As with other comorbidities, central obesity is a more potent predictor of dyslipidemia than BMI.[73,74]

OBSTRUCTIVE SLEEP APNEA

In a large population in which sleep studies were performed, obesity was a major risk factor for the prevalence of sleep-disordered breathing (apnea and hypopnea). For each one standard deviation increase in BMI, WHR, or body mass, the odds ratios for the presence of obstructive sleep apnea (OSA) were 4.2, 3.4, and 2.0, respectively.[75] In a Swedish cohort of men, risk of CVD was increased in OSA, even independent of BMI and blood pressure.[76] Known sequelae of OSA include important risk factors for CVD such as hypertension, altered cardiovascular variability,[77] endothelial dysfunction,[78,79] and insulin resistance, which in turn may lead to dyslipidemia and diabetes.[59,80] It is highly plausible, but unproven of course, that the majority of the effect of obesity in worsening cardiovascular risk is mediated through OSA. Interestingly, OSA patients have a greater proportion of visceral fat than obese controls without sleep apnea.[60] In this study, indices of sleep-disordered breathing were correlated with visceral fat, not with BMI or total fat. When blood pressure was measured using 24-hour ambulatory monitors, nocturnal desaturation was associated with a rise in daytime blood pressure, independent of BMI.[81] Night/day ratios of blood pressure were increased in this study (nondipping phenomenon) in patients with severe OSA compared with ratios of participants with mild disease. In a longitudinal study of more than 700 patients in the Wisconsin Sleep Cohort Study, a significant dose

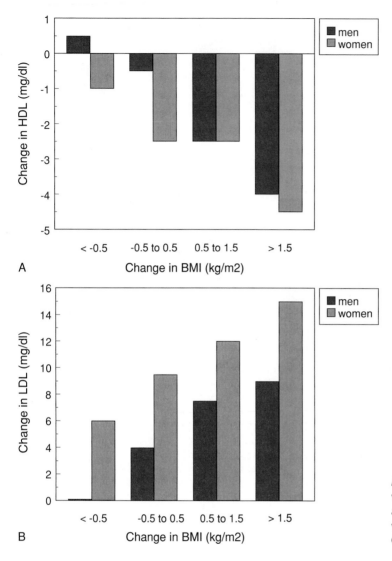

A

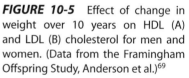

B

FIGURE 10-5 Effect of change in weight over 10 years on HDL (A) and LDL (B) cholesterol for men and women. (Data from the Framingham Offspring Study, Anderson et al.)[69]

response was found between measures of sleep-disordered breathing at baseline and the presence of hypertension at 4-year follow up.[82] In a cross-sectional study of 2677 adults in Toronto who underwent sleep studies, OSA was a significant predictor of both systolic and diastolic blood pressures, independent of age, BMI, and sex. Each additional apnea per hour increased the chance of hypertension by 1%, and each 10% decrease in oxygen saturation during the sleep study increased the odds by 13%.[83] Perhaps the strongest evidence that sleep apnea may mediate some of the effect of obesity on hypertension comes from a canine model of OSA. Artificial OSA resembling the human condition resulted in sustained daytime hypertension after 3 months. In contrast, repeated arousals from sleep without airway occlusion did not result in daytime hypertension.[84]

THE TREATMENT OF OBESITY TO LOWER CARDIOVASCULAR RISK

The overall strategy recommended by the National Obesity Education Initiative (2) for the evaluation and treatment of overweight and obese patients is presented in the treatment algorithm below (Fig. 10-6). This includes evaluation based on BMI and waist circumference cutpoints and recommended initial actions for management

Treatment Algorithm*

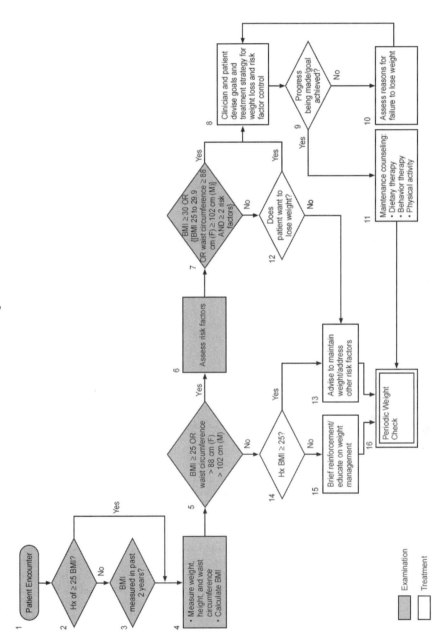

* This algorithm applies only to the assessment for overweight and obesity and subsequent decisions based on that assessment. It does not reflect any initial overall assessment for other conditions and diseases that the physician may wish to do.

FIGURE 10-6 Algorithm for the evaluation and treatment of overweight and obese patients. From the National Institutes of Health Obesity Education Initiative.[2]

according to these cutpoints and other factors such as desire to lose weight and interim progress made. The role of specific interventions for obesity treatment, including surgery, diet and exercise, pharmacotherapy, and behavioral approaches follows in subsequent sections of this chapter.

Effect of weight control on risk reduction

Weight loss studies in obese persons generally focus on surrogate endpoints of CVD. Nutrition intervention trials have been performed in patients not selected for enrollment because of elevated BMI, but because of high coronary risk or need for secondary prevention of myocardial infarction. In one interesting randomized trial, after myocardial infarction, Indian patients were randomized to either (1) a diet low in saturated fat and rich in fruits and vegetables with frequent weight loss advice or (2) a "usual care" group. The diet group lost more weight and had a large reduction in cardiac events and lower mortality than the controls over 1 year.[85] In France, randomization to a Mediterranean diet (replacing animal fat with polyunsaturated vegetable oil rich in omega-3 fats and increasing legumes, fruits, vegetables, and bread) reduced all-cause mortality, coronary death, and recurrent myocardial infarction in survivors of a first heart attack.[86] Reduced CVD mortality was seen in a Norwegian trial in which the diet of myocardial infarction patients was altered to increase polyunsaturated fat at the expense of saturated fat.[87] Therefore, it is prudent to consider that implementation of these dietary strategies might be particularly beneficial in obese patients at increased coronary risk, even if failure of weight loss (the usual situation) occurs.

Many studies have been performed that focus on the effects of weight loss through dietary restriction (with or without exercise) on control of hypertension and dyslipidemia. In general, the vast majority of studies have shown that weight loss in obese persons results in improvement in blood pressure, dyslipidemia, and diabetes. Almost all of these diet studies are short term, and rates of recidivism with regain of weight are substantial; only a small minority of dieters are capable of sustained success. Those who exercise concurrently, however, appear better able to maintain weight loss.

Consequently, many obese people have had recurrent cycles of loss followed by regain of weight. Recent articles have demonstrated that a history of weight cycling in itself may be a risk factor for cardiac events, although this is controversial.[88,89] In a prospective longitudinal study of more than 33,000 women in Iowa who were sent questionnaires over a 30-year period, increasing cardiovascular risk factors were observed across the quartiles of increasing weight cycling.[90] To some extent, however, this was confounded by unhealthy behaviors in those who cycled frequently, although statistical significance remained when these behaviors were factored out. Therefore, methods of weight control that have prolonged results, such as bariatric surgery, are of immense value to the overweight population for permanent reduction of coronary risk factors.

Methods of weight loss

BARIATRIC SURGERY

Bariatric surgery has had the best success in achieving long-term weight loss; often, more than 50% of the excess weight can be lost over the first 2 years.[91] Because of the serious nature of the intervention, most series include only persons with BMIs greater than 35 kg/m^2. Adjustable gastric banding is largely replacing vertical banded gastroplasty; both of these procedures may be performed laparoscopically (Fig. 10-7). These procedures work by gastric restriction, and do not have a malabsorptive component. Generally, therefore, weight loss is lower than with procedures that reroute ingested food in addition to restriction. Distal small bowel bypass surgery has mostly been abandoned because of unpleasant diarrhea, higher rates of surgical complications, and development of micronutrient deficiencies. Roux-en-Y gastric bypass results in very dramatic weight loss, because the gastric remnant limits food intake, and the roux limb creates an element of malabsorption (Fig. 10-8A). Modifications of this procedure include newer and somewhat controversial surgeries such as biliopancreatic diversion (Fig. 10-8B). Both of these operations result in mixing of food with biliary and pancreatic secretions only in the ileum, hence the additional malabsorption component.

An NIH consensus conference in 1991 recommended that surgery should be the treatment of choice for patients with BMIs greater than 40 kg/m^2 or greater than 35 kg/m^2 with major obesity-related comorbidities.[92] A novel potential means of improvement in metabolic syndrome is omentectomy, which removes a substantial portion of fat in patients with visceral obesity. Fifty patients with obesity who were undergoing gastric banding were randomized to a routine procedure or the addition of omentectomy.[93] After 2 years, weight loss and WHR were similar for the groups, but glucose tolerance and insulin sensitivity were significantly better in the omentectomy group, independent of change in BMI and lipids. This might suggest, as discussed above, that removal of a major source of portal vein free fatty acids has improves insulin sensitivity.[94] Pilot studies are underway to investigate the effect of laparoscopic omentectomy alone in improving metabolic syndrome.

In a randomized trial of gastric restriction surgery versus dieting alone, weight maintenance was found to be more successful after gastroplasty than after dieting.[95] By reaching 75% reduction of their excess weight (over a

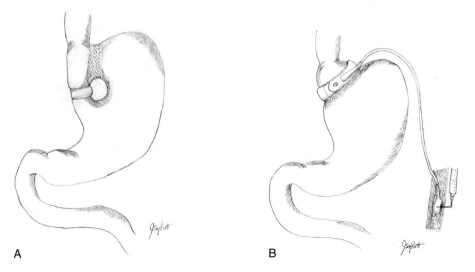

FIGURE 10-7   Bariatric surgical techniques-restrictive types. Vertical banded gastroplasty (A) involves creation of a small gastric pouch by staple partition or transection of the stomach. A band is places around the outlet to slow food movement. Laparoscopic adjustable gastric banding (B) allows adjustment of the stomach orifice by inserting or removing saline from the reservoir.

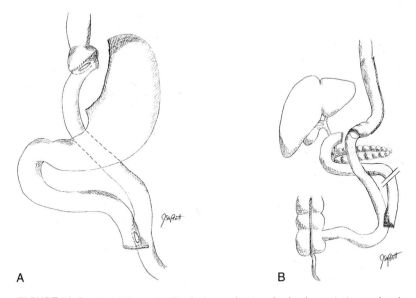

FIGURE 10-8   Bariatric surgical techniques that involve both restriction and malabsorption. Laparoscopic Roux-en Y Gastric Bypass (A) involves creation of a small gastric pouch by stapling and transecting the proximal stomach. The pouch is anastomosed to the jejunum. The length of the biliopancreatic limb can vary from 15–100 cm. The "Roux" or "alimentary" limb can vary in length from 40–300 cm. In biliopancreatic diversion with a duodenal switch (B), following a sleeve gastrectomy, the ileum is anastomosed just below the preserved pylorus, while the intestinal limb that drains the bile and pancreatic juices is anastomosed to the terminal ileum.

mean of 10 months), those who had undergone surgery experienced dramatic changes in their metabolic profiles: HDL-C increased by 24% and a fasting insulin decreased by 62%.[96] Gastric restriction is also effective therapy for hypertension associated with obesity, with preoperative hypertension resolving in 66% at least 1 year later and the amount of weight lost predicting the degree of reduction in blood pressure.[97] Cardiac ventricular compliance and function were significantly improved in a group of 12 obese persons studied before and after surgery with an average weight loss of 55 kg.[98] Similarly, a gastric stapling procedure produced improvements in cardiac chamber size and left ventricular function in a study of 34 patients.[29] Although there have been no long-term randomized trials of reduction of morbidity and mortality with this approach, observational studies have demonstrated that the incidence of diabetes, hypertension, and dyslipidemia can be reduced significantly.[99–104]

Gastric bypass also has significant effects on sleep apnea. In 100 patients who underwent sleep apnea evaluation before and after surgery, profound improvements were seen with weight loss in both clinical symptoms of daytime sleepiness and respiratory disturbance on overnight polysomnography.[105] In an Australian cohort of 313 patients undergoing laparoscopic gastric banding, 123 were reassessed after an average weight loss of 48% at 12 months. Habitual snoring was reduced from 82% preoperatively to 14% postoperatively. Similarly, observed sleep apnea was reduced from 33 to 2%, and daytime sleepiness from 39 to 4%.[106]

As can be seen from the various studies below, dietary therapy can lower risk factors for coronary disease. A variety of different types of diet have been advocated. However, as no diet has ever been demonstrated to have long-lasting effectiveness in maintaining weight loss, the changes in cardiac risk that have been demonstrated are merely proof of principle. The goal of finding a permanent solution to obesity through nonsurgical means is laudable, but currently has failed.

DIET AND EXERCISE

Hypocaloric dieting, whether or not a low-fat diet is employed, invariably produces both weight loss and a decrease in abdominal adiposity, at least over the short term. Sadly, most participants regain the lost weight after a certain period in clinical trials. Surveys of dieters suggest that maintenance of 10% weight loss is possible for 5 years or more in many Americans, but experimental data do not always concur.[107] In general, hypocaloric diets allow 1000 to 1200 kcal per day. A more stringent approach is the very low calorie diet that permits only 400 to 500 kcal per day. Initial weight loss is more rapid, although the amount of weight lost over a year is the same with both plans. After 26 weeks of a very low calorie diet in one

typical study, 20 kg was lost versus 10 kg on low calorie diet; however, as with all diet programs, weight regain was the rule, and at 52 weeks the mean weight loss was about 11 kg irrespective of initial therapy.[108] The very low calorie diet is probably more likely to be associated with dropout and failure of adherence. Adoption of an exercise program without a hypocaloric diet has produced weight loss in some but not all trials. To summarize a number of studies comparing modalities of weight loss, the combination of low-calorie diet and aerobic exercise can be more successful than either strategy alone.

The issue of how low a diet should be in fat content is unclear. It is usually easier to consume fewer calories on an ad libitum regime when fat is minimized; this can become self-defeating if palatability decreases. In addition, contrary to common belief, reduction of the fat content of the diet without attention to calories does not result in weight loss.[109] Whether consumption of a low-fat diet independent of caloric restriction can influence visceral adiposity has not been examined. In addition, no macronutrient food choice has been associated with improved endothelial function. Addition of a daily portion of fish did result in improved control of lipids, blood pressure, and insulin sensitivity compared with hypocaloric dieting alone.[110,111] Diets comparing low- with higher-glycemic-index food plans have been studied only in short-term trials. One study suggested that obese children lost more weight with a low-glycemic-index diet than with a low-fat diet,[112] with the suggestion from a later study that satiety was increased on the former diet.[113] No differences were observed between diets in adults, although low-glycemic-index diets were associated with more favorable cardiovascular risk profiles.[114,115]

Recent interest in low-carbohydrate diets has resulted in publication of several randomized controlled trials that lasted 6 to 12 months. Samaha and co-workers enrolled 132 severely obese persons for 6 months. Although 40% dropped out, the low-carbohydrate group lost significantly more weight (6 ± 9 kg) than the low-fat group (2 ± 4 kg) and had lower TG levels and better insulin sensitivity.[116] Similarly, in a 6-month study by Brehm and colleagues, 53 obese women (20% dropout) randomized to a low-carbohydrate diet lost more weight (8.5 ± 1 kg) than those randomized to the low-fat diet (4 ± 1 kg), although lipids and blood pressure did not differ between the groups.[117] However, early success in low-carbohydrate diets might reflect the novelty of the type of diet, a phenomenon that might not be expected to last. Not surprisingly, in the only published study longer than 6 months, 63 patients were enrolled but 40% dropped out by 12 months. Although early on, the high-fat/ high-protein group lost more weight than the "traditional low-fat" diet group, the difference was no longer significant at 1 year. HDL-C was higher ($11 \pm 20\%$ vs $2 \pm 11\%$) and TGs were lower ($-17 \pm 23\%$ vs $1 \pm 40\%$) in the experimental group at the end of the study, although total cholesterol and LDL-C showed a trend to be higher in the controls, significant at the earlier time points of the trial.[118] The groups did not differ with respect to blood pressure and insulin sensitivity. The rates of dropout from these studies, along with evidence in the 12-month study of weight regain, are disheartening for obesity specialists. The possibility of seeing hard clinical endpoints such as CVD morbidity in any nutritional trial of weight loss appears virtually impossible, although we eagerly await data from the Diabetes Prevention Program.[119]

The importance of incorporating regular physical activity concurrently with a dietary program is well documented. One recent study showed that, although diet combined with various types of exercise or no exercise provided weight losses ranging from 13.5 to 17.4 kg over 48 weeks, participants regained 35 to 55% of their weight in the year after treatment. However, those who reported exercising regularly in the 4 months preceding the follow-up assessment regained significantly less weight than the nonexercisers.[108] In addition, a recent meta-analysis of studies published in the past 25 years has shown that, on average, a 15-week diet or diet-plus-exercise program produces a weight loss of about 11 kg, with an approximately 6.6-kg loss maintained after 1 year in the diet-only group and an 8.6-kg weight loss maintained in the diet-plus-exercise group.[120]

Another interesting aspect to exercise, as yet unexplored, is the finding that sustained aerobic activity is associated with reductions in visceral adiposity, independent even of changes in WHR and BMI.[121] In contrast, hypocaloric dieting generally increases fat loss from all depots, subcutaneous and visceral, so that exercise-induced weight loss might finally be associated with a more substantial lowering of cardiovascular risk than hypoenergetic diets.

Chapter 12 provides additional details regarding physical activity recommendations.

PHARMACOTHERAPY

Use of medication to reduce appetite may be effective in the short term, but lost weight is regained when medications are discontinued; thus there are no good long-term data. The implication is that such drugs would most likely need to be taken for a protracted period.

Sibutramine is a serotonin and norepinephrine reuptake blocker and has been approved by the Food and Drug Administration (FDA) for weight control in those with marked adult weight gain or a BMI of 27 kg/m^2 or greater. There is a dose-related effect on weight loss, but not all studies have shown good efficacy.[122,123] Sibutramine increases satiety and thermogenesis of brown adipose tissue in animal models, but has been associated with worsening or new systemic hypertension and,

for this reason, should not be recommended for the treatment of obesity.[124–126]

Orlistat, a newly approved inhibitor of intestinal and pancreatic lipases, works by inhibiting fat absorption from the gut. Several trials involving 1 to 2 years on treatment demonstrate efficacy and favorable effects on cardiovascular risk factors at a dose of 120 mg three times daily, compared with placebo.[127–135] From a meta-analysis of 11 studies of orlistat versus placebo, significant improvements were seen in systolic blood pressure (−1.8 mm Hg), diastolic blood pressure (−1.6 mm Hg), and LDL-C (−10.4 mg/dL), although HDL-C also fell (−0.8 mg/dL).[136]

In a short-term study of children, side effects were minimized by avoiding a high-fat diet,; thus weight loss ensued.[137] Often, however, symptoms of fat malabsorption dominate, and dropout rates are fairly high in clinical practice. There is also a suggestion from the literature that breast cancer rates might be increased in orlistat-treated patients; this is being addressed in a specific trial. To sum up, the degree of weight loss (from 2 to 4% more than with placebo) is probably too small to justify inconvenient dosing along with the multiplicity of side effects.

Following the discovery that leptin, an adipocyte-derived hormone, signals the hypothalamus of nutritional sufficiency, trials using injected, exogenous recombinant leptin (rL) were undertaken. In general, obese persons have elevated leptin concentrations, proportional to the excess fat mass, but may be leptin resistant. Leptin therapy in a small study of obese persons resulted in absolute weight changes across the doses studied between −0.7 and −7.1 kg, with the greatest average weight loss in the cohort receiving the highest dose (placebo [n = 12], −1.3 kg; 0.30 mg/kg rL dose [n = 8], −7.1 kg). The authors concluded that the therapy appeared to be effective and that further research was needed in larger studies.[138] However, additional research has not yet been presented, which leads one to conclude that this treatment was ineffective in longer-term studies. Pegylated recombinant leptin is modified so that it can be administered as once weekly therapy with good pharmacokinetic responses.[139] However, when it was used over an 8-week period in obese women, weight loss was not different from that obtained with placebo.[140]

Ciliary derived neurotrophic factor (CNTF) is an endogenous neuropeptide that signals through leptin-dependent pathways. In a clinical trial using genetically engineered recombinant CNTF, mean weight loss from baseline was 0.1 kg for placebo and −1.5, −4.1, and −3.4 kg for the 0.3, 1.0, and 2.0 μg/kg CNTF dosage groups (P < 0.001, test for trend). However, the dropout rate for this injection therapy was 29% at 12 weeks, suggesting poor general public acceptability. Notably, by 1 year after discontinuation of the study drug, weight curves had almost converged again.[141] However, larger clinical trials using this drug are anticipated.

Topiramate is an antiepileptic was noted to effect weight loss. Investigation into its molecular mechanism of action showed increased hypothalamic leptin and activation of neuropeptide Y pathways.[142] In clinical trials performed to look at obesity, healthy obese subjects lost more weight than with placebo at 24 weeks (−2.6% in placebo vs −4.8 to −6.3% in the various topiramate dosing groups).[143] The drug was also reasonably effective in short-term (14 weeks) treatment of binge eating associated with obesity.[145] Although the search is underway for drugs "without toxicity" that can be used as anorexigens, it is difficult to embrace this approach without evidence that pharmacotherapy has long-lasting beneficial effects.

Recent experience with the popular combination fenfluramine/phenteramine and its possible association with cardiac valvular disease has led to caution in the medical treatment of obesity.[146] The Food and Drug Administration has issued a final regulation declaring dietary supplements containing ephedrine alkaloids (MaHuang) adulterated under the Federal Food, Drug, and Cosmetic Act because they present an unreasonable risk of illness or injury under the conditions of use recommended or suggested in labeling.

Ephedrine alkaloids are members of a large family of pharmacological compounds called sympathomimetics. Sympathomimetics mimic the effects of epinephrine and norepinephrine, which occur naturally in the human body. Multiple studies demonstrate that dietary supplements containing ephedrine alkaloids, like other sympathomimetics, raise blood pressure and increase heart rate. These products expose users to several risks, including the consequences of increased blood pressure (e.g., serious adverse events such as stroke, heart attack, and death) and increased morbidity and mortality from worsened heart failure and pro-arrhythmic effects. Based on the best available scientific data and the known pharmacology of ephedrine alkaloids and similar compounds, we conclude that dietary supplements containing ephedrine alkaloids pose short-term and long-term risks. This is clearest in long-term use, where sustained increased blood pressure in any population will increase the risk of stroke, heart attack, and death, but there is also evidence of risk from shorter-term use in patients with heart failure or underlying coronary artery disease.

BEHAVIOR THERAPY

Behavior therapy (BT) is a treatment modality that recognizes the enormous frustrations encountered by obese patients undertaking weight loss. Behavioral approaches seek to identify and modify eating, activity, and thinking haits that contribute to the weight problem, and provide a set of skills to regulate weight.[147] Clues that

trigger overeating and inactivity are identified and extinguished. Cognitive therapy teaches patients to correct negative thoughts that occur when goals are not met. Specific goals are identified, and behavioral treatment shows patients how to meet these goals. BT is best thought of as a package comprising several components such as self-monitoring, nutrition education, stimulus control, slow eating, physical activity, problem solving, and relapse prevention. Changes in lifestyle activity such as using stairs instead of elevators and parking as far as possible from building entrances are recommended as part of a strategy to avoid weight regain.[148] The combination of BT with a very low energy diet produced better 5-year weight loss results than BT alone.[149] However, the combination of BT and a hypocaloric diet was superior over 1 year to dieting alone, yet by 5 years after the intervention, most subjects in the study had returned to their pretreatment weight, again emphasizing the recalcitrant nature of the obesity problem.[150]

Effect of weight loss on obesity comorbidities

DYSLIPIDEMIA

Weight reduction through caloric restriction has been associated with significant reductions in LDL-C in many studies. A meta-analysis of more than 70 randomized controlled trials found a correlation between fall in lipids and amount of weight lost.[151] This paper reported reductions per kilogram body mass lost of 1.9 mg/dL for total cholesterol, 0.8 mg/dL for LDL-C, and 1.3 mg/dL for TGs. The effects of diet and weight loss on changes in HDL-C have been more variable. It is clear that the institution of a diet low in saturated fat causes a fall in HDL-C as well as LDL-C.[152,153] However, when such a diet is prolonged, and weight loss occurs and is maintained, HDL-C returns to baseline and may subsequently rise.[154,155] The ultimate effect in most studies is a sizable improvement (decrease) in the LDL-C/HDL-C ratio. In the meta-analysis mentioned above, active weight loss caused a 0.27 mg/dL fall in HDL-C per kilogram lost. However, during weight stabilization at the lower weight, each kilogram lost led to a 0.35 mg/dL increase in HDL-C.[151] Many of the studies of dietary intervention for hyperlipidemia in the literature were carried out over weeks to months without long-term follow up. Although such studies have demonstrated sizable reductions in lipids (TG reductions between 2 and 36%, LDL-C reductions between 3 and 32%, and HDL-C changes from −7 to +18% compared with control groups), such short-term data are of little practical use to the clinician facing an overweight or obese patient with a lifelong health problem. What is notable is that, in those studies in which results have been analyzed by gender, the increase in

HDL-C produced by dietary restriction alone is consistently less for women than for men. In one typical example, moderately overweight sedentary persons were assigned randomly to one of three interventions: control; a hypocaloric diet comprising 55% carbohydrate, 30% total fat (with saturated fat ≤10%), and cholesterol below 300 mg/dL; or the same diet in combination with exercise. This study lasted 1 year and resulted in significant weight loss and reduction in body fat in both intervention groups.[156] However, the combined program effected greater loss of weight and fat. For men, exercise plus diet increased HDL-C significantly more than diet alone. In contrast, HDL-C decreased in the women who dieted, although exercise prevented that fall in the combination group.

Reduction in HDL-C has unfortunately been a consistent finding, especially in women who start a diet that is low in saturated fat.[154] Often this decrease is of sufficient magnitude that the overall effect on lipid status is a worsening (increase) of the LDL-C/HDL-C ratio. What remains unclear is whether this is bad for cardiovascular health. In women, HDL-C has been shown in some analyses to be a stronger risk factor for coronary disease than LDL-C.[157,158] However, if it is lowered in conjunction with an LDL-C-lowering diet, the overall effect may be beneficial. Although it is true that, within a population, the HDL-C level is clearly inversely correlated with the chance of developing CHD, ecological studies[159] demonstrate that populations with naturally low-fat diets have lower levels of both LDL-C and HDL-C, and correspondingly lower rates of heart attack and cardiac death.

The efficacy of aerobic exercise alone in altering lipid profiles has been controversial. One meta-analysis indicated that exercise training alone without weight loss yielded no overall change in HDL-C.[160] Another review more than 15 years later concluded that the studies in this field are inadequate.[161] Weight loss was compared with exercise training in a study of 170 obese, middle-aged men over a 9-month period randomized to diet with weight loss, exercise without weight loss, or a control group.[162] The diet group lost 10% of their body weight; the exercisers lost body fat without alteration in BMI. A reduction was seen in the dieters' LDL-C (7%), fasting insulin (18%), and TGs (18%), whereas HDL-C rose 13%. Exercise alone had a lesser benefit on these parameters: LDL-C and fasting insulin, no change; TGs, 7% decrease; and HDL-C, 5% increase, although only the LDL-C level was different from that of controls. In the subsequent multivariate analysis, the major independent predictor of improvement in HDL-C was the amount of body fat lost. Interestingly, older men saw fewer beneficial changes than younger men. In a different study of middle-aged men matched for age, endurance training was carried out over 9 months with improvements

in maximum oxygen consumption.[163] When stratified for body weight, HDL-C rose by the end of the program in lean and moderately obese participants (BMI <30), but did change in those with a BMI of 31 to 37. Thus, especially in the obese population, weight loss may be mandatory in addition to exercise to improve the lipid profile. Chronic exercise training that produces weight loss may have additional beneficial effects in reducing the tendency of LDL-C to become oxidized.[164,165]

There have been fewer published trials of the effect of weight loss on lipid profiles in obese children; however, in general the results are close to those observed in adults.[166,167] In one study, 32 children received dietary and exercise counseling over a period of 1 year and were observed over the second year.[168] An average of 15 kg was lost initially and maintained for 2 years. Fasting hyperinsulinemia was reduced, and favorable effects were seen on HDL-C and the total cholesterol/HDL-C ratio. Other studies of weight reduction in adolescents indicate that those with abdominal obesity exhibit more beneficial changes in the atherogenic risk factor profile than do those with gluteal-femoral obesity.[169]

HYPERTENSION

For hypertension, even moderate weight loss in overweight and obese persons can effect reductions in both systolic and diastolic blood pressures. There are several large studies in which normotensive but overweight individuals have reduced their blood pressure and incidence of hypertension with a hypocaloric diet.[170-174] These trials are described more fully in Table 10-3. With successful dieting and weight reduction, left ventricular mass has been shown to regress.[175] One possible confounding variable is that hypocaloric diets are often low in sodium. However, it is clear that when comparisons have been made between overweight subjects randomized to low-salt versus low-calorie diets, salt reduction is relatively ineffective without weight loss.[176] Several studies have compared weight reduction with pharmacotherapy for hypertension. In general, blood pressures were lower with drug treatment; however, it is clear that the addition of lifestyle modification reduced the need for medication and had an overall effect of reducing vascular risk.[177]

Also notable about these trials, so many of which were relatively long-term, was the fact that regain of lost weight was the rule—not unexpectedly—with return of blood pressure toward baseline values. In one study involving hypertensive obese persons, the "weight loss" group differed in weight from controls only at 3 months, and both groups had similar body mass for the remaining 30 months of the trial. Nonetheless, this short-term weight loss resulted in use of significantly smaller numbers of medications to achieve blood pressure targets.[178]

TABLE 10-3 Effect of Weight Loss on Blood Pressure and Incidence of Hypertension as Compared with "Usual Diet" Group in Recent Clinical Trials

Reference	Trial name	Number of patients	Duration (mo)	Weight loss vs usual care (kg)	BP Difference from "Usual diet" (mm Hg)	Percent remaining normotensive vs placebo
77	TOHP*	2250	48	1.9	1.1/1	62% vs 56%
76	HCP	189	48	1.8	0.6/1.5	39% vs 5%
75	HPT	841	36	3.4	2.4/1.8	61.3% vs 71.8%†
73	TAIM	878	6	4.76	2.8/2.5	

*TOHP, Trials of Hypertension Prevention; HCP, Hypertension Control Program; HPT, Hypetension Prevention Trial; TAIM, Trial of Antihypertensive Interventions and Management Study.
†Not significant.

Recently, a clinical trial evaluating the effects of dietary patterns on blood pressure (Dietary Approaches to Stop Hypertension [DASH]) was published. DASH showed that the addition of low-fat dairy foods and generous helpings of fruits and vegetables to the diet was associated with lowering of both systolic and diastolic blood pressures (by 5.5 and 3.0 mm Hg, respectively, in the entire sample, and by 11.4 and 5.5 mm Hg, respectively, in those with preexisting hypertension, relative to the control diet low in fruits, vegetables, and diary products, all P < .001).[179] The DASH diet maximized palatability, without undue perturbation of cultural dietary norms. Participants in the treatment group received the same salt allowance as the control group. Striking improvements in blood pressure were seen with the diet intervention. Such a diet is probably one that could be maintained for long periods with reasonable compliance.

In a modification of this approach, the PREMIER study randomized untreated hypertensive patients (n = 810) to standard behavioral modification, behavior plus DASH diet, or "advice only." After 6 months, the DASH diet did not have additional blood pressure-reducing effects different from those of lifestyle changes.[180] However, for obese patients with hypertension as their main cardiac risk factor, in whom weight loss through a hypocaloric regime with exercise has failed repeatedly, consideration should be given to the institution of a diet such as DASH, rather than further half-hearted attempts to lose weight (see also Chapter 6).

DIABETES MELLITUS

The patient with type 2 diabetes has everything to gain by weight reduction. Such persons are almost uniformly overweight. Dietary therapy is one of the cornerstones of blood sugar management. Weight loss not only lessens hyperglycemia but, in some patients with diabetes, and with sufficient weight loss, can make possible the discontinuation of insulin or oral therapy.[181] Diabetes-related mortality was shown to be reduced in a cohort of women

who intentionally lost weight over a 12-year period.[182] Conversely, little of the improvement in CVD endpoints seen with lifestyle modification and intensive therapy in a Scandinavian population with type 2 diabetes was related to improved glycemia or weight control.[183] In this multifactorial intervention, despite diet and lifestyle recommendations, the intensively treated patients did not lose more weight than controls. Reductions in CVD were most likely related to greater use of antihypertensive and hypolipidemic drugs.

In normoglycemic overweight persons, several randomized trials of lifestyle modification versus standard dietary advice produced measurable improvements in glucose and insulin levels with weight loss.[162,184,185] When glucose tolerance is already impaired, diet or diet plus exercise can reduce the incidence of diabetes in overweight persons.[121,186,187] However, the long-term effect of these lifestyle interventions on sustained prevention of diabetes or any CVD endpoints is not proven. This area is discussed in more detail in Chapter 9.

OBSTRUCTIVE SLEEP APNEA

The most successful therapy for OSA is bariatric surgery. Only a few nutrition intervention studies have been published, and most have been smaller than the surgery studies discussed above. Weight loss through diet was shown to be associated with decreases in upper airway collapsibility in OSA.[188,189] In other studies, the numbers of nocturnal desaturations and episodes of apnea were reduced.[190,191] While the results pale in comparison with the resolution in OSA observed after weight loss surgery, no weight loss threshold was determined below which no improvement in respiratory disturbance was found in one observational study.[192]

INFLAMMATORY STATES

The finding that obesity, especially visceral obesity, gives rise to endothelial dysfunction,[193-195] as well as to a state of inflammation, may also be contributory to the link between obesity and CVD.[196] Soluble adhesion molecules such as E-selectin were correlated, on regression analysis, with BMI,[197] and were reduced by hypocaloric diet and weight loss.[198] CRP is an independent risk factor for CVD, and is positively associated with adiposity and insulin resistance.[199] In obese patients treated with diet or gastric bypass, CRP fell in parallel with weight loss, although whether CRP is an important mediator of the cardiovascular risk of obesity remains undetermined.[200–202] TNF-α and IL-6 also fall with deliberate weight loss.[202,203] Weight loss through dieting, either with[204] or without[205] physical activity, also results in improvement in endothelial dysfunction. Because treatment of obesity itself is so unsuccessful, an interesting approach is to treat the inflammatory state induced by obesity, as a means of preventing the CVD comorbidities. Under development are antioxidant drugs that inhibit the expression of some of the inflammatory markers, which should improve endothelial function in part by inhibiting production of reactive oxygen species.[206]

Weight control in children

Sibutramine has been used with some short-term success for weight loss versus placebo, both in combination with behavior therapy, although almost 40% had side effects, mainly a rise in blood pressure.[207] Bariatric surgery has also been successfully performed in obese adolescents, with good results similar to those in adults, such as resolution of many cardiovascular risk factors.[106] Most published studies examine the effect of hypocaloric dieting, with or without exercise, on weight in children. Usually, weight maintenance (in the face of ongoing increases in height) is an adequate goal, and a multidisciplinary approach involving parents is recommended. The most successful childhood dieters are those with an involved parent.[208]

Conclusions

Obesity is a rampant problem with serious health consequences, being linked to sleep apnea, hypertension, dyslipidemia, diabetes, and the promotion of a pro-inflammatory milieu. Weight loss by whatever means is clearly associated with less comorbidity; however, there are few good long-term studies in the medical literature. There remains the challenge of how to reduce the increasing prevalence of obesity and its sequelae in both children and adults. Unfortunately, because rates of recidivism are so high after initial periods of success, particularly if initial weight loss occurs rapidly, emphasis must be placed on lifestyle alterations that are personally and culturally acceptable, if there is to be any chance of permanency. Perhaps the greatest challenge for weight loss practitioners is to target obese children and adolescents,

who will grow up to become the obese hypertensive, diabetic, hypercholesterolemic patients of tomorrow's physicians. Finally, both a population approach and an individual approach are needed. The population-based effort should focus on the community, including schools and the media; the individual approach should consist of a multidisciplinary strategy involving physicians, exercise specialists, dietitians, nurses, and other health care personnel.

REFERENCES

1. Krauss RM, Winston M, Fletcher BJ, et al. Obesity: impact on cardiovascular disease. *Circulation* 1998;98:1472–1476.

2. National Institutes of Health. Obesity Education Initiative. Clinial guidelines on the identification, evaluation, and treatment of overweight and obese adults. Executive summary. Bethesda, MD, 1998.

3. Kuczmarski RJ, Carroll MD, Flegal KM, et al. Varying body mass index cutoff points to describe overweight prevalence among U.S. adults: NHANES III (1988 to 1994). *Obes Res* 1997;5:542–548.

4. Flegal KM, Carroll MD, Ogden CL, et al. Prevalence and trends in obesity among US adults, 1999–2000. *JAMA* 2002;288:1723–1727.

5. Steinberger J, Daniels SR. Obesity, insulin resistance, diabetes, and cardiovascular risk in children: an American Heart Association scientific statement from the Atherosclerosis, Hypertension, and Obesity in the Young Committee (Council on Cardiovascular Disease in the Young) and the Diabetes Committee (Council on Nutrition, Physical Activity, and Metabolism). *Circulation* 2003;107:1448–1453.

6. Troiano RP, Flegal KM, Kuczmarski RJ, et al. Overweight prevalence and trends for children and adolescents: the National Health and Nutrition Examination Surveys, 1963 to 1991. *Arch Pediatr Adolesc Med* 1995;149:1085–1091.

7. Ogden CL, Troiano RP, Briefel RR, et al. Prevalence of overweight among preschool children in the United States, 1971 through 1994. *Pediatrics* 1997;99:E1.

8. Ogden CL, Flegal KM, Carroll MD, et al. Prevalence and trends in overweight among US children and adolescents, 1999–2000. *JAMA* 2002;288:1728–1732.

9. Chu NF, Rimm EB, Wang DJ, et al. Clustering of cardiovascular disease risk factors among obese schoolchildren: the Taipei Children Heart Study. *Am J Clin Nutr* 1998;67:1141–1146.

10. Hoffmans MD, Kromhout D, de Lezenne Coulander C. The impact of body mass index of 78,612 18-year-old Dutch men on 32-year mortality from all causes. *J Clin Epidemiol* 1988;41:749–756.

11. Estelles A, Dalmau J, Falco C, et al. Plasma PAI-1 levels in obese children: effect of weight loss and influence of PAI-1 promoter 4G/5G genotype. *Thromb Haemost* 2001;86:647–652.

12. Urbina EM, Gidding SS, Bao W, et al. Association of fasting blood sugar level, insulin level, and obesity with left ventricular mass in healthy children and adolescents: the Bogalusa Heart Study. *Am Heart J* 1999;138:122–127.

13. Kimm SY, Glynn NW, Kriska AM, et al. Decline in physical activity in black girls and white girls during adolescence. *N Engl J Med* 2002;347:709–715.

14. Manson JE, Stampfer MJ, Hennekens CH, et al. Body weight and longevity: a reassessment. *JAMA* 1987;257:353–358.

15. Bender R, Trautner C, Spraul M, et al. Assessment of excess mortality in obesity. *Am J Epidemiol* 1998;147:42–48.

16. Manson JE, Willett WC, Stampfer MJ. Body weight and mortality among women. *N Engl J Med* 1995;333:677–685.

17. Fontaine KR, Redden DT, Wang C, et al. Years of life lost due to obesity. *JAMA* 2003;289:187–193.

18. Manson JE, Colditz GA, Stampfer MJ, et al. A prospective study of obesity and risk of coronary heart disease in women. *N Engl J Med* 1990;322:882–889.

19. Lee IM, Manson JE, Hennekens CH, et al. Body weight and mortality: a 27-year follow-up of middle-aged men. *JAMA* 1993;270:2823–2828.

20. Willett WC, Manson JE, Stampfer MJ, et al. Weight, weight change, and coronary heart disease in women. Risk within the 'normal' weight range. *JAMA* 1995;273:461–465.

21. Prineas RJ, Folsom AR., Kaye SA. Central adiposity and increased risk of coronary artery disease mortality in older women. *Ann Epidemiol* 1998;3:35–41.

22. Terry R.P., Page W.F., Haskell WL. Waist hip ratio, body mass index and premature mortality in US army veterans during a 23-year follow-up study. *Int J Obes* 1992;16:417–422.

23. Rexrode KM, Hennekens CH, Willett WC, et al. A prospective study of body mass index, weight change, and risk of stroke in women. *JAMA* 1997;277:1539–1545.

24. Harris TB, Ballard-Barbasch R, Madans J, et al. Overweight, weight loss, and risk of coronary heart disease in older women: the NHANES I Epidemiologic Follow-up Study. *Am J Epidemiol* 1993;137:1318–1327.

25. Harris TB, Launer LJ, Madans J, et al. Cohort study of effect of being overweight and change in weight on risk of coronary heart disease in old age. *BMJ* 1997;314:1791–1794.

26. Nelson RG, Sievers ML, Knowler WC, et al. Low incidence of fatal coronary heart disease in Pima Indians despite high prevalence of non-insulin-dependent diabetes. *Circulation* 1997;81:987–995.

27. Hubert HB, Feinleib M, McNamara PM, et al. Obesity as an independent risk factor for cardiovascular disease: a 26-year follow-up of participants in the Framingham Heart Study. *Circulation* 1983; 67:968–977.

28. Zarich SW, Kowalchuk GJ, McGuire MP, et al. Left ventricular filling abnormalities in asymptomatic morbid obesity. *Am J Cardiol* 1991;68:377–381.

29. Alpert MA, Terry BE, Kelly DL. Effect of weight loss on cardiac chamber size, wall thickness and left ventricular function in morbid obesity. *Am J Cardiol* 1985;55:783–786.

30. Reeder BA, Senthilselvan A, Despres JP, et al, for the Canadian Heart Health Surveys Research Group. The association of cardiovascular disease risk factors with abdominal obesity in Canada. *Can Med Assoc J* 1997;157(suppl 1):S39–S45.

31. Vanhala MJ, Pitkajarvi TK, Kumpusalo EA, et al. Obesity type and clustering of insulin resistance-associated cardiovascular risk factors in middle-aged men and women. *Int J Obes Relat Metab Disord* 1998;22:369–374.

32. Zhu S, Wang Z, Heshka S, et al. Waist circumference and obesity-associated risk factors among whites in the Third National Health and Nutrition Examination Survey: clinical action thresholds. *Am J Clin Nutr* 2002;76:743–749.

33. Solerte SB, Fioravanti M, Pezza N, et al. Hyperviscosity and microproteinuria in central obesity: relevance to cardiovascular risk. *Int J Obes Relat Metab Disord* 1997;21:417–423.

34. Lo Presti R, Sinagra D, Montana M, et al. Haemorheological profile in metabolic syndrome. *Clin Hemorheol Microcirc* 2002;26:241–247.

35. Rexrode KM, Carey VJ, Hennekens CH, et al. Abdominal adiposity and coronary heart disease in women. *JAMA* 1998;280:1843–1848.

36. Freedman DS, Williamson DF, Croft JB, et al. Relation of body fat distribution to ischemic heart disease. The National Health and Nutrition Examination Survey I (NHANES I) Epidemiologic Follow-up Study. *Am J Epidemiol* 1995;142:53–63.

37. Walker SP, Rimm EB, Ascherio A, et al. Body size and fat distribution as predictors of stroke among US men. *Am J Epidemiol* 1996 ;144:1143–1150.

38. Mittelman SD, Van Citters GW, Kirkman EL, et al. Extreme insulin resistance of the central adipose depot in vivo. *Diabetes* 2002;51:755–761.

39. Wajchenberg BL, Giannella-Neto D, Da Silva ME, et al. Depot-specific hormonal characteristics of subcutaneous and visceral adipose tissue and their relation to the metabolic syndrome. *Horm Metab Res* 2002;34:616–621.

40. Staiger H, Tschritter O, Machann J, et al. Relationship of serum adiponectin and leptin concentrations with body fat distribution in humans. *Obes Res* 2003;11:368–372.

41. Funahashi T, Nakamura T, Shimomura I, et al. Role of adipocytokines on the pathogenesis of atherosclerosis in visceral obesity. *Intern Med* 1999;38:202–206.

42. Atzmon G, Yang XM, Muzumdar R, et al. Differential gene expression between visceral and subcutaneous fat depots. *Horm Metab Res* 2002;34:622–628.

43. Ravelli AC, van der Meulen JH, Michels RP, et al. Glucose tolerance in adults after prenatal exposure to famine. *Lancet* 1998;351:173–177.

44. Roseboom TJ, van der Meulen JH, Osmond C, et al. Plasma lipid profiles in adults after prenatal exposure to the Dutch famine. *Am J Clin Nutr* 2000;72:1101–1106.

45. Roseboom TJ, van der Meulen JH, Osmond C, et al. Coronary heart disease after prenatal exposure to the Dutch famine, 1944–45. *Heart* 2000;84:595–598.

46. Yajnik C: Interactions of perturbations in intrauterine growth and growth during childhood on the risk of adult-onset disease. *Proc Nutr Soc* 2000;59:257–265.

47. Fall CH, Osmond C, Barker DJ, et al. Fetal and infant growth and cardiovascular risk factors in women. *BMJ* 1995;310:428–432.

48. Hsueh WA, Buchanan TA. Obesity and hypertension. *Endocrinol Metab Clin North Am* 1998;23:405–427.

49. Huang Z, Willett WC, Manson JE, et al. Body weight, weight change, and risk for hypertension in women. *Ann Intern Med* 1998;128:81–88.

50. Dyer AR, Elliott P, for the INTERSALT Co-operative Research Group. The INTERSALT study: relations of body mass index to blood pressure. *J Hum Hypertens* 1989;3:299–308.

51. Gillum RF, Mussolino ME, Madans JH. Body fat distribution and hypertension incidence in women and men: the NHANES I Epidemiologic Follow-up Study. *Int J Obes Relat Metab Disord* 1998;22:127–134.

52. MacMahon SW, Blacket RB, Macdonald GJ, et al. Obesity, alcohol consumption and blood pressure in Australian men and women: the National Heart Foundation of Australia Risk Factor Prevalence Study. *J Hypertens* 1984;2:85–91.

53. Bose K, Ghosh A, Roy S, Gangopadhyay S. Blood pressure and waist circumference: an empirical study of the effects of waist circumference on blood pressure among Bengalee male jute mill workers of Belur, West Bengal, India. *J Physiol Anthropol Appl Hum Sci* 2003;22:169–173.

54. Duclos M, Corcuff JB, Etcheverry N, et al. Abdominal obesity increases overnight cortisol excretion. *J Endocrinol Invest* 1999;22:465–471.

55. Hales CN, Barker DJ, Clark PM, et al. Fetal and infant growth and impaired glucose tolerance at age 64. *BMJ* 1991;303:1019–1022.

56. Forouhi NG, Jenkinson G, Thomas EL, et al. Relation of triglyceride stores in skeletal muscle cells to central obesity and insulin sensitivity in European and South Asian men. *Diabetologia* 1999;42:932–935.

57. Perseghin G, Scifo P, De Cobelli F, et al. Intramyocellular triglyceride content is a determinant of in vivo insulin resistance in humans: a ^{1}H–^{13}C nuclear magnetic resonance spectroscopy assessment in offspring of type 2 diabetic parents. *Diabetes* 1999;48:1600–1606.

58. Jacob S, Machann J, Rett K, et al. Association of increased intramyocellular lipid content with insulin resistance in lean nondiabetic offspring of type 2 diabetic subjects. *Diabetes* 1999;48:1113–1119.

59. Ip MS, Lam B, Ng MM, et al. Obstructive sleep apnea is independently associated with insulin resistance. *Am J Respir Crit Care Med* 2002;165:670–676.

60. Vgontzas AN, Papanicolaou DA, Bixler EO, et al. Elevation of plasma cytokines in disorders of excessive daytime sleepiness: role of sleep disturbance and obesity. *J Clin Endocrinol Metab* 1997;82:1313–1316.

61. Knowler WC, Pettitt DJ, Savage PJ, et al. Diabetes incidence in Pima Indians: contributions of obesity and parental diabetes. *Am J Epidemiol* 1981;113:144–156.

62. Lee ET, Howard BV, Savage PJ, et al. Diabetes and impaired glucose tolerance in three American Indian populations aged 45–74 years: the Strong Heart Study. *Diabetes Care* 1995;18:599–610.

63. Larsson B, Bjorntorp P, Tibblin G. The health consequences of moderate obesity. *Int J Obes* 1981;5:97–116.

64. Colditz GA, Willett WC, Stampfer MJ, et al. Weight as a risk factor for clinical diabetes in women. *Am J Epidemiol* 1990;132:501–513.

65. Chan JM, Rimm EB, Colditz GA, et al. Obesity, fat distribution, and weight gain as risk factors for clinical diabetes in men. *Diabetes Care* 1994;17:961–969.

66. Despres JP, Nadeau A, Tremblay A, et al. Role of deep abdominal fat in the association between regional adipose tissue distribution and glucose tolerance in obese women. *Diabetes* 1989;38:304–309.

67. Nestel PJ, Whyte HM, Goodman DS. Distribution and turnover of cholesterol in humans. *J Clin Invest* 1969;48:982–991.

68. Schreibman PH, Dell RB. Cholesterol localization, synthesis and turnover. *J Clin Invest* 1975;55:986–993.

69. Despres JP, Moorjani S, Tremblay A, et al. Relation of high plasma triglyceride levels associated with obesity and regional adipose tissue distribution to plasma lipoprotein-lipid composition in premenopausal women. *Clin Invest Med* 1989;12:374–380.

70. Denke MA, Sempos CT, Grundy SM. Excess body weight: an under-recognized contributor to dyslipidemia in white American women. *Arch Intern Med* 1994;154:401–410.

71. Anderson KM, Wilson PW, Garrison RJ, et al. Longitudinal and secular trends in lipoprotein cholesterol measurements in a general population sample: the Framingham Offspring Study. *Atherosclerosis* 1987;68:59–66.

72. Reaven GM, Chen YD, Jeppesen J, et al. Insulin resistance and hyperinsulinemia in individuals with small, dense low density lipoprotein particles [see comments]. *J Clin Invest* 1993;92:141–146.

73. Okosun IS, Cooper RS, Prewitt TE, Rotimi CN. The relation of central adiposity to components of the insulin resistance syndrome in a biracial US population sample. *Ethn Dis* 1999;9:218–229.

74. Jabbar A, Irfanullah A, Akhter J, Mirza YK. Dyslipidemia and its relation with body mass index versus waist hip ratio. *J Pak Med Assoc* 1997;47:308–310.

75. Young T, Palta M, Dempsey J, et al. The occurrence of sleep-disordered breathing among middle-aged adults. *N Engl J Med* 1993; 328:1230–1235.

76. Peker Y, Hedner J, Norum J, et al. Increased incidence of cardiovascular disease in middle-aged men with obstructive sleep apnea: a 7-year follow-up. *Am J Respir Crit Care Med* 2002;166:159–165.

77. Narkiewicz K, van de Borne PJ, Pesek CA, et al. Selective potentiation of peripheral chemoreflex sensitivity in obstructive sleep apnea. *Circulation* 1999;99:1183–1189.

78. Kato M, Roberts-Thomson P, Phillips BG, et al. Impairment of endothelium-dependent vasodilation of resistance vessels in patients with obstructive sleep apnea. *Circulation* 2000;102:2607–2610.

79. Kraiczi H, Caidahl K, Samuelsson A, et al. Impairment of vascular endothelial function and left ventricular filling: association with the severity of apnea-induced hypoxemia during sleep. *Chest* 2001;119:1085–1091.

80. Punjabi NM, Sorkin JD, Katzel LI, et al. Sleep-disordered breathing and insulin resistance in middle-aged and overweight men. *Am J Respir Crit Care Med* 2002;165:677–682.

81. Pankow W, Nabe B, Lies A, et al. Influence of sleep apnea on 24-hour blood pressure. *Chest* 1997;112:1253–1258.

82. Peppard PE, Young T, Palta M, et al. Prospective study of the association between sleep-disordered breathing and hypertension. *N Engl J Med* 2000;342:1378–1384.

83. Lavie P, Herer P, Hoffstein V: Obstructive sleep apnoea syndrome as a risk factor for hypertension: population study. *BMJ* 2000;320:479–482.

84. Brooks D, Horner RL, Kozar LF, et al. Obstructive sleep apnea as a cause of systemic hypertension: evidence from a canine model. *J Clin Invest* 1997;99:106–109.

85. Singh RB, Rastogi SS, Verma R, et al. Randomised controlled trial of cardioprotective diet in patients with recent acute myocardial infarction: results of one year follow up. *BMJ* 1992;304:1015–1019.

86. de Lorgeril M, Salen P, Martin JL, et al. Mediterranean diet, traditional risk factors, and the rate of cardiovascular complications after myocardial infarction: final report of the Lyon Diet Heart Study. *Circulation* 1999;99:779–785.

87. Hjermann I, Velve Byre K, Holme I, et al. Effect of diet and smoking intervention on the incidence of coronary heart disease: report from the Oslo Study Group of a randomised trial in healthy men. *Lancet* 1981;2:1303–1310.

88. Prentice AM, Jebb SA, Goldberg GR, et al. Effects of weight cycling on body composition. *Am J Clin Nutr* 1992;56:209S–216S.

89. Phinney SD. Weight cycling and cardiovascular risk in obese men and women. *Am J Clin Nutr* 1992;56:781–782.

90. Folsom AR, French SA, Zheng W, et al. Weight variability and mortality: the Iowa Women's Health Study. *Int J Obes Relat Metab Disord* 1996;20:704–709.

91. Macgregor AM, Rand CS. Gastric surgery in morbid obesity: outcome in patients aged 55 years and older. *Arch Surg* 1993;128:1153–1157.

92. Consensus Development Conference Panel. NIH conference: gastrointestinal surgery for severe obesity. *Ann Intern Med* 1991;115:956–961.

93. Thorne A, Lonnqvist F, Apelman J, et al. A pilot study of long-term effects of a novel obesity treatment: omentectomy in connection with adjustable gastric banding. *Int J Obes Relat Metab Disord* 2002;26:193–199.

94. Barzilai N, She L, Liu BQ, et al. Surgical removal of visceral fat reverses hepatic insulin resistance. *Diabetes* 1999;48:94–98.

95. Andersen T, Backer OG, Stokholm KH, et al. Randomized trial of diet and gastroplasty compared with diet alone in morbid obesity. *N Engl J Med* 1984;310:352–356.

96. Wolf AM, Beisiegel U, Kortner B, et al. Does gastric restriction surgery reduce the risks of metabolic diseases? *Obes Surg* 1998;8:9–13.

97. Foley EF, Benotti PN, Borlase BC, et al. Impact of gastric restrictive surgery on hypertension in the morbidly obese. *Am J Surg* 1992;163:294–297.

98. Alaud-din A, Meterissian S, Lisbona R, et al. Assessment of cardiac function in patients who were morbidly obese. *Surgery* 1990;108:809–818; discussion 818–812.

99. Long SD, O'Brien K, MacDonald KG Jr, et al. Weight loss in severely obese subjects prevents the progression of impaired glucose tolerance to type II diabetes: a longitudinal interventional study. *Diabetes Care* 1994;17:372–375.

100. Benotti PN, Bistrain B, Benotti JR, et al. Heart disease and hypertension in severe obesity: the benefits of weight reduction. *Am J Clin Nutr* 1992;55:586S–590S.

101. Lardinois F, Jacquet P, Belachew M. Gastroplasty as a surgical treatment of obesity: experience of over 400 operations. *Acta Chir Belg* 1994;94:75–79.

102. Pontiroli AE, Pizzocri P, Giacomelli M, et al. Ultrasound measurement of visceral and subcutaneous fat in morbidly obese patients before and after laparoscopic adjustable gastric banding: comparison with computerized tomography and with anthropometric measurements. *Obes Surg* 2002;12:648–651.

103. Arribas del Amo D, Elia Guedea M, Aguilella Diago V, et al. Effect of vertical banded gastroplasty on hypertension, diabetes and dyslipidemia. *Obes Surg* 2002;12:319–323.

104. Sugerman HJ, Sugerman EL, DeMaria EJ, et al. Bariatric surgery for severely obese adolescents. *J Gastrointest Surg* 2003;7:102–107.

105. Rasheid S, Banasiak M, Gallagher SF, et al. Gastric bypass is an effective treatment for obstructive sleep apnea in patients with clinically significant obesity. *Obes Surg* 2003;13:58–61.

106. Dixon JB, Schachter LM, O'Brien PE. Sleep disturbance and obesity: changes following surgically induced weight loss. *Arch Intern Med* 2001;161:102–106.

107. McGuire MT, Wing RR, Hill JO. The prevalence of weight loss maintenance among American adults. *Int J Obes Relat Metab Disord* 2001;23:1314–1319.

108. Wadden TA, Foster GD, Letizia KA: One-year behavioral treatment of obesity: comparison of moderate and severe caloric restriction and the effects of weight maintenance therapy. *J Consult Clin Psychol* 1994;62:165–171.

109. Ernst ND, Obarzanek E, Clark MB, et al. Cardiovascular health risks related to overweight. *J Am Diet Assoc* 1997;97:S47–S51.

110. Bao DQ, Mori TA, Burke V, et al. Effects of dietary fish and weight reduction on ambulatory blood pressure in overweight hypertensives. *Hypertension* 1998;32:710–717.

111. Mori TA, Bao DQ, Burke V, et al. Dietary fish as a major component of a weight-loss diet: effect on serum lipids, glucose, and insulin metabolism in overweight hypertensive subjects. *Am J Clin Nutr* 1999;70:817–825.

112. Spieth LE, Harnish JD, Lenders CM, et al. A low-glycemic index diet in the treatment of pediatric obesity. *Arch Pediatr Adolesc Med* 2000;154:947–951.

113. Ball SD, Keller KR, Moyer-Mileur LJ, et al. Prolongation of satiety after low versus moderately high glycemic index meals in obese adolescents. *Pediatrics* 2003;111:488–494.

114. Jarvi AE, Karlstrom BE, Granfeldt YE, et al. Improved glycemic control and lipid profile and normalized fibrinolytic activity on a low-glycemic index diet in type 2 diabetic patients. *Diabetes Care* 1999;22:10–18.

115. Heilbronn LK, Noakes M, Clifton PM: The effect of high- and low-glycemic index energy restricted diets on plasma lipid and glucose profiles in type 2 diabetic subjects with varying glycemic control. *J Am Coll Nutr* 2002;21:120–127.

116. Samaha FF, Iqbal N, Seshadri P, et al. A low-carbohydrate as compared with a low-fat diet in severe obesity. *N Engl J Med* 2003;348:2074–2081.

117. Brehm BJ, Seeley RJ, Daniels SR, et al. A randomized trial comparing a very low carbohydrate diet and a calorie-restricted low fat diet on body weight and cardiovascular risk factors in healthy women. *J Clin Endocrinol Metab* 2003;88:1617–1623.

118. Foster GD, Wyatt HR, Hill JO, et al. A randomized trial of a low-carbohydrate diet for obesity. *N Engl J Med* 2003;348:2082–2090.

119. Knowler WC, Barrett-Connor E, Fowler SE, et al. Reduction in the incidence of type 2 diabetes with lifestyle intervention or metformin. *N Engl J Med* 2002;346:393–403.

120. Miller WC, Koceja DM, Hamilton EJ: A meta-analysis of the past 25 years of weight loss research using diet, exercise or diet plus exercise intervention. *Int J Obes Relat Metab Disord* 1997;21:941–947.

121. Thomas EL, Brynes AE, McCarthy J, et al. Preferential loss of visceral fat following aerobic exercise, measured by magnetic resonance imaging. *Lipids* 2000;35:769–776.

122. McNulty SJ, Ur E, Williams G. A randomized trial of sibutramine in the management of obese type 2 diabetic patients treated with metformin. *Diabetes Care* 2003;26:125–131.

123. Bray GA, Ryan DH, Gordon D, et al. A double-blind randomized placebo-controlled trial of sibutramine. *Obes Res* 1996;4:263–270.

124. James WP, Astrup A, Finer N, et al, for the STORM Study Group. Effect of sibutramine on weight maintenance after weight loss: a randomised trial. Sibutramine Trial of Obesity Reduction and Maintenance. *Lancet* 2000;356:2119–2125.

125. McMahon FG, Fujioka K, Singh BN, et al. Efficacy and safety of sibutramine in obese white and African American patients with hypertension: a 1-year, double-blind, placebo-controlled, multicenter trial. *Arch Intern Med* 2000;160:2185–2191.

126. Dujovne CA, Zavoral JH, Rowe E, et al. Effects of sibutramine on body weight and serum lipids: a double-blind, randomized, placebo-controlled study in 322 overweight and obese patients with dyslipidemia. *Am Heart J* 2001;142:489–497.

127. Hollander PA, Elbein SC, Hirsch IB, et al. Role of orlistat in the treatment of obese patients with type 2 diabetes: a 1-year randomized double-blind study. *Diabetes Care* 1998;21:1288–1294.

128. Davidson MH, Hauptman J, DiGirolamo M, et al. Weight control and risk factor reduction in obese subjects treated for 2 years with orlistat: a randomized controlled trial. *JAMA* 1999;281:235–242.

129. Rossner S, Sjostrom L, Noack R, et al, for the European Orlistat Obesity Study Group. Weight loss, weight maintenance, and improved cardiovascular risk factors after 2 years treatment with orlistat for obesity. *Obes Res* 2000;8:49–61.

130. Finer N, James WP, Kopelman PG, et al. One-year treatment of obesity: a randomized, double-blind, placebo-controlled, multicentre study of orlistat, a gastrointestinal lipase inhibitor. *Int J Obes Relat Metab Disord* 2000;24:306–313.

131. Bakris G, Calhoun D, Egan B, et al. Orlistat improves blood pressure control in obese subjects with treated but inadequately controlled hypertension. *J Hypertens* 2002;20:2257–2267.

132. Hanefeld M, Sachse G: The effects of orlistat on body weight and glycaemic control in overweight patients with type 2 diabetes: a randomized, placebo-controlled trial. *Diabetes Obes Metab* 2002;4:415–423.

133. Kelley DE, Bray GA, Pi-Sunyer FX, et al. Clinical efficacy of orlistat therapy in overweight and obese patients with insulin-treated type 2 diabetes: a 1-year randomized controlled trial. *Diabetes Care* 2002;25:1033–1041.

134. Derosa G, Mugellini A, Ciccarelli L, et al. Randomized, double-blind, placebo-controlled comparison of the action of orlistat, fluvastatin, or both an anthropometric measurements, blood pressure, and lipid profile in obese patients with hypercholesterolemia prescribed a standardized diet. *Clin Ther* 2003;25:1107–1122.

135. Krempf M, Louvet JP, Allanic H, et al. Weight reduction and long-term maintenance after 18 months treatment with orlistat for obesity. *Int J Obes Relat Metab Disord* 2003;27:591–597.

136. Padwal R, Li SK, Lau DC. Long-term pharmacotherapy for overweight and obesity: a systematic review and meta-analysis of randomized controlled trials. *Int J Obes Relat Metab Disord* 2003;27:1437–1446.

137. Norgren S, Danielsson P, Jurold R, et al. Orlistat treatment in obese prepubertal children: a pilot study. *Acta Paediatr* 2003;92:666–670.

138. Heymsfield SB, Greenberg AS, Fujioka K, et al. Recombinant leptin for weight loss in obese and lean adults: a randomized, controlled, dose-escalation trial. *JAMA* 1999;282:1568–1575.

139. Hukshorn CJ, Saris WH, Westerterp-Plantenga MS, et al. Weekly subcutaneous pegylated recombinant native human leptin (PEG-OB) administration in obese men. *J Clin Endocrinol Metab* 2000;85:4003–4009.

140. Hukshorn CJ, van Dielen FM, Buurman WA, et al. The effect of pegylated recombinant human leptin (PEG-OB) on weight loss and inflammatory status in obese subjects. *Int J Obes Relat Metab Disord* 2002;26:504–509.

141. Ettinger MP, Littlejohn TW, Schwartz SL, et al. Recombinant variant of ciliary neurotrophic factor for weight loss in obese adults: a randomized, dose-ranging study. *JAMA* 2003;289:1826–1832.

142. Husum H, Van Kammen D, Termeer E, et al. Topiramate normalizes hippocampal NPY-LI in flinders sensitive line 'depressed' rats and upregulates NPY, galanin, and CRH-LI in the hypothalamus: implications for mood-stabilizing and weight loss-inducing effects. *Neuropsychopharmacology* 2003;28:1292–1299.

143. Bray GA, Hollander P, Klein S, et al. A 6-month randomized, placebo-controlled, dose-ranging trial of topiramate for weight loss in obesity. *Obes Res* 2003;11:722–733.

144. McElroy SL, Arnold LM, Shapira NA, et al. Topiramate in the treatment of binge eating disorder associated with obesity: a randomized, placebo-controlled trial. *Am J Psychiatry* 2003;160:255–261.

145. Connolly HM, Crary JL, McGoon MD, et al. Valvular heart disease associated with fenfluramine–phentermine. *N Engl J Med* 1997;337:581–588.

146. Rules and regulations. *Federal Register* 2004;69:6787–6854.

147. Wadden TA, Foster GD. Behavioral treatment of obesity. *Med Clin North Am* 2000;84:441–461.

148. Perri MG, McAllister DA, Gange JJ, Jordan RC, McAdoo G, Nezu AM. Effects of four maintenance programs on the long-term management of obesity. *J Consult Clin Psychol* 1988;56:529–534.

149. Pekkarinen T, Mustajoki P. Comparison of behavior therapy with and without very-low-energy diet in the treatment of morbid obesity: a 5-year outcome. *Arch Intern Med* 1997;157:1581–1585.

150. Wadden TA, Sternberg JA, Letizia KA, et al. Treatment of obesity by very low calorie diet, behavior therapy, and their combination: a five-year perspective. *Int J Obes* 1989;13(suppl 2):39–46.

151. Dattilo AM, Kris-Etherton PM: Effects of weight reduction on blood lipids and lipoproteins: a meta-analysis. *Am J Clin Nutr* 1992;56:320–328.

152. Cole TG, Bowen PE, Schmeisser D, et al. Differential reduction of plasma cholesterol by the American Heart Association Phase 3 Diet in moderately hypercholesterolemic, premenopausal women with different body mass indexes. *Am J Clin Nutr* 1992;55:385–394.

153. Nicklas BJ, Katzel LI, Bunyard LB, et al. Effects of an American Heart Association diet and weight loss on lipoprotein lipids in obese, postmenopausal women. *Am J Clin Nutr* 1997;66:853–859.

154. Leenen R, van der Kooy K, Meyboom S, et al. Relative effects of weight loss and dietary fat modification on serum lipid levels in the dietary treatment of obesity. *J Lipid Res* 1993;34:2183–2191.

155. Schaefer EJ, Lichtenstein AH, Lamon-Fava S, et al. Body weight and low-density lipoprotein cholesterol changes after consumption of a low-fat ad libitum diet. *JAMA* 1995;274:1450–1455.

156. Wood PD, Stefanick ML, Williams PT, et al. The effects on plasma lipoproteins of a prudent weight-reducing diet, with or without exercise, in overweight men and women. *N Engl J Med* 1991;325:461–466.

157. Miller M, Kwiterovich PO Jr. Isolated low HDL-cholesterol as an important risk factor for coronary heart disease. *Eur Heart J* 1990;11(suppl H):9–14.

158. Rifkind BM. High-density lipoprotein cholesterol and coronary artery disease: survey of the evidence. *Am J Cardiol* 1990;66:3A–6A.

159. Connor WE, Cerqueira MT, Connor RW, et al. The plasma lipids, lipoproteins, and diet of the Tarahumara indians of Mexico. *Am J Clin Nutr* 1978;31:1131–1142.

160. Tran ZV, Weltman A, Glass GV, et al. The effects of exercise on blood lipids and lipoproteins: a meta-analysis of studies. *Med Sci Sports Exerc* 1983;15:393–402.

161. Stefanick ML. Physical activity for preventing and treating obesity-related dyslipoproteinemias. *Med Sci Sports Exerc* 1999;31:S609–S618.

162. Katzel LI, Bleecker ER, Colman EG, et al. Effects of weight loss vs aerobic exercise training on risk factors for coronary disease in healthy, obese, middle-aged and older men: a randomized controlled trial. *JAMA* 1995;274:1915–1921.

163. Nicklas BJ, Katzel LI, Busby-Whitehead J, et al. Increases in high-density lipoprotein cholesterol with endurance exercise training are blunted in obese compared with lean men. *Metabolism* 1997;46:556–561.

164. Houmard JA, Bruno NJ, Bruner RK, et al. Effects of exercise training on the chemical composition of plasma LDL. *Arterioscler Thromb* 1994;14:325–330.

165. Vasankari TJ, Kujala UM, Vasankari TM, et al. Reduced oxidized LDL levels after a 10-month exercise program. *Med Sci Sports Exerc* 1998;30:1496–1501.

166. Widhalm K, Maxa E, Zyman H. Effect of diet and exercise upon the cholesterol and triglyceride content of plasma lipoproteins in overweight children. *Eur J Pediatr* 1978;127:121–126.

167. Epstein LH, Kuller LH, Wing RR, et al. The effect of weight control on lipid changes in obese children. *Am J Dis Child* 1989;143:454–457.

168. Nuutinen O, Knip M. Weight loss, body composition and risk factors for cardiovascular disease in obese children: long-term effects of two treatment strategies. *J Am Coll Nutr* 1992;11:70–714.

169. Wabitsch M, Hauner H, Heinze E, et al. Body-fat distribution and changes in the atherogenic risk-factor profile in obese adolescent girls during weight reduction. *Am J Clin Nutr* 1994;60:54–60.

170. Wassertheil-Smoller S, Oberman A, Blaufox MD, et al. The Trial of Antihypertensive Interventions and Management (TAIM) Study: final results with regard to blood pressure, cardiovascular risk, and quality of life. *Am J Hypertens* 1992;5:37–44.

171. The Treatment of Mild Hypertension Group. A randomized, placebo-controlled trial of a nutritional-hygienic regimen along with various drug monotherapies: the Treatment of Mild Hypertension Research Study. *Arch Intern Med* 1991;151:1413–1423.

172. The Hypertension Prevention Trial Research Group. Three-year effects of dietary changes on blood pressure: Hypertension Prevention Trial. *Arch Intern Med* 1990;150:153–162.

173. Stamler R, Stamler J, Grimm R, et al. Nutritional therapy for high blood pressure: final report of a four-year randomized controlled trial—the Hypertension Control Program. *JAMA* 1987;257:1484–1491.

174. The Trials of Hypertension Prevention Collaborative Research Group. Effects of weight loss and sodium reduction intervention on blood pressure and hypertension incidence in overweight people with high-normal blood pressure: The Trials of Hypertension Prevention, phase II. *Arch Intern Med* 1997;157:657–667.

175. Himeno E, Nishino K, Nakashima Y, et al. Weight reduction regresses left ventricular mass regardless of blood pressure level in obese subjects. *Am Heart J* 1996;131:313–319.

176. Eliahou HE, Erdberg A, Blau A. Energy restriction or salt restriction in the treatment of overweight hypertension. Which one? A point of view. *Clin Exp Hypertens A* 1990;12:795–802.

177. Fagerberg B, Berglund A, Andersson OK, et al. Weight reduction versus antihypertensive drug therapy in obese men with high blood pressure: effects upon plasma insulin levels and association with changes in blood pressure and serum lipids. *J Hypertens* 1992;10:1053–106.

178. Jones DW, Miller ME, Wofford MR, et al. The effect of weight loss intervention on antihypertensive medication requirements in the Hypertension Optimal Treatment (HOT) study. *Am J Hypertens* 1999;12:1175–1180.

179. Appel LJ, Moore TJ, Obarzanek E, et al, for the DASH Collaborative Research Group. A clinical trial of the effects of dietary patterns on blood pressure. *N Engl J Med* 1997;336:1117–1124.

180. Appel LJ, Champagne CM, Harsha DW, et al. Effects of comprehensive lifestyle modification on blood pressure control: main results of the PREMIER clinical trial. *JAMA* 2003;289:2083–2093.

181. Paisey RB, Harvey P, Rice S, et al. An intensive weight loss programme in established type 2 diabetes and controls: effects on weight and atherosclerosis risk factors at 1 year. *Diabet Med* 1998;15:73–79.

182. Williamson DF, Pamuk E, Thun M, et al. Prospective study of intentional weight loss and mortality in never-smoking overweight US white women aged 40–64 years. *Am J Epidemiol* 1995;141:1128–1141.

183. Gaede P, Vedel P, Larsen N, et al. Multifactorial intervention and cardiovascular disease in patients with type 2 diabetes. *N Engl J Med* 2003;348:383–393.

184. Nilsson PM, Lindholm LH, Schersten BF. Life style changes improve insulin resistance in hyperinsulinaemic subjects: a one-year intervention study of hypertensives and normotensives in Dalby. *J Hypertens* 1992;10:1071–1078.

185. Hjermann I, Leren P, Norman N, et al. Serum insulin response to oral glucose load during a dietary intervention trial in healthy coronary high risk men: the Oslo study. *Scand J Clin Lab Invest* 1980;40:89–94.

186. Pan XR, Li GW, Hu YH, et al. Effects of diet and exercise in preventing NIDDM in people with impaired glucose tolerance: the Da Qing IGT and Diabetes Study. *Diabetes Care* 1997;20:537–544.

187. Tuomilehto J, Lindstrom J, Eriksson JG, et al. Prevention of type 2 diabetes mellitus by changes in lifestyle among subjects with impaired glucose tolerance. *N Engl J Med* 2001;344:1343–1350.

188. Schwartz AR, Gold AR, Schubert N, et al. Effect of weight loss on upper airway collapsibility in obstructive sleep apnea. *Am Rev Respir Dis* 1991;144:494–498.

189. Suratt PM, McTier RF, Findley LJ, et al. Effect of very-low-calorie diets with weight loss on obstructive sleep apnea. *Am J Clin Nutr* 1992;56:182S–184S.

190. Smith PL, Gold AR, Meyers DA, et al. Weight loss in mildly to moderately obese patients with obstructive sleep apnea. *Ann Intern Med* 1985;103:850–855.

191. Suratt PM, McTier RF, Findley LJ, et al. Changes in breathing and the pharynx after weight loss in obstructive sleep apnea. *Chest* 1987;92:631–637.

192. Fisher D, Pillar G, Malhotra A, et al. Long-term follow-up of untreated patients with sleep apnoea syndrome. *Respir Med* 20096:337–343.

193. Hashimoto M, Akishita M, Eto M, et al. The impairment of flow-mediated vasodilatation in obese men with visceral fat accumulation. *Int J Obes Relat Metab Disord* 1998;22:477–484.

194. Arcaro G, Zamboni M, Rossi L, et al. Body fat distribution predicts the degree of endothelial dysfunction in uncomplicated obesity. *Int J Obes Relat Metab Disord* 1999;23:936–942.

195. Al Suwaidi J, Higano ST, Holmes DR Jr, et al. Obesity is independently associated with coronary endothelial dysfunction in patients with normal or mildly diseased coronary arteries. *J Am Coll Cardiol* 2001;37:1523–1528.

196. Yudkin JS, Stehouwer CD, Emeis JJ, et al. C-reactive protein in healthy subjects: associations with obesity, insulin resistance, and endothelial dysfunction: a potential role for cytokines originating from adipose tissue? *Arterioscler Thromb Vasc Biol* 1999;19:972–978.

197. Matsumoto K, Sera Y, Abe Y, et al. High serum concentrations of soluble E-selectin correlate with obesity but not fat distribution in patients with type 2 diabetes mellitus. *Metabolism* 2002;51:932–934.

198. Ito H, Ohshima A, Inoue M, et al. Weight reduction decreases soluble cellular adhesion molecules in obese women. *Clin Exp Pharmacol Physiol* 2002;29:399–404.

199. Weyer C, Yudkin JS, Stehouwer CD, et al. Humoral markers of inflammation and endothelial dysfunction in relation to adiposity and in vivo insulin action in Pima Indians. *Atherosclerosis* 2002;161:233–242.

200. Tchernof A, Nolan A, Sites CK, et al. Weight loss reduces C-reactive protein levels in obese postmenopausal women. *Circulation* 2002;105:564–569.

201. Kopp HP, Kopp CW, Festa A, et al. Impact of weight loss on inflammatory proteins and their association with the insulin resistance syndrome in morbidly obese patients. *Arterioscler Thromb Vasc Biol* 2003;23:1042–1047.

202. Esposito K, Pontillo A, Di Palo C, et al. Effect of weight loss and lifestyle changes on vascular inflammatory markers in obese women: a randomized trial. *JAMA* 2003;289:1799–1804.

203. Samuelsson L, Gottsater A, Lindgarde F. Decreasing levels of tumour necrosis factor alpha and interleukin 6 during lowering of body mass index with orlistat or placebo in obese subjects with cardiovascular risk factors. *Diabetes Obes Metab* 2003;5:195–201.

204. Sciacqua A, Candigliota M, Ceravolo R, et al. Weight loss in combination with physical activity improves endothelial dysfunction in human obesity. *Diabetes Care* 2003;26:1673–1678.

205. Ziccardi P, Nappo F, Giugliano G, et al. Reduction of inflammatory cytokine concentrations and improvement of endothelial functions in obese women after weight loss over one year. *Circulation* 2002;105:804–809.

206. Wasserman MA, Sundell CL, Kunsch C, et al. Chemistry and pharmacology of vascular protectants: a novel approach to the treatment of atherosclerosis and coronary artery disease. *Am J Cardiol* 2003; 91:34A–40A.

207. Berkowitz RI, Wadden TA, Tershakovec AM, et al. Behavior therapy and sibutramine for the treatment of adolescent obesity: a randomized controlled trial. *JAMA* 2003;289:1805–1812.

208. Epstein LH, Valoski A, Wing RR, et al. Ten-year outcomes of behavioral family-based treatment for childhood obesity. *Health Psychol* 1994;13:373–383.

Nutrition

Penny M. Kris-Etherton
Kirsten F. Hilpert
Ronald M. Krauss

KEY POINTS

- Dietary patterns associated with reduced cardiovascular risk include fruits and vegetables, whole grains, cereal fiber, low-fat meats, poultry, seafood, and low-fat dairy products. Nuts and legumes also have cardioprotective effects.

- In controlled clinical trials, different diet strategies have been found to be effective in decreasing cardiovascular morbidity and mortality and important risk factors. These diets vary with respect to the type and amount of fat.

- Dietary strategies for decreasing blood pressure include the Dietary Approaches to Stop Hypertension (DASH) diet, weight reduction, and sodium restriction.

- Dietary guidelines for health recommend a diet low in saturated fat, trans fat, and cholesterol and moderate in total fat. Weight control, sodium restriction, and a program of physical activity are important in reducing cardiovascular risk.

- Traversing the gap between knowledge and clinical application requires a multidisciplinary approach to cardiovascular risk factor reduction.

INTRODUCTION

Diet is the cornerstone in the prevention and treatment of cardiovascular disease (CVD). There is a longstanding history of evolving dietary guidance that has targeted major modifiable risk factors (ie, dyslipidemia and hypertension) to reduce the risk of CVD. There are numerous risk factors for CVD beyond elevated cholesterol and hypertension that are diet-responsive (Table 11-1). Although there is keen interest in the clinical significance of emerging CVD risk factors, focusing on the "Big 4" conventional CVD risk factors (cigarette smoking, diabetes, hyperlipidemia, and hypertension) can impact risk profoundly, especially as 87 to 100% of patients present with at least one of these risk factors.[1,2] For three of these factors, diet is the first treatment recommendation, and, consequently, nutrition can play a key role in reducing risk.

The predominant CVD risk factors responsive to diet are diabetes, overweight/obesity, hyperlipidemia, hypertension, thrombosis, and elevated homocysteine levels[3] (Table 11-1). In addition, there is an expanding list of new risk factors that can be affected by diet.[4] Intervention efforts that focus on markedly impacting these major risk factors can precipitously reduce CVD. Hu and Willett have proposed that an "optimal diet" that targets major CVD risk factors could prevent the majority of cardiovascular disease in Western populations.[3] What is the "optimal diet" for maximally reducing CVD risk? This diet provides a wide selection of foods and nutrients that represent dietary patterns that target multiple CVD risk factors. It features certain foods/nutrients such as fruits and vegetables, whole grains, nuts and legumes, fish (preferably fatty), poultry and lean meats, low-fat and fat-free dairy products, and liquid vegetable oils. The nutrient attributes of a healthful dietary pattern are that it

TABLE 11-1 Established and New Diet-Responsive Cardiovascular Disease Risk Factors

Established CVD risk factors	New CVD risk factors
Total cholesterol	Small, dense LDL
LDL-C	Lipoprotein(a)
HDL-C	Remnant lipoproteins
LDL-C/HDL-C	Apolipoproteins A1 and B
Triglycerides (TGs)	HDL lipoprotein subtypes
Blood pressure	Oxidized LDL
Thrombotic tendency	Hemostasis/thrombosis markers
Insulin resistance/ diabetes	Cardiac rhythm
Obesity	Adhesion molecules Endothelial function Inflammatory markers Oxidative stress Homocysteine

SOURCE: Adapted, with permission, from Hu and Willett[3] and Hackam and Anand.[4]

is low in saturated and *trans* fatty acids and cholesterol, rich in vitamins and minerals, controlled in calories, high in dietary fiber, moderate in unsaturated fats including omega-3 fatty acids, and controlled in dietary sodium and sugar. Together with an optimal diet, other lifestyle interventions, including smoking cessation, alcohol consumption in moderation (if alcohol is consumed), and physical activity for at least 30 minutes daily can largely eliminate coronary heart disease (CHD) in individuals 70 years of age and younger.[5]

This chapter summarizes the epidemiologic and clinical trial literature that describes healthful dietary patterns and their effects on major controllable CVD risk factors. Current dietary recommendations, both food-based and nutrient-based, are discussed with the objective of encouraging greater application in practice to achieve unprecedented progress in the primary and secondary prevention of CHD.

DIETARY PATTERNS AND CVD RISK

Several large, recent epidemiologic studies with both men and women,[6–10] as well as smaller studies with women,[11,12] have defined healthful dietary patterns that are associated with reduced CVD risk and all-cause mortality. These studies are described briefly in Table 11-2 and consistently demonstrate that a healthful dietary pattern is associated with a reduction in CVD events and risk. The common cardioprotective food-based dietary

patterns are listed in Table 11-3. Characteristics of these dietary patterns include a wide variety of fruits and vegetables, whole grains, cereal fiber, low-fat meats, poultry, seafood, and low-fat dairy products. In addition, some studies have demonstrated the benefits of moderate alcohol consumption, olive oil and other unsaturated oils, soy protein, and nuts. These dietary patterns are higher in micronutrient and fiber density, and lower in saturated fat, *trans* fatty acids, sugar, and glycemic load. Some have higher dietary calcium, folate, and vitamin E. In addition, total fat can vary in a healthful dietary pattern as long as it is low in saturated fat and *trans* fatty acids. Dietary patterns associated with increased CVD risk are listed in Table 11-4 and are characterized by being high in sugar, saturated fat, and *trans* fat, and low in dietary fiber and micronutrients, as well as nutrient density.

SELECTED FOODS AND CVD RISK

A dietary pattern is reflective of constituent foods. Historically, epidemiologic studies evaluating individual foods formed the basis for subsequent dietary pattern research, followed by dietary recommendations. A number of individual foods have been associated with a decreased risk of CVD. These include whole grains, legumes, wine/alcohol, fruits and vegetables, nuts, and fish.

Whole grains

Whole grains include wheat, brown rice, corn, oats, rye, barley, triticale, sorghum, bulgar, kasha, couscous, and millet. In addition to being rich in fiber (Table 11-5), whole grains deliver minerals, vitamins, phenols, phytoestrogens, omega-3 fatty acids, and resistant starch, and are cholesterol-free.[13–15] These and other unknown factors in whole grains may be protective or may act synergistically to exert cardioprotective effects.

In 1998, Jacobs and colleagues conducted the first comprehensive assessment of whole-grain intake in relation to ischemic heart disease (IHD) using the Iowa Women's Health Study database.[16] About 35,000 postmenopausal women completed a 127-item food frequency questionnaire that allowed researchers to distinguish between refined grain and whole-grain consumption. Overall, the intake of refined grains (4.0–30.0 servings/wk) was higher than that of whole grains (1.5–22.5 servings/wk). A significant inverse association of whole grain intake with risk of IHD death was observed. After age and energy adjustment, the relative risks (RRs) from lowest to highest category of intake by quintiles were 1.0, 0.84, 0.58, 0.45, and 0.60 (*P* for trend = .0002). In fact, the risk of IHD death after a 9-year follow-up was reduced by one third in women eating greater than one serving of whole-grain foods per

TABLE 11-2 Dietary patterns of US Populations and CVD Risk: Epidemiologic Studies

Author	Population	Markers of CVD	Outcome
Trichopoulou et al[6]	Greek component of the European Prospective Investigation into Cancer and Nutrition Study (n = 28,572 adults, 20–86 y)	Total and coronary mortality	Greater adherence to the Mediterranean diet was associated with a reduction in total mortality (adjusted hazard ratio for death = 0.75, 95% CI = 0.64–0.87, P <.001) and coronary mortality (adjusted hazard ratio = 0.67, 95% CI = 0.47–0.94).
McCullough et al[7]	Health Professional's Follow-up Study (N = 38,615 men, 40–75 Y) and the Nurses Health Study (n = 67,271 women, 30–55 y)	CVD events defined as fatal or nonfatal infarction, fatal or nonfatal stroke, or sudden death after 8 y (men) and 12 y (women).	High Alternate Healthy Eating Index (AHEI) scores were associated with lower risk of CVD events in men (RR = 0.61, 95% CI = 0.49–0.75, P <.001) and women (RR = 0.72, 95% CI = 0.60–0.86, P <.001).
Michels and Wolk[8]	Women in the prospective Mammography Screening Cohort in Sweden (n = 59,038)	All-cause and CHD mortality	Women who reported regularly consuming 16 or 17 healthy foods had 42% lower all-cause mortality compared with women who regularly consumed only 0–8 healthy foods (95% CI = 32–50%, P for trend <.0001). For CHD death, there was a 57% decrease in CHD mortality in women who consumed 16 or 17 healthy foods vs women who consumed <8 healthy foods (95% CI = 39–70%, P for trend <0.0001).
Millen et al[11]	Framingham Study, women (n = 1423) without CVD at baseline, 43–51 y	Carotid atherosclerosis and CVD risk factors measured after 12 y	Prevalence of carotid atherosclerosis was lower (6.8%) in the Heart Healthy Group compared with the most unhealthy dietary pattern (Empty Calorie Diet Group) (17.8%), measured after 12 y of follow-up. Compared with the Heart Healthy Group, the ORs were 60% higher for the Light Eating Group (OR = 1.60, 95% CI = 1.01–2.53), and approximately 50% higher in the Wine and Moderate Eating Group and the High Fat Group.
Fung et al[12]	Health Professional's Follow-up Study (n = 466 men), 40–75 y at baseline.	Various CVD risk factors after 8 y	Prudent Diet Pattern was positively correlated with plasma folate (r =.31, P <.0001) and inversely correlated with insulin (r = −.25, P <.01) and homocysteine (r = −.19, P <.01).
Kant et al[9]	Women (n = 42,354) in the Breast Cancer Detection Demonstration Project	All-cause, CHD, and stroke mortality measured after 5.6 y	Multivariate-adjusted RR (95% CI) for subjects in the highest food score quartile (the best) for all-cause mortality was .69 (P <.001); for CHD mortality it was .67 (P <.03); and for stroke it was .58 (P <.02). Recommended Food Score based on number of recommended foods from the 1995 Dietary Guidelines.
Stampfer et al[10]	Women in the Nurses' Health Study (n = 84,129), 30–55 y	Coronary death and nonfatal infarctions after 14 y	Women who best adhered to a healthy lifestyle (diet, exercise, and abstinence from smoking) had the lowest RR (0.17; 95% CI = 0.07–0.41) for coronary events.

RR, relative risk; OR, odds ratio; CI, confidence interval.

TABLE 11-3   Cardioprotective Food-Based Dietary Patterns: Epidemiologic Studies

Dietary pattern	Characteristics
Alternate Healthy Eating Pattern[7]	Higher in vegetables, fruits, nuts, soy protein, cereal fiber, ratio of white to red meat, P/S ratio; moderate alcohol consumption; lower in trans fat *Comments:* Multivitamin was scored higher
RFS* (Dietary Guidelines Pattern)[7]	RFS based on the food recommendations of the Dietary Guidelines (fruits, vegetables, whole grains, low-fat dairy, and lean meats)
Heart healthy diet[11]	Higher in fruits, vegetables, low-fat dairy and other lower-fat foods including whole grains, skinless poultry, and fish *Comments:* Characterized by more servings of lower-fat, nutrient-dense foods; fewer higher-fat, less nutrient-dense foods; lower total SFA and higher micronutrient and fiber density; higher in calcium and folate
Prudent Diet Pattern[12]	Higher in fruit, vegetables, whole grains, and poultry *Comments:* Individuals with higher Prudent Diet scores exercised more, watched less TV, used more vitamin E supplements, and were less likely to smoke
RFS (Dietary Guidelines pattern)[9]	RFS based on fruits, vegetables, whole grains, low-fat dairy, and lean meats *Comments:* Similar results obtained when alcohol, smoking duration, and number of cigarettes smoked/day were controlled
Healthful diet[10]	High in cereal fiber and seafood and moderate alcohol consumption (at least 0.5 drink/day) *Other lifestyle practices:* regular physical activity and abstinence from smoking *Comments:* Healthful Diet included adequate folate, high P/S ratio, and low trans fat and glycemic load
Traditional Mediterranean diet[6]	High intake of vegetables, legumes, fruits, nuts, unrefined cereals, olive oil, moderately high intake of fish, low to moderate intake of dairy products (mostly cheese or yogurt), low intake of meat and poultry, and regular but moderate alcohol intake, primarily from wine consumed during meals
Healthy diet[8]	High variety of fruits, vegetables, whole-grain breads, cereals, fish, and low-fat dairy products

*RFS, Recommended Food Score; SFA, saturated fatty acids; P/S, polyunsaturated fat/saturated fat.

day, compared with those who rarely consumed whole-grain foods. There was little evidence of an association between total refined grains and IHD.

The association between whole-grain intake and IHD also was evaluated in a study of Seventh-Day Adventists in the early 1990s.[17,18] Individuals who preferred whole wheat bread experienced a 44% reduction in risk of non-fatal IHD and a 11% reduction in risk of fatal IHD compared with those who preferred white bread, after adjustment for several nondietary risk factors as well as seven other foods.[18] In addition, a new report using the Physicians' Health Study database of 86,190 US physicians found that whole-grain breakfast cereal intake, but not total or refined grain intake, was inversely associated with total and CVD-specific mortality.[19] Furthermore, two complementary reports from the Nurses' Health Study provide additional evidence of the cardioprotective effect of diets rich in whole grains. After adjusting for age, smoking, body mass index (BMI), alcohol in-

take, mutivitamin and vitamin E use, physical activity, and types of dietary fat intake, Liu and colleagues found that women consuming three servings of whole grains per day had a 25% lower risk of heart attack and death than those consuming less than one serving per week.[20] A similar reduction in the risk of ischemic stroke was associated with whole-grain intake, but not total grain intake, in this cohort.[21] Other large epidemiologic studies also have reported a strong inverse correlation between cereal fiber (refined or whole-grain) and CHD,[22] as well as between total dietary fiber intake and CHD.[23,24]

Several studies suggest that the cardioprotective benefit of regular whole-grain consumption may be conferred via favorable effects on risk factors associated with CVD, including hypertension,[25,26] type 2 diabetes,[27,28] and other metabolic risk factors.[10,29] Therefore, it is prudent to recommend consumption of at least two to three servings of whole grains per day to decrease risk of chronic disease (Table 11-6).

TABLE 11-4 Food-Based Dietary Patterns Associated with Increased CVD Risk: Epidemiologic Studies

Light eating[11]	Wine and moderate eating[11]	High fat[11]	Empty calorie[11]	Western[12]	Not recommended food score[8]
Low sweets	Low desserts	High sweets	High sweetened drinks	High red meat	High meat, meat stew
Low animal fat	High snack foods	High animal fat	High red meats	High processed meats	High processed meats
Low vegetable fats	High eggs	High vegetable fats	High desserts	High fat dairy	High organ meats
Low refined grains	High wine	High refined grains	Low fruits	High sugar drinks	Fried potatoes, fries, chips
Low calories	High alcohol	High margarine	Low vegetables	High sugar sweets	Cheese, butter, margarine
	High dietary cholesterol	Fewer low-fat foods	High sugar	High sugar desserts	White bread, pancakes, waffles
	Low calcium	High total fat	High total fat		Cookies
		High saturated fat	High saturated fat		Ice cream, candy, sugar
			Low fiber		
			Low micronutrients		

TABLE 11-5 Food Sources of Soluble Fiber

Food source	Total fiber (g)	Soluble fiber (g)	kcal/serving
Grains—cereals ($\frac{1}{2}$ cup)			
Oatmeal	2	1	73
Barley	4	1	97
Grains—breads (1 slice)			
Rye	1.5	1	83
White	0.5	0	67
Whole wheat	2	0.5	69
Grains—Rice, Pasta ($\frac{1}{2}$ cup)			
Brown rice	2	0	109
White rice	0.5	0	121
Macaroni	1	0.5	100
Whole wheat macaroni	2	0.5	87
Fruits (1 medium)			
Apple with skin	3.5	1	81
Apple without skin	2.5	1	73
Banana	3	0.5	109
Orange	3	2	70
Peach	2	1	42
Pear, Bartlett	4	2	100
Dried plums ($\frac{1}{4}$ cup)	6	3	101
Blackberries ($\frac{1}{2}$ cup)	4	1	38
Vegetables ($\frac{1}{2}$ cup)			
Green beans	2	1	22
Broccoli	1.5	0.5	26
Brussels sprouts	4.5	3	30
Cauliflower	2	0.5	14
Carrots	2	1	35
Collard greens, cooked	2.8	1.5	10
Soybeans, green, cooked	4	1.5	127
Squash, winter, cooked	1.5	0.5	40
Sweet potato w/ skin	4	1.5	103
Beans, peas, and legumes cooked ($\frac{1}{2}$ cup)			
Black beans	5.5	2	120
Kidney beans	6	3	110
Lima beans	6.5	3.5	85
Navy beans	6	2	130
Pinto beans	7	2	117
Lentils	8	1	115
Chick peas	6	1	135
Green peas	4.5	1.5	68
Soynuts, roasted ($\frac{1}{4}$ cup)	8	3.5	105

Legumes (including soy protein)

Despite being low in fat/saturated fat and excellent sources of protein, dietary fiber, and a variety of micronutrients and phytochemicals, legumes (peas, beans, lentils, soybeans, and other podded plants) have not been widely studied with respect to their relationship to CHD. A new report, which used the National Health and Nutrition Examination Survey (NHANES) I Epidemiologic Follow-up Study database, found that legume consumption was inversely associated with risk of CHD and CVD.[30] After adjustment for age, sex, race, energy,

TABLE 11-6 How to Identify a Serving of Whole-Grain Foods

Whole-grain food	Serving size	Identifying whole-grain foods
Cereal	1 oz ready-to-eat $\frac{1}{2}$ cup, cooked	First ingredient must be a whole grain, ie, wheat, oats, barley) or the "whole-grain" seal or health claim must be printed on the package
Bread	1 slice, 1 small roll, $\frac{1}{2}$ bagel, English muffin, or pita	First ingredient must be a whole-grain flour or the "whole-grain" seal or health claim must be printed on the package
Rice and pasta	$\frac{1}{2}$ cup, cooked	Brown rice and whole-grain pasta only

history of diabetes, physical activity, education level, alcohol intake, and cigarette smoking, individuals who consumed legumes at least four times a week had a 22% lower risk of CHD (RR = 0.78. 95% CI = 0.68–0.90) and an 11% lower risk of CVD (RR = 0.89. 95% CI = 0.80–0.98) compared with those consuming legumes less than once a week. Similarly, the Seven Countries Study examined the association between dietary patterns and 25-year mortality from CHD in 16 cohorts from seven countries.[31] Univariate analysis revealed a significant negative correlation for legumes ($r = -.82$, 95% CI $= -.93$ to $-.53$). Furthermore, an increase in legume consumption of 30 g (from 25 to 55 g) was predicted to decrease CHD mortality by 28%, suggesting that modest dietary changes may have a substantial impact on population health. A review of several observational studies in China found an inverse association between legume intake and CHD ($r = -.29$, $P < .05$) and stroke ($r = -.32$, $P < .05$).[32] In contrast, combined data from the Nurses' Health Study and the Health Professionals Follow-up Study,[33] as well as the Adventist Health Study,[17] revealed no association between legume consumption and CHD risk.

Soybeans are unique because they are the only legumes containing nutritionally relevant levels of isoflavones (one serving of soy foods provides ~25–40 mg isoflavone).[34] A recent observational study in Japan evaluated the effect of several foods in relation to nonfatal acute myocardial infarction (MI).[35] Dietary intake of 632 individuals who suffered an MI was compared with the intake of age-, sex-, and residence-matched controls ($n = 1214$). Consumption of tofu, the most commonly eaten soy food in Japan, was inversely associated with MI in women. Women who consumed four or more servings of tofu per week cut their MI risk by half compared with those who ate fewer than two servings per week ($P < .01$).

Many components of legumes could contribute to their potential cardioprotective effects. For example, one proposed mechanism for soy is its hypocholesterolemic effect. A meta-analysis of 38 clinical trials reported that consumption of 31 to 47 g of soy protein daily reduced total cholesterol, low-density lipoprotein cholesterol (LDL-C), and triglycerides by 9.3, 12.9, and 10.5%, respectively.[36] In clinical studies, legumes, excluding soy, have also been shown to decrease cholesterol,[37–39] possibly due to their high soluble fiber content. In addition, soy and isoflavones have been shown to reduce LDL oxidation; inhibit atherosclerotic lesion progression, cell adhesion, and proliferation in vivo; and improve vascular dilation in animal models.[40]

Wine/alcohol

A J-shaped relationship exists between alcohol consumption and total mortality, where moderate intake is associated with reduced risk for CHD and higher intake is associated with elevated risk.[41] Compared with abstinence, several studies have consistently found that moderate alcohol consumption (1–3 drinks/d) is associated with a decreased risk of CHD.[42] A review evaluating the differential effects of wine, beer, and spirits on the risk of CHD suggests that there is no additional cardioprotective effect of wine over other types of alcohol.[43] A recent study followed 38,077 male health professionals for 12 years to determine the effect of alcohol on MI.[44] Men who consumed alcohol 3 to 4 days per week had a RR of 0.63 (95% CI = 0.55–0.84) compared with men who drank less than once per week. The decreased risk was similar for men who consumed alcohol 5 to 7 days per week. Overall, an increase of 12.5 g/d in alcohol intake decreased the relative risk of MI by 22% and was independent of type of beverage.

In an analysis of the Health Professionals Follow-up Study, men who drank more than 1 drink per week had a reduced risk of ischemic stroke (RR = 0.77. 95% CI = 0.63–0.94) compared with those who drank less.[45] Similar results were found in a case–control study examining several subject groups (young adults, elderly, Caucasians, African-Americans, and Hispanics)[46] and in the Nurses' Health Study.[47] A recent meta-analysis reported that consumption of a small quantity of alcohol (less than 12 g/d) reduced the RR of total stroke and ischemic stroke (RR = 0.83; 95% CI = 0.75–0.91 and RR = 0.80. 95% CI = 0.76–0.96, respectively) compared with abstainers.[48] Consumption of 12 to 24 g/d also reduced the risk of ischemic stroke by 28%.

In support of the beneficial effect of moderate alcohol consumption on CHD, ethanol has been shown to improve lipid and hemostatic profile by increasing high-density lipoprotein cholesterol (LDL-C) and decreasing fibrinogen levels. Moderate alcohol consumption also may beneficially affect insulin sensitivity, platelet aggregation, endothelial function, and inflammation.[49–53] But heavy consumption of alcohol also is a major cause of hypertension, and is related to stroke, as well as certain kinds of cancer, cirrhosis, pancreatitis, accidents, suicides, and homicides. Although a direct link between alcohol consumption and reduction in CHD risk is not firmly established, there will unlikely ever be a randomized controlled trial to test this hypothesis. Despite this, there are recommendations from the American Heart Association Medical/Scientific Statement on Alcohol and Heart Disease that can be made for the patient who is considering beginning or continuing to drink alcohol.[54]

- Consult a physician regarding the risks and benefits of alcohol consumption. Those with a personal or family history of alcoholism, hypertriglyceridemia, pancreatitis, liver disease, certain blood disorders, heart failure, or uncontrolled hypertension, as well as those who are pregnant or on medications that may interact with alcohol, should abstain from its use.
- Moderate alcohol consumption (one to two drinks per day) may be considered safe. One "drink equivalent" is equal to a 12-oz bottle of beer, 4-oz glass of wine, or a 1.5-oz shot of 80-proof spirit, all of which contain the same amount of alcohol.
- Alcohol should never be consumed when operating machinery or motor vehicles.
- The risks and benefits of alcohol consumption should be reviewed periodically as part of regular medical care, and revised as appropriate in the event of excess consumption, problem drinking, or changes in health status that may contraindicate alcohol use.
- Alcohol use in adolescents and young adults should be carefully assessed and monitored, with appropriate advice given to prevent deleterious habits of consumption.

Fruits and vegetables

There is strong epidemiologic evidence that a diet rich in fruits and vegetables lowers CVD risk. A recent report using pooled data from the Nurses' Health Study and the Health Professionals Follow-up Study found that persons in the highest quintile of fruit and vegetable intake

(≥8 servings/d) had a relative risk of CHD of 0.80 (95% CI = 0.69–0.93) compared with those in the lowest quintile of intake (<3 servings/d).[33] Furthermore, an increase of one serving of fruits and vegetables daily translated into a 4% decrease in CHD risk. Green leafy vegetables and vitamin C-rich fruits and vegetables were the strongest protectors of heart health. A separate analysis of this population also revealed a 6% lower risk for ischemic stroke with each one-serving increase in fruits and vegetables daily.[55] In addition, an inverse association between CVD risk and fruit and vegetable intake was noted in the Women's Health Study.[56] After multiple statistical adjustments, the RR of CVD was 0.45 (95% CI = 0.22–0.91) when comparing the highest and lowest quintiles of fruit and vegetable intake. The risk for MI also was lower when comparing extreme quintiles. Similar results were found in the Physicians' Health Study, which followed more than 22,000 physicians over 12 years.[57] Men who consumed two or more servings of vegetables per day had a 22% lower risk of CHD than men who ate less than one serving per day (RR = 0.77, 95% CI = 0.60–0.98). For each additional serving per day of vegetables, the risk of CHD decreased 17% (RR = 0.83, 95% CI = 0.71–0.98). Using the NHANES Epidemiologic Follow-up Study, Bazzano and co-workers reported that consuming fruits and vegetables three or more times daily versus less than once daily was associated with 27 and 24% lower mortality from CVD and IHD, respectively.[58] Stroke mortality and incidence also decreased by 42 and 27%, respectively. Investigations in China[32] and Japan[35] report similar results.

Current fruit and vegetable consumption is very low in the United States. Americans are consuming only 1.5 servings of vegetables and 0.7 serving of fruits daily.[59] Therefore, this observational evidence, coupled with clinical data from the Dietary Approaches to Stop Hypertension (DASH) trial[60] and DASH–Sodium trial,[61] supports recommendations to increase fruit and vegetable intake to at least 5 to 9 servings a day. In fact, greater quantities are acceptable and even recommended by most nutritionists.

Nuts

Strong and consistent evidence from several large-scale epidemiologic studies suggest that there is an inverse association between the frequent consumption of nuts and the risk of heart disease. The Adventist Health Study followed more than 31,000 non-Hispanic white subjects for 6 years to evaluate the relationship between nut consumption and first event of MI or IHD.[17,62–65] The RRs of MI and IHD in individuals who ate nuts more than four times per week were half that of those who ate nuts less than once per week. In addition, persons who consumed nuts one to four times per week had a

22% reduced risk of MI compared with those who ate less. Another analysis of this cohort found that high nut consumption reduced the lifetime risk of CHD by 31% compared with those who rarely ate nuts.[18] Studies of subgroups within the Adventist population also revealed that African-Americans and the oldest-old ($\geq$84 years of age) who consumed nuts frequently also experienced about a 40 to 45% decrease in risk of CHD mortality.[66,67]

The Nurses' Health Study, a prospective study of more than 86,000 female nurses, found that those consuming at least 5 oz of nuts weekly had a 35% reduction in nonfatal MI compared with those eating less than 1 oz of nuts per month (RR = 0.65, 95% CI = 0.47–0.89).[68] In a study of postmenopausal women, the RR of CHD mortality in those who consumed nuts two to four times per week compared with those who rarely consumed nuts was 0.43 ($P = .06$).[69]

In the Physicians' Health Study, as the intake of nuts increased, the risk of sudden cardiac death decreased.[70] Men who consumed nuts two or more times per week had 47 and 30% reduced risk of sudden cardiac death and total CHD death, respectively.

Taken together, the observational evidence suggests that consuming nuts (ie, almonds, brazil nuts, cashews, hazelnuts, macadamia nuts, pecans, pistachios, walnuts, as well as legumes) more than once per week significantly lowers the RR for development of CHD in men and women. Consuming nuts five or more times weekly results in an 18 to 51% reduction in CHD in all persons. In addition, emerging evidence from the Nurses' Health Study supports a role for nuts in preventing type 2 diabetes.[71] The multivariate RRs for developing type 2 diabetes for women who consumed a 1-oz serving of nuts less than once per week, one to four times per week, and five or more times per week were 0.92 (95% CI, 0.85 to 1.00), 0.84 (95% CI, 0.76 to 0.93), and 0.73 (95% CI = 0.60–0.89), respectively (P for trend < .001).[71]

Most nuts are rich sources of monounsaturated fatty acids; walnuts are high in polyunsaturated fatty acids, especially linoleic acid and α-linolenic acid (ALA). Nuts are also good sources of dietary fiber, arginine, potassium, copper, magnesium, vitamin E, and flavonoids (Table 11-7). Clinical studies demonstrate that the cardioprotective effect of nuts is due to favorable effects on plasma lipids and lipoproteins, LDL oxidation, nitric oxide formation, platelet aggregation, vascular smooth muscle proliferation, and homocysteine levels.[72]

Fish (including fish oils)

There is compelling evidence from epidemiologic and secondary prevention studies that the consumption of fish, especially oily fish high in omega-3 fatty acids, has a protective effect against heart disease.[73] Several observational studies have found that men who ate at least some fish weekly had a mortality from CHD lower than that of men who did not eat fish.[74–78] A recent study in which 1822 men were followed up to 30 years found that men who consumed 35 g or more of fish per day had a RR of CHD mortality of 0.62 (95% CI = 0.40–0.94) compared with men who consumed none.[77] Risk of death from MI also was reduced by 42% in these men. Similarly, Kromhout and colleagues found that men who consumed 30 g of fish per day had a 50% lower CHD mortality than men who rarely ate fish.[75] Data from the Nurses' Health Study, in which 84,688 women were followed for 16 years, revealed an inverse association of fish intake and omega-3 fatty acids with CHD mortality.[78] Compared with women who seldom ate fish (less than once per month), women who consumed fish one to three times per month, once per month, two to four times per week, and more than five times per week had 21, 29, 31, and 34% lower risks for CHD death, respectively (P for trend = .001). A separate analysis of this cohort found that a higher dietary intake of alpha-linolenic acid (ALA) was associated with a lower RR of fatal IHD.[79] The RR was 0.55 (95% CI = 0.32–0.94) in women in the highest quintile of fish consumption (1.36 g/d) compared with women in the lowest quintile (0.71 g/d).

Consumption of fish also has been associated with reduced sudden cardiac death. A strong inverse relationship was reported between fish intake and risk of sudden death from cardiac causes in the Physicians' Health Study.[80] Specifically, men who consumed fish at least once weekly had a 52% lower risk of sudden cardiac death (RR = 0.48, 95% CI = 0.24–0.96) compared with men who consumed less. Another report from this cohort relating blood levels of long-chain omega-3 fatty acids and risk of sudden cardiac death provides further support of a cardioprotective effect.[81] Compared with men with blood levels of omega-3 fatty acids in the lowest quartile, RR of sudden death was substantially lower among men with levels in the third and fourth quartiles (RR = 0.28, 95% CI = 0.09–0.87, and RR = 0.19, 95% CI = 0.05–0.71, respectively). In a population-based, nested, case–control study, an intake of 5.5 g per month of eicosapentaenoic acid (EPA) and docosahexaenoic acid (DHA) (equivalent to one fatty fish meal per week) was associated with a 50% reduction in primary cardiac death, compared with individuals who did not consume these fatty acids.[82] Both the Health Professionals Follow-up Study[83] and the NHANES Epidemiologic Follow-up Study[84] found a significant inverse relationship, whereas the Nurses' Health Study found only an inverse trend between stroke and fish intake.[85] In contrast, the Chicago Western Electric Study[86] and the Physicians' Health Study[87] failed to find any protective effect of fish on stroke risk.

The American Heart Association (AHA) has made recommendations about fish and omega-3 fatty acid

TABLE 11-7 Nutrient Profile of Selected Nuts (1-oz Serving)

	Almonds	Brazil nuts	Cashew nuts	Hazelnuts	Macadamia nuts	Peanuts	Pecans	Pine nuts	Pistachio nuts	English walnuts
kcal	164	186	163	178	304	161	196	191	158	185
Total fat (g)	14.4	18.8	13.1	17.2	21.5	14.0	20.4	19.4	12.6	18.5
SFA* (g)	3.9	4.3	2.6	1.3	3.4	1.9	1.8	1.4	1.5	1.7
PUFA (g)	3.5	5.8	2.8	2.2	0.4	4.4	6.1	9.7	3.8	13.4
MUFA (g)	9.1	6.9	7.7	12.9	16.7	6.9	11.6	5.3	6.6	2.5
Protein (g)	6.0	4.1	4.3	4.2	2.2	7.3	2.6	3.9	5.8	4.3
Dietary fiber (g)	3.3	2.1	0.85	2.8	2.4	2.4	2.7	1.0	2.9	1.9
Vitamin E (mg, α-tocopherol)	7.3	1.6	0.3	4.3	0.2	2.4	0.4	2.6	0.7	0.20
Folic acid (µg DFE)	8.2	6.2	19.6	32	3.1	68	6.2	19	14.5	28
Vitamin B-6 (mg)	0.04	0.03	0.07	0.16	0.08	0.1	0.06	0.03	0.48	0.15
Niacin (mg)	1.1	0.1	0.4	0.5	0.7	3.4	0.3	1.0	0.4	0.3
Magnesium (mg)	78	107	74	46	37	48	34	1.2	34	45
Copper (mg)	0.3	0.5	0.6	0.5	0.2	0.3	0.3	0.4	0.4	0.5
Zinc (mg)	1.0	1.2	1.6	0.7	0.4	0.9	1.3	1.8	0.6	0.9
Potassium (mg)	206	187	160	193	105	200	116	169	291	125

*SFA, saturated fatty acids; PUFA, polyunsaturated fatty acids; MUFA, monounsaturated fatty acids.

SOURCE: USDA Nutrient Database for Standard Reference, Release 16, July 2003.

TABLE 11-8 Energy, Fat, and EPA + DHA Content of Selected Fish and Seafood

Fish Type (per 3-oz cooked serving)	kcal	Total fat (g)	SFA* (g)	EPA + DHA (g)	Amount of fish required to equal ~300 mg/d EPA + DHA (g)
Herring					
Pacific	213	15.12	3.548	1.81	14.1
Atlantic	173	9.85	0.354	1.71	14.9
Halibut					
Atlantic and Pacific	119	2.50	0.354	0.395	64.6
Greenland	203	15.08	2.637	1.001	25.5
Swordfish	132	4.37	1.195	0.696	36.6
Pollock					
Atlantic	100	1.07	0.145	0.46	55.4
Walleye	96	0.95	0.196	0.398	64.1
Flounder/sole	99	1.30	0.309	0.426	59.9
Grouper	100	1.11	0.254	0.211	120.9
Catfish					
Farmed	129	6.82	1.521	0.15	170.0
Wild	89	2.42	0.632	0.2	127.5
Cod					
Pacific	89	0.69	0.088	0.24	106.3
Atlantic	89	0.73	1.43	0.13	196.2
Haddock	95	0.79	0.142	0.2	127.5
Tuna					
Light, canned in water	99	0.70	0.199	0.26	98.1
White, canned in water	109	2.53	0.673	0.73	34.9
Fresh	156	5.34	1.37	0.278	91.7
Salmon					
sockeye	184	9.33	1.629	1.05	24.3
pink	127	3.76	0.608	1.09	23.4
chum	131	4.11	0.915	0.68	37.5
chinook	196	11.37	2.732	1.48	17.2
Atlantic—farmed	175	10.50	2.128	1.83	13.9
Atlantic—wild	155	6.91	1.068	1.56	16.3
Mackerel					
Atlantic	223	15.14	3.55	1.022	25.0
Pacific	171	8.60	2.449	1.571	16.2
Spanish	134	5.37	1.531	1.059	24.1
King	114	2.18	0.395	0.341	74.8
Trout, rainbow					
Farmed	144	6.12	1.789	0.98	26.0
Wild	128	4.95	1.376	0.84	30.4
Lobster					
Northern	83	0.50	0.091	0.071	359.2
Spiny	122	1.65	0.258	0.408	62.5
Oyster					
Pacific	139	3.91	0.867	1.17	21.8
Eastern wild	116	4.17	0.496	0.47	54.3
Eastern farmed	67	1.80	0.581	0.37	68.9

(continued)

TABLE 11-8 (Continued)

Fish Type (per 3-oz cooked serving)	kcal	Total fat (g)	SFA* (g)	EPA + DHA (g)	Amount of fish required to equal ~300 mg/d EPA + DHA (g)
Crab					
Alaska King	82	1.31	0.113	0.351	72.6
Blue	87	1.50	0.194	0.403	63.3
Dungeness	94	1.05	0.143	0.335	76.1
Shrimp, mixed species	84	0.92	0.246	0.27	94.4
Clam	126	1.66	0.16	0.24	106.3
Crayfish	74	1.11	0.185	0.137	186.1
Bass					
Freshwater	124	4.02	0.851	0.648	39.4
Striped	105	2.54	0.552	0.821	31.1
Blue fish	135	4.62	0.996	0.84	30.4
Turbot	98	0.88	0.178	0.181	140.9
Carp	138	6.10	1.18	0.383	66.6
Mullet, Stripped	128	4.13	1.26	0.279	91.4
Perch					
Ocean Atlantic	103	1.78	0.266	0.318	80.2
Mixed species	96	1.00	0.201	0.276	92.4
Pike					
Northern	96	0.75	0.128	0.117	217.9
Walleye	101	1.33	0.271	0.338	75.4
Pompano	179	10.32	3.824	0.135	188.9
Rockfish (Pacific)	103	1.71	0.403	0.377	67.6
Sea bass	105	2.18	0.557	0.648	39.4
Snapper	109	1.46	0.31	0.273	93.4
Sturgeon (mixed pieces)	115	4.03	0.997	0.31	82.3

*SFA, saturated fatty acids; EPA, eicosapentaenoic acid; DHA, docosahexaenoic acid.

SOURCE: USDA Nutrient Database for Standard Reference, Release 16, July 2003.

consumption for both healthy individuals and persons with CVD. For healthy individuals, two servings per week of fish (particularly fatty fish) are recommended.[88] Fish, especially oily species like salmon, mackerel, lake trout, herring, sardines, and albacore tuna, provide significant amounts of the two kinds of omega-3 fatty acids shown to be cardioprotective, EPA and DHA. Two servings of fatty fish per week provide approximately 2.0 g of EPA and DHA (using an average of 1.0 g EPA + DHA/3-oz serving of fatty fish). This provides approximately 0.286 g of EPA + DHA per day, an amount that is slightly greater than the current dietary recommendations for omega-3 fatty acids from the Food and Nutrition Board of the National Academies (1.6 and 1.1 g ALA/d are recommended for men and women, respectively, and up to 10% can come from EPA + DHA per

day).[89] Table 11-8 lists the amounts of different types of seafood needed to provide about 300 mg/d EPA + DHA. The AHA also recommends eating plant-derived omega-3 fatty acids. Tofu and other forms of soybeans (ie, soybean oil); walnuts and flaxseeds and their oils; and canola oil all contain ALA. For patients with documented CHD, the AHA recommends about 1 g of EPA + DHA (combined) per day from either fish or fish oil supplements in consultation with a physician. As discussed in the AHA Science Advisory on Fish Consumption, Fish Oil, Omega-3 Fatty Acids and CVD, this recommendation is based on secondary prevention studies (see below).[73]

An EPA + DHA supplement may be useful in patients with hypertriglyceridemia. Two to four grams of EPA + DHA per day can lower triglyceride levels 20 to

TABLE 11-9   Clinical Nutrition Studies That Demonstrate a Cholesterol-Lowering Effect of Diet and a Reduction in Coronary Heart Disease Endpoints

Study	Subjects	Study design/duration	Intervention	Results*	
				Serum cholesterol reduction	CHD† endpoints
High PUFA			**Reduce SFA, increase PUFA**		
Los Angeles Veteran Study[92]	846 men; primary and secondary prevention	Parallel, double-blind/8 y	40% total fat, 17% PUFA, 8% SFA	−13%	−20% in CHD −30% in CVD events
Oslo Diet-Heart Study[93]	206 male; 1 to 2 years following their first MI	Parallel/5 y	39% total fat, 21% PUFA, 9% SFA	−14%	−25% incidence of major CHD relapses (myocardial reinfarction, new angina pectoris) significantly reduced; incidence of sudden death not different between experimental and control groups
Finnish Mental Hospital Study[94]	676 men without CHD	Crossover/6 y	35% total fat, 13% PUFA, 9% SFA	−15%	−44% (appearance of certain ECG patterns and occurrence of coronary deaths)
Finnish Mental Hospital Study[95]	591 women without CHD	Crossover/6 y	35% total fat, 13% PUFA, 9% SFA	−13%	Serum cholesterol-lowering diet: incidence of CHD: 25.0/1000 person-years
Minnesota Coronary Survey[114]	4,393 male and 4,664 women (institutionalized)	Parallel/4.5 y of enrollment; mean duration 1 y	38% total fat, 15% PUFA, 9% SFA, PUFA:SFA ratio = 1.6	−14.5% (NR)	NC
MRC[97]	393 male MI patients	Parallel/4 y	46% total fat; PUFA:SFA ratio = 1.8; 85 g soybean oil daily	−15%	−12%; cholesterol reduction not related to occurrence of CHD death or relapse
LOW fat			**Reduce total fat**		
Ornish[99,100]	28 males and females with moderate to severe CHD	Parallel/1 y	Intensive lifestyle changes 10% total fat vegetarian diet Moderate aerobic exercise Stress management training Smoking cessation Group psychosocial support	−37.2% (LDL-C)	−91% in frequency of anginal episodes −1.75% average diameter stenosis (4.5% relative improvement)

Dietary patterns

Indian Experiment of Infarct Survival[101]	406 male and female MI patients	Parallel/1 y	23.8% total fat, 7.2% SFA, 8.0% MUFA, 8.6% PUFA; advised to eat fruit, vegetables, pulses, nuts, and fish Goal: 400 g/d of fruits and vegetables Other health-related advice (given to both groups): smoking cessation, reduce alcohol intake, stress reduction counseling, physical activity	TC: Intervention, 0.74 mmol/L; control, −0.32 mmol/L LDL-C: Intervention, −0.54 mmol/L; control, −0.24 mmol/L	Cardiac Events: 50 (test) vs 82 (control) Total mortality: 21 (test) vs 38 (control)
Indo-Mediterranean[102]	1000 patients with angina pectoris, MI, or surrogate risk factors for CAD	Parallel/2 y	Recommended: 30% total fat; <10% SFA, <300 mg cholesterol; 250–300 g fruit, 125–150 g vegetables, 25–50 g walnuts or almonds, 400–500 g whole grains, 3 or 4 servings per day of mustard seed or soybean oil Control Diet: NCEP Step 1	TC: intervention, −0.70 mmol/L; control, −0.18 mmol/L LDL-C: intervention, −0.64 mmol/L; control, −0.15	Adjusted rate ratio: 0.48 Total cardiac endpoints include nonfatal MI, fatal MI, sudden cardiac death
Pritikin Program[109,110]	21 males	26-d residential program	Pritikin diet: high-complex-carbohy-drate, high-fiber, low-fat, low-cholesterol diet. Total fat: <10% Fiber: 35–40 g/1000 kcal Cholesterol: <25 mg/d	TC: −20%	NR
Dietary Portfolio of Cholesterol-Lowering Foods[111,112]	46 healthy hyperlipidemic patients (25 men and 21 post-menopausal women)	Parallel/ 1 mo	Therapeutic vegetarian low-fat diet; based on NCEP Step II diet (<7% en SFA, <200 mg/d cholesterol) + 1.0 g plant sterols/1000 kcal, 9.8 g viscous fibers/1000 kcal, 21.4 g soy protein/1000 kcal, 14 g whole almonds/1000 kcal (Portfolio Diet) OR + lovastatin 20 mg/d	LDL-C: Portfolio Diet, −28.6%; lovastatin, −30.9%; control, −8.0%	NR

40%. Patients taking more than 3 g of these fatty acids from supplements should do so only under a physician's care. Very high ("Eskimo") intakes could cause excessive bleeding in some people.

Some types of fish may contain significant levels of methylmercury, polychlorinated biphenyls, dioxins, and other environmental contaminants. Specific guidance on fish consumption can be found on web sites at the Environmental Protection Agency[90] and the Food and Drug Administration.[91]

CONTROLLED CLINICAL TRIALS (WITH AND WITHOUT CHOLESTEROL LOWERING) EVALUATING EFFECTS OF DIETARY FAT AND DIETARY PATTERNS ON CVD MORBIDITY AND MORTALITY AND RISK FACTORS

Studies with cholesterol lowering

Extensive evidence, principally from pharmacologic studies, has shown that lowering LDL-C decreases CHD mortality. For example, a 1% reduction in LDL-C reduces hard CHD events (MI and CHD death) by approximately 1 to 2%, the latter being achieved with prolonged treatment.[41]

A number of diet studies have achieved an appreciable cholesterol-lowering response resulting in a reduction in CVD events. These studies have implemented different dietary approaches to achieve a marked cholesterol-lowering effect. The common approaches that have been used are: low-saturated-fatty-acid (SFA), high-polyunsaturated-fatty-acid (PUFA) diets; a low-SFA, low-fat diet; and a dietary pattern approach that has a favorable fatty acid profile and emphasizes fruits, vegetables, grains, legumes, and soy products. Despite the evidence showing that cholesterol lowering is associated with a reduction in CVD events, there are studies that have shown a beneficial effect in CVD events without a cholesterol-lowering response (see below).

DIETS HIGH IN POLYUNSATURATED FATTY ACIDS

A number of studies have evaluated the effectiveness of a PUFA, blood cholesterol-lowering diet on incidence of CHD[92–97] (Table 11-9). These studies have shown that high-PUFA diets reduce LDL-C levels by 13 to 15%. The reduction in serum cholesterol levels was associated with a 12 to 44% reduction in CVD endpoints. Thus, the relationship between the diet-induced decrease in serum cholesterol levels and the decrease in incidence of CVD is comparable to the relationship observed in pharmacologic studies; that is, coronary events are reduced 2% for every 1% reduction in total cholesterol.[98] No studies

have shown decreases in CVD due to cholesterol lowering with MUFA or omega-3 fatty acids.

LOW-FAT DIET AND INTENSIVE LIFESTYLE PROGRAM

In the Lifestyle Heart Trial, patients with moderate to severe CHD participated in an intensive intervention program that combined a low-fat, vegetarian diet with aerobic exercise, stress management training, smoking cessation, and group psychosocial support[99,100] (Table 11-9). Participants consumed a 10% fat (PUFA:SFA > 1) vegetarian diet that was rich in fruits, vegetables, grains, legumes, and soybean products. After 1 year, LDL-C was reduced by 37%. This was accompanied by a 91% decrease in the frequency of anginal episodes and a 2% reduction in the average diameter of stenosis. Average diameter of stenosis at baseline decreased by 3.1 percentage points in the intervention group and increased by 11.8 percentage points in the control group after 5 years; there were fewer cardiac events in the intervention group (0.89 events per patient in the intervention group vs 2.25 in the control group). Of the participants who remained in the program for 5 years, 82% experienced further atherosclerotic regression.

DIETARY PATTERNS

Several controlled clinical studies have evaluated the effects of different cardioprotective dietary patterns compared with usual care dietary practices on CVD events in participants with coronary artery disease[101,102] (Table 11-9). In the Indian Experiment of Infarct Survival Study,[101] all subjects were instructed to eat a low-fat, low-saturated-fat diet; however, approximately half of these individuals also were instructed to eat fruit, vegetables, nuts, and fish, with the goal of eating 400 g/d fruits and vegetables. Both groups were given advice regarding smoking cessation and limiting of alcohol intake and stress reduction counseling, and were encouraged to increase their physical activity. After 1 year of treatment, individuals in the experimental diet group experienced a significant reduction not only in total cholesterol and LDL-C ($P < .01$), but also in cardiac events ($P < .001$) and total mortality ($P < .01$). In the Indo-Mediterranean Diet Heart Study,[102] there were significantly fewer cardiac events and a similar reduction in total cholesterol levels after 2 years of intervention in participants on a Step 1 Prudent Diet high in ALA provided by mustard or soybean oil (Table 11-9). Individuals were instructed specifically to consume 25 to 50 g/d walnuts or almonds and three to four servings per day of mustard seed or soybean oil. Thus, the consumption of omega-3 fatty acids from mustard or soybean oils, walnuts, whole grains, and leafy vegetables may have a beneficial effect similar to that of omega-3 fatty acids derived from marine sources. Further studies are needed, however, that are designed specifically to test ALA effects.

Studies without cholesterol-lowering

Several clinical studies have reported a reduction in CHD endpoints without any change in serum cholesterol levels[103–108] (Table 11-10). The Diet and Reinfarction Trial (DART)[103] tested the effect of three dietary factors: (1) type and amount of fat, (2) fish intake, and (3) fiber consumption (18 g/day) in a cohort of 2033 MI patients for 2 years. Although there were no decreases in serum cholesterol levels in any treatment group, the group consuming the fatty fish experienced a significant decrease in both total mortality (29%) and coronary mortality (33%).

Similar beneficial findings have been reported in the Gruppo Italiano per lo Studio della Sopravvivenza nell'Infarto Miocardio (GISSI) secondary prevention trial with fish oil supplements.[104–106] MI patients ($n = 11,324$) were randomly assigned to one of four treatment groups for a 3.5-year study period: (1) omega-3 PUFA (0.85 g/d EPA and DHA), (2) omega-3 PUFA + vitamin E, (3) vitamin E (300 mg synthetic α-tocopherol), (4) no supplement. There was no reduction in serum cholesterol levels; however, sudden death and cardiovascular death were reduced 45 and 30%, respectively, in individuals receiving the omega-3 PUFA supplement. Both total mortality ($RR = 0.59$, $P = .037$) and risk of sudden death ($RR = 0.47$, $P = .048$) were significantly reduced following 3 and 4 months of treatment, respectively. In addition, a significant, although delayed, pattern was observed for cardiovascular ($RR = 0.64$, $P = .024$), cardiac ($RR = 0.61$, $P = .036$), and coronary ($RR = 0.62$, $P = .040$) deaths following 6 to 8 months of treatment. No added effect of vitamin E was observed.

The results of the Indian Experiment of Infarct Survival indicate that the addition of fish oil (1.08 g/d EPA and 0.72 g/d DHA) or mustard oil (2.9 g/d ALA) to a low-fat diet reduces total cardiac events by 30 and 19%, respectively, despite no reduction in serum cholesterol levels.[107] In this study, subjects followed a diet that was high in fruits, vegetables, nuts, whole grains, and legumes.

In the Lyon Diet Heart Study, participants following a Mediterranean-style, National Cholesterol Education Program (NCEP) Step 1 diet that was high in ALA provided by a special margarine and rapeseed oil had a marked reduction (50–70%) in recurrent heart disease[108] (see Table 11-10). This study was conducted in 423 MI patients, with a mean follow-up of 3.8 years. Individuals following the Mediterranean diet replaced animal fat with vegetable oil rich in ALA, increased consumption of fruits, vegetables, legumes, and fiber, and reduced consumption of meats, butter, and cream. Total fat was

similar for both groups ($\sim$31% of total energy). There was no reduction in serum cholesterol in subjects on the Mediterranean diet compared with the Step 1 diet. There were, however, significant reductions in all-cause death (-56%), cardiac mortality (-65%), nonfatal MI (-70%), and cancer (-61%).

STUDIES DEMONSTRATING MAXIMAL CHOLESTEROL LOWERING

Some studies have shown a much greater reduction in serum cholesterol beyond the typical 11 to 15% when diet intervention is optimized[109–112] (see Table 11-9). The Pritikin Program recommends consumption of a diet high in complex carbohydrates and low in fat ($<10\%$) and cholesterol (<25 mg/d), and includes daily exercise. Following this 26-day residential program, participants ($n = 21$) experienced a 21% reduction in total cholesterol levels.[109] Similar results (19% reduction) were reported in individuals 70 years of age and older following the Pritikin diet.[110]

Weight loss is an effective means of enhancing the effects of dietary modification on risk factors for CVD. Lichtenstein and colleagues found that the decrease in serum total cholesterol and LDL-C was enhanced in individuals on a low-fat, energy-restricted diet compared with a low-fat (15% kcal total fat) or reduced fat d (29% kcal total fat) diet with no energy restriction.[113] Reductions in total cholesterol (15%) and LDL-C (23%) were greater in those on the low-fat diet when accompanied with energy restriction than in those on the low-fat diet alone (total cholesterol = 7%, LDL-C = 14%).

A recent study by Jenkins and colleagues reported that the Portfolio diet (a diet that targets multiple dietary factors/constituents) reduces cholesterol to an extent comparable to that attained with low-dose pharmacologic therapy.[111,112] Healthy, hyperlipidemic individuals ($n = 46$) were randomized to one of three treatments: the control diet, a therapeutic vegetarian low-fat diet, based on the NCEP Step 2 diet ($< 7\%$ kcal SFA, < 200 mg/d cholesterol) ($n = 16$); a Step 2 diet plus 20 mg/d lovastatin ($n = 14$); the Portfolio diet, low in saturated fat (6% of kilocalories) and cholesterol (54 mg/1000 kcal) and high in plant sterols (1.0 g/1000 kcal), viscous fibers (9.8 g/1000 kcal), soy protein (21.4 g/1000 kcal), and almonds (14 g/1000 cal) ($n = 16$). The Portfolio diet decreased LDL-C 29%, compared with an 8% reduction in the control group. The lovastatin group experienced a reduction in LDL-C (31%) similar to that of the Portfolio diet group. This study demonstrates that a traditional cholesterol-lowering diet can be markedly enhanced to achieve LDL-C lowering similar to that produced by first-generation statin drugs.

Other studies have shown that a healthy dietary pattern can significantly reduce recurrent cardiac events. The Ornish diet[99,100] is very low in fat and very

TABLE 11-10 Clinical Nutrition Studies That Demonstrate a Reduction in Coronary Heart Disease Endpoints, with No Cholesterol Reduction

Study	Subjects	Study design/duration	Intervention	Results* Serum cholesterol reduction	Results* CHD[†] endpoints
DART[103]	2033 MI patients	Parallel/2 y	Fat: reduce total fat intake to 30% en and increase PUFA:SFA ratio to 1.0 Fish: two weekly portions (200–400 g) of fatty fish Fiber: increased intake of cereal fiber to 18 g/d	Fat: −3.5% TC Fish: +2.1% TC (NS) Fiber: NC	Fish group: −29% in total mortality; −33% in coronary mortality
GISSI[104–106]	11,324 MI patients	Parallel/3.5 y	1 g/d EPA + DHA (EPA:DHA = 1:2) 300 mg vitamin E EPA + DHA + 300 mg vitamin E	NC	−45% in sudden death, −30% in CVD mortality
Indian Experiment of Infarct Survival[107]	360 MI patients	Parallel/1 y	Low-fat diet + Fish oil: 1.08 g/d EPA and 0.72 g/d DHA OR Mustard oil: 2.9 g/d ALA	TC: fish oil, −0.25 mmol/L (NS); mustard oil, −0.23 mmol/L (NS)	Total cardiac events: fish oil, −30%; mustard oil, −19%
Lyon Diet Heart Study[108]	423 MI patients	Parallel/3.8 y of mean follow-up	Mediterranean-type diet Total fat: 30.4%; SFA 8.0%, PUFA 4.6%, 0.84% ALA; 18.6 g fiber; 203 mg cholesterol	NC	All-cause mortality: −56%, Cardiac mortality: −65%, Nonfatal MI: −70%

* All results are significant, P <.05 unless noted as NS (nonsignificant).
[†] CHD, coronary heart disease; DART, Diet and Reinfarction Trial; MI, myocardial infarction; % en, percentage of total energy intake; PUFA, polyunsaturated fatty acids; SFA, saturated fatty acids; TC, total cholesterol; GISSI, Gruppo Italiano per lo Studio della Sopravvivenza nell' Infarto Miocardio Trial; EPA, eicosapentaenoic acid; DHA, docosahexaenoic acid; ALA, α-linolenic acid; CVD, cardiovascular disease; LDL-C, low-density lipoprotein cholesterol; NC, no change; NR, not reported.

TABLE 11-11   Cardioprotective Food-Based Dietary Patterns: Controlled Clinical Trials

Indo-mediterranean diet	Lyon diet: mediterranean-type blood cholesterol-lowering diet	Lifestyle heart diet	Portfolio diet
Rich in whole grains (at least 400–500 g whole grains), fruits, vegetables, walnuts and almonds, legumes, rice, maize, wheat, and 3 or 4 servings/d mustard seed or soybean oil	Mediterranean-type diet that contains more bread, more root vegetables and green vegetables, more fish, fruits at least once daily, less red meat (replaced with poultry), and margarine supplied by the study to replace butter and cream; exclusive use of rapeseed oil and olive oil recommended for salads and food preparation	Low-fat, plant-based diet that uses fruits, vegetables, whole grains, beans, and soy products in their natural forms, moderate quantities of egg whites and nonfat dairy or soy products, and only small amounts of sugar and white flour	Low-fat vegetarian diet containing a dietary portfolio that includes a plant sterol ester-enriched margarine, oats, barley, and psyllium, soy milk and soy meat analogs, fruits and vegetables, and whole almonds; eggplant and okra also used as additional sources of viscous fiber

high in complex carbohydrates whereas the Indo-Mediterrnean[102] and Lyon[108] diets provided moderate amounts of total fat from unsaturated fats with emphasis on omega-3 fatty acids. Despite differences in macronutrient composition, all diets were high in fruits, vegetables, whole grains, and legumes, and low in red meat and full-fat dairy products (Table 11-11). This dietary pattern forms the foundation for the inclusion of additional foods that contribute other important cardioprotective nutrients/factors such as soluble fiber, omega-3 fatty acids, alcohol in moderation, soy protein, nuts, plant stanols/sterols, and many micronutrients (eg, folate, calcium, magnesium, potassium, vitamin E).

CONTROLLED CLINICAL TRIALS EVALUATING EFFECTS OF DIET AND OTHER DIETARY FACTORS ON BLOOD PRESSURE

Dietary strategies for blood pressure lowering

A typical reduction of 5 mm Hg in diastolic blood pressure (DBP) from drug treatment is estimated to reduce the incidences of CHD events and cerebrovascular disease by 1 and 45%, respectively.[114] It is well known that the risk of CVD increases with progressive elevations in blood pressure beginning at normal levels. An increment of 20 mm Hg in systolic blood pressure (SBP) or 10 mm Hg in DBP doubles CVD risk in people with a blood pressure of 115/75 mm Hg or greater[115] National guidelines recommend nonpharmacologic therapies (ie,

lifestyle modifications) as first-line of therapy to prevent and treat hypertension. These include weight reduction if needed, dietary sodium restriction, increased physical activity, moderation of alcohol consumption, and adoption of the DASH eating plan, all of which have been shown to effectively lower blood pressure.[115]

Dietary patterns

The DASH eating plan is based on the seminal DASH trial[60] and DASH–Sodium trial.[61] The DASH trials were unique in that they tested the effects of modifying dietary patterns in people with DBPs of 80 to 95 mm Hg and SBPs less than 160 mm Hg.

In the DASH trial, participants ($n = 459$) were fed a control diet for a 3-week run-in period. The control diet paralleled the macronutrient content of the typical American diet (low in fruits and vegetables, high in saturated and total fat)[60,61,116–120] (Table 11-12). The amount of calcium, potassium, and magnesium were in the 25th percentile of the US diet. Participants then were randomly allocated to one of three intervention diets for 8 weeks: the control diet, the fruit and vegetable diet, or the DASH diet. The fruit and vegetable diet provided approximately 10 servings of fruits and vegetables per day, was high in potassium, magnesium, and fiber, but was similar to the control diet in macronutrient content. The DASH diet was high in fruits and vegetables (approximately 9 servings), low-fat dairy products, whole grains, fish, poultry, and nuts, and was low in red meat and sweets. The DASH diet was reduced in saturated fat, total fat, and cholesterol, and moderately high in protein,

TABLE 11-12 Clinical Nutrition Studies That Demonstrate a Blood Pressure-Lowering Effect

Study	Subjects	Study design/duration	Intervention	Results* SBP† (mm Hg)	DBP (mm Hg)
Dietary Patterns					
DASH[60,116,117]	n = 459 DBP 80–95 mm Hg SBP <160 mm Hg 29% had stage 1 HTN	Parallel/8 wk	Combination diet vs control diet	−5.5 all subjects −11.6 in HTN −3.5 in NTN	−3.0 all subjects −5.3 in HTN −2.2 in NTN
			Fruit and vegetable diet vs control diet	−2.8 all subjects −7.2 in HTN	−1.1 all subjects (NS) −2.8 in HTN
			Combination diet vs fruit and vegetable diet	−2.7 all subjects −4.1 in HTN	−1.9 all subjects −2.6 in HTN
DASH–Sodium[61,118,119]	n = 412 DBP 80–95 mm Hg SBP <160 mm Hg 41% had stage 1 HTN	Crossover within two parallel arms/4 wk	Combination diet with 1.5, 2.4, or 3.0 g Na	−3.0 from high to low Na, all subjects	−1.6 from high to low Na, all subjects
			Control diet with 1.5, 2.4, or 3.0 g Na	−6.7 from high to low Na, all subjects	−3.5 from high to low Na, all subjects
			Combination diet vs control diet at		
			High Na	−5.9 all subjects	−2.9 all subjects
			Medium Na	−5.0 all subjects	−2.5 all subjects
			Low Na	−2.2 all subjects	−1.0 all subjects (NS)
			Combination low-Na diet vs control high-Na diet	−8.9 all subjects −11.5 in HTN −7.1 in NTN	−4.5 all subjects −5.7 in HTN −3.7 in NTN
Vanguard Study[120]	n = 158 HTN, HTHL, and NTN	Parallel/10 wk	Prepared meal plan (meets published recommendations) vs self-selected diet with nutrition counseling	−6.2 all subjects	−4.2 all subjects
			Prepared meal plan vs baseline	−7.0 in HTN −10.0 in HTHL	−6.0 in HTN −6.0 in HTHL
			Self-selected diet vs baseline	−9.0 in HTN −5.0 in HTHL	−6.0 in HTN −3.0 in HTHL
Weight Loss					
TAIM (121)	n = 787 Overweight HTN	Placebo-controlled/6 mo	Weight loss (> 4.4 kg) + placebo vs baseline	Not reported	−11.6
			Chlorthalidone (25 mg/d) vs baseline		−11.1
			Atenolol (50 mg/d) vs baseline		−12.4
			Weight loss (> 4.4 kg) + atenolol (50 mg/d) vs baseline		−18.4

(continued)

Study	Patients	Design/duration	Intervention		
TOHP[125]	n = 564, Overweight DBP 80–89 mm Hg	Parallel/18 months	Weight loss (> 4.4 kg) + chlorthalidone (25 mg/d) vs baseline		−15.4
			Weight loss of 4.7 kg for men and 1.6 kg for women vs usual care	−2.8 in men; −1.1 in women	−3.1 in men; −2.0 in women
Su et al[126]	n = 22, Overweight, 11 with HTN and 11 without HTN	Parallel/3 mo	Caloric restriction and light exercise with weight loss averaging 8 kg vs usual care	−12.0 in NTN; −14.0 in HTN	−7.0 in NTN; −12.0 in HTN
Ikeda et al[124]	n = 24, Obese HTN	Controlled/4 wk	Caloric restriction with weight loss averaging 7 kg vs baseline	−21.0	−15.0
Weight Loss and Na Restriction					
TOHP Phase[122]	n = 2382, Overweight, SBP < 140 mm Hg DBP 83–89 mm Hg	Parallel/6 mo	Weight loss (>4.4 kg) vs usual care	−3.7	−2.7
			Sodium reduction (1800 mg/d) vs usual care	−2.9	−1.6
			Weight loss (>4.4 kg) + sodium reduction (80 mmol/d) vs usual care	−4.0	−2.8
TONE[127]	n = 975, 60–80 years old on 1 BP drug, overweight/obese, SBP < 145 mm Hg, DBP < 85 mm Hg	Parallel/15–36 mo	Weight loss (3.5–4.5 kg) vs baseline	−4.0	−1.1
			Sodium reduction (900 mg/d) vs baseline	−3.4	−1.9
			Weight loss (3.5–4.5 kg) + sodium reduction (900 mg/d) vs baseline	−5.3	−3.4
TOHP Phase I follow-up[129]	n = 181, Participants of TOHP Phase I SBP <160 mm Hg DBP 80–89 mm Hg	Parallel/18 mo	Weight loss (3.5 kg) vs usual care	−5.8	−3.2
			Sodium reduction vs usual care	−3.3	−1.7 (NS)
Fish Oil					
Bao et al[130]	n = 63, Overweight with medication-treated HTN	Parallel/16 wks	Weight loss (5.6 kg) vs usual	−5.5	−2.2
			Fish meal (3.65 g omega-3 fatty acid) vs usual	−6.0	−3.0
			Weight loss and fish meal vs usual	−13.0	−9.3

TABLE 11-12 (Continued)

Study	Subjects	Study design/duration	Intervention	Results* SBP† (mm Hg)	DBP (mm Hg)
Mori et al[131]	n = 59 Overweight NTN	Parallel/6 wks	DHA (4 g/d) vs olive oil placebo (4 g/d)	−5.8	−3.3
			EPA (4 g/d) vs olive oil placebo (4 g/d)	No change	No change
Whole Grains					
Pins et al[132]	n = 88 Medication-treated HTN	Parallel/12 wks[b]	Oat cereal (11.7 g fiber, 6.2 soluble fiber)	−6.0 in first 4 wk	−3.0 (NS)
			Wheat cereal (3.5 fiber, <1.1 soluble fiber)	No change	No change
Keenan et al[133]	n = 18 HTN hyperinsulinemic	Parallel/6 wk	Oat cereal (5.52 g/d β-glucan) vs baseline	−7.5	−5.5
			Low-fiber cereal (< 1.0 g/d) vs baseline	No change	No change
Saltzman et al[134]	n = 43 Normal and overweight NTN	Parallel/8 wk	Weight loss (4 kg) vs control	−1.0	−3.0
			Weight loss + oats (45 g) vs. control	−6.0	−4.0
			Weight loss vs weight loss + oats	−5.0	−1.0 (NS)
Soy Protein					
Teede et al[135]	n = 179	Placebo-controlled/ 12 wk	Soy protein isolate (40 g, 118 mg isoflavones) vs baseline	−7.5	−4.3
			Soy protein isolate (40 g) vs casein (40 g)	−5.9	−2.4
Rivas et al[136]	n = 40 HTN, 50% were medication-treated	Placebo-controlled/ 12 wk	Soy milk (18 g protein, 143 mg isoflavone) vs cow milk placebo	−17.0	−12.0
Burke et al[137]	n = 41 Medication-treated HTN	Parallel/8 wk	High protein (25% kcal, 66 g soy protein isolate) + low fiber (15 g/d) vs low protein (12.5% kcal) + low fiber	−2.9 (NS)	−2.5 (NS)
			Low protein + high fiber (15 g/d fiber, 12 g soluble fiber as psyllium) vs low protein + low fiber	−2.4 (NS)	−1.9 (NS)
			High protein + high fiber vs low protein + low fiber	−10.5	−3.6 (NS)

*All results are significant, $P < .05$, unless noted as NS (nonsignificant).
†DASH, Dietary Approaches to Stop Hypertension; DBP, diastolic blood pressure; HTN, hypertensive; NTN, normotensive; NS, nonsignificant; HTHL, hypertensive hyperlipidemic; TAIM, Trial of Antihypertensive Interventions and Management Study; TOHP, Trials of Hypertension Prevention; TONE, Trial of Nonpharmacologic Interventions in the Elderly; DHA, docosahexaenoic acid, EPA, eicosapentaenoic acid.
‡Three weeks of baseline feeding, 3 weeks of blood pressure medication reduction, and 3 weeks of maintenance.

calcium, potassium, and magnesium. All three diets contained about 3000 mg of sodium per day and body weight was maintained throughout the study.

Both intervention diets reduced blood pressure compared with the control diet. The DASH diet significantly lowered SBP by 5.5 mm Hg and DBP by 3.0 mm Hg compared with the control diet.[60] Although to a lesser degree, the fruit and vegetable diet also significantly lowered blood pressure by 2.8/1.1 mm Hg compared with the control diet. In subjects with stage 1 hypertension (140/90 to 159/95 mm Hg, 29% of the total sample), the combination diet decreased SBP by 11.6 mm Hg and DBP by 5.3 mm Hg.[116] Normotensive subjects had a significant reduction in blood pressure but to a much lesser extent (3.5/2.2 mm Hg). Hypertensive African-Americans had the most robust response to the combination diet, reducing blood pressure by 13.2/6.1 mm Hg compared with the control diet.[116] The reductions in blood pressure occurred within 2 weeks of consuming the DASH diet and rival the effects of blood pressure-lowering medications. The DASH diet also controlled hypertension in 70% of the hypertensive group.[117] It is estimated that CHD and stroke could be reduced by 15 and 27%, respectively, if Americans followed the DASH diet.[60]

To explore the additional effect of sodium reduction in the context of the combination diet, the DASH–Sodium trial was conducted.[61] There were three levels of sodium intake: high = 3,300 mg/d, which is similar to average US intake; intermediate = 2400 mg/d, which is the upper level of current recommendations; and low = 1500 mg/d.

Reduction in sodium intake reduced blood pressure (from high sodium to low sodium: decreases of 3.0/1.6 mm Hg on the combination diet and 6.7/3.5 mm Hg on the control diet).[61] Compared with the combination diet, the sodium-related decrease in blood pressure was greater in those on the control diet. However, the lowest mean blood pressure was experienced by those consuming the combination diet with the lowest level of sodium. Although these effects were significant in all subgroups, hypertensive individuals, those older than 45 years of age, women, and African-Americans appeared to especially benefit from the combined interventions.[118] These results indicate that the DASH diet is beneficial throughout a range of sodium intakes and that the combined effects of the DASH diet and sodium restriction are superior.

Potential limitations of the DASH study are that it was short-term and was done under "artificial" conditions and not in a free-living setting. Effectiveness of the DASH dietary pattern, as well as adherence to the diet among free-living persons over the long term, is not known. Because of multiple differences between diets, the nutrients or foods responsible for lowering blood pressure cannot be determined from the DASH trials. Other unanswered questions include how the diet will affect persons with higher levels of blood pressure and if the diet will be an effective adjunct to antihypertensive therapy. Overall, the results of the DASH trials are consistent with observational evidence and offer strong support for recommending the DASH diet, which is compatible with other dietary recommendations for the reduction of CVD, cancer, and osteoporosis.

To answer some of the above questions, the PREMIER study tested the effects of implementing the DASH diet in combination with other recommendations for lowering blood pressure in a free-living population.[119] This was a multicenter, randomized, parallel-arm, free-living trial in 810 adults with above-optimal blood pressure (120–159 mm Hg systolic and 80–95 mm Hg diastolic blood pressure) and not taking antihypertensive medication. Participants were randomly allocated to one of three intervention groups for 6 months. The interventions included: (1) an advice only group, which included one 30-minute personalized session with a registered dietitian, (2) an established recommendations group, which included 18 sessions promoting weight loss of at least 15 lbs. if needed, 180 min/wk of moderate intensity exercise, limited sodium intake (≤100 mEq) and moderate alcohol consumption (≤1 oz. for men, ≤0.5 oz. for women), or (3) an established recommendations plus DASH diet group, which included the established recommendations in conjunction with information on the DASH dietary plan. The advice only group experienced a substantial decrease in blood pressure from baseline (−6.6/−3.8 mm Hg), while the established group and the established plus DASH group showed larger decreases of −10.5/5.5 and −11.1/−6.4 mm Hg, respectively. While both interventions resulted in significant reductions compared with the advice only group, the addition of the DASH diet did not significantly lower blood pressure compared to the established recommendation group. However, the prevalence of hypertension at 6 months was lowest in the DASH plus group (12%). The DASH plus group consumed more fruits and vegetables (7.8 servings/d), compared with the established recommendations group, but the number of servings of these foods were still lower than in the original DASH studies (9.6 servings of fruits and vegetables).[60] Therefore, the free-living population may not have experienced the best possible blood pressure-lowering effects of the DASH diet. In addition, multiple behavioral changes may lower blood pressure through the same biological pathways, thus when used in combination they may not demonstrate an additive effect. The researchers also suggest that initiation of several lifestyle modifications may overwhelm individuals and thus reduce their overall effectiveness. This study is important because its sample population represents about 50% of US adults.

The beneficial effect observed in the advice only group suggests that physicians can play a vital role in lowering patients' blood pressure in a clinical setting. Adjunct counseling on the DASH diet and established recommendations offers promise in optimizing blood pressure without the use of drug therapy.

The Vanguard study compared the effects of weight loss and diet modification on blood pressure[120] (see Table 11-12). Both interventions significantly lowered blood pressure in all subjects. Independent of weight loss, dietary changes consistent with the DASH dietary pattern (ie, increased dietary potassium, calcium, and magnesium) caused a further decrease in blood pressure.

Weight reduction

A modest weight loss (5–10%) has been shown to decrease blood pressure in both hypertensive[121–124] and normotensive[125–127] individuals. In addition, weight loss can decrease the need for anithypertensive drugs and/or the dosage of such drugs. The Trial of Antihypertensive Interventions and Management Study examined the effects of weight loss alone or in combination with antihypertensive drugs on DBP in 787 overweight hypertensive subjects[121] (see Table 11-12). Weight loss of 5% or greater reduced DBP 11.6 mm Hg, which was equivalent to the decrease in response to drug therapy. Weight loss in combination with drug therapy further reduced blood pressure. Other studies have show that hypertensive individuals who have lost and maintained weight loss for an extended period can normalize blood pressure and prevent the need for drug therapy.[123,128]

Weight reduction and sodium reduction

The Trial of Hypertension Prevention (TOHP), Phase II, evaluated the effect of weight loss alone, sodium reduction alone, and the combination of the two in overweight normotensive subjects.[122] Blood pressure significantly decreased at 6 months in all three groups (see Table 11-12). After 36 months, the effects on blood pressure declined, but were still significant for the weight loss group (1.3/0.9 mm Hg) and the sodium reduction group (1.2/0.7 mm Hg), but not for the combined group. Despite decreased compliance with the interventions over time, the incidence of hypertension decreased by about 20% in all three groups over a 3- to 4-year follow-up. In addition, a study in overweight older adults on monotherapy to control blood pressure evaluated the effects of weight loss and sodium reduction.[127] In the group that lost weight (~10 lb) and decreased sodium intake to 900 mg/d, about 50% were able to discontinue drug therapy compared with about one third of those in a single intervention group.

The TOHP, Phase I Follow-up study was the first to demonstrate the long-term effects of two 18-month interventions, weight loss and sodium reduction.[129] After 7 years, short-term weight loss was significantly associated with a 77% decrease in incidence of hypertension, and sodium reduction was associated with a nonsignificant 35% reduction in incidence. The proportion of the weight loss group on antihypertensive drugs was also significantly lower than the proportion of the control group at follow-up.

Other dietary factors that affect blood pressure

Although benefits of certain dietary patterns cannot be attributed to a single dietary factor, certain foods and nutrients confer hypotensive effects. Identifying particular foods that show benefit is important in defining the optimal diet. Several dietary constituents that show promise are fish and fish oil,[130,131] whole grains,[132–134] and soy protein[135–137] (see Table 11-12). In the majority of these studies, SBP was lowered by approximately 4 to 11 mm Hg and DBP was reduced by 2 to 9 mm Hg, with greater responses observed in some studies.[130,136]

EFFECT OF DIET ON OTHER ESTABLISHED CVD RISK FACTORS
Overweight and obesity (including role of low-carbohydrate diets)

The question as to whether diet composition per se is a factor that affects the efficacy of weight loss continues to be an active area of research. Studies of individuals who have achieved long-term weight loss indicate that behavioral changes to control dietary fat intake, increase physical activity (especially strenuous activity), and maintain a greater frequency of self-weighing are important.[138] It is still not clear whether alternate dietary strategies, such as very low carbohydrate and/or high-protein diets may be more effective, based on their metabolic effects or influence on ingestive behavior. Only recently have studies been carried out specifically to test the efficacy of such dietary approaches.[139–140] Results to date suggest that at least over periods up to 6 months, average weight loss is higher for diets with very low carbohydrate content, for example, less than 35 g/d, than for diets containing more conventional amounts of carbohydrate that are restricted in total fat.[141] Possible explanations for this include restricted food choices and the possibility that satiety is favorably affected by higher dietary content of protein and/or lower content of carbohydrates, especially simple sugars and rapidly digested starches with lower glycemic effects. The safety and overall health effects of carbohydrate-restricted diets are not known. These diets restrict many of the foods associated with cardiovascular and overall health, including fruits, vegetables, and whole grains, and they are high in saturated and *trans* fats and cholesterol. The effects of these diets on LDL-C levels are variable, with studies showing beneficial or adverse effects.[139,142] A recently published systematic review of low-carbohydrate diets showed that among obese patients weight loss was associated with longer diet duration and restriction of calorie content, but not with reduced carbohydrate content. Such diets had no significant adverse effect on serum lipids, fasting glucose, insulin levels, or blood pressure. The Authors concluded that there was insufficient evidence to make recommendations for or against the use of low-carbohydrate diets.[143]

It is not clear that diets very low in carbohydrate or fat can be maintained long term. With respect to low-fat diets, however, this appears to be possible for highly motivated individuals.[138,144] This has not yet been demonstrated for low-carbohydrate, high-protein diets.

HDL-C

Although low HDL-C is a recognized independent risk factor for coronary artery disease, it has not been ascertained whether changes in HDL-C, in particular those induced by diet, are predictive of changes in risk.[41] There are two general categories of nutritional effect on HDL-C: those due to changes in dietary fatty acid composition, and those due to factors that also affect plasma triglyceride levels, as described in the next section. Because dietary fatty acids affect LDL-C and HDL-C, these effects should be assessed jointly to evaluate risk status. Thus, the ratio of LDL-C or total cholesterol to HDL-C is a powerful predictor of CHD risk because it reflects two significant components of risk.

When carbohydrates replace SFA (a diet that is reduced in total and saturated fat), the plasma cholesterol to HDL-C ratio does not change (for review, see Ref. 89). In contrast, the ratio is decreased when *cis* unsaturated fatty acids replace saturated fatty acids. When *trans* fatty acids replace a mixture of carbohydrates and *cis* unsaturated fatty acids, the ratio increases. In fact, *trans* fatty acids increase the ratio by about twofold compared with SFA.

Triglycerides and the atherogenic dyslipidemia of obesity, diabetes, and the metabolic syndrome

Atherogenic dyslipidemia typically presents in patients with type 2 diabetes mellitus, metabolic syndrome, and excess adiposity.[145] The triad of lipid abnormalities in these conditions consists of elevated plasma triglyceride (>~150 mg/dL), reduced HDL-C, and a relative excess of small, dense LDL particles with total

LDL-C levels that may be normal. Adiposity and dietary carbohydrate[146] are the key nutrition-related factors that contribute to atherogenic dyslipidemia. In general, simple sugars and rapidly hydrolyzed starches have a greater triglyceride-raising effect than more complex carbohydrates and those consumed in conjunction with higher intake of fiber. The triglyceride-raising effects of carbohydrates tend to correlate with their glycemic effects.[147] Dietary carbohydrate-induced increases in plasma triglycerides are often accompanied by decreases in HDL-C and increases in small, dense LDL particles.[144] Thus, limiting sugars and high glycemic and triglyceride-raising carbohydrates is advisable for patients with this type of dyslipidemia.

EMERGING CVD RISK FACTORS AFFECTED BY DIET

Several risk factors for CVD beyond elevated cholesterol and hypertension have been identified. These emerging risk factors include C-reactive protein, small, dense LDL particles, lipoprotein(a), homocysteine, and platelet function (see Table 11-1). Of interest is how these risk factors can be modified by diet.

C-Reactive protein

C-reactive protein (CRP) has been shown to be a strong independent risk factor for CVD. Diet has been shown to affect CRP levels in a variety of ways. A strong positive association between high-sensitivity CRP and a high dietary glycemic load was observed in 244 healthy middle-aged women in the Women's Health Study.[148] In 76 male dyslipidemic patients, dietary supplementation with ALA for 3 months significantly decreased CRP by 38% ($P = .0008$), independent of changes in lipids, whereas supplementation with linoleic acid had no effect.[149] The presence of increased CRP diminished the total cholesterol- and LDL-C-lowering effect of a DASH style reduced-fat/low-cholesterol diet in a study conducted by Erlinger and colleagues.[150] A recent study compared the effects of a dietary portfolio of cholesterol-lowering foods with the effects of both a control, very low saturated fat diet and a control diet plus 20 mg/d lovastatin.[151] The control, statin, and dietary portfolio groups had reductions in CRP of 10.0, 33.3, and 28.2%, respectively. These reductions were significant only for the statin group ($P = .002$) and the dietary portfolio group ($P = .02$). More importantly, there were no differences between the dietary portfolio and statin groups with respect to these reductions in CRP, suggesting that this dietary portfolio lowered CRP to the same extent as a statin.

A reduction in CRP was observed following a multidisciplinary program aimed at reducing body weight in obese women through lifestyle changes.[152] Premenopausal obese women were randomly assigned to either the intervention group ($n = 60$)—receiving detailed advice about how to achieve a weight reduction of 10% or greater by following a low-energy Mediterranean-style diet—or to the control group ($n = 60$)—receiving general information about healthy food choices. Both CRP and BMI were reduced more in the intervention group than in the control group ($P = .008$ and $P < .001$, respectively). In a study of obese postmenopausal women ($n = 25$), weight loss significantly reduced CRP levels by 32%.[153] The average weight loss was 16% (14.5 ± 6.2 kg). Correlations were observed between CRP levels and changes in body weight ($r = .44$, $P < .03$), total body fat mass ($r = .47$, $P < .02$), and HDL-C ($r = -.56$, $P < .004$). Various dietary manipulations appear to be helpful in lowering CRP levels, including reducing glycemic load, adding omega-3 fatty acids, implementing dietary patterns such as the DASH diet and Portfolio diet, and losing weight.

Small, dense LDL particles

Krauss[154] and Austin and colleagues[155] have defined three subclass LDL patterns. These include the large LDL subclass pattern A (>26.2 nm), the small LDL subclass pattern B (<25.5 nm), and an intermediate subclass in which neither LDL subclass is predominant. Recently, NCEP ATP-III defined small, dense LDL particles as an emerging risk factor for CAD.[41] These smaller, more dense LDL particles have been associated with a threefold greater risk of MI than larger, more buoyant particles.[156]

Dietary effects on LDL subclass patterns were explored in a randomized crossover study of 105 normolipidemic men who consumed a high-fat diet (46% kcal total fat) and a low-fat diet (24% kcal total fat) each for 6 weeks.[157] LDL-C was reduced on the low-fat diet for both subclasses; however, this reduction was significantly greater ($P = .003$) for individuals with pattern B, approximately twofold compared with individuals with pattern A. Additionally, 41% of the men with pattern A on the high-fat diet converted to pattern B on the low-fat diet. The effects of further reductions in dietary fat were studied in men who had shown pattern A on both the high- and low-fat diets ($n = 38$) in the previous study.[158] A diet providing 10% of calories from total fat consumed for 10 days resulted in a conversion to pattern B in 12 men; 26 men remained pattern A. Reductions in LDL-C did not differ in either group from previous values attained with the low-fat diet (24% kcal total fat). Therefore, dietary fat intake appears to be a strong determinant of pattern B, and a low-fat diet may induce this trait in susceptible individuals.

Consequently, a moderate-fat diet (defined as 25–35% of calories) that is at the upper end of this fat range (ie, 30–35% of calories) and also low in saturated fat and cholesterol (ie, consistent with ATP-III guidelines) is recommended to prevent expression of pattern B phenotype.

Lipoprotein(a)

Lipoprotein (a) (Lp(a)), an LDL-C particle linked to apolipoprotein(a), is a suggested independent risk factor for CHD.[159–163] Although Lp(a) is thought to be controlled by genetic factors, several studies have shown that Lp(a) levels can be modulated by the type of fat consumed.[164–167] Fish oil has been shown to reduce Lp(a) concentrations in hypertriglyceridemic patients.[166] The combination of a high dose (12 g/d) of fish oil (8.5 g of omega-3 fatty acids) and a low-fat (30% kcal total fat), low-calorie diet resulted in a 14% reduction in plasma Lp(a) levels in one study.[168]

A study examining the effects of trans fatty acids levels commonly found in US diets on Lp(a) found that a diet rich in saturated fat (16.2% of total calories) reduced Lp(a) levels by 8 to 11% compared with a diet rich in oleic acid (16.7% of total calories), a moderate-trans-fatty-acid diet (3.8% of total calories), and a high-trans-fatty-acid diet (6.6% of total calories).[169] No statistically significant differences among Lp(a) levels were observed between the moderate-trans-fat diet, the high-trans-fat diet, and the diet rich in oleic acid. Elevations in Lp(a) have been observed in several other studies in which trans fatty acids were increased,[164,165,170] as well as in studies with higher stearic acid content as a percentage of fat calories.[171,172] The Dietary Effects on Lipoproteins and Thrombogenic Activity (DELTA) study observed a stepwise increase in plasma Lp(a) concentrations as saturated fat in the diet was reduced from 15.0 to 9.0 to 6.1%. As the level of saturated fat in the diet decreased from 15 to 6% of total calories, Lp(a) levels increased approximately 15%.[173]

Platelet function

Omega-3 fatty acids have been shown to decrease platelet aggregation.[174,175] In platelets, the synthesis of thromboxane A2 from arachidonic acid, which causes platelet aggregation and, ultimately, vasoconstriction, is inhibited by EPA in fish oil. Large amounts of fish oil or large numbers of capsules containing fish oil extracts are often used in studies investigating the effects of omega-3 fatty acids on platelet aggregation.[176] However, the effects on platelet aggregation when fish is the source of omega-3 fatty acids have been reported as well in a few studies.[177–179]

The effects of fish or fish oil, within the context of a high-fat (40% of total calories) or low-fat (30% of total calories) diet, on platelet aggregation and platelet thromboxane were studied in men ($n = 120$) with increased risk of CVD.[175] Subjects were randomly assigned to one of two low-fat groups (30% kcal total fat) that received either a fish or placebo capsule, or to one of five high-fat groups (40% kcal total fat) that received either 6 or 12 fish oil capsules daily, fish (equivalent to 6 fish oil capsules), a combination of fish and fish oil, or placebo capsules for 12 weeks. Platelet aggregation was reduced in all groups consuming omega-3 fatty acids. No differences were observed in collagen-induced platelet aggregation or platelet thromboxane between fish and fish oils on a high- or low-fat diet. No effect on platelet activating factor-induced platelet aggregation was observed following the low-fat diet; however, a small effect on platelet responses to collagen ($P < .05$) was observed. Fish also was associated with a greater reduction of platelet aggregation (10.3%, $P < .0001$) when incorporated into a lower fat (30% energy), rather than a higher fat (40% energy) diet.

Homocysteine

Elevated serum homocysteine has been suggested as an independent modifiable risk factor for CHD.[180] A recent meta-analysis of observational studies, including a total of 5073 IHD events and 1113 stroke events, revealed that a lower homocysteine level (about 3 μmol/L) was associated with an 11% lower risk of IHD and 19% lower risk of stroke.[181] Dietary folic acid plus vitamins B_6 and B_{12} is the primary intervention for elevated homocysteine. In 1998, the US Food and Drug Administration (FDA) required all enriched grain products to contain 140 μg of folic acid per 100 g of product. Data from the Framingham Offspring Study has shown a substantial improvement in folate status due to the fortification of enriched grain products with folic acid.[182] Plasma folate and total homocysteine concentrations were measured in 350 subjects whose follow-up examination occurred after fortification and a control group consisting of 756 subjects whose follow-up examination occurred before fortification. High homocysteine concentrations (>13 μmol/L) were reduced from 18.7 to 9.8% and low folate concentrations (<7 nmol/L) were reduced from 22 to 1.7% (both P's < .0001). No statistically significant changes in folate or homocysteine concentrations were observed in the control group.

The effects of breakfast cereals fortified with three levels of folic acid, and also containing the Recommended Daily Allowance for vitamins B_6 and B_{12}, were examined in men and women ($n = 75$) with CAD.[183] Cereal that contained an amount of folic acid (127 μg) approximately equal to the FDA enrichment policy increased plasma folate by 31% ($P=.045$), but only decreased plasma homocysteine by 3.7% ($P = .24$). However, the cereals that provided 499 and 665 μg of folate decreased homocysteine by 11% ($P < .001$) and 14% ($P= .001$),

respectively, suggesting that higher folate intakes have greater benefits for the population studied.

DIETARY GUIDELINES FOR HEALTH

Dietary recommendations have been made for the prevention and treatment of coronary disease by numerous agencies and organizations such as the National Academies,[89] the National Institutes of Health/National Heart, Lung and Blood Institute (NIH/NHLBI),[41] the US Department of Agriculture and Department of Health and Human Services,[184] the AHA,[88,185] and the American Diabetes Association.[186] Guidance has been made for macronutrients (fat, protein, carbohydrates)/micronutrients and other dietary constituents, and also as food-based dietary recommendations. In general, the recommendations of the groups/organizations are similar (Table 11-13). The guidance for dietary fat intake is very consistent, ranging between 20 and 35% of calories; protein intake is between 10 and 35% of calories; and total carbohydrates constitute the remainder of the diet, ranging from 45 to 65% of calories. Specific recommendations have been made for fatty acid classes: to decrease saturated and *trans* fat to less than 10% of calories and less than 7% of calories for high-risk populations, and to consume adequate amounts of unsaturated fatty acids including linoleic acid and ALA. The recommendation for MUFA is based on achieving total fat recommendations. Dietary cholesterol should be less than 300 mg/d; for high-risk individuals, less than 200 mg/d is recommended. All recommendations advise achieving and maintaining a healthy weight and participating in regular physical activity.

Food-based recommendations have been made by the AHA[88] (Table 11-14) that emphasize a diet rich in whole grains, fiber, fruit, vegetables and legumes, lean meat, fish and poultry, and low-fat dairy products. These dietary guidelines target major risk factors including overweight/obesity, high blood cholesterol, and high blood pressure, and provide guidance about healthy eating patterns to decrease these risk factors.

In addition, the American Heart Association does not recommend antioxidant supplements to reduce the risk of CVD.[187] A review of research conducted on antioxidants between 1994 and 2002 has shown that antioxidant supplements largely have no effect on primary or secondary prevention of CVD.[187] Thus, the American Heart Association continues to recommend a diet rich in fruits, vegetables, whole grains, fish, poultry, lean meat, and low fat dairy products as a means to derive antioxidant vitamin benefits. CVD risk reduction can be achieved by the long-term consumption of a diet that meets the AHA Dietary Guidelines and that promotes the long-term maintenance of a healthy body weight

TABLE 11-13 Macronutrient Recommendations/Guidelines*

	National Academy of Science Dietary-reference intakes[89]	American Diabetes Association[186]	NHLBI NCEP ATP-III[41]	USDA dietary guidelines[184]	AHA dietary guidelines[88,185]
Total fat (%)	20–35	< 30	25–35	< 30	< 30
Saturated fat (%)	Low as possible	< 10 < 7 (high risk)	< 7	< 10	< 10 <7 (high risk)
MUFA (%)	—	—	≤20	—	Unsaturated for SFA
PUFA (%)	5–10	~ 10	≤10%	—	Unsaturated for SFA
Omega-6 linoleic acid (%)	5–10%	—	—	—	—
Omega-3 linoleic acid (%)	0.6–1.2	—	—	—	2 servings fatty fish/wk
Trans fat	Low as possible	Minimize intake	Keep intake low	Reduce intake	TFA + SFA < 10%
Cholesterol (mg/d)	Low as possible	< 300 < 200 (high risk)	< 200	< 300	< 300
Carbohydrate (%)	45–65	60–70	50–60	6–11 servings	≥6 servings, include 3 servings whole grains
Protein	10–35	≤20	15	2–3 servings	50–100 g/d
Fiber (g/d)	21–38	—	20–30	≥6 servings grain products daily	> 25

*Values are expressed as percentages of calories unless indicated otherwise.

achieved through balancing energy intake with regular physical activity.

TREATMENT GUIDELINES FOR HYPERCHOLESTEROLEMIA, HYPERTENSION, AND WEIGHT CONTROL

Guidelines have been issued by the NIH/NHLBI for the prevention and treatment of high blood cholesterol,[41] high blood pressure,[115] and overweight and obesity.[188] Resources are available from NIH/NHLBI and the AHA to facilitate implementation of these treatment guidelines.

Therapeutic lifestyle changes

NCEP ATP-III recommends a multifactorial approach to reducing the risk of CHD. The Therapeutic Lifestyle Changes (TLC) diet/approach is recommended to achieve the LDL-C goal. The components of TLC are:

- Reduced intakes of saturated fats and *trans* fats (<7% energy) and cholesterol (<200 mg/d)
- Therapeutic dietary options for enhancing LDL-C lowering (plant stanols/sterols [2 g/d] and increased viscous [soluble] fiber [10–25 g/d])
- Weight reduction
- Increased regular physical activity

The cumulative estimate of LDL-C lowering that could be expected with implementation of TLC (including a 10-lb weight loss) is 20 to 30%.

Treatment guidelines for high blood pressure (JNC-7)

The treatment guidelines of the Joint National Committee on Prevention, Detection, Evaluation, and Treatment

TABLE 11-14 Food-Based Dietary Recommendations

Population goal	Major guidelines
Overall healthy eating pattern	Include a variety of fruits, vegetables, grains, low-fat or nonfat dairy products, fish, legumes, poultry, lean meats
Appropriate body weight	Match energy intake to energy needs, with appropriate changes to achieve weight loss when indicated
Desirable cholesterol profile	Limit foods high in saturated fat and cholesterol; substitute unsaturated fat from vegetables, fish, legumes, nuts
Desirable blood pressure	Limit salt and alcohol; maintain healthy body weight and diet with emphasis on vegetables, fruits, and low-fat or nonfat dairy products.

SOURCE: Adapted, with permission, from Krauss et al.[88]

of High Blood Pressure[115] define the goals of therapy for hypertension as a SBP less than 140 mm Hg and a DBP less than 90 mm Hg. For hypertensive diabetic patients or patients with renal disease, the target is less than 130/80 mm Hg. Newly defined is the category *prehypertension*, which is classified as a SBP of 120 to 139 mm Hg and a DBP of 80 to 89 mm Hg.

Lifestyle modifications are the cornerstone of the treatment of hypertension and include:

- Reduce weight for those who are overweight or obese. A 10-kg weight loss has been associated with a 5 to 20 mm Hg reduction in SBP.
- Consume the DASH diet, which has been associated with an 8 to 14 mm Hg reduction in SBP.
- Limit sodium intake to no more than 2.4 g sodium (6 g sodium chloride). Reduction in dietary sodium may lower SBP 2 to 8 mm Hg.
- Engage in regular aerobic physical activity for 30 minutes per day, most days of the week. This type of activity may lower SBP 4 to 9 mm Hg.
- Consume alcohol in moderation for those who already drink alcohol (no more than two drinks per day for men and one drink [1 oz ethanol = 24 oz beer, 10 oz wine, or 3 oz 80-proof whiskey] per day for women and lighter-weight men). Moderate alcohol consumption has been shown to lower SBP 2 to 4 mm Hg.

Lifestyle modifications not only lower blood pressure but also enhance antihypertensive drug efficacy and, pos-

sibly, alleviate the need for drug therapy. On a population level, even a small decrease in DBP of 2 mm Hg has been estimated to reduce the prevalence of hypertension, the risk of CHD, and the risk of stroke by 17, 6, and 15%, respectively.[189]

Clinical guidelines on the identification, evaluation, and treatment of overweight and obesity in adults

The recommended goals and strategies for weight loss and weight maintenance are presented in the Evidence Report.[188] A weight loss target and timeline must be individualized although a 10% weight loss over a 6-month period is reasonable for many patients. An energy deficit of 500 to 1000 calories per day that is achieved through decreased food consumption and increased physical activity is recommended. The weight loss diet recommended should be consistent with good health (low in saturated fat and cholesterol) and teach patients new eating habits they can follow for a lifetime. Thus, a weight maintenance program is essential to help patients maintain their weight loss. Frequent follow-up and monitoring provide the support and encouragement required for successful weight loss.

It is evident that weight loss depends on a calorie deficit. Because of the obesity epidemic, there is significant interest in various diet approaches to achieve weight loss. This has resulted in a plethora of weight loss diets that differ in many ways, but most notably in their macronutrient profile. The low-carbohydrate, ketogenic diet (ie, high-protein diet) has gained widespread popularity. Examples include the Atkins diet, the Zone diet, the South Beach diet, among others. In an extensive analysis assessing the efficacy of low-carbohydrate diets, Bravata and co-workers found that they were associated with reduced calorie intake and weight loss that was the result of a decreased calorie intake.[190] Other studies have reported that decreasing fat (approximately 25% of calories from fat) facilitates decreasing calories and, hence, weight loss.[191] Another recent study reported that a moderate-fat (35% of calories) diet resulted in a more favorable, long-term weight loss than did a low-fat diet.[192] Thus, collectively these studies demonstrate that macronutrient profile can be changed in different ways to achieve weight loss. Of note, though, is that the overall nutrient profile of the diet should be nutritionally adequate and consistent with current dietary guidelines for heart health. This is the basis of the AHA Science Advisory on dietary protein and weight reduction, which does not recommend high-protein diets because individuals who follow these diets could be at risk for compromised vitamin and mineral intake, as well as potential cardiac, renal, bone, and liver problems.[193]

PHYSICAL ACTIVITY IN PARTNERSHIP WITH A HEALTHY DIET TO REDUCE CVD RISK

Physical activity recommendations have been made to prevent chronic disease. This guidance works synergistically with dietary recommendations to lower CVD risk. The Surgeon General's Report on Physical Activity and Health, the AHA,[194,195] the American College of Sports Medicine,[194,196] the Dietary Guidelines,[197] and the NCEP[41] recommend that adults accumulate at least 30 minutes of moderate physical activity on most, if not all, days of the week. These national groups recommend 60 minutes of moderate physical activity daily for weight control during the adult years.

Assessing diet, physical activity, and lifestyle practices for heart health

Collecting information about dietary patterns, physical activity practices, and other lifestyle practices is important for individualizing interventions for heart health. A very brief dietary questionnaire can be used to assess intake of saturated fat and cholesterol. The CAGE Questionnaire is presented in Table 11-15.[41] This questionnaire is useful in reinforcing diet messages by the physician during follow-up visits. A more extensive questionnaire, MEDFICTS (Table 11-16), has been developed for systematic dietary assessment, typically carried out by a nutrition professional.[41] This questionnaire also can be used to teach patients the principles of a cholesterol-lowering diet.

THE GAP BETWEEN KNOWLEDGE AND CLINICAL APPLICATION

Despite impressive advances that have been made to date in nutrition, physical activity, and other lifestyle behaviors that can markedly reduce the risk of CVD, perhaps by as much as 90%, it is apparent that "both health providers and members of the public are not applying what we know" to achieve significant decreases in CVD morbidity and mortality.[198] For example, using data from the Fourth National Health and Nutrition Examination Survey (NHANES-IV) 1999 to 2000, Ford and colleagues reported that although virtually all hypercholesterolemic population groups, including men and women of different ethnicity, aged 20 and older had their cholesterol levels checked (ie, on average > 60%), far fewer were aware that they had hypercholesterolemia (ie, about 35%), only about 10 to 15% were being treated for elevated cholesterol levels (see Fig. 11-1), and alarmingly fewer than 10% had achieved a total cholesterol less than 200 mg/dL.[199] It is of further concern that population cholesterol levels have decreased only about 1% between NHANES-III (1988–1994) and NHANES-IV (1999–2000).[199] This latter observation is a graphic reminder of the shortcomings of the application of science to public health.

This gap in applying existing scientific knowledge, as well as treatment guidelines, is looming as a significant barrier to further, major reductions in CVD risk. Physicians and other health care professionals, as well as patients, share the responsibility for the effective application of clinical medicine. Another major contributor to the problem is the lack of patient compliance. For instance, between 29 and 56% of patients discontinue antihypertensive therapy by 12 months.[198] It is vitally important that health care professionals effectively acquire and disseminate the latest and most appropriate clinical knowledge in practice. This will require new approaches for disseminating the vast amount of new information. In addition, with new information in hand, health care professionals must be skilled in communicating this to their patients in a way that results in long-term compliance. NCEP ATP-III has emphasized the importance of strategic approaches to lifestyle interventions to achieve long-term adherence.[41] The behavior literature offers effective strategies to health care professionals that can be most helpful in enhancing patient adherence to lifestyle intervention strategies to decrease CVD risk.

TABLE 11-15 Dietary CAGE Questionnaire for Assessing Saturated Fat and Cholesterol Intake

C—Cheese (and other sources of dairy fats: whole milk, 2% milk, ice cream, cream, whole-fat yogurt)
A—Animal fats (hamburger, ground meat, frankfurters, bologna, salami, sausage, fried foods, fatty cuts of meat)
G—Got it away from home (high-fat meals either purchased and brought home or eaten in restaurants)
E—Eat (extra) high-fat commercial products: candy, pastries, pies, doughnuts, cookies

SOURCE: Reproduced, with permission, from NCEP ATP-III.[41]

THE IMPORTANCE OF A MULTIDISCIPLINARY APPROACH IN DIETARY MANAGEMENT FOR CVD RISK REDUCTION

The role of the physician

Interventions that have produced the greatest improvements in patient adherence and outcomes involve a multidisciplinary team. A multidisciplinary team should include a physician, nurse, pharmacist, exercise physiologist, and registered dietitian. Additional counselors may be used for smoking cessation and stress management.

TABLE 11-16 MEDFICTS Dietary Assessment Questionnaire

Sample Dietary Assessment Questionaire
MEDFICTS*

In each food category for both Group 1 and Group 2 foods check one box from the "Weekly Consumption" column (number of servings eaten per week) and then check one box from the "Serving Size" column. If you check Rarely/Never, do not check a serving size box. See next page for score.

Food Category	Weekly Consumption			Serving Size			Score
	Rarely/ never	3 or less	4 or more	Small <5 oz/d 1 pt	Average 5 oz/d 2 pts	Large >5 oz/d 3 pts	

Meats

- Recommended amount per day: ≤5 oz (equal in size to 2 decks of playing cards).
- Base your estimate on the food you consume most often.
- Beef and lamb selections are trimmed to 1/8" fat.

Group 1. 10g or more total fat in 3 oz cooked portion

Beef – Ground beef, Ribs, Steak (T-bone, Flank, Porterhouse, Tenderloin), Chuck blade roast, Brisket, Meatloaf (w/ground beef), Corned beef **Processed meats** – ¼ lb burger or lg. sandwich, Bacon, Lunch meat, Sausage/knockwurst, Hot dogs, Ham (bone-end), Ground turkey **Other meats, Poultry, Seafood**–Pork chops (center loin), Pork roast (Blade, Boston, Sirloin), Pork spareribs, Ground pork, Lamb chops, Lamb (ribs), Organ meats†, Chicken w/skin, Eel, Mackerel, Pompano	☐	☐ 3 pts	☐ 7 pts x	☐ 1 pt	☐ 2 pts	☐ 3 pts	—

Group 2. Less than 10g total fat in 3 oz cooked portion

Lean beef – Round steak (Eye of round, Top round), Sirloin‡, Tip & bottom round‡, Chuck arm pot roast‡, Top Loin‡ **Low-fat processed meats** – Low-fat lunch meat, Canadian bacon, "Lean" fast food sandwich, Boneless ham **Other meats, Poultry, Seafood** – Chicken, Turkey (w/o skin)§, most Seafood†, Lamb leg shank, Pork tenderloin, Sirloin top loin, Veal cutlets, Sirloin, Shoulder, Ground veal, Venlson, Veal chops and ribs‡, Lamb (whole leg, loin, fore-shank, sirloin)‡	☐	☐	☐ x	☐	☐	☐ 6 pts	—

Eggs – Weekly consumption is the number of times you eat eggs each week | Check the number of eggs eaten each time

				≤1	2	≥3	
Group 1. Whole eggs, Yolks	☐	☐ 3 pts	☐ 7 pts x	☐ 1 pt	☐ 2 pts	☐ 3 pts	—
Group 2. Egg whites, Egg substitutes (½ cup)	☐	☐	☐	☐	☐	☐	—

FIG MEDFICTS assessment tool.
* MEDFICTS was orginally developed for and printed in the Second Adult Treatment Panel of the National Cholesterol Educational Program.

(continued)

TABLE 11-16 *(Continued)*

Food Category	Weekly Consumption			Serving Size			Score
	Rarely/ never	3 or less	4 or more	Small <5 oz/d 1 pt	Average 5 oz/d 2 pts	Large >5 oz/d 3 pts	

Dairy

Milk – Average serving 1 cup
Group 1. Whole milk, 2% milk, 2% buttermilk, Yogurt (whole milk)

| | ☐ | ☐ 3 pts | ☐ 7 pts x | ☐ 1 pt | ☐ 2 pts | ☐ 3 pts | ____ |

Group 2. Fat-free milk, 1% milk, Fat-free buttermilk, Yogurt (Fat-free, 1% low fat)

| | ☐ | ☐ | ☐ | ☐ | ☐ | ☐ | ____ |

Cheese – Average serving 1 oz
Group 1. Cream cheese, Cheddar, Monterey Jack, Colby, Swiss, American processed, Blue cheese, Regular cottage cheese ($1/2$ cup), and Ricotta ($1/4$ cup)

| | ☐ | ☐ 3 pts | ☐ 7 pts x | ☐ 1 pt | ☐ 2 pts | ☐ 3 pts | ____ |

Group 2. Low-fat & fat-free cheeses, Fat-free milk mozzarella, String cheese, Low-fat, Fat-free milk & Fat-free cottage cheese ($1/2$ cup) and Ricotta ($1/4$ cup)

| | ☐ | ☐ | ☐ | ☐ | ☐ | ☐ | ____ |

Frozen Desserts – Average serving $1/2$ cup
Group 1. Ice cream, Milk shakes

| | ☐ | ☐ 3 pts | ☐ 7 pts x | ☐ 1 pt | ☐ 2 pts | ☐ 3 pts | ____ |

Group 2. Low-fat ice cream, Frozen yogurt

| | ☐ | ☐ | ☐ | ☐ | ☐ | ☐ | ____ |

Frying Foods - Average servings: see below. This section refers to method of preparation for vegetables and meat.

Group 1. French fries, Fried vegetables ($1/2$ cup), Fried chicken, fish, meat (3 oz)

| | ☐ | ☐ 3 pts | ☐ 7 pts x | ☐ 1 pt | ☐ 2 pts | ☐ 3 pts | ____ |

Group 2. Vegetables, not deep fried ($1/2$ cup), Meat, poultry, or fish— prepared by baking, broiling, grilling, poaching, roasting, stewing: (3 oz)

| | ☐ | ☐ | ☐ | ☐ | ☐ | ☐ | ____ |

In Baked Goods – 1 Average serving

Group 1. Doughnuts, Biscuits, Butter rolls, Muffins, Croissants, Sweet rolls, Danish, Cakes, Pies, Coffee cakes, Cookies

| | ☐ | ☐ 3 pts | ☐ 7 pts x | ☐ 1 pt | ☐ 2 pts | ☐ 3 pts | ____ |

Group 2. Fruit bars, Low-fat cookies/cakes/pastries, Angel food cake, Homemade baked goods with vegetable oils, breads, bagels

| | ☐ | ☐ | ☐ | ☐ | ☐ | ☐ | ____ |

Convenience Foods

Group 1. Canned, Packaged, or Frozen dinners: e.g., Pizza (1 slice), Macaroni & cheese (1 cup), Pot pie (1), Cream soups (1 cup), Potato, rice & pasta dishes with cream/cheese sauces ($1/2$ cup)

| | ☐ | ☐ 3 pts | ☐ 7 pts x | ☐ 1 pt | ☐ 2 pts | ☐ 3 pts | ____ |

Group 2. Diet/Reduced calorie or reduced fat dinners (1), Potato, rice & pasta dishes without cream/cheese sauces ($1/2$ cup)

| | ☐ | ☐ | ☐ | ☐ | ☐ | ☐ | ____ |

(continued)

TABLE 11-16 (Continued)

Food Category	Weekly Consumption			Serving Size			Score
	Rarely/ never	3 or less	4 or more	Small <5 oz/d 1 pt	Average 5 oz/d 2 pts	Large >5 oz/d 3 pts	
Convenience Foods							
Table Fats Average serving:1 Tbsp							
Group 1. Butter, Stick margarine, Regular salad dressing, Mayonnaise, Sour cream (2 Tbsp)	☐	☐ 3 pts	☐ 7 pts	x ☐ 1 pt	☐ 2 pts	☐ 3 pts	___
Group 2. Diet and tub margarine, Low-fat & fat-free salad dressing, Low-fat & fat-free mayonnaise	☐	☐	☐	☐	☐	☐	___
Snacks							
Group 1. Chips (potato, corn, taco), Cheese puffs, Snack mix, Nuts (1 oz), Regular crackers (½ oz), Candy (milk chocolate, caramel, coconut) (about 1½ oz), Regular popcorn (3 cups)	☐	☐ 3 pts	☐ 7 pts	x ☐ 1 pt	☐ 2 pts	☐ 3 pts	___
Group 2. Pretzels, Fat-free chips (1 oz), Low-fat crackers (½ oz), Fruit, Fruit rolls, Licorice, Hard candy (1 med piece), Bread sticks (1–2 pcs), Air popped or low-fat popcorn (3 cups)	☐	☐	☐	☐	☐	☐	___

Total from page 1 ___

[†] Organ meats, shrimp, abalone, and squid are low in fat but high in cholesterol.
[‡] Only lean cuts with all visible fat trimmed. If not trimmed of all visible fat, score as if in Group 1.
[*] Score 6 pts if this box is checked.
[§] All parts not listed in group 1 have <10g total fat.

Total from page 2 ___

Final Score ___

To Score: For each food category, multiply points in weekly consumption box by points in serving size box and record total in score column. If Group 2 foods checked, no points are scored (except for Group 2 meats, large serving = 6 pts).

Example:

☐	☐ 3 pts	☑ 7 pts	x	☐ 1 pt	☐ 2 pts	☑ 3 pts	21 pts

Add score on page 1 and page 2 to get final score.

Key:
≥ 70   Need to make some dietary changes
40–70   Heart-Healthy Diet
<40   TLC Diet

Although this may be the ideal model, it often is not practical in many primary care settings. Consequently, it is important for physicians to assume a leadership role in promoting lifestyle interventions with their patients.

Because treatment begins in the physician's office, dietary guidance should be given at this time and subsequently. Nutrition counseling is estimated to occur in only 25% of all office visits to family physicians.[200] Rea-

sons for this include short visit times, the lack of nutrition teaching in medical schools, and poor compliance of patients with physicians' dietary prescriptions.[201] In addition, links between diet and disease are complicated, and often are difficult to explain to patients.[202]

The short duration of patient encounters in the primary care setting remains a reality. However, simply "priming" patients in a primary care setting can produce

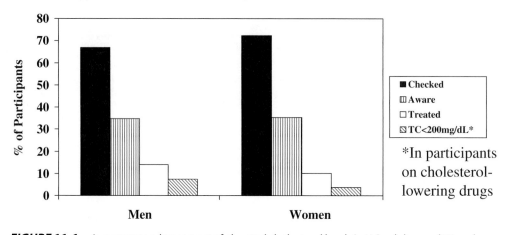

FIGURE 11-1 Awareness and treatment of elevated cholesterol levels in U.S. adults aged 20 and over. (Adapted, with permission, from Ford et al.[198])

significant changes in risk factor modification. Kreuter and colleagues sought to identify the differences in the ways patients respond to printed behavior change materials based on whether their primary care physician had previously advised them to change the same behavior.[203] Patients who reported receiving physician advice to quit smoking, eat less fat, or get more exercise prior to receiving printed materials on the same topics were more likely to remember the material, share it with a friend or family member, and perceive the material as applying to them, compared with patients who did not report receiving advice from their primary care physician.

In a study designed to evaluate the effectiveness of a training program for physician-delivered nutrition counseling, alone and in combination with an office-support program, researchers determined that brief physician nutrition counseling can produce beneficial changes in diet, weight, and blood lipids.[204] Physicians were randomized into one of three groups: (1) usual care, (2) physician nutrition counseling training, and (3) physician nutrition counseling training plus an office-support program. Results at the 1-year follow-up demonstrate that patients in the most intensive treatment group experienced a decrease in percentage of energy from saturated fat (10.3% kcal), weight (2.3 kg), and LDL-C (3.8 mg/dL), compared with the usual care group,[204] indicating the potential benefit of a multidisciplinary approach.

The role of the registered dietitian

A registered dietitian or qualified nutrition professional is a key member of the multidisciplinary team because nutrition is a cornerstone for the prevention and treatment of CVD. On physician referral, a patient may seek individualized dietitian intervention, referred to as medical nutrition therapy (MNT), for the treatment of hypercholesterolemia and hypertension. Medical nutrition therapy uses patient-centered counseling that targets the diet of the patient to treat hypercholesterolemia. A study conducted by Henkin and associates reported a significantly greater LDL-C-lowering effect at 3 months in hypercholesterolemic patients who were counseled (two to four times, over the 3 months) by a dietitian versus a physician ($-11.4 \pm 1.3\%$ vs $-6.6 \pm 1.4\%$), respectively ($P < .004$).[204] Moreover, a significantly greater percentage of subjects counseled by a dietitian achieved a 10% or greater reduction in LDL-C (65% vs 35%, respectively). Thus, the study by Henkin and associates has demonstrated significant benefits of dietitian intervention for LDL-C lowering.[205] Comparable effects have been observed in several other studies in which dietitians were used. Katzel and co-workers showed reductions in total cholesterol levels associated with increased time spent with a dietitian.[206] In this study involving elderly men with silent myocardial ischemia, a Step 1 isocaloric diet was compared with a Step 1 hypocaloric diet for 3 months. Triglycerides, LDL-C, and LDL-C/HDL-C ratio were decreased 44, 18, and 19%, respectively. Sikand and colleagues found that nutrition intervention provided by registered dietitians reduced total cholesterol by 13% ($P < .001$), LDL-C by 15% ($P < .0001$), triglycerides by 11% ($P < .05$), and HDL-C by 4% ($P < .05$) in an 8-week study in which a group of hypercholesterolemic subjects were provided nutrition therapy before the initiation of cholesterol-lowering medications.[207] More than half of the subjects (51%) were no longer candidates for drug therapy following dietary counseling. Furthermore, the results of Henkin and associates underscore the importance of long-term follow-up by a dietitian, as the cholesterol-lowering effects were diminished by approximately 50% in both groups at 12 months.[205]

Because of the importance of nutrition in the prevention and treatment of CVD and the relative shortage of registered dietitians for MNT, it is essential nutrition be more widely integrated in the curricula of other health professions. A signature program (Nutrition Academic Award Program) has been launched by NIH/NHBLI to integrate more nutrition into medical school curricula. Presently, 15 medical schools are part of this pioneering program. This is a program with great promise; however, additional novel educational programs will be needed.

Both the AHA and NCEP support nutrition therapy as an essential component of the treatment of dyslipidemia. The observational and clinical trial evidence clearly indicates that lipid profiles are improved through implementation of nutrition therapy. Thus, from a health care perspective, including associated costs, the services of a registered dietitian can beneficially affect CVD health and, as is apparent, also reduce health care costs including Medicare costs, because CVD is highly prevalent in this cohort. Registered dietitians currently are the primary group of health care professionals with the necessary type of education and training to provide a level of nutrition service that should be considered a covered benefit for Medicare beneficiaries.

The projected reduction attainable by providing additional MNT is not only of clinical significance from the perspective of a reduction in CVD events, but also in terms of health care costs. The economic cost of CVD is greater than $350 billion annually in the United States.[13] Evaluation of the cost-effectiveness of nutrition therapy by a registered dietitian involves taking into account both direct and indirect costs and is thus quite complex. However, even a 1% decrease in LDL-C has been shown to decrease CVD risk by ≈1.5%. In the study by Henkin and associates, those subjects counseled by a dietitian achieved a 10% or greater reduction in LDL-C or, according to the previous statement, a 15% CVD risk reduction.[205] MNT has been shown to be a cost-effective intervention in the treatment of patients with hypercholesterolemia in a study by Sikand and co-workers, in which an average of three individualized visits with a registered dietitian (1 hour each) over an 8-week period resulted in a savings of $3.03 in drug therapy for each dollar spent on MNT.[208]

SUMMARY

Our current understanding of the role that diet plays in reducing elevated blood cholesterol and hypertension, major CVD risk factors, has positioned us to make unprecedented strides to substantially lower CVD morbidity and mortality. Importantly, the emerging era integrates multiple dietary strategies that beneficially impact many CVD risk factors, with the consequent outcome of even greater benefits of diet. A cardioprotective diet should emphasize fruits and vegetables, whole grains, legumes, lean meats, poultry and fish (especially fatty fish), low-fat dairy products, food sources of unsaturated fats, and alcohol in moderation (for those who drink). Achieving and maintaining a healthy body weight and a regular program of physical activity also are important to achieve the maximal reduction in CVD risk possible. Many dietary guidelines have been issued by different agencies/organizations to reduce risk of CVD and other chronic diseases. However, there remains a large gap between science knowledge and its application to the reduction of CVD on a population basis. Health care professionals and health care teams must strive to narrow this gap and assume a central role in effectively translating new science to prevention and treatment activities. Successful implementation of lifestyle practices that include diet and physical activity will help achieve a major public health goal, a marked reduction in the burden of CVD.

ACKNOWLEDGMENTS

The authors thank Amy Binkoski, Amy Griel, Gigi Meyer, and Dr. Terry Etherton for assistance in the preparation of this chapter.

REFERENCES

1. Greenland P, Knoll MD, Stamler J, et al. Major risk factors as antecedents of fatal and nonfatal coronary heart disease events. *JAMA* 2003;290:891–897.

2. Khot UN, Khot MB, Bajzer CT, et al. Prevalence of conventional risk factors in patients with coronary heart disease. *JAMA* 2003;290:898–904.

3. Hu FB, Willett WC. Optimal diets for prevention of coronary heart disease. *JAMA* 2002;288:2569–2578.

4. Hackam DG, Anand SS. Emerging risk factors for atherosclerotic vascular disease: a critical review of the evidence. *JAMA* 2003;290:932–940.

5. Kromhout D, Menotti A, Kesteloot H, et al. Prevention of coronary heart disease by diet and lifestyle: evidence from prospective cross-cultural, cohort, and intervention studies. *Circulation* 2002;105:893–898.

6. Trichopoulou A, Costacou T, Bamia C, et al. Adherence to a Mediterranean diet and survival in a Greek population. *N Engl J Med* 2003;348:2599–2608.

7. McCullough ML, Feskanich D, Stampfer MJ, et al. Diet quality and major chronic disease risk in men and women: moving toward improved dietary guidance. *Am J Clin Nutr* 2002;76:1261–1271.

8. Michels KB, Wolk A. A prospective study of variety of healthy foods and mortality in women. *Int J Epidemiol* 2002;31:847–854.

9. Kant AK, Schatzkin A, Graubard BI, et al. A prospective study of diet quality and mortality in women. *JAMA* 2000;283:2109–2115.

10. Stampfer MJ, Hu FB, Manson JE, et al. Primary prevention of coronary heart disease in women through diet and lifestyle. *N Engl J Med* 2000;343:16–22.

11. Millen BE, Quatromoni PA, Nam BH, et al. Dietary patterns and the odds of carotid atherosclerosis in women: the Framingham Nutrition Studies. *Prev Med* 2002;35:540–547.

12. Fung TT, Rimm EB, Spiegelman D, et al. Association between dietary patterns and plasma biomarkers of obesity and cardiovascular disease risk. *Am J Clin Nutr* 2001;73:61–67.

13. American Heart Association. Heart disease and stroke statistics—2003 update. Dallas, Tex: American Heart Association; 2002.

14. Slavin J, Jacobs D, Marquart L. Whole-grain consumption and chronic disease: protective mechanisms. *Nutr Cancer* 1997;27:14–21.

15. Slavin JL, Martini MC, Jacobs DR, et al. Plausible mechanisms for the protectiveness of whole grains. *Am J Clin Nutr* 1999;70:459S–463S

16. Jacobs DR Jr, Meyer KA, Kushi LH, et al. Whole-grain intake may reduce the risk of ischemic heart disease death in postmenopausal women: the Iowa Women's Health Study. *Am J Clin Nutr* 1998;68:248–257.

17. Fraser GE, Sabate J, Beeson WL, et al. A possible protective effect of nut consumption on risk of coronary heart disease: the Adventist Health Study. *Arch Intern Med* 1992;152:1416–1424.

18. Fraser GE. Associations between diet and cancer, ischemic heart disease, and all-cause mortality in non-Hispanic white California Seventh-Day Adventists. *Am J Clin Nutr* 1999;70:532S–538S.

19. Liu S, Sesso HD, Manson JE, et al. Is intake of breakfast cereals related to total and cause-specific mortality in men? *Am J Clin Nutr* 2003;77:594–599.

20. Liu S, Stampfer MJ, Hu FB, et al. Whole-grain consumption and risk of coronary heart disease: results from the Nurses' Health Study. *Am J Clin Nutr* 1999;70:412–419.

21. Liu S, Manson JE, Stampfer MJ, et al. Whole grain consumption and risk of ischemic stroke in women: a prospective study. *JAMA* 2000;284:1534–1540.

22. Rimm EB, Ascherio A, Giovannucci E, et al. Vegetable, fruit, and cereal fiber intake and risk of coronary heart disease among men. *JAMA* 1996;275:447–451.

23. Wolk A, Manson JE, Stampfer MJ, et al. Long-term intake of dietary fiber and decreased risk of coronary heart disease among women. *JAMA* 1999;281:1998–2004.

24. Pietinen P, Rimm EB, Korhonen P, et al. Intake of dietary fiber and risk of coronary heart disease in a cohort of Finnish men: the Alpha-Tocopherol, Beta-Carotene Cancer Prevention Study. *Circulation* 1996;94:2720–2727.

25. Ascherio A, Rimm EB, Giovannucci EL, et al. A prospective study of nutritional factors and hypertension among US men. *Circulation* 1992;86:1475–1484.

26. He J, Klag MJ, Whelton PK, et al. Oats and buckwheat intakes and cardiovascular disease risk factors in an ethnic minority of China. *Am J Clin Nutr* 1995;61:366–372.

27. Montonen J, Knekt P, Jarvinen R, et al. Whole-grain and fiber intake and the incidence of type 2 diabetes. *Am J Clin Nutr* 2003;77:622–629.

28. Fung TT, Hu FB, Pereira MA, et al. Whole-grain intake and the risk of type 2 diabetes: a prospective study in men. *Am J Clin Nutr* 2002;76:535–540.

29. McKeown NM, Meigs JB, Liu S, et al. Whole-grain intake is favorably associated with metabolic risk factors for type 2 diabetes and cardiovascular disease in the Framingham Offspring Study. *Am J Clin Nutr* 2002;76:390–398.

30. Bazzano LA, He J, Ogden LG, et al. Legume consumption and risk of coronary heart disease in US men and women: NHANES I Epidemiologic Follow-up Study. *Arch Intern Med* 2001;161:2573–2578.

31. Menotti A, Kromhout D, Blackburn H, et al, for the Seven Countries Study Research Group. Food intake patterns and 25-year mortality from coronary heart disease: cross-cultural correlations in the Seven Countries Study. *Eur J Epidemiol* 1999;15:507–515.

32. Zhao W, Chen J. Implications from and for food cultures for cardiovascular disease: diet, nutrition and cardiovascular diseases in China. *Asia Pac J Clin Nutr* 2001;10:146–152.

33. Joshipura KJ, Hu FB, Manson JE, et al. The effect of fruit and vegetable intake on risk for coronary heart disease. *Ann Intern Med* 2001;134;1106–1114.

34. Wang HJ MP[JP1]. Isoflavone content in commercial soybean foods. *J Agric Food Chem* 1994;42:1666.

35. Sasazuki S. Case–control study of nonfatal myocardial infarction in relation to selected foods in Japanese men and women. *Jpn Circ J* 2001;65:200–206.

36. Anderson JW, Johnstone BM, Cook-Newell ME. Meta-analysis of the effects of soy protein intake on serum lipids. *N Engl J Med* 1995;333:276–282.

37. Anderson JW, Gustafson NJ. Hypocholesterolemic effects of oat and bean products. *Am J Clin Nutr* 1988;48:749–753.

38. Anderson JW, Gustafson NJ, Spencer DB, et al. Serum lipid response of hypercholesterolemic men to single and divided doses of canned beans. *Am J Clin Nutr* 1990;51:1013–1019.

39. Van Horn L. Fiber, lipids, and coronary heart disease: a statement for healthcare professionals from the Nutrition Committee, American Heart Association. *Circulation* 1997;95:2701–2704.

40. Anderson JJ, Anthony MS, Cline JM, et al. Health potential of soy isoflavones for menopausal women. *Public Health Nutr* 1999;2:489–504.

41. Expert Panel on Detection, Evaluation, and Treatment of High Blood Cholesterol in Adults. Executive Summary of the Third Report of The National Cholesterol Education Program (NCEP) Expert Panel on Detection, Evaluation, And Treatment of High Blood Cholesterol in Adults (Adult Treatment Panel III). *JAMA* 2001;285:2486–2497.

42. Rotondo S, de Gaetano G. Protection from cardiovascular disease by wine and its derived products: epidemiological evidence and biological mechanisms. *World Rev Nutr Diet* 2000;87:90–113.

43. Rimm EB, Klatsky A, Grobbee D, et al. Review of moderate alcohol consumption and reduced risk of coronary heart disease: is the effect due to beer, wine, or spirits? *BMJ* 1996;312:731–736.

44. Mukamal KJ, Conigrave KM, Mittleman MA, et al. Roles of drinking pattern and type of alcohol consumed in coronary heart disease in men. *N Engl J Med* 2003;348:109–118.

45. Berger K, Ajani UA, Kase CS, et al. Light-to-moderate alcohol consumption and risk of stroke among U.S. male physicians. *N Engl J Med* 1999;341:1557–1564.

46. Sacco RL, Elkind M, Boden-Albala B, et al. The protective effect of moderate alcohol consumption on ischemic stroke. *JAMA* 1999;281:53–60.

47. Stampfer MJ, Colditz GA, Willett WC, et al. A prospective study of moderate alcohol consumption and the risk of coronary disease and stroke in women. *N Engl J Med* 1988;319:267–273.

48. Reynolds K, Lewis B, Nolen JD, et al. Alcohol consumption and risk of stroke: a meta-analysis. *JAMA* 2003;289:579–588.

49. Klatsky AL: Commentary: could abstinence from alcohol be hazardous to your health? *Int J Epidemiol* 2001;30:739–742.

50. Rimm EB, Williams P, Fosher K, et al. Moderate alcohol intake and lower risk of coronary heart disease: meta-analysis of effects on lipids and haemostatic factors. *BMJ* 1999;319:1523–1528.

51. Mukamal KJ, Jadhav PP, D'Agostino RB, et al. Alcohol consumption and hemostatic factors: analysis of the Framingham Offspring cohort. *Circulation* 2001;104:1367–1373.

52. Gaziano JM, Buring JE, Breslow JL, et al. Moderate alcohol intake, increased levels of high-density lipoprotein and its subfractions, and decreased risk of myocardial infarction. *N Engl J Med* 1993;329:1829–1834.

53. Mezzano D, Leighton F, Martinez C, et al. Complementary effects of Mediterranean diet and moderate red wine intake on haemostatic cardiovascular risk factors. *Eur J Clin Nutr* 2001;55:444–451.

54. Pearson TA. Alcohol and heart disease: AHA Medical/Scientific Statement. *Circulation* 1996;94:3023–3025.

55. Joshipura KJ, Ascherio A, Manson JE, et al. Fruit and vegetable intake in relation to risk of ischemic stroke. *JAMA* 1999;282:1233–1239.

56. Liu S, Manson JE, Lee IM, et al. Fruit and vegetable intake and risk of cardiovascular disease: the Women's Health Study. *Am J Clin Nutr* 2000;72:922–928.

57. Liu S, Lee IM, Ajani U, et al. Intake of vegetables rich in carotenoids and risk of coronary heart disease in men: the Physicians' Health Study. *Int J Epidemiol* 2001;30:130–135.

58. Bazzano LA, He J, Ogden LG, et al. Fruit and vegetable intake and risk of cardiovascular disease in US adults: the first National Health and Nutrition Examination Survey Epidemiologic Follow-up Study. *Am J Clin Nutr* 2002;76:93–99.

59. Lanza E, Jones DY, Block G, et al. Dietary fiber intake in the US population. *Am J Clin Nutr* 1987;46:790–797.

60. Appel LJ, Moore TJ, Obarzanek E, et al, for the DASH Collaborative Research Group. A clinical trial of the effects of dietary patterns on blood pressure. *N Engl J Med* 1997;336:1117–1124.

61. Sacks FM, Svetkey LP, Vollmer WM, et al, for the DASH–Sodium Collaborative Research Group. Effects on blood pressure of reduced dietary sodium and the Dietary Approaches to Stop Hypertension (DASH) diet. *N Engl J Med* 2001;344:3–10.

62. Sabate J. Nut consumption, vegetarian diets, ischemic heart disease risk, and all-cause mortality: evidence from epidemiologic studies. *Am J Clin Nutr* 1999;70:500S–503S.

63. Fraser GE. Nut consumption, lipids, and risk of a coronary event. *Clin Cardiol* 1999;22:III11–III15.

64. Sabate J. Does nut consumption protect against ischaemic heart disease? *Eur J Clin Nutr* 1993;47 Suppl 1:S71–S75.

65. Fraser GE, Lindsted KD, Beeson WL. Effect of risk factor values on lifetime risk of and age at first coronary event: the Adventist Health Study. *Am J Epidemiol* 1995;142:746–758.

66. Fraser GE, Sumbureru D, Pribis P, et al. Association among health habits, risk factors, and all-cause mortality in a black California population. *Epidemiology* 1997;8:168–174.

67. Fraser GE, Shavlik DJ. Risk factors for all-cause and coronary heart disease mortality in the oldest-old: the Adventist Health Study. *Arch Intern Med* 1997;157:2249–2258.

68. Hu FB, Stampfer MJ, Manson JE, et al. Frequent nut consumption and risk of coronary heart disease in women: prospective cohort study. *BMJ* 1998;317:1341–1345.

69. Prineas RJ, Kushi LH, Folsom AR, et al. Walnuts and serum lipids. *N Engl J Med* 1993;329:359; author reply 359–360.

70. Albert CM, Gaziano JM, Willett WC, et al. Nut consumption and decreased risk of sudden cardiac death in the Physicians' Health Study. *Arch Intern Med* 2002;162:1382–1387.

71. Jiang R, Manson JE, Stampfer MJ, et al. Nut and peanut butter consumption and risk of type 2 diabetes in women. *JAMA* 2002;288:2554–2560.

72. Kris-Etherton PM, Zhao G, Binkoski AE, et al. The effects of nuts on coronary heart disease risk. *Nutr Rev* 2001;59:103–111.

73. Kris-Etherton PM, Harris WS, Appel LJ. Fish consumption, fish oil, omega-3 fatty acids, and cardiovascular disease. *Circulation* 2002;106:2747–2757.

74. Stone NJ. Fish consumption, fish oil, lipids, and coronary heart disease. *Circulation* 1996;94:2337–2340.

75. Kromhout D, Bosschieter EB, de Lezenne Coulander C. The inverse relation between fish consumption and 20-year mortality from coronary heart disease. *N Engl J Med* 1985;312:1205–1209.

76. Kromhout D, Feskens EJ, Bowles CH. The protective effect of a small amount of fish on coronary heart disease mortality in an elderly population. *Int J Epidemiol* 1995;24:340–345.

77. Daviglus ML, Stamler J, Orencia AJ, et al. Fish consumption and the 30-year risk of fatal myocardial infarction. *N Engl J Med* 1997;336:1046–1053.

78. Hu FB, Bronner L, Willett WC, et al. Fish and omega-3 fatty acid intake and risk of coronary heart disease in women. *JAMA* 2002;287:1815–1821.

79. Hu FB, Stampfer MJ, Manson JE, et al. Dietary intake of alpha-linolenic acid and risk of fatal ischemic heart disease among women. *Am J Clin Nutr* 1999;69:890–897.

80. Albert CM, Hennekens CH, O'Donnell CJ, et al. Fish consumption and risk of sudden cardiac death. *JAMA* 1998;279:23–28.

81. Albert CM, Campos H, Stampfer MJ, et al. Blood levels of long-chain n-3 fatty acids and the risk of sudden death. *N Engl J Med* 2002;346:1113–1118.

82. Siscovick DS, Raghunathan T, King I, et al. Dietary intake of long-chain n-3 polyunsaturated fatty acids and the risk of primary cardiac arrest. *Am J Clin Nutr* 2000;71:208S–212S.

83. He K, Rimm EB, Merchant A, et al. Fish consumption and risk of stroke in men. *JAMA* 2002;288:3130–3136.

84. Gillum RF, Mussolino ME, Madans JH. The relationship between fish consumption and stroke incidence: the NHANES I Epidemiologic Follow-up Study (National Health and Nutrition Examination Survey). *Arch Intern Med* 1996;156:537–542.

85. Iso H, Rexrode KM, Stampfer MJ, et al. Intake of fish and omega-3 fatty acids and risk of stroke in women. *JAMA* 2001;25:304–312.

86. Orencia AJ, Daviglus ML, Dyer AR, et al. Fish consumption and stroke in men: 30-year findings of the Chicago Western Electric Study. *Stroke* 1996;27:204–209.

87. Morris MC, Manson JE, Rosner B, et al. Fish consumption and cardiovascular disease in the Physicians' Health Study: a prospective study. *Am J Epidemiol* 1995;142:166–175.

88. Krauss RM, Eckel RH, Howard B, et al. AHA dietary guidelines: revision 2000: a statement for healthcare professionals from the Nutrition Committee of the American Heart Association. *Circulation* 2000;102:224–2299.

89. National Academy of Sciences and the Institutes of Medicine. Dietary reference intakes: energy, carbohydrate, fiber, fat, fatty acids, cholesterol, protein, and amino acids. Washington, DC: National Academies Press; 2002.

90. US Environmental Protection Agency. Fish Advisories web page. Available at: http://www.epa.gov/waterscience/fish/. Accessed on June 8, 2004.

91. US Food and Drug Administration, Center for Food Safety and Applied Nutrition, Office of Seafood. Mercury Levels in Seafood Species. Available at: http://www.cfsan.fda.gov/~frf/sea-mehg.html. Accessed on June 8, 2004.

92. Dayton S, Pearce ML, Hashimoto S, et al. A controlled clinical trial of a diet high in unsaturated fat. *Circulation* 1969;40:1–2.

93. Leren P The Oslo-Diet Heart Study: eleven-year report. *Circulation* 1970;42:935–942.

94. Turpeinen O, Karvonen MJ, Pekkarinen M, et al. Dietary prevention of coronary heart disease: the Finnish Mental Hospital Study. *Int J Epidemiol* 1979;8:99–118.

95. Miettinen M, Turpinen O, Karvonen MJ, et al. Dietary prevention of coronary heart disease in women: the Finnish Mental Hospital Study. *Int J Epidemiol* 1983;12:17–25.

96. Frantz ID, Dawson EA, Ashman PL, et al. Test of effect of lipid lowering by diet on cardiovascular risk: the Minnesota Coronary Survey. *Arteriosclerosis* 1989;9:129–135.

97. Morris JN, Ball KP, Antonis A, et al. Controlled trial of soyabean oil in myocardial infarction. *Lancet* 1968;2:693–699.

98. Holme I. Cholesterol reduction and its impact on coronary artery disease and total mortality. *Am J Cardiol* 1995;76:10C–17C.

99. Ornish D, Scherwitz LW, Billings JH, et al. Intensive lifestyle changes for reversal of coronary heart disease. *JAMA* 1998;280:2001–2007.

100. Ornish D, Brown SE, Scherwitz LW, et al. Can lifestyle changes reverse coronary heart disease? The Lifestyle Heart Trial. *Lancet* 1990;336:129–133.

101. Singh RB, Rastogi SS, Verma R, et al. Randomised controlled trial of cardioprotective diet in patients with recent acute myocardial infarction: results of one year follow up. *BMJ* 1992;304:1015–1019.

102. Singh RB, Dubnov G, Niaz MA, et al. Effect of an Indo-Mediterranean diet on progression of coronary artery disease in high risk patients (Indo-Mediterranean Diet Heart Study): a randomized single-blind trial. *Lancet* 2002;360:1455–1461.

103. Burr ML, Fehily AM, Gilbert JF, et al. Effects of changes in fat, fish, and fibre intakes on death and myocardial reinfarction: Diet and Reinfarction Trial (DART). *Lancet* 1989;2:757–761.

104. Valagussa F, Franzosi MG, Geraci E, et al. Dietary supplementation with Ω-3 polyunsaturated fatty acids and vitamin E after myocardial infarction: results of the GISSI-Prevenzione trial. *Lancet* 1999;354:447–455.

105. Marchioli R, Barzi F, Bomba E, et al. Early protection against sudden death by ?-3 polyunsaturated fatty acids after myocardial infarction: time course analysis of the results of the Gruppo Italiano per lo Studio della Sopravvivenza nell'Infarto Miocardico (GISSI)-Prevenzione. *Circulation* 2002;105:1897–1903.

106. Barzi F, Woodward M, Marfisi RM, et al. Mediterranean diet and all-causes mortality after myocardial infarction: results from the GISSI-Prevenzione trial. *Eur J Clin Nutr* 2003;57:604–611.

107. Singh RB, Niaz MA, Sharma JP. Randomized, double-blind, placebo-controlled trial of fish oil and mustard oil in patients with suspected acute myocardial infarction: the Indian Experiment of Infarct Survival-4. *Cardiovasc Drug Ther* 1997;11:485–491.

108. de Lorgeril M, Salen P, Martin J-L, et al. Mediterranean diet, traditional risk factors, and the rate of cardiovascular complications after myocardial infarction: final report of the Lyon Diet Heart Study. *Circulation* 1999;99:779–785.

109. Rosenthal MB, Barnard RJ, Rose DP, et al. Effects of a high-complex-carbohydrate, low-fat, low-cholesterol diet on serum levels of serum lipids and estradiol. *Am J Med* 1985;78:23–27.

110. Weber F, Barnard RJ, Roy D. Effects of a high-complex-carbohydrate, low-fat diet and daily exercise on individuals 70 years of age and older. *J Gerontol* 1983;38:155–161.

111. Jenkins DJA, Kendall CWC, Faulkner D, et al.: A dietary portfolio approach to cholesterol reduction: combined effects of plant sterol, vegetable proteins, and viscous fibers in hypercholesterolemia. *Metabolism* 2002;51:1596–1604.

112. Jenkins DJA, Kendall CWC, Marchie A, et al. The effects of combining plant sterols, soy protein, viscous fibers, and almonds in treating hypercholesterolemia. *Metabolism* 2003;52:1478–1483.

113. Lichtenstein AH, Ausman LM, Carrasco W, et al. Short-term consumption of a low-fat diet beneficially affects plasma lipid concentrations only when accompanied by weight loss: hypercholesterolemia, low-fat diet, and plasma lipids. *Arterioscler Thromb* 1994;14:1751–1760.

114. Collins R, Peto R, MacMahon S, et al. Blood pressure, stroke, and coronary heart disease: Part 2. Short-term reductions in blood pressure: overview of randomised drug trials in their epidemiological context. *Lancet* 1990;335:827–838.

115. Chobanian AV, Bakris GL, Black HR, et al, for the National Heart, Lung, and Blood Institute Joint National Committee on Prevention, Detection, Evaluation, and Treatment of High Blood Pressure and the National High Blood Pressure Education Program Coordinating Committee. The Seventh Report of the Joint National Committee on Prevention, Detection, Evaluation, and Treatment of High Blood Pressure: the JNC 7 report. *JAMA* 2003;289:2560–2572.

116. Svetkey LP, Simons-Morton D, Vollmer WM, et al. Effects of dietary patterns on blood pressure: subgroup analysis of the Dietary Approaches to Stop Hypertension (DASH) randomized clinical trial. *Arch Intern Med* 1999;159:285–293.

117. Conlin PR, Chow D, Miller ER, 3rd, et al. The effect of dietary patterns on blood pressure control in hypertensive patients: results from the Dietary Approaches to Stop Hypertension (DASH) trial. *Am J Hypertens* 2000;13:949–955.

118. Vollmer WM, Sacks FM, Ard J, et al. Effects of diet and sodium intake on blood pressure: subgroup analysis of the DASH–sodium trial. *Ann Intern Med* 2001;135:1019–1028.

119. Appel LF, Champagne CM, Harsha DW, et al. Effects of comprehensive lifestyle modification on blood pressure control: main results of the PREMIER clinical trial. *JAMA* 2003;289:2083–2093.

120. Resnick LM, Oparil S, Chait A, et al. Factors affecting blood pressure responses to diet: the Vanguard study. *Am J Hypertens* 2000;13:956–965.

121. Wassertheil-Smoller S, Blaufox MD, Oberman AS, et al. The Trial of Antihypertensive Interventions and Management (TAIM) Study: adequate weight loss, alone and combined with drug therapy in the treatment of mild hypertension. *Arch Intern Med* 1992;152:131–136.

122. The Trials of Hypertension Prevention Collaborative Research Group. Effects of weight loss and sodium reduction intervention on blood pressure and hypertension incidence in overweight people with high-normal blood pressure: the Trials of Hypertension Prevention, phase II. *Arch Intern Med* 1997;157:657–667.

123. Stamler R, Stamler J, Grimm R, et al. Nutritional therapy for high blood pressure: final report of a four-year randomized controlled trial—the Hypertension Control Program. *JAMA* 1987;257:1484–1491.

124. Ikeda T, Gomi T, Hirawa N, et al. Improvement of insulin sensitivity contributes to blood pressure reduction after weight loss in hypertensive subjects with obesity. *Hypertension* 1996;27:1180–1186.

125. Stevens VJ, Corrigan SA, Obarzanek E, et al. Weight loss intervention in phase 1 of the Trials of Hypertension Prevention: the TOHP Collaborative Research Group. *Arch Intern Med* 1993;153:849–858.

126. Su HY, Sheu WH, Chin HM, et al. Effect of weight loss on blood pressure and insulin resistance in normotensive and hypertensive obese individuals. *Am J Hypertens* 1995;8:1067–1071.

127. Whelton PK, Appel LJ, Espeland MA, et al, for the TONE Collaborative Research Group. Sodium reduction and weight loss in the treatment of hypertension in older persons: a randomized controlled trial of nonpharmacologic interventions in the elderly (TONE). *JAMA* 1998;279:839–846.

128. Langford HG, Blaufox MD, Oberman A, et al. Dietary therapy slows the return of hypertension after stopping prolonged medication. *JAMA* 1985;253:657–664.

129. He J, Whelton PK, Appel LJ, et al. Long-term effects of weight loss and dietary sodium reduction on incidence of hypertension. *Hypertension* 2000;35:544–549.

130. Bao DQ, Mori TA, Burke V, et al. Effects of dietary fish and weight reduction on ambulatory blood pressure in overweight hypertensives. *Hypertension* 1998;32:710–717.

131. Mori TA, Bao DQ, Burke V, et al. Docosahexaenoic acid but not eicosapentaenoic acid lowers ambulatory blood pressure and heart rate in humans. *Hypertension* 1999;34:253–260.

132. Pins JJ, Geleva D, Keenan JM, et al. Do whole-grain oat cereals reduce the need for antihypertensive medications and improve blood pressure control? *J Fam Pract* 2002;51:353–359.

133. Keenan JM, Pins JJ, Frazel C, et al. Oat ingestion reduces systolic and diastolic blood pressure in patients with mild or borderline hypertension: a pilot trial. *J Fam Pract* 2002;51:369.

134. Saltzman E, Das SK, Lichtenstein AH, et al. An oat-containing hypocaloric diet reduces systolic blood pressure and improves lipid profile beyond effects of weight loss in men and women. *J Nutr* 2001;131:1465–1470.

135. Teede HJ, Dalais FS, Kotsopoulos D, et al. Dietary soy has both beneficial and potentially adverse cardiovascular effects: a placebo-controlled study in men and postmenopausal women. *J Clin Endocrinol Metab* 2001;86:3053–3060.

136. Rivas M, Garay RP, Escanero JF, et al. Soy milk lowers blood pressure in men and women with mild to moderate essential hypertension. *J Nutr* 2002;132:1900–1902.

137. Burke V, Hodgson JM, Beilin LJ, et al. Dietary protein and soluble fiber reduce ambulatory blood pressure in treated hypertensives. *Hypertension* 2001;38:821–826.

138. Foster GD, Wyatt HR, Hill JO, et al. A randomized trial of a low-carbohydrate diet for obesity. *N Engl J Med* 2003;348:2082–2090.

139. Westman EC, Yancy WS, Edman JS, et al. Effect of 6-month adherence to a very low carbohydrate diet program. *Am J Med* 2002;113:30–36.

140. Bonow RO, Eckel RH. Diet, obesity, and cardiovascular risk. *N Engl J Med* 2003;348:2057–2058.

141. Grundy SM. Hypertriglyceridemia, atherogenic dyslipidemia, and the metabolic syndrome. *Am J Cardiol* 1998;81:18B–25B.

142. Larosa JC, Fry AG, Muesing R, et al. Effects of high-protein, low-carbohydrate dieting on plasma lipoproteins and body weight. *J Am Diet Assoc* 1980;77:264–270.

143. Bravata DM, Sanders L, Huang J, et al. Efficacy and safety of low-carbohydrate diets: a systematic review. *JAMA* 2003;289:1837–1850.

144. Parks EJ, Hellerstein MK. Carbohydrate-induced hypertriacylglycerolemia: historical perspective and review of biological mechanisms. *Am J Clin Nutr* 2000;71:412–433.

145. Jenkins DJ, Kendall CW, Augustin LS, et al. Glycemic index: overview of implications in health and disease. *Am J Clin Nutr* 2002;76:266S–273S.

146. Krauss RM. Dietary and genetic effects on low-density lipoprotein heterogeneity. *Annu Rev Nutr* 2001;21:283–295.

147. Liu S, Willett WC, Stampfer MJ, et al. A prospective study of dietary glycemic load, carbohydrate intake, and risk of coronary heart disease in US women. *Am J Clin Nutr* 2000;71:1455–1461.

148. Lui S, Manson JE, Buring JE, et al. Relation between a diet with a high glycemic load and plasma concentrations of high-sensitivity C-reactive protein in middle-aged women. *Am J Clin Nutr* 2002;75:492–498.

149. Rallidis LS, Paschos G, Liakos GK, et al. Dietary alpha-linolenic acid decreases C-reactive protein, serum amyloid A and interleukin-6 in dyslipidaemic patients. *Atherosclerosis* 2003;167:237–242.

150. Erlinger TP, Miller ER 3rd, Charleston J, et al. Inflammation modifies the effects of a reduced-fat low-cholesterol diet on lipids: results from the DASH–Sodium Trial. *Circulation* 2003;108:150–154.

151. Jenkins DJ, Kendall CW, Marchie A, et al. Effects of a dietary portfolio of cholesterol-lowering foods vs. lovastatin on serum lipids and C-reactive protein. *JAMA* 2003;290:502–510.

152. Esposito K, Pontillo A, Di Palo C et al. Effect of weight loss and lifestyle changes on vascular inflammatory markers in obese women: a randomized trial. *JAMA* 2003;289:1799–1804.

153. Tchernof A, Nolan A, Sites CK, et al. Weight loss reduces C-reactive protein levels in obese postmenopausal women. *Circulation* 2002;105:564–569.

154. Krauss RM: Dietary and genetic effects on low-density lipoprotein heterogeneity. *Ann Rev Nutr* 2001;21:283–295.

155. Austin MA, Breslow JL, Hennekens CH, et al. Low-density lipoprotein subclass patterns and risk of myocardial infarction. *JAMA* 1998;260:1917–1921.

156. Gardner CD, Fortmann SP, Krauss RM. Association of small, dense lipoprotein particles with incidence of coronary artery disease in men and women. *JAMA* 1996;276:875–881.

157. Dreon DM, Fernstrom HA, Miller B, et al. Low-density lipoprotein subclass patterns and lipoprotein response to a reduced-fat diet in men. *FASEB J* 1994;8:121–126.

158. Dreon DM, Fernstrom HA, Williams PT, et al. A very-low-fat diet is not associated with improved lipoprotein profiles in men with a predominance of large, low-density lipoproteins. *Am J Clin Nutr* 1999;69:411–418.

159. Hoefler G, Harnoncourt F, Paschke E, et al. Lipoprotein Lp(a): a risk factor for myocardial infarction. *Arteriosclerosis* 1988;8:398–401.

160. Rosengren A, Wilhelmsen L, Eriksson E, et al. Lipoprotein (a) and coronary heart disease: a prospective case-control study in a general population sample of middle aged men. *Br Med J* 1990;301:1248–1251.

161. Schaefer EJ, Lamon-Fava S, Jenner JL, et al. Lipoprotein (a) levels and risk of coronary heart disease in men: the Lipid Research Clinics Coronary Primary Prevention Trial. *JAMA* 1994;271:999–1003.

162. Bostom AG, Gagnon DR, Cupples LA, et al. A prospective investigation of elevated lipoprotein (a) detected by electrophoresis and cardiovascular disease in women: the Framingham Heart Study. *Circulation* 1994;90:1688–1695.

163. Rhoads GG, Dahlen G, Berg K, et al. Lp(a) lipoprotein as a risk factor for myocardial infarction. *JAMA* 1986;256:2540–2544.

164. Mensink RP, Zock PL, Katan MB et al. Effect of dietary cis and trans-fatty acids on serum lipoprotein (a) levels in humans. *J Lipid Res* 1992;33:1493–1501.

165. Nestel P, Noakes M, Belling B et al. Plasma lipoprotein lipid and lp(a) changes with substitution of elaidic acid for oleic acid in the diet. *J Lipid Res* 1992;33:1029–1036.

166. Beil FU, Terres W, Orgass M, et al. Dietary fish oil lowers lipoprotein(a) in primary hypertriglyceridemia. *Atherosclerosis* 1991;90:95–97.

167. Almendingen K, Jordal O, Kierulf P, et al. Effects of partially hydrogenated fish oil, partially hydrogenated soybean oil, and butter on serum lipoproteins and Lp(a) in men. *J Lipid Res* 1995;36:1370–1384.

168. Herrmann W, Biermann J, Kostner GM. Comparison of effects of N-3 to N-6 fatty acids on serum level of lipoprotein(a) in patients with coronary artery disease. *Am J Cardiol* 1995;76:459–462.

169. Clevidence BA, Judd JT, Schaefer EJ, et al. Plasma lipoprotein (a) levels in men and women consuming diets enriched in saturated, cis-, or trans-monounsaturated fatty acids. *Arterioscler Thromb Vasc Biol* 1997;17:1657–1661.

170. Lichtenstein AH, Ausman LM, Carrasco W, et al. Hydrogenation impairs the hypolipidemic effect of corn oil in humans: hydrogenation, trans-fatty acids, and plasma lipids. *Arterioscler Thromb* 1993;13:154–161.

171. Tholstrup T, Marckmann P, Vessby B, et al. Effect of fats high in individual saturated fatty acids on plasma lipoprotein[a] levels in young healthy men. *J Lipid Res* 1995;36:1447–1452.

172. Hornstra G, van Houwelingen AC, Kester ADM, et al. A palm-oil enriched diet lowers serum lipoprotein[a] in normocholesterolemic volunteers. *Atherosclerosis* 1991;90:91–93.

173. Ginsberg HN, Kris-Etherton P, Dennis B et al. Effects of reducing dietary saturated fatty acids on plasma lipids and lipoproteins in healthy subjects The Delta Study, Protocol 1. *Arterioscler Thromb Vasc Biol* 1998;18:441–449.

174. Agren JJ, Vaisanen S, Hanninen O, et al. Hemostatic factors and platelet aggregation after a fish-enriched diet or fish oil or docosahexaenoic acid supplementation. *Prostaglandins Leukot Essent Fatty Acids* 1997;57:419–421.

175. Mori TA, Beilin LJ, Burke V, et al. Interactions between dietary fat, fish, and fish oils and their effects on platelet function in men at risk of cardiovascular disease. *Arterioscler Thromb Vasc Biol* 1997;17:279–286.

176. Kristensen SD, Schmidt EB, Dyerberg J. Dietary supplementation with n-3 polyunsaturated fatty acids and human platelet function: a review with particular emphasis on implications for cardiovascular disease. *J Intern Med Suppl* 1989;225:141–150.

177. Bradlow BA, Chetty N, van der Westhuyzen J, et al. The effects of a mixed fish diet on platelet function, fatty acids and serum lipids. *Thromb Res* 1983;29:561–568.

178. Goodnight SH, Harris WS, Connor WE. The effects of dietary omega 3 fatty acids on platelet composition and function in man: a prospective, controlled study. *Blood* 1981;58:880–885.

179. Thorngren M, Gustafson A. Effects of 11-week increase in dietary eicosapentaenoic acid on bleeding time, lipids and platelet aggregation. *Lancet* 1981;2:1190–1193.

180. Boushey CJ, Beresford SA, Omenn GS et al. A quantitative assessment of plasma homocysteine as a risk factor for vascular disease. Probable benefits of increasing folic acid intakes. *JAMA* 1995;274:1049–1057.

181. Homocysteine Studies Collaboration. Homocysteine and risk of ischemic heart disease and stroke: a meta-analysis. *JAMA* 2002;288:2015–2022.

182. Jacques PF, Selhub J, Bostom AG et al. The effect of folic acid fortification on plasma folate and total homocysteine concentrations. *N Engl J Med* 1999;340:1449–1454.

183. Malinow MR, Duell PB, Hess DL, et al. Reduction of plasma homocyst(e)ine levels by breakfast cereal fortified with folic acid in patients with coronary heart disease. *N Engl J Med* 1998;338:1009–1015.

184. Nutrition and Your Health: Dietary Guidelines for Americans. 5th ed. USDA Home and Garden Bulletin No. 232. 2000.

185. Kris-Etherton PM, Harris WS, Appel LJ. AHA Scientific Statement: fish consumption, fish oil, omega-3 fatty acids and cardiovascular disease. *Circulation* 2002;106:2747–2757.

186. American Diabetes Association. Evidence-based nutrition principles and recommendations for the treatment and prevention of diabetes and related complications. *Diabetes Care* 2003;26:S51–S61.

187. Kris-Etherton PM, Lichtenstein AH, Howard BV, et al. Antioxidant vitamin supplements and cardiovascular disease. *Circulation* 2004;110:637–641.

188. Clinical guidelines on the identification, evaluation and treatment of overweight and obesity in adults: the evidence report. Bethesda, Md: National Institutes of Health, National Heart, Lung and Blood Institute; 1998.

189. Cook NR, Cohen J, Hebert PR, et al. Implications of small reductions in diastolic blood pressure for primary prevention. *Arch Intern Med* 1995;155:701–709.

190. Bravata DM, Sanders L, Huang G, et al. Efficacy and safety of low-carbohydrate diets: a systematic review. *JAMA* 2003;289:1837–1850.

191. Bray GA, Lovejoy JC, Most-Windhauser M, et al. A 9-month randomized clinical trial comparing fat-substituted and fat-reduced diets in healthy, obese men: the Ole Study. *Am J Clin Nutr* 2002;76:928–934.

192. McManus K, Antinoro L, Sacks F. A randomized controlled trial of a moderate-fat, low-energy diet compared with a low fat, low-energy diet for weight loss in overweight adults. *Int J Obes Relat Metab Disord* 2001;25:1503–1511.

193. St Jeor ST, Howard BV, Prewitt TE, et al. Dietary protein and weight reduction: a statement for health care professionals from the Nutrition Committee of the Council on Nutrition, Physical Activity, and Metabolism of the American Heart Association. *Circulation* 2001;104:1869–1874.

194. Thompson PD, Buchner D, Pina IL, et al. AHA Scientifc Statement: exercise and physical activity in the prevention and treatment of atherosclerotic cardiovascular disease: A statement from the Council on Clinical Cardiology (Subcommittee on Exercise, Rehabilitation, and Prevention) and the Council on Nutrition, Physical Activity, and Metabolism (Subcommittee on Physical Activity). *Circulation* 2003;107:3109–3116.

195. Fletcher GF, Balady GJ, Amsterdam EA, et al. Exercise standards for testing and training: a statement for healthcare professionals from the American Heart Association. *Circulation* 2001;104:1694–1740.

196. Pate RR, Pratt M, Blair SN, et al. Physical activity and public health: a recommendation from the Centers for Disease Control and Prevention and the American College of Sports Medicine. *JAMA* 1995;273:402–407.

197. Troiano RP, Macera CA, Ballard-Barbash R. Be physically active each day: how can we know? *J Nutr* 2001131:451S–460S.

198. Lenfant C. Clinical research to clinical practice: lost in translation? *N Engl J Med* 2003;349:868–874.

199. Ford ES, Mokdad AH, Giles WH, Mensah GA. Serum total cholesterol concentrations and awareness, treatment, and control of hypercholesterolemia among U.S. adults: findings from the National Health and Nutrition Examination Survey, 1999 to 2000. *Circulation* 2003;107:2185–2189.

200. Eaton CB, Goodwin MA, Stange KC. Direct observation of nutrition counseling in community family practice. *Am J Prev Med* 2002;23:174–179.

201. Truswell AS: Family physicians and patients: is effective nutrition interaction possible? *Am J Clin Nutr* 2000;71:6–12.

202. vanWeel C. Dietary advice in family medicine. *Am J Clin Nutr* 2003;77(suppl):1008S–1010S.

203. Kreuter MW, Chheda SG, Bull FC: How does physician advice influence patient behavior? *Arch Fam Med* 2000;9:426–433.

204. Ockene IS, Herbert JR, Ockene JK, et al. Effect of physician-derived nutrition counseling training and an office-supported program on saturated fat intake, weight, and serum lipid measurements in a hyperlipidemic population: Worcester Area Trial for Counseling in Hyperlipidemia (WATCH). *Arch Intern Med* 1999;159:725–731.

205. Henkin Y, Shai I, Zuk R et al. Appropriateness of the National Cholesterol Education Program dietary guidelines in general practice: a new look at old guidelines. *Am J Med* 2000;109:549–555.

206. Katzel LI, Coon PJ, Dengel J, et al. Effects of an American Heart Association Step I Diet and weight loss on lipoprotein lipid levels in obese men with silent myocardial ischemia and reduced high-density lipoprotein cholesterol. *Metabolism* 1995;44:307–314.

207. Sikand G, Kashyap ML, Yang I. Medical nutrition therapy lowers serum cholesterol and saves medication costs in men with hypercholesterolemia. *J Am Diet Assoc* 1998;98:889–894.

208. Sikand G, Kashyap ML, Wong ND et al. Dietitian intervention improves lipid values and saves medication costs in men with combined hyperlipidemia and a history of niacin non-compliance. *J Am Diet Assoc* 2000;100:218–224.

Physical activity

Nathan D. Wong
Stanley L. Bassin
William Haskell

KEY POINTS

- One third to one half of US adults are physically inactive. The amount of physical activity during leisure time and work is inversely associated with cardiovascular morbidity and mortality

- Increased levels of physical activity lead to improvements in blood pressure, glucose intolerance, diabetes, high-density lipoprotein cholesterol, triglycerides, and obesity.

- Current recommendations suggest adults participate in 30 minutes or more of moderate-intensity physical activity on most, if not all, days of the week for the primary prevention of cardiovascular disease.

- In persons with cardiovascular disease, or in those with symptoms suggestive of cardiovascular disease or at high risk for cardiovascular disease, as long as the individual is stable, health care providers should perform a symptom-limited exercise test followed by a careful prescription of activity based on the results of the test.

- Health care providers should routinely prescribe exercise and increased physical activity for their patients in accordance with recommendations of the American Heart Association, Centers for Disease Control and Prevention, and American College of Sports Medicine.

- Physical activity should begin sooner, rather than later, within the life span, for increased health and longevity.

- Parents, schools, and community organizations need to provide a supportive environment that encourages and integrates physical activity into the daily lifestyle. Children must be introduced to the principles and skills of regular physical activity and the community must provide opportunities for activity.

INTRODUCTION

Over the last few decades, studies have shown a sedentary lifestyle to be associated with an increased risk of hypertension, coronary heart disease (CHD),[1] cardiovascular disease (CVD),[2-5] and all-cause mortality.[5,6] Physical activity as part of daily living is associated with a decreased risk for CVD, stroke, diabetes, obesity, and all-cause mortality.[7] Even those who are moderately active have lower mortality rates than those who are least active. Unfortunately, the US population is becoming increasingly sedentary, with recent estimates indicating that only 15% of Americans older than 18 years of age get regular vigorous activity (three times a week for at least 20 minutes), and 60% reporting no regular leisure-time activity (with 25% not active at all).[8] There is great potential for reducing CVD risk in those initially sedentary who become moderately active,[6] but those who remain sedentary have the highest risk for CVD and all-cause mortality.[1]

TABLE 12-1   Prevalence of Physical Inactivity by Gender and Race/Ethnicity

Population group	Prevalence (% reporting no leisure-time physical activity)
White males	32.5
White females	36.2
African-American males	44.1
African-American females	55.2
Hispanic males	48.9
Hispanic females	57.4
Asian/Pacific Islander males	30.9
Asian/Pacific Islander females	45.4

SOURCE: NHIS (1997–1998), CDC/NCHS; data are age-adjusted for Americans aged 18 and older.

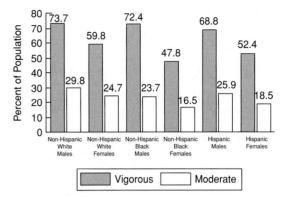

FIGURE 12-2   Percentage of students in grades 9 to 12 who participated in sufficient vigorous or moderate physical activity during the past 7 days by race/ethnicity and sex: United States, 2001. (Reproduced, with permission, from the American Heart Association.[9])

Recent data demonstrate that one third to one half of Americans aged 18 and older report no leisure-time physical activity (Table 12-1); furthermore, the prevalence of moderate-to-vigorous physical activity is reportedly least in Mexican-Americans, non-Hispanic African-Americans, and those who were classified as obese (Fig. 12-1).[9] Further, among American youth in grades 9 to 12, participation in vigorous physical activity in the past 7 days was least in females and those of non-Hispanic, African-American, or Hispanic race/ethnicity (Fig. 12-2),[9] a consequence of significant reductions in required physical education in schools.

EVIDENCE RELATING PHYSICAL ACTIVITY TO CARDIOVASCULAR DISEASE AND ALL-CAUSE MORTALITY

Multiple prospective studies published over the past 35 years have shown a strong, consistent, and graded relation between self-reported occupational[10–15] and leisure-time physical activity and CVD events, CVD mortality, and all-cause mortality.[2–7,16–38]

Occupational physical activity

Initial observations among London busmen suggested a relation between increased levels of occupational physical activity and risk of myocardial infarction.[10] These investigators found that the most highly active conductors on London's double-decker buses were at lower risk of coronary heart disease (CHD) and tended to suffer fewer severe heart attacks than those who worked sitting at the wheel. Other studies of occupationally physically active cohorts, such as farmers[11] and railroad trackmen and clerks,[12,13] have also generally shown lower CHD risk with higher levels of physical activity, but have not addressed potential confounders such as other CHD risk factors. Large meta-analyses have summarized these earlier studies and confirm an inverse relation between physical activity and CHD risk.[14,15]

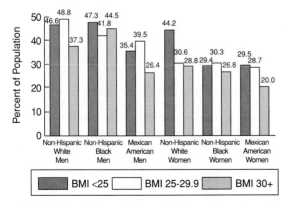

FIGURE 12-1   Prevalence of moderate or vigorous physical activity in Americans aged 20 and older by sex, race/ethnicity, and BMI. (Reproduced, with permission, from the American Heart Association.[9])

Leisure-time physical activity

Recent studies documenting an inverse relation of leisure-time physical activity with CHD incidence and mortality, as well as all-cause mortality, are summarized in Table 12-2. Paffenbarger and colleagues' landmark investigations showed habitual physical activity to be inversely related to the risk of CHD in approximately 17,000 male college alumni aged 35 to 74 years.[16] Their more recent report showed those expending 2000 kcal or more per week (compared to those expending less) to have a 28 percent reduced risk of death from all causes ($p < .0001$) over a follow-up period of 12 to 16 years.[17] Morris and co-workers showed, among 3590 middle-aged male civil servants followed for 10 years, nearly a threefold higher incidence of both fatal myocardial infarction ($P < .001$) and sudden death ($P < .01$) among sedentary men as compared with men who participated in vigorous exercise sports.[3,18]

A number of other recent reports provide further evidence regarding the inverse relation between self-reported physical activity and CHD morbidity and mortality and total mortality. The Finnish Twin Cohort showed, among 7925 men and 7977 women who were initially healthy, a significantly reduced rate of death in those who were classified as conditioning exercisers.[27] Among middle-aged Finnish men, those with an estimated leisure-time physical activity energy expenditure less than 800 kcal/wk, as compared with 2100 kcal/wk, were found to be at an approximately threefold greater risk for both cardiovascular and all-cause mortality after adjustment for age, smoking, and certain social characteristics.[28] These investigators also demonstrated, in middle-aged men and women, a significant inverse relation of physical activity with 10-year incidence of CHD.[29]

Several studies also have reported an inverse relation of physical activity with CHD to be independent of major, potentially confounding risk factors. A 20-year follow-up of 7142 men in Goteborg, Sweden, aged 47 to 55 years at baseline and without symptomatic CHD, showed, after adjustment for a wide range of risk factors, the most active men (as compared with the least active men) to have a significant (28%) reduction in the risk of CHD death and 30% reduction in total mortality.[31] The Israeli Ischemic Heart Disease Study of nearly 8500 government employees showed self-reported leisure-time physical activity (but not work-related physical activity) also to be related to a significant (21%) reduction in CHD mortality and a 9% reduction in all-cause mortality.[32] These findings persisted after adjustment for potential confounding risk factors. Finally, the Alameda County Study, involving follow-up of 6131 adults for 28 years, showed that

those at the 75th percentile (compared with those at the 25th percentile) of physical activity, after adjusting for other risk factors, had a 19% lower risk of CVD mortality and a 16% lower risk of all-cause mortality.[33] More recently, Manson and co-workers reported that among 73,743 postmenopausal women aged 50 to 79, those with higher quintiles of reported energy expenditure (expressed as MET score) had increasingly reduced age and risk factor-adjusted relative risks for CVD events (0.89, 0.81, 0.78, and 0.72 for those in the 2nd thru 5th vs 1st) quintiles).[34] Lee and colleagues showed, among 7337 men, perceived exercise exertion to be inversely related to risk of CHD (relative risks of 0.86, 0.69, and 0.72 for those perceiving their exertion as moderate, somewhat strong, and strong, compared with weak).[35]

The possibility that the greatest cardiovascular benefits from physical activity may occur at moderate levels of exercise has also been noted. Sixteen-year follow-up data on 12,138 middle-aged men at high risk of CHD participating in the Multiple Risk Factor Intervention Trial (MRFIT) revealed men in the least active decile (0–9 min/d) of leisure-time physical activity to have significant, excess age-adjusted CHD and all-cause mortality of 29 and 22%, respectively, as compared with those in deciles 2 to 4 (10–36 min/d).[30] Higher deciles of activity, however, were not associated with further reductions in mortality. Of note is a report from the Nurses' Health Study that in 5125 nurses with diabetes, there was a strong inverse association between self-reported physical activity and incidence of CVD that was independent of other risk factors.[36] These findings suggest that cardiovascular benefits may be maximized at moderate levels of physical activity without further benefit at higher activity levels.

Other data suggest that the association of increased levels of physical activity with CHD incidence and mortality may be due to risk factor differences between exercisers and nonexercisers. In 8006 Japanese-American men initially aged 45 to 68 years and followed for 23 years, those in the highest tertile of physical activity had a significantly (17%) lower risk of incident CHD and 26% lower CHD mortality[37]; however, these findings were attenuated after adjustment for cardiovascular risk factors. Also, among both men and women, aged 45 to 64 years, enrolled in the Atherosclerosis Risk in Communities (ARIC) study,[38] significant CHD risk reductions of 18 to 27% (depending on gender and physical activity measure used) were noted, but were attenuated after adjustment for other risk factors. Of importance, because the protection afforded by physical activity may be mediated through some of these risk factors, weakened relationships after such adjustment do not mean that physical activity is *not* protective.

TABLE 12-2   Selected Studies of Association Between Self-Reported Physical Activity or Measured Fitness and Cardiovascular Disease and Total Mortality

Author	Population	Findings
Self-Reported Physical Activity		
Paffenbarger et al, 1986[17]	16,936 US male college alumni aged 35–74 followed for 12–16 y	28% lower risk of all-cause mortality among those expending 2000 kcal/wk or more vs less ($P < .0001$)
Kujala et al, 1998[27]	7925 men and 7977 women in Finland followed for 17 y	RR (95% CI) for all-cause mortality = 0.57 (0.45–0.74) in conditioning exercisers and 0.71 (0.62–0.81) in occasional exercisers vs sedentary
Haapanen et al, 1996[28]	1072 men in Finland aged 35–63 followed for 11 y	RR = 2.74 (1.46–5.14) for all-cause mortality and 3.58 (1.45–8.85) for cardiovascular mortality for those expending <800 kcal/wk vs >2100 kcal/wk
Haapanen et al, 1997[29]	1340 men and 1500 women aged 35–63 followed for 10 y	RR = 1.98 (1.22–3.23) for those in lowest vs highest tertile of physical activity
Leon et al, 1997[30]	12,138 middle-aged US men followed for 16 y	29% reduction in CHD mortality and 22% reduction in all-cause mortality for those least vs moderately active
Rosengren et al, 1997[31]	7142 men in Sweden aged 47–55 followed for 20 y	RR = 0.72 (0.56–0.92) for CHD death and RR = 0.70 (0.61–0.80) for total mortality in most vs least active
Eaton et al, 1995[32]	8463 Israeli government employees followed for 21 y	RR = 0.79 (0.66–0.95) for CHD mortality and 0.91 (0.83–0.99) for all-cause mortality in those with greatest vs least leisure-time physical activity; no relation to work-related physical activity
Hu et al, 2001[36]	5125 female nurses with diabetes followed for 14 y	RR = 1.0, 1.02, 0.87, 0.61, and 0.55 ($P = .001$) for trend for CVD events adjusted for other risk factors in those with <1, 1–1.9, 2–3.9, 4–6.9, and ≥7 h/wk physical activity, respectively
Kaplan et al, 1996[33]	6131 US adults followed for 28 y	RR = 0.84 (0.77–0.92) for all-cause mortality and 0.81 (0.71–0.93) for CVD mortality comparing those in 75th vs 25th percentile of activity, risk factor-adjusted
Manson et al, 2002[34]	73,743 postmenopausal women aged 50–69 (Women's Health Initiative)	Adjusted RR = 0.89, 0.81, 0.78, and 0.72 ($P = .001$ for trend) for those in the 2nd through 5th (compared with 1st quintile) of energy expenditure in MET score for cardiovascular events
Lee et al, 2003[35]	7337 men (mean age 66) followed for 7 y	Adjusted RR for CHD 0.86, 0.69, and 0.72 (P for trend = .02) for those perceiving their exercise intensity exertion as moderate, somewhat strong, or strong compared with weak
Rodriguez et al, 1994[37]	8006 Japanese-American men aged 45–68 followed for 23 y	RR = 0.83 (0.70–0.99) for CHD incidence and 0.74 (0.5–0.97) for CHD mortality, attenuated after adjustment for risk factors
Folsom et al, 1997[38]	7459 US men and women aged 45–64 followed for 4–7 y	RR = 0.73 for women and RR = 0.82 for men for CHD incidence/standard deviation increment in physical activity, risk factor-adjusted; no relation to occupational physical activity

(continued)

TABLE 12-2 (Continued)

Author	Population	Findings
	Measured Physical Fitness	
Blair et al, 1989[4]	10,224 men and 3120 US women followed for 8 y by the Cooper Clinic	RR (95% CI) for all-cause mortality in those in lowest vs highest fitness quintile=1.58 (1.32–1.89) in men and 1.94 (1.30–2.88) in women, risk factor-adjusted
Ecklund et al, 1988[23]	4276 men aged 30–69 in the Lipid Research Clinics Mortality Follow-up Study followed for 10 y	RR (95% CI) 2.7 for CVD mortality (1.4–5.1) and 3.2 (1.5–6.7) for CHD death per increment of 35 beats/min at submaximal treadmill testing
Slattery et al, 1988[22]	3043 white middle-aged men aged 22–79 followed for up to 20 y	RR = 1.43 (age-adjusted) and 1.20 (age- and risk factor-adjusted) for CHD death per 30 beats/min at submaximal treadmill testing
Gulati et al, 2003[40]	5721 asymptomatic older women followed for 8 y	RR of death for METS achieved of <5, 5–8, and >8 were 3.1 (2.0–4.7), 1.9 (1.3–2.9) and 1.0, respectively

Fitness level and cardiovascular risk

Physical fitness measured by an exercise treadmill test has also been shown to be inversely related to all-cause mortality among more than 10,000 men and 3000 women followed for an average of slightly more than 8 years.[4] Age-adjusted all-cause mortality rates (per 10,000 person-years) declined significantly across fitness quintiles (least fit to most fit), from 64.0 to 18.6 in men and from 39.5 to 8.5 in women. Comparing those in the lowest with those in the highest quintile, relative risks (and 95% confidence intervals) were 1.58 (1.32–1.89) for men and 1.94 (1.30–2.88) for women, after adjusting for other coronary risk factors. In addition, an 8.5-year follow-up of 4276 men initially aged 30 to 69 who participated in the Lipid Research Clinics Mortality Follow-up Study provides further support of this trend. In these individuals, a lower level of physical fitness was associated with a higher risk of death (per increment of 35 beats/min in heart rate during submaximal treadmill testing) from CVD (relative risk [RR] = 2.7, $P < .01$) or CHD (RR = 3.2, $P < .01$).[23] Finally, in 3043 US railroad workers followed for up to 20 years, an increment of 30 beats/min heart rate on submaximal treadmill testing was associated with an age-adjusted RR for CHD of 1.43 (1.20 after adjusting for other risk factors).[24] More recently, Myers and colleagues showed, in 6213 men referred for treadmill testing, that peak exercise capacity measured in metabolic equivalents (METs) was the strongest predictor of death, more powerful than other established risk factors.[39] Finally, a recently reported cohort of 5721 asymptomatic women who underwent symptom-limited stress testing demonstrated, after 8 years of follow-up, adjusted hazard ratios for death associated with MET levels less than 5, 5 to 8, and greater than 8 were 3.1 (2.0–4.7), 1.9 (1.3–2.9) and 1.0, respectively.[40]

CARDIOVASCULAR BENEFITS OF PHYSICAL ACTIVITY AND FITNESS

A wide range of studies conducted in youth, women, men, older persons, and different ethnic groups document increased levels of physical activity to be related to decreased or improved cardiovascular risk factors. Many of the benefits of exercise training from endurance and resistance activities diminish within 2 weeks, and disappear entirely within 2 to 8 months if physical activity is significantly reduced.[8] The magnitude of the effect of physical activity depends on the characteristics of the intervention, individual variation, and whether the exercise produces a reduction in body weight. In some persons, the effect on risk factors can be large, reducing the need for other interventions; however, usually the effect on risk factors is much less than that achieved by pharmacologic intervention.[41] In a meta-analysis of 52 exercise training trials of at least 12 weeks' duration involving 4700 subjects, an average increase in high-density lipoprotein cholesterol (HDL-C) levels of 4.6% and decreases in triglyceride and low-density lipoprotein cholesterol (LDL-C) levels of 3.7 and 5.0%, respectively, were reported.[42] In addition, at least 44 randomized trials involving 2674 participants have collectively shown average reductions in systolic and diastolic blood pressures of 3.4 and 2.4 mm Hg, respectively, as a result of exercise training. Moreover, reductions were substantially greater in hypertensive subjects and did not seem to depend on frequency or intensity of the exercise.[43] Further, beneficial effects of physical activity are also seen on insulin resistance, glucose intolerance, and postprandial hyperglycemia, with a review of nine trials among 337 patients with type II diabetes reporting an average reduction in hemoglobin A_{1c} of 0.5 to 1%.[44]

In children and young adults aged 9 to 24, the Young Finns Study ($n = 2358$) demonstrated level of physical activity to be positively associated with overall HDL-C and HDL_2-C levels and negatively associated with triglycerides, apolipoprotein B, and insulin levels in males. In females, only a negative association with triglyceride levels was noted.[45] An inverse association of physical activity with obesity, but not blood pressure, was also observed. Among more than 1500 Singapore youth aged 6 to 18, self-reported physical activity was significantly correlated (inversely) with total cholesterol and triglycerides in boys and with body fat and body mass index in girls.[46] Amount of television watched as a marker of physical inactivity (among other unhealthful behaviors) has been shown to be significantly associated with body weight in both boys and girls and, additionally with body mass index and systolic blood pressure in boys,[47] in a study of more than 1000 youth in Belgium. In another study, amount of television watched was the strongest indicator of the likelihood of having total cholesterol levels 200 mg/dL or higher after adjusting for other risk factors, including a family history of premature heart disease or hyperlipidemia.[48] Increasing usage of computers and the Internet could also be associated with reduced physical activity and should be the subject of future investigation.

Numerous studies document the relation of increased physical activity or fitness levels with an improved cardiovascular risk factor profile in adults. The Cooper Clinic showed increases in treadmill time to be associated with beneficial changes in several cardiovascular risk factors.[49] Others have demonstrated aerobic exercise to be associated with decreases of 8 to 10 mm Hg in systolic and diastolic blood pressures.[50,51] The Pawtucket Heart Study found, in 381 men and 556 women, that both estimated maximal oxygen consumption and self-reported physical activity were significantly associated with blood pressure, body mass index, and HDL-C.[52] Other studies in Chinese adults,[53] Japanese men,[54] and a pooled analysis among three European cohorts consisting of a total of 402 men aged 69 to 90 years demonstrated a significant protective relation of physical activity with certain cardiovascular risk factors.[55]

Recent studies of women have demonstrated important protective associations of level of physical activity and cardiovascular risk factors. Increased levels of HDL-C seen as a result of exercise are related to reductions in body weight, and those who exercise at higher levels also have greater increases in HDL-C.[56–58] In the Postmenopausal Estrogen/Progestins Intervention Trial,

among 851 women aged 45 to 64, leisure-time self-reported physical activity was positively associated with levels of HDL-C ($P = .001$) and inversely associated with insulin and fibrinogen levels (both P's $< .05$). Moderate and heavy leisure-time activities were associated with the highest HDL-C levels.[59] A large cohort of 4576 Dutch women aged 49 to 70 showed blood pressure (systolic/diastolic) to be inversely associated with time spent in sports after adjustment for age, education, and smoking (128.9/77.8 mm Hg in the highest sports tertile and 132.1/79.0 mm Hg in the lowest sports tertile). Body mass index, waist/hip ratio, and waist circumference were also inversely related to certain physical activities.[60] Finally, intraabdominal adipose tissue, determined by computed tomography, appears to be negatively related to level of physical activity.[61]

Other benefits of physical activity

Improved exercise performance with training is the result of (1) increased ability to use oxygen in deriving energy for work, and (2) increased maximum ventilatory oxygen uptake related to increasing both maximum cardiac output and the ability of muscles to extract and use oxygen from blood. Beneficial changes in hemodynamic, hormonal, metabolic, neurologic, and respiratory function also occur with increased exercise capacity.[1]

Physical activity may favorably affect body fat distribution, whereas physical inactivity results in fewer kilocalories expended, leading to obesity.[8] In overweight persons, regular physical activity enhances the effects on blood lipoprotein levels of a diet low in saturated fat and cholesterol.[62] Exercise training has beneficial effects on insulin sensitivity.[63] There may also be a beneficial effect in the prevention of other diseases, including certain cancers and osteoporosis.[64] Finally, longitudinal studies have shown that exercise training appears to result in improvement in psychologic functioning, including reducing depression,[65–67] improving self-confidence and self-esteem,[68] and attenuating cardiovascular and neurohumoral responses to mental stress.[69] Physical activity also improves health-related quality of life by enhancing psychologic well-being and improving physical functioning in those impaired by poor health.[8]

Assessment of physical activity and fitness

SELF-REPORT TECHNIQUES

Diaries, logs, recall surveys, retrospective quantitative histories, and global self-reports are frequently used to give an overall estimate of physical activity, often taking into account intensity, duration, frequency, and type of activity[8]:

1. Diaries detail nearly all physical activity performed in a given (usually short) period and usually involve a summary index derived by multiplying the total duration of time spent in an activity by the estimated rate of energy expenditure or intensity, or listing the accumulated time across all activities.

2. Logs provide a record of participating in specific types of activities. Both diaries and logs are frequently time-intensive to complete and analyze.

3. Recall surveys are generally useful for assessing physical activity in large populations because they are easy to administer, not costly, and generally acceptable to study participants. They are used for time frames ranging from 1 week to a lifetime and may assess either precise or more general estimates of usual participation.

4. A retrospective quantitative history is the most comprehensive type of physical activity recall survey, requiring detailed information on frequency and duration of participation for a given list of activities performed for up to the past year.

5. Global self-reports involve asking respondents to rate their level of physical activity in relation to the adult population in general or to a specific age/gender group. One drawback is that there is often actually greater variation inherent in persons giving similar ratings.[8]

Appendixes 12-1 and 12-2 provide examples of self-reported physical activity surveys practical to administer to a general adult population.

DIRECT MONITORING

Physical activity can also be measured more directly by behavioral observation, the use of mechanical or electronic devices, or physiologic measurements. Although not subject to the limitations of memory and biases, as in self-reporting, these methods are usually quite expensive and burdensome on participants and staff and have been traditionally used mainly for small-scale studies or for the validation of self-report questionnaires.

Mechanical or electronic measurement involves devices such as those used to monitor heart rate and can provide a continuous recording of a physiologic process, representing both the duration and the intensity of activity. Estimated daily energy expenditure for a given physical activity can be obtained; however, there are limitations. The heart rate–energy expenditure curve is different for each individual and variable for low-intensity physical activities. Furthermore, wearing of such monitors for extended periods can be inconvenient. Other methods involve the use of motion sensors, such as pedometers and accelerometers, and physiologic measures of energy expenditure, such as calorimetry, where measurement of expired air is obtained.[8]

MEASUREMENT OF PHYSICAL ACTIVITY INTENSITY

The intensity of physical activity can be characterized using qualitative terms such as light or low, moderate or mild, hard or vigorous, and very hard or strenuous.[8] For example, one validated instrument, as used in the Coronary Artery Risk Development in Young Adults (CARDIA) study,[70] allows for the calculation of estimated energy expenditure (EEE) for each of several activity groups based on known intensities in metabolic units or METs (ratio of metabolic rate during activity to resting metabolic rate) (Table 12-3; see Appendix 12-2). From the frequency and duration spent on each activity, the EEE per year can be calculated by summing across all activity groups, plus the energy spent in sleep (assigned a MET value of 1.0), plus the EEE from light activities (assigned a MET value of 1.5). The EEE per year is then estimated by subtracting all the time not spent in moderate (MET grouping 3.5–5.0) or vigorous (MET grouping $\geq$ 6.0) activity.

Assessment of physical fitness

Physical fitness assessment is more highly developed and relies on measurements of endurance (or cardiorespiratory fitness), muscular fitness, and body composition, often with excellent accuracy and reliability. Maximal oxygen uptake or aerobic power is the most established criterion of cardiorespiratory fitness and is measured in healthy persons during large-muscle dynamic activity such as walking, running, and cycling. It is most accurately determined by measuring expired air composition and respiratory volume during maximal exertion, but requires expensive equipment, trained technicians, and cooperation from the participant. It can also be estimated from peak exercise workload during a maximal exercise test without measuring respiratory gases; this requires a calibrated exercise device, adherence to a protocol, and cooperation from the participant.[8]

RECOMMENDATIONS FOR PHYSICAL ACTIVITY IN ADULTS

Recommendations for primary prevention of coronary heart disease in healthy persons

In 1996, the National Institutes of Health convened a consensus development conference[71] that resulted in the following recommendations:

1. All Americans should engage in regular physical activity at a level appropriate to their capacity, needs, and interests.

TABLE 12-3   1-Year Physical Activity Recall: Activity Groups and Metabolic Equivalent (MET) values

Activity groups and sample activities*	METs
Vigorous home-related activities (eg, snow shoveling, moving or lifting heavy objects [>9 kg], chopping wood)	6.0
Vigorous work-related activities (eg, lifting and carrying heavy loads [>9 kg], digging ditches, heavy carpentry, heavy construction, heavy ranching [eg, working irrigation ditches])	8.0
Jogging, running, vigorous hiking, cross-country skiing	8.0
Vigorous racket sports	8.0
Vigorous bicycling (>16 km/h), rowing machine, jumping rope	8.0
Swimming, other vigorous water activities (eg, water skiing)	6.0
Vigorous exercise class, jazzercise, vigorous dancing	6.0
Other strenuous sport (eg, downhill skiing, roller skating, soccer, basketball)	7.0
Vigorous conditioning exercises (eg, vigorous calisthenics, universal workout, weight lifting)	6.0
Less strenuous home maintenance, gardening	5.0
Indoor household chores (eg, painting, cleaning bathroom), child care	4.5
Less strenuous work-related activities (eg, waitressing, nursing, lifting, carrying >9 kg)	4.5
Less strenuous home exercise, calisthenics	4.0
Less strenuous sports (eg, hunting, badminton)	4.0
Bowling, golf	3.5
Other brisk walking (not covered in previous questions), hiking	4.0

*"Vigorous" activities were defined as those with a MET level of 6 or greater.

SOURCE: Adapted, with permission, from Sidney et al.[70]

2. Children and adults alike should set a goal of accumulating at least 30 minutes of moderate-intensity physical activity on most and preferably all days of the week.

3. For those with known cardiovascular disease, cardiac rehabilitation programs that combine physical activity with reduction in other risk factors should be more widely used.

These recommendations were based on the premise that most Americans are increasingly becoming sedentary. They have little or no physical activity in their daily lives because of changes in the work and home environments. The evidence to date suggests physical inactivity to be a major risk factor for CVD. Also, even moderate levels of physical activity can confer strong benefits, and those already meeting goals can derive additional benefit by becoming more physically active or including more vigorous activity.[72] Public health recommendations have evolved from emphasizing vigorous aerobic activity for cardiorespiratory fitness to moderate levels of activity for a wide variety of health benefits. Cardiorespiratory endurance activities should be supplemented with strength-development exercises at least twice per week to improve

musculoskeletal health and maintain the ability to perform normal activities.[8]

Health care professionals should personally engage in an active lifestyle to familiarize themselves with the issues involved in maintaining lifelong physical activity and to set a good example for patients and the public.[39]

A physical activity history is a necessary part of the medical history, and health care professionals should include the patient's habitual physical activity as part of the medical record. Health care providers need to emphasize the importance of physical activity as primary or adjunctive therapy for such medical conditions as hypertension, hypertriglyceridemia, glucose intolerance, and obesity.[39] Although it is not necessary that all individuals beginning a moderate-intensity and moderately progressive exercise program undergo an exercise stress test, a consensus group from the American Heart Association and American College of Cardiology[73], while not recommending routine testing in asymptomatic individuals, indicated there was some evidence (although not well-established) to support exercise testing before the initiation of a *vigorous* exercise program in healthy men aged 45 years and older and women aged 55 years and older. More recently published standards by the American Heart Association indicate that exercise testing may be useful for men older than 40 with one or more risk factors, providing information as a guide for more aggressive risk factor intervention. However, further study was indicated before exercise testing in asymptomatic women and the elderly (aged >75 years) could be recommended.[74]

In the health care setting or at the work site, only trained and experienced personnel should discuss physical activity and provide exercise prescriptions for patients and their families. Untrained, but well-intentioned personnel frequently offer unsubstantiated information and are not prepared to supervise or monitor patient activity. Physicians and their staff have the responsibility to promote and monitor their patients' regular physical activity as much as they work to reduce other CHD risk factors. Although many delegate the task of providing these services to other members of the health care team, physicians must set up and support the agenda and determine what is medically appropriate. Exercise specialists, including appropriately trained nurses, and trained personnel in community institutions (eg, YMCAs, boys and girls clubs) can also work with the physician in physical activity assessment, prescription, and monitoring. Medical training programs should begin now to prepare physicians to recommend physical activity and to assess it as part of every medical history.[1] Consideration should be given to intensity, duration, and frequency, as well as mode and progression of all types of physical activity programs.[75] Sedentary men older than 40 and women older than 50 are advised to consult a physician before beginning a vigorous physical activity program.[8]

The President's Council on Physical Fitness and Sports provides, as an initial classification, five different levels of physical activity (Table 12-4).[75] These include activities that are universally recommended and depend on the individual's current level of activity. For those pursuing a modest level of activity, recommendations are provided for additional activity based largely on the individual's specific health, fitness, and/or performance goals.

Activities for everyone promote general health and well-being and can be done as part of the individual's daily living routine. Examples include walking rather than riding whenever possible, climbing stairs instead of taking an elevator, and parking further away from one's destination (eg, workplace or store).

For sedentary individuals who currently engage in no physical activity, or those who cannot walk 30 minutes continuously without discomfort or pain (those unable to walk can substitute other activities, such as moving in a wheelchair and swimming), 30 minutes of moderate-intensity activity is recommended, in addition to the universally recommended activities mentioned above. This may involve walking, yard work, cycling, or low-impact exercise broken into two to four 10-minute segments during the workday and/or in the morning or evening.

TABLE 12-4   Model for Physical Activity Recommendations

Activities recommended for everyone
Activities for sedentary individuals

Activities for moderately active individuals interested in health
  Cardiovascular
  Bone
  Low back
  Psychological

Activities for moderately active individuals interested in physical fitness
  Aerobic fitness
  Relative leanness
  Muscular strength and endurance
  Flexibility

Activities for vigorously active individuals interested in performance
  Sport (s)
  Physical task(s)

SOURCE: Data from the Department of Health and Human Services.[75]

A moderately active individual, in contrast, should be able to accumulate 30 minutes of activity daily (eg, 30 minutes of walking continuously without pain or discomfort) in addition to those activities recommended for sedentary individuals. Such an individual would typically not be able to jog 3 miles (or walk 6 miles at a brisk pace, cycle 12 miles, or swim $\frac{3}{4}$ mile) continuously without discomfort or undue fatigue. These individuals should be encouraged to include 30 minutes of moderate-intensity activity in their daily routine (Table 12-5).

TABLE 12-5   Physical Activity for Health Goals

Health goal	Recommended activity
Cardiovascular	Accumulate at least 30 min of moderate-intensity activities daily Include longer duration and/or higher intensity
Bone	Weight-bearing activities Resistance exercises
Low Back	Static stretching in midtrunk and thigh regions Abdominal curl-ups
Psychologic	Enjoyable activities and fun atmosphere

SOURCE: Data from the Department of Health and Human Services.[75]

TABLE 12-6 Physical Fitness Goals and Recommended Activities*

Physical fitness goal	Recommended activity
Aerobic fitness	20–30 min of vigorous-intensity activity, 3–5 d/wk
Relative leanness	
Too little fat	Eat more calories, especially carbohydrates Include resistance exercise
Too much fat	Reduce calories, especially fat Increase duration of aerobic activities Include resistance exercise
Muscular strength/endurance	Include resistance exercise: one or two sets, 10–15 reps, each muscle group 2 or 3 d/wk
Flexibility	Daily static stretching, 10–30 s, two or three times, each joint

*These activities should be considered only **after** an individual is doing the activities listed in Table 12-5. These activities should be done *in addition* to Table 12-5 activities.

SOURCE: Data from the Department of Health and Human Services.[75]

TABLE 12-7 Recommended Activity for Performance Goals*

Performance goal	Recommended activity
Sport or physical task(s)	Develop and/or maintain fitness levels Interval training Motor tasks related to performance Specific skills related to performance Strategy and mental readiness

* These activities should be considered only **after** an individual is doing the activities recommended in Tables 12-5 and 12-6. These activities should be done *in addition* to activities in Tables 12-5 and 12-6.

SOURCE: Data from the Department of Health and Human Services.[75]

Moderately active individuals with fitness goals should continue to accumulate the recommended 30 minutes of daily activity as described above. In addition, specific types of activity should be considered, depending on the goal desired (Table 12-6). For example, if aerobic fitness is desired, at least 20 minutes of high-intensity activity should be preceded and followed by 5 to 10 minutes of moderate-intensity activity, 3 to 4 days per week. The heart rate during these vigorous activities should be 70 to 85% of the age-predicted maximum, calculated as follows: target heart rate = (0.70 to 0.85) × (220 beats/min – age in years). For example, a 40-year-old individual would have an estimated maximum heart rate of 180 beats/min, with a target heart rate of 126 to 153 beats/min. Other goals, such as achieving muscular strength and endurance, require resistance activities to maintain muscle mass.

A vigorously active individual can run 3 miles (or walk fast 6 miles, cycle 12 miles, or swim $\frac{3}{4}$ mile) continuously within his or her target heart rate, three to four times per week, without discomfort or pain (Table 12-7). For those with performance goals, a variety of sport and performance activities should be considered depending on level of interest, such as soccer, basketball, racquetball, and high-intensity exercise to music, in addition to 30 minutes of daily moderate-intensity activity and in-cluding vigorous activity at the target heart rate on days when no sport/performance activities are planned.

The long-term success of any physical activity program is determined by compliance. While one is on business or vacation, there must be a plan for incorporating physical activities, as other aspects of the trip (meals, social functions, etc). Although many lodging facilities do provide exercise or fitness facilities, this is not always the case. Exercise facilities may not always be convenient or available; as a substitute, one can bring portable exercise equipment, such as walking or jogging shoes.[75]

Important influences on physical activity patterns both in adults and in younger people include confidence in one's ability to engage in certain activities (self-efficacy), enjoyment of the activity, support from others, positive beliefs concerning the benefits of physical activity, and lack of any perceived barriers to being physically active.[8]

Physical activity in secondary prevention

Among patients with myocardial infarction, exercise-based cardiac rehabilitation can have significant benefits in reducing cardiac and total mortality by approximately 30%. However, a meta-analysis of 51 randomized controlled trials of exercise-based cardiac rehabilitation with a mean follow-up of 2.4 years recently demonstrated that exercise-based cardiac rehabilitation was ineffective in reducing the incidence of new myocardial infarction.[76] Important benefits of physical activity also extend to patients with peripheral arterial disease and claudication, where exercise programs have been shown to substantially increase average walking distance to pain onset, as well as average distance to maximal tolerated pain.[77] In persons with CVD or diabetes, or at high risk for these diseases, consultation with a physician is recommended before beginning a new physical activity program.[8] For promotion of physical activity in those who have recently suffered a cardiac event, walking is the recommended mode of early and continuous activity, unless it is recommended that the individual attend supervised exercise classes, where other activities can be provided. Limited walking can begin with gradual increases in duration until 5 to 10 minutes of continuous movement is achieved. In the first 2 weeks after myocardial infarction or coronary artery bypass surgery, the emphasis should be on offsetting the effects of bed rest or prior periods of physical inactivity. Initial activities should be supervised, with symptoms, rating of perceived exertion, heart rate, and blood pressure monitored. When safety and tolerance have been documented, activity can be performed in an unsupervised manner. Such activity is usually safe; however, patients should be instructed regarding precautions—such as awareness of chest discomfort, faintness, and dyspnea—and should appropriately consult their physicians.[73]

After the patient's condition has stabilized, usually 2 to 6 weeks after the coronary event, a symptom-limited exercise test is performed; this is essential prior to beginning a physical activity program. In most cases, a conditioning program can be initiated, with careful prescription of activity based on the results of the exercise test and professional consultation. Conditioning generally involves large-muscle-group activities, initially performed for 10 minutes, with the goal of building up to 20 to 30 minutes at a time. Supervised group sessions are generally recommended to enhance participation, ensure tolerability, confirm progress, and provide medical supervision in high-risk situations. Low-risk persons who are highly motivated and understand the principles of exercise training may undertake unsupervised home programs.[75]

In the absence of ischemia or significant arrhythmias (low-risk patients), exercise intensity should approximate 50 to 80% of the maximal oxygen capacity based on the exercise test, or 20 beats/min above resting heart rate until such a test is performed. The exercise training heart rate should be 50 to 75% of the heart rate reserve, as follows: [(maximal heart rate – resting heart rate) × 50 to 75%] + resting heart rate. Activities can be prescribed on the basis of the work intensity at which this training heart rate is achieved after 5 to 10 minutes at the same workload (steady state). Widely available heart rate counters can be used as aids to monitor levels of physical exertion.[75]

The intensity of exercise can also be judged by the individual using a perceived exertion rating scale consisting of 15 categories ranging from 6 to 20, with a verbal description at every odd number beginning with 7 (very, very light) and progressing to 19 (very, very hard). As a

general guideline, less than 12 is perceived as light intensity (40–60% of maximal heart rate), 12 to 13 as moderate intensity (60–75% of maximal heart rate), and 14 to 16 as high intensity (75–90% of maximal heart rate). Several training sessions using this perceived exertion scale are needed to validate an activity's difficulty. Normally, individuals may begin at moderate intensity, although some may need to begin at light intensity. After safe levels have been established, increments 5 minutes in duration can be made each week. With increased strength and decreases in exercise heart rate with conditioning, intensity levels can eventually be increased and some resistance exercises added.[75]

In moderate- to high-risk individuals, such as those with ischemia or arrthythmias, an exercise test and medical supervision are essential. The conditioning work intensity is derived from the heart rate associated with the abnormality, with the recommended peak training heart rate usually 10 beats/min below the heart rate where the abnormality occurs. If exercise continues to a high level of effort, a heart rate of 50 to 60% of the maximum can be used if it falls at least 10 beats below where the abnormality occurs. Ideally, these individuals should be enrolled in a cardiac rehabilitation program in which they can be risk-stratified appropriately, and exercise testing should be repeated at least annually.[75]

Recommendations for physical activity in youth

School-based activity programs for children and adolescents that have targeted related outcomes such as obesity and CVD risk factors have been successful.[78–82] Some of the studies, such as the large Child and Adolescent Trial for Cardiovascular Health (CATCH) Trial,[83] the Cardiovascular Health in Children (CHIC) study,[84] and others,[85–87] were highly effective in increasing physical activity and the amount of time spent in school physical education (PE).

Physical activity should begin early in the school years and continue throughout an individual's lifetime. The school years are most important for developing healthy attitudes toward physical activity. This is a time when children assume more responsibility for their own choices. Schools must designate PE programs with trained teachers for all grades. Recreational sports, including running, dancing, swimming, and certain resistance exercises using free weights or specific equipment, can be used with supervision. There must also be a supportive environment conducive to physical activity both at school and in the home.[88]

Interventions that target physical education in elementary schools can increase the amount of time that students spend in physical activity.[8] The CHIC-I study

TABLE 12-8 Physical Activity for Children: Guidelines Summary

Guideline 1	Elementary school-aged children should accumulate at least 30 to 60 min of age-appropriate physical activity from a variety of physical activities on all, or most, days of the week.
Guideline 2	Accumulation of more than 60 min, and up to several hours per day, of age- and developmentally appropriate activity is encouraged for elementary school-aged children.
Guideline 3	Some of the child's physical activity each day should be in periods lasting 10–15 min, or longer, and include moderate to vigorous physical activity. This activity will typically be intermittent in nature, involving alternating moderate-to-vigorous activity with brief periods of rest and recovery.
Guideline 4	Extended periods of inactivity are inappropriate for children.
Guideline 5	A variety of physical activities are recommended for elementary school-aged children.

SOURCE: Adapted, with permission, from National Association of Sport and Physical Education.[89]

was able to improve physiologic outcomes (eg, reduce body fat, decrease cholesterol concentrations, and increase aerobic power) in elementary school children.[84] The CHIC-II study was effective in reducing body fat and blood pressure in middle school youth.[89] One of the main reasons the CHIC interventions were successful in affecting physiologic variables is the increased amount of time spent in actual moderate-to-vigorous physical activity in school (20 minutes in elementary schools and 30 minutes in middle schools). Children at higher levels of cardiovascular risk may see significant benefits in the reduction or control of risk factors from physical activity of appropriate quantity and intensity. The increasing trend of obesity demonstrates that a greater effort needs to be made to promote participation in physical activity. The recent increase in type 2 diabetes in children and adolescents is an alarming manifestation of the broader problem of physical inactivity, poor diet, and obesity afflicting young people. Premature development of CVD, even in the absence of diabetes, is linked to childhood

obesity and physical inactivity. But when, in susceptible pediatric populations, these conditions are accompanied by frank diabetes, intensive and costly medical therapy must be instituted, and long-term chronic disease is almost certain. A preventive strategy that breaks the cycle of physical inactivity and obesity in children can potentially improve long-term cardiovascular and metabolic health in a larger population of children and adolescents.

The President's Council on Physical Fitness and Sports has also published guidelines for physical activity in children[75,89] (Table 12-8). These guidelines are intended to aid teachers, coaches, parents, and others who work with children, helping children to make decisions that are in their best interest. Guidelines 1 and 2 specify more activity for children than for adults because children are inherently active, require activity for normal growth and development, and need time in activity to develop lifetime physical activity skills. Because children are by nature active intermittently, and not necessarily captivated by longer, sustained exercise, as are adults, Guideline 3, specifying intermittent exercise, is provided. The rationale of Guideline 4, which discourages extended periods of inactivity for children, is based on the observation that children become less active over time, and childhood inactivity tracks to adulthood inactivity. Therefore, avoiding long periods of inactivity and engaging in frequent periods of activity during the day would, it is hoped, prevent inactivity in adults. Finally, Guideline 5 encourages a wide variety of physical activities that build on all parts of health-related physical fitness, including cardiovascular fitness, strength, muscular endurance, flexibility, and healthy body composition.

Summary guidelines (Table 12-9)[90] specific for adolescents have also been published. Although these

TABLE 12-9 Physical Activity for Adolescents: Guidelines Summary

Guideline 1	All adolescents should be physically active daily, or nearly every day, as part of play, games, sports, work, transportation, recreation, physical education, or planned exercise, in family, school, and community activities.
Guideline 2	Adolescents should engage in three or more sessions per week of activities that last 20 min or longer at a time and require moderate to vigorous levels of exertion.

SOURCE: Adapted, with permission, from Sallis et al.[90]

TABLE 12-10 Guidelines for Promoting Physical Activity Among Youth

Policy	Schools and communities should establish policies that promote enjoyable, lifelong physical activity among young people.
Environment	Schools and communities should provide physical and social environments that encourage and enable safe and enjoyable physical activity.
Physical education	Schools should implement physical education programs that emphasize enjoyable participation in physical activity and that help students develop the knowledge, attitudes, motor skills, behavioral skills, and confidence needed to adopt and maintain physically active lifestyles.
Health education	Schools should implement health education programs that help students develop the knowledge, attitudes, behavioral skills, and confidence needed to adopt and maintain physically active lifestyles.
Extracurricular activities	Schools should provide extracurricular physical activity programs that meet the needs and interests of all students.
Parental involvement	Parents and guardians should be in physical activity instruction programs and in extracurricular and community physical activity programs, and they should be encouraged to support their children's participation in enjoyable physical activity.
Personnel training	Schools and communities should provide training for education, coaching, recreation, and health care personnel that imparts the knowledge and skills needed to effectively promote enjoyable, lifelong physical activity among young people.
Health services	Health care professionals should assess physical activity patterns among young people, counsel them about physical activity, refer them to appropriate programs, and advocate for physical activity instruction and programs for young people.
Community programs	Communities should provide a range of developmentally appropriate community sports and recreation programs that are attractive to all young people.
Evaluation	Schools and communities should regularly evaluate physical activity instruction, programs, and facilities.

SOURCE: Adapted, with permission, from Centers for Disease Control and Prevention.[91]

guidelines are more similar to adult guidelines than the guidelines for children, much of the activity for teens is associated with school and community activities. A wide variety of activities should be encouraged to provide a foundation that can serve for a lifetime.

A comprehensive set of guidelines for the promotion of physical activity among young people and adolescents have also been published (Table 12-10),[91] suggesting initiatives that can be implemented in schools and communities and paying attention to the roles of parents, community organizations, and health care professionals. These guidelines are based on the premise that youth are most likely to develop physically active lifestyles if they are provided with experiences they enjoy and can be successful at, and which are developmentally appropriate and matched to the individual or group's interests.

REFERENCES

1. Fletcher GF, Balady G, Blair SN, et al. Statement on exercise: benefits and recommendations for physical activity programs for all Americans: a statement for health professionals by the Committee on Cardiac Rehabilitation of the Council on Clinical Cardiology, American Heart Association. *Circulation* 1996;94:857–862.

2. Powell KE, Thompson PD, Caspersen CJ, Kendrick JS. Physical activity and the incidence of coronary heart disease. *Annu Rev Public Health* 1987;8:253–287.

3. Morris JN, Clayton DJ, Everitt MG, et al. Exercise in leisure time: coronary attack and death rates. *Br Heart J* 1990;63:325–334.

4. Blair SN, Kohl HW III, Paffenbarger RS Jr, et al. Physical fitness and all-cause mortality: a prospective study of healthy men and women. *JAMA* 1989;262:2395–2401.

5. Lee IM, Hsieh CC, Paffenbarger RS Jr: Exercise intensity and longevity in men: the Harvard Alumni Health Study. *JAMA* 1995;273:1179–1184.

6. Blair SN, Kohl HW III, Barlow CE, et al. Changes in physical fitness and all-case mortality: a prospective study of healthy and unhealthy men. *JAMA* 1995;273:1093–1098.

7. Pate RR, Pratt M, Blair SN, et al. Physical activity and public health: a recommendation from the Centers for Disease Control and Prevention and the American College of Sports Medicine. *JAMA* 1995;73:402–407.

8. *Physical Activity and Health: A Report of the Surgeon General.* Washington, DC: US Department of Health and Human Services, Centers for Disease Control and Prevention, National Center for

Chronic Disease Prevention and Health Promotion, The President's Council on Physical Fitness and Sports; 1996.

9. *Heart Disease and Stroke Statistics—2003 Update.* Dallas: American Heart Association; 2003.

10. Morris JN, Kagan A, Pattison DC, Gardner MJ. Incidence and prediction of ischaemic heart disease in London busmen. *Lancet* 1966;2:552–559.

11. Pomrehn PR, Wallace RB, Burmeister LF. Ischemic heart disease mortality in Iowa farmers: the influence of lifestyle. *JAMA* 1982;248:1073–1076.

12. Taylor HL, Blackburn H, Keys A, et al. Coronary heart disease in seven countries: IV. Five-year follow-up of employees of selected U.S. railroad companies. *Circulation* 1970;41(suppl 1): 20–39.

13. Menotti A, Puddu V. Ten-year mortality from coronary heart disease among 172,000 men classified by occupational physical activity. *Scand J Work Environ Health* 1979;5:100–108.

14. Berlin JA, Colditz GA. A meta-analysis of physical activity in the prevention of coronary heart disease. *Am J Epidemiol* 1990;132:612–628.

15. Karvonen MJ. Physical activity in work and leisure time in relation to cardiovascular diseases. *Ann Clin Res* 1983;14(suppl 34):118–123.

16. Paffenbarger RS Jr, Wing AL, Hyde RT. Physical activity as an index of heart attack risk in college alumni. *Am J Epidemiol* 1978;108:161–175.

17. Paffenbarger RS, Hyde RT, Wing AL, Hsieh C-C. Physical activity, all-cause mortality, and longevity of college alumni. *N Engl J Med* 1986;314:605–613.

18. Morris JN, Everitt MG, Pollard R, Chave SPW. Vigorous exercise in leisure-time: protection against coronary heart disease. *Lancet* 1980;2:1207–1210.

19. Leon AS, Connett J, Jacobs DR, Rauramaa R. Leisure-time physical activity levels and risk of coronary heart disease and death: the Multiple Risk Factor Intervention Trial. *JAMA* 1987;258:2388–2395.

20. Pekkanen J, Marti B, Nissinen A, et al. Reduction of premature mortality by high physical activity: a 20-year follow-up of middle-aged Finnish men. *Lancet* 1987;1:1473–1477.

21. Ekelund LG, Haskell WL, Johnson JL, et al. Physical fitness as a predictor of cardiovascular mortality in asymptomatic North American men: the Lipid Research Clinics Mortality Follow-up Study. *N Engl J Med* 1988;319:1379–1384.

22. Slattery ML, Jacobs DR, Nichaman MZ. Leisure time physical activity and coronary heart disease death: the US Railroad Study. *Circulation* 1989;79:304–311.

23. Shaper AG, Wannamethee G. Physical activity and ischemic heart disease in middle-aged British men. *Br Heart J* 1991;66: 384–394.

24. Paffenbarger RS Jr, Hyde RT, Wing AL, et al. The association of changes in physical activity level and other lifestyle characteristics with mortality among men. *N Engl J Med* 1993;328:538–545.

25. Lakka TA, Venalainen JM, Rauramaa R, et al. Relation of leisure-time physical activity level and cardiorespiratory fitness to the risk of acute myocardial infarction in men. *N Engl J Med* 1994; 339:1549–1554.

26. Blair SN, Kampert JB, Kohl HW, et al. Influences of cardiorespiratory fitness and other precursors on cardiovascular disease and all-cause mortality in men and women. *JAMA* 1996;276:205–210.

27. Kujala UM, Kaprio J, Sarna S, Koskenvuo M. Relationship of leisure-time physical activity and mortality. *JAMA* 1998;279: 440–444.

28. Haapanen N, Miilunpalo S, Vuori I, et al. Characteristics of leisure time physical activity associated with decreased risk of premature all-cause and cardiovascular disease mortality in middle-aged men. *Am J Epidemiol* 1996;143:870–880.

29. Haapanen N, Miilunpalo S, Vuori I, et al. Association of leisure time physical activity with the risk of coronary heart disease, hypertension, and diabetes in middle-aged men and women. *Int J Epidemiol* 1997;26:739–747.

30. Leon AS, Myers MJ, Connett J. Leisure time physical activity and the 16-year risks of mortality from coronary heart disease and all-causes in the Multiple Risk Factor Intervention Trial (MRFIT). *Int J Sports Med* 1997;18(suppl 3):S208–S215.

31. Rosengren A, Wilhelmsen L. Physical activity protects against coronary death and deaths from all causes in middle-aged men: evidence from 20-year follow-up of the primary prevention study in Goteborg. *Ann Epidemiol* 1997;7:69–75.

32. Eaton CB, Medalie JH, Flocke SA, et al. Self-reported physical activity predicts long-term coronary heart disease and all-cause mortalities: twenty-one-year follow-up of the Israeli Ischemic Heart Disease Study. *Arch Fam Med* 1995;4:323–329.

33. Kaplan GA, Strawbridge WJ, Cohen RD, Hungerford LR. Natural history of leisure-time physical activity and its correlates: associations with mortality from all-causes and cardiovascular disease over 28 years. *Am J Epidemiol* 1996;144:793–797.

34. Manson JE, Greenland P, LaCroix AZ, et al. Walking compared with vigorous exercise for the prevention of cardiovascular events in women. *N Engl J Med* 2002;347:716–725.

35. Lee IM, Sesso HD, Oguma Y, Paffenbarger RS Jr. Relative intensity of physical activity and risk of coronary heart disease. *Circulation* 2003;107:1110–1116.

36. Hu FB, Stampfer MJ, Solomon C, et al. Physical activity and risk of cardiovascular events in diabetic women. *Ann Intern Med* 2001;134:96–105.

37. Rodriguez BL, Curb JD, Burchfiel CM, et al. Physical activity and 23-year incidence of coronary heart disease morbidity and mortality among middle-aged men: the Honolulu Heart Program. *Circulation* 1994;89:2540–2544.

38. Folsom AR, Arnett DK, Hutchinson RG, et al. Physical activity and incidence of coronary heart disease in middle-aged women and men. *Med Sci Sports Exerc* 1997;29:901–909.

39. Myers J, Prakash M, Froelicher V, et al. Exercise capacity and mortality among men referred for exercise testing. *N Engl J Med* 2002;346:793–801.

40. Gulati M, Pandey DK, Arnsdorf MF, et al. Exercise capacity and risk of death in women: the St James Women Take Heart Project. *Circulation* 2003;108:1554–1559.

41. Thompson PD, Buchner D, Pina IL, et al. Exercise and physical activity in the prevention and treatment of atherosclerotic cardiovascular disease: a statement from the Council on Clinical Cardiology (Subcommittee on Exercise, Rehabilitation, and Prevention) and the Council on Nutrition, Physical Activity, and Metabolism (Subcommittee on Physical Activity). *Arterioscler Thromb Vasc Biol* 2003;3:e42–e49.

42. Leon AS, Sanchez O. Meta-analysis of the effects of aerobic exercise training on blood lipids [abstract]. *Circulation* 2001;104(suppl II):II-414–II-415.

43. Fagard RH. Exercise characteristics and the blood pressure response to dynamic physical training. *Med Sci Sports Exerc* 2001; 33(6 suppl):S484–S492.

44. Thompson PD, Crouse SF, Goodpaster B, et al. The acute versus the chronic response to exercise. *Med Sci Sports Exerc* 2001;3(6 suppl):S438–S445.

45. Raitakari OT, Taimela S, Porkka KV, et al. Associations between physical activity and risk factors for coronary heart disease: the Cardiovascular Risk in Young Finns Study. *Med Sci Sports Exerc* 1997;29:1055–1061.

46. Schmiedt GJ, Walkuski JJ, Stensel DJ. The Singapore Youth Coronary Risk and Physical Activity Study. *Med Sci Sports Exerc* 1998;30:105–113.

47. Guillaume M, Lapidus L, Bjorntorp P, Lambert A. Physical activity, obesity, and cardiovascular risk factors in children: the Belgian Luxembourg Child Study II. *Obes Res* 1997;5:549–556.

48. Wong ND, Hei TK, Qaqundah PY, et al. Television viewing as a marker for pediatric hypercholesterolemia. *Pediatrics* 1992;90:75–79.

49. Blair SN, Cooper KH, Gibbons LW, et al. Changes in coronary heart disease risk factors associated with increased treadmill time in 753 men. *Am J Epidemiol* 1983;118:352–359.

50. Hagberg JM, Montain SJ, Martin WH III, Ehsani AA. Effect of exercise training in 60–69 year old persons with essential hypertension. *Am J Cardiol* 1989;64:348–353.

51. Jennings GL, Deakin G, Dewar E, et al. Exercise, cardiovascular disease and blood pressure. *Clin Exp Hypertens [A]* 1989;11:1035–1052.

52. Eaton CB, Lapane KL, Garber CE, et al. Physical activity, physical fitness, and coronary heart disease risk factors. *Med Sci Sports Exerc* 1995;27:340–346.

53. Hong Y, Bots ML, Pan X, et al. Physical activity and cardiovascular risk factors in rural Shanghai, China. *Int J Epidemiol* 1994;23:1154–1158.

54. Hsieh SD, Yoshinaga H, Muto T, Sakurai Y. Regular physical activity and coronary risk factors in Japanese men. *Circulation* 1998;97:661–665.

55. Bijnen FC, Feskens EJ, Caspersen CJ, et al. Physical activity and cardiovascular risk factors among elderly men in Finland, Italy, and The Netherlands. *Am J Epidemiol* 1996;143:553–561.

56. Tran ZV, Weltman A. Differential effects of exercise on serum lipid and lipoprotein levels seen with changes in body weight: a meta-analysis. *JAMA* 1985;254:919–924.

57. King AC, Haskell WL, Young DR, et al. Long-term effects of varying intensities and formats of physical activity on participation rates, fitness, and lipoproteins in men and women aged 50 to 65 years. *Circulation* 1995;91:2596–2604.

58. Williams PT. High-density lipoprotein cholesterol and other risk factors for coronary heart disease in female runners. *N Engl J Med* 1996;334:1298–1303.

59. Greendale GA, Bodin-Dunn L, Ingles S, et al. Leisure, home, and occupational physical activity and cardiovascular risk factors in postmenopausal women: the Postmenopausal Estrogens/Progestins Intervention (PEPI) study. *Arch Intern Med* 1996; 156:418–424.

60. Pols MA, Peeters PH, Twisk JW, et al. Physical activity and cardiovascular disease risk profile in women. *Am J Epidemiol* 1997;146:322–328.

61. Hunter GR, Kekes-Szabo T, Treuth MS, et al. Intra-abdominal adipose tissue, physical activity and cardiovascular risk in pre- and postmenopausal women. *Int J Obesity Rel Metab Disord* 1996;20:860–865.

62. Wood PD, Stefanick ML, Williams PT, Haskell WL. The effects on plasma lipoproteins of a prudent weight-reducing diet, with or without exercise, in overweight men and women. *N Engl J Med* 1991;325:461–465.

63. King DS, Dalsky GP, Clutter WE, et al. Effects of exercise and lack of exercise on insulin sensitivity and responsiveness. *J Appl Physiol* 1988;64:1942–1946.

64. Lee IM. Physical activity, fitness, and cancer. In: Bouchard C, Shephard RJ, Stephens T, eds. *Physical Activity, Fitness, and Health: International Proceedings and Consensus Statement.* Champaign, IL: Human Kinetics; 1994:814–831.

65. Blumenthal JA, Emery CF, Madden DJ, et al. Cardiovascular and behavioral effects of aerobic exercise training in healthy older men and women. *J Gerontol* 1989;44:M147–M157.

66. Kavanaugh T, Shephard RJ, Tuck JA, Quershi S. Depression following myocardial infarction: the effects of distance running. *Ann NY Acad Sci* 1977;301:1029–1038.

67. Martinsen EW, Medhus A, Sandvik L. Effects of aerobic exercise on depression: a controlled study. *Br Med J (Clin Res Ed)* 1985;291–109.

68. Folkins CH, Sime WE. Physical fitness training and mental health. *Am J Psychol* 1981;36:373–389.

69. Blumenthal JA, Fredrikson M, Kuhn CM, et al. Aerobic exercise reduces levels of cardiovascular and sympatho-adrenal responses to mental stress in subjects without prior evidence of myocardial ischemia. *Am J Cardiol* 1990;65:93–98.

70. Sidney S, Jacobs DR, Haskell WL, et al. Comparison of two methods of assessing physical activity in the Coronary Artery Risk Development in Young Adults (CARDIA) study. *Am J Epidemiol* 1991;133:1231–1245.

71. NIH Consensus Development Panel on Physical Activity and Cardiovascular Health. Physical activity and cardiovascular health. *JAMA* 1996;276:241–246.

72. Fletcher GF. American Heart Association Medical/Scientific Statement: How to implement physical activity in primary and secondary prevention. *Circulation* 1997;96:355–357.

73. Gibbons RJ, Balady GJ, Beasley JW, et al. ACC/AHA Guidelines for Exercise Testing: a report of the American College of Cardiology/American Heart Association Task Force on Practice Guidelines (Committee on Exercise Testing). *J Am Coll Cardiol* 1997;30:260–311.

74. Fletcher GF, Balady GJ, Amsterdam EA, et al. Exercise standards for testing and training: a statement for healthcare professionals from the American Heart Association. *Circulation* 2001;104:1694–1710.

75. Department of Health and Human Services. Physical activity for young people. *President's Council Physical Fitness Sports Res Digest* 1998;Series 3(3):1–7. Washington, DC: DDHS; 1998.

76. Jolliffe JA, Rees K, Taylor RS, et al. Exercise-based rehabilitation for coronary heart disease. *Cochrane Database Syst Rev* 2001;1:CD001800.

77. Gardner AW, Poehlman ET. Exercise rehabilitation programs for treatment of claudication pain: a meta-analysis. *JAMA* 1995;274:975–980.

78. Gortmaker SL, Peterson K, Wiecha J, et al. Reducing obesity via a school-based interdisciplinary intervention among youth. *Arch Pediatc Adolesc Med* 1999;153:409–418.

79. Marcus AC, Wheeler RC, Cullen JW, Crane LA. Quasi-experimental evaluation of the Los Angeles Know Your Body program: knowledge, beliefs, and self-reported behaviors. *Prev Med* 1987;16(6):803–815.

80. Simons-Morton BG, Parcel GS, Baranowski T, et al. Promoting physical activity and a healthful diet among children: results of a school-based intervention study. *Am J Public Health* 1991; 81(8):986–991.

81. Stone EJ, McKenzie TL, Welk GJ, Booth ML. Effects of physical activity interventions in youth: review and synthesis. *Am J Prev Med* 1998;15(4):298–315.

82. Tell GS, Vellar OD. Physical fitness, physical activity, and cardiovascular disease risk factors in adolescents: the Oslo Youth Study. *Prev Med* 1988;17(1):12–24.

83. Luepker RV, Perry CL, McKinlay SM, et al. Outcomes of a field trial to improve children's dietary patterns and physical activity: the Child and Adolescent Trial for Cardiovascular Health (CATCH). *JAMA* 1996;275:768–776.

84. Harrell JS, McMurray RG, Gansky SA, et al. A public health vs a risk-based intervention to improve cardiovascular health in elementary school children: the Cardiovascular Health in Children Study. *Am J Public Health* 1999;89:1529–1535.

85. Burke V, Milligan RA, Thompson C, et al. A controlled trial of health promotion programs in 11-year-olds using physical activity "enrichment" for higher risk children. *J Pediatr* 1998;132(5):840–848.

86. Donnelly JE, Jacobsen DJ, Whatley JE, et al. Nutrition and physical activity program to attenuate obesity and promote physical and metabolic fitness in elementary school children. *Obes Res* 1996;4(3):229–243.

87. Keenan DP, Achterberg C, Kris-Etherton PM, et al. Use of qualitative and quantitative methods to define behavioral fat-reduction strategies and their relationship to dietary fat reduction in the Patterns of Dietary Change Study. *J Am Diet Assoc* 1996;96:1245–1250,1253; quiz 1251–1252.

88. McMurray RG, Harrell JS, Bangdiwala SI, Bradley CB, Deng S, Levine A. A school-based intervention can reduce body fat and blood pressure in young adolescents. *J Adolesc Health* 2002;31:125–132.

89. *Physical Activity for Children: A Statement of Guidelines.* Reston, VA: National Association for Sport and Physical Education; 1998.

90. Sallis JF, Patrick K, Long BL. An overview of the international consensus conference on physical activity guidelines for adolescents. *Pediatr Exerc Sci* 1994;6:299–301.

91. Centers for Disease Control and Prevention. Guidelines for school and community programs to promote lifelong physical activity among young people. *MMWR* 1997;46(RR-6): 1–36.

APPENDIX 12-1 THE AEROBICS CENTER LONGITUDINAL STUDY PHYSICAL ACTIVITY QUESTIONNAIRE

Activity component(s) assessed:
Leisure and household
Time frame of recall:
Past 3 mo
Original mode of administration:
Self-administered by mail
Primary source of information:
Dr. Steven N. Blair
Cooper Institute for Aerobics Research
12330 Preston Road
Dallas, TX 75230
Primary reference:
Kohl, H. W., S. N. Blair, R. S. Paffenbarger, Jr., C. A. Macera, and J. J. Kronenfeld. A mail survey of physical activity habits as related to measured physical fitness. *Am J. Epidemiol.* 127:1228–1239, 1988.

Reliability and Validity Studies

TABLE 1 Validation studies of the Aerobics Institute Longitudinal Study Questionnaire

References	Method	Sample	Summary results	
Kohn et al. (1)	Relationships between treadmill time and various physical activity parameters from the survey (Pearson correlations)	374 male patients of the Cooper Clinic with an average age of 47.1 years	Racket sports	0.01
			Bicycling	0.06
			Swimming	−0.11
			Other strenuous sports	0.19*
			Frequency of sweating	0.51*
			Runners, joggers, and walkers	
			Miles/workout	0.35*
			Workouts/wk	0.29*
			Average time/mile	−0.39*
Oliveria et al. (3)	Relationships between weekly energy expenditure from physical activity and maximal exercise treadmill time (correlation coefficients†)	7570 predominantly white, married, college-educated men between the ages of 20 and 80 yr	Baseline physical activity	0.41
			Follow-up physical activity in 1982	0.32

* $P < 0.05$.
† No p value reported.
SOURCE: Reprinted with permission from Dr. Steven N. Blair, Cooper Institute for Aerobics Research, Dallas, TX.

In this section we would like to ask you about your current physical activity and exercise habits that you perform regularly, at least once a week. Please answer as accurately as possible. Circle your answer or supply a specific number when asked.

Exercise /Physical Activity

1. For the last three months, which of the following moderate or vigorous activities have you performed regularly? *(Please circle YES for all that apply and NO if you do not perform the activity; provide an estimate of the amount of activity for all marked YES. Be as complete as possible.)*

Walking
NO YES → How many sessions per week? _____
How many miles (or fractions) per session? _____
Average duration per session? _____ (minutes)

What is your usual pace of walking? *(Please circle one)*

CASUAL or STROLLING (<2 mph)	AVERAGE or NORMAL (2 to 3 mph)	FAIRLY BRISK (3 to 4 mph)	BRISK or STRIDING (4 mph or faster)

Stair Climbing
NO YES   ⟶   How many flights of stairs do you   _____
                    climb UP each day? (1 flight = 10 steps)

Jogging or Running
NO YES   ⟶   How many sessions per week?   _____
                 How many miles (or fractions) per session?   _____
                 Average duration per session?   _____ (minutes)

Treadmill
NO YES   ⟶   How many sessions per week?   _____
                 Average duration per session?   _____
                 Speed? _____(mph) Grade?_____(%)

Bicycling
NO YES   ⟶   How many sessions per week?   _____
                 How many miles per session?   _____
                 Average duration per session?   _____ (minutes)

Swimming Laps
NO YES   ⟶   How many sessions per week?   _____
                 How many miles per session?
                    (880 yds = 0.5 miles)   _____
                 Average duration per session?   _____ (minutes)

Aerobic Dance/Calisthenics/Floor Exercise
NO YES   ⟶   How many sessions per week?   _____
                 Average duration per session?   _____ (minutes)

Moderate Sports (e.g. Leisure volleyball, golf (not riding), social dancing, doubles tennis)
NO YES   ⟶   How many sessions per week?   _____
                 Average duration per session?   _____ (minutes)

Vigorous Racquet Sports (e.g. Racquetball, singles tennis)
NO YES   ⟶   How many sessions per week?   _____
NO YES   ⟶   Average duration per session?   _____ (minutes)

Other Vigorous Sports or Exercise Involving Running (e.g. Basketball, soccer)
NO YES   ⟶   Please specify: _____
                 How many sessions per week?   _____
                 Average duration per session?   _____ (minutes)

Other Activities
NO YES   ⟶   Please specify: _____
                 How many sessions per week?   _____
                 Average duration per session?   _____ (minutes)

Weight Training (Machines, free weights)
NO YES   ⟶   How many sessions per week?   _____
                 Average duration per session?   _____ (minutes)

Household Activities (Sweeping, vacuuming, washing clothes, scrubbing floors)
NO YES $\longrightarrow$ How many hours per week? _____

Lawn Work and Gardening
NO YES $\longrightarrow$ How many hours per week? _____

2. How many times a week do you engage in vigorous physical activity long enough to work up a sweat? _____
   (*times per week*)

Instructions:

Instructions for the recipient are listed on the first page of the questionnaire.

Calculations:

Scoring has been done by assigning MET values to reported activities as shown below (1). The scores can also be converted to kilocalories (3).

$$(\text{sessions/wk}) \times (\text{min/session}) \times (\text{h/min}) \times (\text{METs}) = \text{MET-h/wk}$$

Example:

Hypothetical raw data from the ACLS questionnaire:
   Bicycling: 3 sessions/wk, 10 miles/session, 30 min/session
Swimming: 2 session/wk, 1 mile/session, 60 min/session
      Bicycling is assigned a MET value of 4.0, and swimming is assigned a MET value 10.0 (1).
   Bicycling: (3 sessions/wk) × (30 min/session) × (1 h/60 min × 4.0 METs) = 6.0 MET-h/wk
Swimming: (2 sessions/wk) × (60 min/session) × (1 h/60 min × 10.0 METs) = 20.0 MET-h/wk
   Total = 26.0 MET-h/wk

Other Studies Using the Questionnaire

In addition to the references cited above, at least one additional study has used the ACLS Questionnaire (2).

REFERENCES

1. Kohl, H.W., S. N. Blair, R. S. Paffenbarger, Jr., C. A. Macera, and J. J. Kronenfeld. A mail survey of physical activity habits as related to measured physical fitness. *Am. J. Epidemiol.* 127:1228–1239, 1988.

2. Macera, C. A., K. L. Jackson, D. R. Davis, J. J. Kronenfeld, and S. N. Blair. Patterns of non-response to a mail survey. *J. Clin. Epidemiol.* 43:1427–1430, 1990.

3. Oliveria, S. A., H. W. Kohl, III, D. Trichopoulos, and S. N. Blair. The association between cardiorespiratory fitness and prostate cancer. *Med. Sci. Sports Exerc.* 28:97–104, 1996.

APPENDIX 12-2 CARDIA PHYSICAL ACTIVITY HISTORY

Activity component(s) assessed:
Leisure, job, and home/household
Time frame of recall:
Past 12 mo
Original mode of administration:
Interviewer—administered in person or by telephone
Primary source of information:
Dr. David R. Jacobs, Jr.
Division of Epidemiology,
University of Minnesota
1300 South 2nd Street, Suite 300,
Minneapolis, MN 55454
Primary reference:
Jacobs, D. R. Jr., L. P. Hahn, W. L. Haskell, P. Pirie, and S. Sidney. Reliability and validity of a short physical activity history: CARDIA and the Minnesota Heart Health Program. *J. Cardiopulm. Rehab.* 9:448–459, 1989.

Reliability and Validity Studies

TABLE 6 Reliability Studies of the CARDIA Physical Activity History

References	Methods	Sample	Summary results	
Jacobs et al. (1)	Relationships between moderate intensity, heavy intensity, and total activity units at baseline and 2-wk retest (Pearson correlations[†])	129 men and women between the ages of 18 and 74 yr; 46% male, 80% employed, 19% homemaker, 37% high school graduate or less education	Moderate Heavy Total	0.77 0.79 0.84
Jacobs et al. (2)	Relationships between moderate intensity, heavy intensity, and total activity units at first test and 1-mo retest (correlation coefficients)	28 men and 50 women, predominantly Caucasian between the ages of 20 and 59 yr	Moderate Heavy Total	0.66* 0.91* 0.88*

*$p < 0.05$.
[†]No *p* value reported.

CARDIA PHYSICAL ACTIVITY HISTORY

Now I'll be asking you about some specific activities and the amount of time you spend doing each. Only include the time spent actually doing the activity. For example, sitting by the pool does not count as time swimming; sitting in a chair lift does not count as time skiing.

First I'll ask you about vigorous activities. Vigorous activities increase your heart rate or make you sweat when doing them or make you breathe hard or raise your body temperature. If you do an activity but not vigorously, please include it later when I ask you about other non-strenuous sports.

1. The first vigorous activity is running or jogging. Did you run or jog in the past 12 months for at least one hour total time in any month? For instance, you might have done three 20-minute sessions in the month. (VIGOROUS BACKPACKING, HIKING, MOUNTAIN CLIMBING)

_____ Yes ➔   2. How many months did you do this activity?   _____

_____ No ↓   3. (How many of these months/In this month)
                         did you do this activity for at least 1 hour a week?   _____

                     4. (How many of these months/In this month)
                         did you do this activity for at least 2 hours a week?   _____

5. Did you do vigorous racquet sports in the past 12 months for at least one hour total time in any month? (TENNIS, BADMINTON, PADDLE BALL, RACQUETBALL, HANDBALL, SQUASH)

_____ Yes ➔   6. How many months did you do this activity?   _____

_____ No ↓   7. (How many of these months/In this month)
                         did you do this activity for at least 1 hour a week?   _____

                     8. (How many of these months/In this month)
                         did you do this activity for at least 3 hours a week?   _____

9. Did you bicycle faster than 10 miles an hour or exercise hard on an exercise bicycle (in the past 12 months for at least one hour total time in any month)? (ROWING MACHINE)

_____ Yes ➔   10. How many months did you do this activity?   _____

_____ No ↓   11. (How many of these months/In this month)
                         did you do this activity for at least 1 hour a week?   _____

                     12. (How many of these months/In this month)
                         did you do this activity for at least 2 hours a week?   _____

13. Did you swim in the past 12 months for at least one hour total time in any month? (SNORKELING, SCUBA DIVING)

_____ Yes ➔   14. How many months did you do this activity?   _____

_____ No ↓   15. (How many of these months/In this month)
                         did you do this activity for at least 1 hour a week?   _____

                     16. (How many of these months/In this month)
                         did you do this activity for at least 2 hours a week?   _____

17. Did you do a vigorous exercise class or vigorous dancing (in the past 12 months for at least one hour total time in any month)? (JAZZERCISE, JANE FONDA-TYPE WORKOUT, AEROBIC DANCING, BALLET)

_____ Yes ➔   18. How many months did you do this activity?   _____

_____ No ↓   19. (How many of these months/In this month)
                         did you do this activity for at least 1 hour a week?   _____

                     20. (How many of these months/In this month)
                         did you do this activity for at least 3 hours a week?   _____

21. Did you do a vigorous job activity such as lifting, carrying, or digging in the past 12 months for at least one hour total time in any month? (LOADING TRUCKS, STACKING LUMBER)

_____ Yes ➔   22. How many months did you do this activity?   _____

_____ No ⬇   23. (How many of these months/In this month)
            did you do this activity for at least 2 hour a week?   _____

           24. (How many of these months/In this month)
            did you do this activity for at least 5 hours a week?   _____

25. Did you do home or leisure activity such as snow shoveling, moving heavy objects, or weight lifting (in the past 12 months for at least one hour total time in any month)? (SHOVELING SAND OR GRAVEL, NAUTILUS WORKOUT, MOVING FURNITURE)

_____ Yes ➔   26. How many months did you do this activity?   _____

_____ No ⬇   27. (How many of these months/In this month)
            did you do this activity for at least 1 hour a week?   _____

           28. (How many of these months/In this month)
            did you do this activity for at least 3 hours a week?   _____

29. Did you do other strenuous sports such as basketball, football, skating, or skiing in the past 12 months for at least one hour total time in any month? (MARTIAL ARTS, SOCCER, RUGBY, LAND OR WATER SKIING, ICE OR ROLLER SKATING)

_____ Yes ➔   30. How many months did you do this activity?   _____

_____ No ⬇   31. (How many of these months/In this month)
            did you do this activity for at least 1 hour a week?   _____

           32. (How many of these months/In this month)
            did you do this activity for at least 3 hours a week?   _____

Now, I'd like to ask you about more leisurely activities.

33. Did you do nonstrenuous sports such as softball, shooting baskets, volleyball, ping pong, leisurely jogging, swimming or biking which we haven't included before (in the past 12 months for at least one hour total time in any month)? (HORSEBACK RIDING, FISHING FROM BANK OR BOAT, ARCHERY, NONVIGOROUS ROWING OR SAILING, NONVIGOROUS BIKING)

_____ Yes ➔   34. How many months did you do this activity?   _____

_____ No ⬇   35. (How many of these months/In this month)
            did you do this activity for at least 1 hour a week?   _____

           36. (How many of these months/In this month)
            did you do this activity for at least 3 hours a week?   _____

37. Did you take walks or hikes or walk to work in the past 12 months for at least one hour total time in any month? (STREAM FISHING, HUNTING)

_____ Yes ➔   38. How many months did you do this activity?   _____

_____ No ⬇   39. (How many of these months/In this month)
            did you do this activity for at least 2 hour a week?   _____

           40. (How many of these months/In this month)
            did you do this activity for at least 4 hours a week?   _____

41. Did you bowl or play golf (in the past 12 months for at least one hour total time in any month)?

_____ Yes ➜ 42. How many months did you do this activity? _____

_____ No ⬇ 43. (How many of these months/In this month)
did you do this activity for at least 1 hour a week?
_____ Always use motorized cart _____

44. (How many of these months/In this month)
did you do this activity for at least 3 hours a week?
_____ Always use motorized cart _____

45. Did you do home exercises or calisthenics in the past 12 months for at least one hour total time in any month?
(NONVIGOROUS EXERCISE OR ROWING MACHINE)

_____ Yes ➜ 46. How many months did you do this activity? _____

_____ No ⬇ 47. (How many of these months/In this month)
did you do this activity for at least 1 hour a week? _____

48. (How many of these months/In this month)
did you do this activity for at least 3 hours a week? _____

49. Did you do home maintenance and gardening, including carpentry, painting, raking or mowing (in the past
12 months for at least one hour total time in any month)? (HANGING WALLPAPER, WEEDING, GARDENING)

_____ Yes ➜ 50. How many months did you do this activity? _____

_____ No ⬇ 51. (How many of these months/In this month)
did you do this activity for at least 2 hour a week? _____

52. (How many of these months/In this month)
did you do this activity for at least 5 hours a week? _____

53. List sports or other activities not elsewhere classified

SPORT: _____

54. Have you already counted this in any other category?

_____ Yes (if yes, do not record here) _____ No

55. How many months? _____ 56. Average hrs. in those months? _____

57. List sports or other activities not elsewhere classified

SPORT: _____

58. Have you already counted this in any other category?

_____ Yes (if yes, do not record here) _____ No

59. How many months? _____ 60. Average hrs. in those months? _____

TABLE 7   Validation Studies of the CARDIA Physical Activity History

References	Method	Sample		Summary results			
Jacobs et al. (1)	Relationships between total activity units and four skinfolds (SKIN), caloric intake (CAL), treadmill test (TRM), and HDL cholesterol (HDL-C) (Pearson correlations[†])	5069 men and women between the ages of 18 and 30 yr. 52% Black, 54% female; 40% ≤ 12 yr of education		SKIN	CAL	TRM	HDL-C
			Men	− 0.12	0.21	0.25	0.11
			Women	− 0.15	0.07	0.36	0.13
Jacobs et al. (2)	Relationships between moderate and heavy intensity activity units and maximum oxygen consumption (Vo_2max) % body fat (BF), Caltrac (CAL; MET-min/d), and total 4-wk activity history (FWH; MET-min/d) (Spearman correlations)	28 men and 50 women predominantly Caucasian between the ages of 20 and 59 yr		Vo_{2max}	BF	CAL	FWH
			Moderate	0.08	− 0.09	0.11	0.08
			Heavy	0.63*	0.35*	0.31*	0.54*

*$p < 0.05$.
[†]No p value reported.
SOURCE: Reprinted with permission from Dr. David R. Jacobs, Jr., Division of Epidemiology, Univ. of Minnesota, Minneapolis, MN.

Instructions

Instructions are listed on the questionnaire. Individuals are asked to specify any activities from a list of 13 activity categories that they participated in for at least 1 h (total time) during any of the last 12 mo (1). For specific activities, the individual reports the number of months of participation and the number of months of frequent participation. Frequent participation is defined as follows.

2 h or more for activity categories A (jogging or running), C (cycling), and D (swimming)

3 h or more for activity categories B (vigorous racket sports), E (vigorous exercise class or vigorous dancing), F (home or leisure activity such as snow shoveling, moving, lifting), H (strenuous sports such as basketball, football, skating, and skiing), I (nonstrenuous sports, bowling, golf), and L (home exercises, calisthenics)

4 h or more for category J (walks or hikes)

5 h or more for activity categories G (vigorous job activity) and M (home maintenance)

Calculations

Exercise units = sum (for moderate, heavy, or all activities) of:

$$(intensity) \times [(months\ of\ infrequent\ activity)\ (3 \times months\ of\ frequent\ activity)]$$

Exercise units can be computed for moderate, heavy, or all activities separately: 100 exercise units is approximately equivalent to engaging in a heavy intensity activity (such as jogging) for 4 mo of the year. The intensity levels are listed in Table 8.

TABLE 8 Intensity levels for Activities in the CARDIA Physical Activity History

	Intensity (METS/min)*	Cutpoint for frequent participation (h/wk)
Heavy intensity activities		
A. Jog or run	8	2
B. Vigorous racket sports	8	3
C. Bicycle faster than 10 mi/h	6	2
D. Swimming	6	2
E. Vigorous exercise class or vigorous dancing	6	3
F. Nonjob activity such as shoveling, weight lifting, and moving heavy objects	6	3
G. Vigorous job activity such as lifting, carrying, or digging	5	5
H. Other strenuous sports such as basketball, football, skating, or skiing	8	3
Moderate intensity activities		
J. Take walks or hikes or walk to work	4	4
K. Bowling or golf	3	3
L. Home exercises, calisthenics	4	3
M. Home maintenance and gardening, including carpentry, painting, raking, or mowing	4	5

*Approximately equal to kilocalories for a 70-kg man.

SOURCE: Reprinted by permission of the publisher from Jacobs, D. R. Jr., L. P. Hahn, W. L. Haskell, P. Pirie, and S. Sidney. Reliability and validity of a short physical activity history: CARDIA and the Minnesota Heart Health Program. J. Cardiopul. Rehabil. 9:448–459, 1989. Copyright 1989 by Lippincott-Raven Publishers.

Example

Activities of a hypothetical individual:

Weight-lifting: < 3 h/wk for 2 mo and ≥ 3 h/wk for 1 mo
Golf: < 3 h/wk for 3 mo
Walking: < 4 h/wk for 6 mo and ≥ 4 h/wk for 6 mo
Moderate score: $4 \times [6 + (3 \times 6)]$ for walks $+ 3 \times (3 + 0)$ for golf $= 105$
Heavy score: $6 \times [2 + (3 \times 1)]$ for weight lifting $= 30$
Total score: $105 + 30 = 135$ exercise units

REFERENCES

1. Jacobs, D. R. Jr., L. P. Hahn, W. L. Haskell, P. Pirie, and S. Sidney. Reliability and validity of a short physical activity history: CARDIA and the Minnesota Heart Health Program. *J Cardiopul Rehabil* 9:448–459, 1989.

2. Jacobs, D. R. Jr., B. E. Ainsworth, T J. Hartman, and A. S. Leon. A simultaneous evaluation of 10 commonly used physical activity questionnaires. *Med Sci Sports Exerc* 25:81–91, 1993.

3. Sidney, S., D. R. Jacobs, Jr., W. L. Haskell, et al. Comparison of two methods of assessing physical activity in the Coronary Artery Risk Development in Young Adults (CARDIA) Study. *Am J Epidemiol* 133:1231–1245, 1991.

4. Slattery, M. L. and D. R. Jacobs, Jr. Assessment of ability to recall physical activity of several years ago. *Ann Epidemiol* 5:292–296, 1995.

Thrombosis, inflammation, and infection

13

Nathan D. Wong
Paul M. Ridker

KEY POINTS

- *Numerous epidemiologic studies document a relationship between elevated fibrinogen levels and increased risk of coronary heart disease. Measurement of fibrinogen is not routinely recommended, however, as assays for accurate measurement are not widely available, nor are there clinical trials documenting a beneficial role for drugs that selectively lower fibrinogen levels.*

- *Primary and secondary prevention trials have documented the efficacy of aspirin in preventing coronary heart disease events, with more recent data on clopidogrel showing additive benefits over aspirin in secondary prevention. Aspirin remains a standard of care in secondary prevention and is recommended for higher-risk adults without known coronary heart disease.*

- *Of key inflammatory markers for coronary heart disease, C-reactive protein has the most data available from prospective studies documenting its role as an independent risk factor. It is also widely available at reasonable cost with standardized assays for its measurement. The Centers for Disease Control and Prevention and the American Heart Association recently defined normative levels for C-reactive protein and recommended its utility in possibly screening adults with intermediate cardiovascular risk.*

- *Observational studies have shown mixed results regarding the relationship between various infectious pathogens (Chlamydia pneumoniae, Helicobacter pylori, and cytomegalovirus) and cardiovascular disease. More recently, clinical trials examining the efficacy of antibiotic treatment in reducing the risk of recurrent events in persons with known coronary heart disease have been negative, casting doubt on the usefulness of such therapy in secondary prevention of coronary heart disease.*

INTRODUCTION

Epidemiologic studies performed over the past two decades have suggested possibly important roles for thrombosis, local or systemic inflammation, and chronic infection in the initiation and progression of coronary heart disease (CHD).[1,2] The possibility that infectious serology may play a role in this inflammatory process has also been an evolving area of investigation.[3] This chapter reviews the evidence relating thrombotic factors to CHD risk, as well as the role of antithrombotic and antiplatelet agents (especially aspirin) in the primary and secondary prevention of CHD. The state of knowledge regarding inflammatory and infectious factors, including possible prevention therapies, is also discussed.

THROMBOSIS

Thrombus formation is a critical factor in the precipitation of unstable angina, acute myocardial infarction, and thrombotic coronary occlusion during or following coronary angioplasty.[4] Although coronary atherosclerosis is present in most instances of coronary thrombosis,[5] a thrombus often develops at sites of coronary artery stenosis of only mild to moderate severity.[6,7] The concept of evolving coronary thrombosis in unstable angina and in occlusive thrombosis producing myocardial infarction has been established from early studies.[8–11] Occlusive coronary thrombosis is an early event in more than 80% of transmural myocardial infarctions.[12] Roughly 95% of sudden death victims can be shown to have coronary thrombosis, plaque injury, or both.[13]

The chronic inflammatory nature of atherosclerosis eventually leads to breakdown of connective tissue and plaque fissuring and rupture, activating platelets and stimulating formation of thrombin. The platelets undergo a "release reaction," culminating in the synthesis of thromboxane A_2, an extremely potent vasoconstrictor and inducer of platelet aggregation. Platelet aggregation becomes irreversible, accompanied or followed by thrombin generation, incorporation of fibrin and red blood cells, and formation of a red thrombus.[4] Markers of platelet activation, such as thromboxane A_2, are often elevated in the course of unstable coronary artery disease.[14]

Fibrinogen

Fibrinogen appears to contribute to atherosclerosis by several mechanisms: (1) by promoting atherosclerosis, (2) as an essential component of platelet aggregation, (3) in relation to fibrin deposited and the size of the clot, both of which are directly related to the plasma fibrinogen level, and (4) as a result of increasing plasma viscosity.[15] Recent evidence also suggests that the association of fibrinogen with CHD may relate to its role in inflammation.[16]

Observational data indicate that patients with angina pectoris frequently have higher levels of fibrinogen and that plasma levels of fibrinogen increase with severity of CHD.[17] The Leigh Clinical Research Unit[18] showed, in 297 men followed for 7 years, that plasma fibrinogen was the strongest independent indicator of future coronary occlusion. The Northwick Park Heart Study[19] demonstrated higher baseline levels of fibrinogen in those who subsequently experienced a nonfatal or fatal cardiovascular event. Studies done in Goteborg,[20] Framingham,[21] and Caerphilly,[22] taken together, show about a 1.6-fold increased incidence of CVD for each standard deviation increase in fibrinogen levels independent of other risk factors. A recently reported prospective study among 10,600 men living in France and Northern Ireland revealed a significant independent relation of fibrinogen levels with risk of CHD. Fibrinogen levels and CHD risk were higher in Belfast than in France, and 30% of this excess risk was due to fibrinogen.[23] Others have also

reported increased fibrinogen levels measured after angioplasty to be significantly associated with restenosis, where those with a fibrinogen measurement of greater, versus less, than 3.5 g/L had twofold or greater restenosis rates, depending on how restenosis was defined.[24]

Among the largest studies to report a prospective relationship between fibrinogen and CHD is the Atherosclerosis Risk in Communities (ARIC) study, involving 14,477 adults aged 45 to 64 years, followed for 5.2 years. Elevated levels of fibrinogen were associated with significantly increased relative risks for CHD of 1.76 in men and 1.54 in women, which were attenuated (to 1.48 and 1.21, respectively) after adjustment for other risk factors.[25] The Scottish Heart Health Study, involving 5095 men and 4860 women,[26] showed fibrinogen to be an independent risk factor for new coronary events in both men and women, with and without prior CHD, with hazard ratios ranging from 1.93 to 4.86, comparing the highest with the lowest quintile of fibrinogen level. Hazard ratios ranged from 2.2 to 3.4 for coronary death and all-cause mortality in men and women. The Prospective Cardiovascular Munster (PROCAM) study in 2116 healthy men showed the incidence of coronary events to be 2.4-fold greater in the upper versus lower tertile of fibrinogen levels, which remained significant after adjustment for other risk factors.[27] Also, cross-sectional analysis of 3571 elderly Japanese-American men showed a significant association between fibrinogen levels and CHD after adjustment for major risk factors, with the highest prevalence (34%) of CHD seen in past and current smokers in the highest quintile of fibrinogen.[28] A recent study among nearly 700 hypercholesterolemic men free of clinical CHD demonstrated increased fibrinogen levels (upper vs lowest fibrinogen tertile) to be significantly associated with an increased likelihood of atherosclerotic lesions in the carotid, femoral, aorta, and coronary arteries (odds ratios of 2.2–3.6).[29] A recent meta-analysis of 18 studies involving 4018 CHD cases showed a combined relative risk (RR) for CHD of 1.8 (95% confidence interval [CI] = 1.6–2.0) comparing the top (mean = 0.35 g/dL) and bottom (mean = 0.25 g/dL) tertiles of fibrinogen levels (Fig. 13-1).[30]

Fibrinogen levels increase with age and body mass index, and are also associated with higher cholesterol levels. Smoking can reversibly elevate fibrinogen levels; individuals who exercise, eat vegetarian diets, and consume alcohol have been noted to have lower levels.[31] The Caerphilly and Speedwell studies[22] showed that those with the highest levels of blood viscosity or fibrinogen face more than four times the risk of CHD as compared with those with lower levels.

Plasma fibrinogen is also a marker of increased risk for stroke, but risk may be attenuated when adjusted for standard risk factors. One study involving fibrinogen levels measured after the acute-phase following a stroke

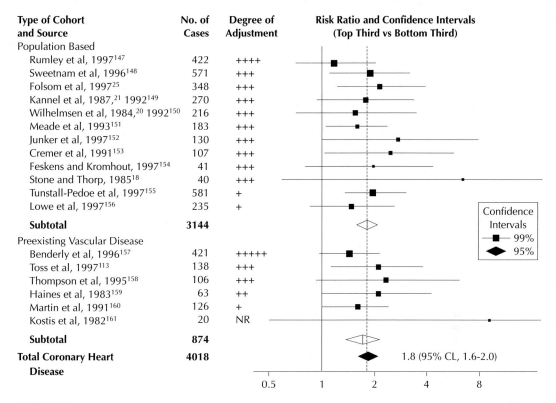

Type of Cohort and Source	No. of Cases	Degree of Adjustment	Risk Ratio and Confidence Intervals (Top Third vs Bottom Third)
Population Based			
Rumley et al, 1997[147]	422	++++	
Sweetnam et al, 1996[148]	571	+++	
Folsom et al, 1997[25]	348	+++	
Kannel et al, 1987,[21] 1992[149]	270	+++	
Wilhelmsen et al, 1984,[20] 1992[150]	216	+++	
Meade et al, 1993[151]	183	+++	
Junker et al, 1997[152]	130	+++	
Cremer et al, 1991[153]	107	+++	
Feskens and Kromhout, 1997[154]	41	+++	
Stone and Thorp, 1985[18]	40	+++	
Tunstall-Pedoe et al, 1997[155]	581	+	
Lowe et al, 1997[156]	235	+	
Subtotal	**3144**		
Preexisting Vascular Disease			
Benderly et al, 1996[157]	421	+++++	
Toss et al, 1997[113]	138	+++	
Thompson et al, 1995[158]	106	+++	
Haines et al, 1983[159]	63	++	
Martin et al, 1991[160]	126	+	
Kostis et al, 1982[161]	20	NR	
Subtotal	**874**		
Total Coronary Heart Disease	**4018**		1.8 (95% CL, 1.6–2.0)

Confidence Intervals
■ 99%
◆ 95%

0.5   1   2   4   8

FIGURE 13-1   Prospective studies relating fibrinogen to coronary artery disease. (From Danesh et al.,[30] with permission.)

demonstrated a twofold increased risk in those with levels above 3.6 g/L after adjustment for other risk factors.[20]

In smokers, cigarette smoking cessation is associated with lower fibrinogen levels. There is also evidence that exercise may lower levels of fibrinogen,[32] as well as plasma viscosity.[33] With respect to pharmacologic therapy, one recent study among patients with familial combined hyperlipidemia and CHD showed combined simvastatin–ciprofibrate therapy to lower plasma fibrinogen levels significantly by 24%,[34] suggesting that a hydroxymethylglutarate coenzyme A reductase–fibrate combinations may be helpful. HMGCoA reductase inhibitors may serve to reduce coronary event risk, partly by inhibiting platelet aggregation and maintaining a favorable balance between prothrombotic and fibrinolytic mechanisms. Some studies involving these medications report reductions in platelet aggregation, reduced plasma viscosity, and lowered fibrinogen levels; however, these findings are not consistent.[35] The Postmenopausal Estrogen/ Progestin Interventions (PEPI) study did show estrogen replacement therapy in postmenopausal women to reduce levels of fibrinogen.[36] In addition, the Benzafibrate Infarction Prevention (BIP) study demonstrated

fibrinogen levels to be decreased, but coronary event risk not to be reduced by therapy with benzafibrate.[37] Despite these promising data, measurement of fibrinogen remains complicated and its clinical utility limited.[38]

The consistent relationship of increased fibrinogen levels with the occurrence of initial and recurrent cardiovascular events has argued for its inclusion as a major risk factor for cardiovascular disease (CVD) and the need for intervention trials aimed at testing the efficacy of lowering fibrinogen in individuals at high risk for CVD.[39] But while plasma fibrinogen contributes to risk over and above established risk factors, it is difficult, because of the lack of clinical trials on drugs that selectively lower plasma fibrinogen levels, to determine whether high fibrinogen levels are a cause or a consequence of CVD.[15]

Factors VII and VIII

There are mixed reports regarding a possible role of coagulation factor VIIc in CVD. The PROCAM study in 2116 healthy male subjects showed no association between factor VIIc and coronary events, although a trend toward higher factor VIIc levels was noted when fatal events were taken into account.[28] A study of 401 consecutive patients undergoing coronary angiography did not reveal an association between factor VIIc and previous myocardial infarction. Levels of activated factor VIIa, however, were lower in those with a previous myocardial infarction and in those who had undergone a prior coronary angioplasty.[40] Among elderly subjects in the Cardiovascular Health Study, fibrinogen and, to a lesser extent, factor VIII, but not factor VII, were associated with evidence of subclinical CVD on the basis of a variety of examination and ultrasound measures.[41]

Factor V Leiden

Another factor related to hypercoagulability is factor V Leiden, a single point mutation in the gene coding for coagulation factor V, which results in a form of factor V that is resistant to degradation by activated protein C, leading to a hypercoagulable state. It is present in approximately 4 to 6% of the US population. A review of published case–control and prospective cohort studies shows factor V Leiden to be associated with a three- to sixfold increase in the risk for primary and recurrent venous thromboembolism, with risks being higher in those with other risk factors such as advanced age, hyperhomocysteinemia, and deficiencies of protein C and protein S.[42] Data from the Physicians' Health Study demonstrate a greater risk associated with venous thromboembolism among affected versus unaffected individuals with advancing age.[43] With respect to arterial thrombosis, the same study did not show factor V Leiden to be related to future risk of myocardial infarction or stroke.[44] Further, the Cardiovascular Health Study did not show factor V Leiden to be associated with the future risk (over 3.4 years of follow-up) of myocardial infarction, angina, stroke, or transient ischemic attack.[45] The lack of a demonstrated association of factor V Leiden mutation with arterial thrombosis and the unknown effect of more intense or prolonged anticoagulant therapy raises the question of the utility of screening for this disorder.[42]

Endogenous fibrinolytic capacity: tissue plasminogen activator and plasminogen activator inhibitor 1

Systemic fibrinolytic balance between thrombosis and hemorrhage is mediated by two proteins, endogenous tissue-type plasminogen activator (tPA) and a fast-acting inhibitor, plasminogen activator inhibitor type 1 (PAI-1).[1] PAI-1 has also been shown to be expressed most frequently in fibrous and calcified plaques and to be increased with the severity of coronary atherosclerotic lesions.[46]

Some studies have linked high levels of tPA and PAI-1 with increased cardiovascular risk.[1] In healthy persons, the only controlled prospective study relating baseline levels of tPA and PAI-1 demonstrated no association between baseline fibrinolytic state and the risk of venous thrombosis.[47] Among patients with coronary artery bypass surgery, those with subsequent graft occlusion within 10 days had significantly higher PAI-1 levels than those without occlusion and also had reduced fibrinolytic response and tPA activity.[48] Among diabetic patients with CHD, a disproportionate elevation of PAI-1 is observed as compared with nondiabetic patients with CHD, thus providing further evidence of an association of increased PAI-1 with insulin resistance and diabetes.[49]

Other observations reveal a relationship between PAI-1 deficiency and bleeding, whereas high levels are associated with frank arterial thrombosis.[50] Plasma PAI-1 is increased among young survivors of myocardial infarction, and other studies show elevated PAI-1 or tPA levels in those with angina, severe CHD, and recurrent ischemia, which may be accompanied by endothelial dysfunction.[1]

The Physician's Health Study showed plasma levels of endogenous tPA to be significantly higher among those who experienced a first myocardial infarction (RR = 2.81, 95% CI = 1.47–5.37) or stroke (RR = 3.51, 95% CI = 1.72–7.17) among those in the fifth versus first quintile.[51,52] A nested case–control study within the Rotterdam study reported increased levels of tPA antigen to be associated with an increased risk of myocardial infarction (odds ratio [95% CI] = 1.7 [0.9–3.3], 2.3 [1.2–4.4], and 2.0 [1.0–3.8] for the second, third, and fourth quartiles compared with the first), but these risks were attenuated after adjustment for other risk factors.[53] With respect to possible interventions to treat impaired fibrinolysis, some studies involving angiotensin-converting enzyme inhibitors do show significant reductions in PAI-1 or tPA antigen levels; however, these findings are by no means consistent.[35,54,55]

The possible role of activation of the endogenous fibrinolytic system as a marker of future CVD risk is partly supported by studies of D-dimer, a breakdown product of fibrinogen, which has been noted to be elevated in those with the highest risk of myocardial infarction.[56,57] In the Physicians' Health Study,[57] those with D-dimer concentrations above the 95th percentile (≥107 ng/mL) were at more than twice the risk of myocardial infarction than those with levels at or below the 50th percentile (<38 ng/mL). Recently, Lowe and co-workers showed, in the prospective Caerphilly Study cohort, that those with levels of D-dimer in the top quintile had an adjusted relative odds of ischemic heart disease events of 3.5 (95% CI = 1.8–6.9).[58]

PLATELET SIZE, FUNCTION, AND AGGREGATION

Platelet hyperreactivity, as measured by spontaneous platelet aggregation (SPA), has been noted to be a marker for survival and secondary coronary events after myocardial infarction. SPA-positive individuals were found to have a fivefold greater risk of death in one limited study of 120 patients.[59] This was consistent with previous observations of a shortened bleeding time being the best clinical marker of platelet reactivity. Cross-sectional data from the Caerphilly Collaborative Heart Disease Study showed a strong relationship between platelet function and past history of myocardial infarction.[58] Platelet reactivity may be reduced by consumption of diets with a high ratio of polyunsaturated to saturated fat[61] and increased n-3 fatty acids[62] and by smoking cessation.[1]

Platelet size (volume) has also been shown to be a sensitive marker of future thrombotic risk. Platelet volume measured 6 months after myocardial infarction in 1716 men was greater in those who suffered a recurrent infarction or death.[63] A Norwegian study of 487 men reported that those with the highest platelet counts had a significant 2.5-fold increased risk of cardiovascular mortality.[64] A more recent case–control study, however, indicated platelet volume not to differ between patients with and those without previous myocardial infarction.[65]

ASPIRIN AND OTHER ANTIPLATELET THERAPY

Aspirin

In platelets, aspirin prevents the formation of thromboxane A_2, thereby preventing platelet aggregation. Aspirin has also been reported to improve endothelial function, which can then improve vasodilation, reduce thrombosis, and help to inhibit progression of atherosclerosis.[66] There is evidence from epidemiologic studies of a protective effect for coronary events; there is also clinical trial evidence in both primary and secondary prevention (Table 13-1).

The largest trial of primary prevention is the Physicians' Health Study,[67] in which more than 22,000 male physicians aged 40 to 84 were assigned to 325 mg aspirin or placebo every other day for 5 years. A highly significant 44% reduction (2.55/1000 vs 4.4/1000 per year, $P < .0001$) in risk of myocardial infarction was observed, in conjunction with a nonsignificant increased incidence of stroke (2.18/1000 vs 1.79/1000 per year). Overall,

TABLE 13-1 Major Clinical Trials of Aspirin Use and Cardiovascular Disease

Reference	Population/intervention	Result
Primary Prevention		
US Physicians' Health Study[67]	22,071 male physicians aged 40–84 years, 325 mg every other day	44% decrease in risk of MI, 13% increase in risk of stroke (NS)
British Doctors' Study[68]	5,139 male physicians aged 50–78 years, 500 mg/day	3% decrease in risk of MI (NS), 13% increase in risk of stroke (NS)
Hypertension Optimal Treatment (HOT)[74]	18,790 hypertensive patients (53% male), 75 mg/day	15% ↓ CVD events, 36% ↓ MI, 2% ↓ risk of stroke (NS), 7% ↓ risk of mortality (NS)
Women's Health Study[71]	40,000 female health professionals, 100 mg every other day	Ongoing
Secondary Prevention		
Antiplatelet Trialists' Collaboration[85]	54,000 patients with CVD (10 trials post-MI) 273 mg/d (mean dosage)	31% decrease in risk of nonfatal MI, 42% decrease in risk of nonfatal stroke, 13% decrease in risk of total vascular mortality
International Study of Infarct Survival[84]	17,187 patients with evolving MI Aspirin arm: 160 mg/d	49% decrease in risk of reinfarction, 26% decrease in risk of nonfatal stroke, 23% decrease in risk to total vascular mortality

CVD, cardiovascular disease; MI, myocardial infarction; NS, nonsignificant.

bleeding was more common in aspirin users, as was bleeding requiring transfusion. The British Doctors' Study of 5000 male physicians aged 50 to 78 years, taking 500 mg aspirin per day or placebo for 6 years, demonstrated little effect on either myocardial infarction or stroke.[68] Although the Physicians' Health Study and the British Doctors' Study provide evidence of the efficacy of aspirin in men, results from trials done specifically in women are not yet available.

The largest prospective cohort study reported involving aspirin use is the Nurses' Health Study of 87,678 US registered nurses aged 34 to 65, free of diagnosed coronary heart disease, stroke, and cancer at baseline.[69] Among women who took one to six aspirins per week, there was a significant 32% lower risk of first myocardial infarction among those aged 50 or older. No benefit or harm was seen with respect to stroke risk among them or among women taking more than six aspirins per week. In older women, however, the Cardiovascular Health Study demonstrated frequent or infrequent aspirin use in women to be associated with an 80% increased risk of ischemic stroke (RR = 1.8, 95% CI = 1.2–2.8) and a fourfold increased risk of hemorrhagic stroke (95% CI = 1.6–10.0) after adjustment for other risk factors.[70] These findings did not hold in men, however.

The currently ongoing Women's Health Study involving low-dose aspirin use (100 mg every other day) among 40,000 female nurses aged 45 and older will provide data on the efficacy of aspirin use in women.[71] In view of the higher baseline risk of stroke versus myocardial infarction (MI) in women and overall risk/benefit considerations, recommendations regarding low-dose aspirin use for primary prevention in women must await the results of this trial.[72,73] In the Hypertension Optimal Treatment (HOT) study,[74] among the nearly 9400 hypertensive patients (47% women) randomized to 75 mg/d aspirin as compared with a nearly equivalent number assigned to placebo, all major cardiovascular events were reduced by 15% ($P = .03$) and MI by 36% ($P = .002$), but there was no effect on stroke. Unfortunately, nonfatal bleeds remained nearly twice as common in the aspirin group (RR = 1.8, $P < .001$).

A recently reported meta-analysis of 16 trials with 55,462 subjects, involving a mean dosage of 273 mg/d aspirin and mean duration of treatment of 37 months, showed aspirin use to be associated with an absolute reduction in risk of MI of 137 events/10,000 persons (95% CI = 107–167) and, for ischemic stroke, a RR of 39 events/10,000 persons (95% CI = 17–61) (both P's < .001). A significant increase in risk of hemorrhagic stroke of 12 events/10,000 persons (95% CI = 5–20, $P < .001$), however, was reported.[75]

For secondary prevention, six large, randomized, double-blind clinical trials of use of aspirin alone after MI have been conducted.[76–81] Five of these trials used dosages of 300 to 1500 mg of aspirin daily and showed favorable trends for a reduction in total mortality. The Aspirin Myocardial Infarction Study (AMIS) revealed a trend against aspirin for mortality, but a nonsignificant reduction in risk of recurrent MI.[80] In patients with unstable angina, the VA Cooperative Trial in 1266 men showed aspirin to be associated with a 51% reduction in death and acute MI (from 10.1% to 5%).[82] The Montreal Heart Institute Study reported a 72% lower risk.[83] Aspirin has also been shown to be necessary in the acute phase following MI, when thrombolytic therapy is used. The best evidence for this derives from the Second International Study of Infarct Survival (ISIS-2),[84] in which a 40% reduction in the risk of 5-week vascular mortality was noted in those on the combination of aspirin and streptokinase, as compared with only a 23% reduction in those given streptokinase and a 21% reduction in those receiving aspirin alone.

The Antiplatelet Trialists' Collaboration reported an updated meta-analysis of 145 randomized trials conducted in 70,000 high-risk patients with occlusive vascular disease and 30,000 low-risk patients from the general population, most commonly using aspirin as an antiplatelet agent.[85] Among the high-risk patients receiving antiplatelet therapy, significant reductions were seen in overall mortality (18%), nonfatal MI (35%), and nonfatal stroke (31%). Among 20,000 patients with a history of MI, there was a 29% lower risk of new vascular events in those receiving aspirin (10.6%) versus the control regimen (14.4%) (see Table 13-1).

Other antiplatelet therapy

Ticlopidine is a platelet antiaggregatory agent that inhibits the formation of arterial thrombi, prolongs bleeding time, and normalizes shortened platelet survival. The Canadian American Ticlopidine Study (CATS) reported a 30.2% reduction in the risk of stroke, MI, or vascular death among 1053 patients assigned to ticlopidine or placebo 1 to 17 weeks after thromboembolic stroke.[86] The Ticlopidine Aspirin Stroke Study (TASS) showed a slight advantage of ticlopidine over aspirin in reducing death from any cause or nonfatal stroke (20% vs 23% of patients), over 6 years.[87] In a recent trial of 1809 African-American men and women with a prior ischemic stroke, there was no difference in the primary outcome of recurrent stroke, MI, or vascular death (hazard ratio = 1.22, 95% CI = 0.94–1.57) after 6.5 years, and the blinded phase of the study was halted. A trend ($P = .08$) for fatal or nonfatal stroke favoring aspirin over ticlopidine was reported, however.[88]

Clopidogrel, a new thienopyridine derivative similar to ticlopidine, also inhibits platelet aggregation. As shown in the trial of Clopidogrel versus Aspirin in Patients at Risk of Ischaemic Events (CAPRIE), among more than 19,000 patients with either ischemic stroke, MI, or peripheral vascular disease followed for nearly 2 years, there was a significant 8.7% reduction in risk (95% CI = 0.3–16.5) favoring clopidogrel over aspirin.[89] The overall safety profile in the clopidogrel group was at least as good as in those on aspirin. More recently, its use in the Clopidogrel in Unstable Angina to Prevent Recurrent Events (CURE) trial, which involved 12,562 patients with acute coronary syndromes without ST segment elevation who were given aspirin, the additional use of clopidogrel was associated with a 20% lower risk ($P <$ .001) of cardiovascular death, nonfatal MI, or stroke, although a greater risk of major bleeding, compared with those on placebo and aspirin alone.[90]

Recommendations for aspirin/antiplatelet therapy

Antiplatelet therapy is effective in reducing vascular events, including nonfatal MI, stroke, and vascular death, in patients with preexisting coronary artery disease or stroke. Aspirin is effective in dosages of 75 to 325 mg. When thrombolytic therapy is used, concomitant aspirin therapy provides substantial additional risk reduction.[84] In such high-risk patients, aspirin reduces vascular events by about one fourth, nonfatal MI by one third, nonfatal stroke by one third, and vascular death by one sixth. For secondary prevention of stroke, there is evidence that ticlopidine may be more effective than aspirin, but its greater cost and more frequent and serious adverse effects warrant its careful consideration only for select groups of stroke patients.[4] For aspirin-intolerant patients, clopidogrel may be an option and has been shown to be efficacious in patients with MI, stroke, and peripheral vascular disease.[88] As the benefits are clear and aspirin use is clearly recommended post–MI, based on these data, utilization rates appear to be 95% or higher overall, but slightly less in men, the elderly, and those with health maintenance organization insurance.[91] The argument has been made that some 5000 to 10,000 additional lives annually could be saved if aspirin were administered to all patients after acute MI.[92]

The efficacy of lower dosages of aspirin is under investigation to determine the optimal dose of aspirin that provides cardiovascular benefits while minimizing side effects, such as gastrointestinal bleeding. The ability of 100 mg alternate-day aspirin to inhibit platelet function has been documented, with decreases in mean thromboxane and prostacyclin levels to 7.5 and 15.6% of baseline, respectively (both P's < .001).[93] In the HOT study, although showing the continued efficacy of low-dose (75 mg/day) aspirin therapy in reducing cardiovascular events and MI with no increase in stroke, nonfatal bleeds remained twice as common.[74] The clinical efficacy of this dosage in the primary prevention of cardiovascu-

lar events is being evaluated in the ongoing Women's Health Study.[71] Data from the Physicians' Health Study suggest that alternate-day aspirin could yield lower benefits. While those with excellent adherence (at least 95% of prescribed tablets) experienced a significant 51% reduction in the risk of MI, poor adherers (less than 50% of prescribed tablets) had a nonsignificant 17% reduction in risk.[94] Others have argued that dosages in secondary prevention as low as 30 mg/d may be sufficient for the prevention of MI through inhibition of thromboxane synthesis, arguing for more extensive clinical trials on low-dose formulations.[95]

In those free of CHD and younger than 50 years, aspirin is not recommended, considering evidence of no benefit in those younger than 50 years of age and an increased risk of bleeding and transfusion and trend toward more hemorrhagic stroke.[72] Aspirin use may be considered, however, in those older than 50 years of age who have at least an additional risk factor for CHD and who are free of contraindications to its use, based on evidence of increasing benefits with advancing age and presence of hypertension, diabetes, cigarette smoking, and lack of exercise.[67,69] More recently, groups such as the American Diabetes Association have recommended aspirin use in diabetics with at least one other coronary risk factor or preexisting CHD.[96]

INFLAMMATION AND C-REACTIVE PROTEIN

Local and systemic inflammation may play a role in the initiation and progression of atherosclerosis. Proinflammatory cytokines such as interleukin-1 and tumor necrosis factor α (TNF-α), along with intercellular adhesion molecule 1, selectins, interleukin-6, and serum amyloid A, have been implicated in atherogenesis. In addition, C-reactive protein (CRP), an acute-phase reactant for underlying systemic inflammation, the levels of which increase 100-fold or more in response to severe bacterial infection, physical trauma, or other inflammatory conditions, may have an important role (Fig. 13-2)[97]

Studies over the past two decades show CRP to be significantly higher in patients with MI or CHD[98–100] and, more recently, demonstrate the predictive value of CRP for subsequent coronary events in patients with preexisting CHD.[100–102] In a recent review comprising 18 studies, RRs for future cardiovascular events ranged from approximately 2 to 4, comparing the risk in persons in the highest versus the lowest quartiles of CRP levels (Fig. 13-3).[103]

In the Physicians' Health Study,[104] CRP was measured in 543 initially healthy men who developed MI or stroke and in an equivalent number of controls not reporting events. Baseline CRP was significantly

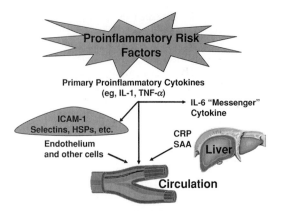

FIGURE 13-2 Imflammatory Pathways in Atherogenesis. (From Libby and Ridker[97] with permission.) IL-1, interleukin-1; TNF-α, tumor necrosis factor α; IL-6, interleukin-6; HSP, heat shock protein; ICAM-1, intercellular adhesion molecule-1; CRP, C-reactive protein; SAA, serum amyloid A.

higher in those experiencing than those not experiencing subsequent MI (1.51 mg/L vs 1.13 mg/L) or ischemic stroke (1.38 mg/L vs 1.13 mg/L). In comparing those in the highest versus lowest quartile for CRP, the RR was 2.9 for MI and 1.9 for stroke. In a second report from the Physicians' Health Study, CRP provided significantly better prediction of first MI when added to models including total cholesterol and high-density lipoprotein cholesterol (HDL-C) alone, further suggesting its utility in the prediction of CHD.[105]

A recent report from the Women's Health Study[106] showed substantially higher baseline CRP levels in women developing CVD events than in those remaining disease-free, with a 7.4-fold increased risk of MI or stroke (4.8-fold for any CVD event) among those with the highest levels of CRP. A more recent report from this cohort indicated that the combination of hs-CRP and total cholesterol/HDL-C ratio to be a stronger indicator of future CVD event risk than either alone, low-density lipoprotein cholesterol (LDL-C), or other lipid and inflammatory factors (Fig. 13-4).[107] The same investigators also recently examined event-free survival by CRP and LDL-C categories in all 27,939 women, providing the largest follow-up analysis in relation to hs-CRP measures of any study. Although those with high CRP and high LDL-C expectedly had the worst prognosis, outcome was as bad or worse for persons with high CRP and low LDL-C as for those with low CRP and high LDL-C (Fig. 13-5),[108] suggesting the presence of an important group of high-risk persons not currently under lipid treatment guidelines. Moreover, this report also showed CRP to provide incremental information for predicting

CVD event risk at all levels of LDL-C and Framingham Risk Score (see Fig. 13-6). Further, among women with the metabolic syndrome, measures of CRP provided incremental prognostic information for the prediction of CVD events,[109] suggesting its utility for risk assessment in such individuals, many of whom are at intermediate risk for CVD events.

From population-based studies, evidence of an association of CRP with an increased risk of CHD mortality derives from the Multiple Risk Factor Intervention Trial (MRFIT), a nested case–control study of 98 cases of MI, 148 CHD deaths, and 491 controls that showed that over 17 years of follow-up, deaths from CHD among smokers were 4.3-fold greater (95% CI = 1.74–10.8) among those in the highest versus the lowest quartile of CRP.[110] In 936 men who participated in the MONICA Augsburg Cohort Study, the RR associated with a one standard deviation increase in log CRP level was 1.67 (95% CI = 1.29–2.17), which was essentially unaffected after adjustment for age and smoking.[111] Further, a nested case–control study of postmenopausal subjects of the Women's Health Initiative showed the highest versus lowest quartile of CRP measures to be associated with a significant, approximately twofold increased risk of CHD events.[112]

CRP measurement may also be an effective means for risk stratification of those with acute coronary syndromes. CRP levels are associated with a poor prognosis in patients with unstable angina or non-Q-wave MI; risks of death within 5 months were 2.2, 3.6, and 7.5% by increasing tertile of CRP level (<2, 2–10 and >10 mg/L, respectively; $P < .01$).[113] In 97 cases of sudden cardiac death among those enrolled in the Physician's Health Study, only baseline CRP levels (and not lipids or homocysteine) were associated with a greater risk (2.8-fold) of sudden cardiac death in a nested case–control analysis.[114] In another prospective cohort study of 1458 patients undergoing coronary angioplasty, an increased C-reactive protein level was a significant independent predictor of death or nonfatal MI (RR = 3.6, $P = .0001$).[115]

The role of different therapies for reducing inflammation and subsequent CHD risk is under investigation. One promising report demonstrated a possible nonlipid, anti-inflammatory effect of the HMGCoA reductase therapy pravastatin.[116] An approximate 20% reduction in CRP levels associated with statin treatment has been demonstrated.[117]

The role of circulating adhesion molecules as cellular mediators of inflammation is of increasing interest. In a nested case–control comparison of the Atherosclerosis Risk in Communities (ARIC) longitudinal cohort study, increased levels of endothelial leukocyte adhesion molecule 1 (E-selectin) and intercellular adhesion molecule 1 (ICAM-1) were measured in patients with incident CHD or carotid artery atherosclerosis as compared

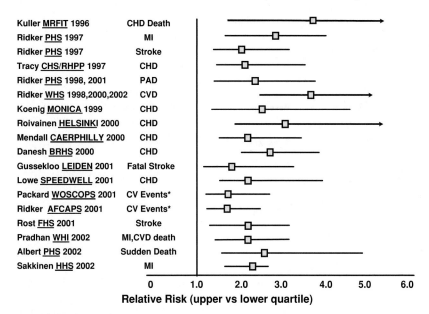

FIGURE 13-3   Prospective studies relating baseline CRP levels to the risk of first cardiovascular events. CHD, coronary heart disease; MI, myocardial infarction; PAD, pulmonary artery disease; CV, cardiovascular; MRFIT, Multiple Risk Factor Intervention Trial; PHS, Physicians' Health Study; CHS, Cardiovascular Health Study; RHPP, Rural Health Promotion Project; WHS, Women's Health Study; MONICA, MONItoring trends and determinants in Cardiovascular disease; HELSINKI, Helsinki Heart Study; CAERPHILLY, Caerphilly Heart Study; BRHS, British Regional Heart Study, LEIDEN, Leiden Heart Study; SPEEDWELL, Speedwell Heart Study; WOSCOPS, West of Scotland Coronary Prevention Study; AFCAPS, Air Force Coronary Atherosclerosis Prevention Study; FHS, Framingham Heart Study; WHI, Women's Health Initiative; HHS, Honolulu Heart Study. (From Ridker[103] with permission.)

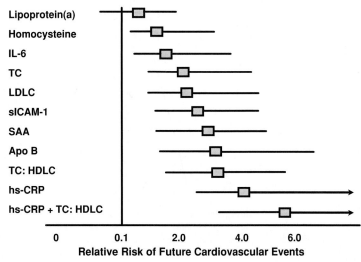

FIGURE 13-4   Risk factors for future cardiovascular events associated with highest vs. lowest quartile of individual risk factors: Women's Health Study. (From Ridker et al.[107] with permission.)

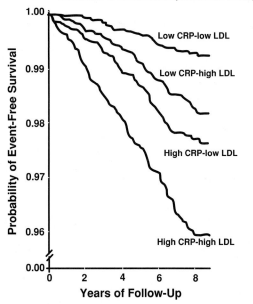

FIGURE 13-5 Cardiovascular event-free survival using combined CRP and LDL-C measurements. (From Ridker et al.[108] with permission.)

with control subjects.[118] In the Physicians' Health Study, baseline levels of soluble ICAM-1 in the highest quartile (>0.260 ng/mL) were associated with an 80% increased risk of future MI (RR = 1.8, 95% CI = 1.1–2.8) after multivariate adjustment for risk factors.[119] In the Women's Health Initiative, a nested case–control study

showed levels of interleukin-6 to be independently associated with an approximate twofold odds of CHD events, even after adjustment for other lipid and nonlipid risk factors, including C-reactive protein.[112] Of interest is the prospective cohort study on myocardial infarction (PRIME study), in which a nested case–control comparison demonstrated only interleukin-6 to be independently associated with MI and coronary death in models containing CRP and fibrinogen as well as other risk factors.[120]

Recommendations regarding the measurement of C-reactive protein and other inflammatory factors

The American Heart Association and Centers for Disease Control and Prevention issued a statement[121] evaluating whether certain markers of inflammation should be used to define high-risk patients, which patients should be tested, and the indications for using certain tests. Among those under consideration were adhesion molecules, cytokines, acute-phase reactants (including fibrinogen, serum amyloid A, and C-reactive protein), white blood cell count (WBC), and other factors, including erythrocyte sedimentation rate.

Required criteria for the clinical acceptability of a new marker included: (1) ability to standardize the assay and control variability of measurement, (2) independence from established risk factors, (3) association with clinical endpoints in observational studies and clinical trials, (4) presence of population norms to guide interpretation, (5) ability to improve overall prediction beyond standard risk factors, (6) generalization of results to various population groups, and (7) acceptable cost. Currently, assays

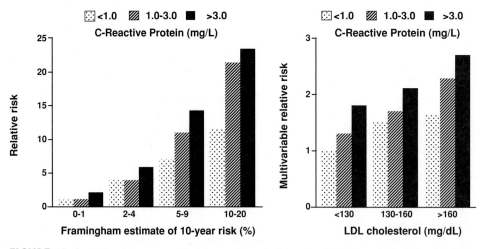

FIGURE 13-6 CRP adds prognostic information at all levels of LDL-C and at all levels of the Framingham Risk Score. (From Ridker et al.[108] with permission.)

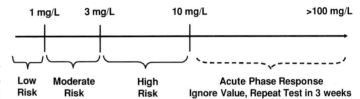

FIGURE 13-7 Clinical application of hs-CRP for cardiovascular risk reduction: categories of risk. (From Ridker, with permission.)

are available only for acute-phase reactants and WBC, and a program to standardize CRP testing using recommended high-sensitivity measurement is underway at the Centers for Disease Control and Prevention. Although most of the risk markers under consideration satisfy few of these criteria, hs(high sensitivity)-CRP appears to have the strongest evidence supporting most or all of these criteria. This has led the panel to provide the following recommendations regarding the measurement and assessment of hs-CRP (Fig. 13-7)[121]:

1. hs-CRP is not suitable for screening the entire adult population.

2. hs-CRP may be appropriate for screening those at intermediate risk from global risk assessment (10–20% risk of CHD in 10 years) and may help direct further evaluation and therapy in the primary prevention of CVD.

3. Other inflammatory markers should not be measured for the determination of risk in addition to hs-CRP;

4. In patients with stable coronary disease or acute coronary syndromes, hs-CRP measurement may be a useful independent marker of prognosis for recurrent events, including death, MI, and restenosis, after percutaneous interventions.

5. Patients with persistently unexplained marked elevations of hs-CRP (>10 mg/L) after repeated testing should be evaluated for noncardiovascular etiologies.

6. Measurement should be done twice, and the results averaged (except repeating if markedly elevated, >10 mg/L), with averaged values classified as follows: low <1 mg/L, average 1.0 to 3.0 mg/L, and high >3 mg/L.

INFECTION AND CARDIOVASCULAR DISEASE

Local or systemic infections resulting from gram-negative bacteria such as *Chlamydia pneumoniae* and *Helicobacter pylori*, as well as from viruses, including cytomegalovirus (CMV) and herpes simplex virus, have been implicated in the development of atherosclerosis, partly by stimulating inflammation.[122] Systemic antibody titers reflect previous exposure to infectious pathogens with persistently

positive serology and represent markers for chronic, persistent infection. More than a dozen retrospective serologic studies have reported a positive relationship between infectious pathogens and CHD, including angiographic restenosis; however, these studies are subject to substantial bias and confounding. In contrast, prospective studies in which the exposure is ascertained before the onset of cardiovascular events have not provided strong evidence of an association. These prospective studies are summarized in Table 13-2.

Saikku and colleagues first reported a relationship between *C. pneumoniae* and CHD and acute MI in 1988.[123] They found that 68% of patients with acute MI had elevated IgG and/or IgA titers against *C. pneumoniae,* as compared with only 17% of control subjects. An overall association of 70 to 100% between *C. pneumoniae* and atherosclerosis is derived from immunocystochemistry and staining techniques. *C. pneumoniae* is uncommon in childhood, but increases in prevalence to 70% in men and 50% in women.[124] It has been detected in fatty streaks and in atheromatous lesions from autopsy,[125] as well as in plaques from the coronary and carotid arteries in several studies, including those in young adults with atherosclerosis.[126,127] One study of 60 autopsies showed 36 of 42 severe atherosclerotic cases to be seropositive, as compared with only 1 of 18 with mild disease.[128] The Helsinki Heart Study reported an odds for developing CHD of 2.6 (not significant) in those with elevated *C. pneumoniae* antibody titers versus controls.[129] A recently reported prospective follow-up of the Physicians' Health Study, however, casts doubt on the prospective relationship of *C. pneumoniae* to CHD risk.[130] Chlamydial IgG seropositivity (as an indicator of *C. pneumoniae* with CHD exposure) was virtually identical among those subsequently experiencing first MI and age- and-smoking-matched controls. In addition, there was no relationship between *C. pneumoniae* and CRP.

H. pylori seropositivity also shows mixed results with respect to CHD (see Table 13-2). Whincup and co-workers showed an association of *H. pylori* with MI (odds ratio [OR] = 1.8), but this diminished to 1.3 (not significant) after adjustment for risk factors.[131] Three other prospective studies have also not documented a relationship between *H. pylori* seropositivity and CHD death[132,133] or MI.[134] Most recently, within

TABLE 13-2 Summary of Major Prospective Studies of Infectious Pathogens and Coronary Artery Disease

Reference	Patients, endpoint	Controls	RR (95% CI)
	Chlamydia pneumoniae		
Saikku et al, 1992[129]	103, CHD	103	2.3 (0.9–6.2)[†]
Ridker et al, 1998[130]	343	343	1.1 (0.8–1.5)[†]
	Helicobacter pylori		
Whincup et al, 1996[131]	135, MI	136	1.31 (0.70–2.43)[†]
Strandberg et al, 1997[132]	127, CVD death	497	1.07 (0.73–1.5)
Aromaa et al, 1996[134]	441, MI	842	1.29 (0.94–2.00)
Wald et al, 1997[133]	648, CHD death	1296	1.06 (0.86–1.31)[†]
Folsom et al, 1998[135]	217, CHD	498	0.85 (0.43–1.69)[†]
Strachan et al, 1998[136]	1796 (total)		
	IHD incidence		1.05 (0.80–1.39)[‡]
	All-cause death		1.46 (1.12–1.92)[‡]
	Fatal IHD		1.54 (1.03–2.30)[‡]
	Cytomegalovirus		
Ridker et al, 1998[142]	643, MI/stroke	643	0.94 (0.7–1.2)[†]
	Herpes Simplex Virus		
Ridker et al, 1998[142]	643, MI/stroke	643	0.72 (0.6–0.9)[†]

*CHD, coronary heart disease; MI, myocardial infarction; CVD cardiovascular disease; IHD, ischemic heart disease.
[†]Adjusted for other coronary risk factors.
[‡]Did not retain statistical significance when adjusted for other risk factors.

the large, longitudinal ARIC study, there was no association of *H. pylori* seropositivity with incident CHD over a 3.3-year follow-up period among middle-aged men and women.[125] The smaller, but longer-term Caerphilly Prospective Heart Disease Study demonstrated, among 1796 men followed for a mean of 13.7 years, no association of incident ischemic heart disease with *H. pylori* (OR = 1.05, 95% CI = 0.80–1.39), but a relationship with all-cause mortality (OR = 1.46, 95% CI = 1.12–1.92) and fatal ischemic heart disease (OR = 1.54, 95% CI = 1.03–2.30).[136] However, those seropositive for both *C. pneumoniae* and *H. pylori* had ORs of 2.6 for coronary artery disease and 2.0 for MI and also tended to have higher CRP levels.[121] Also, in a case–control study, *H. pylori* infection was significantly higher among CHD patients than among matched controls (62% vs 40% , *P* < .01; OR = 2.8, 95% CI = 1.3–7.4) and was mediated through cytotoxin-associated gene A (CagA), an indicator of more virulent *Helicobacter* strains.[137]

Herpes simplex virus and cytomegalovirus (CMV) are associated with mixed results regarding the risk for CHD (see Table 13-2). CMV genomes are observed more frequently in those with severe versus mild or no atherosclerosis.[138] CMV seropositivity has been shown to be a significant risk factor (OR = 3.6) for pretransplant atherosclerosis in a cardiac transplant population.[139] Also, in a transplant study,[140] compared with CMV-negative patients, CMV-positive patients experienced lower 5-year survival (32% vs 68%), higher rate of graft loss due to atherosclerosis (69% vs 37%), and higher death rate due to 50% or greater obstruction (8% vs 1%). The longitudinal ARIC study provides the strongest evidence of association, with a graded relation between odds of intima–media thickness and serum CMV antibody titer, even after adjustment for risk factors.[141] A large, nested case–control study among nearly 1300 participants of the Physicians' Health Study, however, actually showed an unexpected inverse relationship between CMV seropositivity and risk for MI or stroke over 12 years (RR = 0.72, 95% CI = 0.6–0.9), which the authors attributed to chance. Nevertheless, this study does not support a relationship of CMV seropositivity to increased vascular event risk.[142]

Recently published clinical trials have cast doubt on the effectiveness of antibiotic treatment in the prevention of CVD events. Although one clinical trial indicated the benefits of treatment with azithromycin on endothelial function in patients with documented coronary artery disease,[143] results of trials involving the prevention of recurrent coronary events have not been positive. In the ACADEMIC study, involving 302 coronary disease patients seropositive to *C. pneumoniae* and randomized to placebo or azithromycin 500 mg/wk for 3 months (after 500 mg/d for 3 days), there was no significant treatment difference (hazard ratio = 0.89, P = .74) in the primary endpoint of recurrent cardiac events.[144] A much larger recently published multicenter trial in 1439 patients with unstable angina or acute MI, who were randomized to 250 mg daily for up to 6 months, also showed no significant benefit in preventing death, recurrent MI, or recurrent ischemia requiring hospitalization.[145] Finally, the largest published trial to date (WIZARD) randomized 7747 adults with a prior myocardial infarction to 12 weeks of therapy with azithromycin or placebo, and found no significant reduction in the likelihood of reinfarction, revascularization, hospitalization for angina, or death compared with placebo.[146] These findings essentially rule out the likelihood of any significant benefit of short-term antibiotic therapy in the secondary prevention of CVD.

REFERENCES

1. Ridker PM. The pathogenesis of atherosclerosis and acute thrombosis: relevance to strategies of cardiovascular disease prevention. In: Manson JE, Ridker PM, Gaziano JM, Hennekens CH, eds. *Prevention of Myocardial Infarction.* New York: Oxford University Press; 1996:32–54.

2. Ridker PM. Inflammation, infection, and cardiovascular risk: how good is the clinical evidence [editorial]? *Circulation* 1998;97:1671–1674.

3. Libby P, Egan D, Skarlatos S. Roles of infectious agents in atherosclerosis and restenosis: an assessment of the evidence and need for future research. *Circulation* 1997;96:4095–4103.

4. Cairns JA, Lewis D, Meade TW, et al. Antithrombotic agents in coronary artery disease: Fourth ACCP Consensus Conference on Antithrombotic Therapy. *Chest* 1995;108 (suppl):380S–400S.

5. Sanz G, Castanev A, Bertrui A, et al. Determinants of prognosis in survivors of myocardial infarction: a prospective clinical angiographic study. *N Engl J Med* 1982;306:1065–1071.

6. Ambrose J, Tannenbaum M, Alexopoulos D, et al. Angiographic progression of coronary artery disease and the development of myocardial infarction. *J Am Coll Cardiol* 1988;12:56–62.

7. Little WC, Constantinescu M, Applegate RJ, et al. Can coronary angiography predict the site of a subsequent myocardial infarction in patients with mild-to-moderate coronary artery disease? *Circulation* 1988;78:1157–1166.

8. Parkinson J, Bedford DE. Cardiac infarction and thrombosis. *Lancet* 1928;14:195–239.

9. Levine SA, Brown CL. Coronary thrombosis: its various clinical features. *Medicine* 1929;8:245–418.

10. Sampson JJ, Eliaser M. The diagnosis of impending acute coronary artery occlusion. *Am Heart J* 1937;13:676–686.

11. Feil H. Preliminary pain in coronary thrombosis. *Am J Med Sci* 1937;193:42–48.

12. DeWood MA, Spores J, Notske R, et al. Prevalence of total coronary occlusion during the early hours of transmural myocardial infarction. *N Engl J Med* 1980;303:897–902.

13. Davies MJ, Thomas AC. Plaque fissuring: the cause of acute myocardial infarction, sudden ischaemic death, and crescendo angina. *Br Heart J* 1988;60:459–464.

14. Fitzgerald DJ, Roy L, Catella F, et al. Platelet activation in unstable coronary disease. *N Engl J Med* 1986;315:983–989.

15. Heinrich J, Assmann G. Fibrinogen and cardiovascular risk. *J Cardiovasc Risk* 1995;2:197–205.

16. Andreotti F, Burzotta F, Maseri A. Fibrinogen as a marker of inflammation: a clinical view. *Blood Coagul Fibrinolysis* 1999;10(suppl 1):S3–S4.

17. Rainer C, Kawanishi DT, Chandraranta AN, et al. Changes in blood rheology in patients with stable angina pectoris as a result of coronary artery disease. *Circulation* 1987;76:15–20.

18. Stone MC, Thorpe JM. Plasma fibrinogen: a major coronary risk factor. *J R Coll Gen Pract* 1985;35:565–569.

19. Meade TW, Mellows S, Brozovic M, et al. Haemostatic function and ischemic heart disease: principal results of the Northwick Park Heart Study. *Lancet* 1986;2:533–537.

20. Wilhelmsen L, Svardsudd K, Korsan-Bengtsen K, et al. Fibrinogen as a risk factor for stroke and myocardial infarction. *N Engl J Med* 1984;311:501–505.

21. Kannel WB, Wolf PA, Castelli WP, D'Agostino RB. Fibrinogen and risk of cardiovascular disease: the Framingham study. *JAMA* 1987;258:1183–1186.

22. Yarnell JWG, Baker IA, Sweetnam PM, et al. Fibrinogen, viscosity, and white blood cell count are major risk factors for ischemic heart disease: the Caerphilly and Speedwell Collaborative Heart Disease Studies. *Circulation* 1991;83:836–844.

23. Scarabin PY, Arveiler D, Amouyel P, et al. Plasma fibrinogen explains much of the difference in risk of coronary heart disease between France and Northern Ireland: the PRIME Study. *Atherosclerosis* 2003; 166: 103-9.

24. Montalescot G, Ankri A, Vicaut E, et al. Fibrinogen after coronary angioplasty as a risk factor for restenosis. *Circulation* 1995;92:31–38.

25. Folsom AR, Wu KK, Rosamond WD, et al. Prospective study of hemostatic factors and incidence of coronary heart disease: the Atherosclerosis Risk in Communities (ARIC) study. *Circulation* 1997;96:1102–1108.

26. Woodward M, Loew GD, Rumley A, Tunstall-Pedoe H. Fibrinogen as a risk factor for coronary heart disease and mortality in middle-aged men and women: the Scottish Heart Health Study. *Eur Heart J* 1998;19:55–62.

27. Henrich J, Balleisen L, Schulte H, et al. Fibrinogen and factor VII in the prediction of coronary risk: results from the PROCAM study in healthy men (published errarum appears in Arterioscler Thromb 1994;14:392). *Arterioscler Thromb* 1994;14:54–59.

28. Sharp DS, Abbott RD, Burchfiel CM, et al. Plasma fibrinogen and coronary heart disease in elderly Japanese-American men. *Arterioscle Thromb Vasc Biol* 1996;16:262–268.

29. Levenson J, Giral P, Megnien JL, et al. Fibrinogen and its relations to subclinical extracoronary and coronary atherosclerosis in hypercholesterolemic men. *Arterioscler Thromb Vasc Biol* 1997;17:45–50.

30. Danesh J, Collins R, Appleby P, Peto R. Association of fibrinogen, C-reactive protein, albumin, or leukocyte count with coronary heart disease: a meta-analysis of prospective studies. *JAMA* 1998;279:1477–1482.

31. Ernst E. Plasma fibrinogen: an independent cardiovascular risk factor. *J Intern Med* 1990;27:365–372.

32. Stratton JR, Chandler WL, Schwartz RS, et al. Effects of physical conditioning on fibrinolytic variables and fibrinogen in young and old healthy adults. *Circulation* 1991;83:1692–1697.

33. Koenig W, Sund M, Doring A, Ernst E. Leisure-time physical activity but not work-related physical activity is associated with decreased plasma viscosity. *Circulation* 1997;95:335–341.

34. Kontopoulos AG, Athyros VG, Papageorgiou AA, et al. Effects of simvastatin and ciprofibrate alone and in combination on lipid profile, plasma fibrinogen and low density lipoprotein particle structure and distribution in patients with familial combined hyperlipidemia and coronary artery disease. *Coron Artery Dis* 1996;7:843–850.

35. Rosenson RS, Tagney CC. Antiatherothrombotic properties of stations: implications for cardiovascular event reduction. *JAMA* 1998;279:1643–1650.

36. The Writing Group of the PEPI Trial. Effects of estrogen or estrogen/progestin regimens on heart disease risk factors in postmenopausal women. *JAMA* 1995;273:199–208.

37. Behar S, for the Benzafibrate Infarction Prevention Study Group. Lowering fibrinogen levels: clinical update. *Blood Coagul Fibrinolysis* 1999;10:41–43.

38. Ridker PM. Evaluating novel cardiovascular risk factors: can we predict better heart attacks? *Ann Intern Med* 1999;130:933–937.

39. Kannel WB. Influence of fibrinogen on cardiovascular disease. *Drugs* 1997;54(suppl 3):32–40.

40. Danielsen R, Onundarson PT, Thors H, et al. Activated and total coagulation factor VII, and fibrinogen in coronary artery disease. *Scand Cardiovasc* 1998;32:87–95.

41. Tracy RP, Bovill EG, Yanez D, et al. Fibrinogen and factor VIII, but not factor VII, are associated with measures of subclinical cardiovascular disease in the elderly: results from the Cardiovascular Health Study *Arterioscler Thromb Vasc Biol* 1995;15:1269–1279.

42. Price DT, Ridker PM. Factor V Leiden mutation and the risks for thromboembolic disease: a clinical perspective. *Ann Intern Med* 1997;127:895–903.

43. Ridker PM, Glynn RJ, Miletich JP, et al. Age-specific incidence rates of venous thromboembolism among heterozygous carriers of factor V Leiden mutation. *Ann Intern Med* 1997;126:528–531.

44. Ridker PM, Hennekens CH, Lindpaintner K, et al. Mutation in the gene coding for coagulation factor V and the risk of myocardial infarction, stroke, and venous thrombosis in apparently healthy men. *N Engl J Med* 1995;332:912–917.

45. Cushman M, Rosendaal FR, Psaty BM, et al. Factor V Leiden is not a risk factor for arterial vascular disease in the elderly: results from the Cardiovascular Health Study. *Thromb Haemostas* 1998;79:912–915.

46. Padro T, Steins M, Li CX, et al. Comparative analysis of plasminogen activator inhibitor-1 expression in different types of atherosclerotic lesions in coronary arteries from human heart explants. *Cardiovasc Res* 1997;36:28–36.

47. Ridker PM, Vaughan DE, Stampfer MJ, et al. Baseline fibrinolytic state and the risk of venous thrombosis: a prospective study of endogenous tissue-type plasminogen activator and plasminogen activator inhibitor. *Circulation* 1992;85:1822–1827.

48. Rifon J, Paramo JA, Panizo C, et al. The increase of plasminogen activator inhibitor activity is associated with graft occlusion in patients undergoing aorto-coronary bypass surgery. *Br J Haematol* 1997;99:262–267.

49. Sobel BE, Woodcock-Mitchell J, Schneider DJ. Increased plasminogen activator inhibitor type 1 in coronary artery atherectomy specimens from type 2 diabetic compared with nondiabetic patients: a potential factor predisposing to thrombosis and its persistence. *Circulation* 1998;97:2213–2221.

50. Erickson LA, Rici GJ, Lund JE, et al. Development of venous occlusions in mice transgenic for the plasminogen activator inhibitor-1 gene. *Nature* 1990;346:74–76.

51. Ridker PM, Vaughan DE, Stampfer MJ, et al. Endogenous tissue-type plasminogen activator and risk of myocardial infarction. *Lancet* 1993;341:1165–1168.

52. Ridker PM, Hennekens CH, Stampfer MJ, et al. A prospective study of endogenous tissue plasminogen activator and the risk of stroke. *Lancet* 1994;343:940–943.

53. van der Bom JG, de Knijff P, Haverkate F, et al. Tissue plasminogen activator and risk of myocardial infarction: the Rotterdam Study. *Circulation* 1997;95:2623–2627.

54. Ridker PM, Gaboury CL, Conlin PR, et al. Stimulation of plasminogen activator inhibitor in vivo by infusion of angiotensin II: evidence of a potential interaction between the renin–angiotensin system and fibrinolytic function. *Circulation* 1993;87:1969–1973.

55. Vaughan DE, Rouleau JL, Ridker PM, et al, for the HEART Study Investigators. Effects of ramipril on plasma fibrinolytic balance in patients with acute anterior myocardial infarction. *Circulation* 1997;96:442–447.

56. Fowkes FGR, Lowe GDO, Housley E, et al. Cross-linked fibrin degradation products, progression of peripheral arterial disease, and risk of coronary heart disease. *Lancet* 1993;342:84–86.

57. Ridker PM, Hennekens CH, Cerskus A, Stampfer MJ. Plasma concentration of cross linked fibrin degradation product (D-dimer) and the risk of future myocardial infarction. *Circulation* 1994;90:2236–2240.

58. Lowe GD, Yarnell JW, Sweetnam PM, et al. Fibrin D-dimer, tissue plasminogen activator, plasminogen activator inhibitor, and the risk of major ischaemic heart disease in the Caerphilly Study. *Thromb Haemostas* 1998;79:129–133.

59. Trip MD, Manger Cats V, van Capelle FJL, Vreeken J. Platelet hyperreactivity and prognosis in survivors of myocardial infarction. *N Engl J Med* 1990;322:1549–1554.

60. Elwood PC, Renaud S, Sharp DS, et al. Ischemic heart disease and platelet aggregation: the Caerphilly Collaborative Heart Disease Study. *Circulation* 1991;83:38–44.

61. Beswick AD, Fehily AM, Sharp DS, et al. Long-term diet modification and platelet activity. *J Intern Med* 1991;229:511–515.

62. Nelson GL, Schmidt PC, Corlash L. The effect of a salmon diet on blood clotting, platelet aggregation, and fatty acids in normal adult men. *Lipids* 2001;26:87–96.

63. Martin JF, Bath PMW, Burr ML. Influence of platelet size on outcome after myocardial infarction. *Lancet* 1991;338:1409–1411.

64. Traulow E, Erikssen J, Sandvik L, et al. Blood platelet count and function are related to total and cardiovascular death in apparently healthy men. *Circulation* 1991;84:613–617.

65. Halbmayer WM, Haushofer A, Radek J, et al. Platelet size, fibrinogen and lipoprotein(a) in coronary heart disease. *Coron Artery Dis* 1995;6:397–402.

66. Husain S, Andrews NP, Mulcahy D, et al. Aspirin improves endothelial dysfunction in atherosclerosis. *Circulation* 1998;97:716–720.

67. The Steering Committee of the Physicians' Health Study Research Group. Final report on the aspirin component of the ongoing Physicians' Health Study. *N Engl J Med* 1989;321:129–135.

68. Peto R, Gray R, Collins R, et al. Randomized trial of prophylactic daily aspirin in British male doctors. *BMJ* 1988;296:313–316.

69. Manson JE, Stampfer J, Colditz GA, et al. A prospective study of aspirin use and primary prevention of cardiovascular disease in women. *JAMA* 1991;266:521–527.

70. Kronmal RA, Hart RG, Manolio TA, et al for the CHS Collaborative Research Group. Aspirin use and incident stroke in the Cardiovascular Health Study. *Stroke* 1998;29:887–894.

71. Buring JE, Hennekens CH, for the Women's Health Study Research Group. The Women's Health Study: summary of the study design *J Myocardial Ischemia* 1992;4:27–29.

72. Hennekens CH, Dyken ML, Fuster V. AHA scientific statement on aspirin as a therapeutic agent in cardiovascular disease: a statement for healthcare professionals from the American Heart Association. *Circulation* 1997;96:2751–2753.

73. Meade TW. Aspirin, myocardial infarction, and gastrointestinal bleeding. *Lancet* 1999;353:676.

74. Hansson L, Zanchetti A, Carruthers SG, et al, for the HOT Study Group. Effects of intensive blood-pressure lowering and low-dose aspirin in patients with hypertension: principal results of the Hypertension Optimal Treatment (HOT) randomised trial. *Lancet* 1998;351:1755–1762.

75. He J, Whelton PK, Vu B, Klag MJ. Aspirin and risk of hemorrhagic stroke. *JAMA* 1998;280:1930–1935.

76. Elwood PC, Cochrane AL, Burr ML, et al. A randomized controlled trial of acetylsalicylic acid in the secondary prevention of mortality from myocardial infarction. *BMJ* 1974;1:436–440.

77. The Coronary Drug Project Research Group. Aspirin in coronary heart disease. *J Chronic Dis* 1976;29:625–642.

78. Breddin K, Loew D, Lechner K, et al. Secondary prevention of myocardial infarction: a comparison of acetylsalicylic acid, placebo, and phenprocoumon. *Hemostasis* 1980;9:325–344.

79. Elwood PC, Sweetnam PM. Aspirin and secondary mortality after myocardial infarction. *Lancet* 1979;2:1313–1315.

80. Aspirin Myocardial Infarction Study Research Group. A randomized, controlled trial of aspirin in persons recovered from myocardial infarction. *JAMA* 1980;243:661–669.

81. The Persantine-Aspirin Reinfarction Study Research Group. Persantine and aspirin in coronary heart disease. *Circulation* 1980;62:449–461.

82. Lewis HD, Davis JW, Archibald DG, et al. Protective effects of aspirin against acute myocardial infarction and death in men with unstable angina: result of a Veterans Administration Cooperative Study. *N Engl J Med* 1983;309:396–403.

83. Cairns JA, Gent M, Singer J, et al. Aspirin, sulfinpyrazone, or both, in unstable angina: results of a Canadian multicenter clinical trial. *N Engl J Med* 1985;313:1369–1375.

84. ISIS-2 (Secondary International Study of Infarct Survival) Collaborative Group. Randomized trial of intravenous streptokinase, oral aspirin, both, or neither among 17,187 cases of suspected acute myocardial infarction: ISIS-2. *Lancet* 1988;2:349–360.

85. Antiplatelet Trialists' Collaboration. Collaborative overview of randomised trials of antiplatelet therapy: 1. Prevention of death, myocardial infarction, and stroke by prolonged antiplatelet therapy in various categories of patients. *BMJ* 1994;308:81–106.

86. Gent M, Blakely JA, Easton JD, et al. The Canadian American Ticlopidine Study (CATS) in thromboembolic stroke. *Lancet* 1989;1:1215–1220.

87. Hass WK, Easton JD, Adams HP, et al. A randomized trial comparing ticlopidine hydrochloride with aspirin for the presentation of stroke in high-risk patients. *N Engl J Med* 1989;321:501–507.

88. Gorelick PB, Richardson D, Kelly M, et al. Aspirin and ticlopidine for prevention of recurrent stroke in black patients: a randomized trial. *JAMA* 2003;289: 2947–57.

89. CAPRIE Steering Committee. A randomised, blinded, trial of clopidogrel versus aspirin in patients at risk of ischaemic events (CAPRIE). *Lancet* 1996;348:1323–1339.

90. Yusuf S, Zhao F, Mehta SR, et al. Effects of clopidogrel in addition to aspirin in patients with acute coronary syndromes without ST-segment elevation. *N Engl J Med* 2001;45: 494–502.

91. Hill JW, Roglieri JL, Warburton SW. Aspirin treatment after myocardial infarction: are health maintenance organization members, women, and the elderly undertreated? *Am J Managed Care* 1996;4:51–58.

92. Hennekens CH, Jonas MA, Buring JE. The benefits of aspirin in acute myocardial infarction: still a well-kept secret in the United States. *Arch Intern Med* 1994;154:37–39.

93. Ridker PM, Hennekens CH, Tofler GH, et al. Antiplatelet effects of 100 mg alternate day oral aspirin: a randomized, double-blind, placebo-controlled trial of regular and enteric coated formulations in men and women. *J Cardiovasc Risk* 1996;3:209–212.

94. Glynn RJ, Buring JE, Manson JE, et al. Adherence to aspirin in the prevention of myocardial infarction: the Physician's Health Study. *Arch Intern Med* 1994;154:2649–2657.

95. Forster W, Parratt JR. The case of low-dose aspirin for the prevention of myocardial infarction: but how low is low? *Cardiovasc Drugs Ther* 1997;10:727–734.

96. American Diabetes Association. Aspirin therapy in diabetes: position statement. *Diabetes Care* 1997;20:1772–1773.

97. Libby P, Ridker PM. Novel inflammatory markers of coronary risk. *Circulation* 1999;100:1148–1150

98. de Beer FC, Hind CR, Fox KM, et al. Measurement of C-reactive protein concentration in myocardial ischemia and infarction. *Br Heart J* 1982;47:239–243.

99. Pietila K, Marmoinen A, Hermens W, et al. Serum C-reactive protein concentration in myocardial infarct patients with a closed versus an open infarct-related coronary artery after thrombolytic therapy. *Eur Heart J* 1993;14:915–919.

100. Gaspardone A, Crea F, Versaci F, et al. Predictive value of C-reactive protein after successful coronary-artery stenting in patients with stable angina. *Am J Cardiol* 1998;82:515–518.

101. Morrow DA, Rifai N, Antman EM, et al. C-reactive protein is a potent predictor of mortality independently of and in combination with troponin T in acute coronary syndromes: a TIMI11a substudy. Thrombolysis in Myocardial Infarction. *J Am Coll Cardiol* 1998;31:1460–1465.

102. Thompson SG, Kienast J, Pyke SDM, et al. Hemostatic factors and the risk of myocardial infarction or sudden death in patients with angina pectoris. *N Engl J Med* 1995;332:635–642.

103. Ridker PM. Clinical application of C-reactive protein for cardiovascular disease detection and prevention. *Circulation* 2003;107:363–369.

104. Ridker PM, Cushman M, Stampfer MJ, Tracy RP. Inflammation, aspirin, and the risk of cardiovascular disease in apparently healthy men. *N Engl J Med* 1997;336:973–979.

105. Ridker PM, Glynn RJ, Hennekens CH. C-reactive protein adds to the predictive value of total and HDL-cholesterol in determining risk of first myocardial infarction. *Circulation* 1998;97:2007–2011.

106. Ridker PM, Buring JE, Shih J, et al. Prospective study of C-reactive protein and the risk of future cardiovascular events among apparently healthy women. *Circulation* 1998;98:731–733.

107. Ridker PM, Hennekens CH, Buring JE, et al. C-reactive protein and other markers of inflammation in the prediction of cardiovascular disease in women. *N Engl J Med* 2000;342: 836–843.

108. Ridker PM, Rifai N, Rose L, Buring JE, Cook NR. Comparison of C-reactive protein and low-density lipoprotein cholesterol in the prediction of first cardiovascular events. *N Engl J Med* 2002;347:1557–1565.

109. Ridker PM, Buring JE, Cook NR, Rifai N. C-reactive protein, the metabolic syndrome, and risk of incident cardiovascular events: an 8-year follow-up of 14,719 initially healthy American women. *Circulation* 2003; 107: 391–7.

110. Kuller LH, Tracy RP, Shaten J, Meilahn EN. Relation of C-reactive protein and coronary heart disease in the MRFIT nested case–control study: Multiple Risk Factor Intervention Trial. *Am J Epidemiol* 1996;144:537–547.

111. Koenig W, Sund M, Frohlich M, et al. C-reactive protein, a sensitive marker of inflammation, predicts future risk of coronary heart disease in initially healthy middle-aged men: results from the MONICA (Monitoring Trends and Determinants in Cardiovascular Disease) Augsburg Cohort Study, 1984–1992. *Circulation* 1999;99:237–242.

112. Pradhan AD, Manson JE, Rossouw JE, et al. Inflammatory biomarkers, hormone replacement therapy, and incident coronary heart disease: prospective analysis from the Women's Health Initiative observational study. *JAMA* 2002;288: 980–987.

113. Toss H, Lindahl B, Siegbahn A, Wallentin L, for the FRISC Study Group. Prognostic influence of increased fibrinogen and C-reactive protein levels in unstable coronary artery disease: Fragmin during instability in coronary artery disease. *Circulation* 1997;96:4204–4210.

114. Albert CM, Ma J, Rifai N, et al. Prospective study of C-reactive protein, homocysteine, and plasma lipid levels as predictors of sudden cardiac death. *Circulation* 2002; 105: 2574–6.

115. de Winter RJ, Koch KT, van Straalen JP, et al. C-reactive protein and coronary events following percutaneous coronary angioplasty. *Am J Med* 2003;115: 85–90.

116. Ridker PM, Rifai N, Pfeffer MA, et al, for the Cholesterol and Recurrent Events (CARE) Investigators. Inflammation, pravastatin, and the risk of coronary events after myocardial infarction in patients with average cholesterol levels. *Circulation* 1998;98:839–844.

117. Ridker PM, Rifai N, Pfeffer M, et al. Long-term effects of pravastatin on plasma concentration of C-reactive protein. *Circulation* 1999;100:230–235.

118. Hwang S-J, Ballantyne CM, Sharrett AR, et al. Circulating adhesion molecules VCAM-1, ICAM-1, and E-selectin in carotid atherosclerosis and incident coronary heart disease cases: the Atherosclerosis Risk in Communities (ARIC) study. *Circulation* 1997;96:4219–4225.

119. Ridker PM, Hennekens CH, Roitman-Johnson B, et al. Plasma concentration of soluble intercellular adhesion molecule 1 and risks of future myocardial infarction in apparently healthy men. *Lancet* 1998;351:88–92.

120. Luc G, Bard JM, Juhan-Vague I, et al. C-reactive protein, interleukin-6, and fibrinogen as predictors of coronary heart disease: the PRIME study. *Arterioscler Thromb Vasc Biol* 2003; 23:1255–1261.

121. Pearson TA, Mensah GA, Alexander RW, et al. AHA/CDC Scientific Statement: Markers of inflammation and cardiovascular disease: application to clinical and public health practice. A statement for healthcare professionals from the Centers for Disease Control and Prevention and the American Heart Association. *Circulation* 2003;107:499–511.

122. Anderson JL, Carlquist JF, Muhlestein JB, et al. Evaluation of C-reactive protein, an inflammatory marker, and infectious serology as risk factors for coronary artery disease and myocardial infarction. *J Am Coll Cardiol* 1998;32:35–41.

123. Saikku P, Mattila K, Nieminen S, et al. Serological evidence of an association of a novel chlamydia, TWAR, with chronic coronary heart disease and acute myocardial infarction. *Lancet* 1988;1:983–985.

124. Grayston JT, Campbel LA, Kuo CC, et al. A new respiratory pathogen: Chlamydia pneumoniae infection and atherosclerosis. *J Invest Med* 1997;45:168–174.

125. Shor A, Kuo CC, Patton DL. Detection of Chlamydia pneumoniae in coronary arterial fatty streaks and atheromatous plaques. *South Afr Med J* 1992;82:158–161.

126. Kuo CC, Grayston JT, Campbell LA, et al. Chlamydia pneumoniae (TWAR) in coronary arteries of young adults (15–34 years old). *Proc Natl Acad Sci USA* 1995;92:6911–6914.

127. Campbell LA, O'Brien ER, Cappuccio AL, et al. Detection of Chlamydia pneumoniae TWAR in human coronary atherectomy tissues. *J Infect Dis* 1995;172:585–588.

128. Mehta JL, Saldeen TG, Rand K. Interactive role of infection, inflammation, and traditional risk factors in atherosclerosis and coronary artery disease. *J Am Coll Cardiol* 1998;31:1217–1225.

129. Saikku P, Leinonen M, Tenkanen L, et al. Chronic Chlamydia pneumoniae infection as a risk factor for coronary heart disease in the Helsinki Heart Study. *Ann Intern Med* 1992;116:273–278.

130. Ridker PM, Kundsin RB, Stampfer MJ, et al. A prospective study of Chlamydia pneumoniae IgG seropositive and risks

of future myocardial infarction [abstract]. Presented at: the 71st Scientific Sessions, American Heart Association, Dallas, November 1998.

131. Whincup PH, Mendall MA, Perry IJ, et al. Prospective relations between Helicobacter pylori infection, coronary heart disease, and stroke in middle-aged men. *Heart* 1996;75:568–572.

132. Strandberg TE, Tilvis RS, Vuoristo M, et al. Prospective study of Helicobacter pylori seropositivity and cardiovascular diseases in a general elderly population. *BMJ* 1997;314:1317–1318.

133. Wald NJ, Law MR, Morris JK, Bagnall AM. Helicobacter pylori infection and mortality from ischaemic heart disease: negative result from a large, prospective study. *BMJ* 1997; 315:1199–1201.

134. Aromaa A, Knekt P, Reunanen A, et al. Helicobacter infection and the risk of myocardial infarction [abstract]. *Gut* 1996;39(suppl 2):A91.

135. Folsom AR, Nieto J, Sorlie P, et al. Helicobacter pylori seropositivity and coronary heart disease incidence. *Circulation* 1998;98:845–850.

136. Strachan DP, Mendall MA, Carrington D, et al. Relation of Helicobacter pylori infection to 13-year mortality and incident ischemic heart disease in the Caerphilly Prospective Heart Disease Study. *Circulation* 1998;98:1286.

137. Pasceri V, Cammarota G, Patti G, et al. Association of virulent Helicobacter pylori strains with ischemic heart disease. *Circulation* 1998;97:1675–1679.

138. Hendricks MGR, Salimens MMM, Vauboven CPA, Bruggerman CA. High prevalence of latently present cytomegalovirus in arterial walls of patients suffering from grade III atherosclerosis. *Am J Pathol* 1990;136:23–28.

139. Dummer S, Lee A, Breinig MK, et al. Investigation of cytomegalovirus infection as a risk factor for coronary atherosclerosis in the explanted hearts of patients undergoing heart transplantation. *J Med Virol* 1994;44:305–309.

140. Grattan MT, Moreno-Cabral CE, Starnes VA, et al. Cytomegalovirus infection is associated with cardiac allograft rejection and atherosclerosis. *JAMA* 1989;261:3561–3566.

141. Neito FJ, Adam E, Sorlie P, et al. Cohort study of cytomegalovirus infection as a risk factor for carotid intimal–medial thickening, a measure of subclinical atherosclerosis. *Circulation* 1996;94:922–927.

142. Ridker PM, Hennekens CH, Stampfer MJ, Wang F. Prospective study of herpes simplex virus, cytomegalovirus, and the risk of future myocardial infarction and stroke. *Circulation* 1998;98:2796–2799.

143. Parchure N, Zouridakis EG, Kaski JC. Effect of azithromycin treatment on endothelial function in patients with coronary artery disease and evidence of Chlamydia pneumoniae infection. *Circulation* 2002;105:1298–1303.

144. Muhlestein JB, Anderson JL, Carlquist JF, et al. Randomized secondary prevention trial of azithromycin in patients with coronary artery disease: primary clinical results of the ACADEMIC study. *Circulation* 2000;102:1755–1760.

145. Cercek B, Shah PK, Noc M, et al. Effect of short-term treatment with azithromycin on recurrent ischaemic events in patients with acute coronary syndrome in the Azithromycin in Acute Coronary Syndrome (AZACS) trial: a randomised controlled trial. *Lancet* 2003;361:809–813.

146. O'Connor CM, Dunne MW, Pfeffer MA, et al. Azithromycin for the secondary prevention of coronary heart disease events. The WIZARD Study: a randomized controlled trial. *JAMA* 2003;290:1459–1466.

147. Rumley A, Lowe GDO, Norrie J, et al. Blood rheology and outcome in the West of Scotland Coronary Prevention Study. *Br J Haematol* 1997;97(suppl 1):78.

148. Sweetnam PM, Thomas HF, Yarnell JWG, et al. Fibrinogen, viscosity and the 10-year incidence of ischaemic heart disease. *Eur Heart J* 1996;17:1814–1820.

149. Kannel WB. Fibrinogen: a major cardiovascular risk factor. In: Ernst E, Koenig W, Lowe GDO, Meade TW, eds. *Fibrinogen: A "New" Cardiovascular Risk Factor.* Vienna, Austria: Blackwell-MZV; 1992:101–109.

150. Eriksson H, Wilhelmsen L, Welin L, et al. 21-year follow-up of CVD and total mortality among men born in 1913. In: Ernst E, Koenig W, Lowe GDO, Meade TW, eds. *Fibrinogen: A "New" Cardiovascular Risk Factor.* Vienna: Blackwell-MZV; 1992:115–119.

151. Meade T, Ruddock V, Stirling Y, et al. Fibrinolytic activity, clotting factors, and long-term incidence of ischaemic heart disease in the Northwick Park Heart Study. *Lancet* 1993;342:1076–1079.

152. Junker R, Heinrich J, Schulte H, et al. Coagulation factor VII and the risk of coronary heart disease in healthy men. *Arterioscler Thromb Vasc Biol* 1997;17:1539–1544.

153. Cremer P, Nagel D, Bottcher B, Seidel D. Fibrinogen: ein koronärer Risikofaktor. *Diagn Labor* 1991;42:28–35.

154. Feskens EJM, Kromhout D. Fibrinogen and factor VII activity as risk factors for cardiovascular disease in an elderly cohort. *Can J Cardiol* 1997;13(suppl B):282B.

155. Tunstall-Pedoe H, Woodward M, Tavendale R, et al. Comparison of the prediction by 27 different risk factors of coronary heart disease and death in men and women of the Scottish Heart Health Study. *BMJ* 1997;315:722–729.

156. Lowe GDO, Lee AJ, Rumley A, et al. Blood viscosity and risk of cardiovascular events: the Edinburgh Artery Study. *Br J Haematol* 1997;96:168–173.

157. Benderly M, Graff E, Reicher-Reiss H, et al. Fibrinogen is a predictor of mortality in coronary heart disease patients. *Arterioscler Thromb Vasc Biol* 1996;16:351–356.

158. Thompson SG, Kienast J, Pyke SDM, et al. Hemostatic factors and the risk of myocardial infarction or sudden death in patients with angina pectoris. *N Engl J Med* 1995; 332:634–641.

159. Haines AP, Howarth D, North WRS, et al. Haemostatic variables and outcome of myocardial infarction. *Thromb Haemostas* 1983;50:800–803.

160. Martin JF, Bath PMW, Burr ML. Influence of platelet size on outcome after myocardial infarction. *Lancet* 1991;338:1409–1411.

161. Kostis JB, Baughman DJ, Kuo PT. Association of recurrent myocardial infarction with hemostatic factors: a prospective study. *Chest* 1982;81:571–575.

Psychosocial factors and cardiovascular disease prevention

14

Gary G. Bennett
Lisa F. Berkman

KEY POINTS

- There is ample empirical evidence of associations between a number of psychosocial factors (including depression, anxiety, hostility, social networks and support, and occupational stress) and cardiovascular disease morbidity and mortality. Adverse psychosocial characteristics tend to cluster with traditional biologic and behavioral risk factors; the highest levels of psychosocial risk are generally found among the socially disadvantaged.

- The results of large-scale clinical trials of psychosocial interventions have generally been mixed with respect to their impact on cardiovascular disease outcomes.

- Key areas of consideration when evaluating the effectiveness of psychosocial intervention trials are: (1) the timing of the intervention in relation to the course of disease development and accumulated exposure, and (2) the magnitude and appropriateness of the intervention.

- Greater innovation in the consideration of psychosocial influences on cardiovascular outcomes, behavioral risk factors, and intermediary biological processes may enhance clinical efforts to improve both primary and secondary prevention outcomes.

INTRODUCTION

Tucked away in his classic first description of the cardiovascular system, English physician William Harvey observed that, "For every affection of the mind that is attended with either pain or pleasure, hope or fear, is the cause of an agitation whose influence extends to the heart, and there induces change from the natural constitution, in the temperature, the pulse and the rest."[1] Many centuries later, researchers continue to probe Harvey's thesis. Results of this work suggest that many social and psychologic factors not only have the capacity to affect cardiovascular functioning, but also may serve

as risk factors for cardiovascular disease (CVD) incidence and mortality.[2–4] Despite the burgeoning empirical evidence supporting an association between psychosocial factors and CVD, the area remains controversial. Perhaps as a result, CVD prevention approaches that integrate psychosocial factors are not widespread and the results of such efforts are largely mixed.[5]

Over the past 30 years, the term *psychosocial* has been used quite broadly to categorize factors reflecting a host of purely psychologic (ie, anxiety, depression), psychosocial (ie, work stress, discrimination, emotional support), and social-structural (ie, socioeconomic status, social integration, neighborhood effects) constructs.[5] This chapter reviews the empirical evidence linking selected psychosocial factors (including depression, hostility, social support and social network structure, and work

---

[1] Portions of this chapter are adapted, with the author's permission, from previous work.[1,2]

stress) with CVD outcomes, including material in this area that has been adapted from the authors' previous work.[5,6] The discussion also includes a new area that has potential importance, but where the data are more limited—discrimination. Also presented are findings from large-scale intervention trials designed to remediate psychosocial risk, and recommendations to improve the efficacy of future psychosocial intervention/prevention efforts are offered. Throughout, the chapter focuses on those factors that (1) have been empirically associated with CVD endpoints, either onset or mortality, and (2) have the greatest applicability to CVD prevention, including efforts aimed at both primary prevention and secondary prevention.

Numerous psychosocial factors have been associated with CVD and its risk factors, and detailed descriptions of established psychosocial risk factors and their mechanisms have previously been reviewed.[4–6] There also exists a vast and important literature on socioeconomic position (or socioeconomic status) and CHD. Among the important social conditions influencing the course and prognosis of CVD, socioeconomic position ranks among the most important and best documented. Briefly, numerous epidemiologic investigations have documented an association between indices of low socioeconomic position and poor health.[7–12] This association is generally linear in nature and is observed in the United States and abroad.[11,13] To illustrate, the Whitehall Study of British civil servants showed a strong gradient between employment grade and mortality, with the highest risk of mortality found among the lowest occupational classification.[7,9] The literature in this area is extensive, and because socioeconomic position is best conceived of as a social or social-structural factors (as opposed to a purely psychosocial factor), several publications have focused exclusively on these relationships.[8–11,13]

PSYCHOLOGIC STATES

Depression

Major depression is an increasingly significant health problem in the United States. Although the lifetime prevalence of major depression is approximately 14% in the general US population, this is almost certainly an underestimate, given the condition's relatively low rate of detection and treatment.[14] Depression is more common among cardiac patients than in the general population,[15–18] with some estimates suggesting a nearly 30% prevalence rate.[19]

Clinical episodes of major depression are characterized by depressed mood and a combination of other symptoms including weight change, sleep disturbance, insomnia, fatigue, feelings of guilt, worthlessness, and/or hopelessness, loss of interest in favored activities, psy-

chomotor retardation, attentional difficulties, and suicidal ideation.[20] These symptoms may vary in intensity and/or structure during the course of the condition. Major depression may occur in an episodic fashion, but more often the condition recurs in affected individuals.[20]

Among all of the psychosocial factors studied, there is arguably the most evidence of an association between depression and CVD.[21] Several well-designed prospective investigations have demonstrated that depressed cardiac patients are at significantly increased risk for subsequent mortality after an acute myocardial (MI).[17,19,22] Frasure-Smith and colleagues reported that depression was associated with a fourfold increase in mortality during the 6 months immediately following acute MI. The mortality risk from depression among cardiac patients (adjusted hazard ratio = 4.29, 95% confidence interval [CI] = 3.14–5.44) is similar to and independent of other organic risk factors for mortality, including advanced Killip class (adjusted hazard ratio = 3.52, 95% CI = 2.32–4.72) and previous MI (adjusted hazard ratio = 3.32, 95% CI = 1.96–4.68).[22]

The effect of depression on the development of CVD among initially healthy individuals has been the subject of much debate. A recent meta-analysis of published studies,[21] however, suggests that clinical depression is indeed a strong predictor of coronary heart disease (CHD) incidence (relative risk [RR] = 2.69) after adjustment for traditional risk factors. These findings are important because it could be argued that in the absence of such data, people with more severe CVD may be more likely to be depressed as a result of their illness rather than vice versa.

The relationship between depression and CHD does not necessarily rely on the clinical diagnosis of major depression; the presence of depressive symptoms has also been associated with increased risk for cardiac events.[23–26] For example, hopelessness, a symptomatic feature of depression, has been studied extensively as a predictor of adverse cardiovascular functioning.[27–29] This factor has been linked to sudden cardiac death in both observational human studies and animal models. Recent prospective evidence indicates that hopelessness may also be associated with the development of coronary artery disease (CAD), perhaps mediated by increased carotid atherosclerosis.[30] Moreover, the association between depressive symptoms and CAD is graded, such that the magnitude of depressive symptoms is positively related to CAD risk.[21] For example, Ruguilies, in a meta-analysis, also found that among healthy individuals, clinical depression was a stronger predictor of CHD incidence than was depressed mood (RR = 2.69 and 1.49, respectively).[21]

Constellations of subclinical depressive symptomatology may also have pathogenic effects. For example, the "vital exhaustion" construct grew out of clinical and empirical evidence indicating that high levels of fatigue often precede sudden cardiac events such as MI and sudden cardiac death.[31,32] The factor has been linked with adverse acute events in both healthy and cardiac population samples.[31,32] Depression is associated with a variety of adverse lifestyle factors such as increased cigarette smoking and poorer compliance with medical regimens.[33,34] These behaviors may account for some of the association between depression and CVD risk, but a great deal of evidence points to the importance of some direct biologic pathways.

Depression is mediated by a number of potential biologic mechanisms. Depressed individuals demonstrate heightened cardiovascular and neuroendocrine reactivity, as well as reduced heart rate variability and impaired vagal control of the heart rhythm[35,36] (suggesting heightened arrhythmogenic potential). Depression is also associated with increased cortisol secretion and impaired platelet functioning, characterized by the excess release of products such as platelet factor 4 and β-thromboglobulin.[37-42] Interestingly, the combination of hypercortisolemia and enhanced platelet function suggests the proatherogenic effects of depression.[5] Depression may also have immunosuppressive effects.[43,44] Although a number of biologic mechanisms appear to mediate its influence on CHD, it remains unclear which system or combination thereof accounts for the link between depression and CHD.

Depression is assessed using numerous measurement modalities, including standardized self-report instruments, structured and semistructured diagnostic rating scales, and the clinical interview. There is considerable debate about diagnostic strategies of depression, particularly in the clinical setting where assessment approaches vary widely. Commonly used indices include the Beck Depression Inventory[45], the Hamilton Depression Rating Scale[46], the Composite International Diagnostic Interview (CIDI)[47], the Structured Clinical Interview for DSM-III-R (SCID) ,[48,49] and the Center for Epidemiologic Studies Depression Scale[50] (see Appendix).

Anxiety

Anxiety disorders are perhaps the most frequently occurring mental disorders in the United States and abroad.[51-55] Generally, anxiety disorders are characterized by an extreme disturbance of emotional tone resulting in heightened levels of perceived fear and nervousness. Clinically, the anxiety disorders include primarily panic disorder, agoraphobia, generalized anxiety disorder, social phobia, obsessive–compulsive disorder, acute stress disorder, specific phobias, and posttraumatic stress disorder.[20] Anxiety disorders are thought to emerge from a combination of life experiences, psychologic traits, and genetic factors, although the disorders often vary widely in their expression.

In contrast to depression, anxiety is perhaps most clearly related to sudden cardiac death (SCD).[56] A series of investigations conducted among community samples have demonstrated an association between anxiety and SCD, often occurring in a dose-dependent fashion.[57,58] Many of the anxiety disorders, including panic disorder and phobic anxiety, have been related to CVD.[56] Kawachi and colleagues measured symptoms of phobic anxiety among men being followed in the Normative Aging Study. Over a period of 32 years, men reporting two or more phobic anxiety symptoms had an increased risk of fatal CHD (age-adjusted odds ratio [OR] = 3.20) and sudden death (age-adjusted OR = 5.73).[56] As with depression, symptomatic features of anxiety such as "worry" have also been independently associated with CAD in prospective trials.[57]

Interestingly, however, there is no apparent evidence of a relationship between anxiety and MI.[5] Rozanski and co-workers suggest that because anxiety is related to SCD, but not MI, ventricular arrhythmia may be the primary underlying physiologic mechanism.[5] This notion is further supported by the presence of reduced heart rate variability among anxious individuals,[59] suggesting imbalance between sympathetic activation and vagal outflow. Though there is some evidence of higher levels of negative health behaviors among the anxious, the lack of an association between anxiety and MI suggests that this mechanism may not be immediately pathogenic.[5]

Numerous conceptual and methodologic limitations to the anxiety literature impede the discernment of clear patterns. Despite the fact that anxiety disorders tend to be more prevalent among women (for reasons that are largely unclear),[14] most studies have not systematically examined for potential gender differences in the effects of anxiety on CVD outcomes.[56,59,60] Additionally, many studies investigating the relationship between anxiety and CVD have not used clinical diagnostic guidelines for establishing anxious cases. Thus, most work is based on those with varying levels of anxious symptomatology. One then might expect that clinical anxiety disorders would be associated with more deleterious cardiovascular outcomes, and there is some support for this notion, particularly among patients with established CHD.[61,62]

Summary

Taken together, there is considerable evidence of an association between psychologic states and CVD, particularly among established cardiac patients.[4,5] The comments thus far regarding the relationships among anxiety, depression, and CHD perhaps reflect a clinical bias that stresses differentiation of the constructs. Indeed, diagnostic strategies rely on such symptomatic and conditional distinctions to facilitate the assessment process.[20] However, there is strong evidence that anxiety and depressive disorders frequently co-occur, and their symptoms and related personality traits are closely related.[52,63] Thus, many of the symptoms common to both depression and anxiety disorder may be cogent markers of psychosocial risk, independent of a differential diagnosis. Indeed, such conditional differentiation may result in misestimation of the considerable amount of naturally occurring co-morbidity of the conditions in the general population.

PERSONALITY CONSTRUCTS

The study of personality as a determinant of CVD was spurred largely by Friedman and Rosenman's classic work[64] elucidating the type A behavior pattern (TABP). Arguably the most widely known psychosocial risk factor, interest in the TABP increased exponentially after publication of the Western Collaborative Group Study,[65] which found that TABP was related to both CAD risk and recurrent MI. By the late 1970s, through studies like the Recurrent Coronary Prevention Project (to be discussed in greater detail), researchers and clinicians in the area had taken steps to name TABP as an identified risk factor for CVD.[66] Numerous subsequent investigations, however, found no relationship between TABP and CVD,[61–67] which promoted its disaggregation in future investigations.

Hostility

Hostility, characterized in the TABP model as "cynical" and "free-floating," is considered to be the most predictive component of TABP. Hostility is a multidimensional construct that reflects emotional (anger, contempt), behavioral (verbal and physical aggression), and cognitive (cynicism, mistrust) factors.[70] Hostility appears to be most common among those of low socioeconomic status (SES), men, and nonwhites.[71]

Hostility has been shown to predict new coronary events among previously healthy individuals.[72–74] For example, Niaura and colleagues prospectively examined 774 men free from CVD. They found that hostility positively predicted incident CHD after adjustment for traditional risk factors, sociodemographic characteristics, and behavioral patterns.[74]

There is somewhat less evidence that hostility predicts recurrent cardiac events or mortality among those with established CHD.[4,75] However, there is evidence of an association between hostility and acute coronary events.[76] The risk of experiencing these events may be particularly heightened during emotionally charged situations.[77,78] Hostility is associated with heightened cardiovascular reactivity in laboratory settings and higher blood pressure levels in ambulatory assessments.[79] Although lifestyle factors too may be implicated in the link between hostility and CHD, most studies have demonstrated an associa-

tion with CHD that persists after adjustment for health behaviors.[4]

Given its high prevalence among those in lower SES strata,[71] some have argued that hostility might be a primary psychologic mechanism linking low SES with CVD outcomes. Gump and colleagues showed among a sample of African-American and white children that lower SES (measured using both neighborhood and individual indices) was associated with higher hostility levels and elevated cardiovascular reactivity to laboratory stressors.[80] However, this association was limited to African-American children. Among white children, only family SES (independent of neighborhood socioeconomic factors) was associated with heightened cardiovascular reactivity. These findings are notable for numerous reasons: they highlight the potential importance of multilevel assessment of psychosocial risk and identify a clear risk factor and temporal point of intervention for a group that experiences vastly disproportionate levels of CVD later in life.

Though meta-analytic reviews have demonstrated an association between hostility and the development of CHD,[81] more recent work indicates that there is considerable variability in the presence and strength of the association.[75,79] This level of unreliability may stem from difficulty elucidating hostility's predictive role in the context of the other traditional risk factors with which it is associated.[6] For example, Siegler showed that hostility was associated with a variety of such risk factors, including age, dietary patterns, decreased physical activity, and increased alcohol and cigarette smoking.[71] As Krantz and McCeney note, adjustment for these risk factors may also reduce the observable effect of hostility.[6]

There are also significant methodologic complications in hostility's assessment, which can be conducted using either self-report or behavioral indices. The choice of measurement modality may be of considerable importance. Meta-analytic review of early studies showed that the association between hostility and CHD was stronger for behavioral ratings as compared with self-report.[79]

Taken together, it appears that hostility may be a stronger predictor of initial CHD than of its progression, recurrence, or mortality. Inconsistency in the model's predictive power may stem from a number of factors, though the assessment of hostility may present particular difficulty. Despite these complications, the model may hold particular promise in explaining the elevated CHD risk among populations who disproportionately report high levels of hostility, including African-Americans and those in lower socioeconomic strata.

SOCIAL RELATIONS

Over the last 30 years there has accumulated a vast literature linking social networks or social support and morbidity and mortality, especially related to CVD. A complete review of this literature is beyond the scope of this chapter and the reader is referred to several recent reviews covering a broad array of outcomes.[82–89] The intention here is to review the evidence linking social networks and social support with CVD morbidity and mortality.

Thirteen large prospective cohort studies across a number of countries, from the United States to Scandinavian countries to Japan, have shown that people who are isolated or disconnected from others are at increased risk of dying prematurely. In the first of these studies from Alameda County,[90] men and women who lacked ties to others (in this case, based on an index assessing contacts with friends and relatives, marital status, and church and group membership) were 1.9 to 3.1 times more likely to die in a 9-year follow-up period from 1965 to 1974 than were those who had many more contacts. Those who lacked social ties were at increased risk of dying from ischemic heart disease, cerebrovascular and circulatory disease, cancer, a final category including respiratory, gastrointestinal, and all other causes of death.

Another study in Tecumseh, Michigan, found as strong a positive association for men, but not for women, between social connectedness/social participation and mortality risk over a 10- to12-year period.[91] An additional strength of this study was the ability to control for some biological predictors assessed from physical examination (eg, cholesterol, blood pressure, and respiratory function). In the same year, Blazer reported similar results from an elderly sample of men and women in Durham County, North Carolina. He compared three measures of social support and attachment: (1) self-perceived impaired social support, including feelings of loneliness; (2) impaired social roles and attachments; (3) low frequency of social interaction. The relative risks (RRs) for dying associated with these three measures were 3.4, 2.0, and 1.9, respectively.[92]

In the last few years, results from several more studies, one in the United States and three in Scandinavia, have been reported. Using data from Evans County, Georgia, Schoenbach and co-workers used a measure of social contacts modified from the Alameda County Study. They found risks to be significant in older white men and women, even when controlling for biomedical and sociodemographic risk factors, although some racial and gender differences were observed.[93] In Sweden, the Goteborg Study reported that in different cohorts of men born in 1913 and 1923, social isolation proved to be a risk factor for dying, independent of age and biomedical risk factors.[94] The study by Orth-Gomér and Johnson is the only study besides the Alameda County study to report significantly increased risks for women who have been socially isolated.[95] Finally, in a study of 13,301 men and women in eastern Finland, Kaplan and associates have

shown that an index of social connections almost identical to the Social Network Index used in Alameda County predicts cardiovascular mortality risk for men but not for women, independent of standard cardiovascular risk factors.[96]

Several studies of older men and women in the Alameda County Study and the Established Populations for the Epidemiologic Study of the Elderly (EPESE) studies confirm the continued importance of these relationships into late life.[97,98] Furthermore, two studies of large cohorts of men and women in a large health maintenance organization[99] and 32,000 male health professionals[100] suggest that social networks are, in general, more strongly related to mortality than to the incidence or onset of disease. In more recent reports from the US Physicians' Health Study, socially isolated men had an increased risk of fatal CHD in multivariate analyses (RR = 1.82, 95% CI = 1.02–3.23).[101] Two studies in Danish men[102] and Japanese men and women[103] further indicate that aspects of social isolation or social support are related to mortality. Virtually all of these studies find that people who are socially isolated or disconnected from others are at between two and five times the risk of dying from all causes, compared with those who maintain strong ties to friends, family, and community. There is conflicting, albeit limited, evidence that a social network or support is related to the incidence or onset of CVD. Although one study of middle-aged Swedish men found social integration to be related to the incidence of MI,[104] several other studies have reported no associations.[99,100]

In contrast, in the last 6 years, a host of studies have suggested that social ties, especially intimate ties and emotional support provided by those ties, influence survival among people post-MI or with serious CVD. In the first of these, Ruberman and colleagues examined 2320 male survivors of acute MI who were participants in the Beta-Blocker Heart Attack Trial. Patients who were socially isolated were more than twice as likely to die over a 3-year period as those who were less socially isolated.[105] When this measure of social isolation was combined with a general measure of life stress, which included items related to occupational status, divorce, exposure to violent events, retirement, and financial difficulty, the risks associated with high-risk psychosocial status were even greater. Individuals in the high-risk psychosocial categories were four to five times as likely to die as those in the lowest-risk categories. This psychosocial characteristic was associated with death from all causes and sudden death. It made large contributions to mortality risk in both the high-arrhythmia and low-arrhythmia groups.

In a second Swedish study of 150 cardiac patients and patients with high-risk factors for CHD, the finding that lack of support predicts death was confirmed.[106] Patients who were socially isolated had a 10-year mortality rate three times higher than the rate of those who were socially active and integrated. Because these patients were examined extensively for prognostic factors at study entry, it was possible to disentangle effects of psychosocial and clinical characteristics.

In a third study, Williams and co-workers enrolled 1368 patients who were undergoing cardiac catheterization from 1974 through 1980 and found to have significant CAD. They examined survival time until cardiovascular death through 1989. In this study, men and women who were unmarried or without a confidant were more than three times likely to die within 5 years compared with those who had a close confidant or who were married (OR = 3.34, CI = 1.8–6.2). This association was independent of other clinical prognostic indicators and sociodemographic factors, including SES.[107]

Case and colleagues examined the association between marital status and recurrent major cardiac events among patients post-MI who were enrolled in the placebo arm of a clinical trial, the Multicenter Diltiazem Post-Infarction Trial. These investigators reported that living alone was an independent risk factor with a hazard ratio of 1.54 (CI = 1.04–2.29) for recurrent major cardiac events, including both nonfatal infarctions and cardiac deaths.[108]

In a fifth study, the relationship between social networks and support and mortality was examined among men and women hospitalized for MI between 1982 and 1988 who were participants in the population-based New Haven EPESE.[109] Among both men and women, emotional support, measured prospectively, was related to both early in-hospital death and later death over a 1-year period. Among those admitted to the hospital, almost 38% of those who reported no source of emotional support died in the hospital, compared with 11.5% of those with two or more sources of support. The patterns remained steady throughout the follow-up period. In multivariate models that control for sociodemographic factors, psychosocial factors (including living arrangements and depressive symptoms), and clinical prognostic indicators, men and women who reported no emotional support had almost three times the mortality risk compared with subjects who reported at least one source of support (OR = 2.9, 95% CI = 1.2–6.9).

In a study of men and women undergoing coronary bypass surgery or aortic valve replacement, Oxman and colleagues found that being a member of voluntary organizations, including religious organizations, and drawing strength and comfort from religious or spiritual faith were related to survival postsurgery. When these two dimensions were combined, people who endorsed neither of these items, that is, those who did not belong to organizations and who did not draw comfort from their faith, were more than seven times likely to die as those who did.[110]

Among Mexican-Americans and non-Hispanic whites in the Corpus Christi Heart Project, higher levels of social support were associated with longer survival during an average period longer than 3 years.[111] However, when analyzed separately, there was no effect of social support on mortality among whites. However, a considerable mortality risk associated with low social support was noted among Mexican-American men and women (3.38, CI = 1.73–6.62).

These findings in post-MI populations, coupled with the strong data on long-term mortality and relatively weaker data on MI incidence, would suggest that social networks and support may have the greatest impact on determining not the onset of disease, but prognosis and survival.

To date, there have been only a handful of studies related to other cardiovascular diseases. A study of congestive heart failure among older men and women in New Haven reported emotional support to be related to survival for men but not women,[112] and found no association with risk for initial hospitalization.[113]

Several studies have identified a trend toward higher risk of death from stroke among those who are socially isolated,[100,114] although these studies have lacked the statistical power to fully evaluate the associations. However, a number of additional studies have shown that social networks and support (particularly social isolation) are associated with case fatality in the poststroke period. For example, in a study by Vogt and co-workers, social network measures were strong predictors of both cause-specific and all-cause mortality among persons who had incident cases of ischemic heart disease, cancer, and stroke.[99] During 10 years of follow-up of newly diagnosed stroke patients, clinical diagnosis of depression was associated with poor survival.[115] In that study, patients who were both socially isolated and clinically depressed were at particular risk for poststroke fatality. To date, no studies have reported a link between social isolation and incidence of nonfatal stroke. In one study of 32,624 US male health care workers, Kawachi and colleagues reported a trend in the association between risk of nonfatal stroke and social networks. However, it was not possible to conduct multivariate analyses due to inadequate statistical power.[100]

OCCUPATIONAL STRESS

The workplace is a context that provides almost routine exposure to chronic psychosocial stressors. Occupational demands account for a large proportion of the daily stressors encountered by individuals,[116,117] primarily because of the extended time (30–40% of one's waking hours) and effort expended there.[118] Although they may more easily avoid other stressors, most individuals are subject to the demands of the occupational arena.

Job strain

The demand/control or job strain model[119,120] is the dominant theoretical construct of occupational stress.[118]

The model posits that physiologic arousal is influenced "from the joint effects of the demands of a work situation and the range of decision making freedom (discretion) available to the workers facing those demands."[119] Thus, an interaction between workplace decision latitude (job control) and psychologic job demands is hypothesized.[119,120] Jobs with high demands require an excessive amount of work output, usually under a variety of constraints (ie, time pressures, performance expectations, layoff possibilities). Those in jobs with low decision latitude have little control over their assigned tasks, work that is often characterized by its simplicity and repetitive nature. The job strain condition is characterized by jobs with high demands and low perceived control.[119]

The accumulated evidence supports an association between job strain and CVD incidence and mortality,[118,121–124] as well as all-cause mortality,[125,126] though there have been several negative studies as well.[127,128] For example, Falk and associates demonstrated, among a sample of elderly men, that job strain was associated with a nearly doubled risk of mortality.[126] However, mortality risk increased substantially among those with a combination of high job strain and poor social networks (RR = 2.1–4.6 depending on social network index). Similarly, Karasek and co-workers imputed job strain categorizations from the US Health Examination Survey and the Health and Nutrition Examination Survey. They found a higher prevalence of MI among men in both samples with elevated levels of job strain.[129]

There is, however, significant sociodemographic variation in job strain findings. The influence of job strain on CVD risk has been shown to be stronger in workers of low SES[122,130]; however, relatively few studies have investigated the construct among samples including ethnic minorities. Thomas and colleagues' longitudinal comparison of white and African-American physicians revealed that although the incidence of hypertension in African-American men was twice that of the white subjects, the disparity was not explained by job strain.[125] African-Americans in the study had significantly lower workplace demands and significantly higher rates of job control when compared with white participants. Other studies have been largely unable to demonstrate a significant association between job strain and CVD risk factors among African-Americans.[132–134] Curtis and co-workers' investigation of rural African-American men and women showed that among men, high job control was associated with a 50% decrease in hypertension prevalence. In both men and women, however, neither job demands nor composite job strain variables were associated with elevated blood pressure or hypertension prevalence.[133,135]

Further, a number of investigators have shown that the demand/control model may be most applicable to the occupational experiences of men.[136] For example, Riese and

associates found no effect of job strain on traditional biologic CVD risk factors among female nurses.[137] Though there is little evidence suggesting that job strain directly influences the expression of CVD risk among women, there is some evidence that the factor might moderate the effects of other psychosocial risk factors.

Laflamme and co-workers found significantly higher levels of ambulatory blood pressure as a function of high job strain only among women with a university degree.[138] Similarly, Brisson and colleagues reported that high job strain predicted elevated blood pressure only among women who also reported high levels of family responsibilities.[139] The reasons for job strain's lack of external validity among women remain unclear. Some have argued that such occupations may serve as beneficial coping mechanisms for women who have multiple occupational demands.[136] Clearly, this issue deserves further attention.

Effort–reward imbalance

The more recently developed "effort–reward imbalance" (ERI) model is conceptualized as "the reward structure of work and its potential for self-regulation."[116] In short, the construct argues risk is encountered when workplace effort (considered a function of extrinsic job demands and behavioral coping) is not commensurate with both tangible (salary, benefits) and intangible (support) occupational rewards.[116]

Prospective investigations suggest that the ERI model predicts CVD incidence[140,141] and a host of CVD risk factors.[142–145] One study of CHD incidence among male, middle-aged, blue-collar steel workers revealed that CHD incidence was associated with higher ERI after adjustment for age, smoking, body mass index, and physical activity.[144]

An empiric examination comparing the ERI and job strain models with respect to prediction of CHD incidence was conducted among a sample of British male and female civil servants.[140] Both ERI and the job control component of the job strain model were shown to independently predict CHD incidence. In post hoc analyses, ERI retained a significant association with CHD incidence after controlling for job control and hostility. In addition to providing support for the uniqueness of each model, these findings highlight the potentially deleterious effects of chronic exposure to a harsh social work environment.

EMERGING AREAS

Discrimination

There has been increasing interest in investigating racial discrimination as a determinant of health outcomes among historically marginalized American ethnic groups.[63,146–148] Interest in studying racial discrimination emerges from the frequent finding that members of ethnic minority groups (particularly African-Americans) and those of low SES are likely to encounter situations throughout their lives that limit their access to the resources necessary for the maintenance of good health.[146] Furthermore, African-Americans have been found to have higher rates of cardiovascular and cerebrovascular disease and hypertension unexplained by standard risk factors. There has been some debate as to the taxonomic classification of discrimination, but there are at least two broad categories currently under study: institutional and interpersonal discrimination.[149]

Studies examining the impact on minority health of biased institutional practices have only recently emerged. Many of these studies examine how such policies promote residential segregation,[135,150] particularly in locations characterized by lower SES and multiple exposures to toxic agents. Other work has examined bias in medical treatment practices, often showing systemic bias against African-Americans and other ethnic minorities.[151]

Generally speaking, most studies have examined the impact of interpersonal discrimination on a variety of health-related outcomes. This is a prudent approach given that many African-Americans report experiencing regular racial discrimination.[146,152] It should however, be noted that studies in this area are concerned with perceptions of discrimination, and generally do not seek to objectively investigate the validity of the subject's claims. The measurement of racial discrimination has also been the subject of some debate, and assessment strategies vary widely.[149] Further, the overwhelming majority of these studies have been conducted among African-Americans, primarily because of the groups' historical exposure to discriminatory acts. Work examining racial discrimination among majority group members shows no consistent pattern.

Reports of racial discrimination at work and in everyday life have been associated with elevated blood pressure and cardiovascular reactivity to laboratory-based stressors. Krieger's seminal study showed that acceptance and internalization of racial discrimination were associated with increased blood pressure in both working class and professional African-Americans. She also showed that differences in blood pressure between African-Americans and whites were reduced substantially when encounters with discrimination were adjusted for.[148] Other work has linked perceptions of racial discrimination with adverse health behaviors, including cigarette smoking.[153]

At least one study has demonstrated an association between racial discrimination and all-cause morbidity or mortality,[154] and there is mounting evidence that perceived racial discrimination affects a variety of CVD risk factors and intermediary biological pathways.[153,155,156] As primary racial discrimination is a chronic psychosocial stressor for many individuals,[146] the continued investigation of this factor may hold particular promise in discerning determinants of the substantial disparities in CVD outcomes between African-Americans and whites.[63]

Clustering

Although psychosocial risk factors are usually discussed in isolation, they regularly cluster within individuals and among populations, often substantially raising the risk for cardiovascular dysfunction.[157–159] While a large body of evidence suggests that clustering of psychosocial risk factors raises risk among post-MI and other cardiac patients, increasing evidence similarly indicates that this risk might extend to healthy populations. For example, Ruberman and co-workers showed a nearly doubled risk of MI among individuals with high levels of life stress and social isolation.[105] Lynch and colleagues, in data from the Kuopio Ischemic Heart Disease Risk Factor Study, showed that both negative psychosocial factors and adverse lifestyle variables were clustered among men in lower-income strata.[159]

Although these data suggest that psychosocial factors act synergistically to increase risk, there is also evidence that psychosocial factors may cluster with behavioral risk factors to heighten the risk of adverse cardiac outcomes.[5,159] Taken together, it appears that multiple nonlinear relations with other psychosocial variables, sociodemographic characteristics, and organic risk factors may characterize the "causal" pathways linking any individual psychosocial factor with CVD endpoints. Though this model opposes traditional epidemiologic analytic notions, appreciation of the complexity of the interrelations among such risk factors may eventually promote the development of more effective preventive approaches.

PSYCHOSOCIAL INTERVENTIONS: RANDOMIZED CLINICAL TRIALS

Several randomized clinical trials have been aimed at psychosocial altering conditions and CVD. Of these, many have reported equivocal results. For a more detailed description of these trials, including fuller descriptions of the intervention and training, the reader is referred to a recent review by Burg and Berkman.[2] This section describes several large-scale interventions, the major results, and our interpretation of the findings. An overview of these studies is presented in Table 14-1. Much of the section is based on earlier review.[2]

The recurrent coronary prevention project

The goals of the Recurrent Coronary Prevention Project (RCPP) were to use group therapy to reduce type A behavior, and to demonstrate that this approach would effectively reduce type A and cardiac endpoints (eg, reinfarction and cardiac death).[160] Participants in RCPP were randomly assigned to either a cardiac counseling condition ($n = 270$) or a type A counseling condition ($n = 592$). Those in the cardiac counseling group received counseling aimed at increasing knowledge of and adherence to the treatment regimen prescribed by their physician, including efforts to reduce lifestyle risk factors such as diet and exercise; they were invited to attend a total of thirty-three 90-minute-long monthly sessions over the course of the study. Those in the type A counseling group received cardiac counseling and also a comprehensive package designed to address and alter the specific type A behaviors in the participants' behavioral repertoire[161]; they were invited to attend a total of 62 (initially weekly, fading to monthly after 1 year) sessions over the course of the study. Mean attendance for both conditions averaged 67% of sessions.[162]

At study outset, the two groups were found to be equivalent with respect to a range of medical and sociodemographic factors, and approximately 98% were found to exhibit some significant degree of type A behavior.[163] At the end of 3 years, the cardiac counseling group evidenced a combined coronary recurrence rate of 13%, whereas the type A counseling group evidenced a combined coronary recurrence rate of 7.2% ($P < .005$), a difference accounted for by primarily nonfatal events.[162] The latter group also showed a marked reduction in type A behavior. Reductions in type A behavior were found to persist 1 year after termination of treatment.[164] Hence, the RCPP demonstrated the viability of treatment efforts targeting a stress-related cognitive and behavioral factor associated with cardiac endpoints and the significant impact on CHD endpoints of such an intervention.

The enhancing recovery in coronary heart disease study

Funded by the National Heart, Lung and Blood Institute, the Enhancing Recovery in Coronary Heart Disease (ENRICHD) study was a multicenter, randomized, controlled clinical trial designed to determine the impact on subsequent morbidity and mortality in patients with acute MI of treating depression and low perceived social support (LPSS). A total of 2481 patients were recruited for this trial, with diverse representation of gender and racial/ethnic groups. Primary endpoints were cardiovascular mortality and recurrent nonfatal MI; secondary endpoints included all-cause mortality, incidence of revascularization procedures, cardiovascular hospitalizations, and change in risk factor profile. Secondary psychosocial endpoints included severity of depression, degree of social support, and health-related quality of life. Patients were eligible for randomization to a usual care or intervention arm within 28 days of their index cardiac

event if they met DSM-IV criteria for major depression, minor depression with a history of major depression, or dysthymia, or if they achieved a criterion score on the ENRICHD Social Support Instrument (ESSI), a six-item, Likert scored scale composed of items found in other studies to be predictive of morbidity and mortality following MI.[105,109,165,166] A more comprehensive report of the eligibility and recruitment aspects of ENRICHD is provided elsewhere.[167]

A rapid and aggressive treatment approach was necessitated for ENRICHD because the greatest risk for poor outcome is found in the months immediately after the index event.[168] In addition, with its focus on cardiac endpoints rather than treatment efficacy, the intervention needed to rely on the most effective treatment approach described in the literature.[169] Hence, cognitive-behavioral therapy[170,171] and social learning approaches[171,172] were used. In addition, a combination of individual and group treatment was selected, and adjunctive pharmacotherapy was included for participants with more severe or unresponsive depression.

Treatment started with a reliance on individual therapy. This allowed treatment to begin immediately after randomization and very soon after the index myocardial event. Treatment duration ranged from six sessions to a maximum of 6 months, depending on treatment progress. Success in treatment was criterion based and determined largely by both a sufficient reduction in symptoms and a demonstrated capacity for self-therapy.

A patient's course of treatment was completed, where possible, by open membership group therapy. Although individual treatment was rapid and aggressive, the group component provided a cost-effective way to reinforce and extend early progress. A participant could join a group at any point in a 12-session continuum, after completing 3 individual sessions, but no later than 6 months after enrolling in the trial; patients could attend both individual and group therapy concurrently. For some of the ENRICHD sites, there were often too few patients to form a therapy group at any one time, but the curricular nature of the intervention allowed the group material to be presented within the context of individual therapy sessions.

Adjunctive pharmacotherapy, managed by study psychiatrists, was also used for patients with severe depression and for those whose response to treatment was slow. Sertraline, a selective serotonin reuptake inhibitor (SSRI), was used as the initial agent (unless contraindicated), based on its efficacy and safety in patients with CVD. Patients unable to tolerate sertraline, or judged to have an inadequate response to treatment after 4 weeks, were considered for alternative treatment with another SSRI or with nortriptyline. The therapeutic agent was given for 12 months; if treatment beyond 12 months was needed, the patient was referred to community resources.

TABLE 14-1 Selected Clinical Trials Involving Psychosocial and/or Behavioral Interventions to Reduce Cardiovascular Disease Risk

Program	Sample	Intervention	Randomized	Intention to treat	Major outcome(s)	Secondary outcome(s)
Recurrent Coronary Prevention Project[162]	Post-MI cardiac patients (n = 862)	Type A counseling (IX)* vs cardiac counseling (4.5 year program)	Yes	Yes	Lower recurrence of nonfatal MI at 3, 4.5 years During final 3.5 years of IX, fewer cardiac deaths At 1-year follow-up, lower MI recurrence among IX subjects who reduced type A behaviors	During program: reduced type A behavior, hostility, anger, impatience, depression During program: higher life satisfaction, stress management self-efficacy, social support At 1-year follow-up, lower type A behaviors among IX subjects
ENRICHD[173]	Post-MI cardiac patients (n = 2481)	CBT-based individual and group therapy with SSRIs for severely depressed (IX) vs usual care	Yes	Yes	No IX effect on event-free survival	Reduced depression and higher social support
Ischemic Heart Disease Life Stress Monitoring Program[174]	Post-MI cardiac patients (n = 461)	Monthly stress monitoring and home-based nurse visits for highly distressed (IX) vs usual care	Yes	Yes (1 year follow-up) Yes (7-year follow-up)	2-fold higher cardiac mortality among controls At 7 years, fewer MI recurrences in IX group Reduced distress	No effect of IX on general, cardiac, or elective bypass surgery readmissions during program or at follow-up
Montreal Heart Attack Readjustment Trial[175]	Post-MI cardiac patients (n = 1376)	Monthly stress monitoring and home-based nurse visits for highly distressed (IX) vs usual care	Yes	Yes	No IX effect on survival	No effect of IX on psychologic factors
Blumenthal et al[182]	Cardiac patients with myocardial ischemia (n = 107)	Stress management (IX) vs exercise group, usual care	No (noncontrol subjects randomly assigned to either stress management or exercise)	Yes	Lower risk of adverse cardiac event	Reduction in left ventricular wall motion abnormalities during mental stress testing Increased treadmill time Weight loss Fewer ischemic episodes Decreased hostility and psychologic distress

IX, intervention; CBT, cognitive-behavioral therapy; SSRI, selective serotonin reuptake inhibitor.

The problem of LPSS provided a unique opportunity for ENRICHD. Although LPSS is a risk factor for poor medical outcome after acute MI, it is not psychopathologic, and there are no standard treatments with tested efficacy. Cognitive-behavioral therapy and social learning approaches provided a framework for the treatment of LPSS.

The ENRICHD intervention did not increase event-free survival, the primary endpoint of the study.[173] After an average follow-up of 29 months, there was no significant difference in event-free survival between usual care (75.9%) and psychosocial intervention (75.8%). There were also no differences in the primary endpoint, mortality or reinfarction, in any of the psychosocial subgroups, for example, those who were depressed only, had LPSS only, or those who were both isolated and depressed.[173]

There were, however, significant differences and improvement in depression and social support. Improvements in psychosocial outcomes at s6 months favored treatment: mean (SD) change in depression scores using the Hamilton were −10.1 (7.8) in the psychosocial intervention group versus −8.4 (7.7) in the usual care group ($P < .001$). Mean change in LPSS as assessed by the ESSI was 5.1 (5.9) in the intervention group and 3.4 (6.0) in the usual care group ($P < .001$). Over the length of the trial, the relative difference in the psychosocial group, compared with the usual care group, was less than expected due to substantial improvement in the usual care group. Although to some extent this was anticipated with respect to the resolution of depression (and treatment for depression in the usual care group), the limited observational data on social support do not indicate there are increases in support from 6 months to several years post-MI.

The ENRICHD trial results suggest some evidence of a treatment group by sex interaction, with men tending to benefit more from the intervention than women. When adjusted for other significant covariates, this interaction became nonsignificant. Thus, the observed interaction may be due to disparities in conditions associated with gender. However, adverse findings reported for women in the Montreal Heart Attack Readjustment Trial (see below) support the view that there may be something important and consistent about the ENRICHD findings that warrant further study.

The ischemic heart disease life stress monitoring program and the montreal heart attack readjustment trial

Interventions to relieve distress associated with disease and its treatment offer an additional promising avenue for stress reduction in the cardiac population. These approaches typically rely on a wide range of techniques, ranging from relaxation training and group psychoeduca-

tion to more individually tailored approaches. One of the most important distress mitigation approaches demonstrated with cardiac patients has been the Ischemic Heart Disease Life Stress Monitoring Program.[174,175] In this study, 461 male patients recovering from MI were randomized to a stress monitoring intervention or usual care. The hypothesis of this investigation was that targeting life stress through a coordinated program of screening and multimodal intervention would reduce the risk of cardiac recurrence and death. Patients were contacted by telephone on a regular basis and screened for symptoms of stress and distress. Those in the intervention group who showed an increasing trend in symptoms of stress received home nursing interventions consisting of individually tailored combinations of education, support, collaborative problem solving, and referral. Nursing visits were continued until there was a significant reduction in symptoms of stress. After 1 year, follow-up data revealed that the program had a significant impact on stress symptoms and that control patients had twice the risk of death due to cardiac causes as their intervention counterparts.[174] After 7 years, the mortality differences between the two groups were found to persist, with the greatest impact being on sudden cardiac death.[176]

The success of this trial led to the subsequent Montreal Heart Attack Readjustment Trial, designed to treat life stress in a larger cohort of 1376 men and women who had survived MI; this trial, unfortunately, showed no benefit for the intervention group. Indeed, a significant increase in cardiac and all-cause mortality was observed among women in the intervention group.[175] Further analyses of the data, however, revealed that patients who responded to the support intervention within two home visits had improved medical outcomes, whereas those who continued to display high levels of distress worsened.[169] This indicates the importance of interventions that have a significant effect on the presenting psychosocial problem and of using staff who have the background and experience needed to address the complex stress-related problems of patients with CHD. Indeed, interventions with equivocal results may share this problem of failing to intervene sufficiently on the target problem and of not using appropriately trained personnel.[177]

Transient ischemia in CAD

Transient myocardial ischemia is common in patients with CAD. Up to 75% of incidents are asymptomatic, and most often occur in the absence of physical exertion. The presence of this phenomenon may be a significant predictor of both fatal and nonfatal cardiac events.[178,179] Studies have shown that mental stress can trigger ischemic episodes in susceptible individuals,[77,180] and that ischemia induced by mental stress under controlled conditions in the laboratory is associated with an increased likelihood of ischemia in natural settings, during routine daily experience.[161,181] Blumenthal and colleagues evaluated the impact of a stress management intervention (exercise training and usual care) on clinical outcomes and myocardial ischemia in 136 men and women with CAD.[182] Patients underwent baseline and follow-up evaluations at the conclusion of a 4-month intervention, including an assessment of changes in myocardial ischemia during exercise and mental stress testing and during ambulatory electrocardiographic monitoring. Follow-up of adverse events, including nonfatal MI, death, and revascularization secondary to progressive angina, was conducted yearly. Compared with the control group, the stress management group had a lower RR of an event (0.26, 95% CI = 0.07–0.93, $P = .04$), even after adjusting for baseline left ventricular ejection fraction, history of MI, and age. Patients in the stress management group demonstrated a reduction in left ventricular wall motion abnormalities during posttreatment mental stress testing ($P < .004$), and significantly fewer ischemic episodes and angina than those in usual care. In addition, those receiving stress management who had more severe pretreatment wall motion abnormalities during mental and exercise testing showed the greatest improvement ($P < .001$). Patients in the stress management group also showed exhibited the greatest effect with respect to measures of distress ($P < .001$).

In Blumenthal and colleagues' study, the stress management program was based on a cognitive-social learning model of behavior. Within this model, stress is seen as a function of an interaction between the social environment and aspects of an individual's personality traits that predispose to responding to situations in potentially cardiotoxic ways. This model further assumes that emotion and behavior are determined largely by an individual's perceptions of, and automatic thoughts about, routine events experienced throughout the day. The program consisted of sixteen 90-minute-long sessions, conducted in a group of eight patients. Elements from the Recurrent Coronary Prevention Project and the Ischemic Heart Disease Life Stress Monitoring Program described above were incorporated, as was cognitive-behavioral therapy.[170,172] The initial sessions were largely psychoeducational and provided information about coronary disease, the structure and function of the heart, risk factors, and stress. Subsequent sessions involved instruction in specific skills to reduce the affective, behavioral, cognitive, and physiologic components of stress. Patients were additionally taught progressive muscle relaxation techniques and the incorporation of progressive muscle relaxation into their daily routine. Each patient received at least two individual sessions of electromyographic biofeedback training in addition to the 16 group sessions.

Although a number of similarities exist between their work and the RCPP and the Montreal experience,

Blumenthal and co-workers highlighted a number of important considerations for the treatment of stress in cardiac populations. This study demonstrates the potential importance of such an approach on intermediate endpoints such as transient ischemic events and wall motion abnormalities, in addition to mortality-based endpoints. Of perhaps greatest interest was the finding of a positive impact during mental stress testing. In this condition, patients are exposed to provocative and demanding laboratory tasks (eg, time-pressured mental arithmetic, recall of an anger provoking incident). The positive findings related to the stress management intervention hint at a chronic and generalized effect. The implications are not just that the patient learns ways to reduce stress when it is occurring, but rather that the patient learns to approach life circumstances in new ways so that previously provocative (routine daily) events are no longer so. The ability to achieve this with a relatively quick and inexpensive intervention further highlights the importance of such an approach and the potential role that stress reduction and management interventions can play in the treatment of CHD.

CONSIDERATIONS FOR INTERPRETING PSYCHOSOCIAL STUDIES

This review has highlighted the strong and consistent results of observational studies linking depression, anxiety, social networks and support, and work stress with cardiovascular health. In observational studies, two issues are critical to ensure identification of a likely causal link between an exposure and an outcome: (1) that the exposure is not the result of the disease process (health selection), and (2) that the observed association is not due to some other third covariate or sets of covariates confounding the association. In the studies reviewed, careful attention has been paid to both of these issues and the evidence found is compelling. Over the last decade, scientists have devoted enormous attention to sorting out these two issues. At this time, the observational evidence is consistent and strong that depression, anxiety, social isolation, and job stress influence CVD mortality and, in most cases, morbidity. It appears unlikely that these associations, derived from long-term longitudinal studies, are the result of poor health influencing the psychosocial condition (eg, depression, social isolation, job stress). In most of the studies, investigators controlled for baseline health status, prevalent CVD, and, increasingly, severity of illness, comorbidity, and physical functioning.

With respect to the issue of confounding by other covariates, most studies again have included known covariates related to other psychosocial conditions and relevant behaviors and biomedical risks in multivariable analyses. In fact, over the last two decades a very broad range of psychosocial conditions have been hypothesized to play a role in CVD. The majority of findings have either not been replicated, or the specific conditions under investigation have not been related to other constructs. The conditions presented in this chapter are those that, in a manner of speaking, have withstood the test of time. They have been replicated in a number of studies, most of which are prospective cohort studies, and all of which include a broad range of critical covariates.

So then, why are there such considerable differences between the results of the observational studies and those of the clinical trials? One interpretation is that even with the numerous methodologic controls, there is still some unobserved factor accounting for the relationships among depression, social isolation, job stress, and CHD. Although this possibility cannot be ruled out, we think there are several other important issues related to clinical intervention trials that are more likely to account for the discrepancies. The two most important relate to: (1) the timing of the intervention in relation to the course of disease development and accumulated exposure, and (2) the magnitude and appropriateness of the intervention. We believe these two issues may explain more of the discrepancy than the possibility of an unobserved, potentially causal covariate.

In previous work Burg and Berkman advanced a taxonomy of psychosocial interventions.[2] This taxonomy helps us address several of the points related to timing and effectiveness of interventions. The taxonomy cuts across four dimensions and is illustrated in Fig. 14-1.

In this taxonomy, the first axis is related to the definition of the psychosocial risk under investigation. One might think of such conditions along a continuum from clearly psychologic (eg, depression, hostility, vital exhaustion) through those that are psychosocial (eg, social support, work strain) to those that are more purely structural (eg, socioeconomic position, structure of network ties, social capital). The second axis is related to the level at which intervention occurs. Again, this ranges from interventions aimed at the individual, to those aimed at some collective or system (such as small groups, family, or worksite), to larger ones aimed at the community and society. The third axis relates to the point along the spectrum of disease at intervention occurs, for instance, at the level of secondary prevention, at the subclinical level of disease development, or at the level of primary prevention, before any evidence of disease is present. Finally, there is the question posed by Rose, of whether a high-risk strategy should be pursued, with intervention in cases at highest psychosocial risk, as opposed to pursuing a population-based strategy.[183]

Perhaps what is so remarkable about this review of interventions is that these interventions "line up" along the left side of each of these domains. Thus, even when investigators have chosen to intervene on a risk factor that

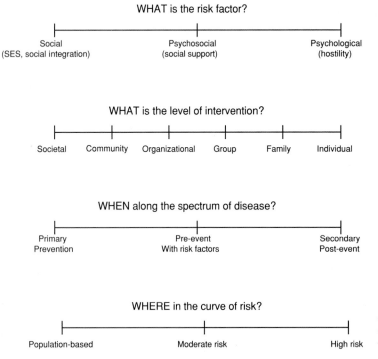

FIGURE 14-1 Taxonomy of psychosocial interventions. (Reproduced from Smith and Ruiz.[2])

is social in nature, they have chosen an individually oriented intervention approach or a high-risk intervention strategy. Research on interventions to reduce the risk of CHD associated generically with "stress" would benefit substantially from greater innovation. Such innovation could apply the taxonomy provided as a structure to rethink the nature of the standard approach and thereby expand the potential for risk reduction.

For instance, if work on interventions were extended based on the results of ENRICHD or the Montreal Heart Attack Readjustment Trial, it would be suspected that intervention occurred too late in the CVD process to be effective. Future interventions might be oriented toward people with cardiovascular risk factors who have not yet experienced an acute event or toward truly primary prevention efforts in the entire population (regulations regarding tobacco consumption are an example of such successful efforts). Before aiming interventions at critical periods of exposure, these periods must be identified. In addition, it is necessary to know the extent to which interventions reverse the effects of accumulated exposures (that may have occurred over decades). For interventions to be successful, more work on the relationship between psychosocial factors and mechanisms or biomarkers of disease processes is needed.

The second obvious issue relating to psychosocial interventions is whether the interventions themselves have been too weak to change the conditions significantly. This is especially important in light of the changes that are reported in the usual care group in many trials. In many behavioral randomized, controlled trials, the subjects in the usual care group change and improve in unanticipated ways, as a result of enrollment in the trial itself, result of communitywide patterns of care, or information that is disseminated during the trial. For example, many cardiologists started prescribing antidepressants during the ENRICHD intervention. Interventions that are too short, not intensive enough, or are lacking the capacity to deal with the complex psychologic and social experiences of subjects may not be able to change disease trajectories. Researchers and clinicians should be particularly skeptical of interventions that do not incorporate change in the sociostructural conditions that may obstruct opportunities for change or that do not provide sufficient resources to individuals to promote change. Thus, women who are widowed and socially isolated may need interventions that impact the structure of their social networks, in addition to skills training related to communication about social support. Men and women in socially disadvantaged positions may require access to resources that lead to opportunities to improve job conditions. In fact, interventions aimed at the social environment (work sites, schools, neighborhoods), rather than solely at individuals, may lead to substantial improvements in cardiovascular health.

CONCLUSION

There is extensive empirical evidence linking psychosocial factors with CVD risk factors, incidence, and mortality. Despite this mounting scientific literature, consideration of psychosocial influences in clinical practice and in the design of prevention efforts is largely forthcoming. Thus, the aim in this chapter was to provide the reader with: (1) the evidence linking psychosocial conditions with cardiovascular health, and (2) the results of several large-scale trials. It is hoped that the juxtaposition of these two sets of findings will provoke cardiologists and those in the fields of behavioral medicine and public health to think more deeply about the range of opportunities to reduce CVD morbidity and mortality.

REFERENCES

1. Harvey W. *On the Motion of the Heart and Blood in Animals.* Chicago: H. Regnery; 1962.

2. Smith TW, Ruiz JM. Psychosocial influences on the development and course of coronary heart disease: current status and implications for research and practice. *J Consult Clin Psychol* 2002;70:548.

3. Rozanski A, et al. Impact of psychological factors on the pathogenesis of cardiovascular disease and implications for therapy [comment]. *Circulation* 1999;99:2192.

4. Krantz DS, McCeney MK. Effects of psychological and social factors on organic disease: a critical assessment of research on coronary heart disease. *Annu Rev Psychol* 2002;53:341.

5. Burg M, Berkman LF. In: *Stress and the Heart: Psychosocial pathways to coronary heart disease.* London: BMS Books; 2002:278–293.

6. Berkman LF. Social integration, social networks, social support and health. In: Berkman LF, Kawachi I, eds. *Social Epidemiology.* Oxford/New York: Oxford University Press; 2000:xxii.

7. Marmot MG, et al. Inequalities in death: specific explanations of a general pattern? *Lancet* 1984;1:1003.

8. Marmot MG, et al. Social/economic status and disease. *Annu Rev Public Health* 1987;8:111.

9. Marmot MG, et al. Health inequalities among British civil servants: the Whitehall II study. *Lancet* 1997;337:1387.

10. Marmot MG, et al. Socioeconomic status and disease. *WHO Reg Publ Eur Ser* 1991;37:113.

11. Adler NE, et al. Socioeconomic status and health: the challenge of the gradient. *Am Psychol* 1994;49:15.

12. Syme SL, Berkman LF. Social class, susceptibility and sickness. *Am J Epidemiol* 1976;104:1.

13. Kaplan GA, Keil JE. Socioeconomic factors and cardiovascular disease: a review of the literature. *Circulation* 1993;88:1973.

14. US Department of Health and Human Services. *Mental Health: A Report of the Surgeon General, Executive Summary.* Rockville, Md: US Public Health Service; 1999.

15. Ziegelstein RC, et al. Patients with depression are less likely to follow recommendations to reduce cardiac risk during recovery from a myocardial infarction. *Arch Intern Med* 2000;160:1818.

16. Schleifer SJ, et al. The nature and course of depression following myocardial infarction. *Arch Intern Med* 1989;149:1785.

17. Penninx BW, et al. Depression and cardiac mortality: results from a community-based longitudinal study [comment]. *Arch Gen Psychiatry* 2001;58:221.

18. Hance M, et al. Depression in patients with coronary heart disease: a 12-month follow-up. *Gen Hosp Psychiatry* 1996;18:61.

19. Frasure-Smith N, et al. Depression and 18-month prognosis after myocardial infarction. *Circulation* 1995;91:999.

20. *Diagnostic and Statistical Manual of Mental Disorders.* Washington, DC: American Psychiatric Association; 1994.

21. Rugulies R. Depression as a predictor for coronary heart disease: a review and meta-analysis. *Am J Prev Med* 2002;23:51.

22. Frasure-Smith N, et al. Depression following myocardial infarction: impact on 6-month survival. *JAMA* 1993;270:1819.

23. Shiotani I, et al. Depressive symptoms predict 12-month prognosis in elderly patients with acute myocardial infarction. *J Cardiovasc Risk* 2002;9:153.

24. Unutzer J, et al. Depressive symptoms and mortality in a prospective study of 2,558 older adults. *Am J Geriatr Psychiatry* 2002;10:521.

25. Mehta KM, et al. Additive effects of cognitive function and depressive symptoms on mortality in elderly community-living adults. *J Gerontol Ser A* 2003;58:M461.

26. Brummett BH, et al. Effect of smoking and sedentary behavior on the association between depressive symptoms and mortality from coronary heart disease. *Am J Cardiol* 2003;92:529, 2003.

27. Furlanetto LM, et al. Association between depressive symptoms and mortality in medical inpatients. *Psychosomatics* 2000;41:426.

28. Stern SL, et al. Hopelessness predicts mortality in older Mexican and European Americans. *Psychosom Med* 2001;63:344.

29. Everson SA, et al. Hopelessness and risk of mortality and incidence of myocardial infarction and cancer. *Psychosom Med* 1996;58:113.

30. Everson SA, et al. Hopelessness and 4-year progression of carotid atherosclerosis: the Kuopio Ischemic Heart Disease Risk Factor Study. *Arterioscler Thromb Vasc Biol* 1997;17:1490.

31. Appels A. Mental precursors of myocardial infarction. *Br J Psychiatry* 1990;156:465.

32. Appels A, Mulder P. Fatigue and heart disease: the association between 'vital exhaustion' and past, present and future coronary heart disease. *J Psychosom Res* 1989;33:27.

33. Carney RM, et al. Major depression and medication adherence in elderly patients with coronary artery disease. *Health Psychol* 1995;14:88.

34. Covey LS, et al. Cigarette smoking and major depression. *J Addict Dis* 1998;17:5.

35. Malhotra S, et al. The relationship between depression and cardiovascular disorders. *Curr Psychiatry Rep* 2000;2:241.

36. Wielgosz AT, Nolan RP. Biobehavioral factors in the context of ischemic cardiovascular diseases. *J Psychosom Res* 2000;48:339.

37. Laghrissi-Thode F, et al. Elevated platelet factor 4 and beta-thromboglobulin plasma levels in depressed patients with ischemic heart disease. *Biol Psychiatry* 1997;42:290.

38. Musselman DL, et al. Exaggerated platelet reactivity in major depression. *Am J Psychiatry* 1996;153:1313.

39. Nemeroff CB, Musselman DL. Are platelets the link between depression and ischemic heart disease? *Am Heart J* 2000;140:57.

40. Joyce PR. Neuroendocrine changes in depression. *Aust NZ J Psychiatry* 1985;19:120.

41. Parker KJ, et al. Neuroendocrine aspects of hypercortisolism in major depression. *Horm Behav* 2003;43:60.

42. Miller AH. Neuroendocrine and immune system interactions in stress and depression. *Psychiatr Clin North Am* 1998;21:443.

43. Kiecolt-Glaser JK, et al. Emotions, morbidity, and mortality: new perspectives from psychoneuroimmunology. *Annu Rev Psychol* 2002;53:83.

44. Kiecolt-Glaser JK, Glaser R. Depression and immune function: central pathways to morbidity and mortality. *J Psychosom Res* 2002;53:873.

45. Beck AT. *Beck depression inventory.* Philadelphia: Center for Cognitive Therapy, 1961.

46. Beck AT, Steer RA, Brown GK. *BDI-II, Beck depression inventory: manual.* 2d ed. Boston: Harcourt Brace; 1996.

47. Hamilton M. Development of a rating scale for primary depressive illness. *Br J Soc Clin Psychol* 1967;6:278–296.

48. World Health Organization. (1993). *CIDI-Auto Version 1.1: Administrator's Guide and Reference.* Sydney: Training and Reference Centre for WHO CIDI.

49. Kessler RC, Andrews G, Mroczek D, et al. (1998). The World Health Organization Composite International Diagnostic Interview Short Form (CIDISF). *International Journal of Methods in Psychiatric Research* 1998;7:171–185.

50. First MB, Spitzer RL, Gibbon M, et al. Structured Clinical Interview for DSM-IV Axis I Disorders, Clinician Version (SCID-CV). Washington, D.C.: American Psychiatric Press, Inc., 1996.

51. Kessler RC, et al. Lifetime and 12-month prevalence of DSM-III-R psychiatric disorders in the United States: results from the National Comorbidity Study. *Arch Gen Psychiatry* 1994;51:8.

52. Kessler RC. The National Comorbidity Survey of the United States. *Int Rev Psychiatry* 1994;6:365.

53. Eaton WW, et al. Panic and panic disorder in the United States. *Am J Psychiatry* 1994;151:413.

54. Regier DA, et al. One-month prevalence of mental disorders in the United States and sociodemographic characteristics: the Epidemiologic Catchment Area study. *Acta Psychiatr Scand* 1993;88:35.

55. Weissman MM, et al. The cross-national epidemiology of panic disorder. *Arch Gen Psychiatry* 1997;54:305.

56. Kawachi I, et al. Symptoms of anxiety and risk of coronary heart disease: the Normative Aging Study. *Circulation* 1994;90:2225.

57. Kubzansky LD, et al. Is worrying bad for your heart? A prospective study of worry and coronary disease in the Normative Aging Study. *Circulation* 1997;95:818.

58. Kubzansky LD, et al. Anxiety and coronary heart disease: a synthesis of epidemiological, psychological, and experimental evidence. *Ann Behav Med* 1998;20:47.

59. Kawachi I, et al. Decreased heart rate variability in men with phobic anxiety (data from the Normative Aging Study). *Am J Cardiol* 1995;75:882.

60. Kawachi I, et al. Prospective study of phobic anxiety and risk of coronary heart disease in men. *Circulation* 1994;89:1992.

61. Denollet J, Brutsaert DL. Personality, disease severity, and the risk of long-term cardiac events in patients with a decreased ejection fraction after myocardial infarction. *Circulation* 1998;97:167.

62. Moser DK, Dracup K. Is anxiety early after myocardial infarction associated with subsequent ischemic and arrhythmic events? *Psychosom Med* 1996;58:395.

63. Williams DR, et al. Racial/ethnic discrimination and health: findings from community studies. *Am J Public Health* 2003;93:200.

64. Friedman M, Rosenman RH. Association of specific overt behavior pattern with blood and cardiovascular findings; blood cholesterol level, blood clotting time, incidence of arcus senilis, and clinical coronary artery disease. *JAMA* 1959;169:1286.

65. Rosenman RH, et al. Coronary heart disease in Western Collaborative Group Study: final follow-up experience of $8\frac{1}{2}$ years. *JAMA* 1975;233:872.

66. Review Panel on Coronary-Prone Behavior and Coronary Heart Disease. Coronary-prone behavior and coronary heart disease: a critical review. *Circulation* 1981;63:1199.

67. Shekelle RB, et al. The MRFIT behavior pattern study: II. Type A behavior and incidence of coronary heart disease. *Am J Epidemiol* 1985;122:559.

68. Ragland DR, Brand RJ Type A behavior and mortality from coronary heart disease. *N Engl J Med* 1988;318:65.

69. Case RB, et al. Type A behavior and survival after acute myocardial infarction. *N Engl J Med* 1985;312:737.

70. Smith TW. Concepts and methods in the study of anger, hostility, and health. In: Siegmam AW, Smith TW, eds. Anger, Hostility, and the Heart. Hillsdale, NJ: Lawrence Erlbaum Associates; 1994:23–42.

71. Siegler IC. Hostility and risk: demographic and lifestyle variables. In: Siegman AW, Smith TW, eds. *Anger, Hostility, and the Heart.* Hillsdale, NJ: Lawrence Erlbaum Associates; 1994.

72. Shekelle RB, et al. Hostility, risk of coronary heart disease, and mortality. *Psychosom Med* 1983;45:109.

73. Barefoot JC, et al. Hostility, CHD incidence, and total mortality: a 25-year follow-up study of 255 physicians. *Psychosom Med* 1983;45:59.

74. Niaura R, et al. Hostility, the metabolic syndrome, and incident coronary heart disease. *Health Psychol* 2002;21:588.

75. Hemingway H, Marmot M. Evidence based cardiology: psychosocial factors in the aetiology and prognosis of coronary heart disease. Systematic review of prospective cohort studies. *BMJ* 1999;318:1460.

76. Moller J, et al. Do episodes of anger trigger myocardial infarction? A case-crossover analysis in the Stockholm Heart Epidemiology Program (SHEEP). *Psychosom Med* 1999;61:842.

77. Gabbay FH, et al. Triggers of myocardial ischemia during daily life in patients with coronary artery disease: physical and mental activities, anger and smoking. *J Am Coll Cardiol* 1996;27:585.

78. Ironson G, et al. Effects of anger on left ventricular ejection fraction in coronary artery disease. *Am J Cardiol* 1992;70:281.

79. Miller TQ, et al. A meta-analytic review of research on hostility and physical health. *Psychol Bull* 1996;119:322.

80. Gump BB, et al. Modeling relationships among socioeconomic status, hostility, cardiovascular reactivity, and left ventricular mass in African American and white children. *Health Psychol* 1999;18:140.

81. Smith TW. Hostility and health: current status of a psychosomatic hypothesis. *Health Psychol* 1992;11:139.

82. Anderson D, et al. Social support, social networks and coronary artery disease rehabilitation: a review. *Can J Cardiol* 1996;12:739.

83. Berkman LF. The role of social relations in health promotion. *Psychosom Med* 1995;57:245.

84. Bowling A. Social support and social networks: their relationship to the successful and unsuccessful survival of elderly people in the community: an analysis of concepts and a review of the evidence. *Fam Pract* 1991;8:68.

85. Ell K. Social networks, social support and coping with serious illness: the family connection. *Social Sci Med* 1996;42:173.

86. Greenwood DC, et al. Coronary heart disease: a review of the role of psychosocial stress and social support. *J Public Health Med* 1996;18:221.

87. Helgeson VS, Cohen S. Social support and adjustment to cancer: reconciling descriptive, correlational, and intervention research. *Health Psychol* 1996;15:135.

88. Seeman TE. Social ties and health: the benefits of social integration. *Ann Epidemiol* 1996;6:442.

89. Eriksen W. The role of social support in the pathogenesis of coronary heart disease: a literature review. *Fam Pract* 1994;11:201.

90. Berkman LF, Syme SL. Social networks, host resistance and mortality: a nine year follow-up study of Alameda County residence. *Am J Epidemiol* 1979;109:186.

91. House JS, et al. The association of social relationships and activities with mortality: prospective evidence from the Tecumseh Community Health Study. *Am J Epidemiol* 1982;116:123.

92. Blazer DG. Social support and mortality in an elderly community population. *Am J Epidemiol* 1982;115:684.

93. Schoenbach VJ, et al. Social ties and mortality in Evans County, Georgia. *Am J Epidemiol* 1986;123:577.

94. Welin L, et al. Prospective study of social influences on mortality: the study of men born in 1913 and 1923. *Lancet* 1985;1:915.

95. Orth-Gomer K, Johnson J. Social network interaction and mortality: a six year follow-up of a random sample of the Swedish population. *J Chronic Dis* 1987;40:949.

96. Kaplan GA, et al. Social connections and mortality from all causes and from cardiovascular disease: prospective evidence from eastern Finland. *Am J Epidemiol* 1988;128:370.

97. Seeman TE, et al. Intercommunity variations in the association between social ties and mortality in the elderly: a comparative analysis of three communities. *Ann Epidemiol* 1993;3:325.

98. Seeman TE, Berkman LF. Structural characteristics of social networks and their relationship with social support in the elderly: who provides support? *Social Sci Med* 1988;26:737.

99. Vogt TM, et al. Social networks as predictors of ischemic heart disease, cancer, stroke and hypertension: incidence, survival and mortality. *J Clin Epidemiol* 1992;45:659.

100. Kawachi I, et al. A prospective study of social networks in relation to total mortality and cardiovascular disease in men in the USA. *J Epidemiol Community Health* 1996;50:245.

101. Eng PM, et al. Social ties and change in social ties in relation to subsequent total and cause-specific mortality and coronary heart disease incidence in men. *Am J Epidemiol* 2002;155:700.

102. Penninx BW, et al. Effects of social support and personal coping resources on mortality in older age: the Longitudinal Aging Study, Amsterdam. *Am J Epidemiol* 1997;146:510.

103. Sugisawa H, et al. Social support networks, social support and mortality among older people in Japan. *J Gerontol* 1994;49:S3.

104. Orth-Gomer K, et al. Lack of social support and incidence of coronary heart disease in middle-aged Swedish men. *Psychosom Med* 1993;55:37.

105. Ruberman W, et al. Psychosocial influences on mortality after myocardial infarction. *N Engl J Med* 1984;311:552.

106. Orth-Gomer K, et al. Social isolation and mortality in ischemic heart disease. *Acta Med Scand* 1988;224:205.

107. Williams LL, et al. Quantitative association between altered plasma esterified omega-6 fatty acid proportions and psychological stress. *Prostaglandins Leukotrienes Essential Fatty Acids* 1992;47:165.

108. Case RB, et al. Living alone after myocardial infarction. *JAMA* 1992;267.

109. Berkman LF, et al. Emotional support and survival following myocardial infarction: a prospective population-based study of the elderly. *Ann Intern Med* 1992;117:1003.

110. T. E. Oxman, et al. Lack of social participation or religious strength and comfort as risk factors for death after cardiac surgery in the elderly. *Psychosom Med* 57:5, 1995.

111. I. Farmer, et al. Higher levels of social support predict greater survival following acute myocardial infarction: The Corpus Christi Heart Project. *Behav Med* 22:59, 1996.

112. Krumholz HM, et al. The prognostic importance of emotional support for elderly patients hospitalized with heart failure. *Circulation* 1998;97:958.

113. Chen YT, et al. Risk factors for congestive heart failure in the elderly: a prospective community-based study. In review.

114. Berkman LF, Breslow L. *Health and Ways of Living: The Alameda County Study*. New York: Oxford University Press; 1983.

115. Morris PL, et al. Association of depression with 10-year post-stroke mortality. *Am J Psychiatry* 1993;150:124.

116. Siegrist J. Adverse health effects of high-effort/low-reward conditions. *J Occup Health Psychol* 1996;1:27.

117. Repetti RL. Short-term effects of occupational stressors on daily mood and health complaints. *Health Psychol* 1993;12:125.

118. Schwartz JE, et al. Work-related stress and blood pressure: current theoretical models and considerations from a behavioral medicine perspective. *J Occup Health Psychol* 1996;1:287.

119. Karasek RA. Job demands, job decision latitude, and mental strain: implications for job redesign. *Administrative Sci Q* 1979;24:285.

120. Karasek R, Theorell T. *Healthy Work: Stress, Productivity, and the Reconstruction of Working Life*. New York: Basic Books; 1990.

121. Haan MN. Job strain and ischaemic heart disease: an epidemiologic study of metal workers. *Ann Clin Res* 1988;20:143.

122. Johnson JV, et al. Combined effects of job strain and social isolation on cardiovascular disease morbidity and mortality in a random sample of the Swedish male working population. *Scand J Work Environ Health* 1989;15:271.

123. Theorell T, et al. The effects of the strain of returning to work on the risk of cardiac death after a first myocardial infarction before the age of 45. *Int J Cardiol* 1991;30:61.

124. Theorell T, Karasek RA. Current issues relating to psychosocial job strain and cardiovascular disease research. *J Occup Health Psychol* 1996;1:9.

125. Astrand NE, et al. Job demands, job decision latitude, job support, and social network factors as predictors of mortality in a Swedish pulp and paper company. *Br J Ind Med* 1989;46:334.

126. Falk A, et al. Job strain and mortality in elderly men: social network, support, and influence as buffers. *Am J Public Health* 1992;82:1136.

127. Reed DM, et al. Occupational strain and the incidence of coronary heart disease. *Am J Epidemiol* 1989;129:495.

128. Alterman T, et al. Decision latitude, psychologic demand, job strain, and coronary heart disease in the Western Electric Study. *Am J Epidemiol* 1994;139:620.

129. Karasek RA, et al. Job characteristics in relation to the prevalence of myocardial infarction in the US Health Examination Survey (HES) and the Health and Nutrition Examination Survey (HANES). *Am J Public Health* 1988;78:910.

130. Johnson JV, Hall EM. Job strain, work place social support, and cardiovascular disease: a cross-sectional study of a random sample of the Swedish working population. *Am J Public Health* 1988;78:1336.

131. Thomas J, et al. Cardiovascular disease in African American and white physicians: the Meharry Cohort and Meharry–Hopkins Cohort studies. *J Health Care Poor Underserved* 1997;8:270.

132. Greenlund KJ, et al. Psychosocial work characteristics and cardiovascular disease risk factors in young adults: the CARDIA study. Coronary Artery Risk Disease in Young Adults. *Social Sci Med* 1995;41:717.

133. Curtis AB, et al. Job strain and blood pressure in African Americans: the Pitt County Study. *Am J Public Health* 1997;87:1297.

134. Albright CL, et al. Job strain and prevalence of hypertension in a biracial population of urban bus drivers. *Am J Public Health* 1992;82:984.

135. Weidner G, et al. Relationship of job strain to standard coronary risk factors and psychological characteristics in women and men of the Family Heart Study. *Health Psychol* 1997;16:239.

136. Riese H, et al. Job strain and risk indicators for cardiovascular disease in young female nurses. *Health Psychol* 2000;19:429.

137. Laflamme N, et al. Job strain and ambulatory blood pressure among female white-collar workers. *Scand J Work Environ Health* 1998;24:334.

138. Brisson C, et al. Effect of family responsibilities and job strain on ambulatory blood pressure among white-collar women. *Psychosom Med* 1999;61:205.

139. Bosma H, et al. Two alternative job stress models and the risk of coronary heart disease. *Am J Public Health* 1998;88:68.

140. Kuper H, et al. When reciprocity fails: effort–reward imbalance in relation to coronary heart disease and health functioning within the Whitehall II study. *Occup Environ Med* 2002;59:777.

141. Peter R, et al. High effort, low reward, and cardiovascular risk factors in employed Swedish men and women: baseline results from the WOLF Study. *J Epidemiol Community Health* 1998;52:540.

142. Siegrist J, et al. Chronic work stress is associated with atherogenic lipids and elevated fibrinogen in middle-aged men. *J Intern Med* 1997;242:149.

143. Appels A, et al. "Chronic workload," "need for control," and "vital exhaustion" in patients with myocardial infarction and controls: a comparative test of cardiovascular risk profiles. *Stress Med* 1997;13:117.

144. Siegrist J, et al. Low status control, high effort at work and ischemic heart disease: prospective evidence from blue-collar men. *Social Sci Med* 1990;31:1127.

145. Clark R, et al. Racism as a stressor for African Americans: a biopsychosocial model. *Am Psychol* 1999;54:805.

146. Nazroo JY. The structuring of ethnic inequalities in health: economic position, racial discrimination, and racism. *Am J Public Health* 2003;93:277.

147. Krieger N. Does racism harm health? Did child abuse exist before 1962? On explicit questions, critical science, and current controversies: an ecosocial perspective. *Am J Public Health* 2003;93:194.

148. Meyer IH. Prejudice as stress: conceptual and measurement problems. *Am J Public Health* 2003;93:262.

149. Acevedo-Garcia D, et al. Future directions in residential segregation and health research: a multilevel approach. *Am J Public Health* 2003;93:215.

150. Acevedo-Garcia D. Residential segregation and the epidemiology of infectious diseases. *Social Sci Med* 2000;51:1143.

151. Schulman KA, et al. The effect of race and sex on physicians' recommendations for cardiac catheterization. *N Engl J Med* 1999;340:618.

152. Jones C. The impact of racism on health. *Ethnicity Dis* 2002;12:S2.

153. Landrine H, Klonoff EA. Racial discrimination and cigarette smoking among blacks: findings from two studies. *Ethnicity Dis* 2000;10:195.

154. Kennedy BP, et al. (Dis)respect and black mortality. *Ethnicity Dis* 1997;7:207.

155. Klonoff EA, Landrine H. Is skin color a marker for racial discrimination? Explaining the skin color–hypertension relationship. *J Behav Med* 2000;23:329.

156. Harrell JP, et al. Physiological responses to racism and discrimination: an assessment of the evidence. *Am J Public Health* 2003;93:243.

157. Williams RB. Lower socioeconomic status and increased mortality: early childhood roots and the potential for successful interventions. *JAMA* 1998;279:1745.

158. Williams RB, et al. Psychosocial risk factors for cardiovascular disease: more than one culprit at work. *JAMA* 2003;290:2190.

159. Lynch JW, et al. Why do poor people behave poorly? Variation in adult health behaviours and psychosocial characteristics by stages of the socioeconomic lifecourse. *Social Sci Med* 1997;44:809.

160. Friedman M, et al. Feasibility of altering type A behavior pattern after myocardial infarction: Recurrent Coronary Prevention Project Study: methods, baseline results and preliminary findings. *Circulation* 1982;66:83.

161. Friedman M, Rosenman RH. *Type A Behavior and Your Heart.* New York: Knopf; 1974.

162. Friedman M, et al. Alteration of type A behavior and reduction in cardiac recurrences in postmyocardial infarction patients: summary results of the Recurrent Coronary Prevention Project. *Am Heart J* 1986;112:653.

163. Friedman M, et al. Alteration of type A behavior and reduction in cardiac recurrences in postmyocardial infarction patients. *Am Heart J* 1984;108:237.

164. Friedman M, et al. Effect of discontinuance of type A behavioral counseling on type A behavior and cardiac recurrence rate in post myocardial infarction patients. *Am Heart J* 1987;114:483.

165. Williams RB, et al. Prognostic importance of social and economic resources among medically treated patients with angiographically documented coronary artery disease. *JAMA* 1992;267:520.

166. Gorkin L, et al. Psychosocial predictors of mortality in the Cardiac Arrhythmia Suppression Trial-1 (CAST-1). *Am J Cardiol* 1993;71:263.

167. ENRICHD Investigators. Enhancing recovery in coronary heart disease patients (ENRICHD): study design and methods. *Am Heart J* 2000;139:1.

168. Carney RM, et al. Psychiatric depression, anxiety, and coronary heart disease: implications for treatment. *Compr Ther* 1989;15:8.

169. Cossette S, et al. Impact of improving psychological distress in post-MI patients [abstract]. *Psychosom Med* 1999;61:93.

170. Beck JS. *Cognitive Therapy: Basics and Beyond.* New York: Guildford; 1995.

171. Bandura *A Social Foundations of Thought and Action: A Social Cognitive Theory.* Englewood Cliffs, NJ: Prentice–Hall;1986.

172. Tobin DL, et al. Self-management and social learning theory. In: Holroyd KA, Creer TL, eds. *Self-Management of Chronic Disease: Handbook of Clinical Interventions and Research.* Orlando, FL: Academic Press; 1986.

173. Berkman LF, et al. Effects of treating depression and low perceived social support on clinical events after myocardial infarction: the Enhancing Recovery in Coronary Heart Disease Patients (ENRICHD) Randomized Trial. *JAMA* 2003;289:3106.

174. Fraser-Smith N, Prince R. The Ischemic Heart Disease Life Stress Monitoring Program: impact on mortality. *Psychosom Med* 1985;47:431.

175. N. Fraser-Smith, et al. Randomized trial of home-based psychosocial nursing intervention for patients recovering from myocardial infarction. *Lancet* 350: 473, 1997.

176. Fraser-Smith N, Prince R. Long-term follow-up of the Ischemic Heart Disease Life Stress Monitoring Program. *Psychosom Med* 1989;51:485.

177. Jones DA, West RR. Psychological rehabilitation after myocardial infarction: multicentre randomized controlled trial. *BMJ* 1996;313:1517.

178. Rocco MB, et al. Prognostic importance of myocardial ischemia detected by ambulatory monitoring in patients with stable coronary artery disease. *Circulation* 1988;78:877.

179. Trauner MA, et al. Prognostic significance of silent myocardial ischemia. *Ann Behav Med* 1994;16:24.

180. Gullette ECD, et al. Mental stress triggers myocardial ischemia during daily life. *JAMA* 1997;277:1521.

181. Blumenthal JA, et al. Mental stress-induced ischemia in the laboratory and ambulatory ischemia during daily life: association and hemodynamic features. *Circulation* 1995;92:2102.

182. Blumenthal JA, et al. Stress management and exercise training in cardiac patients with myocardial ischemia: effects on prognosis and evaluation of mechanisms. *Arch Intern Med* 1997;157:2213.

183. Rose G. *The Strategy of Preventive Medicine.* Oxford: Oxford University Press; 1992.

184. Radloff, L. The CES-D scale: a self-report depression scale for research in the general population. *Applied Psychological Measurement* 1977;1:385–401.

APPENDIX 14-1 CENTER FOR EPIDEMIOLOGIC STUDIES DEPRESSION SCALE (CES-D)[184]

The next set of questions is related on how you *felt or behaved* in the PAST WEEK. Using the scale below, please choose the number which best describes how often you felt or behaved this way DURING THE PAST WEEK.

1 = rarely or none of the time   2 = some or a little of the time

3 = a moderate amount of the time   4 = most or all of the time

 1. You were bothered by things that usually don't bother you.
 2. You did not feel like eating; your appetite was poor.
 3. You felt that you could not shake off the blues even with help from your family and friends.
 4. You felt that you were just as good as other people.
 5. You had trouble keeping your mind on what you were doing.
 6. You felt depressed.
 7. You felt that everything you did was an effort.
 8. You felt hopeful about the future.
 9. You thought your life had been a failure.
10. You felt fearful.
11. Your sleep was restless.
12. You were happy.
13. You talked less than usual.
14. You felt lonely.
15. People were unfriendly.
16. You enjoyed life.
17. You had crying spells.
18. You felt sad.
19. You felt that people disliked you.
20. You could not get "going."

PART IV

Special Populations

Children and adolescents

Dennis M. Davidson

KEY POINTS

- *Genetic and environmental factors may lead to development of atherosclerosis during childhood and to its progression to coronary artery disease during adolescence and young adulthood.*

- *Indicators of risk for early development of atherosclerosis and coronary artery disease include cigarette smoking, dyslipidemia, high blood pressure, physical inactivity, obesity, and diabetes mellitus.*

- *Primary coronary artery disease prevention efforts for all youth should have high priority at home, in the medical office, and at school.*

- *Proper nutrition and vigorous exercise are indicated for those youth identified as being at high risk for coronary artery disease. Those who continue to smoke should be helped to quit.*

- *If hygienic efforts to lower coronary artery disease risk in youth are inadequate, pharmacologic approaches may be considered.*

INTRODUCTION

Among the most important goals of preventive cardiology are to identify and then develop interventions to lower those indicators of coronary artery disease (CAD) risk during childhood and adolescence that are predictive of subsequent development of CAD in adult life. The purposes of this chapter are to: (1) assess the prevalence of different CAD risk factors as reported in cross-sectional studies of children of different ages and ethnicity;

(2) examine longitudinal studies ("tracking") of CAD risk factors in children, including autopsy studies of those who were study participants earlier in their lives; (3) outline current prevention recommendations for optimizing the cardiovascular health of all children; (4) survey recommendations for screening children for high levels of CAD risk factors; and (5) present recommendations for hygienic and pharmacologic treatment of children found to be at high risk for CAD events later in life.

DEVELOPMENT OF ATHEROSCLEROSIS IN YOUTH

In the past five decades, considerable evidence has accumulated to support the contention that atherosclerosis may begin early in life and can progress to an advanced stage by young adulthood. Deposits of cholesterol and cholesterol esters in large arteries are termed *fatty streaks* and are considered to be the earliest precursors of CAD. At certain sites, further lipid accumulation is followed by formation of a fibrous plaque. If plaques rupture, thrombosis may follow, leading to arterial occlusion.[1]

Korean War autopsy studies revealed significant evidence of coronary artery disease (CAD) in 77% of US soldiers, who, on average, were 22 years old.[2] These results were confirmed later in American military men dying in Vietnam.[3] Postmortem examination of American and Finnish schoolchildren revealed fatty streaks and intimal thickening in youth.[4,5] In a large analysis of 4737 subjects aged 10 to 39, coronary fatty streaks were found to develop beginning in the age group 10 to 14; they were present in all those older than 20 in New Orleans and by age 30 in most persons from other populations.[6] Subsequent studies found evidence that such lesions progressed to fibrous plaques.[7,8]

The multicenter Pathobiological Determinants of Atherosclerosis in Youth (PDAY) study evaluated coronary arteries, aortas, and blood and other specimens from approximately 3000 individuals 15 to 34 years old who died of external causes. Investigators correlated the extent of atherosclerosis in the right and left anterior descending coronary arteries with serum lipid concentrations, glycohemoglobin level, history of smoking, and indices of adiposity.[9] Each of these factors was independently associated with the extent of atherosclerosis noted.[10]

It has become clear that both genetic and environmental factors are implicated in the pathogenesis of atherosclerosis and subsequent coronary artery events, such as myocardial infarction and sudden cardiac death.

CAD RISK INDICATORS IN YOUTH

In adults, CAD has been clearly associated with modifiable factors such as cigarette smoking, dyslipidemias (high levels of low-density lipoprotein cholesterol [LDL-C] and low levels of high-density lipoprotein cholesterol [HDL-C]), high blood pressure, physical inactivity, obesity, and diabetes, as well as those factors that are not amenable to change, such as age and a premature family history of CAD.[11]

More recently, investigators have looked for evidence that elevated levels of risk factors in children are closely correlated with high levels of the same indicators in adults who develop CAD. They have systematically examined such indicators of CAD risk as smoking, dyslipidemias,

TABLE 15-1 Coronary Artery Disease Risk Indicators in Children

Genetic

Sociodemographic
  Ethnocultural
  Socioeconomic

Daily environment
  Family
  Friends
  School

Smoking
Physical inactivity

Suboptimal nutrition
  Quality
  Quantity

Obesity

Dyslipidemia
  High LDL cholesterol
  Low HDL cholesterol

High blood pressure
Diabetes/glucose intolerance

high blood pressure, physical inactivity, obesity, and glucose intolerance in children (Table 15-1). The majority of investigations have been cross-sectional in design, measuring levels of these risk factors in groups of children at one point in time, yielding prevalence rates. Others have been longitudinal in design; some of these studies have followed their subjects into adulthood.[12,13] The investigations have examined the reliability and reproducibility of risk factor measurements as well as their consistency in indicating high risk (to "track") over time.

Investigators have also examined several sociobehavioral determinants that may underlie or modify these physiologic factors. Figure 15-1 is a schematic representation of the integration of these parameters.

In the 1970s and 1980s, studies in North America documented the prevalence of CAD risk factors in children of diverse racial and ethnic backgrounds. Investigators in Bogalusa, Louisiana,[14] studied African-American and Caucasian children, and the National Health and Nutrition Examination Survey (NHANES) surveyed children of all major ethnicities 9 to 11 years of age nationwide.[15–17] Several other studies have focused on Latino, Native American, and Alaskan children in the United States[18,19] and indigenous First Nation children in Canada.[20] Studies in Finland have also added to the knowledge base of children's cardiovascular risk factors at different ages.[21]

A review of cross-sectional and longitudinal studies to date follows. Despite our increased knowledge, it is now

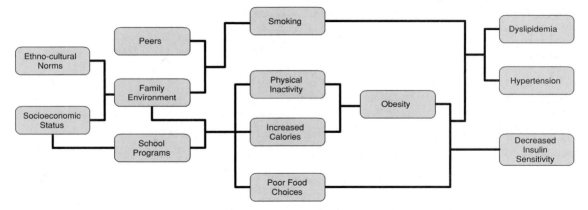

FIGURE 15-1   Contributors to coronary artery disease risk in children.

clear that most of the indicators of CAD risk in children and adolescents have worsened in the past 25 years.[22]

Sociodemographic factors

Winkleby and colleagues analyzed data from 7686 children and young adults that were collected during NHANES-III. They examined risk factor levels categorized by ethnicity (African-American, Caucasian, Mexican-American) and by family socioeconomic status (SES) as represented by years of education of the head of household. Among study participants aged 18 to 24 whose head of household had less than 12 years of education, Caucasians had much higher smoking rates (77% for men, 61% for women) than African-American and Mexican-American youth (35%) with similar SES levels. The rates for low-SES Caucasians were twice as high as those for Caucasians from higher-SES groups and were nearly double the smoking rates for low-SES African-Americans and Mexican-Americans.[17]

Children from underserved populations, those from economically and educationally disadvantaged families, and those who live with little social support are found consistently to have higher levels of CAD risk factors. These observations have been made in North America,[23] Finland,[24] and the United Kingdom.[25]

Family history

Bao and colleagues collected parental history of cardiovascular conditions from 8276 offspring. Children of parents who had experienced myocardial infarction or who were diabetic had significantly higher levels of total cholesterol, LDL-C, insulin, glucose, and body weight, as compared with those without a parental history. Children of hypertensive parents had significantly higher levels of blood pressure than their peers without such a family

history. However, the authors concluded that, because of the young age of parents, parental history information alone is not adequate to identify children needing lipid screening.[26]

In the Coronary Artery Risk Development in Young Adults (CARDIA) study of African-American and Caucasian women and men aged 18 to 30 at baseline, parental risk indicators were consistently associated with increased CAD risk in their offspring. These included hypertension, glucose intolerance, obesity, and hyperlipidemia. Subjects with a parental history of myocardial infarction had higher levels of total cholesterol and blood pressure and lower levels of HDL-C.[27]

Smoking

Several laboratory methods exist to document cigarette smoking, including thiocyanate levels (from serum or saliva), serum cotinine, and breath analysis for carbon monoxide. For large-scale studies, however, self-report is more often used.[28]

More than 1 million adolescents in the United States are daily smokers of cigarettes; two thirds of all persons adopting the smoking habit are under age 18 (most commonly at age 14–15).[29] These and other data are contained in periodic reports from the US Surgeon General.[30] In 2001, the percentage of high school students who had used any tobacco product in the past month ranged from 17% in African-American girls to 43% in non-Hispanic boys.[31] Between 1980 and 2001, the percentage of high school seniors smoking tobacco decreased, notably in African-Americans.[32]

In Bogalusa, Louisiana, African-American children who were smokers appeared to be more influenced by siblings and peers, whereas Caucasian children who adopted smoking were more likely to follow parents' smoking habits.[33] Nearly half of all children were given their first cigarette by family members or smoked it at home.[34]

Children with academic difficulties are more likely to begin smoking than others in their age group.[35] In another study, sixth-graders with "problem behaving" peers were found to be at high risk for smoking onset, but only when parents were "relatively uninvolved" in their children's lives.[36]

It has been estimated that 15 million children under age 18 are routinely exposed to tobacco smoke in their homes in the United States.[37] Studies in the state of Washington found that, when neither parent has ever smoked, the odds that their children will begin smoking are 71% less than in families in which both parents smoke. If both parents have quit, the odds of daily smoking by children are 39% less.[38]

In Muscatine, Iowa, adolescent cigarette smoking was strongly correlated with friends' smoking habits.[39] A Copenhagen, Denmark, study revealed that maternal smoking doubled the likelihood that a child would become a smoker.[40]

In addition to its effect on lung function, smoking has been correlated with atherosclerosis in autopsy studies of adolescents.[41,42] In the PDAY study, serum thiocyanate, which indicates tobacco usage, was also associated with the prevalence of raised atherosclerotic lesions, especially in the abdominal aorta.[43]

Physical inactivity

No direct measures of physical activity are suitable for large-scale studies, and indirect methods are often inconvenient or inaccurate in children. Nevertheless, the best estimates of participation by children in aerobic activity show a dramatic downward trend in recent years.[44] In 2001, although 52% of high school students in the United States were enrolled in a physical education class, only 32% attended regularly.[31]

As with other health behaviors, children are influenced largely by parents and peers in their decisions about habitual physical activity.[45] NHANES-III data indicate that girls and boys who watch more than 4 hours of television daily have greater percentage body fat and greater body mass index.[17] Obarzanek and colleagues reported similar findings after analyzing National Heart, Lung, and Blood Institute (NHLBI) National Growth and Health Study data for physical activity and body fat in African-American and Caucasian girls.[46]

Inactivity also adversely influences lipid levels; in one study, hours watching television were directly correlated with the likelihood the child had a total cholesterol of 200 mg/dL or greater.[47]

Nutrition

Nutritional intake can be measured by such methods as direct observation and measurement of cafeteria leftovers, but food diaries and a 24-hour recall using food models are more adaptable to epidemiologic studies.[48]

Two decades ago, Bogalusa and NHANES data indicated that children in the United States derived 36 to 39% of their calories from fat, with approximately 16% of calories coming from saturated fat (goals for these two indicators are 30 and 10%, respectively). Snacks contributed approximately one fourth of all caloric intake, with a percentage of fat similar to that of the children's regular meals.[49]

Data from the US Department of Agriculture (USDA) Continuing Survey program suggest that children's diets have improved in recent years, but approximately 70% of children still exceed current guidelines for both total and saturated fat intake.[50] USDA investigators reported that only 1% of the US population met recommendations for all food groups in feeding their children, but even that group exceeded fat intake guidelines.[13] In the NHLBI/NHGS, intake of total and saturated fat decreased in girls in the decade following study entry (when girls were 9 or 10). Decreases were greater in Caucasian girls than in their African-American counterparts.[51]

Obesity

Obesity is most conveniently measured using body mass index (BMI), which is calculated as weight in kilograms divided by height in square meters (kg/m^2). BMI is reasonably correlated with body fat estimates from skinfold measurements and underwater weighing, methods more commonly used in small research studies.[52] Obesity and overweight have also been defined by BMI percentile rank (eg, 95th percentile) for each gender.

International scientific groups generally agree that calculation of BMI offers a reasonable index of adiposity in populations of children and adolescents without a significant prevalence of stunted growth. However, BMI should be used more carefully in developing countries and in certain ethnic groups in North American populations.[53] Despite these caveats, body weight and height remain parameters that are easily and reliably assessed and should be measured at most clinical encounters. BMI of 25 kg/m^2 or greater generally defines overweight, with BMI of 30 kg/m^2 or greater indicating obesity. Additionally, waist circumference can also be measured for assessment of abdominal obesity.

In the United States, the prevalence of obesity among boys and girls of all age groups has continued to increase in the past three decades, increasing by 50% in children aged 6 to 11 and nearly doubling in adolescents aged 12 to 19.[54] Findings have been documented in

TABLE 15-2   Trends in Mean Serum Total Cholesterol Levels among US Adolescents 12 to 17 Years of Age by Sex and Race: 1966–1970, 1971–1974, and 1988–1994

Population	NHES-III* (1966–1970)			NHANES-I (1971–1974)			NHANES-III (1988–1994)		
	N	Mean	(SEM)	N	Mean	(SEM)	N	Mean	(SEM)
Male									
African-American	471	171	(1.8)	250	165	(2.5)	389	166	(1.5)
Caucasian	3024	163	(0.7)	806	163	(1.4)	622	155	(1.6)
Total	3514	165	(0.8)	1064	164	(1.3)	1055	157	(1.3)
Female									
African-American	513	172	(1.6)	259	174	(3.5)	456	168	(1.4)
Caucasian	2668	170	(0.9)	796	166	(1.4)	714	163	(1.5)
Total	3196	170	(0.8)	1062	167	(1.3)	1222	164	(1.3)
Total[†]	6710	167	(0.7)	2126	165	(1.0)	2277	160	(1.1)

*NHES, National Health Examination Survey III; NHANES, National Health and Nutrition Examination Survey.
[†]Includes other race groups in addition to Caucasian and African-American.
SOURCE: Centers for Disease Control and Prevention.[66]

large-scale studies, such as the NHLBI National Growth and Health Study[46] and NHANES.[55] In smaller studies, obesity rates in girls were noted to have increased more dramatically than in boys in the past four decades.[56] These findings hold true for various ethnic groups studied in the United States, including African-Americans in Louisiana,[57] Native Americans,[58] and Latinos.[59] Similar findings have been reported in the United Kingdom and Europe.[55] Obesity is often associated with a cluster of other CAD risk factors, including hypertension and dyslipidemias.[45,60]

Lipids

In most of the studies reported herein, Lipid Research Clinic techniques have been used to measure total blood cholesterol (TC), HDL-C, and triglycerides. If serum triglycerides (TG) are <400 mg/dL, LDL-C can be calculated as LDL-C = TC – HDL-C - (TG/5).[61,62] In general, levels of TC and its subfractions are similar in boys and girls until puberty, after which HDL-C decreases significantly in boys.

Differences between children of different ethnic groups within the United States have been studied. In a multiethnic community in Southern California, children of Vietnamese-American, European-American, and Latino origins had similar mean TC concentrations, ranging from 165 to 172 mg/dL.[63] Levels of TC and LDL-C in Navajo children were similar to those of children in the general US population, but their HDL-C was 5 to 10 mg/dL lower and their triglyceride levels were 30 mg/dL higher.[18] In the multicenter (Louisiana, Texas, Minnesota, and California) Child and Adolescent Trial for Cardiovascular Health, TC levels were similar

among Caucasian, African-American, and Hispanic children, but HDL-C levels were higher in African-American boys and girls than in children in the other two ethnic categories.[64] Total and saturated fat levels from food records obtained in the third grade were predictive of serum TC 2 years later.[65]

Table 15-2 summarizes trends in TC levels among adolescents aged 12 to 17 years screened between 1966 and 1994 in three major population-based studies. During this period, there was a general decrease in mean TC levels, from 165 to 157 mg/dL among boys and from 170 to 164 mg/dL among girls. The decline appears to have been greater among Caucasian youth than among African-Americans of similar ages.[66]

Data from NHANES-III (Table 15-3) show that approximately one quarter of children still have borderline-high (170–199 mg/dL) TC, with another 10% being in the elevated (≥200 mg/dL) category. Non-Hispanic African-American children have the highest cholesterol levels, with mean TC levels of 168 mg/dL in boys and 171 mg/dL in girls, compared with non-Hispanic Caucasians, for whom the respective values are 162 mg/dL in boys and 166 mg/dL in girls.[66]

In the PDAY autopsy study of persons aged 15 to 34 dying of external causes, atherosclerotic intimal surface involvement in both the aorta and right coronary arteries was positively correlated with LDL-C and very low density lipoprotein cholesterol (VLDL-C) concentrations and negatively associated with HDL-C levels.[43]

Others investigators have shown coronary artery calcium deposition (as documented by electron beam computed tomography [EBCT]) to be correlated with the severity of atherosclerosis in adults. In a study of 29 youths aged 11 to 23 years with familial

TABLE 15-3 Serum Total Cholesterol Levels among US Children and Adolescents 4 to 19 Years of Age, by Age, Sex, and Race/Ethnicity: NHANES-III, 1988–1994

| Population | N | Mean | (SEM) | Percentile | | | | | | |
				5th	10th	25th	50th	75th	90th	95th
Age[a]										
4–5	1707	162	(0.9)	124	132	144	161	177	194	204
6–8	1367	166	(1.0)	126	134	149	165	182	197	209
9–11	1488	171	(1.0)	131	139	151	168	187	206	222
12–15	1502	161	(1.2)	118	126	141	158	178	197	209
16–19	1435	165	(1.6)	118	124	141	158	182	207	222
12–19	2937	163	(1.0)	118	125	141	158	180	201	217
Total	7499	165	(0.6)	121	130	145	162	181	200	216
Sex and age[a]										
Male										
4–5		161	(1.5)	122	132	143	159	175	191	202
6–8		166	(1.7)	126	134	146	164	183	202	212
9–11		172	(2.0)	135	140	153	170	188	208	226
12–15		158	(1.6)	116	124	140	157	174	192	203
16–19		158	(1.8)	116	122	138	155	174	199	213
12–19		158	(1.2)	116	123	139	156	174	195	206
Total (4–19)		163	(1.0)	119	127	143	161	179	198	212
Female										
4–5		164	(1.3)	125	133	145	162	178	196	206
6–8		166	(1.4)	126	135	149	165	180	196	203
9–11		169	(1.5)	130	137	148	166	185	204	218
12–15		164	(1.9)	122	129	142	159	181	201	218
16–19		171	(2.3)	118	128	145	163	189	217	237
12–19		167	(1.3)	119	128	144	161	185	209	225
Total (4–19)		167	(0.8)	124	132	147	163	184	202	220
Race/ethnicity and sex										
Non-Hispanic African-American										
Male		168	(1.0)	122	132	148	165	186	204	219
Female		171	(1.2)	122	134	149	167	189	213	226
Non-Hispanic Caucasian										
Male		162	(1.2)	118	126	143	160	178	195	207
Female		166	(1.1)	123	132	146	163	182	200	217
Mexican-American										
Male		163	(1.0)	121	129	143	159	180	202	213
Female		165	(1.1)	121	128	144	161	183	201	226

[a]Includes other race/ethnicity groups in addition to non-Hispanic Caucasian, non-Hispanic African-American, and Mexican.

SOURCE: Reproduced, with permission, from Winkleby et al.[17]

hypercholesterolemia (mean LDL-C = 229 mg/dL), 7 had coronary calcium detected by EBCT.[67] Muscatine Study investigators found that coronary risk indicators measured during childhood and adolescence correlated with coronary artery calcification in early adulthood.[68]

In 1973, the Bogalusa Heart Study began following cohorts of African-American and Caucasian children from birth through 17 years of age, noting changes in risk factors as subjects progressed through childhood and adolescence.[14] In several of the cohorts, observations have extended into young adulthood. After 15 years of

surveillance, it was noted that subjects with LDL-C greater than 130 mg/dL at baseline were five times more likely to be hyperlipidemic, and had double the risk of having hypertension, having a low HDL-C level, and being overweight.[69] As part of its longitudinal design, investigators in the Bogalusa Heart Study reviewed autopsy results in participants who died at 7 to 24 years of age. Analyses showed that coronary artery fatty streaks, as well as aortic and coronary fibrous plaques were directly associated with levels of LDL-C measured previously.[70] Investigators also used sonography to document intimal media thickening in carotid arteries of subjects; the degree of thickening correlated with lipids and other risk factors.[71]

The Cardiovascular Risk in Young Finns (CRYF) study was begun in 1980 with a cross-sectional survey of subjects 3, 6, 9, 12, 15, and 18 years of age. Subsequent examinations of these children and adolescents occurred 3 and 6 years thereafter, resulting in a total of 2236 subjects with complete follow-up data on serum lipids. The investigators found reasonably good tracking for TC, HDL-C, and LDL-C values, particularly in boys. They noted that, when subjects were divided into quintiles, those at highest risk (high TC and LDL-C, low HDL-C) at baseline tended to become obese and to smoke cigarettes more frequently than others.[21] A longitudinal study of Finnish children confirmed the tracking of TC levels in children who were followed from 6 months to 15 years of age. Compared with all other children, those in the highest third of TC levels during infancy were six times as likely to be in the highest third of TC measurements as adolescents.[72]

Obesity is associated with lower HDL-C levels and higher serum triglyceride concentrations. In a study of 880 Japanese school children, waist-to-height ratio was the most significant predictor of both HDL-C and triglycerides.[73] Bogalusa study investigators have also noted these associations in their studies of children in Louisiana.[74]

Blood pressure

Measurement of blood pressure in children should be a routine part of the office visit. However, it is subject to several potential sources of error. These include equipment differences, use of different endpoints for measuring systolic blood pressure (SBP) and diastolic blood pressure (DBP), patterns of bias by individual observers, variability among multiple determinations, and physiologic variability. The Working Group on Hypertension Control in Children and Adolescents examined several national data sets to develop normative blood pressure tables and reported measurement standards, including preparation and positioning of the child, cuff size, and inflation and deflation rates.[75]

Blood pressure should be measured in a quiet environment after 3 to 5 minutes in a seated position. The National High Blood Pressure Education Program Working Group has recommended the use of phase V Korotkoff sounds for DBP measurement for children of all ages. The blood pressure should be recorded at least twice on each occasion, using a cuff whose width is approximately 40% of the arm circumference midway between the olecranon and the acromion. Readings are averaged and then compared with tables by age, gender, and height percentile.[75] Table 15-4 lists 95th percentile levels for blood pressure in children and adolescents by age and percentile for height. If the average SBP or DBP is at or above the 95th percentile, measurements to confirm hypertension should be repeated on subsequent visits.[76] A child with average readings below the 95th percentile but at or greater than the 90th percentile is classified as "high normal."[75]

In biracial studies of children in the United States, African-Americans generally have higher mean blood pressures than Caucasians of the same age. These differences persist over time, but after adjustment for body size, the difference is noted to be substantially less.[27]

TABLE 15-4 95th Percentiles of Blood Pressure (Systolic/Diastolic) for Girls and Boys of Selected Ages as Classified by the 5th, 25th, 50th, 75th, and 95th Height Percentiles for Each Gender

	Girls' SBP/DBP* by height percentile					Boys' SBP/DBP by height percentile				
Age	5th	25th	50th	75th	95th	5th	25th	50th	75th	95th
1	101/57	103/62	104/58	105/59	107/60	98/55	101/56	102/57	104/58	106/59
3	104/65	105/69	107/66	108/67	110/68	104/63	107/64	109/65	111/66	113/67
5	107/69	108/73	110/71	111/72	113/73	108/69	110/70	112/71	114/72	116/74
7	110/73	112/75	113/74	114/75	116/76	110/74	113/75	115/76	116/77	119/78
9	114/75	115/76	117/77	118/78	120/79	113/76	116/78	117/79	119/80	121/81
11	118/78	119/79	121/79	122/80	124/81	116/78	119/79	121/80	123/81	125/83
13	121/80	123/81	125/82	126/82	128/84	121/79	124/81	126/82	128/83	130/84
15	124/82	126/83	128/83	129/84	131/86	127/81	129/83	131/83	133/84	135/86
17	126/83	128/83	129/84	130/85	132/86	132/85	135/86	136/87	138/88	140/89

*SBP, systolic blood pressure; DBP, diastolic blood pressure.

SOURCE: Adapted, with permission, from the National High Blood Pressure Education Program Working Group on Hypertension Control in Children and Adolescents.[75]

In studies of children in California[77] and Chicago,[78] SBP and DBP were higher among Asian children than African-Americans, Latinos, and Caucasians. In children of all ethnic groups, a strong correlation exists between obesity and blood pressure.

The CARDIA study comprised 5115 African-American and Caucasian men and women aged 18 to 30 undergoing baseline examination in 1985–1986 at four centers, with follow-up at years 2, 5, 7, and 10. At the 7-year examination, approximately 80% of the original study cohort were evaluated. In this observational study, anthropometric, sociodemographic, health habit, blood pressure, insulin, glucose, and blood pressure measurements were made. Investigators found that, within each gender–race group, average DBP was positively correlated with age, BMI, and alcohol intake; it was negatively correlated with physical activity. African-Americans had higher DBP levels than Caucasians, but the differences were attenuated greatly after accounting for obesity and the factors mentioned above.[27] They also noted that racial differences in SBP were greatly reduced by taking into account experiences of racial discrimination and responses to unfair treatment recorded at the year 7 surveys.[79] In all gender–race groups, an increase in body mass during the first 7 years was associated with altered glucose and insulin metabolism.[80]

Diabetes/glucose intolerance/metabolic syndrome

The prevalence of type II diabetes mellitus (DM) among children has been rising recently in North America, particularly in Native American children in the United States[18,19] and First Nation children in Canada.[20] In Manitoba, for example, First Nation children are seven times more likely to have type II DM than Caucasian children from the same region.[20] Pima Indian children in Arizona are nearly 10 times more likely to have type II DM than other children in the United States.[19] In Cincinnati, Ohio, studies of African-American and Caucasian youth, the rate of new cases of type II DM increased 10-fold from 1982 to 1994.[81]

In recent years, most North American communities have seen remarkable rises in body weight and much less physical activity in their children. CARDIA investigators documented that these same factors—physical inactivity and weight gain—were associated with higher fasting insulin and glucose levels in their study children.[80] Bogalusa investigators found a persistence of elevated insulin levels in their longitudinal study of children, along with an association of insulin resistance with other CAD risk factors. They also noted that children of diabetic parents developed excess body fatness early in childhood and had accelerated onset of insulin

resistance.[82] Studies of obese African-American children, aged 5 to 10, indicated the presence of reduced insulin sensitivity associated with higher BMI, suggesting they may already be in the early stages of development of type II DM.[83]

The American Diabetes Association released a consensus paper on type II DM in children and adolescents, reviewing this subject from the genetic bases for these findings to community approaches to detection and intervention.[81] The American Heart Association released a similar scientific statement.[84] Among other recommendations, the two groups sought to reinforce the efforts of primary care physicians to encourage weight reduction and physical activity as important measures to prevent the onset of diabetes in children.

Recent efforts to examine the prevalence of metabolic syndrome (MetS) among US adolescents have utilized a National Cholesterol Education Program definition modified for age, where the presence of three or more of the following identifies the presence of the metabolic syndrome: (1) triglycerides 110 mg/dl or greater; (2) HDL-C < 40 mg/dl; (3) waist circumference (cm) of ≥90th percentile; (4) fasting glucose of 110 mg/dl or greater; and/or (5) blood pressure ≥90th percentile or on medication for hypertension. With this definition, 6.1% of males and 2.1% of females aged 12–17 were identified to have MetS, translating to in a total of 910,000 adolescents in the U.S. Nearly a third of overweight adolescents have this condition.[85] Others estimate up to 50% of severely obese adolescents to have MetS; each half-unit increase in body mass index was associated with a 55% greater likelihood, and each unit of insulin resistance defined by the homeostatic model was associated with a 12% greater likelihood of MetS.[86] These observations suggest the need for assessment and appropriate management of MetS in youth and adolescents to reduce the risk of future cardiovascular disease and diabetes.

Longitudinal studies of multiple factors

The Dietary Intervention Study in Children (DISC) was begun in 1987 to examine the efficacy and safety of long-term dietary intervention to reduce LDL-C in children with TC levels between the 80th and 98th percentiles for their age and gender. Children with higher levels were considered to be potential candidates for pharmacologic therapy. Mean age of the 362 boys was 9.7 years, and that of the 301 girls, 9.0 years. Subjects were then randomized to either usual care (notification of the children's high cholesterol levels plus educational publications) or the intervention group, which consisted of individual and group sessions with parents and children during the subsequent 3 years, advocating a 28% fat diet (<8% of calories from saturated fat).

The efficacy outcome measure was LDL-C, while measurements of height, ferritin, folate, albumin, HDL-C, triglycerides, sexual maturation, and psychosocial function were among the safety and efficacy outcomes. Levels of LDL-C decreased significantly more in the intervention group (15.4 mg/dL) than in the usual care group (11.9 mg/dL). There were no differences in any of the safety outcome measures, indicating no adverse effects on growth or other function from the reduced-fat diet.[87] Maternal willingness to implement the study diet was significantly correlated to reduced saturated fat intake in children.[88]

In 1988, NHLBI began its 5-year National Growth and Health Study of 2379 nine- and ten-year-old African-American and Caucasian girls at three clinical centers. Anthropometric, nutritional, blood pressure, and serum lipid measurements were done annually. At baseline, it was found that African-American girls were taller and heavier and had higher blood pressure and HDL-C levels. LDL-C and TC were similar in Caucasians and African-Americans.[89] Body fatness correlated with both reduced energy expenditure (and increased television viewing), percentage of saturated fat recorded on 3-day food records, and age.[46]

The Child and Adolescent Trial for Cardiovascular Health (CATCH) was a NHLBI-sponsored multicenter elementary school-based intervention study begun in 1991, which was designed to enhance heart-healthy eating, increased physical activity, and smoking abstention. Serum TC level was the primary physiologic outcome measure; anthropometric, blood pressure, heart rate, and HDL-C measurements were also made and analyzed.[90] At each site, 24 schools were randomly assigned to one of three groups: control, school-based intervention, or school-based plus family-based intervention. Of 5106 children enrolled at baseline, 4019 were reexamined 2½ years later. At that time, no significant differences were noted between the two intervention groups, so their data were pooled for analysis.[91] At the follow-up examination, children who were higher than the 85th percentile for BMI had significantly higher TC, lower HDL-C, and lower performance times on a 9-minute run than less ponderous children. Being overweight and overfat at baseline was the strongest predictor of adiposity 2½ years later.[92]

The effects of dietary composition on lipids have also been documented in children. In cross-sectional studies, CATCH investigators found that dietary fat (total and saturated) was positively correlated with TC, whereas carbohydrate intake was inversely correlated with HDL-C levels.[65] However, during the study period, nutrient intake in the intervention group showed significant improvements in all ethnic groups and in both genders. Analysis in one subsample of the CATCH population revealed that total fat intake decreased from 32.7 to 30.3% of total calories, and saturated fat consumption dropped from 12.8 to 11.4%.[93] Although statistically significant differences in the children's health behaviors were noted at follow-up, both control and intervention groups had a decrease of approximately 1.0-mg/dL in serum TC. The authors speculated that the lack of significant lipid changes may have resulted from the limited intensity of the intervention (40 minutes per week for 12–15 weeks), short duration (2½ years of follow-up), and suboptimal change in parental health behaviors.[91]

CARDIOVASCULAR HEALTH PROMOTION FOR ALL YOUTH

Preventing the development of coronary risk factors, including dyslipidemia, hypertension, obesity, diabetes, and cigarette smoking, remains the top priority in children and adolescents (Table 15-5).[94] An integrated approach to this goal requires efforts at home, in the medical office, and in the school setting.[95]

Smoking prevention

School-based programs to help students avoid adoption of the smoking habit have been successful.[96] Although information-only programs had limited success, those based on social and behavioral approaches were more successful, particularly when parents and community were involved.[30,97] Particularly helpful have been a) more vigorous enforcement of prohibiting cigarette sales to minors, and b) increasing taxes on cigarette sales.[98]

Guidelines for school health programs to prevent tobacco use and addiction are available from the US Department of Health and Human Services. They recommend that all schools: (1) develop and enforce a school policy on tobacco use; (2) provide instruction about the short- and long-term negative physiologic and social consequences of tobacco use, social influences on tobacco use, peer norms regarding tobacco use, and refusal skills; (3) provide tobacco use prevention education in kindergarten through twelfth grade; (4) provide program-specific training for teachers; (5) involve parents or families in support of school-based programs to prevent tobacco use; (6) support cessation efforts among students and all school staff who use tobacco; and (7) assess the tobacco use prevention program at regular intervals.[99]

In the North Karelia Youth Project, seventh-grade students began a 2-year program aimed at preventing smoking adoption. Students learned about social pressures to begin smoking, which are exerted by peers, parents, other adults, and mass media. They were trained by demonstration and role playing to resist such pressure. Cigarette consumption, measured 15 years after the intervention, was significantly reduced.[100]

TABLE 15-5 Schedule for Cardiovascular Health Promotion in All Youth

Age	Family history*	Cholesterol	Obesity	Blood pressure	Diet	Physical activity	Smoking	Actions taken
0–2	Early heart disease† (age ≤55) Parent's total cholesterol ≥240 mg/dL	Parent cholesterol screening	Plot height and weight on growth charts Parent obesity	Family history of hypertension	Diet history *Early foods influence future food preferences*	Parent physical activity *Discourage television and video viewing*	Parental/household smoking? If yes, counsel to quit; referral to smoking cessation	...
2–6	Update family history Early heart disease† (age ≤55) Parent's total cholesterol ≥240 mg/dL	→ Fasting lipids screening → Total cholesterol screening	Plot height, weight, and BMI (kg/m²) on growth charts BMI percentiles	Start routine blood pressure measures at 3 y (determine if >90th or 95th percentile for sex, age, and height)	Diet history *Low-saturated-fat diet† including 1% or nonfat milk Moderate salt intake*	*Encourage active child–parent play Limit sedentary behaviors such as television and video viewing*	Parental/household smoking? If yes, counsel to quit; referral to smoking cessation *Antismoking counseling§*	...
6–10	Update family history Early heart disease† (age ≤55) Parent's total cholesterol ≥240 mg/dL	→ Fasting lipids screening → Total cholesterol screening	Plot height, weight, and BMI (kg/m²) on growth charts BMI percentiles	Blood pressure measures Blood pressure percentiles	Diet history *Low-saturated-fat diet† including 1% or nonfat milk Moderate salt intake*	Physical activity history *Lifestyle and family activities Limit sedentary behaviors such as television and video viewing*	Parental/household smoking? If yes, counsel to quit; referral to smoking cessation *Antismoking counseling§*	...
>10	Update family history Early heart disease† (age ≤55) Parent's total cholesterol ≥240 mg/dL	→ Fasting lipids screening → Total cholestral screening	Plot height, weight, and BMI (kg/m²) on growth charts BMI percentiles	Blood pressure measures Blood pressure percentiles	Diet history *Low-saturated-fat diet† including 1% or nonfat milk Moderate salt intake*	Physical activity history *Lifestyle and family activities Daily moderate to vigrous activity Limit sedentary behaviors*	Parental/household smoking? Access child smoking If yes, counsel to quit; referral to smoking cessation *Antismoking counseling§*	...

Assessment items are in normal typeface; counseling items are in italics.

*Includes parents, grandparents, and blood-related aunts and uncles.

†Documented myocardial infarction, coronary artery disease, angina pectoris, or sudden cardiac death at age 55 years or younger or family history not available.

‡The diet should average <30% (but not <20%) of calories from total fat, <10% of calories from saturated fats, ≤10% of calories from polyunsaturated fats; and the lesser of 300 mg/d or 100 mg cholesterol per 1000 kcal energy intake.

§Includes immediate physical, social, and psychological effects of smoking, risk of addiction, counter-arguing techniques, and resisting social and environmental pressures to smoke.

SOURCE: Reproduced, with permission, from Williams.94

366

A Report of the Surgeon General on preventing to-bacco use among young people emphasizes the community's role. It concludes that:

> A crucial element of prevention is access: adolescents should not be able to purchase tobacco products in their communities. Active enforcement of age-at-sale policies by public officials and community members appears necessary to prevent minors' access to tobacco. Communities that have adopted tighter restrictions have achieved reductions in purchases made by minors. At the state and national levels, price increases have significantly reduced cigarette smoking; the young have been at least as responsive as adults to these price changes. Maintaining higher real prices of cigarettes provides a barrier to adolescent tobacco use but depends on further tax increases to offset the effects of inflation.[30]

The results of this review thus suggest that a coordinated, multicomponent campaign involving policy changes, taxation, mass media, and behavioral education can effectively reduce the onset of tobacco use among adolescents.[30]

Additional information on tobacco use and its relation to cardiovascular risk as well as tobacco prevention and cessation is found in Chapter 5.

Physical activity

At home, parents can serve as role models for engagement in physical activities and maintenance of ideal body weight. With community encouragement, schools can be prompted to modify their environment to increase the activity level of children and adolescents.[45,101] Guidelines for school and community programs are available from the US Department of Health and Human Services.[102]

As with other health behaviors, attitude and self-efficacy are important determinants of adoption of exercise as a routine habit. An exercise "prescription" by the child's physician can complement efforts at home and school to encourage the overweight child to be aerobically active. Additional recommendations and guidelines for improving physical activity in youth are discussed in detail in Chapter 12.

Nutrition

Prevention of obesity through nutritional strategies is a task that begins in utero; it is affected by maternal obesity, weight gain during pregnancy, and diabetes.[103] It continues during infancy and childhood as feeding, eating, and physical activity patterns are established and subsequently through the adolescent years.

The American Heart Association Nutrition Committee recommends the Step 1 diet for normal growth and development in children older than 2 years, and maintains that limiting the amount of fat and cholesterol should be a task for the entire family, not just the parents. After age 2, a gradual transition to a heart-healthy diet can be accomplished by replacing foods rich in fat with grains, fruits, lean meat, and other foods low in fat and high in complex carbohydrates and protein.[104] If, after at least 3 months on the Step 1 diet, minimal goals of therapy are not achieved, progression to the Step 2 diet should be considered.[105]

Williams and colleagues evaluated the Healthy Start program in children aged 2 to 5 who were enrolled in Head Start centers. This education and intervention program successfully reduced saturated fat intake of their preschool children to less than 10% of calories (with total fat intake remaining at approximately 30% of total calories) without compromising intake of essential nutrients.[106]

Obesity

Whitaker and colleagues reported that among overweight children at age 6, those with normal-weight parents have only a 24% chance of remaining overweight, and overweight children with at least one overweight parent have a 62% likelihood of remaining overweight.[107]

In addition to efforts at home and school to provide better nutritional intake for children, health care professionals play a critical role in reducing the prevalence of overweight children. Routine assessment of BMI and dietary intake, coupled with specific nutritional counseling by pediatricians, pediatric nurse practitioners, and registered dietitians, is among the recommended practices carried out in most, but not all, offices. In particular, more attention to development of high blood pressure (for age and size) and elevated blood glucose levels may provide early warning in those children at highest risk.[108]

Dyslipidemia

To prevent dyslipidemia in children older than 2, an average daily intake of 30% or less of total calories should come from fat, with no more than one third of the fat calories coming from saturated fat sources. Because the American Academy of Pediatrics is concerned that some parents may use more restrictive diets, their recommendations carefully state that "a lower intake of fat is not recommended." Further, "skim or low-fat milk should not be used during the first two years of life because of the high protein and electrolyte content and low calorie density of these milks."[109] Again, aerobic exercise and maintenance of an ideal body weight will help prevent dyslipidemias.

Appendix 15-1 lists foods intended to decrease saturated fatty acid and total fat content of school lunches; Appendix 15-2 lists snack-bar foods consistent with the recommended eating pattern; and Appendices 15-3, 15-4, and 15-5 give examples of sample menus based on school or fast-food lunches to comply with the Step 1 and 2 diets while ensuring adequate caloric intake.[105]

Hypertension

High blood pressure is best prevented by ensuring that all children are aerobically active, maintain an ideal body weight, and limit their caloric and sodium intake to recommended levels. Children with a familial history of hypertension should be monitored carefully and often to ensure early detection. Smoking and alcohol should be avoided.

In the 7th report of the Joint National Committee on Prevention, Detection, Evaluation and Treatment of High Blood Pressure (JNC-7),[110] dietary recommendations for treatment are intensified once an adult is identified as "prehypertensive." Although JNC-7 made no similar recommendations for treatment of children, increased attention should be offered to children at high risk for subsequent development of hypertension.

Diabetes/Metabolic Syndrome

Similarly, prevention of diabetes and the metabolic syndrome is best approached through family, school, and community efforts to: (1) promote aerobic physical activity in all children; (2) encourage maintenance of ideal body weight; and (3) make available more appetizing foods that are lower in calories and simple carbohydrates than are presently consumed by our youth.

IDENTIFICATION OF YOUTH AT HIGH RISK FOR CAD

Indicators of CAD risk may be detected by family members and educators and during acquisition of the pediatric history in the physician's office. These indicators include sociodemographic factors, family history of CAD and risk factors, nutrition at home and at school, and smoking status of child and family members. Other risk indicators, such as elevated BMI and blood pressure, should be identified during periodic physical examinations, while glucose and lipid levels require fasting blood analyses.

Dyslipidemias

The AAP, in their statement on cholesterol, concluded that "serum cholesterol level is an imperfect predictor of future coronary vascular disease" and recommended "selective screening of children more than 2 years of age whose risk of developing coronary vascular disease can be identified by family history." They suggested that those with a parent or grandparent with coronary or peripheral artery disease before the age of 55 should have a fasting lipid profile. Those having a parent with a TC level of 240 mg/dL or higher should have a nonfasting total cholesterol determination.[109] In contrast to these recommendations, the British Hyperlipidaemia Association recommends a nonfasting total cholesterol test as the first step for evaluation in all children.[111]

Others have recommended one-time universal screening of children for dyslipidemia,[63,112] noting that 50% or more of children with hypercholesterolemia would be missed using AAP screening criteria.[113,114] Of course, the yield of cases with heterozygous familial hypercholesterolemia would be low,[115] but a high prevalence of children with TC greater than 200 mg/dL is very likely (greater than 10% in several studies),[62,63] suggesting that behavioral intervention in families should be started early after such identification from school-based testing[112] and intervention[93] programs.

The National Cholesterol Education Program (NCEP) for Children and Adolescents proposed two categories of screening indicators: (1) major screening indicators, defined as a family history of early vascular disease or TC of 240 mg/dL or greater; and (2) discretionary indicators, which include smoking, diabetes, hypertension, high fat consumption, and steroid use. The NCEP recommends a scheme for risk assessment based on initial measurement of TC (Fig. 15-2) and for assessment, classification, and follow-up based on lipoprotein analysis (Fig. 15-3).[105] In their study population, Diller and colleagues found that 30% of children with high LDL-C levels were identified solely by the discretionary indicators listed above.[116]

High Blood Pressure

The National High Blood Pressure Education Program Working Group recommended the incorporation of blood pressure measurement into the routine pediatric office examination. A flowchart for BP monitoring and treatment is found in Fig. 15-4.[94]

Glucose Intolerance

A family history of DM is highly correlated with the development of type II DM in youth; more than three quarters of affected children have a first- or second-degree relative who is diabetic. Detection typically occurs during adolescence, consistent with the occurrence of increased insulin resistance after puberty.

BMI in most children with type II DM exceeds the 85th percentile for age, in contrast to children with type I diabetes. In longitudinal studies, changes in BMI are the strongest predictors of insulin and glucose concentrations.[19] The American Diabetes Association recommends screening children considered to be at high risk for development of type II DM.[84] Table 15-6 lists criteria for testing.

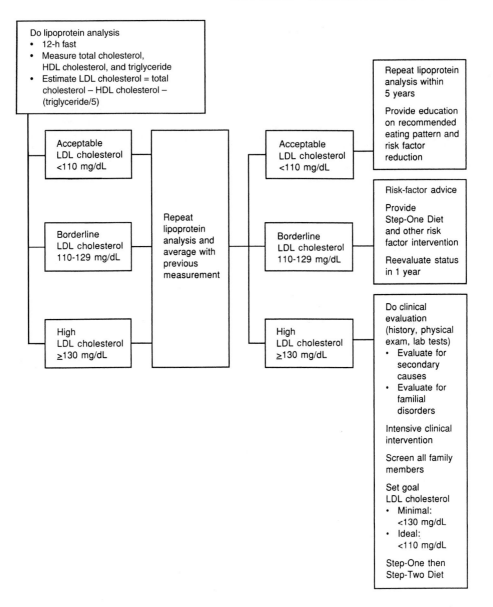

FIGURE 15-2 Risk assessment based on initial measurement of total cholesterol in children. *Defined as a history of premature (before age 55) cardiovascular disease in a parent or grandparent. (Adapted, with permission, from the National Cholesterol Education Program.[103])

MEDICAL INTERVENTION IN YOUTH AT ELEVATED CAD RISK

Treatment in youth should begin with hygienic methods for all indicators of high CAD risk. If these efforts fail to bring blood pressure and/or lipid parameters to acceptable levels, pharmacologic approaches may be considered. Goals for risk intervention and steps for clinical management of key cardiovascular risk parameters as recommended by the American Heart Association are presented in Table 15-7.[117]

Smoking

Most adult smokers begin their habit during adolescence (or earlier).[118] Although smoking cessation

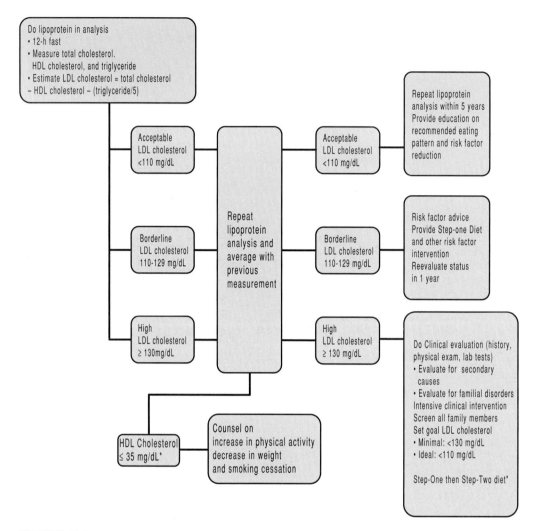

FIGURE 15-3 Classification, education, and follow-up based on lipoprotein readings in children. *For children 10 years or older on the Step 2 diet with an LDL-C level of ≥160 mg/dL and other risk factors or with an LDL-C level of ≥190 mg/dL, pharmacologic intervention should be considered. (Adapted, with permission, from the National Cholesterol Education Program.[105])

programs have low success rates among adolescents, it is important that primary care physicians ask them about their smoking habits. Those currently smoking can be encouraged to quit through the development of positive reinforcement skills, emphasizing the importance of assuming responsibility for one's own health.[119] It has been noted that nicotine dependence is highly prevalent among adolescent smokers.[120] At the community level, efforts at point-of-sale law enforcement and prohibitive pricing of cigarettes may help. Additional recommendations for tobacco prevention and control in youth are provided in Chapter 5.

Obesity

Investigators in children's weight loss studies have shown that more than 80% of participants eventually return to their original weight percentile. Factors favoring success include frequent contact with the intervention team, parental involvement and support in food preparation, adherence to an exercise prescription, and setting of realistic goals. In treating obese children, the American Heart Association recommends that "the primary emphasis of treatment should be prevention of weight gain above that appropriate for expected increases in height.

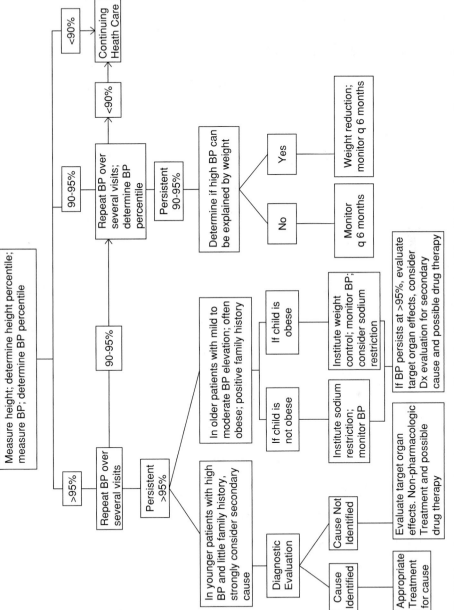

FIGURE 15-4 Flowchart for identification of high blood pressure in children. BP, blood pressure; Dx, diagnosis; q6mo, every 6 months. (Adapted, with permission, from Williams et al.[94])

TABLE 15-6 Criteria for Screening Youth for Type II Diabetes Mellitus

Fasting plasma glucose (preferred) or 2-h postprandial glucose levels should be done in:
• Children who are overweight (BMI > 85th percentile, weight for height > 85th percentile, or weight >120% of ideal for height) and have two or more of these risk factors:
1. First- or second-degree relative with type II DM
2. Non-European ancestry (ie, Native American, African-American, Latino, Asian/Pacific Islander)
3. Signs of insulin resistance or associated conditions (dyslipidemia, hypertension, polycystic ovary syndrome, acanthosis nigricans)
• Children who are overweight but have only one of the above factors may be tested if clinical judgment so indicates

For many children, this may mean limited or no weight gain while linear growth proceeds normally."[121] Behavioral, dietary, pharmacologic, and surgical treatments of childhood obesity have recently been reviewed.[122]

Dyslipidemia

The initial treatment in children above the age of 2 with elevated serum cholesterol levels is dietary management. Although a TC of 170 mg/dL or greater or an LDL-C of 130 mg/dL or greater should trigger dietary intervention (if not already implemented), the Step 1 diet is recommended for all children above the age of 2. It consists of lowering the percentage of fat in the child's diet to less than 30%, with less than 10% of calories coming from saturated fat, and less than 300 mg of cholesterol per day.

The Step 2 diet reduces saturated fat intake to less than 7% of caloric intake and dietary cholesterol intake to less than 200 mg/d.[107] When closely monitored, these diets have been shown not to retard growth and development. In the DISC study, children in the intervention group were encouraged to consume a diet with 28% of calories from total fat and less than 8% from saturated fat. No adverse effects were noted in growth, sexual maturation, or other physiologic parameters.[123]

Figure 15-5 is a schematic diagram of an initiation and follow-up schedule used for dietary intervention.[103] Aerobic exercise is important in maintaining an ideal body weight, which, in turn, contributes to lower cholesterol levels. In children above age 10 with two or more risk factors for CAD, drug therapy may be given if LDL-C remains above 160 mg/dL after at least 6 months of appropriate diet and exercise maintenance. The threshold for drug treatment in children with fewer than two CAD risk factors is 190 mg/dL; for those with either a positive family history of premature cardiovascular disease

(before 55 years of age) or two or more risk factors (after vigorous attempts have been made to control such risk factors), the threshold is 160 mg/dL (Table 15-7).[105,117] The minimum goal is an LDL-C less than 160 mg/dL and ideally less than 130 mg/dL. Traditionally, bile acid sequestrants such as cholestyramine and colestipol have been the first choice for treatment.[124]

Nicotinic acid may be considered if cholesterol-lowering therapy by diet and bile acid sequestrants has failed to optimize lipid levels to therapeutic goals. Considering that nicotinic acid beneficially alters the entire lipid profile, it may be especially helpful for children and adolescents with elevated LDL-C accompanied by hypertriglyceridemia or low HDL-C. Blood uric acid, glucose levels, and liver function should be monitored at each visit, as therapeutic dosages of nicotinic acid are more likely to cause toxicity when used in youth or adolescents.[105]

Results from several multicenter studies suggest that HMGCoA reductase inhibitors are effective and safe for treatment of dyslipidemia in children and adolescents. However, they should not be used in girls and women of childbearing potential until extensive counseling and effective pharmacologic contraception have been employed. The agents are absolutely contraindicated in pregnancy.[81] Investigators using lovastatin[115,125] and simvastatin[126,127] in children and adolescents have noted that measurements of growth and sexual maturation did not differ between treatment and control groups. Despite earlier concerns that pharmacologic treatment of children with dyslipidemia may cause psychologic trauma (from being "labeled" as having a disease), it appears that psychosocial disturbances are rare.[128]

High blood pressure

Obese children who lose weight and successfully maintain a more ideal body weight will have substantial reductions in SBP and DBP (and improvements in lipids as well), so counseling on exercise and decreased caloric intake is essential. Cessation of smoking will likewise reduce blood pressure. The National High Blood Pressure Education Program Working Group recommended a moderate reduction in dietary sodium through elimination of table salt and avoidance of prepared foods with high sodium content. Children whose SBP or DBP remains above the 95th percentile after implementation of hygienic methods can be treated pharmacologically (Table 15-7).

Several classes of antihypertensive drugs have proven to be safe and useful; these include low-dose diuretics, long-acting calcium antagonists, and alpha blockers. Angiotensin-converting enzyme (ACE) inhibitors are considered the agent of choice in diabetic children with microalbuminuria, and are considered by many to be

TABLE 15-7   Guidelines for Cardiovascular Risk Reduction: Intervention for Children and Adolescents with Identified Risk

Risk intervention	Recommendations
	Blood Cholesterol Management

GOALS:
• LDL-C <160 mg/dL
  (<130 mg/dL is even better)
• For patients with diabetes,
  LDL-C <100 mg/dL
	• If LDL-C is above goals, initiate therapeutic lifestyle changes, including diet (<7% of calories from saturated fat; <200 mg cholesterol per day), in conjunction with a trained dietitian.
	• Consider LDL-lowering dietary options (increase soluble fiber by using age [in years] plus 5 to 10 g up to age 15, when the total remains at 25 g/day) in conjunction with a trained dietitian.
	• Emphasize weight management and increased physical activity.
	• If LDL-C is persistently above goals, evaluate for secondary cause (thyroid stimulating hormone, liver function tests, renal function tests, urinalysis).
	• Consider pharmacologic therapy for individuals with LDL-C >190 mg/dL with no other risk factors for CVD; or >160 mg/dL with other risk factors present (blood pressure elevation, diabetes, obesity, strong family history of premature CVD).
	• Bile acid-binding resins or statins are usual first-line agents.
	• Pharmacologic intervention for dyslipidemia should be accomplished in collaboration with a physician experienced in treatment of disorders of cholesterol in pediatric patients.

	Other Lipids and Lipoprotein
GOALS: • Fasting TGs <150 mg/dL • HDL-C >35 mg/dL	• Elevated fasting TGs and reduced HDL-C are often seen in the context of overweight with insulin resistance. Therapeutic lifestyle change should include weight management with appropriate energy intake and expenditure. Decrease intake of simple sugars. • If fasting TGs are persistently elevated, evaluate for secondary causes such as diabetes, thyroid disease, renal disease, and alcohol abuse. • No pharmacologic interventions are recommended in children for isolated elevation of fasting TGs unless this is very marked (treatment may be initiated at TGs >400 mg/dL to protect against postprandial TGs at 1000 mg/dL or greater, which may be associated with an increased risk of pancreatitis).
	Management of Blood Pressure Elevation

GOAL:
• Systolic and diastolic blood
  pressure <95th percentile for
  age, sex, and height
	• Promote achievement of appropriate weight.
	• Reduce sodium in the diet. Emphasize increased consumption of fruits and vegetables.
	• If blood pressure is persistently above the 95th percentile, consider possible secondary causes (eg, renal disease, coarctation of the aorta).
	• Consider pharmacologic therapy for individuals above 95th percentile if lifestyle modification brings no improvement and there is evidence of target organ changes (left ventricular hypertrophy, microalbuminuria, retinal vascular abnormalities). Start blood pressure medication individualized to other patient requirements and characteristics (ie, age, race, need for drugs with specific benefits).
	• Pharmacologic management of hypertension should be accomplished in collaboration with a physician experienced in pediatric hypertension.

	Weight Management
GOAL: • Achieve and maintain BMI <95th percentile for age and sex	• For children who are at risk of overweight (>85th percentile) or obesity (>95th percentile), a weight management program should be initiated with appropriate energy balance achieved through changes in diet and physical activity. • For children of normal height, a secondary cause of obesity is unlikely. • Weight management should be directed at all family members who are overweight, using a family-centered, behavioral management approach. • Weight management should be done in collaboration with a trained dietitian.

(*continued*)

TABLE 15-7 *(Continued)*

Risk intervention	Recommendations
Diabetes Management	
GOALS: • Near-normal fasting plasma glucose (<120 mg/dL) • Near-normal HgA1$_c$ (<7%) (goals for fasting glucose and HgA1$_c$ should take into consideration age and risk of hypoglycemia)	• Management of type 1 and type 2 diabetes in children and adolescents should be accomplished in collaboration with a pediatric endocrinologist. • For type 2 diabetes, the first step is weight management with improved diet and exercise. • Because of risk for accelerated vascular disease, other risk factors (eg, blood pressure, lipid abnormalities) should be treated more aggressively in patients with diabetes.
Cigarette Smoking Cessation	
GOAL: • Complete cessation of smoking for children and parents who smoke	• Advise every tobacco user (parents and children) to quit and be prepared to provide assistance with this (counseling/referral to develop a plan for quitting using available community resources to help with smoking cessation).

SOURCE: Reproduced, with permission, from Kavey et al.[117]

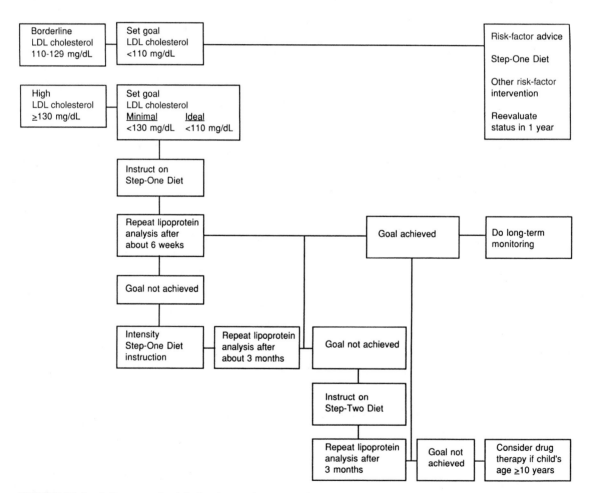

FIGURE 15-5 Follow-up schedule for dietary therapy. (Adapted, with permission, from the National Cholesterol Education Program.[105])

the first-line drug because of their long-term potential to reduce nephropathy. ACE inhibitors and angiotensin receptor blockers should not be used in sexually active adolescents without birth control measures. Beta blockers should be used with caution, as they may mask symptoms of hypoglycemia.[75,81]

Glucose intolerance

Therapeutic goals for the diabetic child are normal values of blood glucose and glycohemoglobin, as well as control of lipid levels, blood pressure, and body weight. Children who are not in diabetic crisis at the time of detection can usually be managed initially with diet and physical activity prescriptions. Dietary counseling should be performed by a registered dietitian experienced in childhood diabetes.[81]

Most children with type II DM will eventually require pharmacologic treatment with one or more of five categories of oral agents that are currently available. Because safety and efficacy data are still sparse for the use of these agents in children, the young diabetic should be referred to a skilled specialist for pharmacologic treatment.[81]

CONCLUSIONS

Atherosclerosis, the precursor of CAD, can begin in childhood. CAD risk factors that can be identified at an early age are correlated with the subsequent development of coronary artery lesions and events. The prevalence of CAD risk factors varies by age and ethnicity. Longitudinal studies demonstrate "tracking" of these indicators, and autopsy studies show correlation of the risk indicators and atherosclerosis.

In contrast to the improvement seen in CAD risk indicators in adults in the past three decades, levels of CAD risk in children have dramatically worsened in the same period. Increased prevalence of dyslipidemia, high blood pressure, and glucose intolerance have been documented in children. Antecedent to these changes have been large decreases in physical activity, greater consumption of fat and simple carbohydrates, and consequent rises in obesity among children. These changes are now being observed in most developed countries. Guidelines have been established for screening children for CAD risk factors, for treatment of those children found to be at high risk, and for the optimization of cardiovascular health for all children. Dietary and other lifestyle approaches remain the cornerstone for the prevention and control of CAD risk factors for most children and adolescents.

To develop effective programs and to reinforce adherence to desirable lifestyles in children and adolescents, a comprehensive, united effort is needed by health care providers and parents at the local level, as well as active involvement of the nation's schools. When primary prevention efforts fail to reduce high levels of risk, pharmacologic and behavioral intervention by medical professionals is indicated.

REFERENCES

1. Ross R. Mechanisms of disease: atherosclerosis—an inflammatory disease. *N Engl J Med* 1999;340:115–126.

2. Enos WF, Beyer JC, Holmes R. Pathogenesis of coronary artery disease in soldiers killed in Korea. *JAMA* 1955;148:912–914.

3. McNamara JJ, Molot MA, Stremple JF, Cutting RT. Coronary artery disease in combat casualties in Vietnam. *JAMA* 1971;216:1185–1187.

4. Strong JP, McGill HC Jr. The natural history of coronary atherosclerosis. *Am J Pathol* 1958;34:209–235.

5. Holman RL, McGill HC Jr, Strong JP, Geer JC. The natural history of atherosclerosis: the early aortic lesions as seen in New Orleans in the middle of the 20th century. *Am J Pathol* 1958;34:209–235.

6. Strong JP. Coronary atherosclerosis in soldiers: a clue to the natural history of atherosclerosis in the young. *JAMA* 1986;256:2863–2866.

7. Hirvonen J, Yla-Herttuala S, Laaksonen H, et al. Coronary intimal thickenings and lipids in Finnish children who died suddenly. *Acta Paediatr Scand* 1985;318(suppl):221–224.

8. McGill HC Jr. Persistent problems in the pathogenesis of atherosclerosis. *Arteriosclerosis* 1984;4:443–451.

9. McGill HC Jr, McMahan CA, Herderick EE, et al. Pathobiological Determinants of Atherosclerosis in Youth (PDAY) research group. Obesity accelerates the progression of coronary atherosclerosis in young men. *Circulation* 2002;105:2712–2718.

10. McGill HC Jr, McMahan CA, Zieske AW, et al. Effects of nonlipid risk factors on atherosclerosis in youth with a favorable lipoprotein profile. *Circulation* 2001;103:1546–1550.

11. Davidson DM. *Preventive Cardiology.* Baltimore: Williams & Wilkins; 1991.

12. Wattigney WA, Webber LS, Srinivisan SR, Berenson GS. The emergence of clinically abnormal levels of cardiovascular disease risk factor variables among young adults: the Bogalusa Heart Study. *Prev Med* 1995;24:617–626.

13. VanHorn L, Greenland P. Prevention of coronary artery disease is a pediatric problem. *JAMA* 1997;278:1779–1780.

14. Berenson GS, Srinivisan SR, Bao W, et al. Association between multiple cardiovascular risk factors and atherosclerosis in children and young adults. *N Engl J Med* 1998;338:1650–1656.

15. Troiano RP, Flegal KM, Kuczmarski RJ, et al. Overweight prevalence and trends for children and adolescents: the National Health and Nutrition Examination Surveys, 1963 to 1991. *Arch Pediatr Adolesc Med* 1995;149:1085–1091.

16. Andersen RE, Crespo CJ, Bartlett SJ, et al. Relationship of physical activity and television watching with body weight and level of fatness among children: results from the Third National Health and Nutrition Examination Survey. *JAMA* 1998;279:938–942.

17. Winkleby MA, Robinson TN, Sundquist J, Kraemer HK. Ethnic variation in cardiovascular disease risk factors among children and young adults: findings from the Third National Health and Nutrition Examination Survey, 1988–1994. *JAMA* 1999;281:1006–1013.

18. Freedman DS, Serdula MK, Percy CA, et al. Obesity, levels of lipids and glucose, and smoking among Navajo adolescents. *J Nutr* 1997;127(10 suppl):2120S–2127S.

19. Fagot-Campagna A, Pettitt DJ, et al. Type 2 diabetes among North American children and adolescents: an epidemiologic review and a public health perspective. *J Pediatr* 2000;136:664–672.

20. Dean H. NIDDM-Y in First Nation children in Canada. *Clin Pediatr* 1998;37:89–96.

21. Porkka KVK, Viikari JSA, Akerblom HK. Tracking of serum HDL-cholesterol and other lipids in children and adolescents: the Cardiovascular Risk in Young Finns Study. *Prev Med* 1991;20:713–724.

22. Morrison JA, James FW, Sprecher DL, et al. Sex and race differences in cardiovascular disease risk factor changes in schoolchildren, 1975–1990: the Princeton School Study. *Am J Public Health* 1999;89:1708–1714.

23. Bronner YL. Nutritional status outcomes for children: ethnic, cultural and environmental contexts. *J Am Diet Assoc* 1996;96:891–903.

24. Leino M, Porkka KV, Raitakari OT, et al. Influence of parental occupation on coronary heart disease risk factors in children: the Cardiovascular Risk in Young Finns Study. *Int J Epidemiol* 1996;25:1189–1195.

25. Batty GD, Leon DA. Socio-economic position and coronary heart disease risk factors in children and young people: evidence from UK epidemiological studies. *Eur J Public Health* 2002;12:263–72.

26. Bao W, Srinivisan SR, Wattigney WA, Berenson GS. The relation of parental cardiovascular disease to risk factors in children and young adults: the Bogalusa Heart Study. *Circulation* 1995;91:365–371.

27. Liu K, Ruth KJ, Flack JM, et al. Blood pressure in young African-Americans and Caucasians: relevance of obesity and lifestyle factors in determining differences: the CARDIA study. *Circulation* 1996;93:60–66.

28. Luepker RV, Pallonen UE, Murray DM, Pirie PL. Validity of telephone surveys in assessing cigarette smoking in young adults. *Am J Public Health* 1989;79:202–204.

29. Youth Risk behavior surveillance—United States, 1999. *MMWR CDC Surveill Summ* 2000; 49:1–32.

30. Centers for Disease Control and Prevention. *Preventing Tobacco Use among Young People. A Report of the Surgeon General.* DHHS Publication S/N 017-001-00491-0. Atlanta, GA: US Department of Health and Human Services, Public Health Service, CDC; 1994.

31. Trends in cigarette smoking among high school students— United States, 1991–2001. *MMWR* 2002;51:409–412.

32. Tobacco use among middle and high school students—United States, 2002. *MMWR* 2003;52:1096–1098.

33. Baugh JG, Hunter SM, Webber LS, Berenson GS. Developmental trends of first cigarette smoking experience of children: the Bogalusa Heart Study. *Am J Public Health* 1982;72:1161–1164.

34. Greenlund KJ, Johnson CC, Webber LS, Berenson GS. Cigarette smoking attitudes and first use among third- through sixth-grade students: the Bogalusa Heart Study. *Am J Public Health* 1997;87:1345–1348.

35. Lee DJ, Trapido E, Rodriguez R. Self-reported school difficulties and tobacco use among fourth- to seventh-grade students. *J School Health* 2002;72:368–373.

36. Simons-Morton BG. Prospective analysis of peer and parent influences on smoking initiation among early adolescents. *Prev Sci* 2002;3:275–283.

37. Centers for Disease Control and Prevention. Exposure of children to second hand smoke. *MMWR* 1997;46:1049–1056.

38. Bricker JB, Leroux BG, Peterson AV Jr, et al. Nine-year prospective relationship between parental smoking cessation and children's daily smoking. *Addiction* 2003;98:585–593.

39. Krohn MD, Naughton MJ, Skinner MF, et al. Social disaffection, friendship patterns and adolescent cigarette use: the Muscatine Study. *J School Health* 1986;5:146–150.

40. Osler M, Clausen J, Ibsen KI, Jensen G. Maternal smoking during childhood and increased risk of smoking in young adulthood. *Int J Epidemiol* 1995;24:710–714.

41. McGill HC Jr, McMahan CA, Malcom GT, et al. Effects of serum lipoproteins and smoking on atherosclerosis in young men and women. *Arterioscler Thromb Vasc Biol* 1997;17:95–106.

42. Strong JP, Malcom GT, McMahan CA, et al. Prevalence and extent of atherosclerosis in adolescents and young adults: implications for prevention from the Pathobiological Determinants of Atherosclerosis in Youth Study. *JAMA* 1999;281:727–735.

43. PDAY Research Group. Relationship of atherosclerosis in young men to serum lipoprotein cholesterol concentrations and smoking: a preliminary report from the Pathobiological Determinants of Atherosclerosis in Youth (PDAY) research group. *JAMA* 1990;264:3018–3024.

44. Kohl HW, Hobbs KE. Development of physical activity behaviors among children and adolescents. *Pediatrics* 1998;101:549–554.

45. Freedman DS, Dietz WH, Srinivisan SR, et al. The relation of overweight to cardiovascular risk factors among children and adolescents: the Bogalusa Heart Study. *Pediatrics* 1999;103:1175–1182.

46. Kimm SY, Barton BA, Obarzanek E, et al. Obesity development during adolescence in a biracial cohort: the NHLBI Growth and Health Study. *Pediatrics* 2002;110:E54.

47. Wong ND, Hei TK, Qaqundah PY, et al. Television viewing and pediatric hypercholesterolemia. *Pediatrics* 1992;90:75–79.

48. Frank GC. Environmental influences on methods used to collect dietary data from children. *Am J Clin Nutr* 1994;59(suppl):207S–211S.

49. Frank GC, Farris RP, Cresanta JL, et al. Dietary trends of 10- and 13-year-old children in a biracial community: the Bogalusa Heart Study. *Prev Med* 1985;14:123–139.

50. American Dietetic Association. Position of the American Dietetic Association: dietary guidance for healthy children aged 2–11 years. *J Am Diet Assoc* 1999;99:93–101.

51. Kronsberg SS, Obarzanek E, Affenito SG, et al. Macronutrient intake of black and Caucasian adolescent girls over

10 years: the NHLBI growth and health study. *J Am Diet Assoc* 2003;103:852–860.

52. Goran MI. Measurement issues related to studies of childhood obesity: assessment of body composition, body fat distribution, physical activity and food intake. *Pediatrics* 1998;101:505–518.

53. Dietz WH, Robinson TN. Use of the body mass index (BMI) as a measure of overweight in children and adolescents. *J Pediatr* 1998;132:191–193.

54. Williams CL, Gulli MT, Deckelbaum RJ. Prevention and treatment of childhood obesity. *Curr Atheroscler Rep* 2001;3:486–497.

55. Troiano RP, Flegal KM. Overweight children and adolescents: description, epidemiology and demographics. *Pediatrics* 1998;101:497–504.

56. Freedman DS, Srinivisan SR, Valdez RA, et al. Secular increases in relative weight and adiposity among children over two decades: the Bogalusa Heart Study. *Pediatrics* 1997;99:420–426.

57. Freedman DS, Khan LK, Mei Z, et al. Relation of childhood height to obesity among adults: the Bogalusa Heart Study. *Pediatrics* 2002;109:E23.

58. Luepker RV, Jacobs DR, Prineas RJ, Sinaiko AR. Secular trends of blood pressure and body size in a multi-ethnic adolescent population: 1986 to 1996. *J Pediatr* 1999;134:668–674.

59. Malina RM, Zavaleta AN, Little BB. Estimated overweight and obesity in Mexican-American school children. *Int J Obesity* 1986;10:483–491.

60. Freedman DS. Clustering of coronary heart disease risk factors among obese children. *J Pediatr Endocrinol Metab* 2002;15:1099–1108.

61. Lauer RM, Clarke WR. Use of cholesterol measurements in childhood for the prediction of adult hypercholesterolemia. *JAMA* 1990;264:3034–3038.

62. Nicklas T, Webber LS, Srinivisan SR, Berenson GS. Secular trends in dietary intake and cardiovascular risk factors in 10-year-old children: the Bogalusa Heart Study (1973–1988). *Am J Clin Nutr* 1993;57:930–937.

63. Davidson DM, Iftner CA, Bradley BJ, et al. Family history predictors of high blood cholesterol levels in 4th grade school children. *J Am Coll Cardiol* 1989;13:36A.

64. Webber LS, Osganian V, Luepker RV, et al. Cardiovascular risk factors among third grade children in four regions of the United States: the CATCH Study. *Am J Epidemiol* 1995;141:428–439.

65. Nicklas TA, Dwyer J, Feldman HA, et al. Serum cholesterol levels in children are associated with dietary fat and fatty acid intake. *J Am Diet Assoc* 2002;102:511–517.

66. *Third Report on Nutrition Monitoring in the United States.* Vol I. Washington, DC: US Government Printing Office; 1995.

67. Gidding SS, Bookstein LC, Chomka EV. Usefulness of electron beam computed tomography in adolescents and young adults with heterozygous familial hypercholesterolemia. *Circulation* 1998;98:2580–2583.

68. Mahoney LT, Burns TL, Stanford W, et al. Coronary risk factors measured in childhood and young adult life are associated with coronary artery calcification in young adults: the Muscatine Study. *J Am Coll Cardiol* 1996;27:277–284.

69. Bao W, Srinivisan SR, Wattigney WA, et al. Usefulness of childhood low-density lipoprotein cholesterol level in predicting adult dyslipidemia and other cardiovascular risks: the Bogalusa Heart Study. *Arch Intern Med* 1996;156:1315–1320.

70. Newman WP, Wattigney W, Berenson GS. Autopsy studies in U.S. children and adolescents: relationship of risk factors to atherosclerotic lesions. *Ann NY Acad Sci* 1991;623:16–25.

71. Berenson GS. Childhood risk factors predict adult risk associated with subclinical cardiovascular disease: the Bogalusa Heart Study. *Am J Cardiol* 2002;90(10C):3L–7L.

72. Fuentes RM, Notkola IL, Shemeikka S, et al. Tracking of serum total cholesterol during childhood: an 8-year follow-up population-based family study in eastern Finland. *Acta Paediatr* 2003;92:420–424.

73. Hara M, Saitou E, Iwata F, et al. Waist-to-height ratio is the best predictor of cardiovascular disease risk factors in Japanese schoolchildren. *J Atheroscler Thromb* 2002;9:127–132.

74. Tershakovec AM, Jawad AF, Stouffer NO, et al. Persistent hypercholesterolemia is associated with the development of obesity among girls: the Bogalusa Heart Study. *Am J Clin Nutr* 2002;76:730–735.

75. National High Blood Pressure Education Program Working Group on Hypertension Control in Children and Adolescents. Update on the 1987 Task Force Report on high blood pressure in children and adolescents: a working group report from the National High Blood Pressure Education Program. *Pediatrics* 1996;98:649–658.

76. Adrogue HE, Sinaiko AR. Prevalence of hypertension in junior high school-aged children: effect of new recommendations in the 1996 Updated Task Force Report. *Am J Hypertens* 2001;14:412–414.

77. Hohn AR, Dwyer KM, Dwyer JH. Blood pressure in youth from four ethnic groups: the Pasadena Prevention Project. *J Pediatr* 1994;125:368–373.

78. Liu K, Levinson S. Comparisons of blood pressure between Asian-American children and children from other racial groups in Chicago. *Public Health Rep* 1996;111(suppl 2):65–67.

79. Krieger N, Sidney S. Racial discrimination and blood pressure: the CARDIA study of young African-American and Caucasian adults. *Am J Public Health* 1996;86:1370–1378.

80. Folsom AR, Jacobs DR Jr, Wagenknecht LE, et al. Increase in fasting insulin and glucose over seven years with increasing weight and inactivity of young adults: the CARDIA study. *Am J Epidemiol* 1996;144:235–246.

81. American Diabetes Association. Type 2 diabetes in children and adolescents. *Diabetes Care* 2000;23:381–389.

82. Srinivasan SR, Frontini MG, Berenson GS. Longitudinal changes in risk variables of insulin resistance syndrome from childhood to young adulthood in offspring of parents with type 2 diabetes: the Bogalusa Heart Study. *Metabolism* 2003;52:443–450.

83. Young-Hyman D, Schlundt DG, Herman L, et al. Evaluation of the insulin resistance syndrome in 5- to 10-year-old overweight/obese African-American children. *Diabetes Care* 2001;24:1359–1364.

84. Steinberger J, Daniels SR. Obesity, insulin resistance, diabetes and cardiovascular risk in children: an American Heart Association Scientific Statement from the Atherosclerosis,

Hypertension, and Obesity in the Young Committee (Council on Cardiovascular Disease in the Young) and the Diabetes Committee (Council on Nutrition, Physical Activity, and Metabolism). *Circulation* 2003;107:1448–1453.

85. Cook S, Weitzman M, Auinger P. Prevalence of a metabolic syndrome phenotype in adolescents. Findings of the third National Health and Nutrition Examination Survey, 1988-1994. *Arch Pediatr Adolesc Med* 2003;157:821–827.

86. Weiss R, Dziura J, Burgert TS, et al. Obesity and the metabolic syndrome. *N Engl J Med* 2004;350:2362–2374.

87. Obarzanek E, Kimm SY, Barton BA, et al. Long-term safety and efficacy of a cholesterol-lowering diet in children with elevated low-density lipoprotein cholesterol: seven-year results of the Dietary Intervention Study in Children (DISC). *Pediatrics* 2001;107:256–264.

88. Reimers TM, Brown KM, Van Horn L, et al. Maternal acceptability of a dietary intervention designed to lower children's intake of saturated fat and cholesterol: the Dietary Intervention Study in Children (DISC). *J Am Diet Assoc* 1998;98: 31–34.

89. NHLBI Growth and Health Study Research Group. Obesity and cardiovascular disease risk factors in African-American and Caucasian girls: the NHLBI Growth and Health Study. *Am J Public Health* 1992;82:1613–1620.

90. Luepker RV, Perry CL, McKinlay SM, et al, for the CATCH Collaborative Group. Outcomes of a field trial to improve children's dietary patterns and physical activity: the Child and Adolescent Trial for Cardiovascular Health. *JAMA* 1996;275:768–776.

91. Webber LS, Osganian SK, Feldman HA, et al. Cardiovascular risk factors among children after a 2 1/2 year intervention: the CATCH Study. *Prev Med* 1996;265:432–441.

92. Dwyer JT, Stone EJ, Yang M, et al. Predictors of overweight and overfatness in a multiethnic pediatric population. *Am J Clin Nutr* 1998;67:602–610.

93. Lytle LA, Stone EJ, Nichaman MZ, et al. Changes in nutrient intakes of elementary school children following a school-based intervention: results from the CATCH Study. *Prev Med* 1996;25:465–477.

94. Williams CL, Hayman LL, Daniels SR, et al. Cardiovascular health in childhood: a statement for health professionals from the Committee on Atherosclerosis, Hypertension, and Obesity in the Young (AHOY) of the Council on Cardiovascular Disease in the Young, American Heart Association [published erratum appears in *Circulation* 2002:106:1178]. *Circulation* 2002;106:143–160.

95. Resnicow K, Robinson TW. School-based cardiovascular prevention studies: review and synthesis. *Ann Epidemiol* 1997;S7:S14–S31.

96. Elder JP, Perry CL, Johnson CC, et al. Tobacco use measurement, prediction, and intervention in elementary schools in four states. *Prev Med* 1996;25:486–494.

97. Forster JL, Murray DM, Wolfson M, et al. The effects of community policies to reduce youth access to tobacco. *Am J Public Health* 1998;88:1193–1198.

98. Rigotti NA, DiFranza JR, YuChiao C, et al. The effect of enforcing tobacco-sales laws on adolescents' access to tobacco and smoking behavior. *N Engl J Med* 1997;337:1044–1051.

99. Centers for Disease Control and Prevention. Guidelines for school health programs to prevent tobacco use and addiction. *MMWR* 1994;43:1–18.

100. Vartiainen E, Paavola M, McAlister A, Puska P. Fifteen-year follow up of smoking prevention effects in the North Karelia Youth Project. *Am J Public Health* 1998;88:81–85.

101. Sallis J, McKenzie T, Alcaraz J, et al. The effects of a 2 year physical education program (SPARK) on physical activity and fitness in elementary school students. *Am J Public Health* 1997;87:1328–1334.

102. Centers for Disease Control and Prevention. Guidelines for school and community programs to promote lifelong physical activity among young people. *MMWR* 1997;46:1–35.

103. Whitaker RC, Dietz WH. Role of the prenatal environment in the development of obesity. *J Pediatr* 1998;132:768–776.

104. Fisher EA, Van Horn L, McGill HC for the Nutrition Committee. Nutrition and children: a statement for healthcare professionals from the Nutrition Committee, American Heart Association. *Circulation* 1997;95:2332–2333.

105. National Cholesterol Education Program. *Report of the Expert Panel on Blood Cholesterol Levels in Children and Adolescents.* NIH Publication 91-2732. Bethesda, Md: National Heart Lung and Blood Institute; 1991.

106. Williams CL, Bollella MC, Strobino BA, et al. "Healthy-start": outcome of an intervention to promote a heart healthy diet in preschool children. *J Am Coll Nutr* 2002;21:62–71.

107. Whitaker R, Wright J, Pepe M, et al. Predicting obesity in young adulthood from childhood and parental obesity. *N Engl J Med* 1997;337:869–873.

108. Barlow SE, Dietz WH, Klish WJ, Trowbridge FL. Medical evaluation of overweight children and adolescents: reports from pediatricians, pediatric nurse practitioners, and registered dietitians. *Pediatrics* 2002;110:222–228.

109. American Academy of Pediatrics Committee on Nutrition. Cholesterol in children. *Pediatrics* 1998;101:141–147.

110. Chobanian AV, Bakris GL, Black HR, et al. Seventh report of the Joint National Committee on Prevention, Detection, Evaluation and Treatment of High Blood Pressure. *Hypertension* 2003;42:1206–1252.

111. Wray R, Neil H, Rees J. Screening for hyperlipidaemia in childhood: recommendations of the British Hyperlipidaemia Association. *J R Coll Physicians Lond* 1996;30:115–118.

112. Berenson GS, Srinivasan SR. Consideration of serum cholesterol in risk factor profiling for all young individuals. *Nutr Metab Cardiovasc Dis* 2001;11(suppl 5):1–9.

113. Davidson DM, VanCamp J, Iftner CA, et al. Family history fails to detect the majority of children with high capillary blood total cholesterol. *J School Health* 1991;61:75–80.

114. Bao W, Srinivisan SR, Wattigney WA, et al. Usefulness of childhood low-density lipoprotein cholesterol level in predicting adult dyslipidemia and other cardiovascular risks. *Arch Intern Med* 1996;156:1315–1320.

115. Stein EA, Illingworth DR, Kwiterovich PO, et al. Efficacy and safety of lovastatin in adolescent males with heterozygous familial hypercholesterolemia. *JAMA* 1999;281:137–144.

116. Diller PM, Huster GA, Leach AD, et al. Definition and application of the discretionary screening indicators according

to the National Cholesterol Education Program for Children and Adolescents. *J Pediatr* 1995;126:345–352.

117. Kavey R-E, Daniels SR, Lauer RM, et al. American Heart Association Guidelines for primary prevention of atherosclerotic cardiovascular disease beginning in childhood. *Circulation* 2003;107:1562–1566. Also published in *J Pediatr* 2003;142: 368–372.

118. Johnston LD, O'Malley PM, Bachman JG. *National Survey Results on Drug Use from the Monitoring the Future Study, 1975–1993.* DHHS Publication PHS 94-3809. Washington, DC: US Public Health Service; 1994.

119. Franzgrote M, Ellen JM, Millsein SG, Irwin CE. Screening for adolescent smoking among primary care physicians in California. *Am J Public Health* 1997;87:131–134.

120. Rojas NL, Killen JD, Haydel KF, Robinson TN. Nicotine dependence among adolescent smokers. *Arch Pediatr Adolesc Med* 1998;152:151–156.

121. Gidding SS, Leibel RL, Daniels S, et al. Understanding obesity in youth. *Circulation* 1996;94:3383–3387.

122. Epstein LH, Myers MD, Raynor HA, Saelens BE. Treatment of pediatric obesity. *Pediatrics* 1998;101:554–570.

123. Obarzanek E, Kimm SY, Barton BA, et al, for the DISC Collaborative Research Group. Long-term safety and efficacy of a cholesterol-lowering diet in children with elevated low-density lipoprotein cholesterol: seven-year results of the Dietary Intervention Study in Children (DISC). *Pediatrics* 2001;107:256–264.

124. Tonstad S, Knudtzon J, Siversten M, et al. Efficacy and safety of cholestyramine therapy in peripubertal and prepubertal children with familial hypercholesterolemia. *J Pediatr* 1996;229:42–49.

125. Kwiterovich PO Jr. Safety and efficacy of treatment of children and adolescents with elevated low density lipoprotein levels with a step two diet or with lovastatin. *Nutr Metab Cardiovasc Dis* 2001;11(suppl 5):30–34.

126. Dirisamer A, Hachemian N, Bucek RA, Wolf F, Reiter M, Widhalm K. The effect of low-dose simvastatin in children with familial hypercholesterolaemia: a 1-year observation. *Eur J Pediatr* 2003;162:421–425.

127. de Jongh S, Ose L, Szamosi T, et al for the Simvastatin in Children Study Group. Efficacy and safety of statin therapy in children with familial hypercholesterolemia: a randomized, double-blind, placebo-controlled trial with simvastatin. *Circulation* 2002;106:2231–2237.

128. Tonstad S. Stratification of risk in children with familial hypercholesterolemia with focus on psychosocial issues. *Nutr Metab Cardiovasc Dis* 2001;11(suppl 5):64–67.

APPENDIX 15-1 Foods to Provide to Decrease Saturated Fatty Acid and Total Fat Content of School Lunches

Milk
Low-fat milk (1%) or skim (nonfat) milk
Protein sources
Lean cuts of meat, such as round steak, round rump, round tip roast, tenderloin roast
Lean ground beef (<15% fat content) or soy protein added to fattier ground beef
Chicken or turkey without skin, baked, broiled, roasted, or boiled
Fresh or frozen fish, baked, broiled, or poached
Tuna fish or salmon
Cooked dry beans and peas, such as Great Northern, kidney, lima, navy, pinto, red, black, and garbanzo beans, black-eyed peas, lentils, and split peas
Low-fat and part-skim cheeses: farmer, cottage, part-skim ricotta and mozzarella
Peanut butter
Bread or bread alternatives
Breads and bread products: bagels, breads, graham crackers, muffins, rolls, and pancakes, including whole-grain or enriched products
Noodles, rice, barley, pasta, and bulgur
Fruits and vegetables
Fresh, frozen, dried, or canned fruit: apricots, cantaloupe, grapefruit, grapes, honeydew melon, peaches, plums, prunes, raisins, tangerines, strawberries
Fresh, frozen, or canned vegetables and salads: broccoli, brussels sprouts, cabbage, carrots, cauliflower, corn, green beans, green pepper, green peas, potatoes, lettuce, okra, spinach, sweet potatoes, tomatoes, winter squash, zucchini
Fats
Reduced-calorie and modified-fat, light, or low-sodium salad dressings and mayonnaise
Margarine
Liquid vegetable oils: canola, corn, cottonseed, olive, peanut, and safflower oils
Desserts/snacks
Baked goods low in fat: modified cakes and cookies, including angel-food cake, fig cookies, ginger snaps, oatmeal cookies, raisin cookies
Ice milk, sherbet, low-fat puddings, low-fat yogurt

SOURCE: Adapted, with permission, from the Child and Adolescent Trial for Cardiovascular Health (CATCH) *Eat Smart School Lunch Program Guide: A Guide for Nutrition Directors, Managers, and Cooks in Elementary School Cafeterias.* In: National Cholesterol Education Program.[103]

APPENDIX 15-2 Snack Food Consistent with Recommended Eating Pattern

1% low-fat or skim milk, low-fat cheese, low-fat or nonfat yogurt (plain or with fruit)
Fresh fruits and vegetables
Dried fruits
Fruit juices and vegetable juices; soda water with fruit juice added
Pretzels, popcorn popped in unsaturated oil, bagels, bagel chips (no fat added), baked tortilla chips
Chef's salads prepared with lean meat or water-packed tuna and low-fat cheese served with low-fat or fat-free salad dressing
Sandwiches made with sliced turkey, lean roast beef, lean ham, low-fat cold cuts, and tuna salad prepared with water-packed tuna and reduced-fat mayonnaise or salad dressing
Peanut butter* and jelly sandwiches
Hamburgers or sloppy joes made with lean, well-drained ground beef or ground turkey
Tacos made with lean, well-drained ground beef and soft corn tortillas with low-fat cheese or a small amount of regular cheese
Beef, chicken, or bean chalupa with baked (not fried) corn tortilla and low-fat cheese or a small amount of regular cheese
Pizza made with lean, well-drained ground beef and low-fat cheese or a small amount of regular cheese
Nachos with baked (not fried) corn tortilla chips and con queso made with low-fat cheese

(*continued*)

APPENDIX 15-2   *(Continued)*

| Cookies, cupcakes, and muffins prepared with unsaturated oil or margarine |
| Frozen yogurt (low-fat and nonfat), ice-milk, frozen fruit bars, sherbet, fruit sorbets, low-fat pudding pops |

*High in total fat; low in saturated fatty acids.

SOURCE: Adapted, with permission, from the Child and Adolescent Trial for Cardiovascular Health (CATCH) *Eat Smart School Lunch Program Guide: A Guide for Nutrition Directors, Managers, and Cooks in Elementary School Cafeterias.* In: National Cholesterol Education Program.[103]

APPENDIX 15-3   Sample Menus for Children 7 to 10 with School Lunch

Typical diet		Step 1 diet		Step 2 diet	
Breakfast at Home		**Breakfast at Home**		**Breakfast at Home**	
Orange juice ($\frac{1}{2}$ cup)		Orange juice ($\frac{1}{2}$ cup)		Orange juice ($\frac{1}{2}$ cup)	
Oatmeal w/maple and brown sugar (1 packet)		Oatmeal w/maple and brown sugar (1 packet)		Oatmeal w/maple and brown sugar (1 packet)	
Whole milk (1 cup)		1% milk (1 cup)		Margarine (2 tsp)	
				Skim milk (1 cup)	
School Lunch		**School Lunch**		**Bag Lunch**	
Oven fried chicken w/skin		Oven fried chicken w/skin		Ham sandwich	
Mashed potatoes ($\frac{1}{2}$ cup)		Mashed potatoes ($\frac{1}{2}$ cup)		Bread (2 slices)	
Green beans w/butter ($\frac{1}{2}$ cup)		Green beans w/butter ($\frac{1}{2}$ cup)		Lean ham (2 oz)	
Canned pear ($\frac{1}{2}$)		Canned pear ($\frac{1}{2}$)		Mayonnaise (2 tsp)	
Whole milk (1 cup)		2% milk (1 cup)		Lettuce, tomato, pickle	
				Banana (1 med)	
				Skim milk (1 cup)	
Snack at Home		**Snack at Home**		**Snack at Home**	
Ham sandwich		Turkey sandwich		Turkey sandwich	
Bread (2 slices)		Bread (2 slices)		Bread (2 slices)	
Ham juncheon meat (1 oz)		Turkey luncheon meat ($1\frac{1}{2}$ oz)		Turkey luncheon meat ($1\frac{1}{2}$ oz)	
Lettuce, tomato, pickle		Low-fat cheese (1 oz)		Low-fat cheese (1 oz)	
Mayonnaise ($\frac{1}{2}$ tbsp)		Lettuce, tomato, pickle		Lettuce, tomato, pickle	
Cola drink (1 can)		Mayonnaise (1 tsp)		margarine (1 tsp)	
		Cola drink (1 can)		Mayonnaise (1 tsp)	
				Cola drink (1 can)	
Dinner at Home		**Dinner at Home**		**Dinner at Home**	
Tuna macaroni casserole (1 serving)		Tuna macaroni casserole* (1 serving)		Tuna macaroni casserole† (1 serving)	
Carrots and peas ($\frac{1}{2}$ cup)		Carrots and peas ($\frac{1}{2}$ cup)		Carrots and peas ($\frac{1}{2}$ cup)	
Roll (1 small)		Roll (1 small)		Margarine (2 tsp)	
Applesauce ($\frac{1}{2}$ cup)		Margarine (1 tsp)		Applesauce ($\frac{1}{2}$ cup)	
Water		Applesauce ($\frac{1}{2}$ cup)		Water	
		Water			
Snack at Home		**Snack at Home**		**Snack at Home**	
Chocolate brownie (2 × 1 in.)		Oatmeal cookies, commercial (4 medium)		Oatmeal cookies, homemade† (4 medium)	
Whole milk (1 cup)		1% milk (1 cup)		Skim milk (1 cup)	
Calories	2008	**Calories**	2005	**Calories**	1966
Fat, % cal	35	**Fat, % cal**	29	**Fat, % cal**	29
SFA, % cal	15	**SFA, % cal**	11	**SFA, % cal**	7
Cholesterol, mg	261	**Cholesterol, mg**	118	**Cholesterol, mg**	126

*Stick margarine used for food preparation.
†Tub margarine used for food preparation.

SOURCE: Adapted, with permission, from the National Cholesterol Education Program.[105]

APPENDIX 15-4 Sample Menus for Girls 11 to 14 with Fast Food Lunch

Typical diet		Step 1 diet		Step 2 diet	
Breakfast at Home		**Breakfast at Home**		**Breakfast at Home**	
Orange juice (1 cup)		Orange juice (1 cup)		Orange juice (1 cup)	
Presweetened cereal (1 cup)		Corn flakes ($\frac{3}{4}$ cup)		Corn flakes ($\frac{3}{4}$ cup)	
Whole milk (1 cup)		1% milk (1 cup)		Skim milk (1 cup)	
				English muffin ($\frac{1}{2}$)	
				Margarine‡ (1 tsp)	
Fast Food Lunch		**Fast Food Lunch**		**Sandwich Shop**	
Cheeseburger		Hamburger ($\frac{1}{4}$ 1b)		Tuna sandwich: Bread (2 slices) Tuna, water	
French fries (1 regular order)		French fries (1 regular order)		pack (3 oz) Tomato, celery, relish	
Catsup (3 packets)		Lettuce, tomato, onion, catsup		Mayonnaise (4 tsp)	
Cola drink (1 small)		Animal crackers ($\frac{1}{2}$ box)		Pretzels ($\frac{3}{4}$-oz bag)	
		Cola drink (1 medium)		Oatmeal cookies, homemade‡ (4)	
				Cola drink (1 medium)	
Snack at Home		**Snack at Home**		**Snack at Home**	
Ginger snaps (2 medium)		Multigrain low-fat crackers (4)		Multigrain low-fat crackers (4)	
Club soda (1 can)		Low-fat cheese ($\frac{3}{4}$ oz)		Low-fat cheese ($\frac{3}{4}$ oz)	
		Club soda (1 can)		Club soda (1 can)	
Dinner at Home		**Dinner at Home**		**Dinner at Home**	
Fried chicken breast, breaded and		Broiled chicken, breast, no skin (3 oz)		Broiled chicken, breast, no skin (3 oz)	
fried in shortening, skin eaten		Boiled potato† (1)		Boiled potato‡ (1)	
Boiled potato* (1)		Broccoli spears† (4)		Broccoli spears‡ (4)	
Broccoli spears* ($\frac{1}{2}$ cup)		Tomato (4 slices)		Tomato (4 slices)	
Roll (1 small)		Bread (1 slice)		Bread (1 slice)	
Margarine† (1 tsp)		Strawberries ($\frac{1}{2}$ cup)		Margarine‡ (2 tsp)	
Iced tea (1 cup)		Nonfat yogurt (1 container)		Strawberries ($\frac{1}{2}$ cup)	
		Water		Nonfat yogurt (1 container)	
				Water	
Snack at Home		**Snack at Home**		**Snack at Home**	
American cheese ($\frac{3}{4}$ oz)		Cupcake, commercial (1)		Cupcake, homemade (1)	
Crackers (4)		1% milk (1 cup)		Skim milk (1 cup)	
Fruit drink ($\frac{1}{2}$ cup)					
Calories	2219	**Calories**	2240	**Calories**	2248
Fat, % cal	35	**Fat, % cal**	29	**Fat, % cal**	27
SFA, % cal	15	**SFA, % cal**	10	**SFA, % cal**	6
Cholesterol, mg	264	**Cholesterol, mg**	188	**Cholesterol, mg**	159

*Seasoned with butter.
†Stick margarine used in food preparation.
‡Tub margarine used in food preparation.
SOURCE: Adapted, with permission, from the National Cholesterol Education Program.[105]

APPENDIX 15-5   Sample Menus for 15- to 19-Year-Old Males with Fast Food Lunch

Typical diet	Step 1 diet	Step 2 diet
Breakfast at Home	**Breakfast at Home**	**Breakfast at Home**
Orange juice (1 cup)	Orange juice (1 cup)	Orange juice (1 cup)
Granola cereal ($\frac{1}{2}$ cup)	Presweetened corn flakes	Presweetened corn flakes
	($\frac{3}{4}$ cup)	($\frac{3}{4}$ cup)
Whole milk (1 cup)	Margarine (1 tsp)	Margarine (2 tsp)
	Bagel (1)	Bagel (1)
	1% milk (1 cup)	Skim milk (1 cup)
Fast Food Lunch	**Sandwich Shop**	**Sandwich Shop**
Hot dog on bun w/chili (1)	Roast beef sandwich	Roast beef sandwich
Potato chips (1 oz)	Tossed salad (2 cups)	Tossed salad (2 cups)
Cola drink (12 fl oz)	Thousand Island dressing	Thousand Island dressing
	(2 tbsp)	(3 tbsp)
	Corn chips (1-oz bag)	Medium cola drink
	Medium cola drink	
Snack at Home	**Snack at Home**	**Snack at Home**
Chocolate candy bar (2 oz)	Ham and cheese sandwich	Turkey and cheese sandwich
Cola drink (12 fl oz)	Bread (2 slices)	Bread (2 slices)
	Low-fat ham (1 oz)	Turkey breast (1 oz)
	Low-fat cheese (1 oz)	Low-fat cheese (1 oz)
	Mayonnaise (2 tsp)	Lettuce, tomato, pickle
	Lettuce, tomato, pickles	Mayonnaise (2 tsp)
	Oatmeal cookies, commercial (4)	Pretzels ($\frac{3}{4}$ oz bag)
	Orange juice (1 cup)	Gingersnaps (5)
		Orange juice (1 cup)
Dinner at Home	**Dinner at Home**	**Dinner at Home**
Beef lasagna (4 × 3 in.)	Chicken cacciatore (3 oz)	Chicken cacciatore (3 oz)
Tossed salad (2 cups)	Green beans ($\frac{1}{2}$ cup)*	Green beans ($\frac{1}{2}$ cup)[†]
Thousand Island dressing (3 tbsp)	Rice, white (1 cup)	Rice, white (1 cup)[†]
French bread (1 slice)	Margarine (1 tsp)	Margarine (1$\frac{1}{2}$ tsp)[†]
Brownies (2 each 2 × 1 in.)	Bread (1 slice)	Bread (1 slice)
Whole milk (1 cup)	Grapes (15)	Grapes (15)
	Nonfat yogurt w/fruit flavor	Nonfat yogurt w/fruit flavor
	(1 cup)	(1 cup)
	Water	Water
Snack at Home	**Snack at Home**	**Snack at Home**
Frozen yogurt (1 cup)	Peanut butter cookies, homemade (6)	Apple pie, homemade,[†] single crust
Cola drink (12 fl oz)	1% milk (1 cup)	($\frac{1}{8}$ or 9-in.)
		Skim milk (1 cup)
Calories 2998	**Calories** 3026	**Calories** 2993
Fat, % cal 36	**Fat, % cal** 30	**Fat, % cal** 29
SFA, % cal 15	**SFA, % cal** 9	**SFA, % cal** 7
Cholesterol, mg 258	**Cholesterol, mg** 224	**Cholesterol, mg** 157

*Stick margarine used for food preparation.
[†]Tub margarine used for food preparation.
SOURCE: Adapted, with permission, from the National Cholesterol Education Program.[105]

Women

16

Karol E. Watson

KEY POINTS

- *Each year in the United States more than 250,000 women die of coronary heart disease.*

- *Symptoms of coronary heart disease differ in men and women, and unfortunately, noninvasive assessment of coronary heart disease in women has proven to be difficult.*

- *Although women with coronary artery disease have risk factor profiles similar to those of men, the quantitative impact of a particular risk factor on overall coronary heart disease risks may be different. For instance, diabetes is an even more powerful risk factor for coronary heart disease in women than it is in men.*

- *Perhaps the biggest change in preventive cardiology for women to occur in the past decade*

has been in the use of postmenopausal hormone replacement therapy. Because of recent clinical trial data it is now recommended that hormone replacement therapy not be initiated for either the primary or secondary prevention of cardiovascular disease.

- *Given the disappointing data on hormone replacement therapy, there has been increasing interest in the potential cardiovascular effects of selective estrogen receptor modulators, which has been promising.*

- *Although the lifetime risk of developing coronary heart disease is at least one in three for women, many women (and some health care providers) are unaware that coronary heart disease is a woman's greatest threat to life.*

INTRODUCTION

Each year in the United States, more than 250,000 women die of coronary heart disease (CHD).[1] Despite this fact, heart disease is still often considered primarily a "man's disease" and is usually diagnosed later and treated less aggressively in women than in men. Though many similarities exist in CHD between the sexes, several important differences exist as well. Important differences include:

- Differences in presentation and symptomatology
- Differences in the accuracy of noninvasive tests
- Differential impact of risk factors
- Influence of reproductive hormones

- Gender disparities in cardiovascular care
- Underestimation of cardiac risk

DIFFERENCES IN PRESENTATION AND SYMPTOMATOLOGY

Follow-up data from the Framingham Heart study have given us great insight into sex-specific patterns of CHD.[2] In the Framingham study, men were found to have about twice the total incidence of morbidity from CHD, but this sex differential diminished significantly after approximately 45 years of age. In general, women lag behind men in first presentation of CHD by about 10 years,[2] but after menopause there is a rapid increase in CHD morbidity and mortality such that CHD rates elderly men and women are similar (Table 16-1). Another important

TABLE 16-1   Mortality Rates (per 100,000 Population) for Diseases of the Heart by Gender

Age range	Mortality rate		Male/Female ratio
	Men	Women	
35–44	41.7	17.6	2.37
45–54	136.6	50.7	2.69
55–64	349.8	151.8	2.30
65–74	851.3	455.9	1.86
75–84	2177.3	1428.9	1.52
>85	6040.5	5506.8	1.10

SOURCE: Data from National Vital Statistics Reports, vol 52, number 9. November 7, 2003.

finding from the Framingham study is that despite there being fewer cases of CHD in women, the case fatality rate for women exceeds that for men (32% vs 27%).[2] Other studies have produced similar findings.[3–5] For instance, in the Global Utilization of Streptokinase and Tissue Plasminogen Activator for Occluded Coronary Arteries (GUSTO-I) trial, women were found to have higher mortality rates after acute myocardial infarction at all ages, with the greatest differences being at the younger ages.[3] Because of the higher case fatality rate, and because the number of elderly women exceeds that of elderly men in the United States, since 1984 the number of cardiovascular deaths for females has exceeded the number of deaths for males.[1]

Symptoms of CHD have been found by several studies to differ in men and women. Men are more likely to have "typical" chest pain consisting of retrosternal location, aggravation by exertion, and relief by rest.[6] Women, on the other hand, are more likely than men to report chest pain during rest, sleep, or periods of mental stress.[7] Women also are more likely to have neck pain, shoulder pain, nausea, vomiting, fatigue, or dyspnea in addition to chest pain during an acute myocardial infarction.[8,9]

DIFFERENCES IN ACCURACY OF NONINVASIVE TESTS

A critical first step toward improving CHD outcomes in women is accurate diagnosis. The mainstay of early diagnosis is noninvasive testing: primarily exercise electrocardiography and exercise imaging studies such as stress echocardiography and myocardial perfusion imaging. Unfortunately, noninvasive assessment of CHD in women has proven to be difficult. Studies have shown that the accuracy of noninvasive testing is lower for women than for men.[10] Exercise electrocardiography (ECG) has been the most studied exercise test in women.

Both specificity and sensitivity for detection of coronary artery disease (CAD) by exercise ECG have been found to be lower in women than in men. In the Coronary Artery Surgery Study (CASS), for instance, the sensitivity of exercise ECG in women was 76%, and the specificity was 64%; in men, the sensitivity was 80%, and the specificity was 74%.[11] Some of the causes for this lower sensitivity and specificity in women are a lower prevalence of multivessel CAD,[12] submaximal performance on treadmill or bicycle stress protocols, and greater incidence of false-positive ST segment depression during stress ECG in women.[13]

Combining a form of imaging (eg, radionuclide or echocardiography) with exercise stress testing provides increased accuracy. Radionuclide perfusion and ventriculography studies identify areas of ischemic or infarcted myocardium because the radioisotope (usually thallium or sestamibi) is taken up only by myocardium with blood flow. Use of radionuclide imaging, however, poses unique problems in women. Breast tissue can cause anterior perfusion artifacts that are actually secondary to attenuation of the radioactivity, not decreased myocardial perfusion. This can lead to a falsely positive test, and is even more problematic in obese patients and in women with dense or extensive breast tissue. Fortunately, in recent years, problems with breast attenuation have decreased with the use of technetium sestamibi and improved attenuation correction algorithms.

Only a small number of studies have examined the accuracy of exercise thallium tests in women, and fewer studies have examined exercise sestamibi. Reported sensitivity and specificity vary between studies, but, in general, are improved compared with exercise ECG.[14–17] The reported sensitivities in women range from 71 to 95%, and the reported specificities range from 61 to 91%.

In exercise echocardiography, ultrasound is used to directly visualize cardiac wall motion. The diagnosis of CAD is made by the observation of wall motion abnormalities at baseline or with exercise. Although stress echocardiography has not been studied as extensively as stress nuclear imaging, results from the available studies suggest sensitivity as high as 88% and specificity as high as 84%.[18]

Pharmacologic stress testing in conjunction with an imaging modality is an alternative to conventional exercise stress testing in patients unable to exercise. Commonly used agents include adenosine, dipyridamole, and dobutamine. Although pharmacologic stress testing may yield comparable diagnostic results in terms of identifying CAD, it is unable to provide other useful information for prognosis or management of CHD. Exercise stress testing can provide information such as functional capacity, heart rate and blood pressure response, and symptom evaluation; therefore, exercise is preferred in all patients able to exercise adequately.

DIFFERENTIAL IMPACT OF RISK FACTORS

Although women with CHD have risk factor profiles similar to those of men, the quantitative impact of a particular risk factor on overall CHD risks may differ between men and women.

Cigarette smoking

In the past several decades, the prevalence of cigarette smoking has declined. The decline, however, has been much more dramatic in men (21% decrease) than in women (6% decrease).[19] Furthermore, although smoking among women overall has declined, the incidence of cigarette smoking among *young* women has actually increased.[20] Of concern, 25% of women still smoke,[21] and smoking is one of the major risk factors for CHD occurring in premenopausal women. In the Framingham Heart Study, smoking was associated with an increased risk of CHD death in all women, particularly in premenopausal women.[22] Younger women appear to be particularly vulnerable to the effects of cigarette smoking and the risk appears to be dose-related. Rosenberg and colleagues demonstrated that angina, myocardial infarction (MI), and CHD deaths were related to the number of cigarettes smoked per day by women, and smoking as few as one to four cigarettes per day raised the relative risk of fatal CHD and nonfatal MI by 2.4-fold.[23] Despite advertising to the contrary, low-nicotine cigarettes do not decrease the risk associated with smoking. In the Framingham Heart Study, smoking filtered cigarettes actually led to an increased risk of CHD as compared with smoking conventional cigarettes.[24] The good news, however, is that research suggests that smoking cessation can normalize the relative risk of CHD after as few as 2 years of abstinence.[25]

Cholesterol

Before age 20, men and women have similar lipid profiles; from 20 to 55 years of age, men tend to have higher total cholesterol levels than women, and after 55 years of age, women's cholesterol levels increase rapidly and may slightly exceed those of men.[26] Women's levels of high-density lipoprotein cholesterol (HDL-C) are typically higher than those of men, and they continue to exceed men's HDL-C levels by approximately 10 mg/dL throughout much of life. Nonetheless, absolute levels of HDL-C decline following menopause, and begin to equalize between the sexes at about age 70.[26] Premenopausal women have lower triglyceride levels than men and postmenopausal women; however, with aging, triglyceride levels increase more in women than they do in men.[27,28]

As is true for men, increased total cholesterol, decreased HDL-C, and increased triglyceride levels are risk factors for CHD in women. HDL-C and triglyceride levels, in fact, appear to be even more powerful predictors of CHD in women.[29] In the Framingham study, for every 10 mg/dL increase in HDL-C, there was a 40 to 50% decrease in CHD events for women.[30] In Framingham, a triglyceride level greater than 150 mg/dL was an independent risk factor for CHD.[30]

Women have now been studied in several large randomized, controlled trials of lipid-lowering therapy. The first large lipid-lowering trial using statin medication was the 4S trial. The 4S trial was a secondary-prevention study of 4444 patients who had angina or prior MI and elevated cholesterol. Overall, after a 5.4-year follow-up, this study showed a relative risk of cardiac death of 0.70 in the subjects randomized to receive the statin.[31] In a subgroup analysis of 420 women in the treatment group (vs 407 on placebo), the relative risk of CHD mortality was 0.86 (95% confidence interval [CI] = 0.42−1.74). Another large statin trial was the Cholesterol and Recurrent Events (CARE) study. The CARE study evaluated 4159 subjects with prior MI but only modestly elevated cholesterol levels, and found that after 5 years of treatment with a statin, both men and women had fewer cardiovascular events.[32] In a substudy of the 576 women enrolled in the CARE trial, it was found that within 6 to 12 months of beginning therapy, women randomized to the statin had a 43% lower risk of death from CHD and a 57% reduction in recurrent MI. Another secondary prevention trial, the large-scale Long-Term Intervention with Pravastatin in Ischaemic Disease (LIPID) study, analyzed a subgroup of 1516 women and found that the benefit women received from lipid-lowering therapy with a statin was similar to the benefit measured in men.[33] The first primary prevention statin trial to include women was the Air Force/Texas Coronary Atherosclerosis Prevention Study (AFCAPS/TEXCAPS).[34] In this study, statin therapy was given to 997 postmenopausal women who had no clinical evidence of CVD, average LDL-C levels, and below-average HDL-C levels. With statin therapy, risk for a first major coronary event was reduced and the reduction was comparable in men and women.

The largest number of women studied in a lipid-lowering trial was evaluated in the Heart Protection Study (HPS). The HPS evaluated individuals at risk for CHD regardless of their baseline cholesterol levels. In HPS, a total of 5082 women were randomized to statin therapy and followed-up for approximately 6 years.[35] This study found a significant 24% reduction in major vascular events for both men and women, with no apparent difference by sex.

All of these studies demonstrate a beneficial role for statin therapy in patients at risk for CHD, regardless of sex.

Hypertension

Men with hypertension outnumber women with hypertension during young adulthood and early middle age, but after the age of menopause, hypertensive women outnumber hypertensive men.[36] The prevalence of hypertension, in fact, reaches as high as 80% in women 75 years of age or older. African-Americans have higher rates of hypertension than do whites for both genders.[37]

Hypertension has long been known to be a significant risk factor for stroke. It is also a significant risk factor for CHD and heart failure. The relative risk for CHD contributed by hypertension was shown to be elevated in the Framingham Heart Study.[38] Another analysis of the Framingham Heart Study found that hypertension was a more important predictor of future heart failure in women than was MI.[39] The opposite was true for men, with prior MI being a stronger predictor of future heart failure than hypertension. This likely reflects the greater prevalence of heart failure with preserved systolic function (diastolic heart failure) in women as compared with men, and the fact that hypertension is a prime contributor to diastolic heart failure.

Another important point is that even within the prehypertensive range, higher blood pressure levels result in greater risk of CVD. Control of hypertension has been shown to reduce the risk of stroke or death in older as well as in younger persons, and in men as well as women, and in those with only stage 1 hypertension as well as stage 2.[41–43]

As is true with men, however, hypertension treatment and control rates for women are not optimal in current clinical practice. Hypertension control rates were evaluated in older women enrolled in the Women's Health Initiative (WHI) study.[44] The WHI observational study cohort consisted of nearly 100,000 postmenopausal women in the United States, both with and without known heart disease. In this study, in two thirds of the hypertensive women, hypertension was not adequately controlled. Though hypertension is less common in younger women, it appears to be even more dangerous. In premenopausal women, hypertension leads to as much as a 10-fold increase in the rate of CHD mortality as compared with the rate of young women without hypertension.[45]

Also of interest in premenopausal women is the potential impact of oral contraceptive agents on the incidence of hypertension. Older formulations of oral contraceptives containing high doses of estrogen induced hypertension in approximately 5% of users.[46] The newer, lower-dose oral contraceptives, however, have been shown to cause only minimal, clinically insignificant elevations in blood pressure.[47,48] Therefore, women with well-controlled hypertension can usually tolerate oral contraceptive agents but should be monitored during therapy. For blood pressure control, diuretics may be a good choice in women taking oral contraceptives, because any mild increase in blood pressure caused by oral contraceptives may be due to volume expansion.[49]

Because of potential teratogenic effects, angiotensin-converting enzyme inhibitors and angiotensin receptor blockers are contraindicated in pregnancy.

Diabetes

Diabetes is an even more powerful risk factor for CHD in women than it is in men. The Framingham Heart Study found that men with diabetes had a 2.4-fold increased risk of developing CHD as compared with men without diabetes; by contrast, women with diabetes had a 5.4-fold increased risk for CHD as compared with women without diabetes.[50] In addition, the Nurses' Health Study reported a 6.3-fold increased risk for total cardiovascular mortality among women with, as compared to those without,[51] diabetes. Notably, in this study, even if a woman had been diagnosed with diabetes less than 4 years, the risk of CHD was significantly elevated. Furthermore, although women typically develop CHD 10 years later in life than do men, women with diabetes have rates of CHD equivalent to those of men of a comparable age; in other words, they lose their gender protection.[52] This means that whatever protection from CHD is afforded premenopausal women appears to be completely lost if that woman has diabetes. Why the risk is markedly increased among women with diabetes is not completely understood; however, it may, at least in part, be due to the fact that diabetes is usually associated with other cardiac risk factors such as obesity, hypertension, low HDL-C, and high triglycerides.

The United Kingdom Prospective Diabetes Study (UKPDS) was a large treatment trial of 5208 patients with type 2 diabetes. The 2693 patients from this group in whom baseline risk factors were assessed were analyzed to determine the risk factors that best predicted CHD in the patients (41.8% women) with type 2 diabetes evaluated in this study.[53] The investigators found that high LDL-C, low HDL-C, and high hemoglobin A_{1c} levels, hypertension, and smoking are all related to the development of CHD. It is, therefore, important that all of these risk factors be addressed in women to reduce the negative impact of diabetes on development of CHD.

Metabolic syndrome

The metabolic syndrome (MetS) is an aggregation of metabolic abnormalities that tend to congregate and that have been shown to greatly increase the risk of CHD.[54] The syndrome, as defined by the National Cholesterol Education Program, is diagnosed when the or more of the following five abnormalities are found in a patient[55]:

- Waist circumference greater than 102 cm (40.2 in.) in men or greater than 88 cm (34.6 in.) in women
- Serum triglyceride level of 150 mg/dL (1.69 mmol/L) or greater
- HDL-C level less than 40 mg/dL (1.04 mmol/L) in men or less than 50 mg/dL (1.29 mmol/L) in women
- Blood pressure greater than 130 mm Hg systolic/greater than 85 mm Hg diastolic
- Serum glucose level of 110 mg/dL (6.1 mmol/L) or greater

The metabolic syndrome illustrates how multiple, subtle risk factors can combine to form a significantly elevated CHD risk. The overall prevalence of MetS is quite high in the United States, with 24% of men and 23.4% of women meeting criteria.[56] The prevalence increases with advancing age, and for certain ethnic populations, the gender gap is significant. Among African-Americans, for instance, women have a 57% higher prevalence of MetS than do men; and among Mexican-Americans, women have a 26% higher prevalence than men.[56] There is evidence that the genetic basis of MetS may be strongly modified by gender. McCarthy and colleagues surveyed 207 single-nucleotide polymorphisms in 110 candidate genes among a patient population enriched for MetS.[57] They found a strong association with a silent polymorphism in the LDL receptor-related protein gene among females, but not males. Other atherosclerosis-related genes associated with MetS only in females included thrombospondin 1, acyl-coenzyme A:cholesterol acyltransferase 2, integrin $\beta3$, and P selectin.

As physical inactivity and excess weight are the primary underlying contributors to the development of MetS, increased exercise and weight loss are essential to reducing or preventing the complications associated with this condition.[55] Counseling women as to the importance of weight loss and exercise is paramount in preventing the CHD and other risks associated with MetS.

Family history

The relationship between a family history of premature CHD and the occurrence of MI has not been studied as extensively in women as it has in men. Some studies have shown a strong association between family history of premature CHD and coronary events in women, whereas others have not.

In a retrospective chart review performed by De and colleagues, female patients aged 45 years or younger with ʜain were studied. Angiographically critical CAD in 29% of the women. The most common

cardiac risk factor was a family history of premature CAD (67%), followed by smoking (55%) and dyslipidemia (55%).[58]

In the Nurses' Health Study, researchers examined nearly 122,000 women between the ages of 30 and 55 years and found that women whose parents had a history of MI prior to 60 years of age had a 5-fold increased risk for fatal CHD, whereas those whose parents had a history of MI *after* age 61 had a 2.6-fold increased risk.[59] Another study followed more than 4000 men and women aged 40 to 79 years longer than 9 years. In this study, a positive family history of premature CHD was significantly associated with an excess risk of cardiovascular and CHD death in men, but not in women.[60] Other data suggest that a positive family history is more potent of a risk factor depending on whom the affected family member is (ie, sibling vs parent or male vs female). One study demonstrated that having a female relative with premature CHD was a more potent risk factor for women than for men. In this study, the risk of early-onset CHD was increased 2.7-fold for female and 1.6-fold for male first-degree relatives of women with confirmed coronary death before age 55.[61]

Obesity

Published research on the effect of obesity on a woman's relative risk for CHD has been contradictory. One large prospective study of 262,019 women and 62,116 men aged 30 to 85 showed that the greater the body mass index, the higher the CVD mortality. This association held up to the age of 75.[62] The Framingham Heart Study noted a twofold increased risk of CHD for obese versus nonobese women.[63] The Nurses' Health Study found that obese women had a similar twofold elevated risk, which persisted after controlling for other risk factors.[64] Several retrospective case–control studies, however, have not found a significant relationship between obesity and CHD. It may be that distribution of body fat is as important as total body fat. Several investigators have found that the waist-to-hip ratio of fat is correlated with CHD events in women better than is total fat.[65] In general, waist circumference, an indicator of both central and general obesity, appears to be a stronger predictor of CHD than does body mass index.

INFLUENCE OF SEX HORMONES

Hormone replacement therapy

Without question, the biggest change in preventive cardiology for women to occur in the past decade has been in the use of postmenopausal hormone replacement therapy. Hormone replacement therapy had been recommended as a measure to prevent CHD in postmenopausal women on the basis of more than 30 observational studies that had suggested that estrogen prevented heart disease in postmenopausal women.[66] Furthermore, multiple beneficial effects of estrogen on surrogate markers such as lipids and vascular reactivity had been documented in clinical and basic science studies.[67–69]

Therefore, when the first large randomized, placebo-controlled clinical trial in women assigned to hormones versus placebo was performed, the results were very surprising. The Heart and Estrogen/Progestin Replacement Study (HERS)[70] began in 1993 and evaluated 2763 women who had an intact uterus and documented CHD, and were assigned to either one tablet daily containing 0.625 mg of conjugated equine estrogen (CEE) plus 2.5 mg of medroxyprogesterone acetate or placebo. The primary outcome evaluated was a combined endpoint of nonfatal MI and CHD death. After an average follow-up of 4.1 years, the study was closed. The investigators found that there was no difference between the two groups in the primary CHD outcome nor in any other cardiovascular endpoint. In fact, in the first year of the trial, there was actually a statistically significant, 52% excess risk of CHD events in women on hormone treatment. The HERS results were not only surprising, but also quite unpopular, and early on the trial was criticized for many reasons. Though most observers were surprised by the HERS results, there had been earlier suggestions that perhaps hormones might cause cardiovascular harm.[71] A review of 22 small published trials in 4124 women measured a 39% increased risk of CVD after use of hormone therapy.[72]

Furthermore, an earlier trial in humans, the Coronary Drug Project,[73] found estrogen to cause more cardiovascular harm than benefit. In this study, *men* with known heart disease were randomly assigned to receive one of five active therapies or placebo. Two arms of this trial studied CEE, at a daily dose of either 2.5 or 5.0 mg. Both of the estrogen arms of this trial were prematurely terminated because the estrogen-treated men had an increased rate of thromboembolic events and MIs. A reanalysis of data from the Coronary Drug Project revealed a significant increase in cardiovascular events in the first 4 months of therapy, a time frame similar to that during the early risks were present in HERS.[74] At the time, little was made of the estrogen findings of the Coronary Drug Project; however, since the publication of HERS, they add to the weight of evidence against hormone therapy in secondary prevention of CHD.

After publication of HERS, other secondary prevention trials were published as well. These trials evaluated different hormone preparations and assessed different outcomes, yet they all also showed no benefit from hormone replacement therapy. The Papworth Hormone-Replacement Therapy Atherosclerosis Survival Enquiry (PHASE)[75] treated subjects with transdermal estradiol plus norethisterone and assessed fatal and nonfatal CHD, including hospitalization for unstable angina, as the primary outcome. They found no benefit with hormone therapy. The Estrogen Replacement and Atherosclerosis (ERA)[76] study treated women with CEE with or without medroxyprogesterone acetate and assessed quantitative coronary angiography as the primary outcome. They again found no benefit from hormones. The Women's Estrogen and Stroke Trial (WEST)[77] treated women with oral 17ß-estradiol, assessed stroke as the primary outcome, and found no benefit with hormones.

Another popular explanation for the lack of benefit of CEE in these trials was that hormone therapy was not carried out long enough. Although evidence was striking for an early cardiovascular hazard with hormone therapy, many felt that with continued hormone treatment, cardiovascular benefit would be revealed. The hypothesis that there may be late benefit from hormone replacement therapy in secondary prevention was refuted by the open-label HERS-II study.[78] In HERS-II, the majority of surviving participants in the original HERS study were followed for a mean of almost 3 additional years. During this follow-up, no cardiovascular benefit was detected in either on-treatment analysis or intention-to-treat analysis.

Although the secondary prevention studies were uniform in their findings of no cardiovascular benefits from hormones, a continued popular explanation for the absent benefit was the belief that in the secondary prevention trials, hormone therapy had been started too late in the course of atherosclerosis to alter the natural history and, thus, too late to show benefit. Therefore, many scientists and clinicians alike waited eagerly for results from a primary prevention study. This study was the Women's Health Initiative (WHI).[79] In the WHI, 16,608 patients were randomized to receive hormone replacement therapy (0.625 mg CEE plus 2.5 mg medroxyprogesterone acetate in a once-daily tablet) or placebo. The trial was scheduled for completion in 2005; however, the Estrogen–progestin component of the trial was halted in July 2002, after a mean of 5.2 years of follow-up, when an interim analysis discovered that the preset boundary for excess invasive breast cancer risk was exceeded in the hormone replacement therapy group. Earlier in the trial, participants were also notified that an increased risk for MI, stroke, and pulmonary embolism had been observed in the combination hormone arm, but that the study was being continued because the potential later benefits might still exceed the risks. The WHI results are summarized in Table 16-2. The excess risk for cardiovascular events had been detected as early as 1999, but the preset boundary for cardiovascular risk had not yet been reached when the study was prematurely terminated in 2002. A recent follow-up report[80] of the cardiovascular results further documented these findings: combined estrogen–progestin therapy was associated with a hazard

TABLE 16-2 Summary of Results from the Women's Health Initiative Study

Outcome	Combined estrogen–progestin clinical trial component			
	CEE* + MPA %	Placebo %	RR %	AR %
CHD	1.93	1.50	↑29	↑0.43
Stroke	1.49	1.05	↑42	↑0.44
PE	0.82	0.38	↑116	↑0.44
DVT	1.35	0.64	↑111	↑0.71
Total CVD	8.16	6.74	↑21	↑1.42
Breast cancer	1.95	1.53	↑27	↑0.42
Colorectal cancer	0.53	0.83	↓36	↓0.3
Hip fracture	0.52	0.77	↓33	↓0.25
All fractures	7.64	9.73	↓22	↓2.09

*CEE, conjugated equine estrogens; MPA, medroxyprogesterone acetate; RR, relative risk; AR, absolute risk; DVT, deep venous thrombosis; PE, pulmonary embolism; CVD, cardiovascular disease.
SOURCE: Adapted, with permission, from the Writing Group for the Women's Health Initiative Investigators.[79]

ratio for CHD of 1.24 (95% CI = 1.00–1.54), with risk especially elevated in the first year (hazard ratio = 1.81, CI = 1.09–3.01), and treatment-related risk held in most subgroups of women. In a similar report on stroke 0.82 (0.4–1.56) risks, the treatment-related hazard ratio was 1.44 (CI = 1.09–1.90) for ischemic strokes and for hemorrhagic strokes, with an excess risk seen in all age groups, those with and without hypertension, prior cardiovascular disease, and hormone, statin, or aspirin use.[81] In the WHI, there was also an estrogen-alone arm, in which women who had had a hysterectomy before joining the trial were randomized to receive either 0.625 mg CEE or placebo. In the estrogen-only arm of the study, although there were significant differences in the incidence of breast or overall cancer between women receiving estrogen and those receiving placebo, unfavorable increases in the risk of stroke (relative risk = 1.39, 95% CI = 1.10–1.77) and overall CVD (relative risk = 1.12, 95% CI = 1.01–1.24) led to discontinuation of this component too in February 2004.[82]

The results of the WHI are consistent with results of the secondary prevention studies, and confirm that hormone replacement therapy should not be started for the primary or secondary prevention of CHD. It should, however, be remembered that the absolute risks conferred by hormone therapy were quite small for any individual woman. In the WHI, 97% of the women had no adverse event. The WHI results suggest that if 10,000 women were treated with the combination hormone regimen for 1 year, there would be 7 excess CHD events, 8 excess strokes, 8 excess pulmonary emboli, 18 excess venous thromboembolic events, and 8 excess breast cancers. By contrast, there would be 6 fewer colorectal cancers and

5 fewer hip fractures.[79] For women on estrogen alone, there would be an excess risk of 12 additional strokes per 10,000 person-years (although a reduction of 6 hip fractures for the same exposure).[82]

Given the currently available data on hormone replacement therapy and CHD, the following recommendations can be made:

- Hormone replacement therapy should not be initiated for either primary or secondary prevention of CVD.
- If a woman develops an acute CVD event while undergoing hormone replacement therapy, discontinuation of the therapy should be considered.
- Initiation and administration of hormone replacement therapy should be based on weighing established benefits against established risks, considering other available options, and taking into account patient preference.

Selective estrogen receptor modulators

Given the disappointing data on hormone replacement therapy, there has been increasing interest in the potential cardiovascular effects of selective estrogen receptor modulators (SERMs). SERMs have been shown to have favorable effects on some cardiovascular risk factors. The SERM raloxifene has been shown to significantly lower total cholesterol, LDL-C, lipoprotein(a), and fibrinogen levels. Raloxifene does not appear to increase triglyceride concentrations as do estrogens; however, it also does not appear to have the same favorable effects on HDL-C as do estrogens.[83] It is not yet known what effect SERMS will have on CHD morbidity and mortality; however, a recent trial suggests potential benefits. The

Multiple Outcomes of Raloxifene Evaluation (MORE) trial was a 4-year osteoporosis treatment study in 7705 postmenopausal women.[84] Patients were randomly assigned to receive raloxifene 60 mg/d ($n = 2557$), raloxifene 120 mg/d ($n = 2572$), or placebo ($n = 2576$) for 4 years. At the study's conclusion, the researchers found that raloxifene therapy did not significantly affect the risk of cardiovascular events in the overall MORE study population. Even more promising was the fact that, in a subset of 1035 MORE participants who were at increased risk for CVD, raloxifene reduced the risk of cardiovascular events by 40%. Furthermore, there was no evidence that raloxifene caused an early increase in the risk of cardiovascular events in either the overall MORE population or the high-risk subset. These preliminary data must be confirmed in larger randomized, controlled trials such as the Raloxifene for the Heart (RUTH) study. In RUTH, 10,101 women with CHD or at risk for CHD are being treated with raloxifene 60 mg/d or placebo and followed for 5 to 7 years.

Oral contraceptives

A link between oral contraceptives (OCs) and acute myocardial infarction was suggested in the 1970's when these agents contained much higher doses of estrogens. Since that time, it has been found that myocardial infarctions are extremely rare in women using newer OCs, containing lower doses of hormones. With current OC therapy, CHD incidence rates rise above 4 per 100,000 per year only among OC users who smoke.[85] In women under the age of 35 who are nonsmokers, are normotensive, and have no other cardiovascular risk factors (diabetes, hyperlipidemia, smoking, etc), there is a very low risk of CHD.

TABLE 16-3   Spectrum of Cardiovascular Disease Risk in Women

Risk group	Framingham global risk (10-y absolute CHD risk)	Clinical examples
High Risk	>20%	• Established CHD* • Cardiovascular disease† • Peripheral arterial disease • Abdominal aortic aneurysm • Diabetes melitus • Chronic kidney disease ‡
Intermediate risk	10 to 20%	• Subclinical CVD§ (eg. coronary calcifiation) • Metabolic syndrome • Multiple risk factors∥ • Markedly elevated levels of a single risk factor¶ • First-degree relative(s) with early-onset (age <55 in men and <65 in women) atherosclerotic CHD
Lower risk	<10%	• May include women with multiple risk factors, metabolic syndrome, or one or no risk factor
Optimal risk	<10%	• Optimal levels of risk factors and heart-healthy lifestyle

*CHD, coronary heart disease; CVD cardiovascular disease.
†Cerebrovascular disease may not confer high risk for CHD if the affected vasculature is above the carotids. Carotid artery disease (symptomatic or asymptomatic with >50% stenosis) confers high risk.
‡As chronic kidney disease deteriorates and progresses to end-stage kidney disease, the risk of CVD increases substantially.
§Some patients with subclinical CVD will have >20% 10-year CHD risk and should be elevated to the high risk-category.
∥Patients with multiple risk factors can fall into any of 3 categories by Framingham scoring.
¶Most women with a single, severe risk factor will have 10-year risk<10%.
SOURCE: Reproduced, with permission, from Mosca et al.[100]

TABLE 16-4 Clinical Recommendations for the Prevention of Cardiovascular Disease in Women

	Lifestyle Interventions	
Cigarette smoking	Consistently encourage women not to smoke and to avoid environmental tobacco.	Class, Level B, GI 1*
Physical activity	Consistently encourage women to accumulate a minimum of 30 min of moderate-intensity physical activity (eg, brisk walking) on most, and preferably all, days of the week.	Class I, Level B, GI 1
Cardiac rehabilitation	Women with a recent acute coronary syndrome or coronary intervention or new-onset or chronic angina should participate in a comprehensive risk-reduction regimen, such as cardiac rehabilitation or a physician-guided home- or community-based program.	Class I, Level B, GI 2
Heart-healthy diet	Consistently encourage an overall healthy eating pattern that includes intake of a variety of fruits, vegetables, grains, low-fat or nonfat dairy products, fish, legumes, and sources of protein low in saturated fat (eg, poultry, lean meats, plant sources). Limit saturated fat intake to <10% of calories, limit cholesterol intake to <300 mg/d, and limit intake of *trans* fatty acids.	Class I, Level B, GI 1
Weight maintanance/reduction	Consistently encourage weight maintenance/reduction through an appropriate balance of physical activity, caloric intake, and formal behavioral programs when indicated to maintain/achieve a BMI† between 18.5 and 24.9 kg/m² and a waist circumference <35 in.	Class I, Level B, GI 1
Psychosocial factors	Women with CVD should be evaluated for depression and refer/treat when indicated.	Class IIa, Level B, GI 2
Omega 3 fatty acids	As an adjunct to diet, omega-3 fatty acid supplementation may be considered in high-risk‡ women.	Class IIb, Level B, GI 2
Folic acid	As an adjunct to diet, folic acid supplementation may be considered in high-risk women (except after revascularization procedure) if a higher-than-normal level of homocysteine has been detected.	Class IIb, Level B, GI 2
	Major Risk Factor Interventions	
Blood pressure—lifestyle	Encourage an optimal blood pressure of <120/80 mm Hg through lifestyle approaches.	Class I, Level B, GI 1
Blood pressure—drugs	Pharmacotherapy is indicated when blood pressure is ≥140/90 mm Hg or an even lower in the setting of blood pressure-related target-organ damage or diabetes. Thiazide diuretics should be part of the drug regimen for most patients unless contraindicated.	Class I, Level A, GI 1
Lipids, lipoproteins	Optimal levels of lipids and lipoproteins in women are LDL-C <100 mg/dL, HDL-C >50 mg/dL, triglycerides <150 mg/dL, and non-HDL-C (total cholesterol minus HDL-Cl) <130 mg/dL and should be encouraged through lifestyle approaches.	Class I, Level B, GI 1
Lipids—diet therapy	In high-risk women or when LDL-C is elevated, saturated fat intake should be reduced to <7% of calories, cholesterol to <200 mg/d, and *trans* fatty acid intake should be reduced.	Class I, Level B, GI 1

(continued)

TABLE 16-4   *(Continued)*

Lipids—pharmacotherapy, high risk[‡]	Initiate LDL-C lowering therapy (preferably a statin) simultaneously with lifestyle therapy in high-risk women with LDL-C ≥100 mg/dL (Class I, Level A)$_{a-1}$, and initiate statin therapy in high-risk women with an LDL-C <100 mg/dL unless contraindicated.	Class I, Level B, GI 1
	Initiate niacin[¶] or fibrate therapy when HDL-C is low, or non-HDL-C elevated in high-risk women.	Class I, Level B, GI 1
Lipids—pharmacotherapy, intermediate risk[§]	Initiate LDL-C-lowering therapy preferably a statin) if LDL-C level is ≥130 mg/dL on lifestyle therapy	Class I, Level B, GI 1
	or	
	Niacin[¶] or fibrate therapy when-HDL-C is low or non-HDL-C elevated after LDL-C goal is reached.	Class I, Level B, GI 1
Lipids—pharmacotherapy, lower risk[‖]	Consider LDL-C-lowering therapy in low-risk women with 0 or 1 risk factor when LDL-C level is ≥190 mg/dL or if multiple risk factors are present when LDL-C is ≥160 mg/dL	Class IIa, Level B, GI 1
	or	
	Niacin[¶] or fibrate therapy when HDL-C is low or non-HDL-C elevated after LDL-C goal is reached.	Class IIa, Level B, GI 1
Diabetes	Lifestyle and pharmacotherapy should be used to achieve near normal HbA$_c$ (<7%) in women with diabetes.	Class I, Level B, GI 1
Preventive Drug Interventions		
Aspirin—high risk[‡]	Aspirin therapy (75 to 162 mg) or clopidogrel if patient is intolerant to aspirin, should be used in high-risk women unless contraindicated.	Class I, Level A, GI 1.
Aspirin—intermediate risk[§]	Consider aspirin therapy (75 to 162 mg) in intermediate-risk women as long as blood pressure is controlled and benefit is likely to outweigh risk of gastrointestinal side effects.	Class IIa, Level B, GI 2
Beta blockers	Beta blockers should be used indefinitely in all women who have had a myocardial infarction or who have chronic ischemic syndromes unless contraindicated.	Class I, Level A, GI 1
ACE inhibitors	ACE inhibitors should be used (unless contraindicated) in high-risk[‡] women.	Class I, Level A, GI 1
ARBs	ARBs should be used in high-risk[‡] women with clinical evidence of heart failure or an ejection fraction <40% who are intolerant to ACE inhibitors.	Class I, Level B, GI 1
Atrial Fibrillation Stroke Prevention		
Warfarin— atrial fibrillation	Among women with chronic or paroxysmal atrial fibrillation, warfarin should be used to maintain the INR at 2.0—3.0 unless they are considered to be at low risk for stroke (<1%) or high risk of bleeding.	Class I, Level A, GI 1
Aspirin—atrial fibrillation	Aspirin (325 mg) should be used in women with chronic or paroxysmal atrial fibrillation with a contraindication to warfain or at low risk for stroke (<1%)	Class I, Level A, GI 1
Class III Interventions		
Hormone therapy	Combined estrogen plus progestin hormone therapy should not be initiated to prevent CVD in postmenopausal women.	Class III, Level A
	Combined estrogen plus progestin hormone therapy should not be continued to prevent CVD in postmenopausal women.	Class III, Level C

(continued)

TABLE 16-4 (Continued)

	Other forms of menopausal hormone therapy (eg, unopposed estrogen) should not be initiated or continued to prevent CVD in postmenopausal women pending the results of ongoing trials.	Class III, Level C
Antioxidant supplements	Antioxidant vitamin supplements should not be used to prevent CVD pending the results of ongoing trials.	Class III, Level A, GI 1
Aspirin—lower risk[‡]	Routine use of aspirin in lower-risk women is not recommended pending the results of ongoing trials.	Class III, Level B, GI 2

*Classification: Class I, intervention useful and effective; Class IIa, weight of evidence is in favor of usefulness/efficacy; Class IIb, usefulness/efficacy is less well established by evidence/opinion; Class III, intervention is not useful/effective and may be harmful. *Levels of evidence:* A, sufficient evidence from multiple randomized trials; B, limited evidence from single randomized trial or other nonrandomized studies; C, based on expert opinion, case studies, or standard of care. *Generalizability Index:* 1, very likely that results generalize to women; 2, somewhat likely that results generalize to women; 3, unlikely that results generalize to women; 0, unable to project whether results generalize to women.
[†]GI, generalizability index; LDL-C, low-density lipoprotein cholesterol; HDL-C, high-density lipoprotein cholesterol; ACE, angiotensin-converting enzyme; and ARB, angiostensin receptor blocker; BMI, body mass index.
[‡]High risk is defined as CHD or risk equivalent, or 10-year abslute CHD risk >20%.
[§]Intermediate risk is defined as 10-year absolute CHD risk 10% to 20%.
[||]Lower risk is defined as 10-year absolute CHD risk <10%.
[¶]Dietary supplement niacin must not be used as a substitute for prescription niacin, and over-the-counter niacin should only be used if approved and monitored by a physician.
Reproduced, with permission, from Mosca et al.[100]

GENDER DISPARITIES IN CARDIOVASCULAR CARE

Numerous studies have found that men are referred for invasive cardiac procedures such as coronary angiography more frequently than are women.[86–92] For instance, in 1987, Tobin and colleagues reported that significant gender bias existed in the referral for coronary arteriography.[86] Of 390 patients referred for nuclear exercise testing, results were abnormal in 31% of the women and in 64% of the men. Despite this objective evidence of ischemia, only 4% of the women with abnormal radionuclide scans were referred for cardiac catheterization compared with 40% of the men. In a review of hospital discharge records, Ayanian and Epstein also noted that men were referred for cardiac catheterization more often than women (15% vs 28%).[87] However, Weintraub and associates found that once catheterization is performed, revascularization appears to occur at equivalent rates for men and women.[88]

Not only are women referred less often for coronary angiography,[88–92] studies also suggest that women are referred less often for noninvasive testing for CAD.[93] Women also appear to receive preventive services, such as cholesterol screening and risk factor modification, less often than do men.[94–96] Understanding and correcting these gender disparities is essential for preventing CHD in women.

UNDERESTIMATION OF RISK

Although the lifetime risk of developing CHD is at least one in three for women,[97] many women (and some health care providers) are unaware that CHD represents a woman's greatest threat to life. Many women perceive the chance of dying from breast cancer as far more likely than their chance of dying from CHD.[98,99] For women to pay optimal attention to cardiac risk factors and risk factor modification, they must first perceive themselves to be at risk; therefore, measures aimed at educating the public as to the actual risks are essential. Although the estimation of global risk as recommended by the Third Adult Treatment Panel of the National Cholesterol Education Program[55] (and discussed extensively in Chapter 1) remains the focus of risk assessment in women, recently released guidelines by the American Heart Association provide details of clinical examples and risk factor conditions that constitute the spectrum of CVD risk in women (Table 16-3).

PREVENTIVE CARDIOLOGY GUIDELINES FOR WOMEN

Several national organizations have issued recommendations for the primary prevention of CHD in the general population and in women, specifically.[55,100–103] The most recently updated American Heart Association

TABLE 16-5 Priorities for Prevention in Practice According to Risk Group

High-risk women (>20% risk)
Class I recommendations:
  Smoking cessation
  Physical activity/cardiac rehabilitation
  Diet therapy
  Weight maintenance reduction
  Blood pressure control
  Lipid control/statin therapy
  Aspirin therapy
  Beta blocker therapy
  ACE inhibitor therapy (ARBs contraindicated)*
  Glycemic control in diabetics
Class IIa recommendation:
  Evaluate/treat for depression
Class IIb recommendations:
  Omega 3 fatty-acid supplementation
  Folic acid supplementation

Intermediate-Risk Women (10–20% risk)
Class I recommendations:
  Smoking cessation
  Physical activity
  Heart-healthy diet
  Weight maintenance/reduction
  Blood pressure control
  Lipid control
Class IIa recommendations:
  Aspirin therapy

Lower-Risk Women (<10% risk)
Class I recommendations
  Smoking cessation
  Physical activity
  Heart-healthy diet
  Weight maintainance/reduction
  Treat individual CVD risk factors as indicated

Stroke Prevention among women with atrial fibrillation
Class I recommendations
  High/intermediate risk of stroke
    Warfarin therapy
  Low risk of stroke (<1%/y) contraindication
    to warfarin
    aspirin therapy

*ACE, angiotensin-converting enzyme; ARB, angiotensin receptors blockers.
SOURCE: Reproduced, with permission, from Mosca et al.[100]

clinical recommendations are summarized in Table 16-4. In addition, these guidelines provide specific priorities for prevention according to risk group (Table 16-5).

CHD is epidemic in women. In the United States, it kills more women than all forms of cancer combined.

Women have poorer outcomes after MI and revascularization procedures than do men. Studies show that women often have more cardiovascular risk factors than do men at the time of their MI or revascularization procedure. Studies also show that women are not always offered life-saving therapies for CHD at the same rate as are men. Although there have been significant technologic advances in the field of cardiovascular medicine, the causes of coronary atherosclerosis are often more amenable to risk factor reduction and use of proven preventive therapies than to high-tech interventions. Prompt recognition, diagnosis, and treatment of cardiovascular risk is essential to reducing the burden of disease in women and men alike.

REFERENCES

1. *American Heart Association 2002 Heart and Stroke Statistical Update.* Dallas, Tex: American Heart Association; 2001.

2. Lerner DJ, Kannel WB. Patterns of coronary heart disease morbidity and mortality in the sexes: a 26-year follow-up of the Framingham population. *Am Heart J* 1986;111:383–390.

3. Weaver WD, White HD, Wilcox RG, et al, for the GUSTO-I Investigators. Comparisons of characteristics and outcomes among women and men with acute myocardial infarction treated with thrombolytic therapy. *JAMA* 1996;275:777–782.

4. Tofler GH, Stone PH, Muller JE, et al, and the MILIS Study Group. Effects of gender and race on prognosis after myocardial infarction: adverse prognosis for women, particularly black women. *J Am Coll Cardiol* 1987;9:473–482.

5. Vaccarino V, Parsons L, Every NR, et al, for the National Registry of Myocardial Infarction 2 Participants. *N Engl J Med* 1999;341:217.

6. Douglas PS, Ginsburg GS. The evaluation of chest pain in women. *N Engl J Med* 1996;334:1311–1315.

7. Pepine CJ, Adams J, Marks RG, et al. Characteristics of a contemporary population with angina pectoris. *Am J Cardiol* 1994;74:226–231.

8. Maynard C, Weaver WD. Treatment of women with acute MI: new findings from the MITI registry. *J Myocardial Ischemia* 1992;4:27–37.

9. Willich SN, Löwel H, Lewis M, et al. Unexplained gender differences in clinical symptoms of acute myocardial infarction [abstract]. *J Am Coll Cardiol* 1993;21:238A.

10. Chen G, Redberg RF. Noninvasive diagnostic testing of coronary artery disease in women. *Cardiol Rev* 2000;8:354–360.

11. Kennedy JW, Killip T, Fisher LD, et al. The clinical spectrum of coronary artery disease and its surgical and medical management: the Coronary Artery Surgery Study. *Circulation* 1982;66:16–23.

12. Morise AP. Comparison of the Diamond–Forrester method and a new score to estimate the pretest probability of coronary disease before exercise testing. *Am Heart J* 1999;138:740–745.

13. Stoletniy LN, Pai RG. Value of QT dispersion in the interpretation of exercise stress test in women. *Circulation* 1997;96:904–910.

14. Friedman T, Greene A, Iskandrian A, et al. Exercise thallium-210 myocardial scintigraphy in women: correlation with coronary angiography. *Am J Cardiol* 1982;49:1632–1637.

15. Fintel D, Links J, Brinker J, et al. Improved diagnostic performance of exercise thallium-210 single photon computed tomography over planar imaging in the diagnosis of coronary artery disease: a receiver operating character analysis. *J Am Coll Cardiol* 1989;13:600–612.

16. Amanullah A, Friedman J, Berman B. Adenosine technetium-99m sestamibi myocardial perfusion SPECT in women: diagnostic efficiency in detection of coronary artery disease. *J Am Coll Cardiol* 1996;27:803–809.

17. Hung J, Chaitman B, Lam J, et al. Noninvasive diagnostic test choices for the evaluation of coronary artery disease in women: Multivariate comparison of cardiac fluoroscopy, exercise electrocardiography, and exercise thallium, myocardial perfusion scintigraphy. *J Am Coll Cardiol* 1984;4:8–16.

18. Marwick T, Anderson T, Williams J, Haluska B, Melin J, Pashkow F, Thomas J. Exercise echocardiography is an accurate and cost-efficient technique for detection of coronary artery disease in women. *J Am Coll Cardiol* 1995;26:335–41.

19. Brochier ML, Arwidson P. Coronary heart disease risk factors in women. *Eur Heart J* 1998;19(suppl A):45–52.

20. Pinilla J, Gonzalez B, Barber P, Santana Y. Smoking in young adolescents: an approach with multilevel discrete choice models. *J Epidemiol Community Health* 2002;56:227–232.

21. Women and smoking: the US Surgeon General's report. *Mayo Clin Womens Healthsource* 2001;5(7):3.

22. Kannel WB, Castelli WP, McNamara PM. Cigarette smoking and risk of coronary heart disease: epidemiologic clues to pathogensis. The Framingham Study. *Natl Cancer Inst Monogr* 1968;28:9–20.

23. Rosenberg L, Kaufman DW, Helmrich SP, et al. Myocardial infarction and cigarette smoking in women younger than 50 years of age. *JAMA* 1985;253:2965–2969.

24. Castelli WP, Garrison RJ, Dawber TR, et al. The filter cigarette and coronary heart disease: the Framingham study. *Lancet* 1981;2:109–113.

25. Wolf PA, D'Agostino RB, Kannel WB, et al. Cigarette smoking as a risk factor for stroke: the Framingham Study. *JAMA* 1988;259:1025–1029.

26. National Center for Health Statistics–National Heart, Lung, and Blood Institute Collaborative Lipid Group. Trends in serum cholesterol levels among US adults aged 20 to 74 years: data from the National Health and Nutrition Examination Surveys, 1960–1980. *JAMA* 1987;257:937–942.

27. Couillard, Bergeron N, Prud'homme D, et al. Gender difference in postprandial lipemia: importance of visceral adipose tissue accumulation. *Arterioscler Thromb Vasc Biol* 19:2448–2455.

28. van Beek AP, Ruijter-Heijstek FC, Erkelens DW, de Bruin TW. Menopause is associated with reduced protection from postprandial lipemia. *Arterioscler Thromb Vasc Biol* 1999;19:2737–2741.

29. Cullen P. Evidence that triglycerides are an independent coronary heart disease risk factor. *Am J Cardiol* 2000;86:943–949.

30. Gordon T, Castelli WP, Hjortland MC, Kannel WB. The prediction of coronary heart disease by high-density and other lipoproteins: an historical perspective. In: Rifkind BM, Levy RI, eds. *Hyperlipidemia: Diagnosis and Therapy.* New York: Grune & Stratton; 1977:71–78.

31. Scandinavian Simvastatin Survival Study Group. The Scandinavian Simvastatin Survival trial (4S): randomized trial of cholesterol lowering in 4444 patients with coronary heart disease. *Lancet* 1994;344:1383–1389.

32. Sacks FM, Pfeffer MA, Moye LA, et al, for the Cholesterol and Recurrent Events Trial Investigators. The effect of pravastatin on coronary events after myocardial infarction in patients with average cholesterol levels. *N Engl J Med* 1996;335:1001–1009.

33. The Long-Term Intervention with Pravastatin in Ischaemic Disease (LIPID) Study Group. Prevention of cardiovascular events and death with pravastatin in patients with coronary heart disease and a broad range of initial cholesterol levels *N Engl J Med* 1998;339:1349–1357.

34. Downs JR, Clearfield M, Weis S, et al. Primary prevention of acute coronary events with lovastatin in men and women with average cholesterol levels: results of AFCAPS/TexCAPS. Air Force/Texas Coronary Atherosclerosis Prevention Study. *JAMA* 1998;279(20):1615–1622.

35. Heart Protection Study Collaborative Group. MRC/BHF Heart Protection Study of cholesterol lowering with simvastatin in 20,536 high-risk individuals: a randomised placebo-controlled trial. *Lancet* 2002;360:7–22.

36. Burt VL, Whelton P, Roccella EJ, et al. Prevalence of hypertension in the US adult population: results from the Third National Health and Nutrition Examination Survey, 1988–1991. *Hypertension* 1995;25:305–313.

37. The Fifth Report of the Joint National Committee on Detection Evaluation and Treatment of Hypertension: JNC V. *Arch Intern Med* 1993;153:154–183.

38. Kannel WB, Wolf PA, McGee DL, et al. Systolic blood pressure, arterial rigidity, and risk of stroke: the Framingham Study. *JAMA* 1981;245:1225–1229.

39. Lloyd-Jones DM, Larson MG, Leip EP, et al. Lifetime risk for developing congestive heart failure: the Framingham Heart Study. *Circulation* 2002;106:3068–3072.

40. MacMahon S, Peto R, Cutler J, et al. Blood pressure, stroke, and coronary heart disease: I. Prolonged differences in blood pressure: prospective observational studies corrected for the regression dilution bias. *Lancet* 1990;335:765–774.

41. Hypertension Detection and Follow-Up Program Research Group. Five-year findings of the Hypertension Detection and Follow-up Program: reduction in mortality of persons with high blood pressure including mild hypertension. *JAMA* 1979;242:2562–2571.

42. Langford H, Stamler J, Wassertheil-Smoller S, Prineas R. All-cause mortality in the Hypertension, Detection, and Follow-up Program: findings in the whole cohort and for persons with less severe hypertension, with and without other traits related to risk of mortality. *Prog Cardiovasc Dis* 1986;29(suppl 1):29–54.

43. SHEP Cooperative Research Group. Prevention of stroke by antihypertensive drug treatment in older persons with isolated systolic hypertension: final results of the Systolic Hypertension in the Elderly Program (SHEP). *JAMA* 1991;265:3255–3264.

44. Wassertheil-Smoller S, Anderson G, Psaty BM, et al. Hypertension and its treatment in postmenopausal women: baseline data from the Women's Health Initiative. *Hypertension* 2000;3:780–789.

45. Cornoni-Huntley J, LaCroix AZ, Havlik RJ. Race and sex differentials in the impact of hypertension in the United States: the National Health and Nutrition Examination Survey I

Epidemiologic Follow-up Study. *Arch Intern Med* 1989;149: 780–788.

46. Tsung SH, Loh WP. A review: adverse effects of oral contraceptives. *J Indiana State Med Assoc* 1979;72(8):578–580.

47. Koltyn KF, Landis JA, Dannecker EA. Influence of oral contraceptive use on pain perception and blood pressure. *Health Care Women Int* 2003;24:221–229.

48. Bassol S, Alvarado G, Arreola RG, et al. A 13-month multicenter clinical experience of a low-dose monophasic oral contraceptive containing 20 microg ethinylestradiol and 75 microg gestodene in Latin American women. *Contraception* 2003;67(5):367–372.

49. Morley Kotchen J, Kotchen TA. Impact of female hormones on blood pressure: review of potential mechanisms and clinical studies. *Curr Hypertens Rep* 2003;5:505–512.

50. Kannel W. Metabolic risk factors for coronary heart disease in women: perspective from the Framingham Study. *Am Heart J* 1987;114:413–419.

51. Manson J, Colditz G, Stampfer M, et al. A prospective study of maturity-onset diabetes mellitus and risk of coronary heart disease and stroke in women. *Arch Intern Med* 1991;1511:1141–1147.

52. Pradhan AD, Skerrett PJ, Manson JE. Obesity, diabetes, and coronary risk in women. *J Cardiovasc Risk* 2002;9(6):323–330.

53. Turner RC, Millns H, Neil HAW, et al, for the United Kingdom Prospective Diabetes Study Group. Risk factors for coronary artery disease in non-insulin dependent diabetes mellitus: United Kingdom Prospective Diabetes Study (UKPDS: 23). *BMJ* 1998;316:823–828.

54. Isomaa B, Almgren P, Tuomi T, et al. Cardiovascular morbidity and mortality associated with the metabolic syndrome. *Diabetes Care* 2001;24:683–689.

55. ATP-III: Executive summary of the Third Report of the National Cholesterol Education Program (NCEP) Expert Panel on Detection, Evaluation, and Treatment of High Blood Cholesterol in Adults (Adult Treatment Panel). *JAMA* 2001;285:2486–2497.

56. Ford ES, Giles WH, Dietz WH. Prevalence of the metabolic syndrome among US adults: findings from the third National Health and Nutrition Examination Survey. *JAMA* 2002;287:356–359.

57. McCarthy JJ, Meyer J, Moliterno DJ, et al. Evidence for substantial effect modification by gender in a large-scale genetic association study of the metabolic syndrome among coronary heart disease patients. *Hum Genet* 2003;114:87–98.

58. De S, Searles G, Haddad H. The prevalence of cardiac risk factors in women 45 years of age or younger undergoing angiography for evaluation of undiagnosed chest pain. *Can J Cardiol* 2002;18:945–948.

59. Colditz GA Stampfer MJ, Willett WC, et al. A prospective study of parental history of myocardial infarction and coronary heart disease in women. *Am J Epidemiol* 1986;123:48–58.

60. Barrett-Connor E, Khaw K. Family history of heart attack as an independent predictor of death due to cardiovascular disease. *Circulation* 1984;69:1065–1069.

61. Hunt SC, Blickenstaff K, Hopkins PN, Williams RR. Coronary disease and risk factors in close relatives of Utah women with early coronary death. *West J Med* 1986;145:329–334.

62. Stevens J, Cai J, Pamuk ER, et al. The effect of age on the association between body-mass index and mortality. *N Engl J Med* 1998;338:1–7.

63. Hubert H, Feinleib M, McNamara P, et al. Obesity as an independent risk factor for cardiovascular disease: a 26-year follow-up of participants in the Framingham Heart Study. *Circulation* 1983;69:1065–1069.

64. Manson J, Colditz G, Stampfer M, et al. A prospective study of obesity and risk of coronary heart disease in women. *N Engl J Med* 1990;322:883–889.

65. Lapidus L, Bengstsson C, Larsson B, et al. Distribution of adipose tissue and risk of cardiovascular disease and death: a 12-year follow-up of participants in the population study of women in Gothenburg, Sweden. *BMJ* 1984;289:1257–1261.

66. Grodstein F, Stampfer MJ, Colditz GA, et al. Postmenopausal hormone therapy and mortality. *N Engl J Med* 1997;336:1769–1775.

67. Williams JK, Adams MR, Klopfenstein HS: Estrogen modulates responses of atherosclerotic coronary arteries. *Circulation* 1990;81:1680–1687.

68. Mendelsohn ME, Karas RH. Protective effects of estrogen on the cardiovascular system. *N Engl J Med* 1999;340:1801–1811.

69. The Writing Group for the PEPI Trial. Effects of estrogen on heart disease risk factors in postmenopausal women. *JAMA* 1995;273:199–208.

70. Hulley S, Grady D, Bush T, et al, for the Heart and Estrogen/Progestin Replacement Study (HERS) Research Group. Randomized trial of estrogen plus progestin for secondary prevention of coronary heart disease in postmenopausal women. *JAMA* 1998;280:605–613.

71. Stampfer MJ, Colditz GA. Estrogen replacement therapy and coronary heart disease: a quantitative assessment of the epidemiologic evidence. *Prev Med* 1991;20:47–63.

72. Hemminki E, McPherson K. Impact of postmenopausal hormone therapy on cardiovascular events and cancer: pooled data from clinical trials. *BMJ* 1997;315:149–153.

73. The Coronary Drug Project Research Group. The Coronary Drug Project: findings leading to discontinuation of the 2.5 mg/day estrogen group. *JAMA* 1973;226:652–657.

74. Wenger NK, Knatterud GL, Canner PL. Early risks of hormone therapy in patients with coronary heart disease [letter]. *JAMA* 2000;284:41–43.

75. Clarke SC, Kelleher J, Lloyd-Jones H, et al. A study of hormone replacement therapy in postmenopausal women with ischaemic heart disease: the Papworth HRT Atherosclerosis Study. *Br J Obstet Gynaecol* 2002;109:1056–1062.

76. Herrington DM, Reboussin DM, Brosnihan KB, et al. Effects of estrogen replacement on the progression of coronary artery atherosclerosis. *N Engl J Med* 2000;343:522–529.

77. Viscoli CM, Brass LM, Kernan WN, et al. Estrogen replacement after ischemic stroke: report of the Women's Estrogen for Stroke Trial (WEST). *N Engl J Med* 2001;345:1243–1249.

78. Grady D, et al. Cardiovascular disease outcomes during 6.8 years of hormone therapy: Heart and Estrogen/Progestin Replacement Study follow-up (HERS II). *JAMA* 2002;288:49–57.

79. Writing Group for the Women's Health Initiative Investigators. Risks and benefits of estrogen plus progestin in healthy postmenopausal women: principal results from the Women's Health

Initiative randomized controlled trial. *JAMA* 2002;288:321–333.

80. Manson JE, Hsia J, Johnson KC, et al, for the Women's Health Initiative Investigators. Estrogen plus progestin and risk of coronary heart disease: final results from the Women's Health Initiative. *N Engl J Med* 2003;349:523–534.

81. Wassertheil-Smoller S, Hendrix SL, Limacher M, et al. Effect of estrogen plus progestin on stroke in postmenopausal women: the Women's Health Initiative: a randomized trial. *JAMA* 2003;289:2673–2684.

82. Writing Group fo the Women's Health Initiative Investigators. Effects of conjugated equine estrogen in postmenopausal women with hysterectomy: the Women's Health Intiative randomized controlled trial. *JAMA* 2004;291:1701–1712.

83. Walsh BW, Kuller LH, Wild RA, et al. Effects of raloxifene on serum lipids and coagulation factors in healthy postmenopausal women. *JAMA* 1998;279:1445–1551.

84. Barrett-Connor E; Grady D, Sashegyi A, et al, for the MORE Investigators. Raloxifene and cardiovascular events in osteoporotic postmenopausal women: four-year results from the MORE (Multiple Outcomes of Raloxifene Evaluation) randomized trial. *JAMA* 2002;287:847–857.

85. WHO Collaborative Study of Cardiovascular Disease and Steroid Hormone Contraception. Acute myocardial infarction and combined oral contraceptives: results of an international multicentre case controlled study. *Lancet* 1997;349:1202–1209.

86. Tobin JN, Wassertheil-Smoller S, Wexler JP, et al. Sex bias in considering coronary bypass surgery. *Ann Intern Med* 1987;107:19–25.

87. Ayanian J, Epstein A. Differences in the use of procedures between women and men hospitalized for coronary heart disease. *N Engl J Med* 1991;325:221.

88. Weintraub W, Kosinski A, Wenger N. Is there a bias against performing coronary revascularization in women? *Am J Cardiol* 1996;78:1154–1160.

89. Schulman K, Berlin J, Harless W, et al. The effect of race and sex on physicians' recommendations for cardiac catheterization. *N Engl J Med* 1999;340:618–626.

90. Roger V, Farkouh M, Weston S, et al. Sex differences in evaluation and outcome of unstable angina. *JAMA* 2000;283:646–652.

91. Rathore S, Chen J, Wang Y, et al. Sex differences in cardiac catheterization: the role of physician gender. *JAMA* 2001;286:2849–2856.

92. Ghali W, Faris P, Galbraith P, et al. Sex differences in access to coronary revascularization after cardiac catheterization: importance of detailed clinical data. *Ann Intern Med* 2002;136:723–732.

93. Shaw L, Miller D, Romeis J, et al. Gender differences in the non-invasive evaluation and management of patients with suspected coronary artery disease. *Ann Intern Med* 1991;120:559.

94. Miller M, Byington R, Hunninghake D, et al. Sex bias and underutilization of lipid-lowering therapy in patients with coronary artery disease at academic medical centers in the United States and Canada. *Arch Intern Med* 2000;160:343–347.

95. Majumdar S, Gurwitz J, Soumerai S. Undertreatment of hyperlipidemia in the secondary prevention of coronary artery disease. *J Gen Intern Med* 1999;14:711–717.

96. McBride P, Schrott H, Plane M, et al. Primary care practice adherence to National Cholesterol Education Program guidelines for patients with coronary heart disease. *Arch Intern Med* 1998;158:1238–1244.

97. Lloyd-Jones DM, Larson MG, Beiser A, Levy D. Lifetime risk of developing coronary heart disease. *Lancet* 1999;353:89–92.

98. Legato MJ, Padus E, Slaughter E. Women's perceptions of their general health, with special reference to their risk of coronary artery disease: results of a national telephone survey. *J Womens Health* 1997;6:189–198.

99. Pilote L, Hlatky MA. Attitudes of women toward hormone therapy and prevention of heart disease. *Am Heart J* 1995;129:1237–1238.

100. Mosca L, Appel LJ, Benjamin E, et al. AHA Guidelines: evidence-based guidelines for cardiovascular disease prevention in women. *Circulation* 2004;109:672–693.

101. US Preventive Services Task Force. Aspirin for the primary prevention of cardiovascular events: recommendation and rationale. *Ann Intern Med* 2002;136:157–160.

102. American Diabetes Association. Standards of medical care for patients with diabetes mellitus. *Diabetes Care* 2003;26:S33–S50.

103. Chobanian AV, Bakris GL, Black HR, et al, and the National High Blood Pressure Education Program Coordinating Committee. The Seventh Report of the Joint National Committee on Prevention, Detection, Evaluation, and Treatment of High Blood Pressure: the JNC 7 report. *JAMA* 2003;289:3560–3572.

Seniors

Seniors

17

Wilbert S. Aronow

KEY POINTS

- *Cigarette smoking, hypertension, left ventricular hypertrophy, dyslipidemia, diabetes mellitus, the metabolic syndrome, obesity, and physical inactivity are risk factors for cardiovascular disease in elderly men and women.*

- *Smoking cessation reduces mortality from coronary heart disease, other cardiovascular disease, and all-cause mortality in elderly men and women.*

- *Treatment with antihypertensive drugs reduces new coronary events, stroke, heart failure, and cardiovascular mortality in elderly men and women with hypertension.*

- *Elderly men and women with coronary heart disease manifest reduced coronary heart disease event rates after treatment with statins and should be treated to a low-density lipoprotein level less than 100 mg/dL (less than 70 mg/dL if very high risk).*

- *Exercise training programs not only are effective in preventing coronary heart disease, but have been found to improve endurance and functional capacity in elderly persons after myocardial infarction.*

INTRODUCTION

Coronary heart disease (CHD) is the most common cause of death in the elderly. CHD, stroke, and peripheral arterial disease (PAD) are more common in the elderly than in younger persons. In 2000, there were 781,000 hospital admissions in the United States with the diagnosis of acute myocardial infarction (MI).[1] Of these, 499,000 (64%) were aged 65 years and older and one third of the 781,000 patients were older than 75.[1,2] As for strokes, more than 70% occur in those aged 75 and older.[3]

Among the elderly, as estimated from the Cardiovascular Health Study, the incidence per 1000 of new and recurrent heart attacks in non–African American men increases from 26.3 in those aged 65 to 74 to 53.6 in those aged 85 and older.[4] Among non–African American women, the incidence increases from 7.8 to 24.2. In African American men, these rates increase from 16.3 to 54.9, and in African American women the

rates range from 13.3 to 18.3, being highest in those aged 75 to 84. The estimated annual rate per 1000 of new and recurrent strokes among the elderly increases from 14.4 among non–African American men aged 65 to 74 to 27.9 among non–African American men aged 85 and older. Among non–African American women in the same age groups, these rates range from 6.2 to 30.6. Among African American men, the rates increase from 11.9 to 40.8; and among African American women, the rates range from 16.1 to 22.4.[4]

All the major risk factors for CHD in younger persons remain important in the elderly, as demonstrated by the Framingham Heart Study, which compared regression coefficients for each major risk factor in those aged 65 to 94 with those for persons aged 35 to 64 (Table 17-1).[5] Although some of the coefficients, such as those for serum cholesterol and smoking, appear to be attenuated in the elderly, the greater absolute risk of CHD associated with any given risk factor in the elderly more than compensates for this. The prevalence of a number of risk factors,

399

TABLE 17-1 Effect of Risk Factors on Coronary Heart Disease Incidence: Framingham Heart Study, 30-Year Follow-up

| | Bivariate (age-adjusted) standardized regression coefficient | | | |
| | Ages 35–64 | | Ages 65–94 | |
Study	Men	Women	Men	Women
Systolic blood pressure	0.338*	0.148*	0.401*	0.286*
Diastolic blood pressure	0.321*	0.363*	0.296*	0.082
Serum cholesterol	0.322*	0.307*	0.121	0.213*
Cigarette smoking	0.259*	0.095	−0.017	−0.034
Blood glucose	0.043	0.206*	0.166*	0.209*
Vital capacity	−0.112†	−0331.*	−0.127	−0.253*
Relative weight	0.190*	0.264*	0.177‡	0.124†

*$P < .001$.
†$P < .05$.
‡$P < .01$.

SOURCE: Reproduced, with permission, from Cupples and D'Agostino.[5]

including diabetes, dyslipidemia, and hypertension, increases dramatically with age, and these are quite common in the elderly. This chapter discusses the significance of these and other risk factors for CHD, stroke, and PAD in the elderly, as well as strategies for risk factor modification for the prevention of cardiovascular disease (CVD) in the elderly.

CIGARETTE SMOKING

The Cardiovascular Health Study demonstrated in 5201 men and women 65 years of age and older that more than 50 pack-years of smoking increased 5-year mortality 1.6 times.[4] The Systolic Hypertension in the Elderly Program pilot project showed that smoking was a predictor of first cardiovascular event and MI/sudden death.[6] At 30-year follow-up of persons 65 and older in the Framingham Heart Study, cigarette smoking was not associated with the incidence of CHD, but was associated with

mortality from CHD.[7] At 12-year follow-up of men 65 to 74 years of age in the Honolulu Heart Program, the absolute excess risk of nonfatal MI and fatal CHD associated with cigarette smoking was 1.9 times higher in older men than in middle-aged men.[8]

At 5-year follow-up of 7178 persons 65 and older in three communities, the relative risk for CVD mortality was 2.0 for male smokers and 1.6 for female smokers.[9] The incidence of CVD mortality in former smokers was similar to the risk in those who had never smoked.[9] At 40-month follow-up of 664 men, mean age 80 years, and at 48-month follow-up of 1488 women, mean age 82 years, current cigarette smoking increased the relative risk of new coronary events (nonfatal or fatal MI or sudden cardiac death) 2.2 times in men and 2.0 times in women (Table 17-2).[10] At 6-year follow-up of older men and women in the Coronary Artery Surgery Study registry, the relative risk of MI or death was 1.5 for persons 65 to 69 years of age and 2.9 for persons 70 and older

TABLE 17-2 Association of Cigarette Smoking with New Coronary Events, New Stroke, and Peripheral Arterial Disease in Elderly Men and Women

| | | | Follow-up (mo) | | Relative risk | |
Study	No.	Mean age	Men	Women	Men	Women
Incidence of new coronary events[10]	2152	81	40	48	2.2	2.0
Incidence of new stroke[15]	2152	81	42	48	1.5	1.9
Prevalence of peripheral arterial disease[23]	869	82	—	—	2.4	2.9

who continued smoking compared with quitters during the year before study enrollment.[11]

A meta-analysis of 32 studies demonstrated that cigarette smoking was a risk factor for stroke in men and women with a relative risk of 1.9.[12] In the Medical Research Council Trial, the incidence of stroke was 2.3 times higher in cigarette smokers than in non-smokers.[13] Nonsmokers who received propranolol as antihypertensive therapy had a reduction in the incidence of stroke, whereas cigarette smokers did not.[13] At 26-year follow-up in the Framingham Study, cigarette smoking increased the incidence of stroke 1.6 times in men and 1.9 times in women.[14] The incidence of stroke in cigarette smokers who smoked more than 40 cigarettes daily was two times higher than in those who smoked fewer than 10 cigarettes daily. The impact of cigarette smoking did not decrease with increasing age. The risk of stroke was substantially decreased within 2 years of quitting smoking, with the incidence of stroke returning to the level of nonsmokers 5 years after cessation of smoking.[14]

At 42-month follow-up of 664 men, mean age 80 years, and at 48-month follow-up of 1488 women, mean age 82 years, current cigarette smoking increased the relative risk of new stroke 1.5 times in men and 1.9 times in women (Table 17-2).[15] In a study of 1063 persons, mean age 81 years, cigarette smoking was associated with a 4.2-fold increased likelihood of significant narrowing in diameter of the extracranial internal or common carotid artery.[16]

Numerous studies have demonstrated that cigarette smoking is a risk factor for PAD in men and women.[17–22] In a study of 244 men and 625 women, mean age 82 years, cigarette smoking increased the prevalence of PAD 2.4 times in men and 2.9 times in women (Table 17-2).[22] At 43-month follow-up of 291 persons, mean age 82 years, with PAD, cigarette smoking was an independent predictor of new coronary events with a relative risk of 1.6.[23]

The impact of passive smoking on CHD risk has also been demonstrated. One study showed that in married women aged 50 to 79, the relative risk for death from CHD in nonsmoking women married to current or former cigarette smokers was 14.9 ($P \leq 0.10$).[24]

Recommendations

Elderly men and women who smoke cigarettes should be strongly encouraged to stop smoking to reduce the development of CHD, stroke, and PAD. Smoking cessation decreases mortality from CHD, other CVD, and all-cause mortality in elderly men and women. The California Tobacco Control Program was associated with declines in cigarette consumption and in mortality from heart disease.[25]

Approaches to smoking cessation include use of nicotine patches or nicotine polacrilex gum, which are available over the counter.[26] If this therapy is unsuccessful, nicotine nasal spray or treatment with the antidepressant drug buproprion should be considered.[26,27] A nicotine inhaler may also be used.[28] The dosage and duration of treatment of each of these pharmacotherapies are considered in detail elsewhere.[28] Concomitant behavioral therapy may also be needed.[29]

HYPERTENSION

Increased peripheral vascular resistance is the cause of systolic and diastolic hypertension in elderly persons. Systolic hypertension in elderly persons is diagnosed if the systolic blood pressure is 140 mm Hg or higher from two or more readings on two or more visits.[30] Diastolic hypertension in elderly persons is similarly diagnosed if the diastolic blood pressure is 90 mm Hg or higher.[30] In a study of 1819 persons, mean age 80 years, living in the community, the prevalence of hypertension was 71% in elderly African Americans, 64% in elderly Asians, 62% in elderly Hispanics, and 52% in elderly whites.[31]

Isolated systolic hypertension in elderly persons is diagnosed if the systolic blood pressure is 140 mm Hg or higher with a diastolic blood pressure of less than 90 mm Hg.[30] Approximately two thirds of elderly persons with hypertension have isolated systolic hypertension.[31] Isolated systolic hypertension is the predominant form of hypertension in the elderly; by age 60, it is present in more than 80% of individuals.[32] Isolated systolic hypertension and diastolic hypertension are both associated with increased CVD morbidity and mortality in elderly persons.[33] Increased systolic blood pressure is a greater risk factor for CVD morbidity and mortality than is increased diastolic blood pressure.[33] The higher the systolic or diastolic blood pressure, the greater the morbidity and mortality from CHD in elderly women and men. The Cardiovascular Health Study demonstrated in 5202 elderly men and women that a brachial systolic blood pressure greater than 169 mm Hg is associated with a 2.4-fold greater 5-year mortality.[4]

At 30-year follow-up of persons 65 years of age and older in the Framingham Heart Study, systolic hypertension was related to a greater incidence of CHD in elderly men and women.[7] Diastolic hypertension correlated with the incidence of CHD in elderly men but not in elderly women.[7] At 40-month follow-up of 664 elderly men and 48-month follow-up of 1488 elderly women, systolic or diastolic hypertension was associated with relative risks of new coronary events of 2.0 in men and 1.6 in women (Table 17-3).[10] Recent data from Framingham also suggest the importance of increased pulse pressure, a measure of large artery stiffness. Among 1924 men and women aged 50 to 79, at any given level of systolic blood pressure

TABLE 17-3 Association of Systolic or Diastolic Hypertension with New Coronary Events, New Stroke, and Peripheral Arterial Disease in Elderly Men and Women

| Study | No. | Mean age | Follow-up (mo) | | Relative risk | |
			Men	Women	Men	Women
Incidence of new coronary events[10]	2152	81	40	48	2.0	1.6
Incidence of new stroke[15]	2152	81	42	48	2.2	2.4
Prevalence of peripheral arterial disease[22]	869	82	—	—	1.7	1.5

of 120 mm Hg or greater, the risk of CHD over 20 years rose with lower diastolic blood pressure, suggesting that higher pulse pressure was an important component of risk.[34] Among 1061 men and women aged 60 to 79 in the Framingham Heart Study, the strongest predictor of CHD risk was pulse pressure (hazard ratio = 1.24).[35]

In addition, antihypertensive drugs have been shown to reduce CVD events in elderly men and elderly women with hypertension (Table 17-4).[36–40] A meta-analysis of 1670 patients with hypertension aged 80 years and older in randomized controlled clinical trials showed that antihypertensive drug therapy reduced stroke 34%, major CVD events 22%, and heart failure 39%.[41] Pahor and colleagues conducted a meta-analysis of nine trials involving 27,743 patients with 120,000 person-years of follow-up which revealed that compared with diuretics, beta blockers, angiotensin-converting enzyme (ACE) inhibitors, and clonidine (15,044 patients), calcium channel blockers resulted in a 25% increase in MI, a 24% increase in heart failure, and a 24% increase in major CVD events in 12,699 patients.[42]

In the Antihypertensive and Lipid-Lowering Treatment to Prevent Heart Attack Trial (ALLHAT), patients of mean age 67 years with hypertension (47% women, 47% white, 36% African American, and 13% Hispanic) were randomized to the alpha blocker doxazosin (9067 patients), the thiazide diuretic chlorthalidone (15,268 patients), the calcium channel blocker amlodipine (9048 patients), or the ACE inhibitor lisinopril (9054 patients).[43,44] At the 3.3-year follow-up, doxazosin was stopped because compared with chlorthalidone, doxazosin increased stroke 19%, combined CVD 25%, heart failure 204%, and angina pectoris 16% (Table 17-5).[43] At the 4.9-year follow-up, compared with chlorthalidone, amlodipine increased heart failure 38% and lisinopril increased combined CVD 10%, stroke 15%, and heart failure 19% (Table 17-5).[44]

The Second Australian National Blood Pressure Study randomized 6083 patients with hypertension, mean age 72 years (range 65 to 84 years), to the thiazide diuretic hydrocholorothiazide or to the ACE inhibitor enalapril.[45] At the 4.1-year follow-up, compared

TABLE 17-4 Recent Trials Showing Reduction in New Coronary Events, Stroke, and Heart Failure in Elderly Persons with Hypertension Treated with Antihypertensive Drugs versus Placebo

Study	Follow-up	Result
Swedish Trial in Old Patients with Hypertension[36] (ages 70–84)	25 mo	Drug therapy caused a 25% decrease in fatal MIs, a 67% reduction in sudden deaths, and a 73% decrease in fatal stroke
Medical Research Council[37] (ages 65–74)	5.8 y	Drug therapy caused a 19% borderline significant reduction in coronary events and a 25% decrease in stroke
Systolic Hypertension in the Elderly Program[38,39] (mean age 72)	4.5 y	Drug therapy caused a 27% decrease in nonfatal MIs plus coronary deaths, a 36% reduction in stroke, and a 49% decrease in heart failure
Systolic Hypertension in Europe[40] (mean age 70)	2.0 y	Drug therapy caused a 27% insignificant decrease in coronary mortality, a 30% insignificant reduction in fatal plus nonfatal MIs, and a 42% reduction in stroke

TABLE 17-5   Results from the Antihypertensive and Lipid-Lowering Treatment to Prevent Heart Attach Trial (ALLHAT) and the Second Australian National Blood Pressure Trial

Study	Follow-up (y)	Result
ALLHAT[43] (mean age 67)	3.3	Compared with chlorthalidone, doxazosin increased stroke 19%, combined CVD 25%, heart failure 204%, and angina 16%
ALLHAT[44] (mean age 67)	4.9	Compared with chlorthalidone, amlodipine increased heart failure 38% and lisinopril increased combined CVD 10%, stroke 15%, and heart failure 19%
Second Australian National Blood Pressure Study[45] (mean age 72)	4.1	Compared with hydrochlorothiazide, enalapril reduced all CVD or death from any cause 11%

with hydrochlorothiazide, enalapril caused a significant reduction in all CVD or death from any cause (Table 17-5), which was seen in elderly men but not in elderly women.[45]

Numerous studies have also demonstrated that both systolic hypertension and diastolic hypertension increase the incidence of stroke in elderly persons.[15,17,30,33,36–38,40,72,73] The higher the systolic or diastolic blood pressure, the higher the incidence of new stroke. At the 30-year follow-up in the Framingham Heart Study, hypertension was the risk factor most strongly correlated with stroke in elderly men and women.[73] At the 42-month follow-up of 664 men, mean age 80 years, and the 48-month follow-up of 1488 women, mean age 82 years, systolic or diastolic hypertension was associated with an increased relative risk of new stroke (2.2 times in men and 2.4 times in women) (Table 17-3).[15]

Many studies have demonstrated that hypertension is a risk factor for PAD.[17,18,20,23] In a study of 244 men and 625 women, mean age 82 years, systolic or diastolic hypertension increased the prevalence of PAD 1.7 times in men and 1.5 times in women (Table 17-3).[23]

Systolic or diastolic hypertension is also a powerful risk factor for heart failure.[74,75] In the Systolic Hypertension in the Elderly Program (SHEP), antihypertensive drug therapy with the step 1 drug chlorthalidone 12.5 to 25 mg daily and the step 2 drug atenolol 25 to 50 mg daily for 4.5 years was associated with a 49% reduction in the development of heart failure in elderly men and women (Table 17-4).[38]

Recommendations

Elderly persons with hypertension should restrict salt intake, reduce weight if necessary, discontinue drugs that increase blood pressure, avoid alcohol and tobacco, increase physical activity, decrease dietary saturated fat and cholesterol, and maintain an adequate dietary potassium, calcium, and magnesium intake.

The Joint National Committee on Detection, Evaluation, and Treatment of High Blood Pressure (JNC-7) recommends as initial drug treatment diuretics or beta blockers, because these drugs have been found to reduce cardiovascular morbidity and mortality in controlled clinical trials.[30] The goal of treatment of hypertension in elderly persons should be the same as in younger persons—to reduce the blood pressure to less than 140/90 mm Hg if possible and ideally toward the optimal level of less than 120/80 mm Hg.[30] Those with a systolic blood pressure of 120 to 139 mm Hg or diastolic blood pressure of 80 to 89 mm Hg, who account for a substantial proportion of elderly persons, are considered to be "prehypertensive," and nonpharmacologic interventions should be implemented as needed to achieve optimal levels or, at least, to prevent the progression of blood pressure levels to hypertensive levels. If the systolic blood pressure is between 130 and 139 mm Hg and the person has target-organ damage, heart failure, renal insufficiency, and/or diabetes mellitus, drug therapy should be prescribed in addition to lifestyle modification.[30]

The choice of medication selected as monotherapy for hypertension should depend on associated medical conditions. In uncomplicated patients, thiazide diuretics or a combination of thiazide diuretics plus beta blockers is recommended as initial therapy in those who do not respond adequately to lifestyle modification.[30] Diuretics are preferred in those with isolated systolic hypertension,[30] followed by the addition beta blockers, ACE inhibitors, and calcium channel blockers as second-, third-, and fourth-line agents. Table 17-6 lists the preferred initial drug or drugs of choice for the treatment of elderly persons with hypertension and associated medical conditions. In many older persons, the initial dose of antihypertensive drug may need to be lower to avoid symptoms of postural hypotension. However, standard doses and multiple drugs are needed in most older persons to reach appropriate blood pressure target goals. Postural hypotension is more frequent in older persons

TABLE 17-6 Preferred Initial Drug or Drugs for Treatment of Elderly Persons with Hypertension and Associated Medical Conditions

Medical condition	Preferred initial antihypertensive drug
Heart failure[46–52]	Diuretics plus ACE inhibitors plus beta blockers
Prior myocardial infarction[53–58]	Beta blockers plus ACE inhibitors
Angina pectoris[59]	Beta blockers
Myocardial ischemia[60]	Beta blockers
Diabetes mellitus[30,61]	ACE inhibitors or angiotensin receptor blockers
Renal insufficiency[30,62]	ACE inhibitors
Abnormal left ventricular ejection fraction[55,63]	ACE inhibitors plus beta blockers
Complex ventricular arrhythmias[64,65]	Beta blockers
Supraventricular tachyarrhythmias[66]	Beta blockers
Hyperthyroidism[67]	Beta blockers
Osteoporosis[68]	Thiazide diuretics
Left ventricular hypertrophy[69,70]	ACE inhibitors or angiotensin receptor blockers
Preoperative hypertension[71]	Beta blockers
Migraine[30]	Beta blockers
Essential tremor[30]	Beta blockers

with systolic hypertension and diabetes, and in persons taking diuretics, nitrates, and alpha blockers. The blood pressure should be monitored in the upright position in these persons. Volume depletion and excessively rapid titration of antihypertensive drugs should be avoided.

Antihypertensive drug therapy has been demonstrated to reduce the incidence of new stroke in elderly persons.[36–38,40,73] Elderly men and women with a systolic blood pressure of 140 mm Hg or greater or a diastolic blood pressure of 90 mm Hg or greater despite nonpharmacologic intervention should be treated with antihypertensive drug therapy to reduce the incidence of new stroke.[30]

Antihypertensive drug therapy may lead to orthostatic hypotension[76] or postprandial hypotension[77] in elderly persons, especially in those who are frail and institutionalized. Management of orthostatic and postprandial hypotension in elderly persons is discussed in detail elsewhere.[78] The dose of antihypertensive drug may need to be reduced or another antihypertensive drug used.

LEFT VENTRICULAR HYPERTROPHY

Left ventricular hypertrophy (LVH) caused by hypertension or other CVD is not only a marker for CVD morbidity and mortality but also a contributor to these events in elderly men and women. Elderly men and women with electrocardiographic LVH[75,79–81] and echocardiographic LVH[75,80,82–88] are at increased risk of developing new

coronary events, stroke, PAD, and heart failure. At the 4-year follow-up of 406 elderly men and 735 elderly women in the Framingham Heart Study, echocardiographic LVH was 15.3 times more sensitive in predicting new coronary events in elderly men and 4.3 times more sensitive in predicting new coronary events in elderly women than was electrocardiographic LVH.[82] At the 37-month follow-up of 360 men and women, mean age 82 years, with hypertension or CHD, echocardiographic LVH was 4.3 times more sensitive in predicting new coronary events and 4.0 times more sensitive in predicting new stroke than was electrocardiographic LVH.[80]

Recommendations

Physicians should try to prevent LVH from developing or progressing in elderly men and women with hypertension or other CVD. Framingham Heart Study data have demonstrated a reduction of CVD events in patients with regression of LVH.[89] The Cornell group has also found, in patients with uncomplicated hypertension followed for 10.2 years, that regression of LVH probably reduces the incidence of new CVD events.[90] At the 10-year follow-up in the Bronx Aging Study, elderly persons in whom electrocardiographic LVH disappeared over time had a lower incidence of CVD morbidity and mortality than elderly persons with persistent LVH.[81] In the Losartan Intervention for Endpoint Reduction (LIFE) substudy, in 1326 patients, mean age 70 years, with isolated systolic hypertension and electrocardiographic LVH at the 4.7-year follow-up, losartan reduced electrocardiographic LVH more than atenololol, and reduced CVD mortality, stroke, new-onset diabetes mellitus, and total mortality.[69]

A meta-analysis of 109 treatment studies found that ACE inhibitors were more effective than other antihypertensive drugs in decreasing left ventricular mass.[69] In an echocardiographic substudy of SHEP, at the 3-year follow-up, the left ventricular mass index decreased by 13% in the active drug treatment group (a diuretic-based drug regimen) and increased by 6% in the placebo group.[91] The Department of Veterans Affairs Cooperative Study Group on Antihypertensive Agents showed, at the 1-year follow-up of 1105 men, that patients treated with captopril, hydrochlorothiazide, or atenolol had a reduction in left ventricular mass, but patients treated with diltiazem, clonidine, or prazosin did not.[92]

Prospective studies using different types of antihypertensive drugs are necessary to determine whether regression of left ventricular mass leads to a reduction in CVD morbidity and mortality in elderly men and women.

DYSLIPIDEMIA

Numerous studies have demonstrated that high serum total cholesterol is a risk factor for new or recurrent coronary events in elderly men and women.[7,10,93–97] Among patients 65 years of age and older with prior MI in the Framingham Heart Study, serum total cholesterol was significantly related to death from CHD and to all-cause mortality.[94] In the Established Populations for Epidemiologic Studies of the Elderly study, after 5 years of follow-up in 4066 older men and women, serum total cholesterol was a risk factor for mortality from CHD, but with apparent adverse effects of lower cholesterol levels being associated with comorbidity and frailty.[98] At the 40-month follow-up of 664 elderly men and the 48-month follow-up of 1488 elderly women, an increment of 10 mg/dL in serum total cholesterol was associated with a modest increase in the relative risk of 1.12 for new coronary events in both men and in women.[10]

Low serum high-density lipoprotein cholesterol (HDL-C) is a risk factor for new coronary events in elderly men and women.[7,10,93,99–102] In the Framingham Heart Study,[93] in the Established Populations for Epidemiologic Studies of the Elderly study,[99] and in a large cohort of convalescent home patients,[10] a low serum HDL-C was a more powerful predictor of new coronary events than was serum total cholesterol. At the 40-month follow-up of 664 elderly men and the 48-month follow-up of 1488 elderly women, a decrement of 10 mg/dL in serum HDL-C increased the relative risk of new coronary events 1.70 times in men and 1.95 times in women.[10]

Hypertriglyceridemia is a risk factor for new coronary events in elderly women but not in elderly men.[10,93] At the 40-month follow-up of elderly men and the 48-month follow-up of elderly women, the level of serum triglycerides was not a risk factor for new coronary events in men and was a very weak risk factor for new coronary events in women.[10]

In an observational prospective study of 488 men and 922 women, mean age 81 years, with prior MI and a serum low-density lipoprotein cholesterol (LDL-C) of 125 mg/dL or higher, 48% of persons were treated with statins (Table 17-7).[103–105] At the 3-year follow-up, compared with placebo, statins reduced CHD death or nonfatal MI by 50%,[103] stroke by 60%,[104] and heart failure by 48%[105] (Table 17-7). In another observational study of elderly persons with prior MI and diabetes, at the 29-month follow-up, compared with placebo, statins reduced CHD death or nonfatal MI by 37% and stroke by 47% (Table 17-7).[106] And among those with symptomatic PAD, at 39 months of follow-up, compared with placebo, statins reduced CHD death or nonfatal MI by 52% in persons with prior MI and by 59% in persons with no prior MI (Table 17-7).[107]

The strongest and most consistent evidence relating cholesterol lowering to coronary event reduction in the elderly derives from recently published secondary prevention studies. At the 5.4-year median follow-up of 4444 men and women (of whom 1021 were 65 to 70 years of age at study entry) with CHD and hypercholesterolemia, compared with placebo, simvastatin decreased serum total cholesterol 25% and serum LDL-C by 35%; it increased serum HDL-C by 8% and decreased total mortality, coronary death, major coronary events, cerebrovascular events, new or worsening angina pectoris, and arterial bruits (Table 17-8).[108–111] In men and women 65 to 70 years of age, simvastatin decreased all-cause mortality by 34%, CHD mortality by 43%, major coronary events by 34%, and any atherosclerosis-related endpoint event by 44%.[104] Reductions in endpoint events were similar in older and younger men and women. The absolute risk reduction for both all-cause mortality and CHD mortality was approximately twice as great in persons 65 years of age and older as in those younger than 65. At a 7.4-year median follow-up, simvastatin reduced all-cause mortality by 30% and CHD mortality by 38% among those 65 to 70 years of age.[106]

Within the Cholesterol and Recurrent Events (CARE) trial involving pravastatin treatment for a period of 5 years in post-MI patients with serum total cholesterol levels less than 240 mg/dL and serum LDL-C levels of 115 to 174 mg/dL, subset analysis of the 1283 patients aged 65 to 74 revealed a 32% lower risk of major coronary events, a 45% lower risk of CHD death, a 39% lower risk of CHD death or nonfatal MI, a 40% lower risk of stroke, and a 32% lower risk of coronary revascularization

TABLE 17-7 Observational Studies Showing Reduction by Statins of Coronary Events, Stroke, and Heart Failure in Elderly Persons with Coronary Heart Disease, Peripheral Arterial Disease, and Diabetes Mellitus

Study	Follow-up	Result
1410 persons, mean age 81 with prior MI[103–105]	3 y	Compared with placebo, statins reduced CHD death or nonfatal MI by 50%, stroke by 60%, and heart failure by 48%
529 persons, mean age 79 with prior MI and diabetes[106]	29 mo	Compared with placebo, statins reduced CHD death or nonfatal MI by 37% and stroke by 47%
660 persons, mean age 80 with symptomatic peripheral arterial disease[107]	39 mo	Compared with placebo, statins reduced CHD death or nonfatal MI by 52% in persons with prior MI and by 59% in persons with no prior MI

TABLE 17-8 Effect of Reducing Increased Serum Total and Low-Density Lipoprotein Cholesterol by Simvastatin, Pravastatin, and Lovastatin versus Placebo in Elderly Persons

Study	Follow-up (y)	Result
Scandinavian Simvastatin Survival Study (4S)[108–110] (prior MI or angina)	5.4	Among persons aged ≥65, simvastatin compared with placebo decreased total mortality by 34%, CHD death by 43%, major coronary events by 34%, nonfatal MI by 33%, cerebrovascular events by 30%, any atherosclerosis-related endpoint by 34%, intermittent claudication by 38%, new or worsening angina by 26%, and bruits by 30%
Cholesterol and Recurrent Events (CARE) trial[112,113] (prior MI)	5.0	Compared with placebo, pravastatin decreased major coronary events by 32%, CHD death by 45%, CHD death or nonfatal MI by 39%, stroke by 40%, and coronary revascularization by 32% in persons aged 65–75
Long-Term Intervention with Pravastatin in Ischaemic Disease (LIPID) Study[114,115] (prior MI or unstable angina)	8.0	Compared with placebo, pravastatin decreased the risk of death due to CHD or nonfatal MI by 22% in persons aged 65–69 and by 20% in persons aged 70–75
Heart Protection Study (HPS)[116] (prior MI, other CHD, cerebrovascular disease, PAD, diabetes, and treated hypertension)	5.0	Compared with placebo, simvastatin reduced first major CVD event by 24% in persons <65 by 23% in persons aged 65–69 and by 18% in persons aged 70–80
Prospective Study of Pravastatin in the Elderly at Risk (PROSPER)[117] (history of, or risk factors for CVD)	3.2	Compared with placebo, pravastatin reduced CHD death or nonfatal MI by 19%
Air Force/Texas Cardiac Atherosclerosis Prevention Study[118,119] (persons free of CHD)	5.2	Compared with placebo, lovastatin reduced the primary endpoint of unstable angina, fatal or nonfatal MI, and sudden cardiac death 37%, including a 29% risk reduction in those >65

versus the placebo group (Table 17-7).[112,113] For every 1000 persons aged 65 to 75 treated for 5 years with pravastatin, 225 cardiovascular hospitalizations would be prevented compared 121 in 1000 younger persons.[113]

The Long-Term Intervention with Pravastatin in Ischaemic Disease (LIPID) study randomized 9014 persons with a history of MI or unstable angina who had initial serum total cholesterol levels of 155 to 271 mg/dL to pravastatin or placebo.[114,115] At the 8-year follow-up, compared with placebo, pravastatin was associated with a reduction in death from CHD or nonfatal MI of 22% in persons aged 65 to 69 at study entry and of 20% in persons aged 70 to 75 at study entry (Table 17-8).[115] Treatment of 1000 persons for 6 years with pravastatin prevented 30 deaths, 28 nonfatal MIs, 9 nonfatal strokes, 23 episodes of coronary artery bypass surgery, 20 episodes of coronary angioplasty, and 82 hospital admissions for unstable angina.[114] The absolute benefits of treatment with pravastatin were greater in groups at higher absolute risk for a major coronary event, including older persons.[114]

The Heart Protection Study randomized 20,536 men and women (5806 of whom were aged 70 to 80) with prior MI (8510 persons), other CHD (4876 persons), and no CHD (7150 persons) and a serum total cholesterol level of 135 mg/dL or higher to simvastatin 40 mg daily or placebo (Table 17-8).[116] These reductions occurred regardless of initial levels of serum lipids, age, or gender. Simvastatin reduced first major CVD event risk by 24% in persons younger than 65, by 23% in persons aged 65 to 69, and by 18% in persons aged 70 to 80 at study entry (Table 17-8).[116]

The Prospective Study of Pravastatin in the Elderly at Risk (PROSPER) trial randomized 5804 men and women aged 70 to 82 with a history of risk factors for CVD and a serum total cholesterol level of 154 mg/dL or higher to pravastatin 40 mg daily or placebo.[117] At the 3.2-year follow-up, the primary endpoint of CHD death, nonfatal MI, or stroke was reduced 15% by pravastatin compared with placebo ($P = .014$). CHD death or nonfatal MI was reduced 19% by pravastatin ($P = .006$). Stroke risk was unaffected but pravastatin reduced the risk for transient ischemic attack by 25% ($P = .051$).

There are also data relating lipid reduction to coronary event reduction in elderly persons without prior CHD. At the 5.2-year follow-up of 6605 men and women (21% aged 66–73 at study entry) with serum LDL-C levels between 130 and 190 mg/dL, serum HDL-C levels below 50 mg/dL, and no clinical evidence of CHD enrolled in the Air Force/Texas Cardiac Atherosclerosis Prevention Study (AFCAPS/TexCAPS), compared with placebo, lovastatin caused a 37% decrease in the primary endpoint of unstable angina pectoris, fatal or nonfatal MI, and sudden cardiac death (Table 17-8).[118] Lovastatin decreased this primary endpoint by 34% in men, 54% in women, 29% in persons older than 65, 59% in smokers, 43% in persons with hypertension, and 43% in persons with diabetes mellitus.[118,119]

The association between statin use and all-cause mortality and incidence of CVD events was investigated at the 7.3-year follow-up of 1250 women and 664 men, aged 65 to 80, with hypercholesterolemia free of CVD in the Cardiovascular Health Study.[120] Thirteen percent of persons reported statin use, which was associated with a reduction in all-cause mortality of 44% and CVD events of 56%.[120]

Recommendations

On the basis of the above data, elderly men and women with CVD who have elevated serum LDL-C levels despite dietary therapy should be treated with hydroxymethylglutaryl coenzyme A (HMGCoA) reductase inhibitor therapy. The serum LDL-C level should be decreased to less than 100 mg/dL.[121] Moreover, among those at very high risk (eg, acute coronary syndrome, or both CVD and diabetes present) an LDL-C goal of less than 70 mg/dL has recently been suggested as a therapeutic option.[122] In addition, HMG-CoA reductase inhibitor therapy should be considered in addition to a prudent diet, regular exercise, and risk factor modification in elderly persons without heart disease who have elevated serum LDL-C levels in the absence of other serious or life-limiting illness such as cancer, dementia, or malnutrition.

Although the data on the association of serum lipids with stroke in men and women are conflicting,[16,73,123–125] a meta-analysis of eight secondary prevention trials and four primary prevention trials that used simvastatin, pravastatin, or lovastatin to decrease serum total cholesterol levels revealed that HMGCoA reductase inhibitor therapy caused a 27% reduction in stroke.[126] These data and data from other studies[103,104,106,108–116] support the use of HMGCoA reductase inhibitor therapy in elderly men and women with elevated serum LDL-C levels despite dietary therapy to reduce the incidence of new stroke as well as CHD events.

There are also conflicting data on the association of increased serum total cholesterol[17–23,125,127,128] and increased serum triglycerides[19–23,125,128] with PAD. However, a low serum HDL-C is associated with PAD.[19,21,23,125,128] In a study of 559 men and 1275 women, mean age 81, there was a 1.24 times higher probability of development of PAD for a 10 mg/dL decrement in serum HDL-C.[125] The Scandinavian Simvastatin Survival Study (4S) showed that compared with placebo, simvastatin reduced new intermittent claudication by 38%, new carotid bruits by 48%, and one or more bruits by 30%.[105]

TABLE 17-9   Association of Diabetes Mellitus with New Coronary Events, New Stroke, and Peripheral Arterial Disease in Elderly Men and Women

Study	No.	Mean age	Follow-up (mo)		Relative risk	
			Men	Women	Men	Women
Incidence of new coronary events[10]	2152	81	40	48	1.9	1.8
Incidence of new stroke[15]	2152	81	42	48	1.5	1.5
Prevalence of peripheral arterial disease[23]	869	82	—	—	2.4	3.0

DIABETES MELLITUS

Diabetes mellitus is a risk factor for new coronary events in elderly men and women.[10,129,130] In the Cardiovascular Health Study, an elevated fasting glucose level (>130 mg/dl) increased 5-year mortality 1.9 times.[4] At the 40-month follow-up of 664 elderly men and the 48-month follow-up of 1488 elderly women, diabetes mellitus increased the relative risk of new coronary events 1.9 times in men and 1.8 times in women (Table 17-9).[10]

Diabetes mellitus is a risk factor for new stroke in elderly men and women.[15,73,131] Diabetes mellitus also increased the prevalence of extracranial carotid arterial disease 1.7 times among 1063 persons (mean age 81).[16] At the 42-month follow-up of men and 48-month follow-up of women, diabetes mellitus increased the relative risk of new stroke 1.5 times in both men and women (Table 17-9).[15]

Diabetes mellitus is also a risk factor for PAD in elderly men and women.[17–20,21–23,132] In a study of 244 elderly men and 625 elderly women, diabetes mellitus increased the prevalence of PAD 2.4 times in men and 3.0 times in women (Table 17-9).[23]

Elderly persons with diabetes mellitus should receive dietary therapy, reduce weight if necessary, and be prescribed appropriate drugs if necessary to control hyperglycemia. The hemoglobin A_{1c} level should be maintained at less than 7%.[133] Other risk factors such as smoking, hypertension,[134] dyslipidemia,[118] obesity, and physical inactivity should be controlled. Given that diabetes is also considered a CHD risk equivalent, the serum LDL-C level should be reduced to less than 100 mg/dL, or less than 70 mg/dL if CVD is also present.[122] Moreover, the American Diabetes Association recommends optimal triglyceride levels below 150 mg/dL and HDL-C levels greater than 45 mg/dL.[135]

METABOLIC SYNDROME

The combination of high serum triglycerides, small LDL particles, low serum HDL-C levels, hypertension, insulin resistance (with or without glucose intolerance), and a prothrombotic state is called the *metabolic syndrome* (also commonly referred to as *syndrome X*).[136,137] More than 40% of adults aged 60 and older have the metabolic syndrome as defined by the National Cholesterol Education Program.[118,138] HMGCoA reductase inhibitor therapy alone or in combination with other lipid-altering therapy, such as fenofibrate or niacin, should be used to reduce the atherogenic lipoproteins.[118,136] Hypertension should be treated in accordance with JNC-7 guidelines.[30] Nondrug therapy for insulin resistance consists of weight control and increased physical activity. Metformin and rosiglitazone may be useful in some persons for reducing insulin resistance.[137] Low-dose aspirin may also be used to reduce the risk from a prothrombotic state.[137]

OBESITY

Obesity was an independent risk factor for new CHD events in elderly men and women in the Framingham Heart Study.[136] Disproportionate distribution of fat to the abdomen assessed by the waist-to-hip circumference ratio has also been shown to be a risk factor for CVD, mortality from CHD, and total mortality in elderly men and women.[139,140] At the 40-month follow-up of elderly men and 48-month follow-up of elderly women, obesity was a risk factor for new CHD events in men and women by univariate analysis but not by multivariate analysis.[10]

The Framingham Heart Study found that relative weight was not a risk factor for new stroke in elderly men, but was a weak risk factor for new stroke in elderly women.[73] Barrett-Connor and Khaw demonstrated no association between body mass index and new stroke in elderly men and women.[132] At the 42-month follow-up of 664 elderly men, obesity was not a risk factor for new stroke.[15] At the 48-month follow-up of 1488 elderly women, obesity was a risk factor for new stroke by univariate analysis but not by multivariate analysis.[15]

The Framingham Heart Study observed that Metropolitan Life Insurance relative weight was not associated with intermittent claudication in women, but was inversely associated with intermittent claudication in men.[17] In a study of 244 elderly men and 625 elderly women, obesity was insignificantly associated with PAD in men, but increased the prevalence of PAD 1.8 times in women.[23]

Obese men and women with CHD, stroke, or PAD must undergo weight reduction. Weight reduction is also the first approach to controlling mild hypertension, hyperglycemia, and dyslipidemia before placing persons on long-term drug therapy. Regular aerobic exercise should be used in addition to diet to treat obesity. Clinical trials are needed to establish the efficacy of long-term drug therapy for treating obesity in the elderly.

PHYSICAL INACTIVITY

Physical inactivity is associated with obesity, hypertension, hyperglycemia, and dyslipidemia. At the 12-year follow-up in the Honolulu Heart Program, physically active men 65 and older had a relative risk of 0.43 for CHD compared with inactive men.[141] Paffenbarger and co-workers demonstrated that persons 65 to 79 years of age with a physical activity index above 2000 kcal/wk had a better survival rate than those with a physical activity index below 2000 kcal/wk.[142] Lack of moderate or vigorous exercise increased 5-year mortality in elderly men and women in the Cardiovascular Heart Study.[4] The relationship between physical inactivity and stroke is unclear.[73,143,144]

Moderate exercise programs suitable for elderly persons include walking, climbing stairs, swimming, and bicycling. However, care must be taken in prescribing any exercise program because of the high risk of injury in this age group. Walking and other low-impact exercises minimize injury. The amount of physical activity should be gradually increased over time. Group or supervised sessions, including aerobics classes, offered by senior health care plans are especially appealing. High-risk individuals should see a physician and exercise professional before beginning an exercise program. Individuals with CVD or symptoms should have an exercise stress test before starting a vigorous exercise program. Exercise training programs not only are beneficial in preventing CHD,[145] but have also been found to improve endurance and functional capacity in elderly persons after MI.[146]

POLYPHARMACY

Elderly persons often take multiple drugs, which can cause drug interactions. Because they take multiple drugs, compliance with individual drugs is more difficult. Memory problems in some elderly persons may interfere with compliance. The cost of multiple drugs may also interfere with compliance. Only essential drugs should be prescribed to elderly persons. The initial dose of drug should be low and the increase in dose should be slow. The dose of drug should be titrated according to the elderly person's response. Appropriate use of cardiovascular drugs in elderly persons requires knowledge of age-related physiologic changes, the effects of concomitant disorders that may alter the pharmacokinetics and pharmacodynamic effects of cardiovascular drugs, and drug interactions. This subject is discussed in detail elsewhere.[147]

SUMMARY

The significant morbidity and mortality from CVD in the elderly warrants that this group receive special attention directed at awareness, detection, and control of important risk factors. Many of these risk factors, particularly smoking, diabetes, hypertension, dyslipidemia, obesity, and physical inactivity, continue to be important predictors of CVD events in the elderly. They are largely modifiable and, in many cases, reversible. Among the many older persons with preexisting CVD, risk factor modification is even more important, as disease will often progress rapidly otherwise. Older persons must be educated to understand that CVD is not an inevitable consequence of aging but is largely preventable and, in some cases, even reversible. As large segments of populations in developed countries rapidly reach older ages, soon to be repeated in developing countries, where life spans have dramatically increased along with the incidence of CVD and other chronic diseases, there is significant opportunity for prevention.

REFERENCES

1. Hall MJ, Owings MF. *National Hospital Discharge Survey. Advanced Data from Vital and Health Statistics, No. 329*. Hyattsville, Md: National Center for Health Statistics; 2002.

2. Gillum RF. Trends in acute myocardial infarction and coronary heart disease death in the United States. *J Am Coll Cardiol* 1993;23:1273–1277.

3. American Heart Association. *1998: Heart and Stroke Statistical Update*. Dallas: American Heart Association; 1998.

4. Fried LP, Kronmal RA, Newman AB, et al. Risk factors for 5-year mortality in older adults: the Cardiovascular Health Study. *JAMA* 1998;279:585–592.

5. Cupples LA, D'Agostino RB. Some risk factors related to the annual incidence of cardiovascular disease and death using pooled repeated biennial measurements. In: Kannel WB, Wolf PA, Garrison RJ, eds. *Framingham Study: 30-Year Follow-Up*. National Institutes of Health Publication No. 87-2703. Springfield, Va: US Department of Commerce, National Technical Information Service; 1987.

6. Siegel D, Kuller L, Lazarus NB, et al. Predictors of cardiovascular events and mortality in the Systolic Hypertension in the Elderly Program pilot project. *Am J Epidemiol* 1987;126:385–399.

7. Kannel WB, Vokonas PS. Primary risk factors for coronary heart disease in the elderly: the Framingham Study.

In: Wenger NK, Furberg CD, Pitt B, eds. *Coronary Heart Disease in the Elderly.* New York: Elsevier Science; 1986:60–92.

8. Benfante R, Reed D, Frank J. Does cigarette smoking have an independent effect on coronary heart disease incidence in the elderly? *Am J Public Health* 1991;81:897–899.

9. LaCroix AZ, Lang J, Scherr P, et al. Smoking and mortality among older men and women in three communities. *N Engl J Med* 1991;324:1619–1625.

10. Aronow WS, Ahn C. Risk factors for new coronary events in a large cohort of very elderly patients with and without coronary artery disease. *Am J Cardiol* 1996;77:864–866.

11. Hermanson B, Omenn GS, Kronmal RA, Gersh BJ. Beneficial six-year outcome of smoking cessation in older men and women with coronary artery disease: results from the CASS registry. *N Engl J Med* 1988;319:1365–1369.

12. Shinton R, Beevers G. Meta-analysis of relation between cigarette smoking and stroke. *BMJ* 1989;298:789–794.

13. Medical Research Council Working Party. MRC trial of treatment of mild hypertension: principal results. *BMJ Clin Res* 1985;291:97–104.

14. Wolf PA, D'Agostino PS, Kannel WB, et al. Cigarette smoking as a risk factor for stroke: The Framingham Study. *JAMA* 1988;259:1025–1029.

15. Aronow WS, Ahn C, Gutstein H. Risk factors for new atherothrombotic brain infarction in 664 older men and 1,488 older women. *Am J Cardiol* 1996;77:1381–1383.

16. Aronow WS, Ahn C, Schoenfeld MR. Risk factors for extracranial internal or common carotid arterial disease in elderly patients. *Am J Cardiol* 1993;71:1479–1481.

17. Stokes J III, Kannel WB, Wolf PA, et al. The relative importance of selected risk factors for various manifestations of cardiovascular disease among men and women from 35 to 64 years old: 30 years of follow-up in the Framingham Study. *Circulation* 1987;75(suppl V):V-65–V-73.

18. Kannel WB, McGee DL. Update on some epidemiologic features of intermittent claudication: the Framingham Study. *J Am Geriatr Soc* 1985;33:13–18.

19. Hughson WG, Mann JI, Garrod A. Intermittent claudication: prevalence and risk factors. *BMJ* 1978;1:1379–1381.

20. Beach KW, Brunzell JD, Strandness DE Jr. Prevalence of severe arteriosclerosis obliterans in patients with diabetes mellitus: relation to smoking and form of therapy. *Arteriosclerosis* 1982;2:275–280.

21. Reunanen A, Takkunen H, Aromaa A. Prevalence of intermittent claudication and its effect on mortality. *Acta Med Scand* 1982;211:249–256.

22. Aronow WS, Sales FF, Etienne F, Lee NH. Prevalence of peripheral arterial disease and its correlation with risk factors for peripheral arterial disease in elderly patients in a long-term health care facility. *Am J Cardiol* 1988;62:644–646.

23. Aronow WS, Ahn C, Mercando AD, Epstein S. Prognostic significance of silent ischemia in elderly patients with peripheral arterial disease with and without previous myocardial infarction. *Am J Cardiol* 1992;69:137–139.

24. Garland C, Barrett-Connor E, Suarez L, et al. Effects of passive smoking on ischemic heart disease mortality of nonsmokers: a prospective study. *Am J Epidemiol* 1985;121:645–650

25. Fichtenberg CM, Glantz SA. Association of the California Tobacco Control Program with declines in cigarette consumption and mortality from heart disease. *N Engl J Med* 2000;343:1772–1777.

26. Benowitz NL. Treating tobacco addiction: nicotine or no nicotine. *N Engl J Med* 1997;337:1230–1231.

27. Hurt RD, Sachs DPL, Glover ED, et al. A comparison of sustained-release bupropion and placebo for smoking cessation. *N Engl J Med* 1997;337:1195–1202.

28. Frishman WH, Ky T, Ismail A. Tobacco smoking, nicotine, and nicotine and non-nicotine replacement therapies. *Heart Dis* 2001;3:365–377.

29. Tonnesen P, Fryd V, Hansen M, et al. Effect of nicotine chewing gum in combination with group counseling on the cessation of smoking. *N Engl J Med* 1988;318:15–18.

30. Chobanian AV, Bakris GL, Black HR, et al. The Seventh Report of the Joint National Committee on Prevention, Detection, Evaluation, and Treatment of High Blood Pressure: the JNC 7 Report. *JAMA* 2003; 289: 2560–2572.

31. Mendelson G, Ness J, Aronow WS. Drug treatment of hypertension in older persons in an academic hospital-based geriatrics practice. *J Am Geriatr Soc* 1999;47:597–599.

32. Franklin SS, Jacobs MJ, Wong ND, L'Italien G, Lapuerta P. Predominance of isolated systolic hypertension among middle-aged and elderly US hypertensives: analysis based on NHANES III. *Hypertension* 2001;37:869–874.

33. Applegate WB, Rutan GH. Advances in management of hypertension in older persons. *J Am Geriatr Soc* 1992;40:1164–1174.

34. Franklin SS, Khan SA, Wong ND, et al. Is pulse pressure useful in predicting risk for coronary heart disease? The Framingham Heart Study. *Circulation* 1999;100:354–360.

35. Franklin SS, Larson MG, Khan SA, et al. Does the relation of blood pressure to coronary heart disease risk change with aging? The Framingham Heart Study. *Circulation* 2001;103:1245–1249.

36. Dahlof B, Lindholm LH, Hansson L, et al. Morbidity and mortality in the Swedish Trial in Old Patients with Hypertension (STOP Hypertension). *Lancet* 1991;338:1281–1285.

37. MRC Working Party. Medical Research Council Trial of treatment of hypertension in older adults: principal results. *BMJ* 1992;304:405–412.

38. SHEP Cooperative Research Group. Prevention of stroke by antihypertensive drug treatment in older persons with isolated systolic hypertension: final results of the Systolic Hypertension in the Elderly Program (SHEP). *JAMA* 1991;265:3255–3264.

39. Kostis JB, Davis BR, Cutler J, et al. Prevention of heart failure by antihypertensive drug treatment in older persons with isolated systolic hypertension. *JAMA* 1997;278:212–216.

40. Staessen JA, Fagard R, Thijs L, et al. Randomised double-blind comparison of placebo and active treatment for older patients with isolated systolic hypertension. *Lancet* 1997;350:757–764.

41. Gueyffier F, Bulpitt C, Boissel J-P, et al. Antihypertensive drugs in very old people: a subgroup meta-analysis of randomised controlled trials. *Lancet* 1999;353:793–796.

42. Pahor M, Psaty BM, Alderman MH, et al. Health outcomes associated with calcium antagonists compared with other first-line antihypertensive therapies: a meta-analysis of randomised controlled trials. *Lancet* 2000;356:1949–1954.

43. ALLHAT Officers and Coordinators for the ALLHAT Collaborative Research Group. Major cardiovascular events in hypertensive patients randomized to doxazosin vs chlorthalidone: the

Antihypertensive and Lipid-Lowering Treatment to Prevent Heart Attack Trial (ALLHAT) *JAMA* 2000;283:1967–1975.

44. ALLHAT Officers and Coordinators for the ALLHAT Collaborative Research Group. Major outcomes in high-risk hypertensive patients randomized to angiotensin-converting enzyme inhibitor or calcium channel blocker vs diuretic: the Antihypertensive and Lipid-Lowering Treatment to Prevent Heart Attack Trial (ALLHAT). *JAMA* 2002;288:2981–2997.

45. Wing LMH, Reid CM, Ryan P, et al. A comparison of outcomes with angiotensin-converting-enzyme inhibitors and diuretics for hypertension in the elderly. *N Engl J Med* 2003;348:583–592.

46. Hunt SA, Baker DW, Chin MH, et al. ACC/AHA guidelines for the evaluation and management of chronic heart failure in the adult: executive summary. A report of the American College of Cardiology/American Heart Association Task Force on Practice Guidelines (Committee to Revise the 1995 Guidelines for the Evaluation and Management of Heart Failure). Developed in collaboration with the International Society for Heart and Lung Transplantation. Endorsed by the Heart Failure Society of America. *J Am Coll Cardiol* 2001;38:2101–2113.

47. Garg R, Yusuf S, for the Collaborative Group on ACE Inhibitor Trials. Overview of randomized trials of angiotensin-converting enzyme inhibitors on mortality and morbidity in patients with heart failure. *JAMA* 1995;273:1450–1456.

48. Aronow WS, Kronzon I. Effect of enalapril on congestive heart failure treated with diuretics in elderly patients with prior myocardial infarction and normal left ventricular ejection fraction. *Am J Cardiol* 1993;71:602–604.

49. MERIT-HF Study Group. Effect of metoprolol CR/XL in chronic heart failure: Metoprolol CR/XL Randomised Intervention Trial in Congestive Heart Failure (MERIT-HF). *Lancet* 1999;353:2001–2007.

50. Packer M, Coats AJS, Fowler MB, et al. Effect of carvedilol on survival in chronic heart failure. *N Engl J Med* 2001;344:651–658.

51. Aronow WS, Ahn C, Kronzon I. Effect of propranolol versus no propranolol on total mortality plus nonfatal myocardial infarction in older patients with prior myocardial infarction, congestive heart failure, and left ventricular ejection fraction ≥40% treated with diuretics plus angiotensin-converting-enzyme inhibitors. *Am J Cardiol* 1997;80:207–209.

52. Aronow WS. Epidemiology, pathophysiology, prognosis, and treatment of systolic and diastolic heart failure in elderly patients. *Heart Dis* 2003;5:279–294.

53. Ryan TJ, Antman EM, Brooks NH, et al. 1999 update: ACC/AHA guidelines for the management of patients with acute myocardial infarction: executive summary and recommendations. A report of the American College of Cardiology/American Heart Association Task Force on Practice Guidelines (Committee on Management of Acute Myocardial Infarction). *Circulation* 1999;100:1016–1030.

54. The Heart Outcomes Prevention Evaluation Study Investigators. Effects of an angiotensin-converting-enzyme inhibitor, ramipril, on cardiovascular events in high-risk patients. *N Engl J Med* 2000;342:145–153.

55. Aronow WS, Ahn C, Kronzon I. Effect of beta blockers alone, of angiotensin-converting enzyme inhibitors alone, and of beta blockers plus angiotensin-converting enzyme inhibitors on new coronary events and on congestive heart failure in older persons with healed myocardial infarcts and asymptomatic left ventricular systolic dysfunction. *Am J Cardiol* 2001;88:1298–1300.

56. Aronow WS, Ahn C. Effect of beta blockers on incidence of new coronary events in older persons with prior myocardial infarction and diabetes mellitus. *Am J Cardiol* 2001;87:780–781.

57. Aronow WS, Ahn C. Effect of beta blockers on incidence of new coronary events in older persons with prior myocardial infarction and symptomatic peripheral arterial disease. *Am J Cardiol* 2001;87:1284–1286.

58. Aronow WS, Ahn C. Incidence of new coronary events in older persons with prior myocardial infarction and systemic hypertension treated with beta blockers, angiotensin-converting enzyme inhibitors, diuretics, calcium antagonists, and alpha blockers. *Am J Cardiol* 2002;89:1207–1209.

59. Tresch DD, Aronow WS. Angina in the elderly. In: Tresch DD, Aronow WS, eds. *Cardiovascular Disease in the Elderly Patient.* 2nd ed. New York City: Marcel Dekker; 1999:213–232.

60. Aronow WS, Ahn C, Mercando AD, et al. Decrease of mortality by propranolol in patients with heart disease and complex ventricular arrhythmias is more an anti-ischemic than an antiarrhythmic effect. *Am J Cardiol* 1994;74:613–615.

61. Brenner BM, Cooper ME, de Zeeuw D, et al. Effects of losartan on renal and cardiovascular outcomes in patients with type 2 diabetes and nephropathy. *N Engl J Med* 2001;345:861–869.

62. Agodoa LY, Appel L, Bakris GL, et al. Effect of ramipril versus amlodipine on renal outcomes in hypertensive nephrosclerosis: a randomized controlled trial. *JAMA* 2001;285:2719–2728.

63. Furberg CD, Hawkins CM, Lichstein E, for the Beta-Blocker Heart Attack Trial Study Group. Effect of propranolol in postinfarction patients with mechanical or electrical complications. *Circulation* 1984;69:761–765.

64. Kennedy HL, Brooks MM, Barker AH, et al. Beta-blocker therapy in the Cardiac Arrhythmia Suppression Trial. *Am J Cardiol* 1994;74:674–680.

65. Aronow WS, Ahn C, Mercando AD, et al. Effect of propranolol versus no antiarrhythmic drug on sudden cardiac death, total cardiac death, and total death in patients ≥62 years of age with heart disease, complex ventricular arrhythmias, and left ventricular ejection fraction ≥40%. *Am J Cardiol* 1994;74:267–270.

66. Aronow WS. Management of the older person with atrial fibrillation. *J Gerontol Med Sci* 2002;57A:M352–M363.

67. Aronow WS. The heart and thyroid disease. In: Gambert SR, ed. *Clinics in Geriatric Medicine. Thyroid Disease.* Philadelphia: WB Saunders; 1995:219–229.

68. LaCroix Z, Ott SM, Ichikawa LE, et al. Low dose thiazide prevents bone loss in older adults: results of a 3-year randomized, double-blind controlled trial. *Bone* 1998;23:S151.

69. Dahlof B, Pennert K, Hansson L. Reversal of left ventricular hypertrophy in hypertensive patients: a metaanalysis of 109 treatment studies. *Am J Hypertens* 1992;5:95–110.

70. Kjeldsen SE, Dahlof B, Devereux RB, et al. Effects of losartan on cardiovascular morbidity and mortality in patients with isolated systolic hypertension and left ventricular hypertrophy: Losartan Intervention for Endpoint Reduction (LIFE) substudy. *JAMA* 2002;288:1491–1498.

71. Mangano DT, Layug EL, Wallace A, et al. Effect of atenolol on mortality and cardiovascular morbidity after noncardiac surgery. *N Engl J Med* 1996;335:1713–1720.

72. Garland C, Barrett-Connor E, Suarez L, Criqui MH. Isolated systolic hypertension and mortality after age 60 years. *Am J Epidemiol* 1983;118:365–376.

73. Wolf PA. Cerebrovascular disease in the elderly. In: Tresch DD, Aronow WS, eds. *Cardiovascular Disease in the Elderly Patient.* New York: Marcel Dekker; 1994:125–147.

74. Levy D, Larson MG, Vasan RS, et al. The progression from hypertension to congestive heart failure. *JAMA* 1996;275:1557–1562.

75. Aronow WS, Ahn C, Kronzon I, Koenigsberg. Congestive heart failure, coronary events and atherothrombotic brain infarction in elderly blacks and whites with systemic hypertension and with and without echocardiographic and electrocardiographic evidence of left ventricular hypertrophy. *Am J Cardiol* 1991;67:295–299.

76. Aronow WS, Lee NH, Sales FF, Etienne F. Prevalence of postural hypotension in elderly patients in a long-term health care facility. *Am J Cardiol* 1988;62:336.

77. Aronow WS, Ahn C. Postprandial hypotension in 499 elderly persons in a long-term health care facility. *J Am Geriatr Soc* 1994;42:930–932.

78. Aronow WS. Dizziness and syncope. In: Hazzard WR, Blass JP, Ettinger WH Jr, Halter JB, Ouslander JG, eds. *Principles of Geriatric Medicine and Gerontology.* 4th ed. New York: McGraw-Hill; 1998.

79. Kannel WB, Dannenberg AL, Levy D. Population implications of electrocardiographic left ventricular hypertrophy. *Am J Cardiol* 1987;60:85I–93I.

80. Aronow WS, Koenigsberg M, Schwartz KS. Usefulness of echocardiographic and electrocardiographic left ventricular hypertrophy in predicting new cardiac events and atherothrombotic brain infarction in elderly patients with systemic hypertension or coronary artery disease. *Am J Noninvas Cardiol* 1989;3:367–370.

81. Kahn S, Frishman WH, Weissman S, et al. Left ventricular hypertrophy on electrocardiogram: prognostic implications from a 10 year cohort study of older subjects: a report from the Bronx Longitudinal Aging Study. *J Am Geriatr Soc* 1996;44:524–529.

82. Levy D, Garrison RJ, Savage DD, et al. Left ventricular mass and incidence of coronary heart disease in an elderly cohort: the Framingham Heart Study. *Ann Intern Med* 1989;110:101–107.

83. Aronow WS, Epstein S, Koenigsberg M, Schwartz KS. Usefulness of echocardiographic left ventricular hypertrophy, ventricular tachycardia, and complex ventricular arrhythmias in predicting ventricular fibrillation or sudden cardiac death in elderly patients. *Am J Cardiol* 1988;62:1124–1125.

84. Aronow WS, Gutstein H, Hsieh FY. Risk factors for thromboembolic stroke in elderly patients with chronic atrial fibrillation. *Am J Cardiol* 1989;63:366–367.

85. Aronow WS, Ahn C, Kronzon I, Gutstein H. Association of plasma renin activity and echocardiographic left ventricular hypertrophy with frequency of new coronary events and new atherothrombotic brain infarction in older persons with systemic hypertension. *Am J Cardiol* 1997;79:1543–1545.

86. Bikkina M, Levy D, Evans JC, et al. Left ventricular mass and risk of stroke in an elderly cohort: the Framingham Heart Study. *JAMA* 1994;272:33–36.

87. Aronow WS, Koenigsberg M, Schwartz KS. Usefulness of echocardiographic left ventricular hypertrophy in predicting new coronary events and atherothrombotic brain infarction in patients over 62 years of age. *Am J Cardiol* 1988;61:1130–1132.

88. Aronow WS, Ahn C, Kronzon I, et al. Association of extracranial carotid arterial disease, prior atherothrombotic brain infarction, systemic hypertension, and left ventricular hypertrophy with the incidence of new atherothrombotic brain infarction at 45-month follow-up in 1,482 older patients. *Am J Cardiol* 1997;79:991–993.

89. Kannel WB, D'Agostino RB, Levy D, et al. Prognostic significance of regression of left ventricular hypertrophy [abstract]. *Circulation* 1988;78(suppl II):II–89.

90. Koren MJ, Savage DD, Casale PN, et al. Changes in left ventricular mass predict risk in essential hypertension [abstract]. *Circulation* 1990;82(suppl III):III-29.

91. Ofili EO, Cohen JD, St. Vrain JA, et al. Effect of treatment of isolated systolic hypertension on left ventricular mass. *JAMA* 1998;279:778–782.

92. Gottdiener JS, Reda DJ, Massie BM, et al. Effect of single-drug therapy on reduction of left ventricular mass in mild to moderate hypertension: comparison of six antihypertensive agents. The Department of Veterans Affairs Cooperative Study Group on Antihypertensive Agents. *Circulation* 1997;95:2007–2014.

93. Castelli WP, Wilson PWF, Levy D, Anderson K. Cardiovascular disease in the elderly. *Am J Cardiol* 1989;63:12H–19H.

94. Wong ND, Wilson PWF, Kannel WB. Serum cholesterol as a prognostic factor after myocardial infarction: the Framingham Study. *Ann Intern Med* 1991;115:687–693.

95. Benfante R, Reed D. Is elevated serum cholesterol level a factor for coronary heart disease in the elderly? *JAMA* 1990;263:393–396.

96. Barrett-Connor E, Suarez L, Khaw K-T, et al. Ischemic heart disease risk factors after age 50. *J Chronic Dis* 1984;37:903–908.

97. Rubin SM, Sidney S, Black DM, et al. High blood cholesterol in elderly men and the excess risk for coronary heart disease. *Ann Intern Med* 1990;113:916–920.

98. Corti M-C, Guralnik JM, Salive ME, et al. Clarifying the direct relation between total cholesterol levels and death from coronary heart disease in older persons. *Ann Intern Med* 1997;126:753–760.

99. Corti M-C, Guralnik JM, Salive ME, et al. HDL cholesterol predicts coronary heart disease mortality in older persons. *JAMA* 1995;274:539–544.

100. Zimetbaum P, Frishman WH, Ooi WL, et al. Plasma lipids and lipoproteins and the incidence of cardiovascular disease in the very elderly: the Bronx Aging Study. *Arterioscler Thromb* 1992;12:416–423.

101. Aronow WS, Ahn C. Correlation of serum lipids with the presence or absence of coronary artery disease in 1,793 men and women aged ≥62 years. *Am J Cardiol* 1994;73:702–703.

102. Lavie CJ, Milani RV. National Cholesterol Education Program's recommendations, and implications of "missing" high-density lipoprotein cholesterol in cardiac rehabilitation programs. *Am J Cardiol* 1991;68:1087.

103. Aronow WS, Ahn C. Incidence of new coronary events in older persons with prior myocardial infarction and serum low-density lipoprotein cholesterol ≥125 mg/dL treated with statins versus no lipid-lowering drug. *Am J Cardiol* 2002;89:67–69.

104. Aronow WS, Ahn C, Gutstein H. Incidence of new atherothrombotic brain infarction in older persons with prior myocardial infarction and serum low-density lipoprotein

cholesterol ≥125 mg/dL treated with statins versus no lipid-lowering drug. *J Gerontol Med Sci* 2002;57A:M333–M335.

105. Aronow WS, Ahn C. Frequency of congestive heart failure in older persons with prior myocardial infarction and serum low-density lipoprotein cholesterol ≥125 mg/dl treated with statins versus no lipid-lowering drug. *Am J Cardiol* 2002;90:147–149.

106. Aronow WS, Ahn C, Gutstein H. Reduction of new coronary events and of new atherothrombotic brain infarction in older persons with diabetes mellitus, prior myocardial infarction, and serum low-density lipoprotein cholesterol ≥125 mg/dL treated with statins. *J Gerontol Med Sci* 2002;57A:M747–M750.

107. Aronow WS, Ahn C. Frequency of new coronary events in older persons with peripheral arterial disease and serum low-density lipoprotein cholesterol ≥125 mg/dl treated with statins versus no lipid-lowering drug. *Am J Cardiol* 2002;90:789–791.

108. Scandinavian Simvastatin Survival Study Group. Randomised trial of cholesterol lowering in 4444 patients with coronary heart disease: the Scandinavian Simvastatin Survival Study (4S). *Lancet* 1994;344:1383–1389.

109. Miettinen TA, Pyorala K, Olsson AG, et al. Cholesterol-lowering therapy in women and elderly patients with myocardial infarction or angina pectoris: findings from the Scandinavian Simvastatin Survival Study (4S). *Circulation* 1997;96:4211–4218.

110. Pedersen TR, Kjekshus J, Pyorala K, et al. Effect of simvastatin on ischemic signs and symptoms in the Scandinavian Simvastatin Survival Study (4S). *Am J Cardiol* 1998;81:333–336.

111. Pedersen TR, Wilhelmsen L, Faergeman O, et al. Follow-up study of patients randomized in the Scandinavian Simvastatin Survival Study (4S) of cholesterol lowering. *Am J Cardiol* 2000;86:257–262.

112. Sacks FM, Pfeffer MA, Moye LA, et al. The effect of pravastatin on coronary events after myocardial infarction in patients with average cholesterol levels. *N Engl J Med* 1996;335:1001–1009.

113. Lewis SJ, Moye LA, Sacks FM, et al. Effect of pravastatin on cardiovascular events in older patients with myocardial infarction and cholesterol levels in the average range: results of the Cholesterol and Recurrent Events (CARE) Trial. *Ann Intern Med* 1998;129:681–689.

114. The Long-Term Intervention With Pravastatin in Ischaemic Disease (LIPID) Study Group. Prevention of cardiovascular events and death with pravastatin in patients with coronary heart disease and a broad range of initial cholesterol levels. *N Engl J Med* 1998;339:1349–1357.

115. The LIPID Study Group. Long-term effectiveness and safety of pravastatin in 9014 patients with coronary heart disease and average cholesterol concentrations: the LIPID trial follow-up. *Lancet* 2002; 359:1379–1387.

116. Heart Protection Study Collaborative Group. MRC/BHF Heart Protection Study of cholesterol lowering with simvastatin in 20,536 high-risk individuals: a randomised placebo-controlled trial. *Lancet* 2002;360:7–22.

117. Shepherd J, Blauw GJ, Murphy MB, et al. Pravastatin in elderly individuals at risk of vascular disease (PROSPER): a randomised controlled trial. *Lancet* 2002:360:1623–1630.

118. Gotto AM. Presentation of the Air Force/Texas Cardiac Atherosclerotic Prevention Study at the Annual Scientific Meeting of the American Heart Association, Dallas, Tex, November, 1997.

119. Downs JR, Clearfield M, Weis S, et al. Primary prevention of acute coronary events with lovastatin in men and women with average cholesterol levels: results of AFCAPS/TexCAPS. *JAMA* 1998;279:1615–1622.

120. Lemaitre RN, Psaty BM, Heckbert SR, et al. Therapy with hydroxymethylglutaryl coenzyme A reductase inhibitors (statins) and associated risk of incident cardiovascular events in older adults: evidence from the Cardiovascular Health Study. *Arch Intern Med* 2002;162:1395–1400.

121. Expert Panel on Detection, Evaluation, and Treatment of High Blood Cholesterol in Adults. Executive Summary of the Third Report of the National Cholesterol Education Program (NCEP) Expert Panel on Detection, Evaluation, and Treatment of High Blood Cholesterol in Adults (Adult Treatment Panel III). *JAMA* 2001;285:2486–2497.

122. Grundy SM, Cleeman JI, Merz CN, et al. Implications of recent clinical trials for the National Cholesterol Education Program Adult Treatment Panel III guidelines. *Circulation* 2004;110:227–239.

123. Iso H, Jacobs DR Jr, Wentworth D, et al. Serum cholesterol levels and six-year mortality from stroke in 350,977 men screened for the Multiple Risk Factor Intervention Trial. *N Engl J Med* 1989;320:904–910.

124. Bihari-Varga M, Szekely J, Gruber E. Plasma high-density lipoproteins in coronary, cerebral and peripheral vascular disease: the influence of various risk factors. *Atherosclerosis* 1981;40:337–345.

125. Aronow WS, Ahn C. Correlation of serum lipids with the presence or absence of atherothrombotic brain infarction and peripheral arterial disease in 1,834 men and women aged ≥62 years. *Am J Cardiol* 1994;73:995–997.

126. Crouse JR III, Byington RP, Hoen HM, Furberg CD: Reductase inhibitor monotherapy and stroke prevention. *Arch Intern Med* 1997;157:1305–1310.

127. Criqui MH, Browner D, Fronek A, et al. Peripheral arterial disease in large vessels is epidemiologically distinct from small vessel disease: an analysis of risk factors. *Am J Epidemiol* 1989;129:1110–1119.

128. Fowkes FGR, Housley E, Riemersma RA, et al. Smoking, lipids, glucose intolerance, and blood pressure as risk factors for peripheral atherosclerosis compared with ischemic heart disease in the Edinburgh Artery Study. *Am J Epidemiol* 1992;135:331–340.

129. Vokonas PS, Kannel WB. Epidemiology of coronary heart disease in the elderly. In: Tresch DD, Aronow WS, eds. *Cardiovascular Disease in the Elderly Patient.* New York: Marcel Dekker; 1994:91–123.

130. Aronow WS, Ahn C. Association of diabetes mellitus using old and new diagnostic criteria with incidence of new coronary events in older men and women. *Am J Cardiol* 2000;85:104–105.

131. Barrett-Connor E, Khaw K-. Diabetes mellitus: an independent risk factor for stroke. *Am J Epidemiol* 1988;128:116–123.

132. Ness J, Aronow WS, Ahn C. Risk factors for symptomatic peripheral arterial disease in older persons in an academic hospital-based geriatrics practice. *J Am Geriatr Soc* 2000;48:312–314.

133. Stratton IM, Adler AI, Neil HAW, et al. Association of glycaemia with macrovascular and microvascular complications of type 2 diabetes (UKPDS 35): prospective observational study. *BMJ* 2000;321:405–412.

134. Adler AI, Stratton IM, Neil HAW, et al. Association of systolic blood pressure with macrovascular and microvascular complications of type 2 diabetes (UKPDS 36): prospective observational study. *BMJ* 2000;321:412–419.

135. Haffner SM, American Diabetes Association. Dyslipidemia management in adults with diabetes. *Diabetes Care* 2004;27 (Suppl 1):S68–S71.

136. Grundy S. Small LDL, atherogenic dyslipidemia, and the metabolic syndrome. *Circulation* 1997;95:1–4.

137. Grundy SM. Hypertriglyceridemia atherogenic dyslipidemia, and the metabolic syndrome. *Am J Cardiol* 1998;81:18B–25B.

138. Ford ES, Giles WH, Dietz WH. Prevalence of the metabolic syndrome among US adults: findings from the third National Health and Nutrition Examination Survey. *JAMA* 2002;287:356–359.

139. Kannel WB, Cupples LA, Ramaswami R, et al. Regional obesity and risk of cardiovascular disease. *J Clin Epidemiol* 1991;44:183–190.

140. Folsom AR, Kaye SA, Sellers TA, et al. Body fat distribution and 5-year risk of death in older women. *JAMA* 1993;269:483–487.

141. Donahue RP, Abbott RD, Reed DM, Yano K. Physical activity and coronary heart disease in middle-aged and elderly men: the Honolulu Heart Program. *Am J Public Health* 1988;78:683–685.

142. Paffenbarger RS Jr, Hyde RT, Wing AL, et al. Physical activity, all-cause mortality, and longevity of college alumni. *N Engl J Med* 1986;314:605–613.

143. Paffenbarger RS Jr, Wing AL. Characteristics in youth predisposing to fatal stroke in later years. *Lancet* 1967;1:753–754.

144. Paffenbarger RS Jr. Factors predisposing to fatal stroke in longshoremen. *Prev Med* 1972;1:522–527.

145. Wenger NK. Physical inactivity as a risk factor for coronary heart disease in the elderly. *Cardiol Elderly* 1994;2:375–379.

146. Williams MA, Maresh CM, Aronow WS, et al. The value of early out-patient cardiac exercise programmes for the elderly in comparison with other selected age groups. *Eur Heart J* 1984;5(suppl E):113–115.

147. Aronow WS. Cardiovascular drug therapy in the elderly. In: Frishman WH, Sonnenblick EH, eds. *Cardiovascular Pharmacotherapeutics*. New York: McGraw–Hill; 1997:1267–1281.

African Americans

18

Keith C. Norris
Charles K. Francis

KEY POINTS

- *Mortality rates from most cardiovascular and related diseases are higher among African Americans than any racial/ethnic group.*

- *Key risk factors for cardiovascular disease such as hypertension and diabetes occur at exceptionally high rates in African Americans and are often related to dietary practices, lifestyle influences, and health beliefs.*

- *The evaluation and treatment of cardiovascular and related diseases in African Americans should minimize perceived racial/ethnic differences in physiology and focus on the implementation of standard evidenced based guidelines with a sensitivity to cultural differences in health beliefs.*

- *The evaluation and treatment of cardiovascular risk factors in African Americans should include a detailed assessment of socio-cultural*

- *and bio-behavioral factors, many of which are modifiable.*

- *Intraracial variations in cardiovascular and related diseases among African Americans highlights the powerful influence of socio-cultural factors.*

- *Community prevention programs that are culturally sensitive have been demonstrated to improve outcomes for many cardiovascular risk factors such as limited physical activity, weight management, blood pressure control, glucose control, and lipid management.*

- *Innovative Public health strategies are needed to effectively implement educational, screening and early prevention programs that address the health beliefs and key cardiovascular risk factors in the African American community.*

Cardiovascular disease (CVD) and its major risk factors are among the 28 focus areas highlighted in Healthy People 2010, the nation's blueprint to increase quality and years of healthy life and eliminate health disparities.[1] The national recognition of CVD as a critical area of racial and ethnic disparity in health status highlights the magnitude and clinical importance of this issue as a significant area of not only individual, but also public health concern. Despite overall declines in age-adjusted CVD morbidity and mortality in African Americans during the past three decades, the rates of illness and death from coronary heart disease, stroke, heart failure and other CVD have not improved to the same extent as they have in whites.[2–4]

Racial and ethnic disparities in health care occur in the context of broad historic and contemporary social and economic inequality. Racial identity, although not a strong predictor, has some impact on health-promoting lifestyles regardless of sociodemographics.[5] Understanding race/ethnicity will assist in unraveling the contribution of biologic, cultural, and/or environmental factors that alter the pharmacodynamics of drug metabolism, therapeutic/toxic ratios, and ultimately treatment response. Also contributing to disparities in the quality of health care among Americans are variations in the ecology of the health care system, such as clinical care, patient preferences, the environment, and persistent racial and ethnic discrimination.[6–8] Additional key factors contributing to racial disparities in cardiovascular health over the last decade include differing rates of improvement and/or control of CVD risk factors. Modifiable risk factors such as hypertension, diabetes, obesity, and a sedentary lifestyle remain more prevalent and severe among African Americans, as well as other racial/ethnic minority populations, which in turn contributes to higher rates of CVD complications.

This chapter will discuss traditional epidemiologic studies as well as data from recent clinical trials that address CVD and CVD risk factors in African Americans. It will also explore—from the perspective of the individual patient, the health care provider, and the community—how these findings may be translated into new strategies to reduce/eliminate racial disparities and improve CVD-related clinical outcomes for all Americans.

EPIDEMIOLOGY OF CARDIOVASCULAR AND RELATED DISEASES IN AFRICAN AMERICANS

CVD is the leading cause of death (nearly one million in 2000) in the United States. More than 60 million people in the United States are estimated to have one or more types of CVD at a cost of over $350 billion annually.[9] From 1990 to 1998, there was a 15% decline in the death rate for white non-Hispanics with CVD, while African American non-Hispanics experienced only an 11% decline.[3] In 2000, death rates from CVD (per 100,000 population) were 28% higher for African American males than for white males (509.6 vs 397.6, respectively) and 39% higher for African American females than for white females (397.1 vs 285.8, respectively).[9]

One longstanding challenge is identifying evidenced-based recommendations for African Americans, who historically have low enrollment in cardiovascular trials. Barriers to minority participation in cardiovascular clinical trials include, but are not limited to, less access to health care, lack of physician recommendation, distrust of medical research, patient compliance issues, cultural beliefs, negative experiences with the health care system, educational and literacy status, transportation costs, and time constraints.[10,11] A better understanding of the prevalence, correlates, and progression of subclinical CVD across racial/ethnic lines is necessary. The existing data for many of the presently known CVD correlates are provided in Table 18-1.

Coronary heart disease

African Americans have the highest overall coronary heart disease (CHD) mortality rates of any ethnic group in the United States.[9,12,13] The 2000 estimated prevalence of CHD for non-Hispanic whites was 6.9% for males and 3.4% for females. For non-Hispanic African Americans, the estimated prevalence was 7.1% for males and 9% for females. Similar trends were noted for the estimated prevalence of angina pectoris across ethnic/racial groups.[9] The 2000 overall CHD death rates (per 100,000 population) were 10% higher in African American males than in white males (262.4 vs 238, respectively) and 29% higher in African American females than in white females (187.5 vs 145.3, respectively).[9] Although reasons for excess CHD mortality among African Americans have not been fully elucidated, it can be accounted for, in part, by socioeconomic factors and by the high prevalence and suboptimal control of coronary risk factors.[4,13]

Temporal trends in the prevalence of nonfatal CHD from 1971 to 1994, as assessed by age-adjusted rates of self-reported myocardial infarction, increased among African Americans as compared with whites.[14] By contrast, the prevalence of age-adjusted electrocardiogram-confirmed myocardial infarction tended to decrease for African Americans.[17] The presence of left ventricular hypertrophy (LVH) reportedly is as much as 50% greater among African Americans and women with CHD.[15] LVH is an independent predictor of mortality after adjusting for other clinical risk factors with prognostic importance equivalent to that of left ventricular ejection fraction.[18] Despite similarities between African Americans and whites in the initial cardiovascular symptoms and time to seek treatment,[16] as well as in the predictive value of most conventional risk factors for CHD,[17,18] marked differences in risk factor prevalence rates and/or genetic constitution call for special attention to improve clinical outcomes.

Congestive heart failure

Congestive heart failure (CHF) is now responsible for nearly one million deaths per year at an annual cost greater than $24 billion.[9] The prevalence of CHF is 50% higher for African American males than for white males (3.5% vs 2.3%) and 100% higher for African American females than for white females (3.1% vs 1.5%).[9] However, the 2000 death rate (per 100,000) for CHF was similar across racial/ethnic lines at 19.5 for white males, 20.4 for African American males, 18.1 for white females, and 19.3 for African American females.[9] Excess hospitalizations among African Americans for CHF reportedly were largely explained by the higher prevalence of CVD risk factors, predominantly hypertension and diabetes.[19]

Race-specific variations in heart failure may be related to the higher prevalence, greater severity, and poorer control rates of hypertension among African Americans.[2] Long-term hypertension trials suggest blood pressure reduction would be the most effective measure for slowing the progression of heart failure.[4] Other explanations for the racial variation in CHF mortality include

TABLE 18-1   Cardiovascular Disease Risk Factors in African-Americans

Major risk factors for CVD*
Diabetes mellitus
Elevated blood pressure (treated or untreated)
Elevated serum total cholesterol or LDL-C
Advancing age
Smoking
Obesity (BMI $\geq$ 30 kg/m^2)
Inactivity
Additional important risk factors for CVD
Evidence of target-organ damage: angina, prior MI or coronary revascularization, left ventricular hypertrophy, heart failure, stroke/transient ischemic attack, peripheral arterial disease, retinopathy, chronic kidney disease (GFR <60 mL/min, proteinuria or microalbuminuria, urine albumin excretion >30 mg/d or >20 mg albumin/g creatinine)
Male or postmenopausal woman
Family history of CVD in women aged <65 or men aged <55
Central obesity (waist circumference >40 in. or 102 cm in men and >35 in. or 88 cm. in women)
Low HDL (<40 mg/dL in men or <50 mg/dL in women)
Elevated triglycerides ($\geq$ 150 mg/dL)
Elevated blood glucose (fasting blood sugar $\geq$ 110 mg/dL)
Low socioeconomic status
Behavioral markers that increase risk for high blood pressure and CVD
Smoking
Overweight (BMI >25 increases risk for developing obesity)[†]
Inactivity
Excessive alcohol intake
High dietary intake of fat and sodium
Low dietary intake of potassium, calcium
Clinical markers associated with high blood pressure and CVD
Low birth weight
Family history of hypertension, diabetes, or premature CVD
High-normal blood pressure (130–139/85–89 mm Hg)
Loss of nocturnal fall in blood pressure
Excessive adult weight gain
Emerging risk factors
Elevated lipoprotein(a) levels
Elevated homocysteine levels
Elevated C-reactive protein levels
Subclinical atherosclerotic disease

*BMI, body mass index; LDL-C, low-density lipoprotein cholesterol: HDL-C, high-density lipoprotein cholesterol; CVD, cardiovascular disease; GFR, glomerular filtration rate; MI, myocardial infarction.
[†]Recent data[155] suggest African-Americans, in contrast to whites, may not have increased mortality risks until BMI >30 kg/m.^{2}
SOURCE: Modified, with permission, from Douglas et al.[54]

neurohormonal differences, delayed treatment due to re-duced access to care, influences of other risk factors on the atherosclerotic processes, and the socioeconomic and cultural environment.

Stroke

Stroke is the third leading cause of death for African Americans behind heart disease and cancer. Increases in stroke prevalence, morbidity, and mortality in African Americans are, perhaps, due to differences in pathogen-esis, stroke management, and risk factor control. The es-timated prevalence of stroke for African American men is 1.8 times, and for women is 2.5 times, that of their white counterparts.[9] The age-adjusted stroke incidence rates (per 100,000) for first-ever strokes are nearly twice as high for African Americans (at 323 for males and 260 for females) than for whites (at 167 for males and 138 for females).[9] Compared with non-Hispanic whites, the relative risk of stroke death is four times higher for non-Hispanic African Americans at ages 35 to 54, three times higher at ages 55 to 64, and almost two times higher at ages 65 to 74.[9]

In the population-based Atherosclerosis Risk in Communities (ARIC) study, subclinical cerebrovascular atherosclerosis, as determined by ultrasound-measured carotid artery intima–media thickness (IMT), was more frequent in African Americans than in whites, primarily because of greater rates of hypertension.[20] By contrast, carotid IMT was increased in African-Caribbeans com-pared with whites, even after controlling for cardiovascu-lar risk factors, suggesting a blood pressure-independent effect.[21] The role of environmental and biologic contri-butions are highlighted in stroke epidemiology, where strong evidence of geographic variations in stroke rates merges with evidence from twin and family studies to show that genetic factors contribute to the risk of stroke and that their role may be at least as important in stroke as in CHD.[4,22]

Chronic kidney disease

Chronic kidney disease (CKD) and end-stage renal dis-ease (ESRD) are two of the most vivid examples of racial differences in cardiovascular-related health out-comes in the United States.[23,24] ESRD is four times more common in African Americans than in their white counterparts, with an adjusted rate of 988 per million in African Americans and 254 per million in whites.[25] African American men between the ages of 24 and 44 are nearly 20 times more likely to suffer from hypertension-related ESRD than are white men.[25] Similarly, at the 15-year examination of 3554 participants in the Coro-nary Artery Risk Development in Young Adults (CAR-DIA) study, the adjusted odds of an elevated creatinine

among African American men was 11.4-fold that of white men, whereas the odds were was only 1.5-fold greater (not significant) for African American women than for white women.[26] The reason(s) for the exceptionally high rates of CKD and ESRD among young African American males is unknown. While socioeconomic status, lifestyle, and clinical factors (diabetes, hypertension) may account for nearly one half of the excess risk of ESRD among African Americans,[27] emerging data continue to identify biologic and genetic factors that may contribute to the increased familial risk of CKD/ESRD noted for African Americans.[28–30] The use of targeted screening can be effective in identifying persons with previously uniden-tified or poorly controlled CKD risk factors, as well as persons with moderately decreased kidney function.[31]

Diabetes and hypertension are responsible for more than 70% of patients treated for ESRD.[25] Patients with diabetes mellitus and hypertension have a 5- to 6-fold greater risk of developing ESRD compared with patients with hypertension alone.[32] With respect to hyperten-sion, it was recently reported that when compared with optimal blood pressure (systolic blood pressure [SBP] < 120 mm Hg, and diastolic blood pressue [DBP] < 80 mm Hg), even high-normal blood pressure (SBP = 130–139 mm Hg, DBP = 85–89 mm Hg) (JNC-IV cate-gories) was associated with a greater than 2-fold increased prevalence of microalbuminuria,[33] a marker of premature cardiovascular mortality. In addition, the adjusted risk of hypertension-associated microalbuminuria was 34% greater for African Americans than for whites.[33]

Peripheral vascular disease

Peripheral vascular disease (PVD) remains a major cause of disability. Amputations among African Americans and Hispanics due to PVD occur at rates two to four times higher than those of whites.[36–38] PVD, diagnosed by an ankle–brachial index less than 0.9, is more frequent among African Americans than among whites and His-panics. However, relative to the prevalence of PVD, the overall prevalence of intermittent claudication is low for African Americans, suggesting treatment may be delayed if the clinician relies on patient symptoms alone.[38] This could influence the extent of vascular disease prior to de-tection and intervention, which along with potential bi-ases in clinician practices may contribute to the 2.5 times greater rate of African Americans who have amputations rather than angioplasty or bypass surgeries.[38]

EPIDEMIOLOGY OF CVD RISK FACTORS IN AFRICAN AMERICANS

Traditional risk factors for CVD include hyperten-sion, hyperlipidemia (especially hypercholesterolemia), smoking, diabetes, sedentary lifestyle, and obesity. The relationship between these risk factors and CVD events seems to be similar in African American and white populations.[17,39,40] Familial aggregation of risk has been demonstrated in both African American and white siblings of persons with premature CHD.[41]

Despite the similarities, differences exist in clinical outcomes due to risk factor prevalence and control. These differences may be a reflection of cultural environment and access to care. A better understanding of the interaction of culture and environment with specific physiologic, clinical, and social risk factors[42] is critical to the identification and treatment of high-risk African Americans and for the development and implementation of effective evidence-based strategies for CVD risk reduction. Several risk factors that contribute to CVD are largely related to lifestyle choices. Because of the high prevalence of multiple cardiovascular risk factors and greater salt sensitivity, therapeutic lifestyle changes have particular relevance for African Americans.[43] Special features of CVD risk factors among African Americans are described in Table 18-2.

The metabolic syndrome

Recognition of the metabolic syndrome (MetS), or the dysmetabolic syndrome as it is sometimes called, is important because of the associated increased risk of CVD morbidity and mortality.[44] As defined by the third report of the National Cholesterol Education Program Adult Treatment Panel (ATP-III), MetS represents a clustering of at least three of five specific cardiovascular risk factors.[17] These include: (1) waist circumference greater than 102 cm in men or greater than 88 cm in women; (2) serum triglyceride level of 150 mg/dL or greater; (3) high-density lipoprotein cholesterol level less than 40 mg/dL in men or 50 mg/dL in women; (4) blood pressure of 130/85 mm Hg or higher; and (5) fasting serum glucose level of 110 mg/dL or higher.[17] Hyperinsulinemia/insulin resistance is another commonly recognized component of MetS and a key feature and powerful predictor of the development of type II diabetes.[40,45] In the ARIC trial, high serum insulin levels, as well as increased body mass index (BMI) and waist/hip ratio, were

---

TABLE 18-2   Special Features of Cardiovascular Disease Risk Factors in African-Americans

LDL-C[17]*	Mean LDL-C levels slightly lower and high LDL-C levels slightly more common in African-American men compared with white men
	LDL-C levels similar in African-American and white women
	Relationship between total cholesterol levels and CHD risk similar in African-American and white men
	African-American men often have relatively high, but still normal baseline level of creatine kinase that should be documented before starting statin therapy
HDL-C[17]	Mean HDL-C levels higher in African-American men than in white men
	Whether higher HDL-C levels in African-American men protect against CHD is not known
	HDL-C levels similar in African-American and white women
Triglycerides[17]	Triglyceride levels lower in African-American men and women than in white men and women
Lipoprotein (a)[17]	Lp(a) levels higher in African-American men and women than in white men and women
	Whether higher Lp (a) in African-Americans increases risk for CHD not known
Hypertension[51,54]	Hypertension more common in African-Americans than whites
	Stage 2 hypertension more common in African-Americans, further increasing risk for CHD and CVD
	LVH more common in African-Americans
	LVH is a powerful predictor of cardiovascular deaths in African-Americans
	Salt sensitivity more common in African Americans than in whites
Obesity[40,155]	Obesity nearly 50% more common in African-American women compared with white women
	Obesity similar in African-American and white men
	Optimal mortality rates associated with BMI of 23–25 kg/m² for whites and 23–30 kg/m² for African-Americans
Diabetes[17,40]	Type 2 diabetes more common in African-Americans than whites
	Higher prevalence of type 2 diabetes in African-Americans appears related to higher prevalence of obesity and increased genetic propensity
Multiple Risk Factors[40]	African-Americans more likely to have at least two risk factors than are whites—related primarily to greater rates of hypertension, obesity, and diabetes, in contrast to lower rates of dyslipidemia

*BMI, body mass index; LDL-C, low-density lipoprotein cholesterol: HDL-C, high-density lipoprotein cholesterol; CVD, cardiovascular disease; GFR, glomerular filtration rate; CHD, coronary heart disease; Lp(a), lipoprotein (a); LVH, left ventricular hypertrophy.

independently predictive of the development of diabetes, hypertension, and/or dyslipidemia in patients who had none of these metabolic abnormalities at baseline.[45] Also, in a cohort of 77 young, healthy, normotensive individuals (aged 23–27, BMI 23–26 kg/m^2) with similar clinical/laboratory profiles, Mexican-Americans, Asian-Americans, and African Americans were noted to have lower levels of insulin sensitivity than whites.[46]

African American women, not men, have a higher prevalence of MetS than whites. African American women and Hispanics have the highest prevalence of MetS in the United States.[47] This is attributable mainly to ethnic and gender variations in the spectrum of risk factors constituting MetS. Whites of European origin appear to have a greater predisposition to atherogenic dyslipidemia, in contrast to African Americans, who have increased rates of elevated blood pressure, obesity, and diabetes, and Hispanics, who have increased rates of obesity and diabetes.[40,47,48] When the clustering of several cardiovascular risk variables of MetS (insulin resistance index, BMI, triglyceride/high-density lipoprotein cholesterol [HDL-C] ratio, blood pressure) were examined in a community-based sample of more than 7000 African American and white children, the risk ratio for clustering of adverse levels of all four variables was 9.8 for whites versus 7.4 for African Americans ($P < .01$).[49] The lower risk ratio in African Americans was due predominantly to a lower triglyceride/HDL-C ratio among the African American children.

Hypertension

Hypertension is the most common diagnosis for ambulatory medical illness.[50] Hypertension is also a key component of MetS and a critical independent risk factor for cardiovascular and related diseases such as stroke, peripheral vascular disease, and renal failure.[51,52] The excess CVD risk exists even for high-normal blood pressure.[53] African Americans suffer disproportionately from hypertension and its sequelae, likely due to a combination of socioeconomic, cultural, and genetic factors.[54] Although blood pressure control for the nation has improved since the first National Health and Nutrition Examination Survey, it is still unacceptably low.[55,56] Data from the National Health and Nutrition Examination Survey 1999–2000 revealed the prevalence of blood pressure control to be only 33% for whites, 28% for African Americans, and 16% for Hispanics.[57]

Diabetes

Diabetes affects nearly 7.3% of African American men and 9.1% of African American women, a rate nearly 50% greater than that of the white population but less than that of Mexican-Americans.[58] The 2000 death rate from diabetes was 25.8 per 100,000 for white males, 47.8 for African American males, 20.6 for white females, and 50.4 for African American females.[9]

The high prevalence of diabetes among African American women, in particular, is due largely to the high prevalence of obesity and the subsequent development of insulin resistance, which has been described as an independent risk factor for hypertension and CVD.[40,59] Thus, significant CVD risk factor clustering occurs intrinsically in patients with type 2 diabetes. One study noted that among 13,446 middle-aged men and women free of CHD at baseline, the relative risk of CHD for people with diabetes, versus those without diabetes, was 3.45 among women and 2.52 among men.[60] Although adjusted rates were slightly lower in African Americans, overall adverse outcomes were greater among African Americans due to a greater prevalence of diabetes.[60]

Evaluation of more than 11,000 participants in the Third National Health and Nutrition Examination Survey (NHANES-III) study noted the likelihood of diabetes was equivalent at high BMI (>32 kg/m^2), but 75% greater for African Americans than for whites at low BMI (<22 kg/m^2).[61] African Americans with diabetes were significantly more likely than non-African Americans with diabetes to have excess risk factors for adverse CVD outcomes, including uncontrolled hypertension, cigarette smoking, and lack of health insurance or a private health care provider.[62]

Dyslipidemia

The benefits of cholesterol lowering for primary and secondary prevention of CHD have been well established.[17] Recently, certain lipid subfractions that may be independently linked with cardiovascular outcomes have received much attention. ARIC investigators reported that mean lipoprotein(a) levels were more than twice as high for African Americans than for whites. They also reported that the levels were an independent risk factor for stroke/transient ischemic attack and CHD in both African Americans and whites, although lipoprotein(a) is less significant as a CHD predictor among African Americans.[63] African Americans were less likely to report serum cholesterol screening than whites.[64] Even when identified as having high cholesterol that required medication, African Americans were less likely than whites to be taking cholesterol-lowering agents.[64] Although data suggest that racial and ethnic groups vary somewhat in baseline risk for CHD (eg, African Americans tend to have higher levels of HDL-C), this evidence was limited and insufficient to lead the ATP-III panel to modify general recommendations for cholesterol management in these populations.[17]

Obesity

Obesity or "severe overweight" is associated with an increased risk of CVD.[65,66] More than 57% of African American men (59.6% of white men), and more than 66% of African American women (45.5% of white women) are considered overweight, with similar trends for children.[9,67] Weight reduction and maintenance of weight loss remain difficult challenges, particularly in African American women. Racial differences in obesity and blood pressure are already present in 9- to 11-year-old children.[68] Obesity was directly associated with atherogenic plasma lipids, SBP, serum glucose and insulin, and prevalence of diabetes mellitus, and independently associated with CVD in young and middle-aged African Americans and whites in the CARDIA and ARIC studies.[69] Weight loss among 3245 white and African American adults who participated in the ARIC study over an average of 9 years was associated with a decrease in blood pressure and with remission of hypertension.[70]

Lifestyle influences on CVD and associated risk factors

PHYSICAL INACTIVITY

Physical inactivity is more prevalent among women than men, among African Americans than whites, among older than younger adults, and among the less affluent than the more affluent.[9] Regular physical activity has been associated with reduced CVD risk factors and improved health outcomes.[71] Recent studies show that among African Americans aged 18 and older, 44.4% of men and 55.2% of women report no activity, versus 32.5% of white males and 36.2% of white females.[9] As with diet, poor patterns for exercise among the younger African American community can contribute to greater risk for CVD with advancing age. Efforts to increase awareness and promote physical activity among children and young adults may help develop low-CVD-risk lifestyles.[72]

DIET

Nutrition plays a significant role in many of the CVD-associated risk factors. Several studies support a relationship between blood pressure and dietary cations, with African Americans generally having greater sodium intake, relative to potassium, and lower calcium intake.[73,74] This may be related to a combination of socioeconomic factors and dietary customs within the African American community that are associated with high salt and high fat intake. Several traditional African American food preparations are believed to be related, in part, to a continuation of cooking practices developed during slavery, when African American slaves often were given leftovers to eat and, thus, used generous amounts of seasonings, salts, and gravies to make the food palatable. Although the challenge of impacting hundreds of years of traditional dietary customs is daunting, subtle modifications, which can be implemented at both the individual and community levels, may improve CVD risk factors and associated outcomes.[75,76]

CIGARETTE SMOKING

Cigarette smoking is associated with a marked increase in CVD risk. This may be due, in part, to smoking-related increases in C-reactive protein, fibrinogen, and homocysteine, important pro-inflammatory and prothrombotic markers.[77] Smoking has been associated with a more than fourfold greater prevalence of severe uncontrolled hypertension among inner-city African Americans.[78] The reported prevalence of smoking among African Americans varies from slightly less[9] to greater than[79] that of whites. The higher rates appear to be related to differences in socioeconomic status.[79] African American males and individuals with less than a high school education are consistently reported as more frequent smokers.[9] Those with less than a high school education and ethnic minorities are also among those least likely to quit smoking.[80] There were lower rates of current and subsequent smoking during a 3-year period of evaluation among 4569 young adults (similar numbers of African Americans and whites) who attended religious services regularly, supporting the role of the church in addressing healthy lifestyles.[81]

PSYCHOSOCIAL FACTORS AND STRESS

Stress may be associated with a variety of neurohormonal changes that contribute to CVD,[82,83] and stress reduction therapies may improve the associated risks.[84,85] Worsening psychosocial stresses arising from indigent lives and disenfranchisement from our health care system are additional putative contributors to increased CVD in African Americans. The increased incidence of hypertension in African Americans has been posited to arise largely due to internalized demands arising from racial or socioeconomic stresses, a phenomenon frequently termed *active coping* or *John Henryism*.[86] Among 334 premenopausal women, African Americans reported more chronic stress and had higher carotid IMT than did whites.[87] African Americans who reported experiencing racial discrimination had marginally more carotid plaque than did those who did not report experiencing racial discrimination, consistent with a vulnerability to chronic stress.[87] Given that the excess of hypertension and other CVD risk factors may be mediated through behavioral factors modifying biologic mechanisms, interventional studies are warranted to assess their efficacy in African American communities.[88,89] In addition, the National Center for Complementary and Alternative Medicine is supporting clinical trials, specialized centers, research training, and investigator-initiated projects addressing CVD and stress reduction techniques.[90]

SPECIAL CONSIDERATIONS: GENDER, HOMOCYSTEINE, AND INFLAMMATORY MARKERS

Postmenopausal African American women are more likely to have excess CVD risk factors.[91] The high rates of diabetes and obesity and the increasing prevalence MetS with advancing age further highlight the need to address CVD risk profiles in postmenopausal women.[47]

Elevated plasma homocysteine levels are becoming more recognized as independent risk factors for coronary and peripheral vascular diseases.[92] Limited data exist with respect to homocysteine levels in African Americans. In an analysis of a subsample of 660 participants with carotid IMT above the 90th percentile or below the 75th percentile in the ARIC study, researchers found age-adjusted homocysteine levels were higher in smokers, men, and African Americans.[93]

Elevated levels of C-reactive protein (CRP), a measure of chronic subclinical inflammation, along with low levels of insulin-like growth factor 1 (IGF-1) and low levels of insulin-like growth factor-binding protein 1 (IGFBP-1), are independently associated with MetS, insulin resistance, and interleukin-6 in predicting CVD risk.[94,95] CRP levels among African Americans vary among reports: levels are lower in some studies[94] and higher in others.[96] Thus, the role of homocysteine levels and inflammatory markers in CVD outcomes for African Americans awaits further study.

Substance abuse can affect adherence to therapy and may have direct effects on blood pressure and the atherosclerotic process.[54,97] Cocaine use in the CARDIA study was related to being African American, male, single, and unemployed.[98] Heavy alcohol use was highest among Hispanics. Alcohol use over a 1-month period was reported by 55% of whites compared with only 39.9% of African Americans, whereas heavy alcohol use was reported by 5.7% of African Americans and 3.8% of whites. Illicit substance abuse during a 1-month period was reported by 8.5% of whites and 9.7% of African Americans.[99] Thus, although not clearly defined, the epidemiology of substance abuse may influence the effectiveness of both pharmacologic and nonpharmacologic therapies and the natural history of CVD.

EVALUATION AND TREATMENT OF CVD IN AFRICAN AMERICANS

Effective risk reduction strategies can markedly reduce the incidence of both primary and secondary cardiovascular events. The American Heart Association recommends that all primary care providers offer their patients counseling to promote physical activity, a healthy diet, and smoking cessation as part of the preventive health examination.[100] Despite the strong body of evidence documenting efficacy, risk reduction therapies continue to be underused or ineffectively implemented.[101] The high prevalence of multiple risk factors for African Americans magnifies the need for early risk factor assessment and family screening and the addressing of these issues in a positive proactive manner at the individual, family, and community levels. Comprehensive changes in health care delivery systems within the African American community are needed to ensure that cardiovascular risk reduction strategies become a routine part of patient care.[6,102]

A thorough assessment by the clinician should include the evaluation of blood pressure, CHD family history, smoking, weight/height, age, level of physical activity, diet, and measurement of lipids (Table 18-3).[51,54,103] General recommendations for CVD prevention include smoking cessation, reduction of dietary fat intake to less than 30% of total energy, attainment of optimal weight, and regular aerobic exercise. An improved understanding of the variations in risk factor prevalence (Table 18-2) and access to care, as well as biologic factors, should lead to improved clinical outcomes. A need still exists to include more African Americans in large randomized prevention studies. Studies such as the Heart Outcomes Prevention Evaluation (HOPE) trial, which demonstrated that angiotensin-converting enzyme inhibitor (ACEI) therapy reduces cardiovascular outcomes, had limited minority enrollment.[104] As a result, ACEI therapy remains debated as an effective therapy in African Americans.

Coronary artery disease

Presenting symptoms of ischemic-type chest pain and their correlation to myocardial infarction differ between races. In a study of 3401 African American and 6600 white patients with symptoms suggestive of acute cardiac ischemia presenting to the emergency room, a diagnosis of acute myocardial infarction was confirmed in only 6% of African American men and 4% of African American women, in contrast to 12% of white men and 8% of white women, respectively.[105] The lower prevalence of confirmed myocardial infarction among African Americans with chest pain may be related to a lesser prevalence of ischemic heart disease and a greater prevalence of left ventricular hypertrophy and/or associated abnormalities in cardiac vasoreactivity.[106] Along those lines, race did not influence brachial artery flow-mediated dilation among 228 hypertensive subjects, yet African Americans had an enhanced response to sublingual nitroglycerin, suggesting racial differences in the responses to medical therapy.[107] East and colleagues reported that there was a 50% greater likelihood of LVH among women and African Americans in a sample of more than 2000 patients diagnosed with CHD. LVH remained an

TABLE 18-3   Key Elements of an Initial Cardiovascular Risk Assessment in African-American Adults

| **History** |
| Family history of HBP*, CVD, or type 2 diabetes mellitus |
| Previous diagnosis of HBP, known duration, levels of BP elevation, and prior treatment |
| Smoking history |
| Current alcohol consumption |
| Leisure-time physical activity |
| Dietary assessment (determine who cooks, dining patterns) |
| Environmental assessment (neighborhood, housing, employment, workplace) |
| Use of street drugs (in particular, cocaine, amphetamines, phencyclidine) |
| Current medications (including over-the-counter medications, supplements, herbal products, home remedies) |
| Medical and psychiatric history (including stress and those illnesses that may affect choice of antihypertensive agent, eg, COPD, erectile dysfunction, depression) |
| Insurance status, ability to purchase prescriptions |
| Home situation, family support structure |
| **Physical examination** |
| Measure height and weight (calculate BMI = weight [kg]/height [m^2]) |
| Observe for central adiposity (waist circumference >40 in. or 102 cm in men and >35 in. or 88 cm in women suggests increased cardiovascular risk) |
| Perform cardiovascular and pulmonary examination |
| Measure blood pressure using appropriate technique |
| Perform funduscopic examination |
| **Laboratory studies** |
| Fasting lipid profile (including total cholesterol, LDL-C, HDL-C, triglycerides) |
| Serum creatinine |
| Morning preferred (or random) urinalysis for protein creatinine ratio (microalbuminuria: urine albumin excretion >30 mg/d or >20 mg albumin/g creatinine, proteinuria >300 mg/d) |
| Fasting plasma glucose |
| Electrocardiogram |
| Echocardiogram (if suspicious of LVH) |
| 24-h urinary sodium excretion if needed to assess dietary sodium intake in more detail (eg, poorly controlled HBP) |

*HBP, high blood pressure; CVD, cardiovascular disease; BMI, body mass index; LDL-C, low-density lipoprotein cholesterol; HDL-C, high-density lipoprotein cholesterol; CHD, coronary heart disease; COPD, chronic obstructive pulmonary disease; LVH, left ventricular hypertrophy.

SOURCE: Modified, with permission, from Douglas et al.[54]

independent predictor of increased mortality after adjusting for other clinical risk factors, and the high prevalence of LVH among African Americans and women partially accounted for racial and gender differences in mortality.[15]

Although similar rates of cardiovascular procedure utilization and subsequent clinical outcomes have been reported for racial/ethnic minorities,[108] the majority of reports suggest lower rates of appropriate cardiovascular intervention and lower survival rates for racial/ethnic minorities, even after adjusting for multiple clinical and demographic variables.[109] A robust analysis of administrative or detailed clinical data published from 1966 to 2000 confirmed that African American patients were less likely than whites to receive cardiac catheterization, percutaneous transluminal coronary angioplasty (PTCA), and coronary artery bypass grafting. Procedure rates also were lower for Hispanic and Asian patients. The review of survey data within this analysis yielded conflicting results regarding patient refusals as a source of racial variation. Less educated patients and patients who were not as experienced with the proposed procedure were more likely to decline PTCA, and physician bias was also associated with racial variation in recommendations for treatment.[109] This is consistent with the Institute of Medicine report on unequal treatment[6] and a recent study among 720 primary care physicians who viewed recorded interviews with actors portraying patients with cardiac symptoms. Women, when compared with men, and African Americans, when compared with whites, were only 60% as likely to be referred for cardiac catheterization, despite a similar clinical picture.[110]

In another analysis of almost 5000 patients, whites were found to be three times as likely to undergo cardiovascular procedures as African Americans prior to the development of ESRD. However, the same cohort had nearly identical rates after developing ESRD, at which time Medicare covered all patients.[111] Leape and coworkers analyzed whether cardiovascular procedures were used when needed rather than comparing crude use rates between ethnic/gender/socioeconomic groups. Although they reported that women, ethnic minorities, and the uninsured did receive needed interventions, the issue of appropriate preventive and early care was not fully addressed.[112] Indeed, researchers using Medicare claims and medical record review of a large and diverse sample of Medicare beneficiaries in five US states found that overuse of PTCA was significantly greater among white men than among other groups.[113] Thus, it is unclear in many instances if whites, who are more likely to have insurance, are being overtreated or if African Americans are receiving inappropriately low levels of care.

Although CVD outcomes for racial/ethnic minorities, women, and the uninsured are still worse in many settings,[7,8] when high-quality medical care is made available, the apparent deleterious effects of race and poverty on adverse cardiovascular related outcomes can be attenuated.[108,111]

Congestive heart failure

CHF in African Americans is characterized by a higher frequency of hypertension as the etiology, a worse prognosis, and often a lesser response to evidenced-based CHF medical therapy compared with CHF in their white counterparts.[114–116] Reported differences in racial response to CHF therapy might be related not only to underlying risk factors and access to care, but also to genetic polymorphisms that may affect response to drug therapy (Table 18-4).[114,117]

Mortality rates among racial groups in Studies of Left Ventricular Dysfunction (SOLVD) after 1-year follow-up were similar, suggesting access to care and appropriate intervention can improve CHF outcomes for African Americans.[118] Unfortunately, at the 34-month follow-up in SOLVD, researchers reported an approximately 30% greater mortality rate among African American versus white subjects after adjusting for age and coexisting medical conditions.[116] A reanalysis of data from the SOLVD prevention and treatment trials using a matched-cohort design with enalapril therapy found no racial difference in mortality rate, but the reduction in the risk of CHF hospitalizations for whites was significantly greater than that for African Americans, which suggests that African Americans with CHF do not benefit as much from ACEI therapy.[19] However, African Americans had higher blood pressure levels, 50% more hypertrophic heart disease, and 50% less aspirin (ASA) use, suggesting the matched cohort design and associated analysis did not compare similar populations.

In a prospective randomized study of more than 1000 participants, of whom 19.8% were African American, the US Carvedilol Heart Failure Study Group reported a similar benefit for both mortality and hospitalization outcomes among African Americans and non-African Americans treated with α-adrenergic blockade.[119] Moreover, in a retrospective study of nearly 30,000 fee-for-service Medicare beneficiaries hospitalized with heart failure in 1998 and 1999, African American Medicare patients hospitalized with heart failure received comparable quality of care. African American Medicare patients had slightly higher rates of readmission, but had lower mortality rates up to 1 year after hospitalization than did white patients, again suggesting that when quality care is provided, racial disparities in CHF outcomes dissipate.[120]

Stroke

Hypertension control remains a key strategy for reducing stroke events, with most hypertension trials showing an even greater reduction in stroke events in comparison to coronary events.[51] While overall stroke mortality rates have been rapidly declining for both African Americans and whites, the magnitude of the relative increased risk of dying from a stroke among African Americans, as compared with whites, has remained largely unchanged.[121] Unlike most CVD outcomes, there appears to be substantially greater variation in response to evidence-based treatment for stroke among African Americans than among whites.

A randomized, double-blind, investigator-initiated, multicenter trial of more than 1800 African Americans with a recent noncardioembolic ischemic stroke followed for up to 2 years found no statistically significant difference between ticlopidine and aspirin in the prevention of recurrent stroke, myocardial infarction, or vascular death. Moreover, there was a trend for reduction of fatal or nonfatal stroke among those in the aspirin group.[122] Based on these data and the risk of serious adverse events with ticlopidine, aspirin appears to be a better treatment for aspirin-tolerant African American patients with noncardioembolic ischemic stroke.

TABLE 18-4   Special Considerations for Cardiovascular Disease Treatment in African-Americans

Clinical entity	Special considerations
Coronary heart disease[51,54]	• Aspirin and beta blockers should be used as indicated. • If hypertension is present, check for LVH (LVH is associated with increased mortality risk and may modify treatment based on further clinical assessment). • Revascularization or surgery should be performed as indicated for the general population.
Congestive heart failure[51,54]	• Class-specific therapy (eg, ACEI, ARB, beta blocker) in combination with diuretic should be used as indicated for the general population. • Hypertension is a particularly powerful risk factor for CHD in African-Americans. • If hypertension is present, check for LVH.
Stroke[51,122]	• Particular attention should be given to maintaining BP <140/90 mm Hg unless not clinically tolerated. • Aspirin should be used as indicated. • Ticlopidine should not be used unless aspirin is contraindicated.
Chronic kidney disease[51,54]	• Elevated BP should be treated to <130/80, especially in the presence of proteinuria or diabetes. • ACEI or ARB in combination with diuretic should be initial therapy; add additional antihypertensive agents as needed to achieve BP goal.
Hypertension[51,54,132]	• Diuretic should be initial therapy. • Second-line agent should be influenced by coexisting medical conditions to achieve BP <140/90 mm Hg (<130/80 if diabetes or chronic kidney disease). • Check 24-h urinary sodium excretion if BP not controlled to assess adherence to low-sodium diet.
Diabetes [40,147]	• Diet, weight reduction (if necessary), insulin, oral hypoglycemics, and/or insulin sensitizers to achieve hemoglobin A_{1C} < 7%.
Hyperlipidemia [17,40]	• Institute lifestyle changes (Table 18–7) and/or lipid-lowering therapy to achieve LDL-C < 100 mg/dL (CHD or CHD equivalents) or <130 mg/dL (≤2 CHD risk factors) as outlined in ATP-III.
Low adherence to prescribed treatment plan [51,54]	• Assess for medication side effects (increased angioedema among African-Americans taking ACEI); check insurance prescription plan and/or ability to pay for prescribed medicines (adjust therapy as needed); assess biobehavioral barriers, assess family support structure (Table 18-6).

*BP, blood pressure; CHD, coronary heart disease; BMI, body mass index; LDL-C, low density lipoprotein cholesterol; HDL-C, high density lipoprotein cholesterol; LVH, left ventricular hypertrophy; ACEI, angiotensin-converting enzyme inhibitor; ARB, angiotensin receptor blocker

In the Losartan Intervention for Endpoint Reduction (LIFE) trial, more than 9000 participants (6% African American) with hypertension and LVH were randomized to atenolol or losartan with diuretic as needed.[123] Although losartan was more effective in reducing CVD events for the cohort, a subanalysis of African Americans revealed no benefit and, actually, an increase in CVD events, including stroke, in comparison to atenolol. This occurred despite the finding that the average blood pressure reduction and left ventricular mass regression were similar in African Americans and non-African Americans with both treatments, but could have been due to a lower percentage of African Americans achieving goal blood pressure (Table 18-5).[124] In the Antihypertensive and Lipid Lowering Therapy to Prevent Heart Attack Trial (ALLHAT), in which 36% of the more than 35,000 randomized participants were African American, there were significant reductions in stroke events with diuretics, ACEIs, with a trend for best outcomes with diuretics

(Table 18-5). In subgroup analyses African Americans were similar to the entire cohort.[125] Lipid lowering in a subset of more than 10,000 ALLHAT cohort participants had no beneficial effect in the cohort as a whole for combined cardiovascular events; however, in subgroup analyses there was benefit in CHD events (relative risk [RR] = 0.73 vs 1.02, P = .03) and a less favorable effect for stroke (RR = 1.12 vs 0.74, P = .03) in African Americans than in non-African Americans (Table 18-5).[126]

The use of carotid endarterectomy in a retrospective review of more than 1000 patients, of whom 133 (13%) were African American and 912 (87%) white, over a 10-year period showed no racial difference in outcomes.[127] The perioperative stroke and death rate was 5.3% for African Americans and 3.1% for whites, which did not reach statistical significance, but was 50% higher in African Americans, suggesting further analyses of carotid endarterectomy in larger numbers of African Americans are needed.

TABLE 18-5 Clinical Trials of Antihypertensive and Lipid–Lowering Treatment to Prevent Heart Attack (ALLHAT)[6,125]

Design	Population*	Drugs	Terminated arm	Final results
Randomized, double–blind, controlled clinical trial Target blood pressure <130/85 mm Hg Primary outcome: composite of fatal and nonfatal cardiac endpoints Follow-up, 6 y	N = 33,357 High-risk hypertensive partic-ipants aged ≥55 36% African American 47% women 36% diabetic	Chlorthalidone vs am-lodipine or lisinopril or doxazosin	Doxazosin arm was terminated by the data and safety monitoring board because doxazosin-treated patients developed CHF† at a greater rate than diuretic-treated patients	Chlorthalidone, lisinopril, and amlodipine did not differ in preventing major coronary events Chlorthalidone was superior to lisinopril in reducing stroke and CHF, and superior to amlodipine in reducing CHF Subgroup analyses: African-Americans were similar to entire cohort

Lipid-lowering treatment to prevent heart attack trial (ALLHAT-LLT)[126]

Design	Population*	Drugs	Terminated arm	Final results
Randomized, double–blind, controlled clinical trial ALLHAT Subset Lipid lowering agent versus usual care Primary outcome: Composite of fatal and nonfatal cardiac end points Follow-up, 6 y	N = 10,355 LDL-C of 120–189 mg/dL (100–119 mg/dL if known CHD) Triglycerides <350 mg/dL Mean age 66 49% women 38% African-American 23% Hispanic 14% history of CHD 35% type 2 diabetes	Pravastatin 40 mg/d vs usual care	Pravastatin reduced total cholesterol levels by 17% vs 8% with usual care Pravastatin reduced LDL-C levels by 28% vs 11% with usual care	All-cause mortality: similar for two groups (RR = 0.99, P = 0.88) 6-y mortality rates for pravastatin; 14.9% vs 15.3% with usual care African-Americans: fared better in CHD events (RR = 0.73 vs 1.02, p =.03), worse for stroke (RR = 1.12 vs 0.74, P =.03)

(continued)

TABLE 18-5 (Continued)

| | Losartan intervention for endpoint reduction (LIFE) [123,124] | | | |
Design	Population*	Drugs	African-American sub analysis	Final results
Randomized, double-blind, controlled clinical trial Target BP <140/90 mm/Hg Primary outcome: death, MI, or stroke composite Average follow-up, 4.8 y	N = 9193 hypertensive participants aged 55–80 with LVH by ECG 6% African-American 54% women 13% diabetic	Losartan vs atenolol HCTZ as second-line agent	Among 566 African-American participants, 11% of atenolol group vs. 17% of losartan group reached primary endpoints	13% reduction in composite outcome for losartan vs atenolol ($P = .021$) and 25% reduction in new-onset diabetes ($P = .001$)
	African-American study of kidney disease and hypertension (AASK) [131,132‡]			
Design	Population*	Drugs	Terminated arm	Final results
Randomized, double-blind, controlled clinical trial Two levels of target BP and three primary antihypertensive agents Primary outcome: rate of decline of GFR Average follow-up, 4y	N = 1094 Nondiabetic African-Americans with hypertensive renal disease, aged 18–70	Amlodipine vs ramipril vs metoprolol as primary therapy 90% received diuretics	Amlodipine arm was terminated by the data and safety monitoring board because of increased clinical composite outcomes of GFR doubling, ESRD, or death	No difference in primary outcome by BP level or BP therapy Ramipril reduced clinical composite (secondary outcome) by 38% compared with amlodipine and by 22% compared with metoprolol

† RR, relative risk; LDL-C, low density lipoprotein cholesterol; HDL-C, high density lipoprotein cholesterol; CHD, coronary heart disease; BP, blood pressure; MI, myocardial infarction; HCTZ, hydrochlorthiazide; LVH, left ventricular hypertrophy; ECG, electrocardiogram; GFR, glomerular filtration rate; CHF, congestive heart failure.

* ALLHAT trial data suggest that α-adrenergic blockers should not be used as first-line agents in high-risk hypertensive patients, and that a thiazide diuretic should be a component of combination therapy in antihypertensive regimens.

‡ AASK trial examined dihydropyridine calcium channel blockers (CCBs). This finding may not apply to nondihydropyridine CCBs.

SOURCE: Modified, with permission, from Douglas et al.[54]

Chronic kidney disease

As is in many other areas of health care, even when African Americans are afflicted at disproportionately high rates, many renal clinical trials contain relatively few African American participants. Indeed, the landmark trial by Lewis and colleagues, which demonstrated the efficacy of ACEIs in reducing the progression of CKD in 409 participants with type I diabetes, included only 15 African Americans.[128] This was critical, because ACEIs were felt to be of limited value in African Americans due to older reports of lesser antihypertensive efficacy.[54] Thus, this study provided no new data to suggest ACEIs might be an effective treatment for African Americans with diabetic nephropathy and hypertension. Additional large studies reporting beneficial effects of ACEIs on clinical outcomes in subjects with CKD also had low minority enrollment.[129,130] The African American Study of Kidney Disease and Hypertension (AASK) is the largest prospective CKD study to focus on, and successfully recruit, African American participants (Table 18-5). The AASK reported that secondary clinical outcomes (including the development of ESRD, doubling of serum creatinine, and death) were lower in the ACEI group in comparison to the beta blocker and dihydropyridine calcium channel blocker (CCB) groups, suggesting that ACEI inhibitors should be used as initial antihypertensive therapy with diuretics in African Americans with hypertensive nephrosclerosis to achieve successful blood pressure control.[131–133]

More recently, in two large multicenter clinical trials, angiotensin receptor blockers (ARBs) have been reported to delay the progression of diabetic nephropathy.[134,135] Results from the nearly 15% of African American participants included in these two studies, although not sufficient for generating independent analyses, strongly suggest that the positive outcomes extended to African Americans as well as non-African Americans.

Thus, emerging data from prospective randomized trials suggest that inhibition of the renin–angiotensin system as the initial therapy, in combination with diuretics for treating hypertensive and diabetic nephropathy—the two leading causes of ESRD in African Americans—confers additional protection beyond blood pressure control.[136] Importantly, these recommendations hold true for African Americans.

EVALUATION AND TREATMENT OF CARDIOVASCULAR RISK FACTORS IN AFRICAN AMERICANS

CVD is influenced by multiple established modifiable and nonmodifiable risk factors, as well as emerging risk factors (Table 18-1). The latter consist of lipoprotein(a), homocysteine, prothrombotic and pro-inflammatory factors, impaired fasting glucose, as well as evidence of subclinical atherosclerotic disease. Specific therapy for these markers has yet to be determined in most cases. The established risk factors are often influenced by lifestyle choices and are direct targets for clinical intervention. Understanding some of the barriers that may impede adherence to lifestyle choices can assist in improving overall CVD care (Table 18-6).

The metabolic syndrome

Evaluation and treatment of the metabolic syndrome (MetS) is a multifactorial process consisting of assessing the patient for high-risk metabolic abnormalities and

TABLE 18-6 Understanding Major Barriers to Adherence in African-Americans

Overweight/obese (body mass index >25/30 kg/m^2)	Cultural concern that a thin body habitus is associated with poor health
High dietary intake of fat and sodium	Cultural food preparation and conditioned tasting likely initiated or exacerbated during slavery when high salt and fat content was needed for preservation and/or palatability of suboptimal food sources
Low dietary calcium intake	Low milk and dairy intake due to high prevalence of lactose intolerance
Inactivity for women	Cultural emphasis on hair styling and relatively high cost of hair maintenance contributes to avoidance of routine exercise with increased heart rate and sweating
Unfilled prescriptions	Higher rates of poverty and lower rates of insurance, high rates of impotence among males
Limited office appointment adherence	Transportation difficulties (many cities have poor mass transportation systems, competing priorities such as child/grandchild care, elder care [often related to extended family home structure] Child and elder care facilities often geographically disconnected from health care and work training locations Inability to leave work to attend health care appointments in many job settings

TABLE 18-7 Therapeutic Lifestyle Changes

Medical target	Practical plan to achieve goal
Weight loss	Lose weight gradually by making permanent changes in daily diet for entire family Initiate 800–1500 kcal/d diet. Set reasonable weight loss goal (1–2 lb/week for first 3–6 m).
Dietary goals Low fat	Eat fewer fast foods and fried foods, and eat more broiled and steamed foods. Eat more grains, fresh fruits, and vegetables. Eat fewer overall fats and use healthier fats, such as olive oil. Eat fewer processed foods and fast foods.
Low sodium High potassium	Read labels and pay attention to sodium and fat content of foods. Reduce high sodium food intake (potato chips, most fast foods and processed foods). Identify low-sodium, high-potassium snacks (eg, dried fruits, bananas, orange juice, raw vegetables). Do not add salt when cooking; instead taste foods first and add salt at the table if needed. Use vinegar, lemon juice, or sodium substitutes such as potassium instead of standard table salt for seasoning. Do not season foods with smoked meats, such as bacon and ham hocks. Eat fewer processed foods and fast foods.
Adequate calcium	Become more aware of food sources that are rich in calcium. If lactose intolerant, try lactose-free milk or yogurt, or drink calcium-fortified juices or soy milk.
Limitation of alcohol	Men: no more than 2 beers, 1 glass of wine, or 1 shot of hard liquor per day. Women: no more than 1 beer or 1 glass of wine per/ day (a shot of hard liquor exceeds these recommendations).
Physical fitness	Increase physical activity as part of the daily routine: eg, if currently sedentary, get off the bus 6 blocks from home or walk in the evening with spouse or friend. Gradually increase time spent at an enjoyable physical activity to 30–45 min 3–5 d/wk.
No tobacco use	For nonsmokers, do not start. For current smokers, attempt smoking cessation, increase tolerance for failure, and be willing to continue the effort until success is achieved. Be aware that smokeless tobacco products (eg, chewing tobacco) also have associated risks.

SOURCE: Modified, with permission, from Douglas et al.[54]

then initiating treatment with specific therapy including diet, exercise, and pharmacologic therapy (Tables 18-4, 18-7). The pharmacologic therapy may comprise statins, ACEIs, and thiazolidinediones to the extent indicated depending on the accompanying MetS factors.[137] The most prevalent features of MetS in African Americans are hypertension, diabetes, and obesity (especially in African American women). Lifestyle choices may heavily influence both the presence and the control of these disorders and need to be addressed in a culturally sensitive manner to achieve effective results. The approach to many of these risk factors in African Americans is discussed in more detail below.

Hypertension

Hypertension has been reported as one of the most important modifiable risk factors for CHD.[51] The Seventh Report of the Joint National Committee on Prevention, Detection, Evaluation, and Treatment of High Blood Pressure (JNC-7) provides updated guidelines for hypertension prevention and management.[51] Extensive investigations have delineated the effectiveness of both nonpharmacologic and pharmacologic therapies and strategies to transcend barriers to optimal outcomes.[138] African Americans have a disproportionate burden of hypertension, and several biologic/genetic factors have been identified that contribute to the development of hypertension and increased end-organ damage, such as salt sensitivity, hyperexpression of transforming growth factor β, vasoregulatory peptides, and others.[139–143]

As outlined by JNC-7, if lifestyle modifications are unable to control blood pressure, pharmacologic intervention with either diuretics or beta blockers is recommended as first-line therapy.[51] Specific CVD risk factors or coexisting diseases may modify the choice to an ACEI (ie, CHF, diabetes), an alpha blocker (ie, prostatic enlargement, hypercholesterolemia), or other agents. Despite studies reporting the lower rates of blood pressure response of African Americans to several antihypertensive agents, in contrast to diuretics and CCBs,[51,54,144] ethnicity should not be the primary criterion for selecting a given class of antihypertensive therapy.[51,54] The clinical decision should be guided by assessment of coexisting risk factors and cultural/socioeconomic factors.[51,54] Restriction of beta blockers[145] and/or possibly ACEIs in African Americans with specific CVD risk factors or previous myocardial infarction could contribute to the increased mortality. ALLHAT demonstrated that chlorthalidone was similar to amlodipine and lisinopril in preventing fatal CHD and nonfatal myocardial infarction and superior in reducing several secondary adverse cardiovascular outcomes, thus supporting prior recommendations for diuretics as first-line therapy for hypertension in African Americans (Table 18-5).[125]

The prevalence, severity, and impact of hypertension are increased in African Americans, who often demonstrate reduced blood pressure responses to monotherapy with beta blockers, ACEIs, or ARBs, compared with diuretics or CCBs. These differential responses are largely eliminated by drug combinations that include adequate doses of a diuretic. Drug-induced side effects can contribute to reduced rates of adherence. It should also be noted that ACEI-induced angioedema occurs two to four times more frequently in African American patients than in other groups.[125] ARBs should be used instead if there is concern over such side effects and interruption of the renin–angiotensin system is warranted. Although there are no specific differences in pharmacologic recommendations for antihypertensive treatment in African Americans, a high sensitivity to differences in the coexisting risk factor, socioeconomic, cultural, and side effect profiles can help in designing the most appropriate comprehensive treatment program.[51]

Diabetes

The strong association between diabetes and adverse cardiovascular events is well-established. The high prevalence of diabetes (diagnosed and undiagnosed) and impaired glucose tolerance among African Americans makes the evaluation and treatment critical for reducing CVD in this population. Although currently it is recommended that diabetes screening begin at age 45, a recent evaluation of the cost-effectiveness of diabetes screening for persons above 25 years noted screening was more cost-ffective among younger persons and African Americans.[146] The threshold for fasting glucose as a diagnostic criterion for diabetes has been lowered from the previous value of 140 mg/dL to the new value of 126 mg/dL.[147]

Fortunately, diabetes care appears to be improving for those with insurance. In an observational study of more than 62,000 diabetic patients, including Asians (12%), African Americans (14%), Hispanics (10%), and whites (64%) in a nonprofit prepaid health care organization, adjusted hazard ratios (relative to that of whites) for African Americans, Asians, and Hispanics were lower for acute myocardial infarction; for Asians and Hispanics, lower for stroke and CHF; for Asians, lower for amputations; and for African Americans, Asians, and Hispanics, higher for ESRD. These data provide additional evidence that uniform medical care coverage markedly improves diabetes complications among ethnic minorities.[148] An analysis of the Insulin Resistance Atherosclerosis Study revealed similar rates of treatment of diabetes, hypertension, hyperlipidemia, albuminuria, and coronary artery disease across race/ethnicity. However, African Americans were twice as likely to have poorly controlled diabetes and both African Americans and Hispanics were three times more likely than whites to have borderline or poorly controlled hypertension.[149] Thus, even when processes of diabetes care were similar, individual health outcomes were worse for minorities, reinforcing the need to address other factors that influence health for many minority patients. Meta-analyses of randomized controlled trials in type 2 diabetes or diabetes subgroups support intensive glucose lowering as essential for the prevention of microvascular disease and the need for concomitant control of lipid and blood pressure levels to reduce CVD.[150]

Dyslipidemia

Accurate assessment of a patient's risk for CHD should include LDL-C, HDL-C, and triglycerides.[17] ATP-III continues to identify elevated LDL-C as the primary target of cholesterol-lowering therapy.[17] It now defines LDL-C levels below 100 mg/dL as optimal, raises categorical low HDL-C from less than 35 mg/dL to less than 40 mg/dL, and lowers the triglyceride classification cut points to give more attention to moderate elevations.

Because of mixed reports regarding lipid abnormalities in African Americans, it is plausible that some health care providers may not focus on this issue as a significant risk factor in comparison to other risk factors such as hypertension and diabetes.[40] There should be an equally high sensitivity for screening high-risk individuals for cholesterol levels and treatment when appropriate.[64] Several of the causes of secondary dyslipidemia that are disproportionately prevalent in African Americans, such as diabetes and CKD, should be sought. Although few prospective randomized trials have enrolled African Americans, the treatment for hyperlipidemia in African Americans should be no different from that for the general population.[17]

It should be noted that the use of statins (pravastatin) alongside blood pressure therapy was ineffective in the overall cohort in comparison to usual care in reducing all-cause mortality (although there was evidence of a significant treatment benefit in the African American subgroup), despite lowering LDL-C levels by 28% in the

ALLHAT substudy of 10,000 participants with elevated LDL-C (Table 18-5).[126] Whether it was the effect of pronounced blood pressure control, the fact that LDL-C improved slightly in the placebo group, the high enrollment of minority participants (>50%), or other factors that played a role in attenuating the efficacy of statin treatment is not clear.[126] The cut points for drug treatment are based primarily on risk–benefit considerations: those at higher risk are likely to get greater benefit. However, cut points for recommended management based on therapeutic efficacy should be balanced against currently accepted standards for cost-effectiveness. Lifestyle changes are the most cost-effective means to reduce risk for CHD. The encouraged use of plant stanols/sterols[17] and water-soluble fiber[151] as therapeutic dietary options to enhance lowering of LDL-C and to reduce CVD risk is particularly important for most minority populations, as many may be uninsured and are less able to afford the relatively expensive cholesterol- lowering agents. Even so, to achieve maximal benefit, many persons may eventually require LDL-C-lowering drugs.

Obesity

Effective intervention strategies for obesity are difficult to implement and particularly challenging in African American women.[152] Measures to decrease sedentary lifestyle (eg, less television viewing) are important to improve obesity and related complications.[153] Such issues as the cultural tolerance for overweight and obesity, as well as the importance of family and social networks in the dissemination of health information, must be considered. Analyzing data from the NHANES-II Mortality Study (1976–1992), researchers reported the optimal BMI (associated with the greatest longevity) was 23 to 25 kg/m^2 for whites and 23 to 30 kg/m^2 for African Americans.[154] Thus, weight reduction for obese African Americans to a goal BMI of 25 kg/m^2, which is particularly difficult to achieve, might be considered highly successful if a BMI less than 30 kg/m^2, rather than 25 kg/m^2, is achieved. Dietary caloric intake and increased physical activity remain the mainstay in weight reduction, particularly in the presence of hypertension.[73,156,157]

Physical inactivity

The need for improved awareness of the benefit of regular physical activity and innovative ways to implement physical activity remains a major challenge for many African American communities.[72] Moderate-intensity exercise has been reported to reduce blood pressure in hypertensive African Americans, while having only a modest effect on serum lipid levels.[158] A 12-week course of moderate-intensity aerobic exercise program and a Tai Chi program of light activity were both effective in reducing blood pressure among 62 sedentary, older adults

(45% African American, 79% women, age ≤60 years) with stage 1 hypertension.[159] Similarly, a weight loss and exercise program for older African Americans with non-insulin-dependent diabetes improved both glycemic and blood pressure control.[160] Among 3234 obese non-diabetic persons (68% women, 45% minorities), a regimen of 150 minutes of physical activity per week was more effective than metformin or placebo in reducing the incidence of diabetes.[161] Also, adults who walked 3 to 4 hours per week at a rate that involved moderate increases in heart and breathing rates had a 50% reduction in mortality across race/ethnicity.[162]

Although measures to decrease sedentary lifestyle (eg, less television viewing) are apparent,[154] community and public health strategies are also needed.[163] Examples include increasing the number and safety of walking areas, eliminating high-calorie fast-food specials, providing simple nutrition information on food labels, teaching the public how to read food labels, and encouraging appropriate school-based programs that promote physical activity. Innovative programs that focus on children may be important in developing physically active lifestyles.[164] Given the marked benefits of several hours of modest physical activity per week for improving multiple CVD risk factors, exercise is an extremely cost-effective approach to reducing CVD risk that should be routinely encouraged in the African American community.

Diet

Reduced dietary sodium intake,[165–168] increased potassium intake,[169,170] and, to a lesser extent, increased dietary calcium[171] have been associated with improvement of hypertension and/or CVD in both African American and white populations. Researchers from the multicenter Dietary Approaches to Stop Hypertension (DASH) study reported that a diet rich in fruit and vegetables with low saturated and total fat content (total fat, 26% of calories; saturated fat, 6% of calories; cholesterol, 151 mg/d; carbohydrate, 55% of calories) was particularly effective in reducing blood pressure, independent of weight loss, in nearly 500 healthy men and women (60% African American) with a baseline SBP less than 160 mm Hg and DBP of 80 to 95 mm Hg.[172] The DASH diet plus reduced sodium intake (≤2300 mg/d) is highly effective in many hypertensive patients, including African Americans and women.[173,174]

For reduction of LDL-C, ATP-III recommends a reduction in the intake of total fat (25–35% of calories), saturated fat (<7% of calories), *trans* fatty acids, cholesterol (<200 mg/d), and carbohydrate (50–60%).[17] It is important to ensure that low-fat diets do not contain excessive amounts of carbohydrate. Low-fat diets containing 60% carbohydrate calories resulted in higher fasting triglyceride and insulin levels than a high-fat diet with 40% carbohydrate calories.[175] The DASH diet or a similar diet with reduced sodium should be recommended for African Americans at risk for CVD (Table 18-7).

Cigarette smoking

A careful evaluation of tobacco use should include the number of cigarettes smoked, the brand, the manner of inhalation, and the number of puffs per cigarette. This allows a detailed assessment and initiates an in-depth dialogue between clinician and patient. This is an important and, it is hoped, more effective approach, as a brief physician-based smoking cessation message was not an effective strategy for use with African American smokers in a large urban public general hospital.[176] In addition to physician counseling and treatment with the nicotine patch,[177] referral to a smoking cessation program may be of benefit for African Americans.[178,179] Unfortunately, the effectiveness of many smoking cessation programs has not been consistently demonstrated, and our understanding of features that enhance effectiveness of such programs is limited.[180−183] Another approach is to integrate several family members willing and motivated to be supportive of smoking cessation.

Despite the suboptimal results of many smoking cessation interventions, a particular approach may work well for a given patient, and thus multiple attempts and strategies to achieve smoking cessation should be pursued. A recent 7-week trial noted that a combination of bupropion SR and brief motivational counseling was more effective than placebo and brief motivational counseling in achieving smoking cessation among 600 African Americans.[184] In addition, those taking bupropion SR had lower rates of depression and lesser weight gain than those taking placebo. Thus, pharmacologic therapy should be tried in those resistant to counseling and smoking cessation programs.

Psychosocial factors and stress

A review of prospective cohort studies suggested moderate support for psychologic factors as predictors of hypertension development, with the strongest support for anger, anxiety, and depression.[185] Fostering rational-cognitive coping skills, which represent the ability to problem-solve effectively and to set priorities, may be particularly beneficial for African American women.[186] Social support satisfaction and higher levels of religious coping also have been associated with lower blood pressure levels among African Americans, though not among whites.[187] This supports the use of churches as an important vehicle for promoting heath care recommendations within the African American community. Castillo-Richmond and co-workers used a randomized controlled clinical trial to evaluate the effects of stress reduction with Transcendental Meditation (TM) or health education on carotid IMT (B-mode ultrasound) in 60 hypertensive African American adults, over a 6- to 9-month period. The TM group experienced a significant decrease compared with an increase in the health education group ($P = .038$). They concluded that compared with health education, stress reduction with the TM program is associated with reduced carotid atherosclerosis in hypertensive African Americans.[188] Although additional prospective studies are needed, the existing literature suggests there is benefit from the use of stress reduction techniques as a complementary strategy to improve CVD outcomes. Tailoring stress reduction techniques to a given patient's level of acceptance can improve adherence and maximize results.

Special considerations: gender, homocysteine and inflammatory markers

Data accumulated from observational studies suggested that postmenopausal women receiving hormone replacement therapy (HRT) had a lower risk for CVD mortality than those not receiving HRT.[189,190] In a randomized primary prevention trial of estrogen plus progestin, 16,608 postmenopausal women who were 50 to 79 years of age at baseline were evaluated. Participants were randomly assigned to receive conjugated equine estrogens (0.625 mg/d) plus medroxyprogesterone acetate (2.5 mg/d) or placebo. The study was terminated early at 5.2 years (planned duration, 8.5 years) because the overall risks exceeded the benefits. Estrogen plus progestin was associated with an increased risk for CHD, stroke, and breast cancer.[191,192] Subgroup analysis provided similar results for whites, African Americans, and Hispanics. Thus, the use of estrogen plus progestin at this time should not be recommended as general preventive care. More recently, the estrogen only arm was also discontinued due to unfavorable increases in the risk of stroke and overall CVD.[193]

The treatment of emerging risk factors for CVD, such as C- reactive protein and homocysteine, is based primarily on association studies and intervention trials examining intermediate outcomes. Although not proven in prospective randomized trials, folate supplementation should be considered in persons with elevated homocysteine levels. Increased levels of homocysteine can be reduced by dietary folate supplementation, and increased dietary folate intake is associated with improved CVD outcomes, suggesting a mechanistic link.[194] However, there is no evidence of racial/ethnic differences as African Americans, whites, and Hispanics with elevated homocysteine levels and low folate levels were more likely have evidence of CVD.[195] Although racial differences in fasting and random homocysteine levels have been observed, the implications are unknown.[196]

The need to address substance abuse is critical to enhancing adherence to treatment recommendations and improving risk factor control rates. In a national survey of more than 40,000 participants, heart disease was reported to occur more often in those having more than five drinks per day for men and two drinks per day for women, relative to less than 1 drink per day.[197] However, African American men reported more heart disease at greater than two drinks per day in comparison to less than 1 drink per day. Thus, recommending modest levels of alcohol intake is affirmed for African Americans and should be stressed along with avoidance of illicit drug use, which may be higher among the underinsured and socioeconomically disadvantaged.

INTRARACIAL VARIATIONS

Examining intraracial variations in CVD can provide unique insights into cultural, environmental, and genetic contributions, with fewer confounders than in examining interracial differences. The rates of incidence of hypertension among middle-class African Americans and whites with similar levels of baseline blood pressure and BMI followed for seven years did not differ.[198] In contrast, among residents of New York City, Southern-born African Americans had substantially higher, and Caribbean-born African Americans substantially lower, CVD mortality rates than African Americans born in the Northeast. African Americans who are members of the Seventh-Day Adventist Church, which encourages both spiritual adherence and a healthy lifestyle, represent a unique opportunity to test the effects of diet, lifestyle, and spirituality on CVD risk within race/ethnicity, but across culture.[199] These findings and similar reports support a role for future studies to examine within race/ethnicity differences to uncover the role of environmental and geographic influences that might be amenable to relatively simple cost-effective interventions.

COMMUNITY PREVENTION PROGRAMS

A 9-year follow-up of blood pressure data from the ARIC study revealed that being socioeconomically disadvantaged at both the neighborhood and individual levels was associated with increased risk of developing hypertension among both whites and African Americans.[200] Using census-derived data, researchers studied blood pressure reactivity in 76 healthy African American adolescents and noted a buffering effect of higher family income and education on the negative consequences of living in low-socioeconomic-status neighborhoods.[201] These reports highlight the need to address cardiovascular health at a community level through multiple dimensions. Community-based strategies for health education and screening are important methods to address multiple cardiovascular risk factors that may not be optimally managed by existing health care resources. Community

resources, for example, libraries, churches, and recreation centers, can assist in providing effective health education and culturally sensitive targeted screenings.[202–205]

One community-based program consisting of exercise, meal planning, weekly support groups, periodic cooking schools, and service coordination improved blood pressure and diabetes control in 75 predominantly African American participants.[206] Schools are also effective in many instances. One semester of aerobic exercise reduced SBP more than the standard physical education in high-risk, predominantly African American, adolescent girls with blood pressure above the 67th percentile. This reinforces physical education in school as a feasible and effective health promotion strategy for high-risk adolescent girls.[207] A comprehensive work site health promotion program among 4000 City of Birmingham employees significantly reduced SBP in African American participants. This study suggests that educational intervention tailored to the specific health perceptions and working conditions of a low-literacy population is feasible and an effective way to improve hypertension control.[208] Another novel approach includes alliance formation, such as the Baltimore Alliance for the Prevention and Control of Hypertension and Diabetes, which was established to promote care to the underserved community and to improve outcomes of hypertension and diabetes in West Baltimore, Maryland. This alliance of university, community health programs, church-based programs, managed care and pharmaceutical company partners, and a health policy and services research group is under evaluation. This unique combination should better address cultural relevance and lead to improved outcomes.[209] Community pharmacists, who are in an ideal position to screen patients at risk for cardiovascular and cerebrovascular disease and refer patients for medical care, can enhance ongoing community screening programs.[210]

The church has been a particularly effective partner for implementing health care strategies in the African American community.[211] Church rosters have been shown to be a low-cost, effective recruitment tool for the recruitment of African Americans. In one study, nearly 50% of eligible church members who were notified by phone participated in a diet and blood pressure survey.[212] Lighten Up, a church-based lifestyle program that includes a baseline health assessment (week 1), eight educational sessions (weeks 2–9) combining study of scripture and a health message, and health checks, was effective in reducing CVD risk factors. Among 133 African Americans, 76% of the participants had two or more modifiable risk factors. After 10 weeks of follow-up, risk factor improvement (weight loss, reduced blood pressure, cholesterol, and triglyceride levels) was greatest among the 60 subjects who attended 75% or more of the educational sessions.[213] Key elements for successful church-based programs include establishing partnerships, identifying positive health values, making available services and access to church facilities, creating community-focused interventions, providing support for health behavior change, and creating supportive social relationships.[214]

Thus, community-based programs at various locations where people congregate, such as churches, barbershops, beauty salons, firehouses, housing projects, schools, and worksites, can play a valuable role in improving cardiovascular health for African Americans.[215] Health care professionals can be a potent force in the development of these programs by defining the scope and function of lay volunteers and by promoting these programs in a variety of other ways. Most important is establishing rapport and trust within the community, such as with leaders of community-based organizations, community service agencies, church representatives, and congregations. This is best accomplished over time and by being a contributor to the community through providing health education and information on an ongoing basis. Ultimately, the effectiveness of disseminating health information, as well as study recruitment, is linked to multiple variables such as trust, study eligibility criteria, roster accuracy, participant time, generalizability of the project, and relevance to the community.

SUMMARY

Both primary and secondary prevention programs targeted at African American populations need to include education at the level of the health care provider, the individual, the immediate family, and the community. Primary prevention education programs, using established groups such as schools, social clubs, and churches to promote risk factor awareness, should be considered. These can be effective sites at which to provide education with respect to appropriate diet, weight control, exercise, blood pressure control, smoking cessation, and alcohol abstinence/moderation in a culturally sensitive manner that can seldom be duplicated in most structured, government-developed programs. When feasible, simultaneous effort should be expended to provide cholesterol, weight, blood pressure, smoking, alcohol, and other risk factor screening, counseling, and/or referral services.

Secondary prevention measures can also be addressed through community programs, as most of these community-based risk reduction strategies will mirror those of primary prevention. Increasing patients' knowledge of evidenced-based interventions to improve cardiovascular risk factors can stimulate them to enter into a more detailed dialogue with their primary care provider and, it is hoped, improve their health. As there is no evidence to support a different secondary prevention goal for African Americans in contrast to whites, it is impor-

tant that health care providers and health management systems make specific secondary prevention therapies and needed cardiovascular interventions widely available.

It is hoped that through the use of innovative individual/family- and community-based approaches to primary and secondary cardiovascular risk prevention, the country will see significant improvements in the health of the African American community.

ACKNOWLEDGMENTS

Dr. Norris is supported by Grant P20 RR011145 from the Research Centers in Minority Institutions Program of the National Center for Research Resources and Grant P20 MD000182 from the National Center on Minority Health and Health Disparities.

REFERENCES

1. *Healthy People 2010* (conference Edition). 2 vols. Hyattsville, Md: US Department of Health and Human Services; 2000.
2. Francis CK. Research in coronary heart disease in blacks: issues and challenges. *J Health Care Poor Underserved* 1997;8:250–269.
3. Keppel KG, Pearcy JN, Wagener DK. Trends in racial and ethnic-specific rates for the health status indicators: United States, 1990–98. *Healthy People 2000 Stat Notes*, 2002;23: 1–16.
4. Cooper R, Cutler J, Desvigne-Nickens P, et al. Trends and disparities in coronary heart disease, stroke, and other cardiovascular diseases in the United States: findings of the national conference on cardiovascular disease prevention. *Circulation* 2000;102;3137–3147.
5. Johnson RL. The relationships among racial identity, self-esteem, sociodemographics, and health-promoting lifestyles. *Res Theory Nurs Pract* 2002;16:193–207.
6. Institute of Medicine. *Unequal Treatment: Confronting Racial and Ethnic Disparities in Health Care.* Washington, DC: National Academy Press; 2002.
7. Philbin EF, McCullough PA, DiSalvo TG, et al. Underuse of invasive procedures among Medicaid patients with acute myocardial infarction. *Am J Public Health* 2001;91:1082–1088.
8. Jha AK, Varosy PD, Kanaya AM, et al. Differences in medical care and disease outcomes among black and white women with heart disease. *Circulation* 2003;108:1089–1094.
9. *Heart Disease and Stroke Statistics—2003 Update.* Dallas, Tex: American Heart Association; 2002.
10. Shavers VL, Lynch CF, Burmeister LF. Racial differences in factors that influence the willingness to participate in medical research studies. *Ann Epidemiol* 2002;12:248–256.
11. Gorelick PB, Harris Y, Burnett B, Bonecutter FJ. The recruitment triangle: reasons why African Americans enroll, refuse to enroll, or voluntarily withdraw from a clinical trial. An interim report from the African American Antiplatelet Stroke Prevention Study (AAASPS). *J Natl Med Assoc* 1998;90:141–145.
12. Clark LT, Ferdinand KC, Flack JM, et al. Coronary heart disease in African Americans. *Heart Dis* 2001;3:97–108.
13. Wong MD, Shapiro MF, Boscardin WJ, et al. Contribution of major diseases to disparities in mortality. *N Engl J Med* 2002;347:1585–1592.

14. Ford ES, Giles WH. Changes in prevalence of nonfatal coronary heart disease in the United States from 1971–1994. *Ethnicity Dis* 2003;13:85–93.

15. East MA, Jollis JG, Nelson CL, et al. The influence of left ventricular hypertrophy on survival in patients with coronary artery disease: do race and gender matter? *J Am Coll Cardiol* 2003;41:949–954.

16. Richards SB, Funk M, Milner KA. Differences between blacks and whites with coronary heart disease in initial symptoms and in delay in seeking care. *Am J Crit Care* 2000; 9(4):237–244.

17. ATP-III. Executive summary of the Third Report of the National Cholesterol Evaluation Program (NCEP) Expert Panel on Detection, Evaluation, and Treatment of High Blood Cholesterol in Adults (Adult Treatment Panel III). *JAMA* 2001;285:2486–2497.

18. Lewington S, Clarke R, Qizilbash N, et al. Age-specific relevance of usual blood pressure to vascular mortality: a meta-analysis of individual data for one million adults in 61 prospective studies. *Lancet* 2002;360:1903–1913.

19. Exner DV, Dries DL, Domanski MJ, et al. Lesser response to angiotensin-converting-enzyme inhibitor therapy in black as compared with white patients with left ventricular dysfunction. *N Engl J Med* 2001;344:1351–1357.

20. Arnett DK, Tyroler HA, Burke G, et al, for the ARIC Investigators. Hypertension and subclinical carotid artery atherosclerosis in blacks and whites: the Atherosclerosis Risk in Communities Study. *Arch Intern Med* 1996;156:1983–1989.

21. Markus H, Kapozsta Z, Ditrich R, et al. Increased common carotid intima–media thickness in UK African Caribbeans and its relation to chronic inflammation and vascular candidate gene polymorphisms. *Stroke* 2001;32:2465–2471.

22. Rastenyte D, Tuomilehto J, Sarti C. Genetics of stroke—a review. *J Neurol Sci* 1998;153:132–145.

23. Martins D, Tareen N, Norris KC. The epidemiology of end-stage renal disease among African Americans. *Am J Med Sci* 2002;323(2):65–71.

24. Norris KC, Agodoa LY. Race and kidney disease: the scope of the problem. *J Natl Med Assoc* 2002;94(8):39S-44S, 2002.

25. US Renal Data System. *USRDS 2003 Annual Data Report: Atlas of End-Stage Renal Disease in the United States.* Bethesda, Md: National Institutes of Health, National Institute of Diabetes and Digestive and Kidney Diseases; 2003.

26. Stehman-Breen CO, Gillen D, Steffes M, et al. Racial differences in early-onset renal disease among young adults: the coronary artery risk development in young adults (CARDIA) study. *J Am Soc Nephrol* 2003;14:2352–2357.

27. Tarver-Carr ME, Powe NR, Eberhardt MS, et al. Excess risk of chronic kidney disease among African American versus white subjects in the United States: a population-based study of potential explanatory factors. *J Am Soc Nephrol* 2002;13:2363–2370.

28. Suthanthiran M, Khanna A, Cukran D, et al. Transforming growth factor-beta 1 hyperexpression in African American end-stage renal disease patients. *Kidney Int* 1998;53:639–644.

29. DeWan AT, Arnett DK, Atwood LD, et al. A genome scan for renal function among hypertensives: the HyperGEN study. *Am J Hum Genet* 2001;68:136–144.

30. Freedman BI. Susceptibility genes for hypertension and renal failure. *J Am Soc Nephrol* 2003;14:S192–S194.

31. Brown WW, Peters RM, Ohmit SE, et al. Early detection of kidney disease in community settings: the kidney early evaluation program (KEEP). *Am J Kidney Dis* 2003;42:22–35.

32. Martins D, Norris KC. Combating diabetic nephropathy with drug therapy. *Curr Diabetes Rep* 2001;1:148–156.

33. Knight EL, Kramer HM, Curhan GC. High-normal blood pressure and microalbuminuria. *Am J Kidney Dis* 2003;41:588–595.

34. Gerstein HC, Mann JF, Yi Q, et al. Albuminuria and risk of cardiovascular events, death, and heart failure in diabetic and nondiabetic individuals. *JAMA* 2001;286:421–426.

35. Hillege HL, Fidler V, Diercks GF, et al. Urinary albumin excretion predicts cardiovascular and noncardiovascular mortality in general population. *Circulation* 2002;106:1777–1782.

36. Dillingham TR, Pezzin LE, Mackenzie EJ. Racial differences in the incidence of limb loss secondary to peripheral vascular disease: a population-based study. *Arch Phys Med Rehabil* 2002;83:1252–1257.

37. Toursarkissian B, Shireman PK, Harrison A. Major lower-extremity amputation: contemporary experience in a single Veterans Affairs institution. *Am Surg* 2002;68:606–610.

38. Lavery LA, Van Houtum WH, Ashry HR, et al. Diabetes-related lower-extremity amputations disproportionately affect blacks and Mexican Americans. *South Med J* 1999;92:593–599.

39. Adeniyi A, Folsom AR, Brancati FL, et al. Incidence and risk factors for cardiovascular disease in African Americans with diabetes: the Atherosclerosis Risk in Communities (ARIC) study. *J Natl Med Assoc* 2002;94:1025–1035.

40. Hall WD, Clark LT, Wenger NK, et al. The metabolic syndrome in African Americans: a review. *Ethn Dis* 2003;13:414-448, 2003.

41. Becker DM, Yook RM, Moy TF, et al. Markedly high prevalence of coronary risk factors in apparently healthy African American and white siblings of persons with premature coronary heart disease. *Am J Cardiol* 1998;82:1046–1051.

42. Davey Smith G, Neaton JD, Wentworth D, et al, for the MRFIT Research Group. Mortality differences between black and white men in the USA: contribution of income and other risk factors among men screened for the MRFIT. Multiple Risk Factor Intervention Trial. *Lancet* 1998;351:934–939.

43. Watson K, Jamerson K. Therapeutic lifestyle changes for hypertension and cardiovascular risk reduction. *J Clin Hypertens (Greenwich)* 2003;5(suppl 1):32–37.

44. Wilson PW, Kannel WB, Silbershatz H, et al. Clustering of metabolic factors and coronary heart disease. *Arch Intern Med* 1999;159:1104–1109.

45. Liese AD, Mayer-Davis EJ, Tyroler HA, et al. Development of the multiple metabolic syndrome in the ARIC cohort: joint contribution of insulin, BMI, and WHR. Atherosclerosis Risk in Communities Study. *Ann Epidemiol* 1997;7:407–416.

46. Chiu KC, Cohan P, Lee NP, et al. Insulin sensitivity differs among ethnic groups with a compensatory response in beta-cell function. *Diabetes Care* 2000;23:1353–1358.

47. Ford ES, Giles WH, Dietz WH. Prevalence of the metabolic syndrome among US adults: findings from the third National Health and Nutrition Examination Survey. *JAMA* 2002;287:356–359.

48. Grundy SM. Obesity, metabolic syndrome, and coronary atherosclerosis. *Circulation* 2002;105:2696–2598.

49. Chen W, Bao W, Begum S, et al. Age-related patterns of the clustering of cardiovascular risk variables of syndrome X from childhood to young adulthood in a population made up of black and white subjects: the Bogalusa Heart Study. *Diabetes* 2000; 49:1042–1048.

50. Cherry DK, Burt CW, Woodwell DA. National ambulatory medical care survey: 2001 summary. *Adv Data* 2003;337:1–44.

51. *Seventh Report of the Joint National Committee on Prevention, Detection, Evaluation, and Treatment of High Blood Pressure. National Institutes of Health, National Heart, Lung, and Blood Institute.* NIH Publication No. 03-5233. May 2003.

52. Hennekens CH. Lessons from hypertension trials. *Am J Med* 1998;104(6A):50S–53S.

53. Vasan RS, Larson MG, Leip EP, et al. Impact of high-normal blood pressure on the risk of cardiovascular disease. *N Engl J Med* 2001;345:1291–1297.

54. Douglas JG, Bakris GL, Epstein M, et al, for the Hypertension in African Americans Working Group of the International Society on Hypertension in Blacks. Management of high blood pressure in African Americans: consensus statement of the Hypertension in African Americans Working Group of the International Society on Hypertension in Blacks. *Arch Intern Med* 2003;163:525–541.

55. Kotchen JM, Shakoor-Abdullah B, Walker WE. Hypertension control and access to medical care in the inner city. *Am J Public Health* 1998;88:1696–1699.

56. Jackson JH 4th, Bramley TJ, Chiang TH, et al. Determinants of uncontrolled hypertension in an African American population. *Ethn Dis* 2002;12(4):S35–S37.

57. Hajjar I, Kotchen TA. Trends in prevalence, awareness, treatment, and control of hypertension in the United States, 1988–2000. *JAMA* 2003;290:199–206.

58. Harris MI, Flegal KM, Cowie CC, et al. Prevalence of diabetes, impaired fasting glucose, and impaired glucose tolerance in US adults: the Third National Health and Nutrition Examination Survey, 1988–1994. *Diabetes Care* 1998;21:518–524.

59. He J, Klag MJ, Caballero B, et al. Plasma insulin levels and incidence of hypertension in African Americans and whites. *Arch Intern Med* 1999;159:498–503.

60. Folsom AR, Szklo M, Stevens J, et al. A prospective study of coronary heart disease in relation to fasting insulin, glucose, and diabetes: the Atherosclerosis Risk in Communities (ARIC) Study. *Diabetes Care* 1997;20:935–942.

61. Resnick HE, Valsania P, Halter JB, et al. Differential effects of BMI on diabetes risk among black and white Americans. *Diabetes Care* 1998;21:1828–1835.

62. Herman WH, Thompson TJ, Visscher W, et al. Diabetes mellitus and its complications in an African American community: project DIRECT. *J Natl Med Assoc* 1998;90:147–156.

63. Sharrett AR, Ballantyne CM, Coady SA, et al, for the Atherosclerosis Risk in Communities Study Group. Coronary heart disease prediction from lipoprotein cholesterol levels, triglycerides, lipoprotein(a), apolipoproteins A-I and B, and HDL density subfractions: the Atherosclerosis Risk in Communities (ARIC) Study. *Circulation* 2001;104:1108–1113.

64. Nelson K, Norris K, Mangione CM. Disparities in the diagnosis and pharmacologic treatment of high serum cholesterol by race and ethnicity: data from the Third National Health and Nutrition Examination Survey. *Arch Intern Med* 2002;162:929–935.

65. Sowers JR. Obesity and cardiovascular disease. *Clin Chem* 1998;44(8, Pt 2):1821–1825.

66. Suk SH, Sacco RL, Boden-Albala B, et al. Abdominal obesity and risk of ischemic stroke: the Northern Manhattan Stroke Study. *Stroke* 2003;34:1586–1592.

67. Flegal KM, Carroll MD, Ogden CL, et al. Prevalence and trends in obesity among US adults, 1999–2000. *JAMA* 2002;288:1723–1727.

68. Figueroa-Colon R, Franklin FA, Lee JY, et al. Prevalence of obesity with increased blood pressure in elementary school-aged children. *South Med J* 1997;90:806–813.

69. Folsom AR, Burke GL, Byers CL, et al. Implications of obesity for cardiovascular disease in blacks: the CARDIA and ARIC studies. *Am J Clin Nutr* 1991;53(6, suppl):1604S–1611S.

70. Juhaeri, Stevens J, Chambless LE, et al. Associations of weight loss and changes in fat distribution with the remission of hypertension in a bi-ethnic cohort: the Atherosclerosis Risk in Communities Study. *Prev Med* 2003;36:330–339.

71. Burnham JM. Exercise is medicine: health benefits of regular physical activity. *J La State Med Soc* 1998;150:319–323.

72. Karanja N, Stevens VJ, Hollis JF, et al. Steps to soulful living (STEPS): a weight loss program for African American women. *Ethn Dis* 2002;12:363–371.

73. The Trials of Hypertension Prevention Collaborative Research Group. Effects of weight loss and sodium reduction intervention on blood pressure and hypertension incidence in overweight people with high-normal blood pressure. The Trials of Hypertension Prevention, phase II. *Arch Intern Med* 1997;157:657–667.

74. McCarron DA, Metz JA, Hatton DC. Mineral intake and blood pressure in African Americans. *Am J Clin Nutr* 1998;68:517–518.

75. Adrogue HJ, Wesson DE. Role of dietary factors in the hypertension of African Americans. *Semin Nephrol* 1996;16:94–101.

76. Gates G, McDonald M. Comparison of dietary risk factors for cardiovascular disease in African American and white women. *J Am Diet Assoc* 1997;97:1394–1400.

77. Bazzano LA, He J, Muntner P, et al. Relationship between cigarette smoking and novel risk factors for cardiovascular disease in the United States. *Ann Intern Med* 2003;138:891–897.

78. McNagny SE, Ahluwalia JS, Clark WS, et al. Cigarette smoking and severe uncontrolled hypertension in inner-city African Americans. *Am J Med* 1997;103:121–127.

79. Kiefe CI, Williams OD, Lewis CE, et al. Ten-year changes in smoking among young adults: are racial differences explained by socioeconomic factors in the CARDIA study? *Am J Public Health* 2001;91:213–218.

80. Royce JM, Corbett K, Sorensen G, et al. Gender, social pressure, and smoking cessations: the Community Intervention Trial for Smoking Cessation (COMMIT) at baseline. *Soc Sci Med* 1997;44:359–370.

81. Whooley MA, Boyd AL, Gardin JM, et al. Religious involvement and cigarette smoking in young adults: the CARDIA (Coronary Artery Risk Development in Young Adults) study. *Arch Intern Med* 2002;162:1604–1610.

82. Kubzansky LD, Kawachi I, Weiss ST, et al. Anxiety and coronary heart disease: a synthesis of epidemiological, psychological, and experimental evidence. *Ann Behav Med* 20(2):47–58, 1998.

83. Bairey Merz CN, Dwyer J, Nordstrom CK, et al. Psychosocial stress and cardiovascular disease: pathophysiological links. *Behav Med* 2002;27(4):141–147.

84. Schneider RH, Nidich SI, Salerno JW, et al. Lower lipid peroxide levels in practitioners of the Transcendental Meditation program. *Psychosom Med* 1998;60:38–41.

85. Schneider RH, Nidich SI, Salerno JW. The Transcendental Meditation program: reducing the risk of heart disease and mortality and improving quality of life in African Americans. *Ethn Dis* 2001;11:159–160.

86. Dressler WW, Bindon JR, Neggers YH. John Henryism, gender, and arterial blood pressure in an African American community. *Psychosom Med* 1998;60:620–624.

87. Troxel WM, Matthews KA, Bromberger JT, et al. Chronic stress burden, discrimination, and subclinical carotid artery disease in African American and Caucasian women. *Health Psychol* 2003;22:300–309.

88. Williams DR, Neighbors H. Racism, discrimination and hypertension: evidence and needed research. *Ethn Dis* 2001;11:800–816.

89. Harrell JP, Hall S, Taliaferro J. Physiological responses to racism and discrimination: an assessment of the evidence. *Am J Public Health* 2003;93:243–248.

90. Wong SS, Nahin RL. National Center for Complementary and Alternative Medicine perspectives for complementary and alternative medicine research in cardiovascular diseases. *Cardiol Rev* 2003;11:94–98.

91. Gerhard GT, Sexton G, Malinow MR et al. Premenopausal African American women have more risk factors for coronary heart disease than white women. *Am J Cardiol* 82:1040–1045, 1998.

92. Refsum H, Ueland PM, Nygard O, et al. Homocysteine and cardiovascular disease. *Annu Rev Med* 1998;49:31–62.

93. Schreiner PJ, Wu KK, Malinow MR, et al. Hyperhomocyst(e)inemia and hemostatic factors: the atherosclerosis risk in communities study. *Ann Epidemiol* 2002;12:228–236.

94. Heald AH, Anderson SG, Ivison F, et al. C-reactive protein and the insulin-like growth factor (IGF)-system in relation to risk of cardiovascular disease in different ethnic groups. *Atherosclerosis* 2003;170:79–86.

95. Pradhan AD, Manson JE, Rossouw JE, et al. Inflammatory biomarkers, hormone replacement therapy, and incident coronary heart disease: prospective analysis from the Women's Health Initiative observational study. *JAMA* 2002;288:980–987.

96. LaMonte MJ, Durstine JL, Yanowitz FG, et al. Cardiorespiratory fitness and C-reactive protein among a tri-ethnic sample of women. *Circulation* 2002;106:403–406.

97. Rose LE, Kim MT, Dennison CR, Hill MN. The contexts of adherence for African Americans with high blood pressure. *J Adv Nurs* 2000;32:587–594,

98. Braun BL, Murray D, Hannan P, et al. Cocaine use and characteristics of young adult users from 1987 to 1992: the CARDIA (Coronary Artery Risk Development in Young Adults) study. *Am J Public Health* 1996;86:1736–1741.

99. *Results from the 2002 National Survey on Drug Use and Health: National Findings.* Office of Applied Studies, NHSDA Series H-22, DHHS Publication SMA 03-3836. Rockville, Md: Substance Abuse and Mental Health Services Administration; 2003.

100. *Guide to Primary Prevention of Cardiovascular Diseases.* Dallas, Tex: American Heart Association; 1997.

101. Missed opportunities in preventive counseling for cardiovascular disease—United States, 1995. *MMWR Morbid Mortal Wkly Rep* 1998;47(5):91–95.

102. Smith SC Jr. Risk reduction therapies for patients with coronary artery disease: a call for increased implementation. *Am J Med* 1998;104(2A):23S–26S.

103. Wood D. European and American recommendations for coronary heart disease prevention. *Eur Heart J* 1998;19(suppl A):A12–A19.

104. The Heart Outcomes Prevention Evaluation Study Investigators. Effects of an angiotensin converting-enzyme inhibitor, ramipril, on cardiovascular events in high-risk patients. *N Engl J Med* 2000;342:145–153.

105. Maynard C, Beshansky JR, Griffith JL, et al. Causes of chest pain and symptoms suggestive of acute cardiac ischemia in African American patients presenting to the emergency department: a multicenter study. *J Natl Med Assoc* 1997;89:665–671.

106. Houghton JL, Smith VE, Strogatz DS, et al. Effect of African American race and hypertensive left ventricular hypertrophy on coronary vascular reactivity and endothelial function. *Hypertension* 1997;29:706–714.

107. Gokce N, Holbrook M, Duffy SJ, et al. Effects of race and hypertension on flow-mediated and nitroglycerin-mediated dilation of the brachial artery. *Hypertension* 2001;38:1349–1354.

108. Maynard C, Wright SM, Every NR, Ritchie JL. Racial differences in outcomes of veterans undergoing percutaneous coronary interventions. *Am Heart J* 2001;142:309–313.

109. Kressin NR, Petersen LA. Racial differences in the use of invasive cardiovascular procedures: review of the literature and prescription for future research. *Ann Intern Med* 2001;135:352–366.

110. Schulman KA, Berlin JA, Harless W, et al. The effect of race and sex on physician's recommendations for cardiac catheterization. *N Engl J Med* 1999;340:618–626.

111. Daumit GL, Hermann JA, Coresh J, et al. Use of cardiovascular procedure among black persons and white persons: a 7-year nationwide study in patients with renal disease. *Ann Intern Med* 1999;130:173–182.

112. Leape LL, Hilbourne LH, Bell R, et al. Underuse of cardiac procedures: do women, ethnic minorities, and the uninsured fail to receive needed revascularization? *Ann Intern Med* 1999;130:183–192.

113. Schneider EC, Leape LL, Weissman JS, et al. Racial differences in cardiac revascularization rates: does "overuse" explain higher rates among white patients? *Ann Intern Med* 2001;135:328–337.

114. Yancy CW. The role of race in heart failure therapy. *Curr Cardiol Rep* 2002;4:218–225.

115. Carson P, Ziesche S, Johnson G, et al. Racial differences in response to therapy for heart failure: analysis of the Vasodilator-Heart Failure Trials. *J Cardiovasc Fail* 1999;5:178–187.

116. Dries DL, Exner DV, Gersh BJ, et al. Racial differences in the outcome of left ventricular dysfunction. *N Engl J Med* 1999;340:609–616.

117. Hajjar, RJ, MacRae, CA. Adrenergic-receptor polymorphisms and heart failure. *N Engl J Med* 2002;347:1196–1199.

118. Bourassa MG, Gurne O, Bangdiwala SI, et al, for the Studies of Left Ventricular Dysfunction (SOLVD) Investigators. Natural history and patterns of current practice in heart failure. *J Am Coll Cardiol* 22(suppl A):14A–19A, 1993.

119. Yancy CW, Fowler MB, Colucci WS, et al, for the U.S. Carvedilol Heart Failure Study Group. Race and the response to adrenergic blockade with carvedilol in patients with chronic heart failure. *N Engl J Med* 2001;344:1358–1365.

120. Rathore SS, Foody JM, Wang Y, et al. Race, quality of care, and outcomes of elderly patients hospitalized with heart failure. *JAMA* 2003;289:2517–2524.

121. Howard G, Howard VJ, for the Reasons for Geographic and Racial Differences in Stroke (REGARDS) Investigators. Ethnic disparities in stroke: the scope of the problem. *Ethn Dis* 2001;11:761–768.

122. Gorelick PB, Richardson D, Kelly M, et al, for the African American Antiplatelet Stroke Prevention Study Investigators. Aspirin and ticlopidine for prevention of recurrent stroke in black patients: a randomized trial. *JAMA* 2003;289:2947–2957.

123. Lindholm LH, Ibsen H, Dahlof B, et al. Cardiovascular morbidity and mortality in patients with diabetes in the Losartan Intervention For Endpoint reduction in hypertension study (LIFE): a randomised trial against atenolol. *Lancet* 2002;359:1004–1010.

124. Merck reports additional subgroup analyses from LIFE study with investigational use of cozaar; results suggest effect of cozaar different in black patient subpopulation in study [press release]. WhiteHouse Station, NJ: Merck & Co., Inc.; April 11, 2002.

125. The ALLHAT Officers and Coordinators for the ALLHAT Collaborative Research Group. Major outcomes in high-risk hypertensive patients randomized to angiotensin converting enzyme inhibitor or calcium channel blocker vs diuretic: the Antihypertensive and Lipid-Lowering Treatment to Prevent Heart Attack Trial (ALLHAT). *JAMA* 2002;288:2981–3007.

126. ALLHAT Officers and Coordinators for the ALLHAT Collaborative Research Group. Major outcomes in moderately hypercholesterolemic, hypertensive patients randomized to pravastatin vs usual care: the Antihypertensive and Lipid-Lowering Treatment to Prevent Heart Attack Trial (ALLHAT-LLT). *JAMA* 2002;288:2998–3007.

127. Conrad MF, Shepard AD, Pandurangi K, et al. Outcome of carotid endarterectomy in African Americans: is race a factor? *J Vasc Surg* 2003;38:129–137.

128. Lewis EJ, Hunsicker LG, Bain RP, et al, for the Collaborative Study Group. The effect of angiotensin-converting-enzyme inhibition on diabetic nephropathy. *N Engl J Med* 1993;329:1456–1462.

129. GISEN Group (Gruppo Italiano di Studi Epidemiologici in Nefrologia). Randomised placebo-controlled trial of effect of ramipril on decline in glomerular filtration rate and risk of terminal renal failure in proteinuric, non-diabetic nephropathy. *Lancet* 1997;349:1857–1863.

130. Heart Outcomes Prevention Evaluation (HOPE) Study Investigators. Effects of ramipril on cardiovascular and microvascular outcomes in people with diabetes mellitus: results of the HOPE study and MICRO-HOPE substudy. *Lancet* 2002:355:253–259.

131. Agodoa LY, Appel L, Bakris GL, et al. for the African American Study of Kidney Disease and Hypertension (AASK) Study Group. Effect of ramipril vs amlodipine on renal outcomes in hypertensive nephrosclerosis: a randomized controlled trial. *JAMA* 2001;285:2719–2728.

132. Wright JT Jr, Bakris G, Greene T, et al, for the African American Study of Kidney Disease and Hypertension Study Group. Effect of blood pressure lowering and antihypertensive drug class on progression of hypertensive kidney disease: results from the AASK trial. *JAMA* 2002;288:2421–2431.

133. Wright JT Jr, Agodoa L, Contreras G, et al. Successful blood pressure control in the African American Study of Kidney Disease and Hypertension. *Arch Intern Med* 2002;162:1636–1643.

134. Brenner BM, Cooper ME, de Zeeuw D, et al. Effects of losartan on renal and cardiovascular outcomes in patients with type 2 diabetes and nephropathy. *N Engl J Med* 2001;345:861–869.

135. Lewis EJ, Hunsicker LG, Clarke WR, et al. Renoprotective effect of the angiotensin-receptor antagonist irbesartan in patients with nephropathy due to type 2 diabetes. *N Engl J Med* 2001;345:851–860.

136. Bakris GL, Williams M, Dworkin L, et al, for the National Kidney Foundation Hypertension and Diabetes Executive Committees Working Group. Preserving renal function in adults with hypertension and diabetes: a consensus approach. *Am J Kidney Dis* 2000;36:646–666.

137. Scott CL. Diagnosis, prevention, and intervention for the metabolic syndrome. *Am J Cardiol* 2003;92(1A):35i–42i.

138. Whelton PK, He J, Appel LJ, et al. Primary prevention of hypertension: clinical and public health advisory from The National High Blood Pressure Education Program. *JAMA* 2002;288:1882–1888.

139. Suthanthiran M, Li B, Song JO, et al. Transforming growth factor-beta1 hyperexpression in African American hypertensives: a novel mediator of hypertension and/or target organ damage. *Proc Natl Acad Sci USA* 2000;97:3479–3484.

140. Thiel BA, Chakravarti A, Cooper RS, et al. A genome-wide linkage analysis investigating the determinants of blood pressure in whites and African Americans. *Am J Hypertens* 2003;16:151–153.

141. Campese VM, Amar M, Anjali C, et al. Effect of L-arginine on systemic and renal haemodynamics in salt-sensitive patients with essential hypertension. *J Hum Hypertens* 1997;11:527–532.

142. Svetkey LP, Chen YT, McKeown SP, et al. Preliminary evidence of linkage of salt sensitivity in black Americans at the beta 2-adrenergic receptor locus. *Hypertension* 1997;29:918–922.

143. Kotchen TA, Broeckel U, Grim CE, et al. Identification of Hypertension-Related QTLs in African American Sib Pairs. *Hypertension* 2002;40:634–639.

144. Veterans Administration Cooperative Study Group on Antihypertensive Agents. Comparison of propranolol and hydrochlorothiazide for the initial treatment of hypertension: I. Results of short-term titration with emphasis on racial differences in response. *JAMA* 1982;248:1996–2003.

145. Gottlieb SS, McCarter RJ, Vogel RA. Effect of beta-blockade on mortality among high-risk and low-risk patients after myocardial infarction. *N Engl J Med* 1998;339:489–497.

146. CDC Diabetes Cost-Effectiveness Study Group. The cost-effectiveness of screening for type 2 diabetes. [published erratum appears in *JAMA* 1999 27;281(4):325]. *JAMA* 25;280(20):1757–1763, 1998.

147. American Diabetes Association. Standards of medical care for patients with diabetes mellitus. *Diabetes Care* 26: S33–50, 2003.

148. Karter AJ, Ferrara A, Liu JY, et al. Ethnic disparities in diabetic complications in an insured population [published erratum appears in *JAMA* 2002;288:46]. *JAMA* 2002;287:2519–2527.

149. Bonds DE, Zaccaro DJ, Karter AJ, et al. Ethnic and racial differences in diabetes care: the Insulin Resistance Atherosclerosis Study. *Diabetes Care* 2003;26:1040–1046.

150. Huang ES, Meigs JB, Singer DE. The effect of interventions to prevent cardiovascular disease in patients with type 2 diabetes mellitus. *Am J Med* 2001;111:633–642.

151. Bazzano LA, He J, Ogden LG, et al. Dietary fiber intake and reduced risk of coronary heart disease in US men and women: the National Health and Nutrition Examination Survey I Epidemiologic Follow-up Study. *Arch Intern Med* 2003;163:1897–1904.

152. Lewis CE, Jacobs DR Jr, McCreath H, et al. Weight gain continues in the 1990s: 10-year trends in weight and overweight from the CARDIA (Coronary Artery Risk Development in Young Adults) Study. *Am J Epidemiol* 2000;151:1172–1181.

153. Hu FB, Li TY, Colditz GA, et al. Television watching and other sedentary behaviors in relation to risk of obesity and type 2 diabetes mellitus in women. *JAMA* 2003;2003;289:1785–1791.

154. Fontaine KR, Redden DT, Wang C, et al. Years of life lost due to obesity. *JAMA* 2003;289:187–193.

155. Kumanyika SK, Espeland MA, Bahnson JL, et al, for the TONE Cooperative Research Group. Ethnic comparison of weight loss in the Trial of Nonpharmacologic Interventions in the Elderly. *Obes Res* 2002;10:96–106.

156. He J, Whelton PK, Appel LJ, et al. Long-term effects of weight loss and dietary sodium reduction on incidence of hypertension. *Hypertension* 2000;35:544–549.

157. Whelton SP, Chin A, Xin X, et al. Effect of aerobic exercise on blood pressure: a meta-analysis of randomized, controlled trials. *Ann Intern Med* 2002;136:493–503.

158. Kokkinos PF, Narayan P, Colleran J, et al. Effects of moderate intensity exercise on serum lipids in African American men with severe systemic hypertension. *Am J Cardiol* 1998;81:732–735.

159. Young DR, Appel LJ, Jee S, et al. The effects of aerobic exercise and T'ai Chi on blood pressure in older people: results of a randomized trial. *J Am Geriatr Soc* 1999;47:277–284.

160. Agurs-Collins TD, Kumanyika SK, Ten Have TR, et al. A randomized controlled trial of weight reduction and exercise for diabetes management in older African American subjects. *Diabetes Care* 1997;20:1503–1511.

161. Knowler WC, Barrett-Connor E, Fowler SE, et al, for the Diabetes Prevention Program Research Group. Reduction in the incidence of type 2 diabetes with lifestyle intervention or metformin. *N Engl J Med* 2002;346:393–403.

162. Gregg EW, Gerzoff RB, Caspersen CJ, et al. Relationship of walking to mortality among US adults with diabetes. *Arch Intern Med* 2003;163:1440–1447.

163. Eyler AA, Matson-Koffman D, Vest JR. Environmental, policy, and cultural factors related to physical activity in a diverse sample of women: the Women's Cardiovascular Health Network Project—summary and discussion. *Women Health* 2002;36:123–134.

164. Stolley MR, Fitzgibbon ML, Dyer A, et al. Hip-Hop to Health Jr., an obesity prevention program for minority preschool children: baseline characteristics of participants. *Prev Med* 36:320–329.

165. Whelton PK, Appel LJ, Espeland MA, et al, for the TONE Collaborative Research Group. Sodium reduction and weight loss in the treatment of hypertension in older persons: a randomized controlled Trial of Nonpharmacologic Interventions in the Elderly (TONE). *JAMA* 1998;279:839–846.

166. Chobanian AV, Hill M. National Heart, Lung, and Blood Institute Workshop on Sodium and Blood Pressure: a critical review of current scientific evidence. *Hypertension* 2000;35:858–863.

167. He J, Ogden LG, Vupputuri S, et al. Dietary sodium intake and subsequent risk of cardiovascular disease in overweight adults. *JAMA* 1999;282:2027–2034.

168. He J, Ogden LG, Bazzano LA, et al. Dietary sodium intake and incidence of congestive heart failure in overweight US men and women: first National Health and Nutrition Examination Survey Epidemiologic Follow-up Study. *Arch Intern Med* 2002;162:1619–1624.

169. Bazzano LA, He J, Ogden LG, et al. Dietary potassium intake and risk of stroke in US men and women: National Health and Nutrition Examination Survey I epidemiologic follow-up study. *Stroke* 2001;32:1473–1480.

170. Whelton PK, He J. Potassium in preventing and treating high blood pressure. *Semin Nephrol* 1999;19:494–499.

171. Hajjar IM, Grim CE, Kotchen TA. Dietary calcium lowers the age-related rise in blood pressure in the United States: the NHANES III survey. *J Clin Hypertens (Greenwich)* 2003; 5:12.

172. Appel LJ, Moore TJ, Obarzanek E, et al. A clinical trial of the effects of dietary patterns on blood pressure. *N Engl J Med* 1997;336:1117–1124.

173. Vollmer WM, Sacks FM, Ard J, et al. Effects of diet and sodium intake on blood pressure: subgroup analysis of the DASH–Sodium Trial. *Ann Intern Med* 2001;135:1019–1028.

174. Sacks FM, Svetkey LP, Vollmer WM, et al, for the DASH–Sodium Collaborative Research Group. Effects on blood pressure of reduced dietary sodium and the Dietary Approaches to Stop Hypertension (DASH) diet. *N Engl J Med* 2001;4;344:3–10.

175. McLaughlin T, Abbasi F, Lamendola C, et al. Carbohydrate-induced hypertriglyceridemia: an insight into the link between plasma insulin and triglyceride concentrations. *J Clin Endocrinol Metab* 2000;85:3085–3088.

176. Allen B Jr, Pederson LL, Leonard EH. Effectiveness of physicians-in-training counseling for smoking cessation in African Americans. *J Natl Med Assoc* 1998;90:597–604,1998.

177. Ahluwalia JS, McNagny SE, Clark WS. Smoking cessation among inner-city African Americans using the nicotine transdermal patch. *J Gen Intern Med* 13(1):1–8.

178. Orleans CT, Boyd NR, Bingler R, et al. A self-help intervention for African American smokers: tailoring cancer information service counseling for a special population. *Prev Med* 1998;27(5, Pt 2):S61–S70.

179. Fisher EB, Auslander WF, Munro JF, et al. Neighbors for a smoke free north side: evaluation of a community organization approach to promoting smoking cessation among African Americans. *Am J Public Health* 1998;88:1658–1663.

180. Pederson LL, Ahluwalia JS, Harris KJ, et al. Smoking cessation among African Americans: what we know and do not know about interventions and self-quitting. *Prev Med* 2000;31:23–38.

181. Moolchan ET, Berlin I, Robinson ML, et al. African American teen smokers: issues to consider for cessation treatment. *J Natl Med Assoc* 2000;92:558–562.

182. Resnicow K, Vaughan R, Futterman R, et al. A self-help smoking cessation program for inner-city African Americans: results from the Harlem Health Connection Project. *Health Educ Behav* 1997;24:201–217.

183. Klonoff EA, Landrine H. Acculturation and cigarette smoking among African Americans: replication and implications for prevention and cessation programs. *J Behav Med* 1999;22:195–204.

184. Ahluwalia JS, Harris KJ, Catley D, et al. Sustained-release bupropion for smoking cessation in African Americans: a randomized controlled trial. *JAMA* 2002;288:468–474.

185. Rutledge T, Hogan B. A Quantitative Review of Prospective Evidence Linking Psychological Factors With Hypertension Development. *Psychosom Med* 2002;64:758–766.

186. Webb MS, Beckstead JW. Stress-related influences on blood pressure in African American women. *Res Nurs Health* 2002;25:383–393.

187. Steffen PR, Hinderliter AL, Blumenthal JA, et al. Religious coping, ethnicity, and ambulatory blood pressure. *Psychosom Med* 2001;63:523–530.

188. Castillo-Richmond A, Schneider RH, Alexander CN, et al. Effects of stress reduction on carotid atherosclerosis in hypertensive African Americans. *Stroke* 2000;31:568–573.

189. Barrett-Connor E, Wenger NK, Grady D, et al. Hormone and nonhormone therapy for the maintenance of postmenopausal health: the need for randomized controlled trials of estrogen and raloxifene. *J Womens Health* 7(7):839–847, 1998.

190. Ferrara A, Quesenberry CP, Karter AJ, et al. Current use of unopposed estrogen and estrogen plus progestin and the risk of acute myocardial infarction among women with diabetes: the Northern California Kaiser Permanente Diabetes Registry, 1995–1998. *Circulation* 2003;107:43–48.

191. Manson JE, Hsia J, Johnson KC, et al, for the Women's Health Initiative Investigators. Estrogen plus progestin and the risk of coronary heart disease. *N Engl J Med* 2003;349:523–534.

192. Rossouw JE, Anderson GL, Prentice RL, et al, for the Writing Group for the Women's Health Initiative Investigators. Risks and benefits of estrogen plus progestin in healthy postmenopausal women: principal results From the Women's Health Initiative randomized controlled trial. *JAMA* 2002;288:321–333.

193. Anderson GL, Limacher M, Assaf AR, et al. Effects of conjugated equine estrogen in postmenopausal women with hysterectomy: the Women's Health Initiative randomized controlled trial. *JAMA* 2004;291:1701–1712.

194. Bazzano LA, He J, Ogden LG, et al. Dietary intake of folate and risk of stroke in US men and women: NHANES I Epidemiologic Follow-up Study. *Stroke* 2002;33:1183–1188.

195. Giles WH, Croft JB, Greenlund KJ, et al. Association between total homocysteine and the likelihood for a history of acute myocardial infarction by race and ethnicity: results from the Third National Health and Nutrition Examination Survey. *Am Heart J* 2000;139:446–443.

196. Estrada DA, Billett HH. Racial variation in fasting and random homocysteine levels. *Am J Hematol* 2001;66:252–256.

197. Hanna EZ, Chou SP, Grant BF. The relationship between drinking and heart disease morbidity in the United States: results from the National Health Interview Survey. *Alcohol Clin Exp Res* 1997;21:111–118.

198. He J, Klag MJ, Appel LJ, et al. Seven-year incidence of hypertension in a cohort of middle-aged African Americans and whites. *Hypertension* 1998;1:1130–1135.

199. Nyenhuis DL, Gorelick PB, Easley C, et al. The Black Seventh-Day Adventist Exploratory Health Study. *Ethn Dis* 2003;13:208–212.

200. Diez Roux AV, Chambless L, Merkin SS, et al. Socioeconomic disadvantage and change in blood pressure associated with aging. *Circulation* 2002;106:703–710.

201. Wilson DK, Kliewer W, Plybon L, et al. Socioeconomic status and blood pressure reactivity in healthy black adolescents. *Hypertension* 2000;35:496–500.

202. Schwartz DG, Mosher E, Wilson S, Lipkus C, et al. Seniors connect: a partnership for training between health care and public libraries. *Med Ref Serv Q* 2002;21(3):1–19.

203. Assaf AR, Coccio E, Gans K, et al. Community-based approaches with implications for hypertension control in blacks. *Ethn Dis* 2002;12(1):S127–S133.

204. Becker DM, Tuggle MB, Prentice MF. Building a gateway to promote cardiovascular health research in African American communities: lessons and findings from the field. *Am J Med Sci* 2001;322:276–281.

205. Keys IR. Take It to Heart: a national health screening and education project in African American communities. A joint project of the NMA and Bayer Corporation. *J Natl Med Assoc* 1999;91(12):649–652.

206. Nine SL, Lakies CL, Jarrett HK, et al. Community-based chronic disease management program for African Americans. *Outcomes Manag* 2003;7(3):106–112.

207. Ewart CK, Young DR, Hagberg JM. Effects of school-based aerobic exercise on blood pressure in adolescent girls at risk for hypertension. *Am J Public Health* 1998;88:949–951.

208. Fouad MN, Kiefe CI, Bartolucci AA, et al. A hypertension control program tailored to unskilled and minority workers. *Ethn Dis* 1997;7(3):191–199.

209. Gerber JC, Stewart DL. Prevention and control of hypertension and diabetes in an underserved population through community outreach and disease management: a plan of action. *J Assoc Acad Minor Phys* 1998;9(3):48–52.

210. J Mangum SA, Kraenow KR, Narducci WA. Identifying at-risk patients through community pharmacy-based hypertension and stroke prevention screening projects. *Am Pharm Assoc* 2003;43(1):50–55.

211. Brown CM: Exploring the role of religiosity in hypertension management among African Americans. *J Health Care Poor Underserved* 2000;11:19–32.

212. Carter-Edwards L, Fisher JT, Vaughn BJ, et al. Church rosters: is this a viable mechanism for effectively recruiting African Americans for a community-based survey? *Ethn Health* 2002;7(1):41–55.

213. Oexmann MJ, Thomas JC, Taylor KB, et al. Short-term impact of a church-based approach to lifestyle change on cardiovascular risk in African Americans. *Ethn Dis* 2000;10(1):17–23.

214. Peterson J, Atwood JR, Yates B. Key elements for church-based health promotion programs: outcome-based literature review. *Public Health Nurs* 2002;19:401–411.

215. Kong BW. Community-based hypertension control programs that work. *J Health Care Poor Underserved* 1997;8(4):409–415.

Hispanic Americans

19

Stanley L. Bassin
Omar F. Duenes

KEY POINTS

- Heart disease and related diseases such as stroke and diabetes constitute the number one cause of death and disability among Hispanic Americans.

- Overweight and obesity are more likely in Mexican-American children and adults than in other ethnic groups.

- Diabetes is three times more prevalent in Hispanics than in whites and continues unabated.

- The rate of smoking is on the rise among Hispanic youth, but is lower for those who participate in school-based education programs.

- Little research has been conducted on the effectiveness of physical activity interventions for Hispanics.

- The Hispanic paradox of traditionally lower mortality rates may need to be reevaluated in the light of acculturation studies.

INTRODUCTION

The largest minority group in the United States approximating 40 million persons of Hispanic origin is still often considered as a single ethnic group. This diverse group includes Cubans, Mexicans, Spaniards, and other Latinos, and more than 4 million are estimated to be living here without legal documents.[1] Approximately 63% of the Hispanic population living in the continental United States, Alaska, and Hawaii is of Mexican origin and reside predominantly in the southwestern United States.[2] Eleven percent are from Puerto Rico, residing on the Eastern Seaboard; 4% are Cuban, living in Florida and New York; and the remaining 22% are of other Hispanic origin, namely, Central America, and live primarily in California and Arizona.[2] Currently, the growth rate of Hispanics in the country is nearly four times that of the African-American population and nearly ten times that of the white population.[3] By 2015, Hispanics are expected to number 97 million and account for nearly one quarter of the US population.[4] Mexican-Americans are projected to be the majority population in the United States in the next decade, with 7 of 10 persons currently under the age of 35; less than half of non-Hispanics are in the same age group. In contrast, three times as many non-Hispanics are older than 65.

Although cardiovascular disease (CVD) and overall mortality rates are lower in Hispanics than in whites (Table 19-1),[5] certain risk factors, that is, diabetes, obesity, and physical inactivity, are among the highest in the Hispanic population, and continue to rapidly increase.[5,6] It is currently unclear why these seemingly paradoxical conditions coexist. There are marked differences in culture, history, and lifestyle among Hispanics. More than one third of all Hispanics are foreign-born. As many as 98% report speaking primarily Spanish at home; only 24% report speaking English very well.[7] A broad diversity exists among Hispanics, despite a shared language, with a core ancestry that can be traced to numerous Spanish-speaking countries, distinct national histories, traditions, and lifestyles. Some diseases that seem to be common among indigenous North Americans also seem to be present among Mexican-Americans, but are not as prevalent in other Hispanics. Hispanics are overrepresented

TABLE 19-1 Age-Adjusted Mortality Rates Among Whites and Hispanics

Cause-specific mortality rate (per 100,000)	Hispanics	Whites
Diseases of the Heart	88.6	131.0
Cerebrovascular disease	19.5	24.4
Malignant neoplasm	77.8	127.6
Respiratory	15.4	40.2
Colorectal	7.3	12.1
Prostate	9.9	13.6
Breast	12.8	20.1
COPD*	8.9	22.1
Pneumonia and influenza	9.7	12.2
Chronic Liver disease	12.6	6.7
Diabetes mellitus	18.8	11.5
HIV/AIDS	16.3	6.0
Unintentional injuries	49.0	29.3
Suicide	6.1	12.0
Homicide and legal intervention	12.4	3.5

*Chronic obstructive pulmonary disease.

SOURCE: Reproduced, with permission, from Morales et al.[4]

as an uninsured and medically underserved population. They are the second lowest (just ahead of African-Americans) of major ethnic groups in earnings, and their health status reflects this level of poverty (Table 19-2).[8] Most do not have a regular doctor in the United States health care system for easy access to medical services. Although the number of Hispanic professionals in the health/mental health care work force is growing, they are not numerically reflective of the Hispanic population.[3]

EPIDEMIOLOGY AND RISK FACTORS

Overview

Although noteworthy research on CVD prevention has been conducted among middle class whites, only recently have sufficient data become available on Hispanics. The Hispanic Health and Nutrition Examination Survey (HHANES) was the first national study to assess the health and nutritional status of the Latin population including mainland Puerto Rico.[9] This report disclosed a larger percentage of Hispanics as being obese, diabetic, hypertensive, and cigarette smokers.

Heart disease and stroke still remain the leading cause of death, both in Hispanic males (27% of all deaths) and in Hispanic females (33% of all deaths).[7] Nevertheless, the death rate (per 100,000 population) appears to be lower for Hispanics (53 per 100,000) than for whites (76 per 100,000).[10]

Nationally, the prevalence of obesity as measured by body mass index (BMI) of 30 kg/m^2 or greater now exceeds 30% in U.S. adults from recent estimates.[11] Hispanics have shown evidence of a greater prevalence of obesity, elevated cholesterol, and triglyceride levels.[12,13] Mexican-Americans are three to five times more likely to have non-insulin-dependent diabetes than whites.[14] The traditional cardiovascular risk factors account for 55% of Mexican-American CVD mortality, but only 46% of CVD mortality in white cohorts.[15] Mortality data reported in the five southwestern states suggest Mexican-American women and all whites are similar, but Mexican-American men have slightly lower rates. On the other hand, mortality following myocardial infarction (MI) is greater among Mexican-Americans than in whites.[3]

The Corpus Christi Heart Project found that Mexican-Americans received fewer cardiovascular medications than whites, and women received fewer than did men.[16] It was also reported that at the 25-month follow-up after hospitalization for MI, age-adjusted all-cause mortality rates among those who survived the initial 28 days were 70% higher among Mexican-American men than among non-Hispanic white men (17.4 and 10.2%, respectively), but were similar in Mexican-American and non-Hispanic white women (17.8 and 18.1%, respectively).[1] This is the first report documenting greater hospitalization rates for MI in Hispanics than in whites for both men and women. The severity of acute MI or post-MI survival rates due to diabetes was also studied. Despite a similar infarction size, diabetic subjects had a poorer prognosis and higher incidence of heart failure than did nondiabetics. It appears that the Hispanic paradox of traditionally lower mortality rates may need to be questioned in the light of acculturation studies.[15] The Hispanic paradox seems to be in need of revision, because today it seems to apply only to Mexican-American men. Strong evidence today indicates that certain risk factors in Hispanics are worse than those in whites (Table 19-3).[4]

Stroke is the third leading cause of death in the United States, surpassed only by heart disease and cancer. The most recent data from the Centers for Disease Control and Prevention show that the age-adjusted stroke death rate for US residents aged 35 and older was 121 per 100,000 during 1991–1998. The age-adjusted stroke death rate for whites in this age group was 117 per 100,000, and that for Hispanics, 79 per 100,000. The geographic band of highest death rates extends from central New Mexico into central Texas (Fig. 19-1).[18] Washington and Texas had the largest number of counties with high rates for men, while New Mexico and California had the greatest stroke rates for women. Most of the lowest stroke death rates were seen in the Northeast states, southern Florida, and Chicago, Illinois. Hispanic men

TABLE 19-2 Health Status, Access to Care, and Health Behaviors Among Latinos and White Non-Latinos

	Latinos (n = 1001)		White non-Latinos (n = 1001)		
	Population prevalence* (%)	SE	Population prevalence* (%)	SE	P †
Perceived health status					
Excellent	28.7	1.5	40.8	1.6	<.01
Good	47.5	2.0	41.2	1.6	
Fair	19.0	1.6	13.9	1.1	
Poor	4.8	0.7	4.1	0.7	
Had disability/health problem	12.1	1.1	16.4	1.2	.02
Mental health (mean)‡	31.3	0.6	29.1	0.5	<.01
Insurance					
Covered by an HMO	18.3	1.3	20.6	1.3	<.01
Covered by fee-for-service/not sure	45.2	1.9	67.7	1.7	
No insurance	36.5	2.0	11.7	1.4	
Had a regular doctor	58.6	2.1	79.9	1.5	<.01
Choice of where to get care					
A great deal	42.9	1.9	60.8	1.6	<.01
Some	25.8	1.6	23.0	1.4	
Very little	22.0	1.6	9.9	1.0	
No choice	9.3	1.2	6.3	1.0	
Barriers to care (at least one)	84.8	1.7	77.7	1.5	<.01
Felt uncomfortable or treated badly in past 12 mo	10.7	1.0	7.8	1.0	.08
Ever thought he/she would have received better care if a different race	13.9	1.5	3.0	0.6	<.01
Used herbal medicine	23.6	1.6	12.3	1.1	<.01
Used traditional healer	2.7	0.5	2.1	0.4	.38
Used home remedy	31.3	1.8	31.4	1.6	.96
Vigorous exercise for at least 20 min					
<3 d/mo	38.0	1.8	33.8	1.6	.20
1–3 d/wk	36.6	1.5	39.9	1.6	
>3 d/wk	25.5	1.5	26.4	1.4	
Maintain a healthy diet					
<3 d/mo	23.2	1.7	17.3	0.3	<.01
1–3 d/wk	26.5	1.6	21.0	1.3	
>3 d/wk	50.4	1.9	61.8	1.6	
Current smoker					
Yes	20.2	1.4	25.9	1.5	.01
No	79.8		74.1		

*Weighted to estimate population prevalences.
†P value between Latino and white non-Latino takes into account the complex survey design.
‡A higher score represents poorer mental health.
SOURCE: Reproduced, with permission, from Wagner and Guendelman.[8]

had greater stroke death rates when compared with Hispanic women. The age-adjusted death rate for stroke was 72 per 100,000 for Hispanic women and 88 per 100,000 for Hispanic men aged 35 years and older, with the largest concentration of both Hispanic women and men observed in the southwestern states and California.[18]

Migration and socioeconomic status have played a strong role in Hispanic mortality and morbidity, with the lowest socioeconomic status having a threefold greater risk of death than those with the highest status.[15] The group with the lowest mortality rate per 1000 persons was US-born Mexican-Americans (5.7%), whereas

TABLE 19-3 Risk Factors of Hispanics Versus Whites

Determinant of health	Risk pattern
Socioeconomic status	
Education	Hispanic > White
Income	Hispanic > White
Occupation	Hispanic > White
Behavioral risk factors	
Tobacco use	White > Hispanic
Diet	White ≥ Hispanic
Alcohol consumption	White > Hispanic
Sedentary lifestyle	White < Hispanic
Access to care	
Insurance	Hispanic > White
Use of care	Hispanic > White
Health status	
Life expectancy	White > Hispanic
Mortality	White > Hispanic
Infant mortality	White > Hispanic

SOURCE: Reproduced, with permission, from Morales et al.[4]

foreign-born Mexican-Americans and whites had comparable rates after accounting for socioeconomic status (3.6 and 3.8%, respectively).

It should be remembered that young, ethnically diverse populations below age 45 who have less than a high school education, lack health insurance, and are subject to governmental recording, which could threaten their residential status, are unlikely to participate in public health screenings. Thus, data on lipid levels, hypertension, and other risk factors are meager among Mexican-American youngsters and adults and may not represent a true population cross section.

Lipids

The best available evidence suggests that behaviors associated with increased CVD are acquired early in life and may accelerate the development of CVD.[19] One of the most influential factors that accounts for a substantial role in heart disease is high blood cholesterol. Among Mexican-Americans aged 20 years and older, 47% of men and 43% of women have total cholesterol levels greater than 200 mg/dL, which contrasts with 52% and 51% in white men and white women, respectively. Total cholesterol levels of 240 mg/dL or greater are present in 18% of Hispanics.[20] Mexican-Americans and non-Hispanic whites had similar mean total cholesterol levels, except for a tendency toward higher mean levels in Mexican-Americans aged 20 to 29 and 70 to 79.[20] Low-density lipoprotein cholesterol (LDL-C) levels of 130 mg/dL or higher were present in 39% of men and 38% of women,

and high-density lipoprotein cholesterol (HDL-C) levels less than 35 mg/dL in 15% of men and 6% of women (Table 19-4).[20]

The largest prospective cardiovascular risk factor study targeting Mexican-Americans is the renowned San Antonio Heart Study. The results revealed that total cholesterol and LDL-C in both sexes and HDL-C in males were similar among Mexican-Americans and non-Hispanic whites, but white women had significantly higher HDL-C levels (49.9 mg/dL in Hispanics vs 55.2 mg/dL in whites). The HDL-C level gap between ethnic groups was diminished after adjustment for obesity. Mexican-Americans of both sexes had higher triglyceride levels than their white counterparts. As adiposity is greater in Mexican-Americans, its linkage with higher triglycerides and central body fat patterning is not surprising.[21]

NHANES-III showed that in the seventh decade of life, average cholesterol levels peak at 219 mg/dL for Mexican-American men and 229 mg/dL for Mexican-American women. These numbers were similar for men, but lower for Mexican-American women in comparison to whites and African-Americans.[20] Substantial levels of obesity in this population do not appear to be associated with the higher levels of serum cholesterol expected.

Relative contributions of the environment and genetics to lipid levels and other risk factors were examined by Hixon and colleagues.[22] They found that lipid and lipoprotein phenotypes, age, gender, and environmental covariates accounted for less than 15% of the total phenotypic variation, whereas genetic factors accounted for double to triple the percentage of phenotypic variation. In the San Antonio Heart Study, standard CVD risk factors accounted for 45% of all-cause mortality and 55% of CVD mortality; there was no evidence of a diminished effect of these risk factors in Mexican-Americans compared to non-Hispanic whites.[23] Valdez studied San Antonio Heart Study subjects and comparable Mexico City residents to further discriminate between genetic and environmental influences.[24] Fasting and 2-hour insulin levels had a genetic component, but fasting and 2-hour glucose levels were consistently higher in Mexican-Americans than in the other two groups. Mexican-Americans and whites residing in Texas had higher levels of triglycerides, lower HDL-C levels, and higher levels of total and LDL-C, regardless of gender. The average Mexico City population diet, which is higher in carbohydrates (65–49%), might have accounted for the differences in lipid levels.

Obesity

Risk factors for CVD include obesity in white populations, high blood pressure in African-Americans, and diabetes in Mexican-Americans and Native Americans.

Smoothed County Stroke Death Rates
1991–1998

Hispanics
Ages 35 Years and Older

New York City

District of Columbia

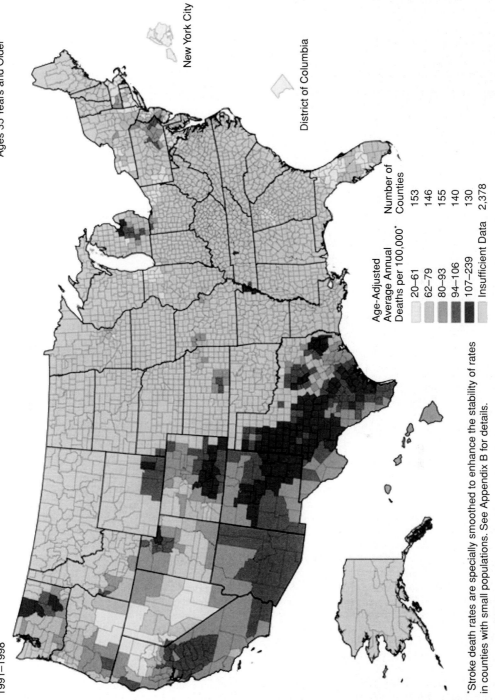

Age-Adjusted Average Annual Deaths per 100,000*	Number of Counties
20–61	153
62–79	146
80–93	155
94–106	140
107–239	130
Insufficient Data	2,378

*Stroke death rates are specially smoothed to enhance the stability of rates in counties with small populations. See Appendix B for details.

FIGURE 19-1 Smoothed country stroke death rates. (Reproduced, with permission, from the *Atlas of Stroke Mortality*.[18])

TABLE 19-4 Percentage of People 20 Years of Age and Older with Low Levels of Serum HDL-C (<35 mg/dL), by Sex, Age, and Race/Ethnicity, 1988–1991

	Total population*			Non-Hispanic white			Non-Hispanic black			Mexican-American		
Sex/age	Sample size	%	SE	Sample size	%	SE	Sample size	%	SE	Sample size	%	SE
Male												
20–29	793	10.3	1.35	202	11.6	2.30	230	5.4	1.51	329	13.4	2.18
30–39	699	14.1	1.65	263	14.6	2.21	194	10.2	2.19	218	11.3	2.50
40–49	600	20.8	2.07	238	23.2	2.79	162	11.4	2.52	174	25.4	3.84
50–59	472	19.8	2.29	258	21.3	2.59	100	10.1[†]	[†]	94	12.2[†]	[†]
60–69	558	20.0	2.12	251	21.2	2.63	129	12.0	2.89	168	20.1	3.60
70–79	458	19.1	2.30	300	19.4	2.32	84	13.0	3.71	69	14.7[†]	[†]
≥80	340	15.4	2.45	291	16.4	2.21	19	—[‡]	—[‡]	25	23.1[†]	[†]
Total	3920	16.3	1.13	1803	17.8	1.32	918	9.2	1.16	1077	15.2	1.67
Female												
20–29	783	4.5	1.10	224	4.8[†]	[†]	232	1.5[†]	[†]	303	4.7	1.27
30–39	740	7.8	1.46	260	8.6	1.95	216	4.1[†]	[†]	239	3.5[†]	[†]
40–49	582	3.4[†]	[†]	221	3.3[†]	[†]	153	5.2[†]	[†]	176	9.1	2.26
50–59	434	6.6	1.77	214	7.5	2.02	115	2.7[†]	[†]	93	7.3[†]	[†]
60–69	549	5.4	1.44	245	5.8	1.69	135	3.5[†]	[†]	157	6.2[†]	[†]
70–79	412	6.2	1.77	261	6.8	1.75	90	3.4[†]	[†]	50	5.3[†]	[†]
≥80	356	7.2	2.04	292	7.6	1.75	38	3.8[†]	[†]	22	7.6[†]	[†]
Total	3856	5.7	0.72	1717	6.2	0.86	979	3.3	0.69	1040	5.5	1.08

*Includes data for race/ethnic groups not shown separately.
†Indicates a statistic that is potentially unreliable because of small sample size or large coefficient of variation.
‡Observed percent is 0.0.
SOURCE: Reproduced, with permission, from the *Third Report on Nutrition Monitoring in the United States.*[21]

Research has demonstrated that more than 60% of American adults are considered overweight or obese, an increase from 45% in 1960.[21,25] More than one third of Americans are considered overweight using a standard of BMI greater than 25 to 30 kg/m², and one-sixth are obese using the definition of a BMI of 30 kg/m² or greater to define obesity.[11] The prevalence of obesity is greater in Mexican-Americans, substantially exceeding the prevalence in whites and matching that in African-Americans.[26,27] Among Mexican-Americans aged 20 to 74, 67% of men and 68% of women are overweight or obese (BMI = ≥25 kg/m²), including 23% of men and 34% of women defined as obese (BMI = ≥30 kg/m²).[21] In California, among Hispanics aged 18 and older, the prevalence of overweight is 35% in men and 43% in women.[28]

Hispanic adults are found to be overweight with a less favorable, centralized distribution of body fat, increasing the risks for diabetes and other CVD.[12,26] The San Antonio Heart Study reported that Mexican-Americans are overweight and have greater adiposity than non-Hispanic white Texans.[29] Mexican-Americans become overweight at an earlier age, and their level of obesity in comparison to other ethnic groups does not change with advancing age. Specifically, Mexican-Americans reach their prevalence peak in obesity prior to age 40, whereas other ethnic groups peak later in life.[30] Both white and Hispanic men show a steady increase in prevalence of overweight; by the fifth decade of life, over 70% are overweight and nearly 30% are obese(Table 19-5). Nearly half of Hispanic women in this age group are obese, compared to a third of white women. From 1988–1994 to 1999–2000, the prevalence of obesity increased from 23% to 29% in Mexican-American men and from 35% to 40% in Mexican-American women.[31]

Surveys on diet and physical activity have shown that Hispanics have excessive dietary intake, low physical activity levels, and a lack of concern about obesity.[29] These findings coincide with other investigations that regard obesity as a problem of energy imbalance, with more

TABLE 19-5 Prevalence of Overweight and Obesity by Age, Sex, and Racial/Ethnic Group: United States, 1999–2000

Sex	Age, y[†]	Sample size, no.				Prevalence of overweight/obesity (BMI ≥ 25), %				Prevalence of obesity (BMI ≥ 30), %			
		All*	Non-Hispanic white	Non-Hispanic black	Mexican American	All*	Non-Hispanic white	Non-Hispanic black	Mexican American	All*	Non-Hispanic white	Non-Hispanic black	Mexican American
Both sexes	≥20	4115	1831	794	1105	64.5	62.3	69.8	73.4‡	30.5	28.7	39.9‡	34.4
Men	≥20	2043	946	374	538	67.2	67.4	60.7	74.7	27.5	27.3	28.1	28.9
	20–39	866	276	125	184	60.5	61.0	52.6	67.5	23.7	22.0	27.4	30.4
	40–59	595	262	127	157	70.0	69.9	63.9	79.1	28.8	28.5	29.9	27.0
	≥60	782	408	122	197	74.1	74.3	69.1	79.6	31.8	34.3	26.4	29.7
Women	≥20	2072	885	420	567	61.9	57.3	77.3‡	71.9	33.4	30.1	49.7‡	39.7
	20–39	640	249	140	180	54.3	49.0	70.8‡	61.6	28.4	24.4	46.2‡	30.6
	40–59	653	249	141	193	66.1	61.0	81.5‡	79.3	37.8	34.2	63.2‡	48.5
	≥60	779	387	139	194	68.1	65.8	81.7†	77.5	35.0	33.3	50.2†	41.0

*Includes racial/ethnic groups not shown separately.
†Estimated prevalences for ages ≥30 years were age-standardized by the direct method to the 2000 Census population using age groups 20–39, 40–59, and ≥60 years.
‡Significantly different from non-Hispanic whites, $p < .05$ (with Bonferroni correction).
Reproduced with permission, from Flegal et al.[31]

calories consumed than expended. Genetic composition may also play a major role in how an individual expresses his or her metabolism in an environment that focuses on consumption of calorie-dense foods. The decrease in physical activity level across all youth makes the population ripe for obesity.[25,32] Within the next two decades, this situation portends an even greater level of adult obesity, and increases the likelihood of a significantly increased prevalence of non-insulin-dependent diabetes.

A critical aspect in determining the level of obesity in an individual is the manner in which weight and adiposity are measured. Diehl and Stern reported that Mexican-Americans should not be judged as obese solely on the basis of being overweight according to BMI standards.[12] Because of their generally shorter stature, excess weight for stature appears to be a poor measure of adiposity for Mexican-Americans.[14,33] The National Obesity Education Initiative guidelines classify those with a BMI of 25 to 29 as "overweight" and those with a BMI greater than 30 as "obese."[34] Experts suggest that a health-determined definition of obesity could be based on the degree of excess body fat associated with increased risk for chronic disease and mortality. Despite their excess weight, the traditional cut points may not be suitable for Hispanics at this time.[35]

Compared with whites, Mexican-Americans have greater upper body adiposity, but the ethnic difference in central adiposity index is greater than what would be expected based on the difference in waist/hip ratio.[36,37] Women, particularly US-born Spanish-speaking women (68.7%), have a higher prevalence of abdominal obesity, and are significantly more likely than their counterparts to have one or more of the following CVD risk factors: high serum insulin, non-insulin-dependent diabetes, high blood lipid levels, and/or hypertension.[38] The failure of lifestyle measures to change fat distribution at either of the two fat deposit sites further substantiates the fact that genetic factors may be the regulating agent in determining body fat distribution.

Excess fat tissue represents an increase in weight. Skinfold thickness recorded by many investigators at central and peripheral sites is a measure of subcutaneous adipose tissue.[37,39–42] Distributions of centrality index (subscapular/triceps) and waist/hip ratio may be used as distinct independent predictors of metabolic diseases for this population.[37] Body fat distribution is an additional component of obesity risk; upper body fat, in particular, has been associated with an increased risk for diabetes.[43] Each of the indices of fat patterning measures separates aspects of intermediate metabolism, for example, lipids, lipoproteins, and triglycerides. Hence, every effort should be made to assess regional areas of body fat dispersal. An expert panel from the National Academy of Sciences suggests that the waist/hip ratio is a very useful measure for determining increased risk for CVD, with a ratio of 0.8

or greater representing an appropriate standard for beginning intervention.[44] If only one adiposity measure is possible, the waist circumference appears to be most practical and to have the best sensitivity for assessing central body fat patterning. The National Obesity Education Initiative[35] indicates a waist circumference exceeding 35 inches in women or 40 inches in men to indentify those at greater cardiovascular risk, even when BMI is in the overweight range.

The growing body of literature suggests obesity acquired during childhood is maintained throughout adulthood.[45] A substantial weight gain is seen among the younger age groups, without a proportional increase in stature, when HHANES-I data for youth height and weight are compared with data collected a decade later.[39,45] The weight increases are progressively higher across all percentiles, with the widest gap seen at the 90th percentile. The excessive weight for stature seems to be related to excessive fat tissue, and not to lean muscle mass.[46] With a positive energy balance, body mass increases to accommodate the increases in energy stores. Hill and Peters suggest that the gain in body mass restores the energy balance at the next level.[32] The growing increase in youth body fatness above the 50th percentile has been associated with adverse changes in lipid and carbohydrate metabolism, leading to adult centralized obesity and increased risk of adult-onset diabetes.[40,47] On average age non-insulin-dependent diabetes mellitus (NIDDM) is diagnosed several years earlier in Mexican-Americans than in whites, which may reflect a longer period of excessive overweight.[48]

Today, overweight is the most common health problem facing US children, and prevalence has increased by more than 50% in the last 10 years, with the sharpest observed increases among boys. NHANES-III (phases I and II) found that young Hispanic males and females (primarily Mexican-Americans) were the groups most likely to be overweight and obese. A recent study from NHANES (1999–2000) shows that the prevalence of overweight is approximately 10% for 2- to 5-year-olds and approximately 15% for 6- to 11-year-olds and 12- to 19-year-olds, with a trend toward an increase in overweight in males (Table 19-6).[4] Overweight children often become overweight adults, and being overweight in adulthood is a health risk. In a sample of nearly 1300 (aged 8–13) children in Los Angeles County, Bassin and co-workers found during a 6-year period that more than 55% were obese, based on skinfold measurement and BMI classification.[46] These findings coincide with findings in adult Hispanics in the Southwest United States.[6,25]

The development of obesity seems to begin even earlier among Mexican-Americans, as compared with non-Hispanic Whites, because of sociocultural and socioeconomic factors linked to diet and physical

TABLE 19-6 Prevalence of Overweight or Risk for Overweight in Children by Sex, Race/Ethnicity, and Age Group: NHANES 1999–2000*

Sex	Age	Overweight or at risk†				Overweight‡			
		All§	Non-Hispanic white	Non-Hispanic African-American	Mexican-American	All	Non-Hispanic white	Non-Hispanic African-American	Mexican-American
Both sexes	2–5	20.6(1.8)	20.5(2.7)	19.3(3.5)	22.7(3.0)	10.4(1.7)	10.1(2.4)	8.4(2.3)	11.1(2.5)
	6–11	30.3(2.4)	26.2(3.6)	35.9(3.0)	39.3(3.0)	15.3(1.7)	11.8(2.4)	19.5(2.0)	23.7(2.0)#
	12–19	30.4(1.9)	26.5(2.4)	40.4(2.2)	43.8(2.6)	15.5(1.2)	12.7(1.7)	23.6(2.1)#	23.4(2.1)#
Male	2–5	20.9(2.4)	21.4(3.7)	12.6(3.1)	26.0(4.9)	9.9(2.2)	8.8(3.2)‖	5.9(2.4)‖	13.0(3.9)
	6–11	32.7(3.7)	29.4(5.7)	34.5(3.6)	43.0(4.2)	16.0(2.3)	12.0(3.0)	17.1(2.8)	27.3(3.1)#
	12–19	30.5(2.1)	27.4(3.0)	35.7(2.8)	44.2(3.0)	15.5(1.6)	12.8(2.4)	20.7(2.6)	27.5(3.0)#
Female	2–5	20.4(3.0)	19.7(4.1)	26.6(6.4)	19.5(4.0)	11.0(2.5)	11.5(3.3)	11.2(3.8)‖	9.2(2.9)‖
	6–11	27.8(3.2)	22.8(4.7)	37.6(3.6)	35.1(4.4)	14.5(2.5)	11.6(3.5)‖	22.2(3.3)	19.6(3.1)
	12–19	30.2(2.8)	25.4(3.3)	45.5(3.0)	43.5(4.2)¶	15.5(1.6)	12.4(2.1)	26.6(2.7)#	19.4(2.8)

*Values are expressed as percentages (SE). NHANES indicates National Health and Nutrition Examination Survey.
†Body mass index for age is at the 85th percentile or higher.
‡Body mass index is at the 95th percentile or higher.
§Includes racial/ethnic groups not shown separately (eg, other category).
‖Does not meet standard of statistical reliability and precision (relative SE >30%).
¶Includes one influential observation. When this observation is deleted, the prevalence (SE) is 39.6 (2.3).
#Significantly different from non-Hispanic whites at *P* < .05 (with Bonferroni adjustment).

SOURCE: Reproduced, with permission, from Ogden et al.[49]

inactivity.[33,50] Popkin and Udry reexamined thousands of ethnically diverse adolescents for body composition and categorized them on the basis of three different generation waves. The data categorized by generation revealed a 24% increase in weight between the first and second generations, and hardly any change between second- and third-generation youth.[51] The major differences in obesity prevalence among Hispanics occurred between teenagers born in another country and those born in the United States. One study looked at acculturation status and observed that Mexican-born women and men living in California had the smallest waist circumference (90.4 and 94.0 cm, respectively); US-born, English-speaking women and men had intermediate waist circumference (93.6 and 97.3 cm); and US-born, Spanish-speaking women and men had the largest waist circumference (96.9 and 97.7 cm).[38] The acculturation process appears to be a very powerful force in the development of obesity.[51]

Data from the San Antonio Heart Study suggest that there are connections between obesity and lifestyle factors, but these are gender- and age-specific. Among men with increasing socioeconomic status, there was an increase in obesity and greater centralized fat. Nevertheless, women in higher socioeconomic classes demonstrated a decrease in obesity and more favorable body fat distribution. Within the same social class, Mexican-Americans were shorter and slightly heavier than non-Hispanic Whites.[10,29] A weak and inconsistent relationship was observed between socioeconomic status and overweight in Hispanic teenage girls and boys, whereas this stronger relationship appears to be much stronger in whites.[10]

Diabetes

Diabetes has ranked among the 10 leading causes of morbidity and mortality in the United States over the last 65 years. Cross-sectional surveys of Hispanic adults have demonstrated a substantial increase compared with whites in the prevalence of NIDDM.[12,42,52] The prevalence of diabetes in Mexican-Americans aged 20 and older is 8% for men and 11% for women. These rates are significantly higher than those for whites. An additional 5% of Mexican-American men and 4% of Mexican-American women may have undiagnosed diabetes. In California, which has the nation's largest Mexican-American population, the prevalence of diabetes was reported as 13%—three times higher than in whites.[53] The San Antonio Heart Study investigators found that approximately 50% of the sample were previously undiagnosed diabetics and were less likely to seek medical care because they had no insurance. Diehl and Stern reported that undiagnosed diabetes in Texas, Colorado, New Mexico, and California significantly

impacts the reported prevalence of diabetes for both men and women. They also pointed out that prevalence rates for NIDDM are related to socioeconomic status, with NIDDM being most prevalent among those at the lowest economic levels.[12] When both social class and obesity were controlled for, Mexican-Americans of both sexes still had a higher prevalence of NIDDM than whites.[54] One of the most interesting investigations of Mexican-Americans by the San Antonio Heart Study involved predicting NIDDM using skin color as an index of Native-American heritage. The highest rate of diabetes has been reported among Native-Americans who inhabit the Southwest. The rate of the disease was related closely to the degree of blending between the two ethnic groups. The authors concluded that NIDDM was highest in the segment of the Mexican-American population that carried a significant Native-American genetic heritage.[55]

The increasing level of childhood obesity places the Mexican-American population at even greater risk of NIDDM. The recent increase in type 2 diabetes in children and adolescents is an alarming manifestation of the broader problem of physical inactivity, poor diet, and obesity afflicting young people throughout the world. Premature development of CVD, even in the absence of diabetes, is linked to childhood obesity and physical inactivity. But when, in susceptible pediatric populations, these conditions are accompanied by frank diabetes, medical therapy is intensive and costly. What makes the situation even more dangerous is that underuse of diabetes screening seems to be related to folk medicine and religious beliefs. In addition to traditional medicine, Hispanic patients not infrequently employ folk healers who use herbs, home medicines, and other potions mixed with prayers to treat the disease (see Table 19-2).[8] Some of the less educated and strongly religious patients believe that it is God's will for them to have diabetes.[56] A greater proportion of the Mexican-American population, compared with whites, are likely to be prediabetic and eventually to become diabetic.

Physical activity

Even though the influence of physical activity in predicting and/or reducing the risk for CVD is well known, only recently has it been scientifically established.[57] Only 24% of Americans are physically active on a regular basis (20 minutes or longer per day three or more times per week). Among Hispanics, 62% of both men and women report a sedentary lifestyle.[2] A substantial number of Hispanics in California (70% of men and 66% of women) report no or irregular physical activity during the last 30 days.[28] California investigators found that substantially more Hispanic men (70%) and women (66%) were physically inactive (reporting no or irregular leisure-time physical activity in the past month), compared with white men (50.2%) and women (50.6%).[27] The report also noted that the less educated are more likely to be physically active than college graduates across adulthood.

Data from NHANES-III document that only 45% of Mexican-Americans claim to be physically active, compared with 61% of whites. In addition, 48% of Mexican-Americans who are underweight exercise three or more times per week, compared with only 41% of those who are overweight (Table 19-7).[21] Participation in physical activity among Mexican-American women is substantially lower than among white women (32% vs 52%, respectively). Ransdell and Wells reported that Mexican-American women older than 40 and having less than a college education seldom exercise. Marital status was a strong predictor of participation in any exercise, as being single was associated with higher exercise levels, and social support was a primary ingredient in encouraging physical activity among women.[58] In youth, physical activity is encouraged and becomes prevalent when viewed as social learning. There has traditionally been a lack of interest in identifying social and cultural determinants, as well as developing appropriate measuring instruments, which has hampered assessment of physical activity during daily living.[59] Data from the Youth National Fitness Test indicate that ethnically diverse populations have not been extensively studied, resulting in reliance on general US population reports. Despite the importance of physical activity in reducing weight, improving the cardiovascular system, and preventing insulin resistance, Mexican-Americans are more likely to be sedentary. Understanding the determinants that encourage Mexican-Americans to participate in physical activity has been a challenge. Physical activity patterns are little known, and predictors of physical activity are hardly explored; thus programs that are generic (American Heart Association, American Diabetes Association) are used. A few community-based programs have made advances (Por la Vida, La Vida Buena); those developed by Stanford Five Cities Project, which targeted Hispanics, and Pawtucket Heart Health, which looked at Puerto Ricans, have reported success.[60] The programs' successes were attributed to forging partnerships with and training lay health advisors (*promotores*) in physical activity and nutrition. Overall little research has been conducted on how effective the interventions have been in reducing cardiovascular risk factors over the long term. In the short term they have been effective.

Cigarette smoking

The adverse effects of smoking have been widely advertised, but the message has not penetrated the Mexican-American community to the extent that it has the white community. Less information is available about Hispanics than about whites and African-Americans regarding short- and long-term trends in smoking. Nationally, the prevalence rates for smoking in Mexican-Americans are 22% for men and 15% for women, but among youth in grades 9 to 12, these rates are markedly higher—36% for males and 32% for females.[61] Hispanic males 12 to 17 years old in California had the highest rate of smoking (49%) of any racial/ethnic group.[61] California smoking prevalence data for adults reveal that Mexican-American women have the lowest prevalence rate. Men are more likely to smoke than women, and Mexican-American men smoke only slightly less than whites (Fig. 19-2).[53] Furthermore, this report suggests that the low smoking rate in Mexican-American adults may not continue.

National and statewide efforts have been launched to prevent youth from smoking experimentation.[62] School-based programs, which target all children, assume that preventing youth from smoking will dampen their interest in smoking during adulthood. HHANES-III found the prevalence of smoking to decline substantially with higher levels of education: those who completed high school or higher education had a lower prevalence. Only a small decline was observed among those with less than a high school education. The reduction in smoking was greater in women than men. On the other hand, youngsters were more inclined to experiment with tobacco use, with the same frequency as in other groups. Smoking had greater acceptance and social support with fewer years of formal education. The social and economic experiences of living in a low-income community with a materialistically and socially conscious culture may have lowered the resistance to smoking,[63,64] and increased the need for stronger and continuous messages. The lower level of education along with increased social pressure results in the vulnerability to tobacco advertising and smoking. Morris and colleagues found that Mexican-American youngsters start to smoke at younger ages than was previously reported.[65] The smoking increase among Mexican-American young people should be viewed with alarm because of its adult health consequences. Substantial attempts should be made to further reduce the prevalence of smoking in all ethnic groups among those with less than a high school education. Without individually tailored intervention strategies for youth, there will likely be an increase in adult tobacco use.

CONCLUSION

During the past half-century, there has been major progress in understanding risk factors for CVD in whites and African-Americans. During the past two decades, there have been increasing efforts to study the Hispanic population, but the research is still sparse. Until there is an increase in the number of scientists and in funding

TABLE 19-7 Percentage of People 20 Years of Age and Older Who Exercised Three or More Times Per Week During Leisure Time, by Age, Race/Ethnicity, and Body Weight Status, 1988–1991

Sex/age/body weight status	Total population*			Non-Hispanic white			Non-Hispanic African-American			Mexican-American		
	Sample size	%	SE	Sample size	%	SE	Sample size	%	SE	Sample size	%	SE
≥20 Years												
Underweight	341	52.2	4.27	132	50.7	5.47	120	63.2	5.76	74	48.2	6.67
Acceptable weight	2,400	62.8	2.24	1,093	64.4	2.44	593	61.8	2.29	625	46.6	2.61
Overweight	1,381	55.1	2.19	593	56.1	2.68	328	58.7	3.09	431	41.1	2.38
Total	4122	59.5	1.79	1818	60.7	2.06	1041	61.0	2.28	1130	44.7	1.59
20-39 years												
Underweight	177	50.0	5.38	55	47.5	6.56	59	73.6	7.67	55	51.6	7.18
Acceptable weight	1,025	64.1	3.23	317	65.0	3.95	283	72.0	3.14	381	48.6	2.39
Overweight	418	59.9	2.99	123	59.2	3.77	132	72.2	4.68	153	44.2	5.95
Total	1620	61.5	2.38	495	61.6	2.91	474	72.2	3.05	589	47.7	1.43
40-59 years												
Underweight	48	66.8	6.92	16	64.2†	†	25	73.8†	†	4	‡	‡
Acceptable weight	606	62.0	2.81	287	64.5	3.31	163	54.6	3.79	124	39.1	5.07
Overweight	480	51.1	2.63	203	53.8	3.24	108	48.2	5.61	155	38.3	8.16
Total	1134	57.9	2.09	506	60.1	2.58	296	53.2	2.69	283	38.2	4.59
≥60 years												
Underweight	116	49.0	6.40	61	53.0	7.41	36	22.6	5.58	15	35.6†	†
Acceptable weight	769	60.4	2.44	489	63.0	2.53	147	38.4	4.83	120	46.0	5.23
Overweight	483	54.0	4.55	267	55.6	5.01	88	45.2	5.97	123	37.3	2.93
Total	1368	57.2	2.65	817	59.5	2.84	271	38.5	3.07	258	41.4	2.66

*Includes data for race/ethnic groups not shown separately.

†Indicates a statistic that is potentially unreliable because of small sample size or large coefficient of variation.

‡Does not meet minimum sample size requirements.

NOTE: Based on self-reported leisure-time physical activity. BMI is an index used to relate weight to stature. Underweight is defined as a BMI ≤15th percentile, acceptable weight as a BMI between 16th and 84th percentiles, and overweight as a BMI ≥85th percentile, based on BMIs for 20- to 29-year-old males.

SOURCE: Reproduced, with permission, from the *Third Report on Nutrition Monitoring in the United States.*[21]

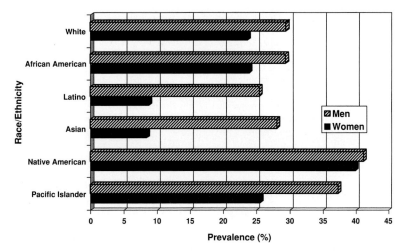

FIGURE 19-2   Prevalence of cigarette smoking among California adults by race and gender, *California Health Interview Survey, 2001*,[53] weighted to the California population. (Data adapted by Tang M, Wong ND, University of California, Irvine.)

committed to the study of Hispanics, comprehension and treatment of CVD in this group will stagnate and, thus, impede a reduction in morbidity and mortality.

The reported advantage Hispanics have with respect to CVD morbidity is disappearing with the growing rate of assimilation. Physicians and health promotion personnel should be taught to consider ancestry and culture when implementing CVD prevention efforts in Hispanics. Further information on Hispanics' major risk factors for heart disease and stroke relative to country of birth, number of generations in the United States, degree of acculturation, traditional diet, and other lifestyle factors is required to improve strategic health policy planning and reduce health care costs, while increasing life expectancy.

REFERENCES

1. Kingston RS, Smith JP. Socioeconomic status and racial and ethnic differences in functional status associated with chronic diseases. *Am J Public Health* 1997;87:805–810.

2. Hajat A, Lucas JB, Kington R. Health outcomes among Hispanic subgroups: data from the National Health Interview Survey, 1992–95. *Vital Health Stat* 2000;310:1–16

3. Ruiz P. Hispanic access to health/mental health services. *Psychiatr Q* 2002;73(2):85–91.

4. Morales LS, Lara M, Kington RS, et al. Socioeconomic, cultural, and behavioral factors affecting Hispanic health outcomes. *J Health Care Poor Underserved* 2002;13:477–501.

5. Sorlie PD, Backlund MS, Johnson NJ, Rogot E. Mortality by Hispanic status in the United States. *JAMA* 1993;270:2464–2468.

6. *Hispanics and Cardiovascular Disease.* Biostatistical Fact Sheets. Dallas, Tex: American Heart Association; 1999.

7. US Bureau of the Census. *Hispanic-Americans Today: Current Population Reports,* Series P-23, No. 183. Washington, DC: US Government Printing Office; 1993.

8. Wagner T, Guendelman S. Heath services utilization among Latinos and white non-Latinos: results from a national survey. J Health Care Poor Underserved 2000;11:179–194.

9. *Plan and Operation of the Hispanic Health and Nutrition Examination Survey 1982–84.* Vital Health Stat [I] 1985; DHHS Publication PHS 85-1321. Hyattsville, Md: US Public Health Service; 1985.

10. National Center for Health Statistics. *Health, United States, 1993.* Hyattsville, Md: US Public Health Service; 1994.

11. Mokdad AH, Ford ES, Bowman BA, et al. Prevalence of obesity, diabetes, and obesity related health risk factors. *JAMA* 2003;289:76–79.

12. Diehl AC, Stern MP. Special health problems of Mexican-Americans: obesity, gall bladder disease, diabetes mellitus and cardiovascular disease. *Adv Intern Med* 1989;34:73–96.

13. Markides KS, Coreil J. The health of Hispanics in the southwestern United States: an epidemiological paradox. *Public Health Rep* 1986;101:253–265.

14. Hazuda HP, Haffner SM, Stern MP, et al. Effects of acculturation and socioeconomic status on obesity and diabetes in Mexican-Americans. *Am J Epidemiol* 1988;128:1289–1301.

15. Wei M, Valdez RA, Mitchel BD, et al. Migration status, socioeconomic status and mortality rates in Mexican-Americans and non-Hispanic whites: the San Antonio Heart Study. *Ann Epidemiol* 1996;6:307–313.

16. Goff DC, Nichaman MZ, Chau W. Greater incidence of hospitalized myocardial infarction among Mexican-Americans than non-Hispanic whites: the Corpus Christi Heart Project, 1988–1992. *Circulation* 1997;March(6):1433–1440.

17. Goff DC Jr, Ramsey DJ, Wear MC. Mortality after hospitalization for myocardial infarction among Mexican-Americans and

non-Hispanic whites: the Corpus Christi Heart Project. *Ethnicity Dis* 1993;3:55–63.

18. *Atlas of Stroke Mortality: Racial, Ethnic, and Geographic Disparities in the United States.* Hyattsville, Md: US Department of Health and Human Services, Centers for Disease Control and Prevention, National Center for Chronic Disease Prevention and Health Promotion; 2003.

19. Berenson GS, Wattigney MS, Tracy RE. Atherosclerosis of the aorta and coronary arteries and cardiovascular risk factors in persons aged 6 to 30 studied at necropsy (the Bogalusa Heart Study). *Am J Cardiol* 1992;70:851–858.

20. *Third Report on Nutrition Monitoring in the United States: Volume I,* Washington, DC: US Government Printing Office; 1995.

21. Haffner SM, Stern MP, Hazuda HP, et al. The role of behavioral variables and fat patterning in explaining ethnic differences in serum lipids and lipoproteins. *Am J Epidemiol* 1986;123:830–839.

22. Hixon JE, Henkel RD, Sharp RM, Comuzzie AG. Genetic and environmental contributions to cardiovascular risk factors in Mexican-Americans: the San Antonio Family Heart Study. *Circulation* 1996;94:2159–2170.

23. Wei M, Mitchell BD, Haffner SM Stern MP. Effects of cigarette smoking, diabetes, high cholesterol and hypertension on all-cause mortality and cardiovascular disease mortality in Mexican-Americans: the San Antonio Heart Study. *Am J Epidemiol* 1996;141:1058–1065.

24. Valdez R, Gonzalez-Villalpando C, Mitchell BD, et al. Differential impact of obesity in related populations. *Obes Res* 1995;3(suppl 2):223s–232s.

25. US Department of Health and Human Services. Update: Prevalence of Overweight Among Children, Adolescents, and Adults—United States, 1988–94. *MMWR* 1997;46:199–202.

26. Pawson IG, Martorel R, Mendoza FE. Prevalence of overweight and obesity in U.S. Hispanic population. *Am J Nutr* 1995;53:15225–15228.

27. Jeffrey RW. Population perspectives on the prevention and treatment of obesity in minority populations. *Am J Clin Nutr* 1991;53:1621–1624.

28. Gazzaniga JM, Kao C, Cowling DW, et al. Cardiovascular disease risk factors among California adults, 1984–1996. Sacramento, CA: CORE Program, University of California San Francisco and California Department of Health Services; 1998.

29. Stern MP, Pugh JA, Gaskell SP, Hazuda HP. Knowledge, attitudes, and behavior related to obesity and dieting in Mexican-Americans and Anglos: the San Antonio Heart Study. *Am J Epidemiol* 1992;115:917–927.

30. Centers for Disease Control and Prevention. Prevalence of overweight for Hispanics: United States, 1982–1984. *JAMA* 1990;263:631–632.

31. Flegal KM, Carroll MD, Ogden CL, Johnson CL. Prevalence and trends in obesity among US adults. *JAMA* 2002;288:1723–1727.

32. Hill JO, Peters JC. Environmental contributions to obesity epidemic. *Science* 1998;28:1371–1374.

33. Malina RM, Little BB, Stern MP, et al. Ethnic and social class differences in selected anthropometric characteristics of Mexican-American and Anglo adults: the San Antonio Heart Study. *Hum Biol* 1983;55:867–883.

34. *National Obesity Initiative Guidelines.* Available at: http://www.nhlbi.nih.gov/guidelines/obesity/ob_home.htm. Accessed June 9, 2004.

35. Mitchell BD, Stern MP, Haffner SM, et al. Risk factors for cardiovascular mortality in Mexican-Americans. *Int J Obes* 1990;14:623–629.

36. Haffner SM, Stern MP, Hazuda HP, et al. Do upper-body and central adiposity measure different aspects of regional body-fat distribution? Relationship to non-insulin-dependent diabetes mellitus, lipids, and lipoproteins. *Diabetes* 1987;36:43–51.

37. Haffner SM, Stern MP, Hazuda HP, et al. Upper body and centralized obesity in Mexican-Americans and Non-Hispanic whites: relationship to body mass index and demographic variables. *Int J Obes* 1986;10:493–502.

38. Sundquist J, Winkleby M. Country of birth, acculturation status and abdominal obesity in a national sample of Mexican-American women and men. *Int J Epidemiol* 2000;29:470–477.

39. Roche AE, Guo S, Bumgartner RN, et al. Reference data for weight, stature, and weight/stature in Mexican-Americans from the Hispanic Health and Nutrition Examination Survey (HHANES) 1982–1984. *Am J Clin Nutr* 1990;51(suppl):217–245.

40. Mueller WH, Joos SK, Havis CL, et al. The Diabetes Alert Study: growth, fatness, fat patterning, adolescence through adulthood in Mexican-Americans. *Am J Phys Anthropol* 1984;64:389–399.

41. Stern SP, Haffner SM. Do anthropometric differences between Mexican-Americans and non Hispanic whites explain ethnic differences in metabolic variables? *Acta Med Scand Suppl* 1989;723:37–44.

42. Joos SK, Mueller WH, Hanis CL, Schull WS. Diabetes Alert Study: weight history and body adiposity in diabetic and non diabetic Mexican-American adults. *Ann Hum Biol* 1984;11:161–171.

43. Kumanyika SK. Special issues regarding obesity in minority populations. *Ann Intern Med* 1993;119(7, pt 2):650–654.

44. *Physical Activity and Health: A Report of the Surgeon General.* Atlanta, Ga: US Department of Health and Human Services, Centers for Disease Control and Prevention, National Center for Chronic Disease Prevention and Health Promotion; 1996.

45. Troiano RP, Flegal KM, Kuczmarski RJ, et al. Overweight prevalence and trends for children and adolescents. *Arch Pediatr Adolesc Med* 1995;149:1085–1091.

46. Bassin SL, Gustin W, Morris GS, et al. Hispanic youth obesity: body fat and cardiovascular risk factors [abstract]. *Circulation* 1995;92:1481.

47. Stern MP, Haffner SM, et al. Hyperinsulinemia in a population at high risk for non-insulin dependent diabetes mellitus. *N Engl J Med* 1986;315:220–224.

48. Raymond CA. Diabetes in Mexican-Americans: pressing problem in a growing population. *JAMA* 1988;259:1772.

49. Ogden CL, Flegal KM, Carroll MD, Johnson CL. Prevalance and trends in overweight among US children and adolescents, 1999–2000. *JAMA* 2002;288:1728–1732.

50. Troiano RP, Flegal KM. Overweight children and adolescents: description, epidemiology and demographics. *Pediatrics* 1998;101(suppl):497–504.

51. Popkin BM, Udry JR. Adolescent obesity increases significantly in second and third generation US immigrants: the National Longitudinal Study of Adolescent Health. *J Nutr* 1998;128:701–706.

52. Stern MP, Haffner SM. Body fat distribution and hyperinsulinemia as risk factors for diabetes and cardiovascular disease. *Arteriosclerosis* 1986;6:123–130.

53. California Health Interview Survey 2001, UCLA Center for Health Policy Research, California Department of Health Services, and Public Health Institute. Available at: http://www.chis.ucla.edu. Accessed on June 9, 2004.

54. Stern MP, Haffner SM. Type II diabetes and its complications in Mexican-Americans. *Diabetes Metab Rev* 1990;6:29–40.

55. Knowler WC, Pettitt DJ, Saad MF, et al. Obesity in the Pima Indians: its magnitude and relationship with diabetes. *Am J Clin Nutr* 1991;53(6, suppl):1543S–1551S.

56. Zaldivar A, Smolowitz J. Perceptions of the importance on religion and folk medicine by non-Mexican-American Hispanic adults with diabetes. *Diabetes Educator* 1994; July 20(4):363–366.

57. Paffenbarger RS, Hyde RT, Wing AL, et al. The association of changes in physical activity level and other lifestyle characteristics with mortality among men. *N Engl J Med* 1993;328:538–545.

58. Ransdell LB, Wells CL. Physical activity in urban white, African-American, and Mexican-American women. *Med Sci Sports Exerc* 1998;3:1608–1615.

59. Moller JH, Taubert KA, Allen HD, et al. Cardiovascular health and disease in children: current status: AHA Medical/Scientific Statement Special Report. *Circulation* 1994;89:923–930.

60. Whitehorse LE, Manzano R. Culturally tailoring a physical activity program for Hispanic Women: recruitment successes of La Vida Buena's Salsa Aerobics. *J Health Educ* 1999;30:18–24.

61. Elder JP, Campbell NR, Litrownik AJ, et al. Predictors of cigarette and alcohol susceptibility and use among Hispanic migrant adolescents. *Prev Med* 2000;31:115–123.

62. Escobedo LG, Anda RF, Smith PF, et al. Sociodemographic characteristics of cigarette smoking initiation in the United States: implications for smoking prevention policy. *JAMA* 1990;264:1550–1556.

63. Escobedo LG, Remington PL. Birth cohort analysis of smoking prevalence among Hispanics in the United States. *JAMA* 1989;261:66–69.

64. Escobedo LG, Peddicord JP. Smoking prevalence in US birth cohorts: the influence of gender and education. *Am J Public Health* 1996;86:231–236.

65. Morris GS, Vo AN, Bassin S, et al. Prevalence and sociobehavioral correlates of tobacco use among Hispanic children: the Tobacco Resistance Activity Program. *J Sch Health* 1993;63(9):391–396.

20

East Asians and South Asians, and Asian and Pacific-Islander Americans

Prakash C. Deedwania
Rajeev Gupta

KEY POINTS

- Cardiovascular disease is a major problem among Asians and Pacific Islanders, causing high morbidity and mortality. Hypertension is the most common risk factor and stroke the predominant form of cardiovascular disease in Chinese and East Asian migrants to the United States, whereas diabetes is the most common risk factor and coronary heart disease the dominant disease among South Asians.

- Traditionally, Asians living in the rural areas of their native countries have a low prevalence of hypertension, coronary heart disease, and other cardiovascular disease. Migration to urban areas within the country or to developed countries of Europe and North America dramatically changes the coronary risk factor profile.

- With urbanization and acculturation, there is a decline in physical activity and increase in the consumption of calorie-dense foods, fat, and salt, resulting in generalized and abdominal obesity.

- The coronary risk factors highly prevalent in migrant Asians include tobacco smoking,

hypertension, diabetes, dyslipidemias, and the metabolic syndrome. Obesity, hypertension, and the metabolic syndrome are particularly prevalent in Pacific Islanders.

- Populationwide interventions, including public education strategies, use of media, and promotion of traditional Asian social lifestyles, are essential in changing dietary habits, physical activity, and tobacco habits,

- High-risk subjects are those with a family history of coronary heart disease, hypertension, or diabetes and those having two or more coronary risk factors such as sedentary lifestyle, obesity, truncal obesity, and metabolic syndrome.

- Appropriate interventions are smoking cessation, physical activity guidelines, weight management, blood pressure control, lipid management, and control of hyperglycemia.

- Barriers to implementing prevention programs among Asians and Pacific Islanders should be identified and overcome.

INTRODUCTION

Cardiovascular disease (CVD) accounts for a large proportion of all deaths and disability worldwide. The Global Burden of Disease (GBD) study reported that

in 1990, there were 5.2 million deaths from CVD in economically developed countries and 9.1 million deaths from the same causes in developing countries.[1] However, in the developed world about one quarter of all deaths occurred in persons younger than 70, whereas in the

TABLE 20-1   Cardiovascular Deaths by Region in 1990: Global Burden of Disease Study, 1990

	No. (x 10^6)	Due to CHD (%)	Due to stroke (%)	Predicted increase by 2002 (%)
Established market economies	3.2	53	25	15
Former socialist economies	2.1	50	31	26
India	2.3	52	20	111
China	2.6	30	50	77
Other Asia and Islands	1.3	34	29	106
Sub-Saharan Africa	0.8	26	47	114
Latin America and Caribbean	0.8	44	32	120
Middle Eastern Crescent	1.3	47	16	129

Table spanning header: *Cardiovascular deaths, 1990*

developing world, more than about half of these deaths occurred in those younger than 70. It has been predicted that by the year 2020, the global CVD burden will increase by almost 75%. Almost all of this increase will occur in developing countries, mainly in Asia and Latin America (Table 20-1).

Individuals living in Asian countries have traditionally had a low prevalence of coronary heart disease (CHD). With the modernization of Asia, there has been an alarming increase in the incidence of CHD. This region is undergoing unprecedented economic growth, rapid technologic changes, urbanization, and major changes in lifestyle. The very high CHD death rates in Singapore,

which are similar to those of the United States and Australia, provide a warning that Asia should expect a surge in CHD similar to that observed in the 1950s and 1960s in the United States and other developed countries. The situation in India is even more alarming. Reddy and Yusuf reported that mortality from CVD was projected to decline in developed countries from 1970 to 2015, whereas it was projected to almost double in the developing countries.[2] In the GBD study, it was reported that of a total of 9.4 million deaths in India in 1990, CVD caused 2.3 million (25%): 1.2 million deaths were due to CHD and 0.5 million to stroke.[3] It has also been predicted that by 2020, there will be a 111% increase in

TABLE 20-2   Mortality due to Cardiovascular Risk Factors in the Americas, Europe, and South Asia: Global Burden of Disease Study, 2000

	Americas VLC, VLA*	Europe VLC, VLA	South Asia HC, HA	Western pacific LC, LA
Total population	160,494/164,689†	201,514/210,376	639,087/602,719	785,055/747,878
Total mortality	1342/1392	2020/2054	6358/5764	5483/4944
High blood pressure	179/191	325/354	668/519	711/758
High cholesterol	161/189	265/282	488/507	222/265
High BMI	135/137	183/197	42/110	163/184
Low fruit/vegetable intake	92/79	95/75	378/311	269/232
Physical inactivity	74/81	103/103	218/185	132/134
Tobacco	352/294	531/145	785/132	661/137
Urban outdoor air pollution	14/14	12/11	72/60	176/179
Indoor smoke	??	??	218/304	137/366

*Mortality stratum as defined by Global Burden of Disease Study: VLC, VLA, very low childhood, very low adult; HC, HA, high childhood, high adult; LC, LA, low childhood, low adult.
†Thousands of deaths, male/female.
Adapted, with permission, from Ezzati et al.[4]

CVD deaths in India. Corresponding increases are more than 77% for China, 106% for other Asian countries, and 15% for economically developed countries. The Comparative Risk Assessment Collaborating Group reported the results of GBD Study 2000.[4] Of the selected 26 risk factors, high blood pressure, tobacco, alcohol intake, and high cholesterol ranked among the major factors contributing to worldwide mortality (Table 20-2). The impact of these risk factors was greater in developed countries, but in terms of absolute numbers these factors were more prevalent in developing countries. All these risk factors contribute to CVD. CVD is already a major cause of death in developing countries, surpassing developed countries in terms of absolute numbers.

This increase in CVD and atherosclerotic CHD in developing countries has been described as an *epidemiologic transition*, a term initially suggested by Omran.[5] At any given time, different countries of the world, and even different sections within a country, are in different phases of this transition, which Gupta has divided into seven phases.[6] Accordingly, tribal (stage 1) to rural (stage 2) to urban (stage 3) transition is associated with escalating sedentary lifestyle and increased intake of calories, fats, and salt (stage 4) and, as a consequence, increases in body mass index, hypertension (stage 5), and CHD (stage 6). The final stage (stage 7) is characterized by improving lifestyles and decline in CHD.

Yusuf and co-workers reclassified the transition into five phases.[7] In the first phase, the predominant forms of CVD are rheumatic heart diseases and other infection- and nutrition-related CVD. As socioeconomic development occurs, in the second phase, infectious burden is reduced, nutrition improves, and diseases related to hypertension become more important. Third, continuing change in diet, adoption of a sedentary lifestyle, and increasing smoking, atherosclerotic diseases increase. The

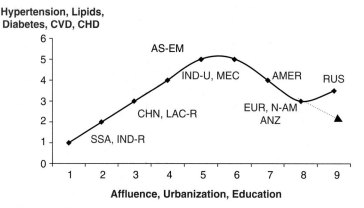

FIGURE 20-1 Stages of epidemiological transition and global changes in cardiovascular prevalence and mortality. With increasing affluence, urbanization and education, there intially a progressive increase in prevalence of hypertension, dyslipidemias, diabetes, CHD, and CVD. This is associated with increase in primordial factors of physical inactivity, smoking, and dietary fat and salt intake. Presently, the populations of sub-Saharan Africa (SSA) and rural India (IND-R) are in very early stages of this transition, while China (CHN) and rural areas of Latin American countries (LAC-R) have progressed to second stage where hypertension is the predominant cardiovascular disease. Population in urban India (IND-U) and the middle east (MEC) have progressed beyond this stage and have a very high morbidity from CHD. A very high CVD morbidity and mortality is present in emigrant Asians (AS-EM). Increasing education and awareness of risk factors among North American (N-AM, AMER), European (EUR), and Australia and New Zealander (ANZ) populations have led to a marked decline in CHD mortality. Due to social and political upheavals in Russia (RUS) and other east European countries, the CVD mortality has increased in these countries, including that epidemiological transition is reversible due to social change.

fourth stage is characterized by increasing public response to the epidemic in the form of increased prevention efforts associated with a decline in mortality. The fifth phase has been added to describe a new development in Eastern Europe, where socioeconomic upheaval has been linked to increased CVD mortality. Rural India is currently in phases I and II of the epidemiologic transition, with CVD manifesting predominantly as nutrition-related CVD, rheumatic heart disease, and hypertension with a low prevalence of CHD. However, urban India has progressed to phases II and III of this transition and there is a massive CHD epidemic. In some parts of rural and urban India and China, transition to stage IV has occurred (Fig. 20-1).

Studies reviewed below from different Asian populations living both within and outside the United States show the status of CVD risk in Asians is becoming increasingly similar to that of Caucasian populations.[8] Consideration must be given to applying the lessons in prevention learned over the past half-century in other populations to prevent the emerging epidemic of CHD in Asian countries and Pacific Islander populations.

RISK FACTORS AND CORONARY DISEASE IN ASIAN POPULATIONS

The World Health Organization (WHO) estimates that death attributable to CVD has increased in parallel with the expanding population in Asia.[1] CVD accounts for a large proportion of disability-adjusted life years lost in these countries, and CHD is expected to rise in parallel with the increase in life expectancy secondary to increases in per capita income and declining infant mortality. Increases in life expectancy would lead to large increases in CHD prevalence. By contrast, in the United Kingdom and Canada, although the CHD mortality rate of Indians compared with other populations remains high, a decline in CHD has been observed over the past 10 years.[9] These data indicate that the high rates of CHD accompanying economic changes are reversible and, perhaps, even avoidable. Therefore, lessons learned from migrant Japanese and Indians may be helpful in developing prevention strategies for other Asians.[10]

Japanese

At the beginning of Seven Countries Study in 1958, Japanese cohorts had the lowest saturated fat intake, the lowest levels of serum cholesterol, and one of the lowest incidences of CHD.[8] In the Japanese rural areas of Tanushimaru, among men aged 40 to 64, mortality rates from myocardial infarction have remained stable at 0.3 to 0.5 per 1000 per year from 1958 to 1992. Overall, in Japan, the crude death rates from CHD increased up to 1972, but remained stable thereafter. Although the age-adjusted death rate from CHD is decreasing, there is an alarming increase in deaths from other heart diseases. This may be related to mortality from hypertensive heart disease. In the Tokyo area, 49.8% of sudden deaths examined at autopsy have been attributed to CHD.

The Ni-Hon-San Study of Japanese living in Japan, Hawaii, and mainland United States provides a classic example of the influence of Western lifestyle and dietary changes on CHD incidence in a low-incidence population.[11] The average annual mortality rates from CHD in Japanese men 55 to 59 years old in the late 1960s were 1.4 per 1000 in Japan, 1.7 per 1000 in Honolulu, and 4.8 per 1000 in San Francisco. Mean levels or prevalence of selected coronary risk factors within each of these three population groups are listed in Table 20-3. There is a trend toward increases in values of all major coronary risk factors, including obesity, systolic blood pressure, and cholesterol and triglyceride levels among those living in Japan, Honolulu, and San Francisco (in order of increasing levels). Although the values of biochemical variables are significantly greater in Japanese living in the United States (Hawaii and California), blood pressure and prevalence of hypertension are not significantly different. Obesity and biochemical risk factors may, in part, explain the greater CHD mortality among Japanese in the United States.

The Honolulu Heart Study is the largest and longest running epidemiologic study of heart disease done in Asian-Americans. It has followed, since 1965, the morbidity and mortality status of 8006 men of Japanese ancestry born between 1900 and 1919 with a series of laboratory and medical examinations, as well as assessment of dietary habits and physical activity.[12] This study has documented many of the same risk factors for CHD found in Caucasian populations, including a strong, recently reported relationship of total cholesterol to CHD and total mortality. Hypertension is also quite common in this population, prevalent in more than half of men aged 60 to 75 and 67% of men aged 75 to 81.

Chinese

Clinicians have long known that CHD has been relatively uncommon in China. However, recent data from a nationwide survey of pathologic material and studies of hospitalized cardiac patients have provided evidence suggesting that the incidence of CHD has increased in the last two decades.[13] A corresponding rise in mean serum cholesterol level has also been noted, although the level attained was still significantly lower than those in the United States and other Western European countries. The changes observed in general disease patterns in China since the late 1950s demonstrate a decline in

TABLE 20-3   Coronary Risk Factor Levels and Prevalence of Obesity in Japanese Men: Ni-Hon-San Study

	Age group	Japan	Honolulu	San Francisco
Total cholesterol (mg/dL)	45–49	179.8 ± 2.2*	219.4 ± .09	223.4 ± 1.3
	50–54	182.5 ± 1.7	219.4 ± 0.7	228.2 ± 1.7
	55–59	181.5 ± 1.7	218.7 ± 1.0	226.8 ± 2.2
Triglycerides (mg/dL)	45–49	142.0 ± 37.2	—	192.0 ± 12.7
	50–54	136.0 ± 19.3	182.0 ± 6.7	182.0 ± 12.6
	55–59	124.0 ± 9.2	180.0 ± 7.5	170.0 ± 14.7
Systolic blood pressure (mm Hg)	45–49	126.0 ± 22.8	131.0 ± 21.8	123.0 ± 18.0
	50–54	130.0 ± 23.4	134.0 ± 24.6	132.0 ± 17.4
	55–59	136.0 ± 25.2	135.0 ± 24.4	139.0 ± 21.8
Diastolic blood pressure (mm Hg)	45–49	81.0 ± 13.7	80.0 ± 13.0	79.0 ± 12.8
	50–54	82.0 ± 13.6	86.0 ± 13.7	84.0 ± 10.0
	55–59	85.0 ± 14.0	82.0 ± 13.0	88.0 ± 13.8
Obesity[†] (%)	45–49	17.8	63.2	38.1
	50–54	23.9	52.6	54.5
	55–59	24.7	50.4	57.6

*Mean ± SD.
[†]Defined as ≥120% of ideal body weight.

mortality from infectious diseases and an increase in average life expectancy at birth. The rates of mortality from heart disease and stroke have apparently increased substantially, and major CVD is now the leading cause of death.[4]

Although the broad generic grouping of CVD is the leading cause of death in both China and the United States, there are important differences in the pattern of specific components of CVD between the two countries.[14] Mortality from CHD constitutes more than 50% of deaths caused by all types of CVD in the United States, but only 20% for urban China and 10% for rural China. Correspondingly, mortality from CHD accounts for about two thirds of all heart disease deaths among Americans, but it accounts for only 50% for urban Chinese and 25% for rural Chinese. CHD death rates per 100,000 people are much higher in the United States than in China. Stroke deaths outnumber coronary deaths in China, whereas the reverse prevails in the United States. Complex biomedical and socioeconomic factors are responsible for these differences.

CVD data on Chinese who have immigrated to the United States are lacking. However, important differences in CHD risk factors between urban and rural Chinese have been noted. People' s Republic of China–United States Cardiovascular and Cardiopulmonary Epidemiology Research Group data in four Chinese samples 35 to 54 years of age show that mean systolic and diastolic blood pressures, lipid (cholesterol, triglycerides) levels, and body mass index are considerably lower in rural subjects as compared with urban subjects.[15]

In addition, hypertension and hypercholesterolemia are less prevalent in rural Chinese. The prevalence of these risk factors was highest in cosmopolitan urban Beijing, followed by semi-urban and rural Beijing, urban Guangzhou, and rural Guangzhou (Table 20-4). The possibility exists that dietary and other lifestyle practices, which differ between northern and southern provinces, and between urban and rural communities, may play a role in these risk factor differences. In fact, a more recent analysis showed that Key's score for dietary fat was significantly related to levels of total cholesterol.[16]

Mean values, as well as the prevalence, of hyperlipidemia are lower in Chinese than in middle-aged populations in Western industrialized countries. The prevalence of hypertension is also lower. In China hypertension is more common in urban subjects within a region. This rural–urban differential suggests a role of dietary and socioeconomic variables in its genesis. In the United Kingdom, compared with their European counterparts, both Chinese men and women had lower total cholesterol and low-density lipoprotein cholesterol (LDL-C) levels, body mass index, and smoking prevalence, although Chinese women had higher blood pressure.[17] In the United States, however, Asian-born Chinese living in New York City's Chinatown had higher total cholesterol levels than both urban and rural Chinese living in Shanghai, China. Asian-born Chinese living in the United States also had cholesterol levels classified as borderline-high (35%) and high (23%) according to the National Cholesterol Education Program, similar to a comparable

TABLE 20-4   Urban–Rural Differences in Coronary Risk Factors in China (34- to 54-Year-Olds)

	Beijing		Guangzhou	
	Urban	Rural	Urban	Rural
Men				
Body mass index (kg/m²)	23.5 ± 3.0	22.3 ± 3.0	20.6 ± 2.4	19.8 ± 2.0
Systolic blood pressure (mm Hg)	123.1 ± 17.6	127.0 ± 20.0	113.3 ± 13.9	114.6 ± 14.3
Diastolic blood pressure (mm Hg)	82.3 ± 11.9	80.9 ± 11.9	75.4 ± 9.5	73.0 ± 9.5
Hypertension* (%)	47.1	39.0	14.2	10.0
Total cholesterol (mg/dL)	184.8 ± 37.8	171.3 ± 38.1	181.6 ± 31.8	158.7 ± 30.9
Triglycerides (mg/dL)	110.1 ± 73.5	116.3 ± 38.1	104.7 ± 85.9	80.9 ± 78.5
High cholesterol† (%)	29.2	21.8	26.3	9.1
Smoking (%)	71.4	77.7	72.7	76.7
Women				
Body mass index (kg/m²)	24.3 ± 3.7	22.7 ± 3.3	21.8 ± 3.0	19.6 ± 2.1
Systolic blood pressure (mm Hg)	123.1 ± 21.6	121.7 ± 19.2	115.7 ± 17.6	109.8 ± 13.7
Diastolic blood pressure (mm Hg)	79.0 ± 11.7	75.9 ± 11.3	75.6 ± 10.5	69.8 ± 8.8
Hypertension* (%)	41.0	27.3	18.2	5.5
Total cholesterol (mg/dL)	187.6 ± 42.4	168.1 ± 40.8	187.5 ± 33.2	154.9 ± 28.7
Triglycerides (mg/dL)	118.4 ± 83.1	108.9 ± 64.9	100.1 ± 89.4	75.7 ± 44.2
High cholesterol† (%)	33.0	18.9	32.1	6.4
Smoking (%)	23.2	30.9	3.2	7.5

*Defined as blood pressure ≥140/90 mm Hg.
†Defined as ≥200 mg/dL.

group of Caucasians screened (32% borderline-high and 36% high).[18]

Koreans

Several studies have documented the prevalence of key cardiovascular risk factors in Korean populations. Among the largest studies, data on more than 180,000 civil service and private school workers in South Korea aged 35 to 59 years who attended insurance examinations showed the prevalence of hypertension to be 29% in men and 16% in women, that of hypercholesterolemia 8.9% in men and 10.4% in women, that of cigarette smoking 57% in men and less than 1% in women, and that of elevated fasting blood sugar (≥126 mg/dL) 4.7% in men and 1.3% in women. Among men, 74% had one or more of the risk factors, compared with 29% of women.[19] In another study involving a population-based survey of more than 4000 Korean adults, a higher prevalence of hypertension was noted (42% in men, 25% in women), which increased by age group from 14% in those aged 18 to 24 to 71% in those aged 75 and older. Only 25% of those with hypertension were aware they had hyper-

tension; of these, 77% were being treated and 24% were under control.[20]

South Asians

The prevalence of CHD is increasing alarmingly in South Asian countries. CVD, especially CHD, is a major contributor to mortality and morbidity in India. Conservative estimates suggest that in 1990, CVD caused 2.39 million deaths and the nation incurred a loss of 28.59 million disability-adjusted life years.[21] Epidemiologic transition, with increasing life expectancy and demographic shifts of the population age profile, combined with lifestyle-related increases in the levels of CVD risk factors, is accelerating the CHD epidemic in India. The present scenario is similar to that of developed countries in the 1930s to 1950s.[10] A doubling of deaths due to CHD between 1985 and 2015 has been projected. In men, the projected death rates per 100,000 population were 145 in 1985, 253 in 2000, and 295 in 2015, and in women these rates were 126, 204, and 239, respectively. CVD, mainly CHD, is likely to account for at least 33.5% of total deaths by the year 2015, and will probably replace infectious diseases as the number one killer of Indians.[19]

CHD prevalence has increased significantly in India since the 1950s. The increase is significantly greater in urban areas than in rural and other parts of Asia.[22,23] CHD prevalence has quadrupled in urban Indian populations and doubled in rural areas in the last 50 years. This increase is associated with a steep increase in major coronary risk factors. The prevalence of hypertension, hypercholesterolemia, diabetes, and smoking has significantly increased in both urban and rural areas. Among civil servants in Kathmandu, Nepal, a CHD prevalence of 4.7% has been reported, with tobacco use noted to be the major risk factor. The prevalence of hypertension ranged from 5 to 6% in rural areas to 8 to 10% in urban areas in the Kathmandu area. As these figures were based on WHO criteria from 1978 defining hypertension as 160/95 mm Hg or greater, the prevalence would be substantially greater by today's standards.[24] In a comparison of urban versus rural areas, obesity was noted to be twice as common (24% vs 12%) and a sedentary lifestyle three times as common (35% vs 11%). South Asian Indians have also been noted to be more prone than Malays or Chinese to central obesity, with insulin resistance and glucose intolerance, as well as higher Lp(a) values, which may relate to their higher propensity to develop the metabolic syndrome.[25] Metabolic syndrome, which comprises multiple metabolic abnormalities, including abdominal obesity, high blood pressure, and high cholesterol, low HDL-C, and high triglyceride levels, is widely prevalent in Asian subjects as well as in emigrant Asians.[26]

A considerable excess of CHD among expatriate South Asian communities has been reported from several countries.[27] During the period 1979–1983, age-standardized CHD mortality was 40% higher in men and women of South Asian extraction than in the general population of England and Wales, irrespective of social class or religious group. The falling CHD mortality rates experienced by most of the Western world over the past two decades contrast sharply with rising CHD mortality in westernized South Asian communities. Among UK-based South Asians, CHD mortality increased by 6% in men and 13% in women in the decade 1970 to 1980. Excess mortality from CHD in South Asians is especially striking in young men.[28]

To determine the coronary risk factors that may be important in Indians, epidemiologic studies were performed

TABLE 20-5 Urban–Rural Difference in Coronary Risk Factor Prevalence in India (%)

	Urban	Rural	X² (P value)
Men	(n = 1415)	(n = 1982)	
Smoking and tobacco use (yes)	548 (38.7)	1006 (50.8)	47.65 (<.001)
Leisure-time activity (yes)	202 (14.3)	363 (18.3)	9.43 (.002)
Diabetes history (yes)	15 (1.1)	4 (0.2)	9.44 (.002)
Hypertension (≥140/90 mm Hg)	417 (29.5)	470 (23.7)	13.88 (<.001)
Hypertension (≥160/95 mm Hg)	146 (10.3)	150 (7.6)	7.51 (.006)
Obesity (BMI ≥27 kg/m²)	161 (11.4)	104 (5.2)	42.30 (<.001)
Truncal obesity (>0.95)	64/252 (25.4)	17/399 (4.3)	61.41 (<.001)
Cholesterol (≥200 mg/dL)	52/199 (26.1)	45/202 (22.3)	0.62 (.433)
HDL-C (<35 mg/dL)	47/199 (23.5)	49/202 (24.2)	0.01 (.97)
Women	(n = 797)	(n = 1166)	
Smoking and tobacco use (yes)	149 (18.7)	54 (4.6)	99.48 (<.001)
Leisure-time activity (yes)	64 (8.0)	88 (7.5)	0.09 (.76)
Diabetes history (yes)	8 (1.0)	2 (0.1)	4.93 (.026)
Hypertension (≥140/90 mm Hg)	267 (33.5)	197 (16.9)	71.40 (<.001)
Hypertension (≥160/95 mm Hg)	97 (12.2)	72 (6.2)	20.87 (<.001)
Obesity (BMI ≥27 kg/m²)	87 (10.9)	74 (6.4)	12.53 (<.001)
Truncal obesity (>0.95)	33/193 (17.1)	5/104 (4.8)	8.08 (.001)
Cholesterol (≥200 mg/dL)	—	22/98 (22.5)	—
HDL-C (<35 mg/dL)	—	40/98 (40.8)	—

in urban and rural populations in Rajasthan.[29] In cross-sectional surveys in randomly selected urban and rural areas of Rajasthan in western India, 3397 men (1415 urban, 1982 rural) and 1963 women (797 urban, 1166 rural) aged 20 years and older were studied. Blood samples were obtained from a random 10%. CHD prevalence diagnosed by history and electrocardiographic changes was greater in urban than in rural areas (men: 6.0% vs 3.4%, women: 10.5% vs 3.7%, $P < .01$). The prevalence of electrocardiographic changes alone was also greater in urban areas (men: 3.5% vs 2.8%, women: 8.4% vs 3.3%, $P < .05$). In urban areas, as compared with rural areas, the prevalence of hypertension (men: 30% vs 24%, women: 33% vs 17%), diabetes history (men: 1.1% vs 0.2%, women: 1.0% vs 0.2%), obesity (11% vs 6%), truncal obesity (men: 26% vs 4%, women: 17% vs 5%), absent moderate-grade leisure-time physical activity (men: 86% vs 82%), high mean total cholesterol (175.8 ± 43 mg/dL vs 165.2 ± 37 mg/dL), high LDL-C (107.6 ± 39 mg/dL vs 96.8 ± 33 mg/dL), and smoking in women (19% vs 5%) was significantly greater ($P < .5$). In rural men, smoking was more prevalent (51% vs 39%) (Table 20-5).

The Indian Council of Medical Research Task Force Project on coronary risk factor prevalence in urban and rural subjects in Delhi also reported a greater prevalence of coronary risk factors (smoking, obesity, truncal obesity, hypertension, diabetes, hypercholesterolemia) in urban subjects.[30] All such studies clearly emphasize that urbanization of traditional rural lifestyles in Asia is associated with increasing coronary risk (Fig. 20-2). Thus, the risk factors that occur more frequently in urban Japanese, Chinese, and South Asians and are associated with a greater prevalence of CHD need to be controlled to prevent CHD (Table 20-6).

TABLE 20-6 Coronary Risk Factors Occurring with Greater Frequency in Urban Asians

Sedentary life style
Obesity
Abdominal obesity
High total cholesterol and LDL-C
High triglyceride levels
Fasting insulin levels, insulin resistance
Metabolic syndrome
Hypertension
Diabetes mellitus

Pacific Islanders

Earlier data on Asian and Pacific Islanders from the National Center for Health Statistics had shown age-adjusted death rates (with heart disease and cancer the two leading causes of death for each Asian or Pacific Islander subgroup) to be greatest for Samoans and Hawaiians (who also had the lowest life expectancy), and the lowest for Asian Indians, Koreans, and Japanese.[31]

Among the few risk factor surveys in native Hawaiians living on Hawaiian Homestead on the island of Molokai, 42% of males were smokers and 14% of those aged 20 to 29 and 46% of those aged 50 to 59 had hypertension. The prevalence of diabetes increased to 23% in those aged 50 to 59 years. In this survey, 63% of women and 66% of men were at least 20% overweight, and 34% of women and 47% of men were severely overweight.[32] In another examination of 574 native Hawaiians aged 30

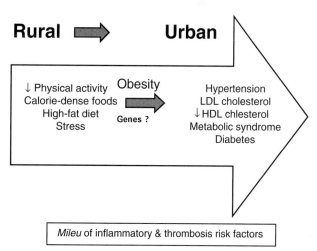

FIGURE 20-2 Urbanization is the proximate coronary risk factor among developing countries of Asia and Africa. As populations move from rural to urban life styles, there is change in dietary habits and physical activity resulting in population-wide increases in important coronary risk factors. These factors act conjointly with multiple thrombosis and inflammatory risk factors in precipitating various manifestations of atherosclerosis.

and older, 66% were overweight or obese and 70% had central adiposity, with significant correlations of fasting insulin with the number of CVD risk factors, indicating the significance of the insulin resistance syndrome in this population.[33,34] Of particular interest is a recent report showing the prevalence of hypertension to be directly related to the degree of Hawaiian ancestry; those who were less than 25%, 25 to 49%, 50 to 74%, 75 to 99%, and 100% Hawaiian, as evaluated by genealogical interview, had prevalences of hypertension of 23.4, 42.2, 46, 51.8, and 34.6%, after adjustment for age, gender, and body mass index.[35]

Dramatic increases in risk factors over recent years are also apparent in certain Pacific Islander populations. Among a study of Western Samoan men examined initially in 1982 and then after 10 years, there were dramatic increases in weight (10.5 kg), abdominal circumference (10.0 cm), and total cholesterol (49.5 mg/dL), with the increases in abdominal obesity strongly related to changes in total and non-HDL-C.[36]

Studies of Asians and Pacific Islanders living in the United States

A study of more than 1700 Asian-Americans living in California showed these individuals to be less knowledgeable about hypertension and less likely to be under treatment or in control than hypertensive persons of other races.[37] The study also noted Filipinos to have the highest prevalence of hypertension (60% of men and 65% of women aged 50 and older), as compared with other Asian groups. A large cross-sectional study of 13,081 Asians living in the United States revealed a higher body mass index and smoking prevalence among US-born men, more hypertension in Chinese US-born men, but no difference in cholesterol levels among those born, versus not born, in the United States.[38] This study also reported body mass index and smoking prevalence to be lowest in Chinese men and women, total cholesterol levels highest in Japanese men and women, and hypertension highest in Filipino men and women.

A study among Southeast Asian refugee children has noted systolic blood pressure among Hmong boys and diastolic blood pressure among Hmong boys and girls and Cambodian girls to be greater than those of African-Americans and whites of the same sexes.[39] Recent data also suggest high smoking rates among certain Asian-American immigrant populations, including Laotians (72%), Cambodians (71%), and native Hawaiians (42%).

Finally, among 205 Koreans aged 60 to 89 residing in Maryland, high blood pressure was the leading risk factor (71%), followed by high blood cholesterol (53%), overweight (43%), sedentary lifestyle (24%), diabetes (18%), and smoking (7%), with two thirds of the sample having multiple cardiovascular risk factors.

WHY IS CHD INCREASING IN ASIANS?

The epidemiologic evolution or transition comprises seven stages characterized by indices of acculturation, urbanization, affluence, saturated fat intake, salt intake, and smoking.[6,7,41] The prevalence of atherosclerotic diseases, CHD, and hypertension initially increases with a rise in these factors, then stabilizes, and finally decreases (see Fig. 20-1). In Asians, the social and economic indices of epidemiologic transition explain the increasing CHD prevalence.[42] The increase in urbanization among Asian countries is greater than in most of the developed countries of Europe, North America, and elsewhere. There is a strong correlation between urbanization and increase in CHD prevalence ($r = .76$) in urban communities. The study of urban–rural and geographic differences can provide useful information regarding pathogenesis of CHD in an ethnic group. The prevalence of CHD is low in rural populations of Asia and has not changed significantly over the years. The prevalence is significantly greater and on the increase in urban populations. The prevalence of major coronary risk factors—sedentary lifestyle, obesity, truncal obesity, hypertension, high total cholesterol and LDL-C, low HD-C, and diabetes—was greater in urban subjects in these studies. This finding has important public health implications as control of these risk factors could lead to control of CVD in Asia.

WHO has reported that the dietary changes that take place as populations in developing countries urbanize and move up the socioeconomic scale are: (1) increase in intake of legumes, vegetables, milk, and, in the case of nonvegetarians, food of animal origin; (2) substitution of coarse grain with polished grains, resulting in decreased fiber intake; (3) increase in intake of edible fat with increasing consumption of saturated hydrogenated fat in the middle class and Indian ghee in more prosperous individuals; (4) increase in intake of calories and sweets; and (5) increase in overall intake relative to expenditure of energy, resulting in obesity.[43] Thus, we hypothesize that the increasing prevalence of CHD in Indians and other Asians can be explained by lifestyle and dietary changes due to epidemiologic transition. The rapid shift from a rural subsistence economy to an urban market-oriented industrial economy is associated with novel health problems. Increases in urbanization, gross domestic product, and the human development index lead to a more affluent lifestyle and, as a consequence, increased dietary intake of calories and saturated fat, causing an increase in blood cholesterol levels. Increased use of transportation increases the prevalence of sedentary lifestyles, contributing to obesity, hypertension, detrimental blood lipid profile, and insulin resistance (see Fig. 20-2).

STRATEGIES FOR PREVENTION

The decline in mortality from CHD in Western countries is due mainly to a decrease in coronary risk factors. This has been achieved by aggressive public education programs regarding control of coronary risk factors. This approach is known as primary prevention or avoidance of the disease. Patients with established heart disease should also be encouraged to use similar measures, in addition to recommended pharmacologic therapies, to decrease the risk of a second heart attack. Primary prevention is based on control of atherosclerosis risk factors. Of major and modifiable coronary risk factors, smoking, sedentary lifestyle, generalized and truncal obesity, hypertension, hypercholesterolemia, and insulin resistance are already widespread in urban and emigrant Asians (Table 20-6).

Do we need more scientific studies before prevention efforts are initiated, or can we learn from the studies performed so far? Migrant studies within a country and transnational migration studies have clearly shown that CHD is a significant problem among Asians. Coronary risk factors such as hypertension, smoking, lack of physical activity, generalized and truncal obesity, and improper diet are fairly widespread.[44] These populations are not very different from Caucasians and other ethnic groups in whom CHD is endemic, although some of the risk factors may be different. Onset of CHD in younger persons is a cause for concern. Also, genetic factors that are modified by environment could be important.

Preventive medicine in Asia is as old as history. The ancient Indian science of *Ayurveda* deals with the influence of lifestyle modifications on health and sickness. Much before Hippocrates, Aristotle, and Galen,[43] a couplet from the *Bhagwad-Gita* emphasized the importance of balanced food, exercise, and other lifestyle variables in disease prevention: "One who observes control over his diet, takes regular exercise, has time to relax, does the right toil in discharge of his duties, observes proper hours of sleep and awakening and is balanced in his actions and reactions, emotions and reason, duties and rewards, conquers disease."[45] This is a summary of the current lifestyle changes recommended to prevent CHD.[46]

The efficacy of traditional medicines, including herbal product mixtures, based on the belief that several individual ingredients may have synergistic effects (eg, hypocholesterolemic, antioxidant, antiplatelet, or other antiatherosclerotic effects), also requires further investigation.[45] Herbal therapies are being investigated with respect to their hypotensive effect, and have been documented to be efficacious in controlling at least milder forms of hypertension.[47] Larger-scale clinical trials are needed to document the effectiveness of these therapies used alone or in combination with established Western pharmacologic therapy to control cardiovascular risk factors and prevent CVD.

POPULATION STRATEGY

We have identified many traditional coronary risk factors as important in Asians. Most of these can be changed through adoption of a healthier lifestyle, as prevention of heart disease necessitates that these changes be established as norms for the entire population. Studies suggest important lifestyle-related changes applicable especially to urban and emigrant populations:

- Control of hypertension can be achieved by reduction of salt, alcohol, and calorie intake, exercise, stress management, and greater intake of calcium, potassium, magnesium, and fiber.
- Control of hypercholesterolemia and decrease in mean LDL-C levels can be achieved by reduced intake of saturated fats, meat, and dairy products and greater intake of polyunsaturated fats and fiber.
- Low HDL-C levels can be influenced by greater intake of monounsaturated fats, fruits and green vegetables, and exercise.
- Generalized and truncal obesity can be reduced by regular exercise.
- Insulin resistance can also be improved by regular physical activity.
- Smoking control requires a variety of measures, including, but not limited to, governmental restrictions on smoking in the workplace and in public, bans on advertising and sponsorship by tobacco companies, enhanced community education programs, and physician-supervised counseling on smoking cessation.

Behavioral and environmental changes relevant to these risk factors include changes in eating patterns, drinking, smoking, physical activity, and other psychosocial factors.

Eating patterns

Production and consumption of the following should be preferred, emphasized, and supported: food of plant origin; cereal grains, vegetables, beans, fruits; fish, poultry, low-fat meat; low-fat milk and dairy products; and liquid polyunsaturated and monounsaturated vegetable oils and soft margarines. Production and consumption of the following should be decreased: high-fat meats and meat products and lard; high-fat dairy products such as whole milk, cheeses, cream, and butter; whole eggs; salt and salty products; sugar and sweet products; and commercially baked products with high fat and high calorie content.

The importance of maintaining cultural beliefs in eating and other lifestyle habits needs to be considered. A study of middle school Chinese children showed that those living in China, as compared with the United States, consumed less meat, dairy products, fat, sweets, and fast foods and more vegetables and fruits.[48] Additionally, Chinese elderly immigrants aged 60 to 96 displayed characteristics similar to those urban Chinese in China. Specifically, they were physically active, seldom obese, consumed a diet low in fat and high in carbohydrates, and had lower lipid levels as compared with elderly whites.[49] Marketing of low-fat food products should be targeted more aggressively to Asian media, and educational materials and dietary assessment tools need to be produced that are culturally sensitive to the diversity of Asian population groups.

Smoking

The smoking habit became epidemic with the growth of the cigarette manufacturing industry. It is thus a recent, widespread, and unnatural behavior, compared with older behaviors. In the whole population, smoking, especially of cigarettes, should be reduced in amount and in frequency with the final aim of eliminating the habit completely.

Smokeless tobacco consumption is another important problem in Asian groups. Both in Chinese and in South Asians, tobacco is consumed in many other forms, for example, *bidi* (tobacco rolled in leaves), Indian pipe (*chillum, hookah*), chewing tobacco in many forms. *Bidi* (tobacco rolled in the *Diospyrus melanoxylon* leaf) is the most common form of tobacco smoked in India. Studies have shown that *bidi* smokers face similar risks of hypertension and CHD as cigarette smokers, despite the fact that *bidi* is less than one fourth tobacco.[50] Smoking and smokeless tobacco consumption need to be curtailed in Asians. Social and economic taboos are needed. Finally, the problem of environmental tobacco exposure cannot be underestimated. One of the most convincing studies of the harmful effect of passive smoking was conducted in China among nonsmoking women with CHD and matched controls.[51] The investigators demonstrates the greater odds of development of CHD by women with husbands who smoked or were exposed to tobacco smoke in the workplace. The nearly twofold greater odds of CHD among women who were exposed to tobacco at work persisted after adjustment for other risk factors, and a linear trend with the amount of tobacco exposure was observed.

Physical activity

Coincident with the switch from hunger and deficient nutrition to gluttony (overeating) in the first two thirds of this century, the mean level of habitual physical activity has also decreased substantially. This has resulted in increased body mass index and obesity. The problem is greater among Asians who have recently undergone this metamorphosis both socially and physically due to the availability of automobiles, television, and computers.[30,52] Obesity contributes to CHD through its effects on blood pressure, cholesterol levels, diabetes mellitus, and insulin resistance. The urbanization of Asian countries has also substantially contributed to decreased levels of physical activity, particularly in the larger cities.

Regular physical activity favorably modifies the CVD risk factors of high blood pressure, blood lipid levels, insulin resistance, and obesity.[53] Several observational and interventional studies performed in developed countries of North America, Europe, and Asia have shown that exercise-training programs significantly reduce overall mortality as well as death caused by myocardial infarction. The highest reduction in mortality (~25%) has been reported to result from formal cardiac rehabilitation programs that also focus on control of other CVD risk factors. It has been shown that there is a quantitative relationship between level of activity and magnitude of cardiovascular benefit. The benefit extends across the full range of activity. A moderate level of physical activity confers optimum health benefits, but this activity must be performed frequently to maintain benefit. It has been recommended that all people increase their regular physical activity to the level appropriate to their capacities and needs. The long-term goal should be at least 30 minutes or longer of moderate-intensity physical activity on most or all days of the week. Intermittent or shorter bouts of physical activity (at least 10 minutes) including occupational, nonoccupational, and tasks of daily living also have similar cardiovascular benefits if performed at moderate intensity (eg, brisk walking, cycling, swimming, home repair, or garden work) with an accumulated duration of at least 30 minutes per day.

Traditionally, South and Southeast Asians have been rural agrarian workers and occupational physical activity levels have been high. Rapid socioeconomic transition in this region has resulted in a change in occupation from farming to formal industry-based jobs; therefore, occupational physical activity has declined. Data supporting these observations are sparse and studies performed in this part of the world have not used internationally acceptable criteria to define physical activity.

Regular physical activity should again become a normal part of everyday adult life, and, similar to the emphasis given in the media and other forms of advertising targeted to Caucasian populations, emphasis on physical activity and exercise needs to be integrated more successfully into the Asian culture. The natural inclination of children and young people to engage in vigorous physical activity should be encouraged, supported, and maintained through the formative years. Enjoyable forms of exercise should be available to everyone.

Psychosocial factors

The importance of psychologic and social factors in contributing to the risk of CHD is obvious.[54] These factors are especially more important in migrant populations, whether the migration is from villages to cities in Asia or from their Asian homelands to developed Western countries. This stress can be gauged indirectly by poor living conditions, low level of education, increasing adult and juvenile crime, smoking and alcohol habits, and breakdown of the family unit among these groups. Not only is the behavior of the individual important, but that of the community as a whole is to be understood in this context. The need for equalizing access to health and social services is important in this regard.

A reassessment of the social value system should be promoted. Social norms that place more value on health, human relations, culture, and preservation of nature should be nurtured. Such changes may result in less tension, aggressive drive, competitiveness, and frustration in individual personality patterns that are believed to enhance CHD risk.

In summary, CHD among Asians can be prevented by controlling intake of tobacco, salt, saturated fats, alcohol, and calories; by increasing both work-related and leisure-time physical activity; by increasing consumption of heart-healthy foods such as fruits and vegetables, high-fiber cereals, oils containing balanced amounts of polyunsaturated and monounsaturated fats (eg, canola oil, soy bean oil), and spices and cereals with high flavonoid content. Stress management techniques, especially yoga, may be important. Reverting to traditional Asian social lifestyles (joint families, small families, good education) is also important.

PUBLIC EDUCATION STRATEGIES

To prevent CVD, it is important to avoid the occurrence of the major risk factors themselves. This is known as primordial prevention. It is not an unrealistic task, but success requires greater efforts at ensuring that the public realizes the magnitude of the problem. Primordial prevention calls for changing the socioeconomic status of the society. Higher social, economic, and cultural status correlates inversely with smoking, abnormal food patterns, and lack of exercise, and is recommended for primordial prevention.[55] To accomplish these goals, WHO recommends the following changes in attitudes, behaviors, and social values.

1. Encouragement of positive health behavior, prevention of adopting risk behavior, elimination of estab-

lished risk behavior, and promotion of the concept of health as a social value.

2. Inclusion of established principles and practices of health and general education in a public health program. Healthy behavior should be made socially acceptable and should be encouraged.

3. Encouragement of cardiovascular health-promotive education in schools; special target groups are children, adolescents, family unit, the underprivileged, and high-risk groups.

4. Close collaboration between health personnel and media representatives so that mass media play a major role in a health education program.

Primordial prevention begins in childhood when health risk behavior begins. Parents, teachers, and peer groups are important in imparting health education to children. Public broadcasting systems, television, and newspapers play an important role in dissemination of health-related information among populations.[56] Suitable strategies to impart information to these print and electronic media should be developed locally.

HIGH-RISK APPROACH

Specific high-risk subjects are those with a family history of CHD, hypertension, or diabetes and those with a sedentary lifestyle, generalized obesity, truncal obesity, metabolic syndrome, and other coronary risk factors.[57] Dyslipidemia is as important in Asians as in other populations.

The effectiveness of the high-risk approach depends directly on practicing physicians and other health care workers. To integrate prevention and treatment at the primary health care level, greater emphasis on prevention must be part of the daily practice of medicine. This requires that physicians take an active interest, that patients be willing to accept and act on preventive advice, and that governments and health insurance programs realize that the cost of preventive services, like that of curative care, should be fully reimbursed. Physicians and other health care providers serving Asian/Pacific Islander populations need to be educated as to specific cultural barriers and the opportunities that would encourage implementation of CVD prevention practices.

Guidelines are needed that specify the measurements and observations to be recorded, the criteria to be used in identifying individuals requiring further evaluation, and management procedures, including both appropriate interventions and goals by which their effectiveness can be monitored. Screening should ordinarily include measurement of height and weight, aerobic fitness, systolic and diastolic blood pressure, total cholesterol, HDL-C, and blood glucose levels. Subjects should be questioned regarding tobacco use and diet. The American

Heart Association recently published updated guidelines for the primary prevention of CHD.[58] These are based on compelling scientific evidence and demonstrate that interventions extend overall survival, improve quality of life, and reduce the incidence of myocardial infarction. The interventions are smoking cessation, lipid management, increased physical activity, weight management, and blood pressure control. There is unequivocal evidence that blood pressure control and lipid management decrease relative and absolute CVD as well as CHD risk.

The American Heart Association also published revised guidelines for secondary prevention of CHD. These are based on compelling scientific evidence in patients with CHD that demonstrates that risk factor interventions extend overall survival, improve quality of life, decrease the need for interventional procedures such as angioplasty and bypass grafting, and reduce the incidence of subsequent myocardial infarction. The interventions include smoking cessation, physical activity guidelines, weight management, blood pressure control, and lipid management.[59] In addition, nutritional guidelines need to be formulated. WHO has formulated certain population nutrition goals that are useful in prevention of CHD.[43] Other chapters discuss guidelines for risk factor modification in depth.

Hypertension control

There is clear scientific evidence that proper control of hypertension reduces CVD risk by 20% and CHD risk by 15%. Hypertension has emerged as a major public health problem among Asians. At a conservative estimate, there are more than 1 billion hypertensives (blood pressure greater than recommended by WHO: systolic blood pressure ≥ 140 and/or diastolic blood pressure ≥ 90 mm Hg) worldwide, more than a quarter of whom are in Asia.[3] Recent lessons learned from studies in Western populations have motivated the Joint National Committee on Prevention, Detection, Evaluation, and Treatment of High Blood Pressure (JNC-7) to define a systolic blood pressure of 120 to 139 mm Hg or diastolic blood pressure of 80 to 89 mm Hg as "prehypertension," indicating the appropriateness of lifestyle management to prevent the further progression of blood pressure to clinical hypertension.[60] The same criteria may apply to Asian populations, particularly those with diabetes and/or metabolic syndrome. Whether all these individuals require therapy is questionable, as about 60 to 70% of those with hypertension suffer from mild hypertension that can be managed by lifestyle changes alone. These changes are increased physical activity, weight control, smoking cessation, reduction of dietary sodium and alcohol intake, and increase in potassium and calcium in diet. Blood pressure not controlled by lifestyle changes

and other nonpharmacologic interventions requires drug treatment.

A large number of antihypertensive drugs are available and are classified into eight major classes: (1) diuretics (thiazides, loop diuretics, potassium-sparing diuretics, aldosterone antagonists), (2) beta blockers, (3) beta blockers with intrinsic sympathomimetic activity, (4) combined alpha and beta blockers, (5) angiotensin-converting enzyme (ACE) inhibitors, (6) angiotensin II antagonists, (7) dihydropyridine calcium channel blockers (CCBs), and (8) nondihydropyridine CCBs. There are some data to suggest that medication changes, dose reductions, and side effects are more common in Asian patients. Similar efficacy, but greater side effects have also been reported among Chinese persons taking certain CCBs or ACE inhhibitors. Drug combinations are recommended when a drug from any of the aforementioned major pharmacologic classes is ineffective in lowering blood pressure. Combination therapy generally minimizes side effects by encouraging use of drugs in low doses, although tolerability data in Asians on combination therapy are limited. In non-Asian populations, an additive effect has been shown when combining: (a) a diuretic with a beta blocker, ACE inhibitor, or alpha blocker; (b) a beta blocker with an alpha blocker or dihydropyridine CCB; and (c) an ACE inhibitor with a dihydropyridine CCB. Not infrequently, more than two drugs may be required to maintain benefit.

Lipid management

Atherogenic dyslipidemia is common among Asians, especially South Asians. This condition is characterized by borderline-high LDL-C (130–160 mg/dL), low HDL-C (<35 mg/dL), high triglycerides (≥150 mg/dL), and increased small, dense LDL particles, and is included in the definition of the metabolic syndrome.[63]

Dietary therapy is important in modifying the lipid profile and reducing coronary risk, but is associated with poor compliance, especially in Asian population groups. High-risk, group-specific measures are therefore important. Reduction of total fat and saturated fat intake is recommended. Total fats should constitute less than 30% of caloric intake, and saturated fats, less than 7%. Consumption of *trans* fatty acid-containing hydrogenated oils and hard margarines should be discouraged and, whenever possible, abandoned. Dietary intake of monounsaturated fats (10–15% of calories) and polyunsaturated fats (7–10% of calories) should be encouraged. Mustard–rapeseed oil and soybean oil are especially rich sources of monounsaturated fats in Asian diets. Also relevant to Indians is increased intake of omega-3 fat-containing oils (mustard–rapeseed oil, fish). Invisible fats that are present in vegetables and cereals are recommended, whereas the intake of animal fats in meat, egg, and poultry is not. Dietary therapy reduces LDL-C by 8 to 15%.[64] In addition, diet therapy also helps to reduce weight, increase vitamin intake, and decrease blood pressure and insulin resistance. Diets severely restricted in total fats (<15%) can increase triglyceride concentrations and reduce HDL-C levels and are not recommended.

Drug therapy in the past included bile acid-binding resins, fibrates, and nicotinic acid. Statins have replaced all these to a large extent. Seven large prospective randomized clinical studies have unequivocally demonstrated that lipid-lowering therapy with statins can both alter the natural history of CHD and drastically reduce clinical events in the range of 30 to 40%.[6] Although none of these trials included sufficient numbers of Asians to demonstrate if treatment benefits are different in these groups, current guidelines do not recommend different approaches to treatment for Asians and non-Asians.[65]

No long-term primary or secondary prevention trials on statins have been conducted in Asian subjects. Such trials need to be undertaken to evaluate whether the benefits observed in Caucasians can be demonstrated in Asian populations as well. Use of colestipol is restricted by abdominal side effects. Nicotinic acid, though useful in increasing HDL-C, is associated with flushing and other side effects. Fibrates are especially relevant in subjects who have raised triglyceride concentrations. A head-on comparison of statins, fibrates, and nicotinic acid should be performed to decide the best choice, as the ability of a drug to increase HDL-C is important in Asian populations. However, until such data become available, statins should be the major drugs used to decrease LDL-C levels in Asians.

Obesity treatment

Obesity, especially truncal obesity, is widespread in urban and migrant Asians.[30] Truncal obesity is associated with insulin resistance, impaired glucose tolerance, and a constellation of metabolic abnormalities that are associated with increased CHD risk. Control of truncal obesity requires regular exercise and diet control. Generalized obesity has emerged as a major problem in Asians. Studies show that 20 to 50% of urban and 5 to 10% of rural Asians have a body mass index of 25 kg/m² or greater. Dietary therapy is the cornerstone of weight reduction. Since the withdrawal of fenfluramines due to reports of severe cardiovascular toxicity, several drugs have become available. These are pancreatic lipase inhibitors (orlistat), central catecholamine pathway stimulants (phentermine), and central serotonin–noradrenaline reuptake

inhibitors (sibutramine). Use of these drugs is recommended only for severe obesity (body mass index >35–40 kg/m²). Use of herbal medications, such as the Ma Huang (Ephedra) and other agents for weight loss, is widespread in Asian populations. These medications have been reported to be toxic and their sale recently banned in the United States.[45]

Other issues

Insulin resistance and diabetes are major concerns among Asians, especially South Asians.[66] Control of diabetes and achievement of normoglycemia are essential for primary prevention of cardiovascular events. In diabetics, aggressive control, using lifestyle measures and pharmacotherapy, of all CVD risk factors is recommended to reduce CHD risk. These measures include blood pressure control to less than 130/85 mm Hg and LDL-C reduction to less than 100 mg/dL. There are no large trials on the relative efficacy and tolerability of hypoglycemic agents in Asians versus non-Asians.

Use of aspirin is associated with a 30 to 40% reduction in CHD events in primary prevention trials and is recommended in high-risk individuals or those with other CHD risk factors such as diabetes and hypercholesterolemia. Antioxidant vitamin supplementation for primary prevention is still controversial. Prospective epidemiologic studies have supported the concept that natural antioxidants, as present in fresh fruits and vegetables, may be more effective compared with supplemental vitamin therapy. Hence, at present, routine use of antioxidant supplements is not recommended. Yoga and other relaxation therapies are in the realm of investigation, and their role needs to be further evaluated in long-term controlled trials. Studies of genetic factors that initiate atherosclerosis and modify therapeutic responses to interventions in Asians are needed.

CONCLUSIONS

The need to contain the epidemic of CVD, as well as combat its impact and minimize its toll in Asians and Pacific Islanders, is obvious and urgent. National strategies to meet this objective must be developed and effectively implemented. Regional and global initiatives by international agencies concerned with health care are required. A large number of social issues that are determinants of health behavior in Asians must be considered before embarking on such a policy (Table 20-7).

Traditional lifestyles that are associated with a lower CHD prevalence in India and many Asian countries (joint family system, good education, religious habits, prayers, small families, social support) should be encouraged. Traditional dietary habits of vegetarianism, fish

TABLE 20-7 Determinants of Health Behavior Among Asians

Educational status, illiteracy
Family structure, breakdown of traditional family system
Peer influence, improper guidance
Caste system and social hierarchy
Lack of media awareness
Lack of motivation to change

consumption, use of plant-based oils for cooking, high-fiber predominantly complex carbohydrate-based diets, antioxidant-containing fruits and vegetables, and physical exercise should be maintained.

Asians are a minority group in most of the developed countries. The high incidence of CHD in emigrants as compared with native populations underlines the importance of population prevention strategies. These strategies should be directed toward prevention of acquisition or augmentation of coronary risk factors in these communities (primordial prevention) and combined with programs to reverse and reduce the increasing prevalence of risk factors observed in urban and migrant communities (primary prevention).

As always, however, the need for prevention should come from within the population. Increasing levels of affluence and acculturation lead to greater recognition that measures for prevention of chronic diseases are useful and cost-effective. In Asians also, greater literacy levels and awareness have led to a decrease in cardiovascular risk factors in the well-educated. Ultimately, it is expected that with proper control of the behavioral and lifestyle risk factors for CHD, Asians can advance to higher phases of the epidemiologic transition, where, through maintenance of a modern lifestyle, return to ancestral low rates of CVD is possible. The roles of literacy and better health education in promoting favorable lifestyles are important, and urgent population and individual measures are needed to control the CHD epidemic among Asians and Pacific Islanders living in Asia and elsewhere.

REFERENCES

1. Murray CJL, Lopez AD. Mortality by cause for eight regions of the world: Global Burden of Disease Study. *Lancet* 1997;349:1269–1276

2. Reddy KS, Yusuf S. Emerging epidemic of cardiovascular disease in developing countries. *Circulation* 1998;97:596–601

3. Rodgers A, Lawes C, MacMahon S. Reducing the global burden of blood pressure related cardiovascular disease. *J Hypertens* 2000;18(suppl 1):S3–S6.

4. Ezzati M, Lopez AD, Rodgers A, et al, and the Comparative Risk Assessment Collaborating Group. Selected major risk factors and global and regional burden of disease. *Lancet* 2002;360:1347–1360.

5. Omran AR. The epidemiological transition: a theory of the epidemiology of population change. *Milbank Mem Fund Q* 1971;49:509–538.

6. Gupta R. Epidemiological transition and increase in coronary heart disease in India. *South Asian J Prev Cardiol* 1997;1:14–22.

7. Yusuf S, Reddy KS, Ounpuu S, Anand S. Global burden of cardiovascular diseases: Part I: General considerations, the epidemiological transition, risk factors and impact of urbanisation. *Circulation* 2001;104:2746–2753.

8. Toshima H, Koga Y, Blackburn H, Keys A. *Lessons for Science from the Seven Countries Study.* Tokyo: Springer-Verlag; 1994.

9. Bhopal R, Unwin R, White M, et al. Heterogeneity of coronary heart disease risk factors in Indian, Pakistani, Bangladeshi, and European origin populations: cross sectional study. *BMJ* 1999;319:215–220.

10. Marmot MG. Coronary heart disease: rise and fall of a modern epidemic. In: Marmot MG, Elliot P, eds. *Coronary Heart Disease Epidemiology: From Aaetiology to Public Health.* Oxford: Oxford University Press; 1992:3–19.

11. Nichaman MZ, Hamilton HB, Kagan A, et al. Epidemiologic studies of coronary heart disease and stroke in Japanese men living in Japan, Hawaii and California: distribution of biochemical risk factors. *Am J Epidemiol* 1975;102:491–501

12. Iribarren C, Reed DM, Burchfiel CM, Dwyer JH. Serum total cholesterol and mortality: confounding factors and risk modification in Japanese-American Men. *JAMA* 1995;273:1926–32.

13. Tao S, Huang Z, Wu W, et al. Coronary heart disease and its risk factors in the People's Republic of China. *Int J Epidemiol* 1989;18(suppl 1):S159–S163.

14. US Department of Health and Human Services, Public Health Service, Centers for Disease Control and Prevention, National Center for Health Statistics. *Population Estimates by Age and Sex: 1990–1994.* Current Population Reports, Series P-27, No. 1127. US Department of Commerce, Bureau of the Census.

15. People's Republic of China–United States Cardiovascular and Cardiopulmonary Epidemiology Research Group. An epidemiological study of cardiovascular and cardiopulmonary disease risk factors in four populations in the People's Republic of China: baseline report from the PRC–USA Collaborative Study. *Circulation* 1992;85:1083–1096.

16. Zhou B, Rao X, Dennis BH, et al. The relationship between dietary factors and serum lipids in Chinese urban and rural populations of Beijing and Guangzhou: PRC–USA Cardiovascular and Cardiopulmonary Research Group. *Int J Epidemiol* 1995;24:528–534.

17. Harland JO, Unwin N, Bhopal RS, White M, Watson B, Laker M, Alberti KG. Low levels of cardiovascular risk factors and coronary heart disease in a UK Chinese population. *J Epidemiol Community Health* 1997;51:636–642.

18. Pinnelas D, et al. Total serum cholesterol levels in Asians living in New York City: results of a self-referred cholesterol screening. *NY State J Med* 1992;92:245–249.

19. Jee SH, Appel LH, Suh I, et al. Prevalence of cardiovascular risk factors in South Korean adults: results from the Korea Medical Insurance Corporation (KMIC) Study. *Ann Epidemiol* 1998;8:14–21.

20. Jo I, Ahn Y, Lee J, et al. Prevalence, awareness, treatment, control and risk factors for hypertension in Korea: the Ansan study. *J Hypertens* 2001;19:1523–32.

21. Reddy KS. Cardiovascular diseases in India. *WHO Stat Q* 1993;46:101–107

22. Gupta R, Gupta VP. Meta-analysis of coronary heart disease prevalence in India. *Indian Heart J* 1996;48:241–245.

23. Gupta R, Rastogi S, Panwar RB, Soangra MR, Gupta VP, Gupta KD. Major coronary risk factors and coronary heart disease epidemic in India. *South Asian J Prev Cardiol* 2003;7:11–40.

24. Pandey MR. Hypertension in Nepal. *Bibl Cardiol* 1997;42:68–76

25. Hughes K, Aw TC, Kuperan P, Choo M. Central obesity, insulin resistance, syndrome X, lipoprotein(a), and cardiovascular risk in Indians, Malays, and Chinese in Singapore. *J Epidemiol Community Health* 1997;51:394–399.

26. Fagan TC, Deedwania PC. The cardiovascular dysmetabolic syndrome. *Am J Med* 1998;105:77S–82S.

27. McKeigue PM, Miller GJ, Marmot MG. Coronary heart disease in South Asians overseas: a review. *J Clin Epidemiol* 1989;42:597–609.

28. Bhopal R. What is the risk of coronary heart disease in South Asians? A review of UK research. *J Public Health Med* 2000;22:375–385.

29. Gupta R, Gupta VP. Urban–rural differences in coronary risk factors do not fully explain greater urban coronary heart disease prevalence. *J Assoc Phys India* 1997;45:683–686.

30. Reddy KS, Prabhakaran D, Shah P, Shah B. Differences in body mass index and waist:hip ratios in North Indian rural and urban populations. *Obes Rev* 2002;3:197–202.

31. Koyert DL, Kung HC. Asian or Pacific Islander mortality, selected states 1992. *Mon Vital Stat Rep* 1997;46(1 suppl):1–63.

32. Curb JD, Aluli NE, Kautz JA et al. Cardiovascular risk factor levels in ethnic Hawaiians. *Am J Public Health* 1991;81:164–167.

33. Aluli NE. Prevalence of obesity in a Native Hawaiian population. *Am J Clin Nutr* 1991;53(6 suppl):1556S–1560S.

34. Mau MK, Grandinetti A, Arakaki RF, et al. The insulin resistance syndrome in native Hawaiians: Native Hawaiian Health Research (NHHR) Project. *Diabetes Care* 1997;20:1376–1380.

35. Grandinetti A, Chen R, Kaholokula JK, et al. *Ethn Dis* 2002;12:221–228.

36. Galanis DJ, Sobal J, McGarvey ST, Pelletier DL, Bausserman L. Ten-year changes in the obesity, abdominal adiposity, and serum lipoprotein cholesterol measures of Western Samoan men. *J Clin Epidemiol* 1995;48:1485–1493.

37. Stavig FR. Hypertension and related health issues among Asians and Pacific Islanders in California. *Public Health Rep* 1988;103:28–37.

38. Klatsky AL, Tekawa IS, Armstrong MA. Cardiovascular risk factors among Asian Americans. *Public Health Rep* 1996;111(suppl 2):62–64.

39. Munger RG. Elevated blood pressure among Southeast Asian refugee children in Minnesota. *Am J Epidemiol* 1991;133:1257–1265.

40. Kim MT, Juon HS, Hill MN, et al. Cardiovascular disease risk factors in Korean American elderly. *West J Nurs Res* 2001;23:269–82.

41. Gillum RF. The epidemiology of cardiovascular disease in Black Americans. *N Engl J Med* 1996;335:1597–1599.

42. Gupta R, Singhal S. Coronary heart disease in India. Letter. *Circulation* 1997;96:3785.

43. WHO Study Group. *Diet, Nutrition, and the Prevention of Chronic Diseases.* Technical Report Series 797. Geneva: World Health Organization; 1990:49–50.

44. Williams B. Westernized Asians and cardiovascular disease: nature or nurture? *Lancet* 1995;345:401–402.

45. Gupta A, Gupta R. Ayurveda, cholesterol and coronary heart disease. *South Asian J Prev Cardiol* 2002;6:86–122.

46. Assman G, Carmena R, Cullen P, et al, for the International Task Force for the Prevention of Coronary Heart Disease. Coronary heart disease: reducing the risk. A worldwide view. *Circulation* 1999;100:1930–1938.

47. Wong ND, Ming S, Zhou HY, Black HR. A comparison of Chinese and Western medical approaches for the treatment of mild hypertension. *Yale J Biol Med* 1991;64:79–87.

48. Sun WY, Chen WW. A preliminary study of potential dietary risk factor for coronary heart disease among Chinese-American adolescents. *J Sch Health* 1994;64:368–371.

49. Choi ES et al. The prevalence of cardiovascular risk factors among elderly Chinese Americans. *Arch Intern Med* 1990;150:413–418.

50. Gajalakshmi V, Peto R, Kanaka TS, Jha P. Smoking and mortality from tuberculosis and other diseases in India: retrospective study of 43000 adult male deaths and 35000 controls. *Lancet* 2003;362:507–515.

51. He Y, Lam TH, Li LS, et al. Passive smoking at work as a risk factor for coronary heart disease in Chinese women who have never smoked. *BMJ* 1994;308:380–384.

52. Zhou B, Wu Y, Yang J, et al. Overweight is an independent risk factor for cardiovascular disease in Chinese populations. *Obes Rev* 2002;3:147–156.

53. Thompson PD, Buchner D, Pina IL, et al. Exercise and physical activity in the prevention and treatment of atherosclerotic cardiovascular disease. *Circulation* 2003;107:3109–3116.

54. Rozanski A, Blumenthal JA, Kaplan J. Impact of psychosocial factors on the pathogenesis of cardiovascular disease and implications for therapy. *Circulation* 1999;99:2192–2217.

55. WHO Study Group. *Primary Prevention of Coronary Heart Disease.* EURO Reports and Studies 98. Geneva: World Health Organisation; 1985.

56. Thompson B, Pertschuk M. Community intervention and advocacy. In: Ockene IS, Ockene JK, eds. *Prevention of Coronary Heart Disease.* Boston: Little, Brown; 1992:493–515.

57. National Cholesterol Education Program. Third report of the National Cholesterol Education Program Expert Panel on detection, evaluation, and treatment of high blood cholesterol in adults. *Circulation* 2002;106:3143–3421.

58. Pearson TA, Blair SN, Daniels SR, et al. AHA guidelines for primary prevention of cardiovascular disease and stroke: 2002 update. *Circulation* 2002;106:388–391.

59. Smith SC, Blair SN, Bonow RO, et al. AHA/ACC scientific statement. AHA/ACC guidelines for preventing heart attack and death in patients with atherosclerotic heart disease: 2001 update. *Circulation* 2001;104:1577–1579.

60. Chobanian AV, Bakris GL, Black HR, et al. The seventh report of the Joint National Committee on Prevention, Detection, Evaluation, and Treatment of High Blood Pressure. *JAMA* 2003;289:2560–2572.

61. Hui KK, Pasic J. Outcome of hypertension management in Asian Americans. *Arch Intern Med* 1997;157:1345–1348.

62. Wong ND. Hypertension in East Asians and Native Hawaiians. In: Izzo JL, Black HR, eds. *Hypertension Primer.* 3rd ed. Dallas, Tex: American Heart Association; 2003.

63. Gupta R, Deedwania PC, Gupta A, et al. Prevalence of metabolic syndrome in an urban Indian population. *Int J Cardiol*, in press.

64. Knoop RH. Drug treatment of lipid disorders. *N Engl J Med* 1999;341:498–511.

65. National Cholesterol Education Program Expert Panel on Detection, Evaluation and Treatment of High Blood Cholesterol in Adults (Adult Treatment Panel III). *Circulation* 2002;106:3143–3421.

66. Misra A, Vikram NK. Insulin resistance syndrome (metabolic syndrome) and Asian Indians. *Curr Sci* 2002;83:1483–1496.

Native Americans

David R. Baines
Thomas K. Welty
Tony Kendrick

21

KEY POINTS

- American Indians and Alaska Natives constitute a small but very diverse population. Cardiovascular disease, once uncommon in this population, is now the leading cause of death in American Indians and Alaska Natives. This has occurred with Westernization of the diet and adoption of more sedentary lifestyles by this population. Although CVD has decreased for all US races, it is increasing in American Indian and Alaskan Native populations.

- The Strong Heart Study, funded by the National Heart, Lung, and Blood Institute at the National Institutes of Health, has shown that overweight and obesity, type 2 diabetes mellitus, cigarette smoking, and binge drinking are more common among American Indians and Alaska Natives.

- Obesity and diabetes continue to increase in prevalence dramatically in American Indians and Alaska Natives. Hypertension is an independent risk factor for cardiovascular disease and its prevalence also is increasing.

- Enhanced screening, identification of high-risk patients, and targeted risk factor reduction programs are needed for Native American communities. As cardiovascular risk factors vary greatly, primary and secondary preventive interventions must be tailored to each community. Some community-based intervention programs have been successful. Involving tribal leadership, traditional healers, and elders and understanding the culture are critical to the success of these programs.

- The federal government is the primary provider of health services for American Indians and Alaska Natives, as a result of tribal population relocation policies to remote and rural areas of the United States and as established through treaties. Funding for health services has historically been inadequate. Investing in health programs that serve Native American communities is essential for raising the health status of American Indians and Alaska Native Americans to the levels enjoyed by other American citizens.

INTRODUCTION

The term *Native American* refers to American Indians and Alaska Native Americans (AI/AN). Native American Hawaiians, although technically Native Americans, are considered under the Asian/Pacific Islander group (discussed in Chapter 20), as they do not have the special trust relationship that AI/AN tribes have with the federal government (Article 1, Section 8, of the US Constitution). However, Native American Hawaiians have many similar health issues.

Although Native American Americans are the first Americans, they are the smallest and most diverse minority group. There are more than 560 federally recognized tribes (or sovereign nations), most located west of the Mississippi River (Fig. 21-1). Each has its own language, traditions, heritage, and culture.[1] The approximately

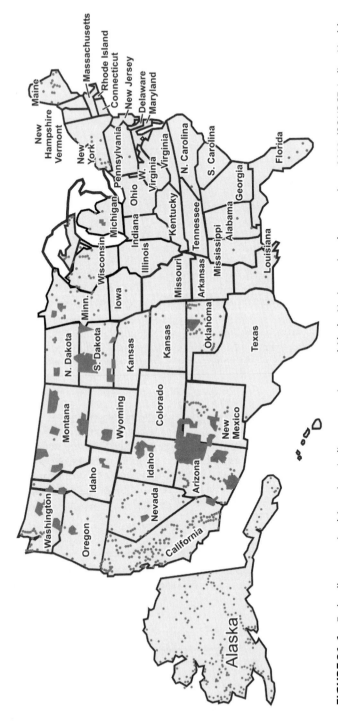
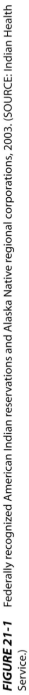

FIGURE 21-1 Federally recognized American Indian reservations and Alaska Native regional corporations, 2003. (SOURCE: Indian Health Service.)

TABLE 21-1   American Indian and Alaska Native Socioeconomic Profile Compared with All US Races, 2002

	American Indian	All US Races
High school graduate	71%	90%
College graduate	11%	15.5%
Average age	28.7	35.3
Life expectancy at birth	70.6	76.5
Years of potential life lost	88.6*	48.4 *
Health per capita expenditure	$1384 †	$5427
Without health insurance	27.1%	14.5%
Annual family income	$32,116	$42,228
Poverty	24.5%	11.7%
Unemployment rate	(AI/AN unemployment statistics are not tracked by the Department of Labor)	5.8%
Home ownership	55%	67.5%
Homes without safe water	11.7%	2.1%
Homes with phones	70%	95%
Persons per household	3.09	2.59
Family size	3.58	3.14

*Rate of years of potential life lost per 1000 persons between birth and 65 years at the time of death.
†Expenditures by the Indian Health Service.
SOURCES: (1) US Census Bureau, *Current Population Survey 2000, 2001, and 2002 Annual Demographic Supplements.* (2) Indian Health Service, *Regional Differences in Indian Health, 2000–2001.*

250 tribes in Alaska are part of three distinct racial aboriginal groups: American Indians (Tsimshian, Tlingit, Haida, and Athabascan tribes), Eskimos, and Aleuts.

In the 2000 census,[2] 2.5 million people reported being solely AI/AN and another 1.6 million people reported being AI/AN in combination with one or more other races. AI/AN reside in every state, with 43% in the West, 17% in the Midwest, 31% in the South, and 9% in the Northeast.[3] Of the 2.5 million who identified solely as AI/AN, 57% lived in urban areas, and of the 4.1 million who reported being AI/AN alone or in combination with one or more other races, 65.5% lived in urban areas.[4]

A demographic overview of AI/AN is provided in Table 21-1. Family income is well below the national average ($32,116 compared with $42,228 for non-Hispanic whites), and 24.5% live in poverty compared with 11.7% for all US races.[5] Unemployment is greater than twice the national average and can exceed 70% in some AI/AN communities. AI/AN have the lowest educational attainment of all minority groups. Only 71% of Native Americans graduate from high school (vs 90% of US All Races), and only 11% have a college degree (vs 15.5% for US All Races). The average Native American family has 3.58 members, which exceeds the national average of 3.14.

The Native American population is relatively young. The median age is 6.6 years younger than the national average (28.7 vs 35.3).[6] This is influenced by a birth rate 1.7 times greater than for all US races and the fact that 30% of deaths occur before age 45, compared with 10% for all US races.[7]

Life expectancy for AI/AN is 5.9 years less than that for all US races: 5.2 years for women and 6.2 years for men.[8] One third of AI/AN are younger than 18 years, compared with 26% for all US races, and 7% of AI/AN are older than 64, compared with 12% for all US races.[2] Most striking is the disparity between the years of potential life lost (YPLL), a measure of premature mortality based on a longevity age of 65 and the age of death before reaching the age of 65. The AI/AN YPLL rate is 88.6/1000 persons between birth and age 65 at the time of death, compared with 48.4/1000 for all US races.[8]

HEALTH STATUS, HEART DISEASE, AND STROKE

Health status

Significant strides have been made in improving the health status of AI/AN over the last 50 years. Nonetheless,

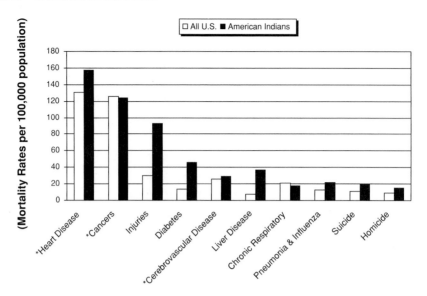

FIGURE 21-2   Mortality rates per 100,000 for the top 10 leading causes of American Indian and Alaska Native Deaths compared with US All races, both sexes, all ages, adjusted to compensate for miscoding of Indian race on death certificates. (SOURCES: *US Department of Health and Human Services, Indian Health Service, Regional Differences in Indian Health, 2000–2001. US Department of Health and Human Services, Indian Health Service, Trends in Indian Health 1998–1999.)

significant disparities continue to exist between AI/AN and other population groups.[8] Statistics for general mortality from all causes for all ages indicate that the AI/AN mortality rate per 100,000 population is 49% higher than that for the rest of the population. The top two leading causes of death were the same for AI/AN as for the rest of the population: diseases of the heart and malignant neoplasms. However, the mortality rate for diseases of the heart in AI/AN was 20% higher than in the general population and the cerebrovascular disease rate was 14% higher (Fig. 21-2). Although the mortality rate for malignant neoplasms in AI/AN was 1% less than that of the general population, it is the second leading cause of AI/AN mortality. Other disparities in mortality rates include alcoholism (638% higher), tuberculosis (400% higher), and diabetes (291% higher).

A study associated with *Healthy People 2000* examined 17 health status indicators and studied the rates of these indicators from 1990 to 1998. Although the disparities for 11 of the indicators decreased somewhat for AI/AN, the remaining 6 increased. The lung cancer death rate increased by 28.1%, the percentage of low-birth-weight infants increased by 10.3%, the suicide death rate increased by 8.1%, the total death rate increased by 3.7%, and the breast cancer death rate increased by 4%. The

health indicator for cardiovascular diseases was subdivided into heart disease deaths and stroke deaths. The stroke death rate increased by 2.6% and the heart disease death rate decreased by 8.4%.[9]

Heart disease

There is a wide variation in mortality rates from heart disease in different areas of the country, corresponding to different tribal rates (Fig. 21-3).[8] Some areas have heart disease rates lower than that for all US races (such as the Indian Health Service [IHS] Albuquerque Area, which includes the states of Colorado and New Mexico, and the IHS Navajo Area, which includes portions of the states of Arizona, Utah, and New Mexico), whereas other areas have much higher rates (such as the IHS Bemidji Area, which includes the states of Minnesota, Wisconsin, and Michigan, and the IHS Aberdeen Area, which includes the states of North Dakota, South Dakota, Nebraska, and Iowa).[7]

An extensive review of the medical literature reveals that coronary heart disease (CHD) was uncommon in American Indians for many decades earlier in the twentieth century.[10–31] These studies were done primarily in the Southwest. More recently, studies have

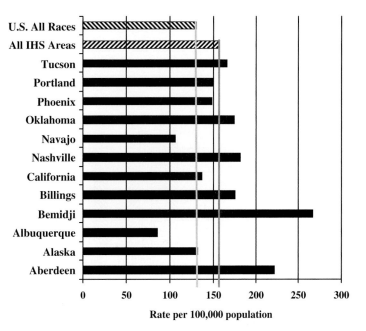

FIGURE 21-3 Age-adjusted heart disease death rate per 100,000 population (calendar year 1996–1998). Death rates were adjusted to compensate for misreporting of American Indian or Alaska Native race on death certificate. (SOURCE: Indian Health Service, Regional Differences in Indian Health, 2000–2001.)

shown that certain tribes had CHD rates that were similar to, or exceeded, those of the US population.[32–34] Currently, CHD is the leading cause of mortality in AI/AN.[5,8,9,35,36] Factors that likely contribute to CHD in AI/AN include: (1) Westernization of the diet; (2) more sedentary lifestyles; (3) increasing obesity; (4) increasing diabetes mellitus; (5) recreational, rather than ceremonial, use of tobacco; (6) poor social and economic status of the population; and (7) lack of consistent and adequate access to health care. There also was a corresponding decrease in infectious diseases, which were the primary cause of mortality in the mid-1900s.[37] From 1991 to 2001, the proportion of deaths from diseases of the heart decreased from 22.7 to 20.1% in AI/AN (a 2.6% reduction), compared with a decrease from 33.2 to 29.0% for all US races (a 4.2% reduction). Thus, diseases of the heart represent a smaller proportion of deaths among AI/AN, but the reduction in the proportion of deaths due to diseases of the heart was less for AI/AN over the last 10 years than it was for all US races.[38]

Until recently, there were no large multicenter studies on American Indians or Alaska Natives. The majority of studies were retrospective and involved tribes in the Southwest. In 1989, the National Heart, Lung, and, Blood Institute funded the Strong Heart Study (SHS), which is currently in its fourth phase (http://strongheart.ouhsc.edu/). The SHS is a large, multicenter, longitudinal epidemiologic study of three American

Indian populations from 13 tribes in Arizona, Oklahoma, North Dakota, and South Dakota. There were more than 4500 participants aged 45 to 74 at the onset of the study who have been followed in subsequent phases. Prior to the SHS, AI/AN represented such small numbers in research studies that they were not identified and were generally grouped in the "other" racial category.

Multiple reports have been issued from this study, focusing primarily on risk factors, disease prevalence, and mortality.[39–58] These reports reveal that risk factors such as cigarette smoking, overweight and obesity, type 2 diabetes mellitus, and binge drinking are substantially more common among American Indian groups than the general population in both genders (Figs. 21-4 and 21-5).

The latest evaluation of risk factors in the SHS cohort[59] indicated that mean blood pressures and hypertension rates increased, hypertension awareness and treatment improved, and smoking rates decreased, but still remained higher than for all US races rate; overweight and obesity rates remained stable, were higher than the national average, and were more pronounced in women.

CVD Risk factors

HYPERTENSION

In 1963, Clifford and colleagues noted a lower prevalence of hypertension among White Mountain Apaches

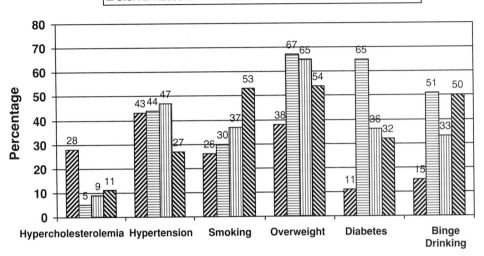

FIGURE 21-4   Cardiovascular disease risk factors for men 45 to 47 years of age, US All Races and Strong Heart Study American Indian male participants, 1989–1991. Hypercholesterolemia, total cholesterol ≥240 mg/dL; Hypertension, SBP ≥140 or DBP ≥90 or taking antihypertensive medications; Smoking, currently smoking cigarettes: Overweight, body mass index ≥27.8; Diabetes, diagnosed with diabetes; Binge Drinking, 5 or more drinks on one occasion in the last year; AZ, Arizona; OK, Oklahoma; SD/ND, South Dakota/North Dakota. Adapted with permission from Welty et al.[45]

compared with US rates and predicted that as the tribe adopted a Western diet and lifestyle, their rates of hypertension and CHD would approach or exceed the rate for all races in the United States.[22] Other studies confirmed the steady increase in the prevalence of hypertension.[27,60–64] Ambulatory visits to IHS facilities related to hypertension are exceeded only by visits for upper respiratory infections, otitis media, and diabetes.[65] Hypertension rates are higher among persons with diabetes than among those who do not have diabetes.[66] When hypertension and diabetes occur concomitantly, they synergistically increase cardiovascular disease (CVD) morbidity and mortality.

The SHS learned that the prevalence of hypertension (defined by a systolic blood pressure ≥ 140 mm Hg or diastolic blood pressure ≥ 90 mmHg, or taking antihypertensive medication) ranged from 27 to 47%[43] and that hypertension is an independent risk factor for both prevalent and incident CHD.[44,67] SHS data also showed that the prevalence of hypertension in Arizona and Oklahoma Indians was higher than in the US population, and South Dakota/North Dakota Indians had lower rates[54] (Figs. 21-4 and 21-5). Although more than 70% of those diagnosed with hypertension were aware of the diagnosis, only slightly more than 50% were receiving treatment

and only 30% had their hypertension under control. Blood pressure level was significantly related to glucose intolerance, age, obesity, and alcohol consumption, but not to plasma insulin.[54,67] The prevalence of definite hypertension increased in the SHS cohort by 7 to 9% in 4 years.[59]

LIPIDS

Like hypertension, hypercholesterolemia was previously uncommon in AI/AN. In 1986, cholesterol was 20 to 40% lower among Navajo myocardial infarction patients than in comparable white patients.[68] More recently, there has been wide variation in studies that investigated lipid levels among AI/AN. Most studies have reported lower levels of total and low-density lipoprotein cholesterol (LDL-C) compared with US whites[12,37,47,69,70]; others have reported comparable[71] or higher levels.[72]

Abnormalities in lipid profiles are also more pronounced in AI/AN women than in men. The higher prevalence of diabetes and obesity in AI/AN women than in men and the menopausal loss of estrogen likely contribute to the higher total and LDL-C and triglyceride levels in women.[73] Estrogen use in postmenopausal SHS participants was low, but was associated with lower levels of LDL-C and higher levels of high-density lipoprotein

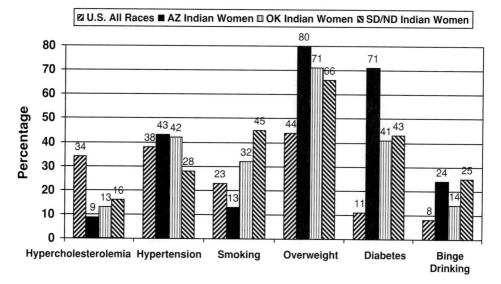

FIGURE 21-5 Cardiovascular disease risk factors for women 45 to 74 years of age, US All Races and Strong Heart Study American Indian female participants, 1989–1991. Hypercholesterolemia, total cholesterol $\geq$240 mg/dL; Hypertension, SBP $\geq$140 or DBP $\geq$90 or taking antihypertensive medications; Smoking, currently smoking cigarettes: Overweight, body mass index $\geq$27.3; Diabetes, diagnosed with diabetes; Binge Drinking, 5 or more drinks on one occasion in the last year; AZ, Arizona; OK, Oklahoma; SD/ND, South Dakota/North Dakota. Adapted with permission from Welty et al.[45]

cholesterol (HDL-C).[74] However, in the light of the results of the Heart and Estrogen/Progestin Replacement Study (HERS)[75] and Women's Health Initiative (WHI) estrogen/progestin results,[76] estrogen replacement therapy is no longer recommended for the primary or secondary prevention of CVD.

For SHS participants, the initial mean total cholesterol ranged from 177 to 199 mg/dL in men and 181 to 202 mg/dL in women. LDL-C levels ranged from 102 to 122 mg/dL in men and from 105 to 120 mg/dL in women (Fig. 21-6). North and South Dakota Indians had higher levels of total cholesterol and LDL-C compared with Arizona and Oklahoma Indians, but lower levels than those of all US races.[45]

At the second SHS examination, mean total cholesterol decreased by 5.3 mg/dL in men over 4years, but remained unchanged in women. Mean LDL-C decreased by 1.7 mg/dL in men, but increased by 1.5 mg/dL in women. Mean HDL-C decreased by more than 9%.[59] Women who entered menopause after the initial exam and who did not start hormone replacement therapy had significant increases in total mean cholesterol, LDL-C, and triglyceride levels (7.3, 10.6, and 7.3 mg/dL respectively). Women who were postmenopausal at the initial exam and did not take estrogen replacement at either

exam had significant increases in LDL-C (3.7 mg/dL) and triglycerides (10.2 mg/dL) and decreases in mean total cholesterol (2.1 mg/dL) and HDL-C (4.9 mg/dL).[59]

Several studies have shown that the strongest independent lipid risk factor for CVD, both in those who have diabetes[70] and those who do not,[77,78] is LDL-C, followed by low HDL-C. Lipoprotein(a) has not been shown to be an independent risk factor in this population[79] and triglycerides have been shown to be an independent CVD risk factor in AI/AN women, but not men.[67]

Diabetes

Like the other CVD risk factors, diabetes was rare before Westernization of lifestyle of the AI/AN population.[10] Since then, there has been an alarming increase in the prevalence of diabetes, and it is now the fourth leading cause of death in this population.[80] The SHS found that triglycerides, obesity, fasting glucose, insulin level, metabolic syndrome, insulin resistance, and degree of American Indian blood were risk factors for developing diabetes.[81–83]

Diabetes has been extensively researched in the Southwest tribes, in whom the rate far exceeds that of the general population. However, the rates vary by tribe. The Pima Indians of Arizona have the highest rates of diabetes

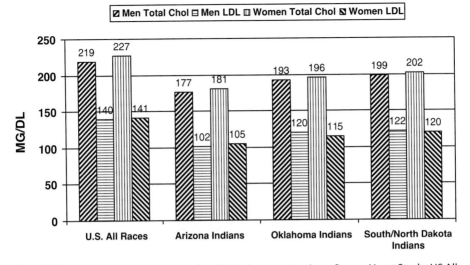

FIGURE 21-6 Mean total cholesterol and LDL-C–concentrations: Strong Heart Study: US All Races, 1988–1991; American Indians, 1989–1991. Adapted with permission from Welty et al.[45]

of any population in the world (500 cases per 1000 adult population).[84] Among the Inuit of the Northwest Territories in Canada, there were only 4 cases per 1000 population.[85] Among Pima participants of the SHS, 65% of men and 71% of women had diabetes and another 15% of men and 14% of women had impaired glucose tolerance. About 33% of men and 40% of women in the Oklahoma, North Dakota, and South Dakota centers had diabetes, and rates of impaired glucose tolerance were similar to those of Arizona Indians[45] (Figs. 21-4 and 21-5). The prevalence of diabetes increased in the SHS cohort over 4 years in all centers and both genders (6–12%)[59] (Fig. 21-7).

Diabetes is a strong risk factor for CHD[44,59,70] in both men and women (Fig. 21-8). Among Navajos, one study found nearly half of all diagnosed myocardial infarctions occurred in persons with diabetes, and the age-adjusted cerebrovascular disease rates were 5.2 times higher for persons with diabetes than for those without.[86] The study also revealed that persons with diabetes had a 10.2 times higher chance of having cerebrovascular disease and a 6.8 times greater risk of having peripheral vascular disease compared with those who did not have diabetes.

The diabetes mortality rate among Native Americans (52.8) is nearly four times that of white Americans (13.5).[8] Kidney disease, mostly due to diabetes, is nearly six times more common among AI/AN than in whites, and among the Pima Indians, the rate of kidney disease is more than 20 times that of the US population.[85] Despite the higher prevalence of diabetes in Pima Indians, the SHS found they had a lower rate of CHD than Sioux

and Oklahoma Indians, possibly because the Pima Indians have significantly lower smoking rates and lower cholesterol levels.[57] Incident diabetes in Pima Indians is positively associated with age, level of obesity, degree of Indian ancestry, and parental diabetes status.[81,87]

Not only is the prevalence of type 2 diabetes increasing in adults, but the prevalence in children is increasing as well.[88,89] Between 1990 and 1998, the total number of young AI/AN diagnosed with diabetes increased by 71% and the prevalence increased by 46%.[86] This is an alarming trend and is felt to be due to increasing obesity and increasing rates of gestational diabetes during pregnancy, that is, exposure to diabetes in utero.[86] Gestational diabetes occurs in 2 to 5% of all pregnancies in the United States,[90] but in 3.4 to 14.5% of all pregnancies among Native Americans.[85] Infants born to mothers with diabetes, or to mothers who develop gestational diabetes, are 9 times more likely to develop diabetes by 19 years of age and 32 times more likely by 24 years of age, compared with children born to mothers without diabetes.[91] The younger a person develops diabetes, the earlier he or she risks developing the complications of diabetes (ie, coronary heart disease, end-stage renal disease, circulatory deficiency).

Fifty-five percent of SHS participants aged 45 to 74 had the metabolic syndrome, as defined by Adult Treatment Panel III.[82] Rates in SHS men and women aged 45 to 49 were over twice as high as those reported in a national survey. SHS men older than 60 had rates similar to national rates, whereas SHS women had rates 1.56 times higher than national rates. Among nondiabetic

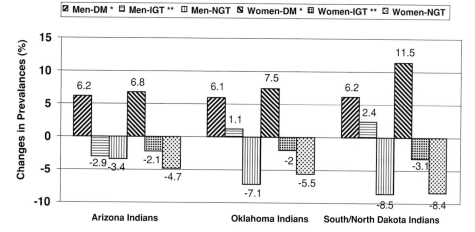

FIGURE 21-7   Changes in diabetes mellitus (DM),* impaired glucose tolerance (IGT),** and normal glucose tolerance (NGT), Strong Heart Study, 1988–1991.* On diabetes medications or after 75-g glucose load, serum glucose of 200 mg/dL or greater.** After 75-g glucose load, serum glucose of 140 to 199 mg/dL. Adapted with permission from Welty et al.[59]

SHS participants who were free of CVD, both metabolic syndrome and insulin resistance predicted diabetes, but neither predicts CVD independent of other CVD risk factors.[83]

OBESITY AND PHYSICAL INACTIVITY

Obesity and physical inactivity are common problems in the Native American population[44,92–94] and have been associated with an increased risk of cerebrovascular disease.[63,70] Whereas the US all-race prevalence of overweight (body mass index [BMI] ≥ 27.8 kg/m^2 for males and ≥ 27.3 kg/m^2 for females) was 38% in men and 44% in women, prevalence rates in American Indian tribes participating in the SHS ranged from 54 to 67% in men and from 66 to 80% in women during the same period. The prevalence of obesity was highest in the Southwest

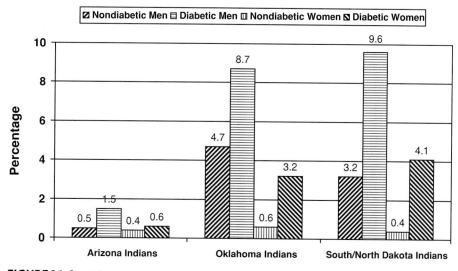

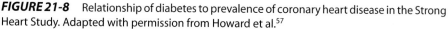

FIGURE 21-8   Relationship of diabetes to prevalence of coronary heart disease in the Strong Heart Study. Adapted with permission from Howard et al.[57]

and Oklahoma tribes as compared with tribes in North Dakota and South Dakota[45] (Figs. 21-4 and 21-5). Although obesity rates did not change in SHS participants over 4 years, the rates remained significantly higher than the national rates.[59] Among SHS participants, obesity was a risk factor for CHD, but no difference was noted in level of risk between generalized and central obesity (waist circumference). These findings differ from those of other studies, possibly because most obese SHS participants had central obesity. Other studies have shown that central obesity correlates more strongly with metabolic risk factors for CHD than BMI. Among nondiabetic SHS participants, central obesity was no more closely associated with CHD factors than was generalized obesity (BMI), and changes in these risk factors with obesity were small. They also noted that obesity is a potent risk factor for diabetes and that may be the major mechanism for increasing CHD risk.[95]

The change from a traditionally active lifestyle, where subsistence living activities such as hunting, fishing, and gathering were the rule, to a sedentary lifestyle has contributed greatly to this problem. American Indians in the SHS reported watching an average of 3 hours of television daily, and 38% of men and 48% of women reported no physical activity during the preceding week.[45]

TOBACCO

Tobacco is considered by many cultures and tribes to be a sacred substance that the Creator gave for ceremonial use. AI/AN men smoke tobacco and the dried leaves, roots, and bark of other plants on ceremonial and important social occasions. Some tribes believe the smoking of tobacco increases the efficacy of prayers and makes a promise or agreement more binding. Recreational use of tobacco by AI/AN began after contact with Europeans and varies by region.[96] The Northern Plains tribes have the highest rates of use and the Southwest tribes the lowest[97,98] (Fig. 21-9). Except for the Southwest tribes, smoking prevalence is consistently higher than in the non-Indian population, but the number of cigarettes smoked per day is smaller.[99,100] A high prevalence of smokeless tobacco use has been noted in Alaska, even for females.[98] Smoking is an independent risk factor for prevalent heart disease in SHS participants,[44,70] except in Arizona where the cigarette consumption per day is very low.[45] Smoking was not associated with incident CHD in SHS participants.[67] The low cigarette consumption and the high passive smoke exposure of Sioux and Oklahoma Indians (>3 hours per day) may contribute to the lack of association of smoking with incident CHD.[45] Smoking cessation was associated with lower daily cigarette consumption, shorter duration of smoking, and history of diabetes among the 21% of SHS participants who quit in a 4-year period.[101]

Tobacco use is very high in AI/AN adolescents,[99,100,102] up to 45% for males and 57% for females.[98] Having a family member who smokes and other stressful life events such as death/loss are linked to increased risk of tobacco use in adolescents. Being

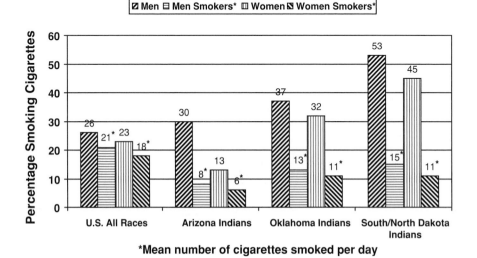

FIGURE 21-9 Cigarette smoking, Strong Heart Study: US All Races, 1987–1991; American Indians, 1989–1991. Adapted with permission from Welty et al.[45]

connected to their traditional culture increased their ceremonial use of tobacco, whereas good family/tribal support and academic orientation lowered the risk of tobacco abuse.[100] Smoking prevention interventions should be targeted at adolescents.[98]

ALCOHOL

Consumption of alcoholic beverages, such as beer, wine, whiskey, brandy, and mixed drinks, is higher for white Americans (55%) than AI/AN (45%). Among users, however, the binge drinking rate is higher for AI/AN (28%) than white Americans (24%).[59,103] Binge drinking (drinking five or more drinks on one occasion) has been associated with high blood pressure[54] and sudden death.[104] Alcohol abuse causes many adverse health effects, including CVD. Among participants in the SHS, the prevalence of current alcohol use was initially found to be between 49 and 60% in men and between 28 and 38% in women.[45] A 4-year follow-up study showed that the prevalence of alcohol use decreased slightly to 40 to 53% in men and 20 to 30% in women.[59]

Although moderate drinking reduces the risk of CVD, SHS participants commonly reported binge drinking (Fig. 21-10). Among drinkers, binge drinking was highly variable, but as many as 94% of men and 87% of women reported binge drinking at least once in the last year.[45] Four-year follow-up in this population demonstrated that despite a reduction in drinking prevalence, binge drinking was still very common among those still drinking (up to 87% of men and 67% of women).[59]

NUTRITION

Over the last 40 years, traditional foods such as wild game, fish, berries, and corn have been replaced by processed and commercially processed foods. Diet is a contributing factor in many health-related issues such as cerebrovascular disease, CHD, diabetes, and obesity, and healthy dietary choices may delay or prevent those conditions. The SHS reported AI/AN mean total fat intake as a percentage of total calories to be consistently above the recommended level of 30%, and fiber intake below the 20 to 30 g/d,[50] but significant variation exists among tribes. Pima Indians had the highest intakes of fat and cholesterol, but also the highest fiber intake among the communities studied.[105] Native communities that retained more of their traditional diet had lower CHD mortality.[106]

Stroke and cerebrovascular disease

Stroke mortality varies, with the Navajo being lower and the IHS areas of Bemidji, Portland (Oregon, Washington, and Idaho), and Billings (Montana and Wyoming) being much higher (Fig. 21-11).[8] Five-year stroke mortality rates among SHS participants were higher for men than women, and heart disease was the leading cause of death, except in Indian women in Arizona. When compared with non-Indian rates in the same state, the all-cause mortality and stroke mortality rates were higher in almost every American Indian age and sex group.[34] The SHS has linked lower socioeconomic status to higher

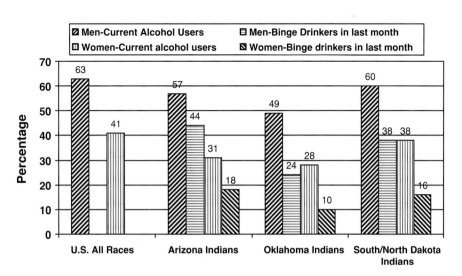

FIGURE 21-10   Alcohol use, Strong Heart Study: US All Races, 1987–1991; American Indians, 1989–1991. Adapted with permission from Welty et al.[45]

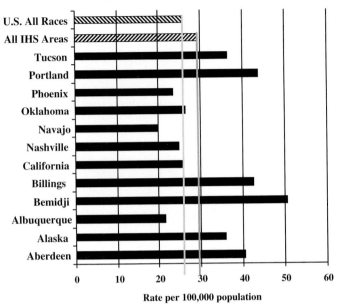

FIGURE 21-11 Age-adjusted cerebrovascular disease death rate per 100,000 population (calendar year 1996–1998). Death rates were adjusted to compensate for misreporting of American Indian or Alaska Native race on death certificate. (SOURCE: Indian Health Service, Regional Differences in Indian Health, 2000–2001.)

rates of cerebrovascular disease.[48] Limited funding available for the IHS, resulting in fewer health services, may also play a role in the rate of cerebrovascular disease, as well as other diseases.

There is very little information on strokes in AI/AN,[107,108] even though it is the fifth leading cause of death. New Mexico Indians had a lower incidence of stroke than Hispanics and non-Hispanic whites.[109] Stroke deaths in AI/AN were more likely to be coded as subarachnoid hemorrhage or lacunar strokes and to have diabetes and heavy alcohol use as risk factors than stroke deaths in Hispanics and non-Hispanic whites.[107] Among New Mexico Indian stroke deaths, hypertension was found in 71%, diabetes in 62%, smoking in 61%, atherosclerotic CVD in 27%, and heavy alcohol use in 43%.[108] Although strokes in AI/AN were more likely to be administratively coded as hemorrhagic than strokes in other ethnic groups, further review showed that only 27% of strokes in American Indians had documented hemorrhage, compared with 37% for non-Hispanic whites and 48% for Hispanics.

PREVENTIVE STRATEGIES

Overview

Enhanced screening, identification of persons at high risk for stroke, and targeted CVD risk factor reduction programs are needed in Native American communities to reduce the incidence of stroke. Local clinics and hospitals that serve Native American communities need resources to conduct community-based screening for hypertension, diabetes, and dyslipidemia and to treat persons who have these conditions as part of a CVD risk factor reduction program. Providers need training in standards for the identification, classification, and management of these conditions, as discussed in depth in earlier chapters of this text. As CVD risk factors vary greatly in Native American communities throughout the country, preventive interventions must be tailored to the community.

Guidelines specific for the management of CVD risk factors among individual Native American groups do not exist. As much as possible, culturally appropriate strategies (see below) should be used to complement proven medical/public health approaches. The IHS Native American Cardiology Program modified national guidelines (available at: http://www.ihs.gov/medicalprograms/cardiology/card/index.cfm) for use in AI/AN communities and supports national collaboration, roundtables, and seminars for providers and tribal leaders, to promote both primary and secondary prevention of CVD.

Broad recommendations regarding promotion of cardiovascular health among Native Americans, titled *Building Healthy Hearts for American Indians and Alaska Natives: A Background Report*, have been published by the National Institutes of Health.[110] This report identified, based on the available epidemiologic data, the following audiences as possible targets for intervention:

1. Cigarette-smoking tribal members living in the Midwestern United States and Alaska

2. Cigarette-smoking youth living on reservations

3. People with diabetes in all tribes, especially those living in the Southwestern and Midwestern United States

4. Those with high blood pressure in tribes with a high prevalence of diabetes

5. Tribal populations with obesity and physical inactivity problems

This report also emphasizes that broad-based community support is needed to implement successful CVD risk reduction programs. Traditional healers, community health representatives, nutrition aides, students in health fields at American Indian colleges, and others should be recruited as volunteers or staff to establish effective community-based programs. Also, school boards, health boards, and community health programs can be channels for incorporating family activities and community events, such as powwows, into the risk reduction program. Finally, the report recommends that Native American professional associations and other professional health groups should incorporate both Western and traditional medicine into training on CVD risk reduction for providers who serve Native American communities.

Although there are no published data on the effectiveness of different risk-reducing therapies among AI/AN, the personal experience of the authors with multiple tribes suggests responses to antihypertensive and lipid-lowering therapy among Native Americans are similar to the responses among white populations. Native Americans do not appear to be salt-sensitive and they have a good response to the major classes of antihypertensive and lipid-lowering therapy. The National Heart, Lung, and Blood Institute has funded the Stop Atherosclerosis in Native Diabetics Study (SANDS), a controlled clinical trial that will determine whether reduction of blood pressure to less than 115/75 mm Hg and of LDL-C to less than 75 mg/dL will slow the progression of carotid atherosclerosis in diabetic Native Americans in Arizona, South Dakota, and Oklahoma.

Increased community awareness regarding healthy lifestyles is an essential component of primary prevention. In an effort to prevent and combat diabetes, advisory groups and coalitions have formed in some tribes to increase community awareness and strengthen the infrastructure necessary to promote healthy lifestyles.[111] Comprehensive obesity-prevention programs are also promising.[112] Group or communitywide strategies may be more effective than individual approaches in this culture- and tradition-based population. Stressing the benefits of therapy for the entire family (eg, diet healthy for all), rather than just for the individual, will likely be more successful because of the extended family and social fabric of Native American communities.

Successful community-based health programs

Pathways, an interventional study of primary prevention of obesity in American Indian children supported by the National Heart, Lung, and Blood Institute, included a cohort of 1704 third to fifth grade children in 41 schools (21 intervention, 20 controls) in seven Indian tribes in Arizona, New Mexico, and South Dakota.[110,113] This is the only randomized controlled study for prevention of obesity in American Indian children ever conducted. Although Pathways documented some improvements in knowledge, attitudes, and beliefs and in dietary intake of healthy foods in interventional schools compared with control schools, mean changes in BMI were similar for children in the interventional and control schools. Further research is needed to identify interventions that can consistently reduce childhood obesity.

The Checkerboard Cardiovascular Curriculum was an intervention designed to increase cardiovascular health knowledge among fifth grade children in rural New Mexico, primarily Pueblo and Navajo Indians and Hispanics. This culturally rich curriculum produced positive results by incorporating information on American Indian traditions about running and exercise and the traditional American Indian and Hispanic diets.[109]

The Zuni Diabetes Project is a community-based exercise and weight control program designed to encourage weight loss and improve glycemic control in people with diabetes. Initiated by the IHS, it was transferred to the Zuni Tribal Wellness Center. It demonstrated that a community-based exercise program can be effective in this population.[110]

The Southwestern Cardiovascular Curriculum is a multifactorial, culturally-oriented curriculum created for American Indian students in rural northwestern New Mexico that is designed to increase knowledge about health and healthy behavior by teaching students about healthier lifestyles and ways to achieve them.[110]

The National Institute of Diabetes and Digestive and Kidney Disorders Diabetes Prevention Program was a randomized controlled trial to determine if diabetes can be prevented or delayed in persons with impaired glucose tolerance. This multicenter project started out with a pilot study in Pima Indians.[110] The study demonstrated a 58% reduction in the incidence of diabetes in the lifestyle group and a 31% reduction in the metformin group.[114,115]

Pima Indians who were exclusively breastfed as infants were less likely to develop diabetes at age 30 to 39 than those who were formula fed or both breastfed and formula fed.[116] The Phoenix Indian Medical Center has promoted breastfeeding as a diabetes prevention initiative (http://www.ihs.gov/nonmedicalprograms/nc4/breastfeed/bf/docs/brstfdgdm.doc).

Effective strategies for researching, assisting, working, and implementing health programs in AI/AN communities are:

1. Incorporate community culture, lifestyle, and values. For Native Americans, the cultural value of family and tribe takes priority over the individual. Interventions that are family centered will be more effective.

2. Gain community support. Historically, Native Americans have been studied without benefiting from the research. This has fostered distrust of researchers in these communities. Involving tribal leadership and community members in all phases of the research will lead to better participation in the project.

3. Develop partnerships within the target community and with other federal, state, and local organizations. A new program implemented within the confines of existing organizations in the community can use infrastructures and viable local networks to reach the target population.

4. Develop and disseminate culturally appropriate materials. Accurate assessment of the target populations' knowledge, values, health beliefs, literacy level, and language preference is essential. Direct community input can enhance this effort to address the needs of the target population.

5. Increase access to health programs. Lack of transportation, lack of safe places to exercise, and lack of affordable healthy foods are frequent problems encountered by AI/AN in remote and rural areas.[110]

CULTURAL ISSUES

Overview

Understanding the culture of a patient can be a major asset in providing effective care. Sir William Osler stated, "It is more important to know what sort of patient has a disease, than what sort of disease a patient has."[117] Provider background can also have a significant impact on health care delivery. Providers of similar background are usually more effective.[118] AI/AN beliefs on health, disease, and healing are often very different from the traditional Western or European concepts. Some understanding of Native American culture can help improve the outcome of the provider–patient encounter. Health in AI/AN culture is not the absence of disease, but rather harmony with oneself (mind, body, spirit), harmony with others, and harmony with one's surroundings or environment. When harmony is lost, illness is able to enter.

Spirituality, or religion, is also inseparable from health in AI/AN culture. Traditional Indian healers use spiritual means to diagnose and heal. They are viewed as healing from the inside of the body because they treat the cause of the illness or whatever led to the loss of harmony. Western medicine is viewed as healing from the outside of the body because they treat the symptoms (eg, headache, dyspepsia). Both methods are viewed as compatible and are not competitive. They have the same goal—a healthy patient! Traditional healers have never felt it is their place to prolong life, but simply to try to make the person's life better, an aspect of healing that is finding its way into the practice of Western medicine as well.

Cultural norms for social interaction are different too. The Native American handshake is gentle, to show respect. The handshake is not a test of strength or a show of domination. Eye contact means a lack of trust. Looking into a person's eyes during an encounter is interpreted as trying to determine if the person is telling the truth. There is no clock fixation and some languages do not have a future tense. There are other differences, but these are a few of the important ones.

Guidelines for those working with patients from another culture

1. Remember, you are the visitor or guest and should not impose your cultural preferences on the patient. Adapt to the patient's ways.

2. Respect the patient. Conduct yourself so as not to be perceived as condescending, paternalistic, or ethnocentric.

3. Be patient. Do not show haste.

4. Speak to your listeners with words and concepts they can understand, and ask them if you explained yourself clearly enough. AI/AN consider it impolite to ask questions, as this would imply that you had done a bad job, and that would be disrespectful.

5. Attend social events and learn by watching. Do not ask a lot of questions, as this would show you are not paying attention.

6. Develop relationships with staff members from the culture. They can help you learn a lot about their ways and their culture.

7. Respect the cultural traditional beliefs and customs of the community.

Lessons taught by elders of the culture

1. Respect the ways of others. Understanding the ways is not necessary to respect them.

2. Healing has a spiritual side. Technologic advances can make it easy to forget this.

3. The healer is not the source of the healing, but simply a conduit through which the healing powers of the Creator reach the patient.

4. Intelligence and the ability to help others are gifts. These need to be treated as gifts if they are to be there when needed.

Qualities of those who are successful in Native American communities

1. They respect their patients, members of the community, and the ways of the people.

2. They are interested in the ways of the people, learning the ways and adapting to the local culture.

3. They care about the people and their families.

4. They are patient.

HEALTH CARE SERVICES AND ISSUES

The federal government is the primary provider of health services for AI/AN, primarily through the IHS. The provision of health services to federally recognized tribes grew out of a special relationship between the federal government and Indian tribes and Native communities that are sovereign nations. This government-to-government relationship is based on Article 1, Section 8, of the US Constitution,[7] and various laws have established and defined the health services that are based in the treaties enacted between tribal governments and the federal government. The remainder of the AI/AN population, approximately 1 million AI/AN belonging to tribes that have not received federal recognition, are covered by Medicare, Medicaid, or private insurance or are uninsured.

The IHS, an agency of the US Department of Health and Human Services (HHS), provides direct and public health services to members of federally recognized tribes, or approximately 1.6 million people. Other agencies of the HHS also work directly with tribes by awarding competitive grants for services, research, and community-based health promotion activities. The IHS administers individual and public health services through a decentralized system of 12 area offices and 155 service units, 60 of which are managed by the IHS and 95 of which are tribally managed. The Indian Health System consists of 49 hospitals, 236 health centers, 176 Alaska village clinics, 133 health stations, and 33 residential treatment centers. In addition, there are 34 independent urban Indian health projects, which receive some of their funding from the IHS, that provide some medical, dental, and other individual health care services for approximately 330,000 urban Indians; some projects provide only outreach and referral. There is a misconception that all AI/AN receive care without charge or that the IHS provides universal coverage for all Native Americans. In reality, health care services have been prepaid by the treaties that transferred land, mineral rights, and resources to the federal government in exchange for health and other services.

The lower health status of AI/AN is also affected by the extent to which health services are available to them. The IHS does not operate in all tribal communities, due to financial and personnel limitations and insufficient workload to justify the presence of a permanent health facility or staff. In the 2003 report *A Quiet Crisis: Federal Funding and Unmet Needs in Indian Country,* issued by the Commission on Civil Rights, the Commission stated that the lack of full funding of federal health programs has violated the treaty agreements with the tribes and, therefore, the civil rights of AI/AN.[119]

An additional factor influencing the health disparities between AI/AN and other Americans is discrimination. In July 2003, President George W. Bush, reaffirmed that the role of the federal government is to bring comfort and compassion to the afflicted[120] and that "we must challenge the soft bigotry of low expectations."[121] Discrimination in health care, as stated by the Director of the HHS Office of Minority Health, Dr. Nathan Stinson, at a health disparity conference in September 2002, is a reflection of bias on the part of caregivers and policymakers.[122] And the President of Moorehouse School of Medicine and former Secretary of Health and Human Services, Dr. Louis Sullivan, has also stated, "there is clear, demonstrable, undeniable evidence of discrimination and racism in our health care system."[123]

Human variables (bias, racism, politics, gender, etc.) virtually always affect human interactions, including the delivery of health services to a socially and culturally diverse population. Inclusion of chapters such as this one in medical publications should sensitize health providers to the fact that providing health care is never bias-neutral; however, increasing one's awareness and cultural understanding is one way to reduce or eliminate the bias barrier to health services and improve the health status of AI/AN.

CONCLUSION

The epidemics of chronic diseases that are currently afflicting all Native American communities developed when these peoples adopted high-fat, high-carbohydrate modern "American" diets and became more sedentary. Their traditional diets and active lifestyles were protective. More research is needed to determine effective community-based interventions that can reduce the prevalence of obesity and diabetes through lifestyle changes, which, in turn, will reduce rates of CHD and end-stage renal disease. To date, no Native American community has reported reductions of these chronic diseases. Rather, these diseases are universally increasing at alarming rates, creating great suffering, premature mortality, and staggering health care costs. Culturally sensitive, community-based interventions, coupled with committed tribal leadership and aggressive clinical programs for CVD risk reduction, are most likely to succeed in stabilizing and eventually reducing the rates of chronic diseases in Native American communities. If Native American communities are able to effectively combat these epidemics, they will make a great contribution to preventive medicine, because most nations are facing similar epidemics of chronic diseases, albeit not nearly as severe. As the rates of obesity and diabetes increase nationally, it is likely that the downward trend in national CVD morbidity and mortality will reverse. Thus, investment in combatting these epidemics in Native American communities may translate into solutions of these problems in communities worldwide.

REFERENCES

1. Bureau of Indian Affairs. Bureau of Indian Affairs Home Page. Department of Interior Web Site, November 2003. Available at: *http://www.doi.gov/bureau-indian-affairs.html*. Accessed June 9, 2004.

2. US Census 2000. Suitland, Md: US Department of Commerce, Economics and Statistics Administration, US Census Bureau.

3. The American Indian and Alaska Native Population 2000—Census 2000 brief. Suitland, Md: US Department of Commerce, Economics and Statistics Administration, US Census Bureau; February 2002.

4. Forquera R. *Urban Indian Health—Issue Brief*. Menlo Park, Calif: The Henry J. Kaiser Foundation; November 2001.

5. Poverty Rates Rise, Household Income Decline, Census Bureau Reports [press release]. Suitland, Md: US Department of Commerce, Economics and Statistics Administration, US Census Bureau; September 24, 2002.

6. Facts for Features: American Indian and Alaska Native Heritage Month November 2002. Suitland, Md: US Department of Commerce, Economics and Statistics Administration, US Census Bureau; October 21, 2002.

7. Trends in Indian Health 1998–1999. Rockville, Md: US Department of Health and Human Services, Public Health Service, Indian Health Service, Office of Public Health; 2000.

8. Regional Differences in Indian Health, 2000–2001. Rockville, Md: US Department of Health and Human Services, Public Health Service, Indian Health Service, Office of Public Health; 2000.

9. Keppel KG, Pearcy JN, Wagener DK. Trends in racial and ethnic-specific rates for the health status indicators: United States, 1990–98. In: *Healthy People Statistical Notes*, No. 23. Hyattsville, Md: National Center for Health Statistics; January 2002.

10. Salsbury CG. Disease incidence among the Navajos. *Southwest Med* 1937;20:230.

11. Kraus BS. *The disease picture in Indian health in Arizona.* Tucson: University of Arizona, 1954;75–109.

12. U.S. Department of Health, Education, and Welfare. Heart disease among Indians in the U.S. Washington, DC: U.S. Government Printing Office, 1957.

13. Gilbert J. Absence of coronary thrombosis in Navajo Indians. *Calif Med* 1955;82:114–115.

14. Page IH, Lewis LA, Gilbert J. Plasma lipids and proteins and their relationship to coronary disease among Navajo Indians. *Circulation* 1956;13:675–679.

15. Smith RL. Recorded and expected mortality among the Navajo with special reference to cancer. *J Natl Cancer Inst* 1956;17:77–89.

16. Adair J. Patterns of health and disease among the Navajos. *Ann Am Acad Pol Soc Sci* 1957;311:80.

17. Smith RL. Cardiovascular, renal, and diabetes deaths among the Navajos. *Public Health Rep* 1957;72:33–38.

18. Leo TF. Cardiovascular survey in a population of Arizona Indians. *Circulation* 1958;18:748.

19. Hesse FG. Incidence of cholecystitis and other diseases among Pima Indians of Southern Arizona. *JAMA* 1959;170:1789–1790.

20. Streeper RB. An electrocardiographic and autopsy study of coronary heart disease in the Navajo. *Dis Chest* 1960;38:305–312.

21. Deuschle K. Interdisciplinary approach to public health on the Navajo Indian reservation–medical and anthropological aspects. *Ann NY Acad Sci* 1960;84:887.

22. Clifford NJ, Kelly JJ, Leo TF, et al. Coronary heart disease and hypertension in the White Mountain Apache Tribe. *Circulation* 1963;28:926–931.

23. Fulmer HS. Coronary heart disease among the Navajo Indians. *Ann Intern Med* 1963;59:740–764.

24. Hesse FG. Incidence of disease in the Navajo Indian—a necropsy study of coronary and aortic atherosclerosis, cholelithiasis, and neoplastic disease. *Arch Pathol* 1964;77:553–557.

25. Kravetz RE. Disease distribution in southwestern American Indians; analysis of 211 autopsies. *Arizona Med* 1964;21:628–634.

26. Sievers ML. Myocardial infarction among southwestern American Indians. *Ann Intern Med* 1967;67:800–807.

27. Ingelfinger JA, Bonnett PH, Liebow IM, et al. Coronary heart disease in the Pima Indians–electrocardiographic findings and postmortem evidence of myocardial infarction in a population with high prevalence of diabetes mellitus. *Diabetes* 1976;25:561–565.

28. Becker TM, Wiggins C, Key CR, et al. Ischemic heart disease mortality in Hispanics, American Indians, and Non-Hispanic Whites in New Mexico, 1958–1982. *Circulation* 1988;78:302–309.

29. Middaugh JP. Cardiovascular deaths among Alaska Natives, 1980–1986. *Am J Public Health* 1990;80:282–285.

30. Rhoades DA, Rhoades ER, Welty TK. The rise of cardiovascular disease, in Rhoades ER (ed): American Indian Health: Innovations in Health Care, Promotion, and Policy. Baltimore: The Johns Hopkins University Press, 2000:151–178.

31. Galloway JM, Goldberg BW, Alpert JS, eds. *Primary Care of Native American Patients–Diagnosis, Therapy, and Epidemiology*. Boston, Butterworth/Heinemann, 1999.

32. Pinkerton RE, Badke FR. Coronary heart disease—an epidemiologic study of Crow and Northern Cheyenne Indians. *Rocky Mountain Med J* 1974;71:577–583.

33. Sievers ML. Diseases of North American Indians. In Rothchild HR, ed. *Biocultural Aspects of Disease.* Academic Press, New York: 1981.

34. Hrabovsky SL, Welty TK, Coulehan JL. Acute myocardial infarction and sudden death in Sioux Indians. *West Med J* 1989;150:420–422.

35. U.S. Department of Health and Human Services. 10 leading causes of death, United States, 2001, American Indians and Alaska Natives. U.S. Department of Health and Human Services, Centers for Disease Control and Prevention, National Center for Injury Prevention and Control, Web-based Injury Statistics Query and Reporting System. Available at: http://www.cdc.gov/ncipc/wisqars/default.htm. Accessed November 4, 2003.

36. Lee ET, Cowan LD, Welty TK, et al. All causes mortality and cardiovascular mortality in three American Indian populations, age 45–74 years, 1984–1988—The Strong Heart Study. *Am J Epidemiol* 1998;147:995–1008.

37. Gillum RF, Gillum BS, Smith, N. Cardiovascular risk factors among urban American Indians: blood pressure, serum lipids, smoking, diabetes, health knowledge, and behavior. *Am Heart J* 1984;107:765–776.

38. U.S. Department of Health and Human Services. 10 leading causes of death, United States, 1991 and 2001, American Indians and Alaska Natives and U.S. all races. U.S. Department of Health and Human Services, Centers for Disease Control and Prevention, National Center for Injury Prevention and Control, Web-based Injury Statistics Query and Reporting System. Available at: http://www.cdc.gov/ncipc/wisqars/default.htm. Accessed December 2, 2003.

39. Lee ET, Welty TK, Fabsitz RR. The Strong Heart Study of cardiovascular disease in American Indians; design and methods. *Am J Epidemiol* 1990;132:1141–1155.

40. Howard BV. Associations of lipoproteins with obesity in American Indians: the Strong Heart Study. In Oomura Y, Tarui S, Shimazu T, eds. *Progress in Obesity Research.* John Libby, 1990: 291–294.

41. Howard BV, Welty TK, Fabsitz RR, et al. Risk factors for coronary heart disease in diabetic and non-diabetic Native Americans: the Strong Heart Study. *J Diabetes Care* 1992;41:4–11.

42. Lowe LP, Tavel D, Wallace RB, et al. Type II diabetes and cognitive function—a population based study on Native Americans. *Diabetes Care* 1994;17:891–896.

43. Lee ET, Howard BV, Savage PJ, et al. Diabetes and impaired glucose tolerance in three American Indian populations aged 45–74 years—the Strong Heart Study. *Diabetes Care* 1995;18:599–610.

44. Howard BV, Lee ET, Cowan LD, et al. Coronary heart disease prevalence and its relation to risk factors in American Indians—The Strong Heart Study. *Am J Epidemiol* 1995; 142:254–268.

45. Welty TK, Lee ET, Yeh J, et al. Cardiovascular disease risk factors among American Indians—the Strong Heart Study. *Am J Epidemiol* 1995;42:269–287.

46. Robbins DC, Knowler WC, Lee ET, et al. Regional differences in albuminuria among American Indians—an epidemic of renal disease. *Kidney Int* 1996;49:557–563.

47. Ribbins DC, Welty TK, Wang WY, et al. Plasma lipids and lipoprotein concentrations among American Indians—comparison with the US population. *Curr Opin Lipidol* 1996;7:188–195.

48. Lee ET, Go OT. Socioeconomic status and cardiovascular health and disease in American Indians—the Strong Heart Study. Proceedings of the National Institutes of Health Conference on Socioeconomic Status and Cardiovascular Disease and Health, November 1995. National Institutes of Health, Bethesda, MD: 1996.

49. Cowan LD, Go OT, Howard BV, et al. Parity, postmenopausal estrogen use and cardiovascular disease risk factors in American Indian women—the Strong Heart Study. *J Women's Health* 1997;6:441–449.

50. Zephier EM, Ballew C, Mokdad A, et al. Intake of nutrients related to cardiovascular disease risk among three groups of American Indians—the Strong Heart Study. *Prev Med* 1997;26: 508–515.

51. Devereux RB, Roman MJ, Paranicas M, et al. Relations of left ventricular mass to demographic and hemodynamic variables in American Indians—the Strong Heart Study. *Circulation* 1997;96:1416–1423.

52. Devereux RB, Roman MJ, Paranicas M, et al. Relations of Doppler stroke volume in normotensive and hypertensive American Indians—the Strong Heart Study. *Am J Hypertens* 1997;10:619–628.

53. Oopik AJ, Dorogy M, Devereux RB, et al. Major electrocardiographic abnormalities among American Indians aged 45–74 years—the Strong Heart Study. *Am J Cardiol* 1996;78: 1400–1405.

54. Howard BV, Lee ET, Yeh JL, et al. Hypertension in adult American Indians—the Strong Heart Study. *Hypertension* 1996;28:256–270.

55. Gray RS, Robbins DC, Wang W, et al. Relation of LDL size to the insulin resistance syndrome and coronary heart disease in American Indians—the Strong Heart Study. *Arterioscler Thromb Vasc Biol* 1997;17:2713–2720.

56. Kataola S, Robbins DC, Cowan LD, et al. Apolipoprotein E polymorphism in American Indians and its relation to plasma lipoproteins and diabetes—the Strong Heart Study. *Arterioscler Thromb Vasc Diol* 1996;16:918–925.

57. Howard BV, Lee ET, Fabsitz RR, et al. Diabetes and coronary heart disease in American Indians—the Strong Heart Study. *Diabetes* 1996;45(Supp13):S6–S13.

58. Welty TK, Coulehan JL. Cardiovascular disease among American Indians and Alaska Natives. *Diabetes Care* 1993;16: 277–283.

59. Welty TK, Rhoades DA, Yeh F, et al. Changes in cardiovascular disease risk factors among American Indians—the Strong Heart Study. *Ann Epidemiol* 2002;12:97–106.

60. Strotz CR, Shorr GI. Hypertension in the Papago Indians. *Circulation* 1973;48:1299–1303.

61. Sievers ML. Historical overview of hypertension among American Indians and Alaska Natives. *Arizona Med* 1977;34: 607–610.

62. Destefano F, Coulehan JL, Wiant MK. Blood pressure survey on the Navajo Indian Reservation. *Am J Epidemiol* 1979;190:335–345.

63. Gillum RF, Prineas RJ, Palta M, et al. Blood pressure of urban Native American school children. *J Hypertens* 1980;2:744–749.

64. Howard BV. Blood pressure in 13 American communities—the Strong Heart Study. *Public Health Rep* 1996;111(suppl2): 47–48.

65. U.S. Department of Health and Human Services Hypertension in Hispanic Americans, American Indians and Alaska Natives, and Asian and Pacific Islanders. Bethesda, MD: U.S. Department of Health and Human Services, National Heart, Lung, and Blood Institute, National Institutes of Health, 1996.

66. Howard, BV for the Strong Heart Study Investigators. Risk factors for cardiovascular disease in individuals with diabetes—the Strong Heart Study. *Acta Diabetologica* 1996;33:180–184.

67. Howard BV, Lee ET, Cowan LD, et al. Rising tide of cardiovascular disease in American Indians—the Strong Heart Study. *Circulation* 1999;99:2389–2395.

68. Coulehan JL, Lerner G, Helzsouer K, et al. Acute myocardial infarction among Navajo Indians, 1976–1983. *Am J Public Health* 1986;76:412–414.

69. Savage PJ, Hamman RF, Bartha G, et al. Serum cholesterol in American (Pima) Indian children and adolescents. *J Pediatr* 1976;58:274–282.

70. Campos-Gutealt D, Ellis J, Aickin M, et al. Prevalence of cardiovascular disease risk factors in a southwestern Native American tribe. *Public Health Rep* 1995;110:742–748.

71. Mendlein JM, Freedman DS, Peter DB, et al. Risk factors for coronary heart disease among Navajo Indians—findings from the Navajo Health and Nutrition Survey. *J Nutr* 1997; 127:2099S–2105S.

72. Sugarman JR, Gilbert TJ, Perry CA, et al. Serum cholesterol concentrations among Navajo Indians. *Public Health Rep* 1992;107:92–99.

73. Folsom AR, Johnson KM, Lando HA, et al. Plasma fibrinogen and other cardiovascular risk factors in urban American Indian smokers. *Ethn Dis* 1993;3:344–350.

74. Cowan D, Oscar TG, Howard BV, et al. Parity, postmenopausal estrogen use, and cardiovascular disease risk factors in American Indian women—the Strong Heart Study. *J Women's Health* 1997;6:441–449.

75. Hulley S, Grady D, Bush T, et al. Randomized trial of estrogen plus progestin for secondary prevention of coronary heart disease in postmenopausal women—Heart and Estrogen/Progestin Replacement Study (HERS) Research Group. *JAMA* 1998;280:605–613.

76. Manson, JE, Hsia J, Johnson KC, et al. for the Women's Health Initiative Investigators. Estrogen plus progestin and risk of coronary heart disease: final results from the Women's Health Initiative. *New Engl J Med* 2003;349:523–534.

77. Howard BV, Robbins DC, Sievers ML, et al. LDL cholesterol as a strong predictor of coronary heart disease in diabetic individuals with insulin resistance and low LDL—the Strong Heart Study. *Arterioscler Thromb Vasc Biol* 2000;20:830–835.

78. Hu D, Jablonski KA, Sparling YH, et al. Accuracy of lipoprotein lipids and apoproteins in predicting coronary heart disease in diabetic American Indians—the Strong Heart Study. *Ann Epidemiol* 2002;12:79–85.

79. Hoy W, Light A, Megill D. Cardiovascular disease in Navajo Indians with type 2 diabetes. *Public Health Rep* 1995;110:87–94.

80. U.S. Department of Health and Human Services Regional Differences in Indian Health, 2000–2001. Rockville, MD: U.S. Department of Health and Human Services, Public Health Service, Indian Health Service, Office of Public Health, 2000.

81. Lee ET, Welty TK, Cowan LD, et al. Incidence of diabetes in American Indians of three geographic areas—the Strong Heart Study. *Diabetes Care* 2002;25:49–54.

82. Resnick HE. Metabolic syndrome in American Indians. *Diabetes Care* 2002;25:1246–1247.

83. Resnick HE, Jones K, Ruotolo G, et al. Insulin resistance, the metabolic syndrome, and risk of incident cardiovascular disease in nondiabetic American Indians—the Strong Heart Study. *Diabetes Care* 2003;26:861–867.

84. Howard BV, Knowler WC, Davis MP, et al. Diabetes and atherosclerosis in the Pima Indians. *M Sinai J Med* 1982;49:169–175.

85. U.S. Department of Health and Human Services Diabetes in America, 2nd ed. NIH publication number 95-1468. U.S. Department of Health and Human Services, National Institute of Diabetes and Digestive and Kidney Diseases, National Institutes of Health. Bethesda, MD, 1995.

86. Gohdes D. Diabetes in North American Indians and Alaska Natives. In *Diabetes in America*, 2nd ed. NIH publication number 95-1468. U.S. Department of Health and Human Services, National Institute of Diabetes and Digestive and Kidney Diseases, National Institutes of Health. Bethesda, MD, 1995.

87. Knowler WC, Pettitt DJ, Saad MF, et al. Diabetes mellitus in the Pima Indians—incidence, risk factors and pathogenesis. *Diabetes Metab Rev* 1990;6:1–27.

88. Dabelea D, Hanson RL, Bennett PH, et al. Increasing prevalence of type II diabetes in American Indian children. *Diabetologia* 1998;41:904–910.

89. Acton KJ, Burrows NR, Moore K, et al. Trends in diabetes prevalence among American Indian and Alaska Native children, adolescents, and young adults. *Am J Public Health* 2002;92:1485–1490.

90. U.S. Preventive Services Task Force. Screening for Gestational Diabetes Mellitus: Recommendations and Rationale. February 2003. Originally in *Obstet Gynecol* 2003;101:393–395. Agency for Healthcare Research and Quality, Rockville, MD. Available at: http://www.ahrq.gov/clinic/3rduspstf/gdm/gdmrr.htm. Accessed November 5, 2003.

91. Pettitt DJ, Aleck KA, Baird HR, et al. Congenital susceptibility to NIDDM. Role of intrauterine environment. *Diabetes* 1988;37:622–628.

92. Gruber E, Anderson MM, Ponton L, et al. Overweight and obesity in Native American adolescents—comparing nonreservation youths with African-American and Caucasian peers. *Am J Prev Med* 1995;11:306–310.

93. Fitzgerald SJ, Kriska AM, Pereira MA, et al. Associations among physical activity, television watching, and obesity in adult Pima Indians. *Med Sci Sports Exerc* 1997;29:910–915.

94. Freedman DS, Sarcula MK, Percy CA, et al. Obesity, levels of lipids and glucose, and smoking among Navajo adolescents. *J Nutr* 1997;127:2120S–2127S.

95. Gray RS, Fabsitz RR, Cowan LD, et al. Relation of generalized and central obesity to cardiovascular risk factors and prevalent coronary heart disease in a sample of American Indians—the Strong Heart Study. *Int J of Obesity* 2000;24:849–860.

96. Spangler JG, Dignan MB, Michielutte R. Correlates of tobacco use among Native American women in western North Carolina. *Am J Public Health* 1997;87:108–111.

97. Kimball EH, Goldberg HI, Oberle MW. The prevalence of selected risk factors for chronic disease among American Indians in Washington State. *Public Health Rep* 1996;111:264–271.

98. Nelson DE, Moon RW, Holtzman D, et al. Patterns of health risk behaviors for chronic disease—a comparison between adolescent and adult American Indians living on or near reservations in Montana. *J Adolescent Health* 1997;21:25–32.

99. Kaplan SD, Lanier AP, Merritt RK, et al. Prevalence of tobacco use among Alaska Natives—a review. *Prev Med* 1997; 26:460–465.

100. LeMaster PL, Connell CM, Mitchell CM, et al. Tobacco use among American Indian adolescents—protective and risk factors. *J Adolesc Health* 2002;30:426–432.

101. Henderson PN, Rhoades D, Henderson JA, et al. Smoking cessation and its determinants among older American Indians: the Strong Heart Study. *Ethn Dis* 2004;14:274–279.

102. Wallace JM, Bachman JB, O'Malley PM, et al. Tobacco, alcohol, and illicit drug use—racial and ethnic differences among U.S. high school seniors, 1976–2000. *Public Health Rep* 2002;117:S67–S75.

103. Substance Abuse and Mental Health Services Administration. Results from the 2002 National Survey on Drug Use and Health: National Findings (Office of Applied Studies, NHSDA Series H-22, DHHS Publication No. SMA 03–3836). Rockville, MD, 2003.

104. May PA. Alcohol abuse and alcoholism among American Indians—an overview. In: Watts TD, Wright R, eds. Alcoholism in minority populations. Springfield, IL: Charles C. Thomas Publisher. 1989:95–119.

105. Smith CJ, Nelson RG, Hardy SA, et al. Survey of the diet of Pima Indians using quantitative food frequency assessment and 24-hour recall. *J Am Diet Assoc* 1996;96:778–783.

106. Dewailly E, Blanchet C, Gringras S, et al. Cardiovascular disease risk factors and n-3 fatty acid status in the adult population of James Bay Creek. *Am J Clin Nutr* 2002;76:85–92.

107. Gillum RF. The epidemiology of stroke in Native Americans. *Stroke* 1995;26:514–521.

108. Frey JL, Jahnke HD, Bulfinch EW. Differences in stroke between white, Hispanic, and Native American patients: the Barrow Neurological Institute stroke database. *Stroke* 1998; 29:29–33.

109. Kttapong VJ, Becker TM. Ethnic differences in mortality from cerebrovascular disease among New Mexico's Hispanics, Native Americans, and non-Hispanic whites, 1958 through 1987. *Ethn Dis* 1993;3:75–82.

110. U.S. Department of Health and Human Services: Building healthy hearts for American Indians and Alaska Natives—a background report. U.S. Department of Health and Human Services, National Institutes of Health, National Heart, Lung, and Blood Institute. Bethesda, MD, 1998.

111. Hood VL, Kelly B, Martinez C, et al. A Native American community initiative to prevent diabetes. *Ethn Health* 1997;2:277–285.

112. Broussard BA, Sugarman JR, Bachman-Carter K, et al. Toward comprehensive obesity prevention programs in Native American communities. *Obesity Res* 1995;3: 289s–297s.

113. Caballero B, Clay T, Davis SM, et al. Pathways: a school-based, randomized controlled trial for the prevention of obesity in American Indian schoolchildren. *Am J Clin Nutr* 2003;78(5):1030–1038.

114. The Diabetes Prevention Program Research Group: The Diabetes Prevention Program (DPP). *Diabetes Care* 2002;25:2165–2171.

115. The Diabetes Prevention Program Research Group. Reduction in the incidence of type 2 diabetes with lifestyle intervention or metformin. *NEJM* 2002;346:393–403.

116. Pettitt DJ, Forman MR, Hanson RL, et al. Breastfeeding and incidence of non-insulin-dependent diabetes mellitus in Pima Indians. *Lancet* 1997;350(9072):166–168.

117. Day TW. Cross cultural medicine at home. *Minn Med* 1992;75:15–17.

118. Moy E, Bartman BA. Physician race and care of minority and medically indigent patients. *JAMA* 1995;273:1515–1520.

119. U.S. Commission on Civil Rights A Quiet Crisis. Federal Funding and Unmet Needs in Indian Country. Washington, D.C. U.S. Commission on Civil Rights. July, 2003.

120. Bush GW. Remarks by the President to the 2003 Urban League Conference, David Lawrence Convention Center, Pittsburgh, Pennsylvania, July 28, 2003. Available at: http://www.whitehouse.gov/news/releases/2003/07/20030728-3.html. Accessed December 6, 2003.

121. Bush GW. Remarks of the President on Education Reform and Parental Options, Kipp D.C. Key Academy, Washington, D.C., July 1, 2003. Available at: http://www.whitehouse.gov/news/releases/2003/07/20030701-3.html. Accessed December 6, 2003.

122. U.S. Department of Health and Human Services National Forum on Health Disparity Issues for American Indians and Alaska Natives Summary Report. U.S. Department of Health and Human Services, Office of Minority Health web site, September 2002. Available at: http://www.omhrc.gov/inetpub/wwwroot/omh/tribal%20colleges/2pgtcu/plans_tcu_002.htm. Accessed December 6, 2003.

123. Mathis R. Moorehouse's medicine man. *Atlanta Tribune Magazine*, April 2001.

PART V

Comprehensive Approaches to Prevention

Primary prevention

22

Matthew A. Wilson
Thomas A. Pearson

KEY POINTS

- *Population studies have documented a slowing of rates of decline in mortality and incidence of coronary heart disease in the 1990s.*

- *The reduction in the case fatality rate coupled with the slower rate of decline in incidence will lead to a doubling of coronary heart disease prevalence from 12.5 million in 2000 to 25 million by 2050.*

- *Proper exercise, weight management, smoking cessation, moderate alcohol consumption, and healthy diet are factors that have been identified with an 83% reduction in coronary heart disease risk.*

- *There are two approaches to primary prevention of cardiovascular disease: the populationwide approach and the high-risk approach.*

- *The populationwide approach can be used to address behavioral risk factors at the community level.*

- *The success of the populationwide approach relies on surveillance, populationwide education, partnerships with community organizations, assurance of health services, environmental change, and policy/legislation.*

- *The populationwide approach should address a brief list of modifiable risk factors: diet, sedentary lifestyle, tobacco use, accessing screening and diagnostic services to detect occult risk factors, and early recognition of symptomatic cardiovascular disease.*

- *The high-risk approach should assess both nonmodifiable and modifiable risk factors to determine individual risk.*

- An individual risk assessment should consist of measuring blood pressure, pulse, height, weight, body mass index, waist circumference, lipid profile, and fasting blood glucose level.

- A global risk score for persons 40 years and older should help identify high-risk individuals and assist in the determination of the appropriate intervention.

- Evidence-based intervention for the primary prevention of cardiovascular disease can be remembered as the ABCs of preventive cardiology: Aspirin, Blood cholesterol, Cigarettes, Diabetes, Exercise, Food, Girth, High blood pressure, and Irregular pulse.

GENERAL APPROACHES TO PRIMARY PREVENTION

A variety of approaches might be considered to reduce the populationwide burden of heart disease, stroke, and peripheral vascular disease. While *secondary prevention* refers to the prevention of death or recurrence of disease in those who are already symptomatic, *primary prevention* pertains to the prevention of the onset of symptomatic disease in persons without prior symptoms of cardiovascular disease (CVD) by means of treatment of risk factors with lifestyle modifications or drugs. An additional approach is *primordial prevention*, in which the factors causative of CVD, or "risk factors" (Fig. 22-1), would be prevented, thereby reducing the likelihood of developing the disease itself and avoiding treatment of risk factors. The distinction between primary and secondary prevention has become increasingly difficult, due to the ability to identify subclinical disease at early stages with increasingly sensitive technologies. These technologies can identify pathophysiologic states, early lesions, or silent disease in persons who have never been symptomatic. Therefore, primary prevention could be redefined as prevention of the atherosclerotic disease process itself, with secondary

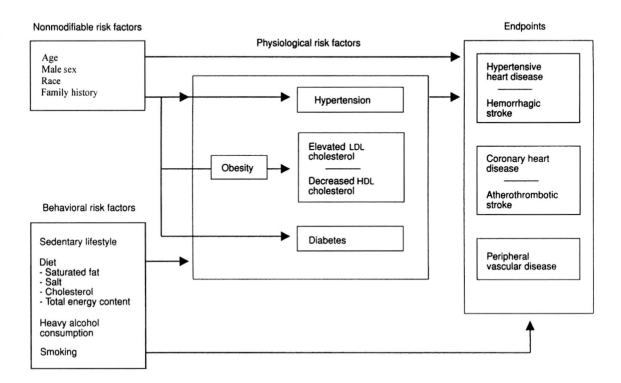

FIGURE 22-1 Relationships between cardiovascular risk factors and cardiovascular disease.

prevention being treatment of the atherosclerotic disease process.[1]

Key to the primary prevention of CVD is the notion of risk factors. A combination of clinical, epidemiologic, and experimental studies have established the role of a number of measurable traits as agents etiologically related to atherosclerotic CVD. In considering these factors as part of an effort to prevent CVD, it may be useful to subclassify them as nonmodifiable, behavioral, and physiologic (see Fig. 22-1).[2] *Nonmodifiable* factors, such as age, sex, race, and family history of CVD, might be used to identify high-risk groups benefiting from special programs. *Behavioral* risk factors, such as a sedentary lifestyle, unhealthful diet, heavy alcohol consumption, and cigarette smoking, might be approached on either

a populationwide or individual basis. These behaviors and all nonmodifiable factors may, in turn, be related to the *physiologic* risk factors (hypertension, obesity, lipid disorders, diabetes) that are generally measured clinically and often managed pharmacologically. The distinction between behavioral and physiologic risk factors takes on added importance in primary prevention: behavioral risk factors can be approached on a populationwide basis and physiologic risk factors are often targets of the high-risk approach (see Fig. 22-1).

In general, there are two approaches to primary prevention: *the populationwide approach* and the *high-risk approach.*[3] Consider the distribution of risk or of a risk factor in the population. In Fig. 22-2,[4] the distribution of serum cholesterol levels in the US population identifies

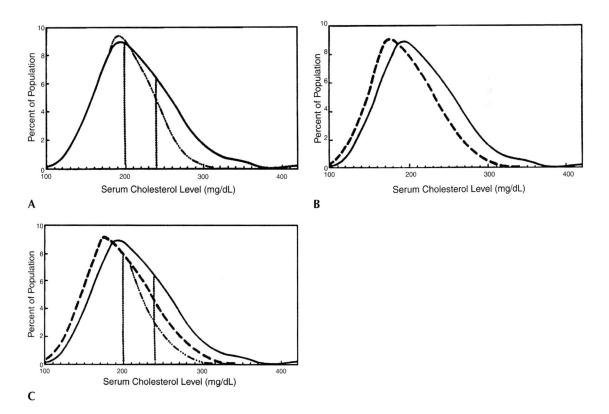

A

B

C

FIGURE 22-2 **A.** Cholesterol distribution in the US population aged 20 to 74 from the *National Health and Nutrition Examination Survey II* (1976–1980) and potential changes in the distribution. Expected shift in population distribution of serum cholesterol values with application of high-risk approach (Adult Treatment Panel Guidelines of National Cholesterol Education Program). Dashed line represents effect of recommendations. **B.** Expected shift in population distribution of serum cholesterol values with application of populationwide approach (Population Panel of the National Cholesterol Education Program). Dashed line represents effect of recommendations. **C.** Anticipated combined effects of a high-risk (dotted-dashed line) approach applied to a populationwide approach (dashed line) of the National Cholesterol Education Program. (Reproduced, with permission, from Carleton et al.[4])

an entire population at higher risk than other populations who have a lower burden of coronary disease, such as the Japanese. Although the difference in averages between two populations are important, there is also a variation in the level of serum cholesterol (the same applies to other risk factors) within a population. Most people are found in the middle of the bell-shaped distribution of values, but a "tail" exists of persons with higher values. One intervention would be the so-called high-risk approach, in which individuals with high values in the "tail" are identified and intensively treated, resulting in reduction of their risk to that of people in the middle of the curve (see Fig. 22-2A). This is, in essence, what a clinician does when a patient's high cholesterol or blood pressure is assessed and drugs are prescribed to reduce the levels into the "normal" range.

The problem with sole reliance on the high-risk approach is that most cases of CVD do not occur in high-risk subjects. Although the rate of CVD is higher for these individuals, high-risk subjects account for a small percentage of those who suffer with CVD. Most cases of CVD occur among those with "average" risk. True reduction in the population burden of CVD may result only from shifting the entire population level of risk factors (see Fig. 22-2B). An example of this approach is the populationwide reductions in serum cholesterol in the 1970s and 1980s in the United States as a result of changes in the American diet. This is the populationwide or public health approach.

The two approaches need not be exclusive. In reality, combinations of high-risk and populationwide approaches are usually employed in practice (see Fig. 22-2C). The purpose of this chapter is to discuss these practical strategies as applied to populations and individuals.

THE NEED FOR EMPHASIS ON PRIMARY PREVENTION

In the United States, coronary heart disease mortality has declined steadily since 1968, and stroke mortality has declined steadily since 1900.[5] Recent data have documented this continued decline in cardiovascular mortality, but at a slower rate since 1990 (Fig. 22-3).[5] To understand these trends, both incidence and case fatality rates must be examined. Case fatality rates for acute coronary syndrome continue to decline, raising the question: "What are the trends in coronary disease incidence?" A population-based study in Worcester, Massachusetts, documents the declining incidence rate for acute myocardial infarction as a measure of coronary heart disease incidence rates until 1990, with no further declines since then (Fig. 22-4).[6] In Olmstead County, Minnesota, coronary incidence rates in males stopped declining in the 1990s; rates for females appear to have increased in this period (Fig. 22-5).[7] One obligatory consequence of this stagnation in the decline of coronary heart disease (CHD) incidence, coupled with continued improvements in case fatality rates, is a corresponding rise in prevalence. Currently, 12.5 million Americans carry the diagnosis of symptomatic CHD; by 2050 the prevalence will at least double to 25 million Americans, a

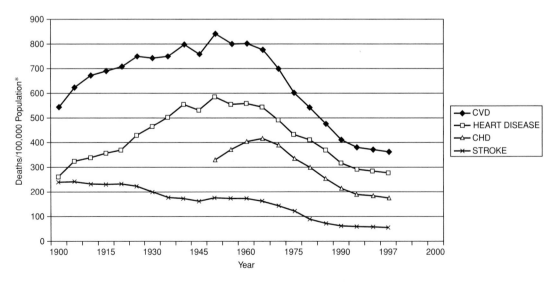

FIGURE 22-3 Death rates for major cardiovascular disease in the United States from 1900 to 1997. Rates are age adjusted to 2000 standard. (Reproduced, with permission, from Cooper et al.[5])

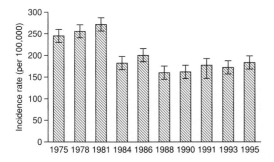

FIGURE 22-4 Temporal trends in the age-adjusted incidence rates of initial acute myocardial infarction: Worcester Heart Attack Study. (Reproduced, with permission, from Goldberg et al.[6])

number that exceeds the entire population of many countries (Fig. 22-6).[8] The contributions of this burden to disability rates, health care costs, and secondary prevention utilization are enormous. The reduction of these ominous trends makes it important to emphasize primary prevention.

THE POPULATIONWIDE APPROACH TO PRIMARY PREVENTION

Conceptual framework for the populationwide approach

The rationale for the populationwide approach to CVD prevention is derived not only from the observation that most cases of CVD have average or slightly above-average risks. Rather, CVD might be considered a disease of Occidental culture, with markedly higher rates of CVD associated with whole populations who adopt a Western lifestyle comprising a high-fat, high-cholesterol diet, tobacco use, and lack of physical activity. Epidemiologic evidence for this cultural basis of CVD is extensive, and is derived from multiple sources, including: comparisons of risk factors and CVD rates between populations, trends in CVD rates, studies of migrants to high-risk societies, and results of public health trials.[9] The basic tenet of the populationwide approach is: If the basis of CVD is social and economic, the solution to the CVD epidemic must be social and economic.[3]

In considering populationwide strategies to control CVD, the major targets are often those populationwide behaviors that can be causative of the physiologic risk factors (eg, a high-fat diet, which contributes to elevated low-density lipoprotein cholesterol [LDL-C] and obesity) as well as directly causative of CVD (eg, cigarette smoking) (see Fig. 22-1). In the United States Nurses Study, women who exercised regularly, were of normal body weight, did not smoke, drank alcohol moderately, and ate a high-quality diet enjoyed an 83% reduction in CHD risk.[10] This suggests those five behaviors account for the vast majority of cases of CVD. A conceptual framework can then be developed as to how these risk factors and risk behaviors might be approached on a populationwide basis (Fig. 22-7). This requires the application of essential public health services such as surveillance, education, organizational partnerships, assurance of personal health services, and legislation/policy[11] in a variety of community settings including work sites, health care facilities, religious organizations, schools, and whole communities.[12] The result is a grid in which a small number of specific behaviors might be targeted for specific interventions in specific community settings, which, in aggregate, make up an entire population (see Fig. 22-7).[13]

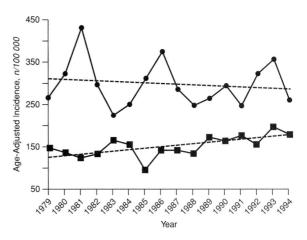

FIGURE 22-5 Trends in the incidence of myocardial infarction from 1979 to 1994 in Olmsted County, Minnesota. Circles represent data for men, and squares, data for women. Incidence is shown on a linear scale and was adjusted, using the direct method, to the age distribution of the total US population in 2000. The heavy dotted lines represent the predicted values for the trends in incidence over time based on a Poisson regression model. (Reproduced, with permission, from Roger et al.[7])

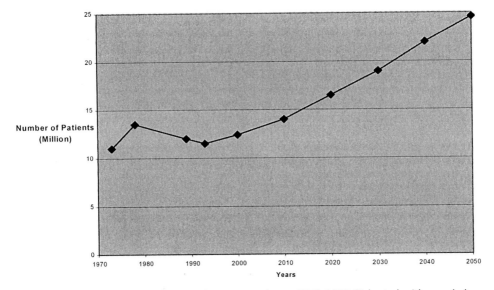

FIGURE 22-6 Projection of US heart disease prevalence, 1970–2050. (Adapted, with permission, from Foote et al.[8])

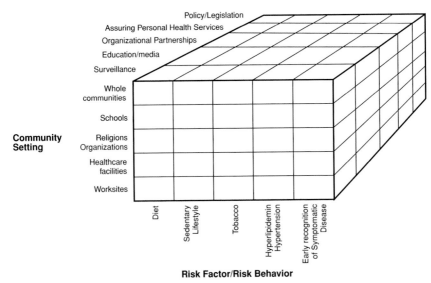

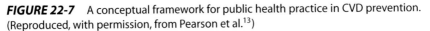

FIGURE 22-7 A conceptual framework for public health practice in CVD prevention. (Reproduced, with permission, from Pearson et al.[13])

Strategies for populationwide prevention of CVD

OVERVIEW

The *American Heart Association Guide for Improving Cardiovascular Health at the Community Level* [14] provides a method of developing comprehensive programs for improving the cardiovascular health of a community. This entails the organization and implementation of programs and dissemination of information at the community level, with multifaceted interventions targeting the community as a whole, schools, religious organizations, health care facilities, and work sites. This dissemination of information should focus on a relatively brief list of modifiable behaviors: diet, sedentary lifestyle, tobacco use, accessing screening and diagnostic services to detect potentially occult risk factors (hypertension, dyslipidemia, diabetes), and early recognition of symptoms of CVD, especially acute coronary syndromes and stroke. Intervention programs should provide surveillance, education, organizational partnerships, personal health services, and communitywide policy and legislation. The American Heart Association Guide provides specific recommendations that may be implemented for each of these strategies (Appendix 22-1). These recommendations are reviewed in this section. One strategy toward a healthier population is to try to change the adult population's behavior; another is to raise children to be healthier. The American Heart Association Scientific Statement on Cardiovascular Health in Childhood[15] recommends strategies and methods for creating a healthy environment for children. The scientific statement establishes a multidisciplinary approach to evaluate children from birth to adolescence, and makes the CVD evaluation a continuous family process.

SURVEILLANCE AND POPULATIONWIDE DATA

A number of strategies are available for influencing populationwide CVD prevention, including surveillance of the burden of CVD in the population.[16] In most countries in Western Europe, North America, and Australia/New Zealand, CVD has been recognized as the leading cause of death for half a century. Only recently, however, has attention been focused on CVD as the major cause of disability and death in developing countries.[17] Data on mortality for CVD can be misleading, as case fatality rates from myocardial infarction, angina, and stroke decline. Morbidity data are much more difficult to obtain and often show little change in incidence (see Figs. 22-4 and 22-5) and an increase in prevalence with an associated increase in health care costs. Risk factor prevalence data are available at the state level in the United States from sources like the Behavioral Risk Factor Survey. These data suggest that certain risk factors such as obesity and diabetes are increasing at rates capable of creating a modern epidemic. Such data may be useful in creating the political and social will to target populationwide behaviors at all levels.[18,19] The data can also be used to support policy and legislative efforts to provide health care services or a healthier environment.

PUBLIC HEALTH EDUCATION/MEDIA

Community interventions have frequently used a variety of different channels of communication to increase awareness of CVD to modify public behaviors. Several community interventions to control CVD have used mass media and print media extensively. A useful consideration in selecting media for intervention is the audience and the message to be conveyed. Flora and co-workers have proposed a framework in which the media might be selected.[20] Selection of a medium might focus on reaching a large number of people minimally or targeting a select group of the population more intensely. The message might serve to alert the audience or get them to contemplate the issue. The recent explosion of electronic communication has exposed a medium that can be considered high reach with internet access to large numbers of people, or it can provide high specificity with directed e-mail. Other types of media, such as posters and church bulletins, can be tailored to the local community.

COMMUNITY ORGANIZATIONS AND PARTNERSHIPS

A cornerstone of the Victoria Declaration on Heart Health was the recognition that a large number of sectors of the community would have to become actively involved if the mass epidemic of CVD were to be controlled.[18] These sectors include: (1) health, media, education, and social science professionals; (2) the scientific research community; (3) governmental agencies concerned with health, education, trade, commerce, and agriculture; (4) the private sector, including health, food, and transportation industries; (5) international organizations and agencies concerned with health and economic development; (6) community health coalitions and voluntary health organizations such as heart associations and foundations; (7) employers and employee organizations, such as unions. Coalition building would be essential to tackle a problem of this magnitude.

ASSURANCE OF PERSONAL HEALTH SERVICES

Strategies should be in place to ensure that services are available to high-risk residents for the purpose of reducing their risk (see below). This may entail interaction with the existing health system, health care providers, clinics, hospitals, and third-party payers, to guarantee access to proven, cost-effective preventive services.

POLICY AND LEGISLATION

Another approach to modification of populationwide behaviors could be the development of policies that affect the environments in which people live and the regulations by which they live.[12] In the United States, government policies involving tobacco have continued to evolve, including taxation, civil litigation, restriction of smoking in various buildings and work sites, control of sales of tobacco to children, and elimination of advertising. These policies are by no means limited to governments, with numerous private companies instituting their own regulations on clean air, increased health care and life insurance premiums for smokers, and even hiring criteria favoring nonsmokers. Similarly, policies related to physical activity might relate to requirements for physical education curricula in the schools, reimbursement for physical activity counseling by health care professionals, corporate and communitywide fitness events or competitions, and development of facilities (eg, gymnasia and walking/biking paths) that would encourage physical activity. Finally, nutrition policy can be effective in changing eating behaviors through price supports and taxation, dietary guidelines, food assistance programs, and school meals.[21] The health care professional may also need to serve as an advocate to advance these policy goals,[19] with timely counseling and evaluation on an individual level and education/policy input on a public level.

Evidence for effectiveness in various settings

INTERVENTIONS IN WHOLE COMMUNITIES

Over the past 30 years, a number of studies aimed at reducing the entire population's risk of CVD have been carried out in Europe, Africa, North America, and Australia.[22] These often include programs in specific community settings, such as work sites, schools, and religious organizations. Although the trials have differed considerably in their approach, a common theme was to change behavior not only in the individual but also in the family, society, and culture targeted for intervention. These communitywide interventions typically used multiple media, provided multiple health education messages, and had multiple target groups.[23,24]

Two early projects provided preliminary evidence for the efficacy of this approach. The Stanford Three Community Study (1972–1975) used two intervention approaches: (1) a mass media campaign (radio, television, print media) and intensive instruction of high-risk residents, and (2) a media campaign alone. The two intervention communities were evaluated against a comparison community with no intervention.[25] The intervention communities demonstrated a 23% reduction in CHD risk score with respect to the comparison community.[26] The North Karelia Project (1972 to present) consisted of a comprehensive, populationwide intervention in the Finnish province of North Karelia, which at the time had one of the highest CVD mortality rates in the world.[27] A similar province was used as a comparison group. The intervention consisted of a public education campaign using radio, newspapers, and other printed material, group education, and environmental interventions. Striking reductions in smoking, dietary fat consumption, blood pressure, and blood cholesterol were observed. Between 1972 and 1978, CHD mortality in North Karelia decreased faster than in the comparison province and Finland as a whole (Fig. 22-8). These two projects provided the basis for a large number of additional programs investigating the process of community interventions for CVD prevention in more detail.[22]

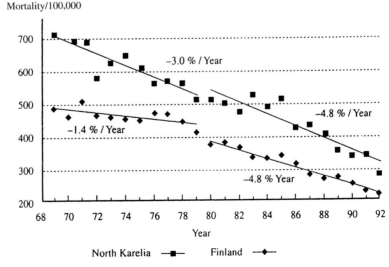

Mortality/100,000

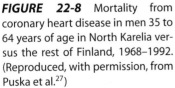

FIGURE 22-8 Mortality from coronary heart disease in men 35 to 64 years of age in North Karelia versus the rest of Finland, 1968–1992. (Reproduced, with permission, from Puska et al.[27])

Three large US trials were initiated to further explore community intervention in theory and in practice[22]: the Stanford Five-City Project (1980–1986),[28] the Minnesota Heart Health Program (1981–1988),[29] and the Pawtucket Heart Health Program (1984–1991).[30] Among the three projects, 13 communities with more than 900,000 people were studied, using a nonrandomized assignment of some communities to intervention and others as comparison communities. A large number of materials were developed and field-tested (Table 22-1). The Stanford Five-City Project demonstrated reductions in smoking, cholesterol, blood pressure, and CHD risk, though the biggest changes occurred early in the comparison.[28] Evaluation of the Minnesota Heart Health Program suggested that physical activity increased and smoking decreased in women.[29] The Pawtucket Heart Health Program also showed a reduction in CHD risk.[30] All programs demonstrated success in organizing and in implementing various aspects of their intervention strategies.

These three large US trials generally had less effect and less sustenance than hypothesized, for reasons that are not entirely clear.[12,22,31] There does seem to be a consensus that community-based interventions (with multiple messages, multiple target groups, and using multiple media) can change the knowledge, attitudes, and behaviors of individuals. Community-based interventions can also encourage environmental changes supportive of healthy lifestyles.[22] Community interventions targeting only one risk factor, however, may be less likely to be successful. The Community Intervention Trial for Smoking Cessation (COMMIT) focused on smoking

TABLE 22-1 Materials Developed for Use in the Minnesota Heart Health Program, the Stanford Five-City Project, and the Pawtucket Heart Health Program

Mass media
Other print (kits, brochures, direct mail)
Events and contests
Screenings
Group and direct education
School programs
Work site interventions
Physician and medical setting programs
Grocery store and restaurant projects
Church interventions
Policies

SOURCE: Reproduced, with permission, from Schooler et al.[22]

cessation among 11 matched community pairs but failed to demonstrate differences in smoking prevalence among intervention and control communities.[32] Quit rates in light to moderate smokers were affected positively, but there was no effect among heavy smokers.[33] Additional analyses suggest that subpopulations, especially those of lower socioeconomic status, may benefit more from these approaches.[34] A large number of subsequent communitywide programs currently underway will continue to enlarge this experience.[22]

INTERVENTIONS IN SCHOOLS AND YOUTH ORGANIZATIONS

Interventions among children attending school offer several advantages to population-based CVD prevention.[35] First, there is good evidence that atherosclerotic disease is well established by the late teenage years, that the risk factors measured in childhood track into adulthood, and that exercise, eating, and smoking behaviors are well established by the early teenage years.[15] Second, school-based programs can involve venues other than the classroom, including school nutrition programs and physical education curricula.[35] Third, school is mandatory, allowing most of the population to be reached. Finally, schoolchildren are an excellent vector for transmitting health messages home to their parents.

Over the past 20 years, a large number of school-based programs to reduce CVD risk have been implemented and evaluated.[35] In general, a variety of theoretical models were employed, with interventions using a wide range of educational techniques, durations and intensities of intervention, and age groups. A meta-analysis of the studies suggests that interventions targeted at smoking behavior and knowledge about CVD and its risk factors were most effective; interventions to improve blood pressure and obesity were least effective; and diet, blood cholesterol, stress, and physical activity interventions were intermediate. Programs with multiple components seemed more effective than single-component interventions.[12] An interesting conclusion was that behavior change may be a more appropriate target in children, whose physiologic measures are changing rapidly during growth and development.

INTERVENTION IN RELIGIOUS ORGANIZATIONS

Religious organizations also offer a number of advantages as sites for primary prevention of CVD. Religious communities often have strong influences on health behavior, and religious organizations offer social support, facilities, volunteers, and networks for communication.[36] Hard-to-reach subpopulations such as specific ethnic and racial groups may be accessed through their religious leaders. Despite this, very few studies have rigorously evaluated communities of faith as a means to reduce CVD risk. In one review, relatively few well-designed studies could be identified.[36] At this point, it can best be concluded that religious organizations offer enormous untapped potential for development of effective CVD prevention programs.

INTERVENTIONS AT WORK SITES

Work sites also offer rich opportunities to influence employee behavior. Increasingly, employers are responsible for the health care costs of their work force, and replacement of skilled workers disabled by or deceased from CVD is an added cost. Managed care organizations that have capitated contracts to provide health services to workers have an additional incentive to prevent, rather than treat, disease. Moreover, work sites can be more than just places to provide health education messages. Environmental interventions such as smoke-free areas and heart-healthy food services can be initiated. The employer can further provide incentives to reduce CVD through reduced health insurance premiums, coverage of athletic center dues, on-site CVD risk reduction programs, and on-site self-measurement of blood pressure and weight.

Well-documented studies of work site CVD prevention programs suggest that brief, low-intensity interventions targeted at the entire work force show little evidence of effectiveness, whereas counseling provided to high-risk employees identified within the entire work force has had the best results.[37,38] As employers and health care providers become increasingly concerned about costs, it is likely that work site programs will expand as a means of identifying and modifying CVD risk in employees.

INDIVIDUAL APPROACHES TO HIGH-RISK POPULATIONS

Health care facilities should be included as important community settings for populationwide CVD risk reduction.[39] Physicians remain among the most credible sources of health information for the population, and the majority of the population has contact with the medical care system at least once a year. Surveys of CVD prevention-related services, such as smoking cessation advice, measurement and treatment of lipid disorders, and physical activity assessment and counseling, are often disappointing.[40,41] A variety of factors at the levels of the patient, physician, health care setting, and community/society may interfere with the provision of these services (Table 22-2).[42]

As a first step in rectifying this problem, the *American Heart Association Guidelines for Primary Prevention of Cardiovascular Disease and Stroke: 2002 Update* provides evidence-based guidance for risk factor assessment, lifestyle modification, and pharmacologic interventions, as well as specific recommendations regarding individual risk factors (Table 22-3).[43] These risk factors might be arranged into the ABCs of Primary Prevention

TABLE 22-2 Barriers to Implementation of Preventive Services

Patient
Lack of knowledge and motivation
Lack of access to care
Cultural factors
Social factors
Physician
Problem-based focus
Feedback on prevention is native or neutral
Time constraints
Lack of incentives, including reimbursement
Lack of training
Poor knowledge of benefits
Perceived ineffectiveness
Lack of skills
Lack of specialist–generalist communication
Lack of perceived legitimacy
Health care settings (hospitals, practices, etc)
Acute care priority
Lack of resources and facilities
Lack of systems for preventive services
Time and economic constraints
Poor communication between specialty and primary care providers
Lack of policies and standards
Community/society
Lack of policies and standards
Lack of reimbursement

SOURCE: Reproduced, with permission, from Pearson et al.[42]

(Table 22-4), to help the health care provider remember the nine things to consider in the asymptomatic patient. Guidelines that highlight preventive cardiology strategies in women have also been issued.[44] All guidelines should be reconciled with the latest evidence-based information, such as is the case with blood pressure guidelines,[45] to create a single, consistent set of recommendations for the busy clinician.

Individual risk assessment

A key recommendation of the AHA Primary Prevention Guidelines is that CVD risk should be assessed in all patients through careful history, physical examination, and selected laboratory testing.[43] Risk factors such as tobacco use, poor diet, alcohol intake, lack of physical activity, and family history of CHD should be routinely evaluated at every visit. Physical parameters such as blood pressure, pulse (for atrial fibrillation), height, weight, body mass index, and waist circumference should be assessed regularly. Physiologic parameters such as lipid profiles and fasting blood glucose levels should be measured in all

TABLE 22-3   Guide to Primary Prevention of Cardiovascular Disease and Stroke

Risk intervention goal	Recommendations
Smoking *Goal:* complete cessation; no exposure to environmental tobacco smoke	Ask about tobacco use status at every visit. In a clear, strong, and personalized manner, advise every tobacco user to quit. Assess the tobacco user's willingness to quit. Assist by counseling and developing a plan for quitting. Arrange follow-up, referral to special programs, or pharmacotherapy. Urge avoidance of exposure to secondhand smoke at work or home.

BP* control
   Normal: <120/<80 mm Hg
   Goal: <140/<90 mm Hg
   Goal with diabetes or chronic kidney disease: <130/ <80 mm Hg
	Promote healthy lifestyle modification. Advocate weight reduction; reduction of sodium intake; consumption of fruits, vegetables, and low-fat dairy products; moderation of alcohol intake; and physical activity in persons with BP ≥120 mm Hg systolic or ≥80 mm Hg diastolic. For persons with renal insufficiency or heart failure initiate drug therapy if BP is ≥130 mm Hg systolic or ≥85 mm Hg diastolic (≥80 mm Hg diastolic for patients with diabetes). Initiate drug therapy otherwise for those with BP ≥140/90 mm Hg. Add BP medications, individualized to other patient requirements and characteristics (eg, age, race, need for drugs with specific benefits).

Dietary intake *Goal:* overall healthy eating pattern	Advocate consumption of a variety of fruits, vegetables, grains, low-fat or nonfat dairy products, fish, legumes, poultry, and lean meats. Match energy intake with energy needs and make appropriate changes to achieve weight loss when indicated. Modify food choices to reduce saturated fats (<10% of calories), cholesterol (<300 mg/day and *trans* fatty acids by substituting grain and unsaturated fatty acids from fish, vegetables, legumes, and nuts. Limit salt intake to <6 g/d. Limit alcohol intake (≤2 drinks/d in men, ≤1 drink/d in women) among those who drink.
Aspirin *Goal:* low-dose aspirin in persons at higher CHD risk (especially those with 10-y risk of CHD ≥10%).	Do not recommend for patients with aspirin intolerance. Low-dose aspirin increases risk for gastrointestinal bleeding and hemorrhagic stroke. Do not use in persons at increased risk for these diseases. Benefits of cardiovascular risk reduction outweigh these risks in most patients at higher coronary risk. Doses of 75–160 mg/d are as effective as higher doses. Therefore, consider 75–160 mg aspirin per day for persons at higher risk (especially those with 10-y risk of CHD of ≥10%).

Blood lipid management
   Primary goal: LDL-C <160 mg/dL if ≤1 risk factor is present; LDL-C <130 mg/dL if ≥2 risk factors are present and 10-y CHD risk is <20%; or LDL-C <100 mg/dL if ≥2 risk factors are present and 10-y CHD risk is ≥20% or if patient has diabetes.
   Secondary goal (if LDL-C is at goal range): If triglycerides are >200 mg/dL, then use non-HDL-C as a secondary goal: non-HDL-C <190 mg/dL for ≤1 risk factor; non-HDL-C <160 mg/dL for ≥2 risk factors and 10-y CHD risk ≤20%; non-HDL-C <130 mg/dL for diabetics or for ≥2 risk factors and 10-y CHD risk >20%
	If LDL-C is above goal range, initials additional therapeutic lifestyle changes consisting of dietary modifications to lower LDL-C: <7% of calories from saturated fat, cholesterol < 200 mg/dL, and, if further LDL-C lowering is required, dietary options (plant stanols/sterols not to exceed 2 g/d and/or increased viscous [soluble] fiber (10–25 g/d), and additional emphasis on weight reduction and physical activity. If LDL-C is above goal range, rule out secondary causes (liver function test, thyroid-stimulating hormone level, urinalysis). After 12 wks of therapeutic lifestyle change, consider LDL-lowering drug therapy if: ≥2 risk factors are present, 10-y risk is >10%, and LDL-C is ≥130 mg/dL; ≥2 risk factors are present, 10-y risk is <10%, and LDL-C is ≥160 mg/dL; or ≤1 risk factor is present and LDL-C is ≥190 mg/dL. Start drugs and advance dose to bring LDL-C to goal range, usually a statin but also consider bile acid-binding resin or niacin. If LDL-C goal not achieved, consider combination therapy (statin+resin, statin+niacin). After LDL-C goal has been reached, consider triglyceride level: if 150–199 mg/dL, treat with therapeutic lifestyle changes. If 200–499 mg/dL, treat elevated non-HDL-C with therapeutic lifestyle changes and, if necessary, consider higher doses of statin or adding niacin or fibrate. If >500 mg/dL, treat with fibrate or niacin to reduce risk of pancreatitis. If HDL-C is <40 mg/dL in men and <50 mg/dL in women, initiate or intensify therapeutic lifestyle changes. For higher-risk patients, consider drugs that raise HDL-C (eg. niacin, fibrates, statins).

(continued)

TABLE 22-3 (Continued)

Risk intenention goal	Recommendations
Other targets for therapy: triglycerides ≥150 mg/dL; HDL-C <40 mg/dL in men and <50 mg/dL in women	
Physical activity *Goal:* At least 30 min of moderate-intensity physical activity on most (and preferably all) days of the week.	If cardiovascular, respiratory, metabolic, orthopedic, or neurologic disorders are suspected, or if patient is middle-aged or older and is sedentary, consult physician before initiating vigorous exercise program. Moderate-intensity activities (40–60% of maximum capacity) are equivalent to a brisk walk (15–20 min per mile). Additional benefits are gained from vigorous-intensity activity (>60% of maximum capacity) for 20–40 min on 3–5 d/wk. Recommend resistance training with 8–10 different exercises, 1–2 sets per exercise, and 10–15 repetitions at moderate intensity ≥2 d/wk. Flexibility training and an increase in daily lifestyle activities should complement this regimen.
Weight management *Goal:* Achieve and maintain desirable weight (BMI 18.5–24.9 kg/m^2). When BMI is ≥25 kg/m^2, waist circumference at iliac crest level ≤40 in. in men, ≤35 in. in women	Initiate weight-management program through caloric restriction and increased caloric expenditure as appropriate. For overweight/obese persons, reduce body weight by 10% in first year of therapy.
Diabetes management *Goals:* Normal fasting plasma glucose (<110 mg/dL) and near-normal HbA$_{1c}$ <7%)	Initiate appropriate hypoglycemic therapy to achieve near-normal fasting plasma glucose or as indicated by near-normal HbA$_{1c}$. First step is diet and exercise. Second-step therapy is usually oral hypoglycemic drugs: sulfonylureas and/or metformin with ancillary use of acarbose and thiazolidinediones. Third-step therapy is insulin. Treat other risk factors more aggressively (eg, change BP goal to <130/80 mm Hg and LDL-C goal to <100 mg/dL).
Chronic atrial fibrillation *Goals:* Normal sinus rhythm or, if chronic atrial fibrillation is present, anticoagulation with INR 2.0–3.0 (target 2.5)	Irregular pulse should be verified by an electrocardiogram. Conversion of appropriate individuals to normal sinus rhythm. For patients in chronic or intermittent atrial fibrillation, use warfarin anticoagulants to INR 2.0–3.0 (target 2.5). Aspirin (325 mg/d) can be used as an alternative in those with certain contraindications to oral anticoagulation. Patients <65 y of age without high risk may be treated with aspirin.

*BP, blood pressure; CHD, coronary heart disease; LDL-C, low-density lipoprotein cholesterol; HDL-C, high-density lipoprotein cholesterol; BMI, body mass index; INR, international normalized ratio.

SOURCE: Adapted, with permission, from Pearson et al.[43]

adults 20 years of age and older. The CVD risk assessment should not be time-consuming or expensive, and is amenable to performance at settings outside of health care facilities, such as work sites and pharmacies. The assessment should be performed at least every 5 years in generally healthy individuals, with more frequent monitoring in high-risk persons. Another key part of the recommendations is the establishment of goals for the various risk factors (see Table 22-3). The definition of "desirable levels" serves as a means of identifying and prioritizing behavioral interventions. These levels provide goals for behavioral and pharmacologic intervention.

The next step in risk factor assessment is calculation of a *global risk* score in persons aged 40 years and older.

The concept here is to factor in the individual contributions of a person's risk factors into an overall risk of CHD. One benefit of this approach is the identification of those who are at high risk not because of a single markedly elevated risk factor, but rather because of the presence of several moderately elevated risk factors. It is likely that a larger proportion of the population at high risk falls into this latter group and not into a group comprising those with a single elevated risk factor.[46] The Third Report of The National Cholesterol Education Program (NCEP) Expert Panel on Detection, Evaluation, and Treatment of High Blood Cholesterol in Adults (Adult Treatment Panel III) provides an updated risk calculator.[47] It includes total serum cholesterol, high-density lipoprotein

TABLE 22-4   The ABCs of Primary Prevention

A	Aspirin
B	Blood cholesterol
C	Cigarettes
D	Diabetes
E	Exercise (physical activity)
F	Food (diet)
G	Girth (obesity)
H	High blood pressure
I	Irregular pulse

cholesterol (HDL-C), systolic blood pressure, age, sex, and smoking grouped into categories; scores are assigned and summed to provide estimates of 10-year risk of myocardial infarction and CHD death (Table 22-5). The AHA Primary Prevention Guidelines recommend that all persons 40 years of age and older have their 10-year risk score calculated every 5 years.[43,45] Diabetes is a CHD risk equivalent, and designates a high risk for CHD. The Joint European Societies have used this multiple-risk approach to develop figures that allow the visual calculation of an absolute risk of developing CHD (myocardial infarction or CHD death) over the next 10 years based on age, sex, smoking, systolic blood pressure, and total cholesterol level.[48] The absolute risk then classifies patients without CHD or diabetes according to their 10-year absolute risk of CHD as low (<10%), intermediate (10–20%), and high (>20%).

It is likely that additional methods for risk assessment will be developed and proven to be cost-effective in the health care setting. In this context, it is useful to differentiate risk factors from risk markers.[49] The term *risk factor* is usually reserved for a characteristic felt to be etiologically related to a disease. The implication is that modification of the factor will prevent the disease's development or progression. Other characteristics may be associated with a disease, but not necessarily in an etiologic fashion. Such characteristics are called *risk markers*, which can be used to identify persons at high risk for the disease in whom aggressive intervention may be worthwhile. A variety of new risk markers have been proposed, including measures of inflammation (eg, C-reactive protein),[48] prothrombotic diathesis (eg, fibrinogen), altered endothelial function (eg, endothelium-dependent brachial reactivity), physiologic evidence of atherosclerosis (eg, ankle–brachial blood pressure index), and noninvasive evidence of atherosclerosis (eg, carotid artery intima–media thickness ratios and coronary calcification detected from computed tomography). Many of these new risk assessment approaches are promising, but have not been fully exam-

ined in primary prevention settings for efficacy or cost-effectiveness.[50] Well-designed clinical studies, such as the ongoing National Institutes of Health-sponsored Multiethnic Study of Atherosclerosis (MESA),[51] will further define the role of a number of screening modalities in cardiovascular risk assessment.

Matching the level of risk with the intensity of the intervention

The use of information about an individual's risk may differ between the patient, the care provider, and the payer for health care services.[52] Traditionally, risk estimation has been used to inform the patient of the importance of changes in risk behaviors or the need for treatment. Increasingly, however, health care providers and payers have used risk stratification to better reserve aggressive (and often expensive) interventions for those at highest risk. Interventions to lower LDL-C serve as a good illustration (Fig. 22-9).[53–55] Clinical trials of HMGCoA reductase inhibitors have demonstrated efficacy in virtually every stratum of risk, from persons with elevated LDL-C levels and myocardial infarction to persons without evidence of coronary disease and relatively normal LDL-C levels. The Air Force/Texas Coronary Atherosclerosis Prevention Study (AFCAPS/TexCAPS) serves as a good example.[55] In the trial, 85% of participants would not have met treatment criteria for the National Cholesterol Education Program (Adult Treatment Panel II),[53] yet there was a statistically significant reduction in coronary endpoints. The primary consideration in the use of these agents then moves to cost-effectiveness rather than efficacy. The rationale is to limit expensive interventions to those among whom the expected reduction in the number of expensive cases of vascular disease is great enough to counterbalance the cost of the preventive intevention.[56]

Guidelines for the National Cholesterol Education Program[47] and the Seventh Report of the Joint National Committee on Prevention, Detection, Evaluation, and Treatment of High Blood Pressure (JNC-7)[45] are based on the concept of risk stratification. These guidelines vary the thresholds for initiation of treatment and the goals of therapy depending on the number of coexisting cardiovascular risk factors, as in the case of LDL-C for initiation and goals of treatment (Table 22-6). Another instance of matching treatment to absolute risk is relevant in the use of aspirin therapy to prevent CHD, in which there is a small but finite risk of gastrointestinal bleeding and hemorrhagic stroke associated with aspirin use. In individuals at lower CHD risk, the risk of aspirin therapy outweighs the benefits, but as the CHD risk increases to 6 to10% or higher per 10 years, the benefits of aspirin therapy outweigh the risks (Table 22-7).[55] This was the rationale for the new recommendations of

TABLE 22-5 NCEP/ATP-III 10-Year Risk Calculator: Estimate of 10-Year Risk for Men and Women (Framingham Point Scores)

Men Age	Points	Women Age	Points
20–34	−9	20–34	−7
35–39	−4	35–39	−3
40–44	0	40–44	0
45–49	3	45–49	3
50–54	6	50–54	6
55–59	8	55–59	8
60–64	10	60–64	10
65–69	11	65–69	12
70–74	12	70–74	14
75–79	13	75–79	16

Men

Total Cholesterol (mg/dL)	Points					Total Cholesterol (mg/dL)	Points				
	Age 20–39	Age 40–49	Age 50–59	Age 60–69	Age 70–79		Age 20–39	Age 40–49	Age 50–59	Age 60–69	Age 70–79
<160	0	0	0	0	0	<160	0	0	0	0	0
160–199	4	3	2	1	0	160–199	4	3	2	1	1
200–239	7	5	3	1	0	200–239	8	6	4	2	1
240–279	9	6	4	2	1	240–270	11	8	5	3	2
≥280	11	8	5	3	1	≥280	13	10	7	4	2

	Points						Points				
	Age 20–39 y	Age 40–49 y	Age 50–59 y	Age 60–69 y	Age 70–79 y		Age 20–39 y	Age 40–49 y	Age 50–59 y	Age 60–69 y	Age 70–79 y
Nonsmoker	0	0	0	0	0	Nonsmoker	0	0	0	0	0
Smoker	8	5	3	1	1	Smoker	9	7	4	2	1

HDL (mg/dL)	Points	HDL (mg/dL)	Points
≥60	−1	≥60	−1
50–59	0	50–59	0
40–49	1	40–49	1
<40	2	<40	2

SBP (mm Hg)	If Untreated	If Treated	SBP (mm Hg)	If Untreated	If Treated
<120	0	0	<120	0	0
120–129	0	1	120–129	1	3
130–139	1	2	130–139	2	4
140–159	1	2	140–159	3	5
≤160	2	3	≥160	4	6

Point Total	10 y Risk (%)	Point Total	10 y Risk (%)
<0	<1	<9	<1
0	1	9	1
1	1	10	1
2	1	11	1
3	1	12	1
4	1	13	2
5	2	14	2
6	2	15	3
7	3	16	4
8	4	17	5
9	5	18	6
10	6	19	8
11	8	20	11
12	10	21	14
13	12	22	17
14	15	23	22
15	20	24	27
16	25	≥25	≥30
≥17	≥30		

SOURCE: Reproduced, with permission, from the Expert Panel on Detection, Evaluation, and Treatment of High Blood Cholesterol in Adults.[47]

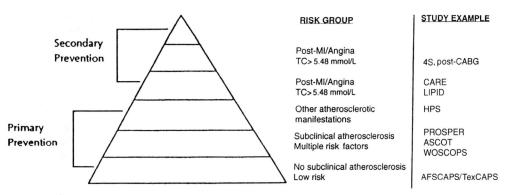

FIGURE 22-9 Pyramid of risk. MI, myocardial infarction; TC, total cholesterol; 4S, Scandinavian Simvastatin Survival Study; post-CABG, post-Coronary Artery Bypass Graft; CARE, Cholesterol and Recurrent Events; LIPID, Long-Term Intervention with Pravastatin in Ischaemic Disease; HPS, Heart Protection Study; PROSPER, Prospective Study of Pravastatin in the Elderly at Risk; ASCOT, Anglo-Scandinavian Cardiac Outcomes Trial; WOSCOPS, West of Scotland Coronary Prevention Study; AFCAPS/TexCAPS, Air Force/Texas Coronary Atherosclerosis Prevention Study. (Reproduced, with permission, from Werner et al.[54])

low-dose aspirin therapy in primary prevention for persons with moderate to high risk of CHD.[43,57]

Strategies to improve primary prevention in clinical settings

A large number of studies have examined interventions in health care practice settings to improve the level of preventive interventions.[39] Although many of the studies have involved patients with CVD in secondary prevention programs, a large number have involved primary care practices and patients prior to onset of symptomatic disease. Both single-risk-factor interventions and multiple-risk-factor modifications have been studied. Although the secondary prevention studies demonstrated greater impact, a number of lessons have been learned about the implementation of primary prevention in clinical settings. First, education and training programs for health care providers can increase the quantity and quality of preventive services, especially when combined with

TABLE 22-6 NCEP/ATP-III LDL-C Thresholds for Initiation and Goals of Treatment

Risk category	LDL-C goal (mg/dL)	LDL-C level at which to initiate therapeutic lifestyle changes (mg/dL)	LDL-C level at which to consider drug therapy (mg/dL)
CHD or CHD risk equivalents (10-y risk > 20%)	<100 (<70 for very high risk)[‡]	≥100	≥100 (<100: drug optional)*
2 + risk factors (10-y risk ≤20%)	<130	≥130	10-y risk 10–20% : ≥130 (100–129 optional) 10-y risk <10% : ≥160
0–1 Risk factor[†]	<160	≥160	≥190 (160–189: LDL-C-lowering drug optional)

Some authorities recommend use of LDL-C-lowering drugs in this category if an LDL-C level of <100 mg/dL cannot be achieved by therapeutic lifestyle changes. Others prefer use of drugs that primarily modify triglycerides and HDL-C, eg, nicotinic acid or fibrate. Clinical judgment also may call for deferring drug therapy in this subcategory.
[†]Almost all people with 0–1 risk factor have a 10-y risk <10%; thus 10-y risk assessment in people with 0–1 risk factor is not necessary.
[‡] Optional goal for those with CHD plus a) multiple risk factors or diabetes, b) severe risk factors or smoking, c) metabolic syndrome or low HDL, or d) recent acute coronary syndrome.[58]

SOURCE: Reproduced, with permission, from the Expert Panel on Detection, Evaluation, and Treatment of High Blood Cholesterol in Adults, and Grundy et al.[47,58]

TABLE 22-7 Estimates of the Type and Magnitude of Benefits and Harm Associated with Aspirin Therapy*

Benefit/Harm	Baseline risk for coronary heart disease over 5 years[†]		
	1%	3%	5%
Total mortality	No effect	No effect	No effect
CHD events[†]	1–4 avoided	4–12 avoided	6–20 avoided
Hemorrhagic strokes[‡]	0–2 caused	0–2 caused	0–2 caused
Major gastrointestinal bleeding events[§]	2–4 caused	2–4 caused	2–4 caused

*These estimates are based on a relative risk reduction of 28% for coronary heart disease events in aspirin-treated patients. They assume risk reductions do not vary significantly by age.
[†]Nonfatal acute myocardial infarction and fatal coronary heart disease. Five-year risks of 1, 3, and 5% are equivalent to 10-y risks of 2, 6, and 10%, respectively.
[‡]Data from secondary prevention trials suggest that increases in hemorrhagic stroke may be offset by reduction in other types of stroke in patients at very high risk for CVD (≥10% 5-y risk).
[§]Rates may be two to three times higher in people older than 70.
SOURCE: Reproduced, with permission, from Hayden et al.[57]

performance feedback and practice guidelines.[42] Second, an important step is the reorganization of the practice setting to an emphasis on prevention, providing the physician with resources and tools both to speed the process and to improve the quality of the intervention. Third, the practice of reorganization often entails formation of a multidisciplinary team, with some members, such as nurses, nutritionists, and counselors, often being more accessible to the patient and more effective than physicians in providing risk factor counseling and other preventive services. They should be given the training, responsibility, and tools to carry out various aspects of the intervention. Thus, a systems approach to primary prevention may increasingly allow the health care system to play a larger role in population-based primary prevention. Chapter 25 provides further details regarding the organization of preventive cardiology services.

CONCLUSIONS

A cornerstone of any approach to reduce the population's burden of CVD must be a primary prevention program aimed at reduction of risk behaviors on a population-wide basis and on the identification, stratification, and selected treatment of high-risk individuals prior to the development of disease. These two approaches should be complementary.

There is cautious optimism that populationwide interventions will influence CVD risk at a relatively low cost. The continued emphasis on and assessment of the burden of CVD and its implications for health are important first steps. Media might be selected according to audience and the type of message that is to be conveyed. A variety of organizations need to get involved; it is unlikely that the health care system, a single voluntary organiza-

tion, or even a governmental body can have substantial impact working alone. The role of regulation and policy in modifying the environment has had increasing relevance, particularly with respect to tobacco and nutrition. These strategies can then be applied to schools, religious organizations, work sites, or even whole countries. Many of the improvements have been widely disseminated as communities search for ways to prevent the CVD epidemic (see Appendix 22-1).

The health care system should benefit from populationwide efforts via health education, environmental intervention, or legislation to reduce the burden of deleterious health behaviors. These changes should facilitate risk factor change in the clinical setting. On the other hand, policymakers, employers, and community leaders look to health care providers to provide advice and leadership. Both the capacity to prevent CVD and the will to implement policies and programs are necessary to reduce CVD in communities *and* health care facilities.[19]

REFERENCES

1. Swan HJC, Gersh BJ, Grayboys TB, Ullyot DJ. Evaluation and management of risk factors for the individual patient (case management). *J Am Coll Cardiol* 1996;27:1030–1047.

2. Pearson TA, Jamison DT, Trejo-Gutierrez J. Cardiovascular disease. In: Jamison DT, Mosley WH, Measham AR, Bobadilla JL, eds. *Disease Control Priorities in Developing Countries.* New York: Oxford University Press; 1993:577–594.

3. Rose G. Sick individuals and sick populations. *Int J Epidemiol* 1989;14:32–38.

4. Carleton RA, Dwyer J, Findberg L, et al. Report of the Expert Panel on Population Strategies for Blood Cholesterol Reduction. *Circulation* 1991;83:2154–2232.

5. Cooper R, Cutler J, Desvigne-Nickens P, et al. Trends and disparities in coronary heart disease, stroke, and other cardiovascular

diseases in the United States: findings of the National Conference on Cardiovascular Disease Prevention. *Circulation* 2000;102:3137–3147.

6. Goldberg RJ, Yarzebski J, Lessard D, Gore JM. A two-decades (1975 to 1995) long experience in the incidence, in-hospital and long-term case-fatality rates of acute myocardial infarction: a community-wide perspective. *J A Coll Cardiol* 1999;33:1533–1539.

7. Roger VL, Jacobsen SJ, Weston SA, et al. Trends in the incidence and survival of patients with hospitalized myocardial infarction, Olmsted County, Minnesota, 1979 to 1994. *Ann Intern Med* 2002;136:341–348

8. Foot DK, Lewis RP, Pearson TA, Beller GA. Demographics and cardiology. *J Am Coll Cardiol* 2000;35(suppl B):66B–80B

9. Blackburn H. Epidemiological basis of a community strategy for the prevention of cardiopulmonary disease. *Ann Epidemiol* 1997;7(suppl):S8–S13.

10. Stampfer MJ, Hu FB, Manson JE, et al. Primary prevention of coronary heart disease in women through diet and lifestyle. *N Engl J Med* 2000;343:16–22.

11. *The President's Health Security Plan: The Clinton Blueprint.* New York: Times Books; 1993.

12. Stone EJ, Pearson TA, Fortmann SP, McKinley JB. Community-based prevention trials: challenges and directions for public health practice, policy, and research. *Ann Epidemiol* 1997;7(suppl):S113–S120.

13. Pearson TA, Wall S, Lewis C, et al. Dissecting the "black box" of community intervention: lessons from community-wide cardiovascular disease prevention programs in the US and Sweden. *Scand J Public Health* 2001;9:69–78

14. Pearson TA, Bazzarre TL, Daniels SR, et al. American Heart Association Scientific Statement: American Heart Association Guide for Improving Cardiovascular Health at the Community Level. *Circulation* 2003;107:645–651.

15. Williams CL, Hayman LL, Daniels SR, et al. American Heart Association Scientific Statement: Cardiovascular Health in Childhood. *Circulation* 2002;106:143–160.

16. Carleton RA, Lasater TM. Population intervention to reduce coronary heart disease. In: Pearson TA, Criqui MH, Luepker RV, et al, eds. *Primer in Preventive Cardiology.* Dallas: American Heart Association; 1994:285–292.

17. Committee on Research, Development, and Institutional Strengthening for Control of Cardiovascular Diseases in Developing Countries. Washington, DC: National Academy Press; 1998.

18. Advisory Board of the International Heart Health Conference. *The Victoria Declaration on Heart Health.* Victoria, British Columbia: Department of Health and Welfare; 1992.

19. Pearson TA, Bales VS, Blair L, et al. The Singapore Declaration: forging the will for heart health in the next millenium. *CVD Prev* 1998;1:182–199.

20. Flora JA, Saphir MN, Schooler C, Rimal RN. Toward a framework for intervention channels: reach, involvement, and impact. *Ann Epidemiol* 1997;7(suppl):S104–S112.

21. Pearson TA. Population strategy. In: Rifkind BM, ed. *Lowering Cholesterol in High Risk Individuals and Populations.* New York: Marcel Dekker; 1995:149–166.

22. Schooler C, Farquhar JW, Fortmann SP, Flora JA. Synthesis of findings and issues from community prevention trials. *Ann Epidemiol* 1997;7(suppl):S54–S68.

23. Shea S, Basch CE. A review of five major community-based cardiovascular disease prevention programs: Part I. Rationale, design, and theoretical framework. *Am J Health Promotion* 1990;4:203–213.

24. Mittelmark MB, Luepker RV, Jacobs DR, et al. Community-wide prevention of cardiovascular disease: education strategies of the Minnesota Heart Health Program. *Prev Med* 1986;15:1–17.

25. Maccoby N, Farquhar JW, Wood PD, Alexander J. Reducing the risk of cardiovascular disease: effects of a community-based campaign on knowledge and behavior. *J Community Health* 1977;3:100–114.

26. Farquhar JW, Wood PD, Breitrose H, et al. Community education for cardiovascular health. *Lancet* 1977;1:1192–1195.

27. Puska P, Tuomilehto J, Nissinen A, Vartiainen E, eds. *The North Karelina Project: 20 Year Results and Experiences.* Helsinki: National Public Health Institute, KTL; 1995.

28. Farquhar JW, Fortmann SP, Flora JA, et al. The Stanford Five-City Project: effect of community-wide education on cardiovascular disease risk factors. *JAMA* 1990;264:359–365.

29. Luepker RV, Murray DM, Jacobs DR, et al. Community education for cardiovascular disease prevention: risk factors changes in the Minnesota Heart Health Program. *Am J Public Health* 1994;84:1383–393.

30. Carleton RA, Lasater TM, Assaf AR, et al. The Pawtucket Heart Health Program: community changes in cardiovascular risk factors and projected disease risk. *Am J Public Health* 1995;85:777–785.

31. Baranowski T, Lin LS, Wetter DW, et al. Theory as mediating variables: why aren't community interventions working as desired? *Ann Epidemiol* 1997; 7(suppl):S89–S95.

32. The COMMIT Research Group. Community Intervention Trial for Smoking Cessation (COMMIT): II. Changes in adult cigarette smoking prevalence. *Am J Public Health* 1995;85:193–200.

33. The COMMIT Research Group. Community Intervention Trial for Smoking Cessation (COMMIT): I. Cohort results from a four-year community intervention. *Am J Public Health* 1995;85:183–192.

34. Winkleby MA. Accelerating cardiovascular risk factor change in ethnic minority and low socioeconomic groups. *Ann Epidemiol* 1997;7(suppl):S96–S103.

35. Resnicow K, Robinson TN. School-based cardiovascular disease prevention studies: review and synthesis. *Ann Epidemiol* 1997;7(suppl):S14–S31.

36. Lasater TM, Becker DM, Hill MN, Gans KM. Synthesis of findings and issues from religious-based cardiovascular disease prevention trials. *Ann Epidemiol* 1997;7(suppl):S46–S53.

37. Jeffery R, Forster J, French S. The Healthy Worker Project: a worksite intervention for weight control and smoking cessation. *Am J Public Health* 1993;83:395–401.

38. Pelletier K. A review and analysis of the health and cost-effective outcome studies of comprehensive health promotion and disease prevention programs at the worksite: 1993–1995 update. *Am J Health Promotion* 1996;19:380–388.

39. Ockene JK, McBride PE, Sallis JF, et al. Synthesis of lessons learned from cardiopulmonary preventive interventions in healthcare practice settings. *Ann Epidemiol* 1997;7(suppl):S32–S45.

40. Kottke TE, Brekke ML, Solberg LI. Making time for preventive services. *Mayo Clin Proc* 1993;68:785–791.

41. Miller M, Konkel K, Fitzpatrick D, et al. Divergent reporting of

coronary risk factors before coronary artery bypass surgery. *Am J Cardiol* 1995;75:736–737.

42. Pearson TA, McBride PE, Houston-Miller N, Smith SC Jr. Organization of preventive cardiology service. *J Am Coll Cardiol* 1996;271039–1047.

43. Pearson TA, Blair SN, Daniels SR, et al, for the American Heart Association Science Advisory and Coordinating Committee. AHA Guidelines for Primary Prevention of Cardiovascular Disease and Stroke: 2002 Update: Consensus Panel Guide to Comprehensive Risk Reduction for Adult Patients Without Coronary or Other Atherosclerotic Vascular Diseases. *Circulation* 2002;106:388–391.

44. Mosca CJ, Appel LJ, Benjamin E, et al. Evidence-based guidelines for cardiovascular disease prevention in women. *Circulation* 2004;109:672–693.

45. Chobanian AV, Bakris GL, Black HR, et al. The Seventh Report of the Joint National Committee on Prevention, Detection, Evaluation, and Treatment of High Blood Pressure: the JNC 7. *JAMA* 2003;289:2560–2572

46. Grundy SM, Balady GJ, Criqui MH, et al, for the American Heart Association. AHA Scientific Statement: primary prevention of coronary heart disease: guidance from Framingham: a statement for healthcare professionals from the AHA Task Force on Risk Reduction. *Circulation* 1998;97:1876–1887.

47. Expert Panel on Detection, Evaluation, and Treatment of High Blood Cholesterol in Adults. Executive Summary of The Third Report of The National Cholesterol Education Program (NCEP) Expert Panel on Detection, Evaluation, and Treatment of High Blood Cholesterol in Adults (Adult Treatment Panel III). *JAMA* 2001;285:2486–2497.

48. De Backer G, Ambrosioni E, Borch-Johnsen K, et al, for the Third Joint Task Force of European and Other Societies on Cardiovascular Disease Prevention in Clinical Practice. European guidelines on cardiovascular disease prevention in clinical practice. *Eur Heart J* 2003;24:1601–1610.

49. Pearson TA, Mensah CA, Alexander RW, et al. Markers of inflammation and cardiovascular disease: application to clinical and public health practice. *Circulation* 2003;107:499–511.

50. Grundy SM, Bazzarre T, Cleeman J, et al. Prevention Conference V: beyond secondary prevention: identifying the high-risk patient for primary prevention: medical office assessment. *Circulation* 2000;101:E3–E11.

51. Bild DE, Bluemke DA, Burke GL, et al. Multi-ethnic study of atherosclerosis: objectives and design. *Am J Epidemiol* 2002;156:871–881.

52. Califf RM, Armstrong PW, Carver JR, et al. 27th Bethesda Conference: matching the intensity of risk factor management with the hazard for coronary disease events. Task Force 5. Stratification of patients into high, medium and low risk subgroups for purposes of risk factor management. *J Am Coll Cardiol* 1996;27:1007–1019.

53. National Cholesterol Education Program. Second Report of the Expert Panel on Detection, Evaluation, and Treatment of High Blood Cholesterol in Adults (Adult Treatment Panel II). *Circulation* 1994;89:1333–1445.

54. Werner RM, Pearson TA. LDL-cholesterol: a risk factor for coronary artery disease—from epidemiology to clinical trials. *Can J Cardiol* 1998;14(suppl B):3B–10B.

55. Downs JR, Clearfield M, Weis S, et al. Primary prevention of acute coronary events with lovastatin in men and women with average cholesterol levels: results of AFCAPS/TexCAPS. Air Force/Texas Coronary Atherosclerosis Prevention Study. *JAMA* 1998;279:1615–1622.

56. Goldman L, Garber AM, Grover SA, Hlatky MA. 27th Bethesda Conference: matching the intensity of risk factor management with the hazard for coronary disease events. Task Force 6. Cost effectiveness of assessment and management of risk factors. *J Am Coll Cardiol* 1996;27:1020–1030.

57. Hayden M, Pignone M, Philips C, Mulrow C. Aspirin for the primary prevention of cardiovascular events: a summary of the evidence for the U.S. Preventive Services Task Force. *Ann Intern Med* 2002;136:161–172.

58. Grundy SM, Cleeman JI, Merz CN, et al. Implications of recent clinical trials for the Natinal Cholesterol Education Program Adult Treatment Panel III guidelines. *Circulation* 2004;110: 227–239.

APPENDIX 22-1   Guide to Improving Cardiovascular Health at the Community Level

Strategies/Goals	Recommendations
Assessment *Goal:* All persons and communities should know that CVD and stroke are the leading causes of death and disability in men and women.	• Data on the burden of CVD and stroke mortality at the local level (city or country) should be collected and made available. • Groups defined by sex, race/ethnicity, socioeconomic status, or geographic location that are at especially high risk of CVD and stroke within each community should be identified. • Levels of major preventable causes of CVD and stroke in the community, including lifestyle behaviors (eg, adverse nutrition, cigarette smoking, sedentary lifestyle) and risk factors (hypertension, atrial fibrillation, diabetes, elevated blood cholesterol, and obesity) should be assessed.
Education GENERAL HEALTH EDUCATION *Goal:* All communities should provide information to their members about the burden, causes, and early symptoms of CVD and stroke.	• Mass media (television, radio, newspapers) should disseminate results of surveillance about the burden of CVD and stroke in the community. • Mass media and local media (eg, pamphlets, brochures) should emphasize the importance of lifestyle behaviors and risk factors to cardiovascular health. • Public education campaigns should make the community aware of guidelines for primary and secondary prevention of CVD and stroke. • Mass and local media should emphasize the early warning signs of myocardial infarction and stroke. • Ongoing education programs should provide training of lay members in cardiopulmonary resuscitation. • All citizens should know how to access the emergency medical care system.
Goal: Communities should provide materials and programs to motivate and teach skills for changing risk behaviors that will target multiple population subgroups.	• A guide to community resources (services and programs) for prevention, diagnosis, and treatment of CVD and stroke should be available. • Communities should support and publicize research-based programs for CVD risk reduction that are targeted to key population subgroups, especially disadvantaged groups and people at all levels of readiness to change. • Communities should promote the use of web site programs for risk reduction by making web site access to such programs available in public libraries and schools. • Food advertising directed to youth should be limited to foods that meet health guidelines. • TV shows for children should promote physical activity during commercial breaks.
SCHOOL AND YOUTH EDUCATION *Goal:* All schools should have research-based, comprehensive, and age-appropriate curricula about cardiovascular health and ways to improve health behaviors and reduce CVD risk.	• School curricula should include lessons about risk factors for CVD and stroke and the extent of heart disease and stroke in the community. • Research-based curricula about effective methods of changing health behaviors should be implemented. • Students should learn skills needed to achieve regular practice of healthful behaviors, and parents should learn how to support their children's healthful behaviors. • Specific curricular materials for healthy nutrition and physical activity should be offered.
Goal: All schools should implement age-appropriate curricula on changing dietary, physical activity, and smoking behaviors.	• Physical education should be required at least three times a week in grades k–12, with an increasing emphasis on lifetime sports/activities. Implementation of research-based curricula is recommended. • Meals provided at schools should include alternatives conducive to cardiovascular health.

(continued)

APPENDIX 22-1   (Continued)

Strategies/Goals	Recommendations
Goal: All schools should provide teaching of early warning signs of myocardial infarction and stroke and appropriate initial steps of emergency care.	• Students should know how to activate the emergency medical system. • Cardiopulmonary resuscitation instruction should be provided to students at appropriate ages.
WORK SITE EDUCATION *Goal:* All work sites should provide materials and services to motivate and assist employees to adopt and maintain heart-healthy behaviors.	• Work sites should promote increased physical activity in the day's work (eg, stair climbing). • Workers should have access to research-based effective materials and services to help them adopt and maintain heart-healthy behaviors.
Goal: All work sites should provide instruction in early warning signs of myocardial infarction and stroke and appropriate initial steps of emergency care.	• Workers should know how to activate the emergency medical system. • Cardiopulmonary resuscitation instruction should be available to all workers.
HEALTH CARE FACILITY EDUCATION *Goal:* All health care facilities should make available research-based, effective educational materials and programs about changing and maintaining risk factors/risk behaviors, ways to prevent CVD and stroke, and early warning signs of CVD and stroke.	• Print and other media should be available in health care facilities to describe CVD and stroke risk factors and their early warning signs. • Guide for primary and secondary prevention should be made available for all patients. • Educational materials should be modified to accommodate for limited literacy, cultural and language diversity, sex differences, and dissemination flexibility.
Community Organization and Partnering *Goal:* All communities will have an action plan for CVD and stroke prevention and control with specific targets and goals.	• Organizations and institutions in the community that can provide services and resources in prevention and care of CVD and stroke must be identified. • Opportunities must be created for citizens of all ages to become involved in community activities for CVD and stroke prevention.
Goal: All communities will provide materials and services for risk behavior and risk factor change that are research based whenever possible.	• Community organizations must be educated about effective research-based materials and services and these should be made available.
Assurance of Personal Health Services *Goal:* The percentage of people at risk who will effectively reduce risk factors to goal levels as established by AHA Guidelines for Primary and Secondary Prevention of Heart Disease and Stroke should be increased.	• Access to screening, counseling, and referral services for CVD and stroke risk factors should be ensured for all persons. • Educational materials should be modified to accommodate for limited literacy and for culture and language diversity. • Tobacco users should be provided with telephone support interventions, including cessation counseling or assistance in attempting to quit or in maintaining abstinence. • Access to rehabilitation and risk factor control programs should be provided for CVD and stroke survivors.

(continued)

APPENDIX 22-1   (Continued)

Strategies/Goals	Recommendations
Goal: The percentage of patients suffering acute coronary syndromes (eg, myocardial infarction, cardiac arrhythmias) or cerebrovascular syndromes (eg, stroke, transient ischemic attack) who receive appropriate acute interventions within the time frame of maximal effectiveness should be increased.	• Emergency first responders must be trained in the use of automatic defibrillators (AEDs) and provided with AEDs in accordance with AHA-recommended guidelines. • High-density public locations and locations in which high-risk activities take place must be equipped with AEDs, and have personnel trained in the use of AEDs, in accordance with AHA-recommended guidelines.
Goal: Training about smoking, physical activity, nutrition, and effective behavior change counseling methods should be provided in medical schools and appropriate residency programs.	• Research-based curricula for the MD, nurse practitioner, PA, and RN degrees emphasizing skill building in behavior change related to smoking, diet, and exercise should be required.
Environmental Change *Goal:* Access to healthy foods should be ensured so that all members of the community can meet national dietary recommendations for saturated fat (<10% of calories), sodium, grains (>6 day, with >3 being whole grain), fruits (>2 servings/day) and vegetables (>3 servings/day)	• Grocery stores and food markets should provide selections of fruits, green and yellow vegetables, and grain products at reasonable cost. • Restaurants should increase offerings of and identify dishes that meet nutritional guidelines and provide nutritional labeling. • Schools should increase access to and identify meals and snacks that contribute to better overall dietary quality and meet dietary guidelines. • Food services at work sites should identify and make available selections low in saturated fat and calories with expended access to fuits, vegetables, and grain products. • Healthful foods should be promoted at all food sources by methods such as point-of-purchase displays. • Communities should support farmer's markets and community gardens.
Goal: Access to safe, appropriate, and enjoyable forms of physical activity should be ensured so that people of all ages can meet national guidelines for moderate and vigorous physical activity.	• Physical education programs should be supported within the school curricula and within community activity centers. • Every community should commit to providing safe and convenient means for walking and bicycling as a means of transportation and recreation. • Buildings should be designed so that stairwells are visible, convenient, and comfortable to use. Use of stairwells should be promoted through signs. • Work sites should provide employer-sponsored physical activity and fitness programs. • Schools should provide access to their physical activity space and facilities for all persons outside of normal school hours.
Goal: A tobacco-free environment should be ensured for all citizens.	• Work sites should have formal smoking policies that prohibit smoking or limit it to a separately ventilated area. • Local or state ordinances should prohibit smoking in public places or limit it to separately ventilated areas. • School facilities, property, vehicles, and school events should be smoke-free and tobacco-free.

(continued)

APPENDIX 22-1   (Continued)

Strategies/Goals	Recommendations
Policy Change *Goal:* Initiation of tobacco use by adolescents and young adults should be reduced.	• Unit price for tobacco products should be increased through local or state excise taxes. • Tobacco advertising and promotions that influence adolescents and young adults must be eliminated. • Laws prohibiting the sale of tobacco products to minors must be enforced, and violators must receive penalties (eg, fines, revoking of retail license). • Tobacco settlement monies should be used for tobacco control and other tobacco-related illnesses, rather than for general funds.
Goal: Adequate reimbursement should be provided for clinical preventive and rehabilitative services	• Insurance coverage should be provided for evidence-based treatments for nicotine dependency and for promoting healthful nutrition and physical activity. • Clinical preventive services and early outpatient cardiac rehabilitation should be covered by health insurance plans.

SOURCE: Reproduced, with permission, from Pearson et al.

Secondary prevention

Robert D. Brook
Philip Greenland

KEY POINTS

- *Secondary prevention comprises medical interventions and therapeutic lifestyle changes that aim to reduce complications, recurrent events, and disease progression in patients with cardiovascular disease.*

- *Many high-risk patients without established cardiovascular disease may be appropriate candidates for secondary prevention strategies (cardiovascular disease risk equivalents).*

- *Treatment of elevated serum lipoproteins reduces cardiovascular events by approximately 30 to 40% and overall mortality by 20% in high-risk patients, and most high-risk patients also benefit from treatment of isolated low high-density lipoprotein cholesterol.*

- *Treatment of high blood pressure with pharmacologic agents reduces cardiovascular events in high-risk patients.*

- *Individuals with certain comorbidities—including left ventricular systolic dysfunction, diabetes, renal insufficiency, microalbuminuria, and systemic atherosclerosis—may receive particular benefit from angiotensin-converting enzyme inhibitors and/or angiotensin receptor blockers.*

- *Most high-risk patients should be on daily low-dose aspirin therapy (75–160 mg/d). Coumadin and clopidogrel are viable alternatives for aspirin-intolerant patients.*

- *A variety of therapeutic lifestyle changes—including dietary modifications, smoking cessation, and increased aerobic exercise—are proven effective secondary prevention strategies.*

- *Estrogen replacement therapy and antioxidants have thus far proven ineffective in reducing cardiovascular events in secondary prevention.*

INTRODUCTION

Secondary prevention of cardiovascular disease (CVD) comprises the medical interventions and therapeutic lifestyle changes that aim to reduce complications, recurrent events, and disease progression in patients with established CVD. Cardiovascular event rates in these patients are approximately five to seven times higher than in apparently healthy individuals.[1,2] In the absence of treatment, the risk for subsequent events is 10% in the first year and 5% per year indefinitely thereafter.[3] Owing to this high absolute risk, secondary prevention is extremely important.

CVD risk equivalents

It is now recognized that several categories of patients without heart disease are at an equally elevated short-term (10-year) risk for coronary events as those with established CVD. The disease states known to confer this high-risk status are termed CVD "risk equivalents" by the National Cholesterol Education Program Adult Treatment Program III (ATP-III)[4] and include patients with:

- Diabetes mellitus
- Symptomatic carotid atherosclerosis

- Aortic aneurysmal disease
- Peripheral vascular disease

In addition, any condition (or combination of CVD risk factors) that elevates the estimated short-term absolute risk for a CVD event to greater than 20% over a 10-year period also places an individual within this high-risk category. For example, due to a very high incidence of CVD events, it has recently been promoted that patients with chronic kidney disease be included within the highest CVD risk equivalent cohort.[5] The overall treatment guidelines and therapeutic intensity that apply to those with established CVD should, in most circumstances, be equally applied to those with CVD risk equivalents.

Patients at intermediate risk (estimated 10-year CVD event rate between 6 and 20%) and with a positive novel risk factor and/or preclinical atherosclerosis screening test may also be appropriate candidates for secondary prevention strategies.[6] An elevated serum C-reactive protein level greater than 3.0 mg/L,[7] an age-adjusted coronary calcium score greater than the 75th percentile,[8] an ankle–brachial index less than 0.9,[9] and a carotid intima–media thickness greater than 1.0 mm[10] all independently increase the relative risk for CVD by two- to sixfold. Accordingly, many intermediate-risk patients with one or more of these other abnormalities may have a short-term absolute CVD risk of greater than 20% per 10 years. In this context, health care providers may be justified in also considering such patients to be CHD risk equivalents and implementing secondary risk prevention therapies.

Risk factor modification in secondary prevention

Risk factor modification is the chief route by which secondary prevention is accomplished. Major national organizations such as the American Heart Association and the American College of Cardiology[11] have advocated specific risk factor modification strategies as the cornerstone of optimal medical care in high-risk patients. Similar emphasis on secondary prevention has been a focus of clinical recommendations outside of the United States as well.[12]

The central importance of risk factor modification in secondary prevention is exemplified by the well-known association between the major risk factors and CVD events. When plotted on a logarithmic scale, this relationship is linear and extends without a lower discernable threshold.[13] Therefore, any given amount of risk factor reduction decreases cardiovascular events by a constant proportion of the preexisting absolute CVD risk, irrespective of the starting level of the risk factor. The major portion of the outcome benefits derived from risk factor modification is thus not determined by the severity of

the risk factor, but by the initial overall absolute CVD risk of an individual. As the absolute risk for subsequent events is markedly elevated (between 2 and 5% per year), high-risk patients stand to benefit tremendously from risk factor reduction. As a further consequence, the number needed to treat to prevent an adverse coronary event is low, ranging between 20 and 40 patients.[13] The lower threshold limit for each risk factor at which to withhold initial therapy or to defer the intensification of treatment remains unknown and awaits clarification from many ongoing trials.

Despite a host of strategies proven to reduce subsequent events, the rate of control of the major CVD risk factors in the United States is unsatisfactory. Only about 20% of high-risk secondary prevention patients have LDL-C treated to a target value less than 100 mg/dL.[4] Blood pressure control rate is similarly poor at about 34%.[14] As the major risk factors account for 75% or more of the risk for developing a CVD event,[15] the foremost focus of secondary prevention should be to achieve optimal risk factor control by all validated means. It has been estimated that the daily use of a "polypill" containing a hydroxymethylglutaryl coenzyme A (HMGCoA) reductase inhibitor (e.g., simvastatin 40 mg), three blood pressure-lowering medications (diuretic, beta blocker, angiotensin-converting enzyme inhibitor at usual doses), folic acid (0.8 mg), and aspirin (75 mg) could reduce recurrent cardiovascular events by 88%.[16]

The subsequent portions of this chapter review approaches toward risk assessment and minimization in persons with preexisting CVD (and/or risk equivalents). The evidence and recommendations for management regarding the risk factors for which interventions are of proven, probable, or possible benefit are outlined.

CARDIOVASCULAR RISK ASSESSMENT AND STRATIFICATION IN PERSONS WITH PREEXISTING CORONARY ARTERY DISEASE

Patients with established CVD, or a CVD risk equivalent, are high-risk patients with absolute ischemic event rates exceeding 2% per year.[4] However, a wide range of absolute risks (from 2 to 5% per year) may exist even among persons with CVD. Further risk assessment may therefore yield clinically useful information. Risk stratification of patients with established CVD involves considering five categories of patients: (1) those with stable coronary heart disease (CHD), (2) those with unstable angina, (3) patients with acute myocardial infarction, (4) those who have undergone coronary artery bypass surgery, and (5) those who have had percutaneous coronary intervention. Although of equal short-term risk, patients with CVD risk equivalents are not included in this discussion as

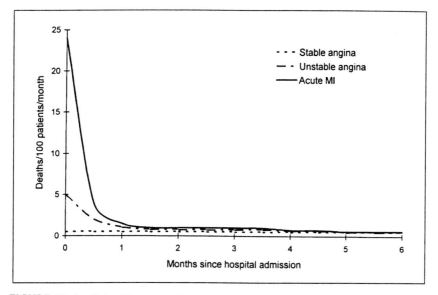

FIGURE 23-1   Risk of future cardiac events as a function of time since the event or procedure. MI, myocardial infarction. (Reproduced, with permission, from Smith et al.[17])

further risk stratification within this category of patients remains untested.

All patients with established CVD have diseased arteries susceptible to plaque fissuring and subsequent thrombosis. Figure 23-1 shows that the patient hospitalized with myocardial infarction or unstable angina is at particularly high risk during the initial month after hospitalization, during which the myocardium is subject to sudden electrical instability or the disrupted plaque may undergo rethrombosis. Figure 23-2 shows that the risk

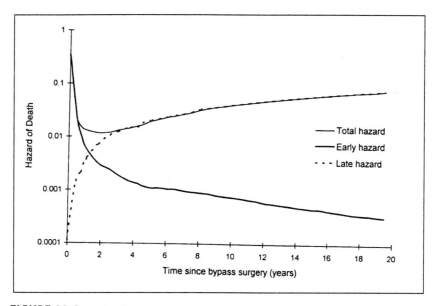

FIGURE 23-2   Risk of occlusion due to thrombosis or mechanical obstruction as a function of time from coronary artery bypass surgery. (Reproduced, with permission, from Smith et al.[17])

after bypass grafting is highest during the first year, when there is an increased risk of graft occlusion.[2,17]

In evaluating the patient with preexisting coronary artery disease for future risk of cardiovascular events, the value of the medical history, physical examination, 12-lead electrocardiogram, and selected laboratory tests merits recognition. The Framingham Heart Study has assembled algorithms for determining the 2-year risk of CHD events, stroke, or cerebrovascular disease death in women (Table 23-1) and men (Table 23-2) with existing CHD. These tables may be useful for initial risk stratification, but they should be considered only approximate guides to risk assessment. Clinical presentation, including the type of chest pain, as well as the presence of any associated comorbidities, also figure into the determination of prognosis (Table 23-3). More detailed information about symptoms, coronary anatomy, left ventricular function, or results from exercise and/or stress imaging testing can provide important incremental risk stratification.

In a community-based study, the generalizability and effectiveness of several post-myocardial infarction (MI) risk stratification tools were recently investigated.[18] It was confirmed that the consideration of multiple comorbidities and the patient's ejection fraction significantly enhanced risk prediction. Nevertheless, due to the high-risk status of all secondary prevention patients, the results from detailed testing and/or comprehensive risk scores rarely impact the course and aggressiveness of therapy. Therefore, their usefulness in clinical practice is currently not well established.

Evidence is also continuing to grow that measuring several novel risk factors and/or pro-inflammatory markers after a CVD event can further enhance risk stratification. In particular, an elevated C-reactive protein (CRP) value has been shown to independently convey an adverse outcome.[7] Post-MI patients with a CRP greater than 10 mg/dL are at particularly high risk. In a similar fashion, higher coronary calcium scores,[19] determined by electron beam computed tomography, and reduced vascular endothelial function[20] both predict worse prognoses in patients with known CVD. Although several small preliminary studies are intriguing, the clinical utility of these modalities requires further testing. In contrast to primary prevention, no recommendations for their measurement presently exist in secondary prevention, primarily because such patients are already regarded as extremely high-risk and should have the most intensive treatment guidelines applied.

Of greatest importance to the practicing physician, the individual major CVD risk factors are known predictors of long-term prognosis in persons with established CVD. Over an average of nearly 10 years of follow-up, systolic blood pressure, total cholesterol, and diabetes remained significant predictors of the risk of reinfarction

or CHD death among subjects who sustained a previous MI in the Framingham Heart Study.[21] Similar findings from other countries[22] and in women[23] support the importance of the traditional risk factors in promoting the recurrence of CVD events and mortality. They also represent appropriate targets of risk-reducing therapies.

RISK FACTOR MODIFICATIONS OF PROVEN OR LIKELY BENEFIT IN PATIENTS WITH CVD

The value of specific risk interventions among patients with coronary or other vascular disease is well recognized. The American Heart Association (AHA) and American College of Cardiology (ACC) consensus panel statement for preventing heart attack and death in patients with atherosclerotic CVD was most recently updated in 2001.[11] Table 23-4 summarizes a suggested global approach to risk factor modification in high-risk patients based on this updated statement.

DYSLIPIDEMIA

Cholesterol as a risk factor in secondary prevention

The prognostic value of serum cholesterol and various other lipoprotein levels in patients with established CVD is proven. In a population-based observational study in survivors of MI, Framingham Heart Study data showed the importance of cholesterol levels in predicting recurrent infarction and total mortality.[24] Survivors of MI with cholesterol levels of 275 mg/dL or greater, compared with MI survivors in the reference range less than 200 mg/dL, were found to have a relative risk of 2.8 for recurrent MI. This association held true for men and women, as well as for the elderly.[24] Similarly, in the Lipid Research Clinics Prevalence study, men with a cholesterol level of 240 mg/dL or greater had a three to four times higher risk of death due to CVD as compared with men whose cholesterol levels were less than 200 mg/dL. Relative risks were also elevated for high low-density lipoprotein cholesterol (LDL-C) and for low high-density lipoprotein cholesterol (HDL-C) (hazard ratios each about 6.0).[25]

The secondary prevention trials using HMGCoA reductase inhibitors (statins) have further demonstrated the important prognostic role of blood lipids in patients with preexisting CVD. In those assigned to placebo in Scandinavian Simvastatin Survival Study (4S)[26] and the Long-Term Intervention with Pravastatin in Ischemic Disease (LIPID) trial,[27] there existed a positive relationship between LDL-C and the subsequent risk of major cardiovascular events. However, once on treatment with a statin medication, LDL-C, HDL-C, and triglycerides

TABLE 23-1   Risk of Coronary Artery Disease Event, Stroke, or Cerebrovascular Disease Death in Women with Existing Coronary Artery Disease

	Points	Total cholesterol (mg/dL)	25	30	35	40	45	50	60	70	80	SBP (mm Hg)	Points
Age													
35	0	160	4	3	3	2	2	1	1	0	0	100	0
40	1	170	4	3	3	2	2	2	1	1	0	110	0
45	2	180	4	3	3	2	2	2	1	1	0	120	1
50	3	190	4	4	3	3	2	2	1	1	1	130	1
55	4	200	4	4	3	3	2	2	2	1	1	140	2
60	5	210	4	4	3	3	3	2	2	1	1	150	2
65	6	220	5	4	4	3	3	2	2	1	1	160	2
70	7	230	5	4	4	3	3	3	2	2	1	170	3
75	7	240	5	4	4	3	3	3	2	2	1	180	3
		250	5	4	4	4	3	3	2	2	1	190	3
		260	5	5	4	4	3	3	2	2	1	200	3
		270	5	5	4	4	3	3	2	2	2	210	4
Other		280	5	5	4	4	3	3	3	2	2	220	4
Diabetes	3	290	5	5	4	4	4	3	3	2	2	230	4
Smoking	3	300	6	5	4	4	4	3	3	2	2	240	4
												250	4

Average 2-Year Risk in Women with CVD

Total points	2-Year probability (%)	Age (years)	Probability (%)
0	0	35–39	<1
2	1	40–44	<1
4	1	45–49	<1
6	1	50–54	4
8	2	55–59	6
10	4	60–64	8
12	6	65–69	12
14	10	70–74	12
16	15		
18	23		
20	35		
22	51		
24	68		
26	85		

*HDL-C, high-density lipoprotein cholesterol; SBP, systolic blood pressure; CVD, cardiovascular disease.

SOURCE: Reproduced, with permission, from Califf et al.[2]

TABLE 23-2 Risk of Coronary Artery Disease Event, Stroke, or Cerebrovascular Disease Death in Men with Existing Coronary Artery Disease

	Points	Total cholesterol (mg/dL)	25	30	35	40	45	50	60	70	80	SBP (mm Hg)	Points
Age													
35	0	160	6	5	4	4	3	2	1	1	0	100	0
40	1	170	6	5	5	4	3	3	2	1	0	110	1
45	1	180	7	6	5	4	4	3	2	1	1	120	1
50	2	190	7	6	5	4	4	3	2	2	1	130	2
55	2	200	7	6	5	5	4	4	3	2	1	140	2
60	3	210	7	6	6	5	4	4	3	2	1	150	3
65	3	220	8	7	6	5	5	4	3	2	2	160	3
70	4	230	8	7	6	5	5	4	3	3	2	170	4
75	4	240	8	7	6	6	5	4	4	3	2	180	4
		250	8	7	6	6	5	5	4	3	2	190	4
		260	8	7	7	6	5	5	4	3	2	200	5
		270	9	8	7	6	6	5	4	3	3	210	5
Other		280	9	8	7	6	6	5	4	4	3	220	5
Diabetes	1	290	9	8	7	7	6	5	4	4	3	230	6
		300	9	8	7	7	6	6	5	4	3	240	6
												250	6

		Average 2-Year Risk in Men with CVD	
Total points	2-Year probability (%)	Age (years)	Probability (%)
0	2	35–39	<1
2	2	40–44	8
4	3	45–49	10
6	5	50–54	11
8	7	55–59	12
10	10	60–64	12
12	14	65-69	14
14	20	70–74	14
16	28		
18	37		
20	49		
22	63		
24	77		

*HDL-C, high-density lipoprotein cholesterol; SBP, systolic blood pressure; CVD, cardiovascular disease.

SOURCE: Reproduced, with permission, from Califf et al.[2]

TABLE 23-3 Risk of Mortality at 1 Year: Clinical History Variables

1. Find points for each risk factor:

Age	Points	Angina, pain type	Points	Comorbid factor	Points*
20	0	Nonanginal pain	3	CVD[†]	20
30	13	Atypical angina	25	PVD	23
40	25	Typical angina		Diabetes	20
50	38	Stable	41	Prior MI	17
60	50	Progressive	46	Hypertension	8
70	62	Unstable	51	Mitral regurgitation	
80	75	Mild	19	Mild	19
90	88	Severe	38	Severe	38
100	100				

2. Sum points for all risk factors:
Age + pain score + comorbidity = point total

3. Look up risk corresponding to point total:

Total points	Probability of death at 1 year (%)	Total points	Probability of death at 1 Year (%)
84	1	184	20
106	2	199	30
120	3	211	40
136	5	220	50
160	10	229	60

*Zero points for each "no."
[†]CVD, cerebrovascular disease; MI, myocardial infarction; PVD, peripheral vascular disease.
SOURCE: Reproduced, with permission, from Califf et al.[2]

tend to lose their predictive power.[28] This should not be interpreted that lipid values are no longer important after starting a medication. In patients both on treatment and on placebo, apolipoprotein B and non-HDL-C continue to predict the risk of subsequent events (usually better than LDL-C).[28] Therefore, lipid values achieved, even on medications, during secondary prevention are important determinants of future CVD risk. Whether follow-up management of patients on therapy is enhanced by measurement of apolipoproteins rather than cholesterol levels is still a matter of debate.

Treatment of LDL-C in secondary prevention

During and prior to the 1980s, secondary prevention trials such as the Coronary Drug Project sought to determine the effect of cholesterol reduction in patients with CVD.[29] Most of the early trials demonstrated modest reductions in cardiovascular events, but no benefits on total mortality. From 1994 until 2003, at least nine large trials with statins have now incontrovertibly established the benefit of cholesterol reduction therapy in high-risk patients (Table 23-5).

To date, in more than 50,000 patients with CVD or a risk equivalent,[30] these trials have demonstrated that a 20 to 40% reduction in LDL-C with a statin medication:

- Reduces the risk of major CVD events by 30 to 40%
- Reduces the risk of overall mortality by approximately 20%
- Reduces the risk of stroke by 10 to 20%

These benefits hold true regardless of age (up to at least 82 years),[31] gender, diabetes status,[32] renal function,[33] and other comorbidities and demographic criteria investigated thus far. Other demonstrated *clinical* benefits include[34]:

- Possible improvement in claudication symptoms[35]
- Reductions in myocardial ischemia[36]
- Reduced requirement for revascularization procedures[30]

TABLE 23-4 Summary of AHA and ACC Recommendations for Secondary Cardiovascular Disease Prevention Version 2001 Update (with Additional Author-Recommended Updates)

Risk Factor Recommendations	
Smoking	
Goal: Strongly encourage patient and family to stop	Counseling, pharmacologic therapy. Complete cessation and formal cessation programs are advocated.
Lipid management	
Primary goal: LDL-C<100 mg/dL (optional goal: <70 mg/dL in very high risk patients[††])[72]	Start AHA Step 2 diet, TLCs * in all patients[†] *LDL<100 mg/dL* LDL-C therapy optional.[‡] Consider adding fibrate/niacin for HDL-C <40[§] or TGs ≥200 mg/dL. *LDL-C 100–129 mg/dL* Intensify LDL-C lowering with statin or resin. Add fibrate or niacin for low HDL-C or high TGs. *LDL-C ≥130 mg/dL* First, intensify LDL-C-lowering therapies.
Secondary goal: non-HDL-C<130 mg/dL (TC−HDL) (optional: <100 mg/dL in very high risk patients[††])[72]	Emphasize TLCs for TGs>150 mg/dL or HDL-C<40 mg/dL. *TG level = 100–499 mg/dL* Consider fibrate or niacin after LDL-C-lowering. *TG level > 500 mg/dL* Consider fibrate or niacin before LDL-C-lowering. Consider omega-3 fatty acids.[‖]
Blood Pressure	
Goal (mm Hg): <140/90 (all patients) <130/80 (for patients with renal insufficiency and diabetes mellitus, JNC-7)	Initiate TLC and DASH diet. Individualize medication for each patient and comorbidities.
Physical activity	
Minimum goal: daily exercise *Optimal goal:* daily exercise	Assess risk; use exercise test to guide therapy. Encourage aerobic activity daily (30 min three or four times per week). Institute medical supervision in certain high-risk patients.
Weight management	
Goal: BMI 18.5–24.9 kg/m^2	Calculate BMI and waist circumference. Advise weight management and exercise as appropriate when BMI≥25 kg/m^2 or waist ≥40 in. (men) and ≥35 in. (women).
Diabetes	
Goal: near-normal fasting glucose HbA$_{1c}$ <7 %	Initiate TLCs in all patients. Institute appropriate hypoglycemic therapy to achieve goals.
Antiplatelet therapy	Start and continue aspirin 75–325 mg/d.
Anticoagulation therapy	Consider clopidogrel or warfarin (INR 2–3) if aspirin contraindicated.[¶]
ACEIs	Treat all patients indefinitely post-MI. Start early in stable high-risk post-MI patients. Consider chronic therapy for all patients with CVD.[#]
Beta blockers	Start in all patients post-MI and with angina. Continue indefinitely.
Additional Recommendations (author updates since 2001)	

(continued)

TABLE 23-4   (Continued)

†A Mediterranean-type diet should be considered in lieu of the AHA Step 2 diet in many patients with CVD as it may be superior in reducing CVD.

‡Strong consideration should be given to starting a statin medication (equivalent to simvastatin 40 mg) daily in all patients with CVD, even if LDL-C is initially <100 mg/dL.

§A medication to raise HDL-C (fibrate/niacin) as much as possible should be considered in all CVD patients with HDL <40 mg/dL, even if non-HDL-C and LDL-C are at goal (isolated low HDL-C).

‖Use of fish oil supplements (omega-3 fatty acids at 1000 mg/d) should be considered in all patients with documented CVD to reduce sudden cardiac death based on clinical trial results.

¶In certain high-risk patients (recent coronary angioplasty/stent, peripheral vascular disease), the combined usage of aspirin and clopidogrel should be considered for at least 1 year.

#The addition of a selective aldosterone receptor blocker (spirinolactone/eplerinone) should be considered in addition to an ACE inhibitor in patients post-MI with a reduced ejection fraction.

- Routine usage of estrogens (hormone replacement therapy) and antiarrhythmia medications is not recommended based on clinical trial results.
- There is no consistent evidence supporting either a beneficial or an adverse effect of antioxidant medications in preventing CVD.
- Recommendations for the usage of folic acid (and other therapies to lower homocysteine) await several ongoing studies.

††Very high risk includes acute coronary syndrome, or CVD plus diabetes or significant risk factors including metabolic syndrome.

†TLCs, therapeutic lifestyle changes; LDL, low-density lipoprotein cholesterol; TG, triglycerides; TC, total cholesterol; HDL, high-density lipoprotein cholesterol; CRI, chronic renal insufficiency; CHF, congestive heart failure; DM, diabetes mellitus; DASH, Dietary Approaches to Stop Hypertension; BMI, body mass index; MI, myocardial infarction, ACEI, angiotensin-converting enzyme inhibitor; HbA$_{1c}$, hemoglobin A$_{1c}$.

- Lower incidence of deep venous thromboses[37]
- Improved kidney/heart transplant survival[34,38]
- Reduction of aortic stenosis progression[39]
- Possible antiarrhythmic effects, including reduction of atrial fibrillation[40]
- Potential improvement in renal insufficiency[41]
- Reductions in blood pressure[42]

Origin of clinical benefits: statin versus LDL-C lowering

Whether some of the clinical benefits outlined above occur due to LDL lowering or to direct "pleiotropic" vascular effects of statins remains unknown.[34] A host of directly beneficial and antiatherosclerotic effects have been demonstrated by these medications. Depending on the statin and dosage used, as well as the experimental techniques involved, these include[34]:

- Improved endothelial function (increased nitric oxide [NO] and NO synthase activity)
- Increased plaque stability and regression of systemic atherosclerosis
- Reduced oxidative stress and pro-inflammatory cytokines (eg, lower superoxide levels, CRP, adhesion molecule expression)
- Anticoagulation effects (increased tissue plasminogen activator inhibitor and reduced plasminogen activator inhibitor 1 levels)

- Inhibition of smooth muscle growth and migration
- Decreased thrombosis (decreased platelet reactivity).

The biologic mechanisms responsible for these pleiotropic effects are related to blockade of the mevalonic acid pathway.[34] By inhibiting the formation of several isoprenoid intermediates, the functions of certain GTP-binding proteins (Ras, Rho) are limited. These G-proteins are responsible for activating many transcription factors and downstream targets that trigger inflammation, cell growth, oxidative stress, and, ultimately, atherogenesis and plaque instability. A few other direct mechanisms not involving the inhibition of Ras/Rho have also been described.

Although pleiotropic effects have been repeatedly demonstrated, the weight of the evidence suggests that the vast majority of the clinical outcome benefits produced by these medications results directly from the resultant LDL lowering.[30,43] At least as far as the proven reduction in major adverse CVD events is concerned, meta-analysis data demonstrate that statins provide no incremental risk reduction beyond that provided by the degree of LDL lowering (equal to all other lipid-lowering medications).[30] Confirming this premise, in the Antihypertensive and Lipid-Lowering Treatment to Prevent Heart Attack Trial (ALLHAT), pravastatin therapy did not significantly reduce the risk of CVD events.[43] This was due to the fact that in the pravastatin limb, cholesterol was lowered by only 9.6% compared with placebo, roughly half the expected reduction. Aggressive

TABLE 23-5 Cholesterol-Lowering Trials with Statins That Enrolled Patients with Cardiovascular Disease or Risk Equivalents

Trial*	Number of subjects	Medication	LDL-C[†] reduction[‡] (%)	CVD event reduction (OR)
4S	4,444	Simvastatin	35.0	0.70
CARE	4,159	Pravastatin	28.0	0.75
LIPID	9,014	Pravastatin	25.0	0.75
HPS	20,536	Simvastatin	38%	0.72
Post-CABG	1,351	Lovastatin	37.0	0.87
LIPS	1,677	Fluvastatin	27.0	0.68
GREACE	1,600	Atorvastatin	46.0	0.46 (RR)
PROSPER	5,804	Pravastatin	34.0%	0.85 (HR)
ALLHAT-LLT	1,475[§]	Pravastatin	17.2	1.03 (HR)

*4S, Scandinavian Simvastatin Survival Study[26]; CARE, Cholesterol and Recurrent Events trial[163]; LIPID, Long-Term Intervention with Pravastatin in Ischemic Disease study[27]; HPS, Heart Protection Study[46]; Post-CABG, Post-Coronary Artery Bypass Grafting study[164]; LIPS, Lescol Intervention Prevention Study[55]; GREACE, Greek Atorvastin and Coronary Heart Disease Evaluation study[165]; PROSPER, Pravastin in Elderly Individuals at Risk of Vascular Disease[31]; ALLHAT-LLT, Antihypertensive and Lipid-Lowering Treatment to Prevent Heart Attack Trial—Lipid-Lowering Trial[43].
[†]LDL-C, low-density lipoprotein cholesterol; CVD, cardiovacular disease; OR, odds ratio; RR, relative risk; HR, hazard ratio.
[‡]Represents percentage LDL-C reduction compared with placebo or usual care.
[§]Number of patients with CVD in ALLHAT-LLT. The percentage HDL-C reduction is given for the entire cohort of patients in the study. The HR of 1.03 is for patients with CVD only.

lifestyle changes and a higher than expected rate of use of cholesterol-lowering medications in the placebo limb likely also explain this finding. As a result, the 9.6% reduction in cholesterol by pravastatin produced a non-significant 9% reduction in CVD event rates. This risk reduction is precisely that expected from the degree of cholesterol lowering regardless of the medications prescribed, and is important to note when discussing the treatment of hyperlipidemia in secondary prevention. The primary goal should be to lower LDL-C in all high-risk patients at least to below 100 mg/dL, with the option of lowering to a goal of <70 mg/dL in those designated as *very high risk* (Table 23-4). Statins are first-line therapy, chiefly because of their favorable characteristics and proven efficacy, not because of putative pleiotropic actions. Other modalities to lower LDL-C, such as bile acid resins (eg, colesavelam), cholesterol absorption inhibitors (eg, ezetimibe, plant stanols), and niacin, if required (alone or in combination with statins), should not be overlooked, especially if elevated triglycerides and/or low HDL-C are also present.

Clinical benefits of lowering LDL-C

The benefits of adhering to LDL-C-lowering therapy are likely much greater than those observed in the clinical trials listed in Table 23-5.[30] First, the mean 30% reduction in CVD events observed over a 5-year period underestimates the overall benefits because little risk reduction occurs during the initial 2 years of therapy.[30] Greater reductions occur in the latter years and after 5 years. Second, because these trials were all intention-to-treat analyses, with patients not taking medications in the active limb and others taking cholesterol-lowering drugs in the placebo limb, the relative clinical efficacy of the statins was reduced. Finally, most of the studies used relatively weak statins and lowered LDL-C by only 20 to 40% (see Table 23-5); newer agents are capable of producing reductions in the range of 60%. Given the linear relationship between LDL-C and CVD events on a log-arithmic scale, greater percentage reductions in LDL-C will very likely yield even greater risk reduction. In fact, it has been estimated that lowering LDL-C by 85 mg/dL in 60-year-old patients with CVD reduces events by nearly 70%.[30] Ongoing studies will provide information regarding the effectiveness of larger degrees of LDL lowering compared with the reductions achieved in previous trials. It is important, however, to note that patients will derive these expected results only if they actually adhere to drug therapy over the long term. It has been estimated in usual clinical practice that compliance rates with statins may be as low as 25 to 40% after only 2 years.[44] In contrast to the aforementioned points, poor adherence to drug therapy may result in a blunting of the anticipated benefits.

Optimal goal LDL-C in secondary prevention

In the past, it had been argued that no additional benefit would be derived from lowering LDL-C beyond 125 mg/dL, or more than 25% from baseline.[45] In contrast, data from the 4S trial[26] did not support this threshold effect. Results from one of the most important clinical trials in cholesterol lowering published in the past few years, the Heart Protection Study, have ended this controversy.[46] In this largest trial to date, 20,536 high-risk adults, aged 40 to 80, with CVD or a risk equivalent were allocated to simvastatin 40 mg/d versus placebo. After 5 years, LDL-C was lowered on average by 38%. This resulted in a 13% reduction in total mortality, an 18% reduction in coronary mortality, and a 24% reduction in all major CVD events (coronary events and mortality, strokes, revascularizations).

The Heart Protection Study confirmed the fact observed from most previous studies that it requires more than 1 year of therapy to witness significant clinical benefits. Important reductions in the incidence of ischemic stroke were also confirmed (decreased by 25%). Several novel findings were also reported. Regardless of comorbidities and the underlying medical condition conferring the high-risk status, all patients significantly benefited from therapy by the same amount. Most striking, the 3500 patients presenting with an initial LDL-C already at goal (<100 mg/dL) received the identical degree of benefit. Reducing LDL-C from 95 to 65 mg/dL was safe, conferred no excess risk of side effects or morbidity, and reduced CVD events by about one quarter. On the basis of these findings, the ATP-III goal LDL-C of less than 100 mg/dL in patients with established CVD is now called into question. All patients with CVD (or high-risk individuals) were shown to benefit from a 38% lowering of LDL-C regardless of the initial values. The implications of this study directly impact the 13 million adults with CVD and LDL-C levels less than 129 mg/dL and the 5 million adults with an initial LDL-C less than 100 mg/dL. Present guidelines state that LDL-C-lowering medications are optional for these groups of individuals.[4] However, based on the results from the Heart Protection Study, all high-risk patients should be treated with a statin to lower LDL-C by approximately 30 to 40%, regardless of their initial cholesterol values.

Further data from meta-analyses suggest that greater reductions in cholesterol will produce superior outcome benefits.[30] The relative odds ratio reduction in clinical CVD events from 49 randomized trials was investigated according to LDL-C reduction achieved. During years 3 to 5, trials that lowered LDL-C by 8 to 27 mg/dL, 28 to 53 mg/dL, and 53 mg/dL or more produced 19, 31, and 50% reductions in CVD events, respectively. These results were achieved regardless of the medications used to attain these reductions in cholesterol.

Finally, several surrogate endpoint experiments also support the benefits of more aggressive LDL lowering. An LDL-C of 76 mg/dL achieved by atorvastatin 80 mg/d versus 110 mg/dL by pravastatin 40 mg/d differentially affected the progression of carotid intima–media thickness over 1 year. The atorvastatin group had a significant 0.034-mm regression compared with the 0.025-mm progression on pravastatin.[47] In an aggressive (LDL-C lowered to 86 mg/dL) versus usual (achieved LDL-C 140 mg/dL) care study, patients with the greater reduction in LDL-C had a smaller progression in coronary plaque volume as determined by intravascular ultrasound.[48] The aggressive treatment produced a significant increase in the echogenicity of coronary plaques compared with usual care. This suggests that lower achieved LDL-C favorably alters plaque characteristics toward stabilization. Finally, CRP has been shown to be reduced more by aggressive versus usual lipid-lowering therapies.[47,49] It is important to note that not all surrogate endpoint studies are in agreement. Aggressive LDL-C lowering has also been shown to be associated with less coronary artery calcium progression than usual care in some, but not all studies.[50,51]

Recently, two important studies were published that strongly support the concept that more aggressive LDL-C lowering beyond the usual goal of 100 mg/dL is beneficial in high risk patients with established coronary disease. In a study using intravascular ultrasound measurements of coronary atherosclerosis, intensively treated patients (achieved LDL-C = 79 mg/dL) had less plaque progression compared to the usual care group (achieved LDL-C = 110 mg/dL).[52] The clinical benefits of aggressive LDL-C lowering were confirmed by the Pravastatin or Atorvastatin Evaluation and Infection Therapy (PROVE-IT) study.[53] In 4162 patients recently hospitalized for an acute coronary syndrome, lowering LDL-C to 62 mg/dL (intensive therapy) compared to 95 mg/dL (standard therapy) reduced the hazard ratio for the primary composite endpoint (total mortality, myocardial infarction, unstable angina requiring hospitalization, revascularization, or stroke) by 16% within a mean of 24 months. This is the first major study outcome evidence that more aggressive lowering of LDL-C beyond the standard goal of 100 mg/dL significantly reduces clinical events.

How early to start cholesterol-lowering medications

The clinical trials performed to date support the benefits of early and aggressive treatment of hyperlipidemia after a CVD event.[54,55] The Lipid-Coronary Artery Disease (L-CAD) study demonstrated a significant reduction in clinical events with early lipid-lowering therapy, compared with usual care after an acute coronary event.[54] The Myocardial Ischemia Reduction with Aggressive Cholesterol Lowering (MIRACL) trial of 3086 patients demonstrated a 16% reduction in combined adverse cardiac events in the early treatment limb (atorvastatin 80 mg/d started 24–96 hours after admission) compared with placebo.[56] Although the benefits were relatively small, they were observed in as little as 16 weeks. The Lescol Intervention Prevention Study (LIPS) extended these findings to include a benefit of early statin therapy in patients undergoing coronary angioplasty.[57] Independent of baseline cholesterol, early use of fluvastatin 80 mg/d postprocedure reduced major adverse cardiac events by 22% compared with placebo.

Most,[55,58,59] but not all,[60] observational studies support early lipid-lowering therapy after a CVD event. However, in addition to reducing clinical complications, the early initiation of medications can increase long-term drug therapy adherence and improve the rate of LDL-C control from 6 to 58% after 1 year.[61] In recognition of these benefits, the AHA/ACC guidelines for therapy after an acute coronary syndrome promote initiation of statin therapy in patients with an LDL-C greater than 100 mg/dL 24 to 96 hours after the onset of unstable angina/non-Q-wave myocardial infarction (class IIa).[62]

Studies on the treatment of metabolic syndrome dyslipidemia (elevated triglycerides and low HDL-C)

The "metabolic syndrome" is a clustering of risk factors causally related to underlying selective tissue insulin resistance, autonomic imbalance, systemic inflammation (increased levels of cytokines/molecules of adipocyte origin), and vascular endothelial dysfunction.[63] The most common etiology is abdominal obesity, although not all overweight adults are insulin resistant.[63] The ATP-III guidelines have provided a clinically useful definition by which patients are diagnosed with metabolic syndrome if they have at least three of the following factors[4]:

- Abdominal obesity (women: >35-in. waist, men: >40-in. waist)
- Borderline or high triglycerides (fasting values ≥150 mg/dL)
- Low HDL-C (women: <50 mg/dL, men: <40 mg/dL)

- Impaired fasting glucose (≥110 mg/dL) (Most patients with overt type 2 diabetes mellitus [even on adequate medical treatment] have significant insulin resistance and the metabolic syndrome.)
- Blood pressure of 130/85 mm Hg or higher (This should also include patients who are on medical treatment for hypertension and who have their blood pressure controlled to below this value.)

Metabolic syndrome is commonly linked to increased numbers of atherogenic apolipoprotein B100 levels, smaller phenotype B LDL particles, and decreased HDL-C levels. Other abnormalities in coagulation, thrombogenicity, arterial vasomotion, and postprandial remnant lipoprotein metabolism have also been described. For these reasons, the roughly 50 million American adults[64] with metabolic syndrome are at an increased risk of CVD independent of traditional risk factor levels.[65]

Although epidemiologic data have demonstrated that elevated triglycerides pose an independent CVD risk,[66] no large outcome trial has directly investigated the clinical impact of lowering triglycerides. On the other hand, a few studies have tested the effect of pharmacologic therapy on raising HDL-C. HDL-C remains a strong, independent predictor of future cardiovascular events in high-risk patients regardless of the LDL-C level achieved, even while on active statin treatment.[67] The Veterans Affairs HDL-C Intervention Trial (VA-HIT) study provides the most powerful support for adding a fibric acid once LDL-C is at goal in the setting of concomitant low HDL-C.[68] Gemfibrozil 1200 mg/d added to traditional therapy increased HDL-C by 6%, whereas LDL-C was not significantly affected (remained below initial values of <140 mg/dL). This resulted in 22 and 31% reductions in recurrent cardiac events and ischemic strokes,[69] respectively. The clinical outcome benefits were statistically shown to be derived most likely from the increase in HDL-C, rather than from the lowering of triglycerides. These results substantiate the stronger observational relationship between HDL-C and CVD (a 3% decrease in CVD risk per 1% increase in HDL-C) than between LDL-C and CVD (a 1% increase in CVD risk per 1.0–1.5% increase in LDL-C).

On the contrary, an 18% increase in HDL-C in the Benzafibrate Infarction Prevention (BIP) trial,[70] did not reproduce the findings of the VA-HIT study. It is possible that the different outcomes can be explained by a high rate of lipid medication usage among patients in the placebo limb of the BIP trial. Furthermore, in a small subset of patients with concomitantly elevated triglycerides, bezafibrate did reduce CVD events by 39.5%.

The HDL-C Atherosclerosis Treatment Study (HATS) provides the most robust evidence for prescribing combination statin–niacin therapy in high-risk patients with metabolic syndrome dyslipidemia.[71]

Although primarily an angiographic regression study of 160 patients over 3 years, HATS demonstrated a marked clinical event reduction by combination therapy. The composite CVD event rate was 90% lower in the simvastatin + niacin group compared with the placebo limb. From previous studies, the expected reduction in events due to simvastatin usage alone is between 30 and 40%. Therefore, HATS strongly supports an additive clinical benefit of LDL-lowering and HDL-C-raising therapies. On the basis of these studies, the addition of niacin to standard statin therapy in an effort to raise HDL-C (if initially <40 mg/dL) should be considered in high-risk patients, even once LDL-C is at goal.

National guidelines and clinical recommendations for treatment of dyslipidemia in secondary prevention

ATP-III has published guidelines for cholesterol-lowering therapy.[4] Goals are based chiefly on levels of LDL-C, the lipoprotein most strongly associated with atherosclerotic disease. Target levels of therapy are based on the risk of cardiovascular events. Increased risk, as assessed by a larger number of risk factors, mandates a lower LDL-C target goal. Patients at the highest risk level are those with established CVD or CVD risk equivalents. It follows that all patients undergoing cholesterol reduction for secondary prevention of CVD fall into this most aggressive LDL-C-lowering category. *The recommended target LDL-C is less than 100 mg/dL in this group of patients.* For many high-risk patients, attainment of this goal may require double- or triple-drug therapy. Because of the high-risk status of these patients, high-dose statin monotherapy, or a combination of medications, is usually warranted and worth the modest increased risk of potential side effects. Clinical symptoms of myalgias and serum liver enzymes should be monitored closely in patients in this situation.[4]

The optimal LDL-C goal for secondary prevention was recently lowered to 50–70 mg/dL in very high risk patients (eg, those with acute coronary syndrome, or CVD plus diabetes or metabolic syndrome)[72] based on the results of the Heart Protection Study[46] and the PROVE-IT trial results.[53] Best available evidence suggests that any patient with CVD or a risk equivalent should be on statin therapy to lower LDL-C by approximately 30 to 40% (equivalent to simvastatin 40 mg/d), regardless of initial LDL-C (even if <100 mg/dL). The optimal LDL-C level remains unclear, but clinical benefit has been shown when LDL-C is lowered to 50–70 mg/dL compared to <100 mg/dL.[53] The recent update to the ATP III guidelines[72] suggest that if the patient is very high risk (Figure 22-3) even more aggressive lipid-lowering therapy should be instituted to achieve an LDL <70 mg/dL.

Once the primary goal of a LDL-C less than 100 mg/dL is met (all patients should be on statin therapy and certain very high risk patients could be optimally treated to an LDL-C <70 mg/dL), the secondary targets of triglycerides and HDL-C should be considered. ATP-III did not promote actual goal values for these lipoproteins in secondary prevention; rather, they promoted the treatment of non-HDL-C. Non-HDL-C (total cholesterol—HDL) represents all apolipoprotein B100-containing atherogenic lipids (LDL-C, intermediate-density lipoproteins, lipoprotein(a), and very low density remnants).[4] It has been found to be superior to LDL-C in predicting future CVD risk on or off therapy in most studies.[28,73,74] It is not uncommon in patients with metabolic syndrome or combined hyperlipidemia, for LDL-C to be at goal (<100 mg/dL), but, because of low HDL-C and/or high triglycerides, for non-HDL-C to remain suboptimal. Goal non-HDL-C is the LDL-C target + 30 mg/dL. Therefore, in secondary prevention, the target for patients with metabolic syndrome or isolated low HDL-C is to achieve a non-HDL-C less than 130 mg/dL. For very high risk patients this goal is a non-HDL-C <100 mg/dL. This can be achieved either by intensifying statin therapy (in some patients) or by adding combination medications (niacin or fibrates) to raise HDL-C, or lower triglycerides, or when clinically prudent.[4] Appropriate caution should be considered when combining statins with other lipid-lowering medications, in particular fibrates, because of the modest increased risk of myositis.[4] However, due to the high-risk status of patients receiving secondary prevention, the risk-to-benefit ratio is usually in favor of attempting combination lipid-lowering medications to achieve target lipid goals when necessary. ATP-III guidelines support the consideration of raising HDL-C should it remain below 40 mg/dL, even with non-HDL-C at goal (isolated low HDL-C), in high-risk patients.[4] However, present AHA/ACC guidelines for therapy after an acute coronary syndrome recommend adding fibrate/niacin therapy (class I) in patients with an isolated low HDL-C.[62] A suggested algorithm for management of dyslipidemia in secondary prevention in outlined in Fig. 23-3.

BLOOD PRESSURE AND HYPERTENSION

Hypertension as a risk factor in secondary prevention

Both systolic and diastolic blood pressures have continuous, graded, independent, and etiologically significant relationships to the development of CVD.[75] Systolic blood pressure and pulse pressure may be of even greater importance than diastolic pressure.[76] In patients with established CVD, hypertension continues to confer an increased risk for the progression of disease and for the recurrence of adverse events.[77]

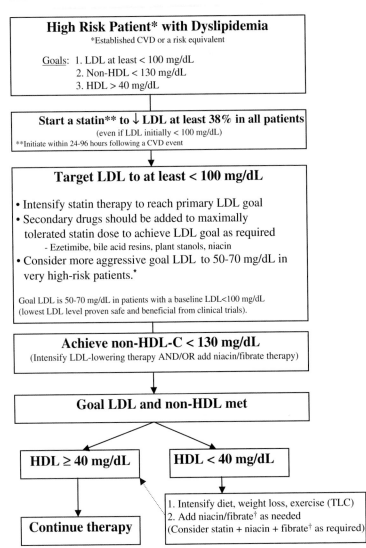

FIGURE 23-3 Algorithm for lipid-lowering therapy in high-risk patients. *Very high risk patients: Established CVD plus 1) multiple risk factors or diabetes; 2) severe risk factors or smoking; 3) metabolic syndrome or low HDL-C; or 4) recent acute coronary syndrome. †Fibrate combination with statin: use with caution.

Clinical trials in hypertension in secondary prevention

Data from placebo-controlled antihypertensive trials in secondary prevention are sparse. Owing to the proven benefits of lowering blood pressure in a vast number of studies involving patients mostly free of established CVD,[78] no trial has specifically investigated the efficacy of hypertension treatment per se in patients exclusively with preexisting CVD. However, one trial demonstrated the benefits of combined angiotensin-converting enzyme inhibitor (ACEI) plus diuretic therapy in prevention of recurrent strokes (28% reduction) and CVD events (26% reduction) in subjects with a previous stroke (PROGRESS Collaborative Group).[79] Early

studies had established that both short- and long-term use of beta blockers improves prognosis after myocardial infarction (MI) over many years of follow-up. Aggregate results show that long-term beta blocker therapy reduces total mortality by approximately 20%, with a pooled relative risk of death of 0.77.[80] The most recent meta-regression analysis confirms these observations of a 23% reduction in events.[81] Whether it is the reduction in blood pressure or the direct cardioprotective actions of beta blockers that matters is difficult to confidently discern. Nevertheless, beta blocker therapy continues to be the standard of care for all patients with a previous MI (with or without heart failure) and/or symptomatic coronary artery disease (CAD). In a similar fashion, convincing clinical trial data support the use of ACEIs in all post-MI patients with impaired cardiac function. A systematic review of the literature suggests that ACEIs reduce CVD events by approximately 23% in high-risk patients with reduced left ventricular function.[82]

Subgroups of large clinical trials and meta-analyses

A subgroup analysis of the Hypertension Detection and Follow-up Program (HDFP) in subjects who had evidence of CVD at the outset of the trial supports the treatment of elevated blood pressure. All CVD patient subgroups in the stepped care group benefited in risk reduction when contrasted with patients in the referred care group.[83] Therefore, this subgroup analysis suggests that hypertension treatment per se is beneficial in patients with established CVD.

The question of which antihypertensive medication(s) should be used in patients with CVD to achieve blood pressure reduction was not addressed by the HDFP. More recently, ALLHAT compared the efficacy of thiazide diuretics versus newer agents (amlodipine, lisinopril, doxazosin) in CVD risk reduction.[84] Approximately 25% of patients were known to have CVD at study onset. The benefits in relation to the primary endpoint (MI and fatal CVD event) were equally observed across all classes of medications. This same finding held true in all subgroups of patients, including those with diabetes (a CHD risk equivalent) and established CVD. There were small differences in secondary study endpoints, the importance of which remains the subject of much debate. For the most part, ALLHAT results support a conclusion that lowering blood pressure is more important than the medication class used. ALLHAT emphasized that most patients with hypertension required two or more medications to reach goal. Patients with diabetes, heart failure, and/or renal insufficiency often required three or four medications. Systolic blood pressure remains much more difficult to control than diastolic, with only two thirds of patients reaching goals in ALLHAT despite multiple medications. The chief message from this landmark trial is that combination drug therapy is required in most high-risk hypertension patients to achieve goal blood pressures and that one of the medications in the regimen should generally be a thiazide diuretic.

A small percentage (8%) of patients in the Second Australian National Blood Pressure Study had established CVD.[85] In this trial of 6083 elderly subjects, ACEIs were found to be slightly superior than thiazide diuretics in reducing total CVD events. In the entire cohort, the hazard ratio of 0.89 for ACEI usage was not significant ($P = .05$). Among elderly men it was 0.83 ($P = .02$). These modest benefits are of uncertain clinical significance in the light of the neutral results reported from the much larger ALLHAT and from several meta-analyses.

The largest meta-analysis to date, including more than 149,000 patients, concluded that the cardiovascular risk reduction provided by all antihypertensive agents is predicted exclusively by the changes in blood pressure.[78] There was no evidence for excess CVD mortality by calcium channel blockers, even in those with preexisting heart disease (also supported by ALLHAT). In addition, ACEIs were found to provide as efficacious in event reduction as older medications. Their conclusion was, "The hypothesis that new antihypertensive drugs ... might influence cardiovascular prognosis over and beyond their antihypertensive effects remains unproven."

Blood pressure-independent effects of new medications

In contrast to the neutral outcome trials, many small studies have suggested that pharmacologic blockade of the renin–angiotensin–aldosterone (RAAS) system is directly protective to the cardiovascular system.[86,87] Due to the observed upregulation of the RAAS within specific tissues (heart/vasculature/atheroma) in many high-risk patients, ACEI usage may yield particular clinical benefit.[86] ACEIs possess a host of pleiotropic antiatherosclerotic effects that appear to be independent of blood pressure lowering, including[86,87]:

- Improvement in endothelial function
- Reduction in oxidative stress (eg, reduced NADP oxidase)
- Decrease in vascular inflammation and adhesion molecules
- Inhibition of mitogenesis
- Regression of atherosclerotic plaque and left ventricular hypertrophy superior to older agents
- Inhibition of proteinuria superior to older agents
- Reduction in new-onset diabetes mellitus
- Improvement in fibrinolysis

As stated earlier, ACEIs are clearly indicated in all individuals with a reduced ejection fraction.[82] However, their benefits may extend beyond this category of patients. The Heart Outcomes Prevention Evaluation (HOPE) study sought to test the efficacy of ACEIs in high-risk patients without heart failure.[88] In 9297 adults with diabetes or vascular disease and a normal ejection fraction, ramipril 10 mg/d reduced combined cardiovascular events (MI, stroke, CVD mortality) by 22%, compared with placebo, after 4.5 years. These benefits were observed in all patient groups and were incremental to all conventional secondary prevention therapies. The investigators claimed that only a small portion of the risk reduction (40% of the stroke and 25% of the CVD benefits) could be attributed to the very small degree of blood pressure lowering (3/2 mm Hg). Further analyses expanded the improvement in outcomes provided by ramipril to include reductions in stroke, fatal/nonfatal MI, worsening or new angina, requirement for coronary revascularizations,[89] and new-onset diabetes.[90]

Whether the benefits observed in the HOPE study are derived from the small reduction of blood pressures even within the nonhypertensive range or from the direct actions of the ACEI itself is a matter of continued debate. The recently completed EUROPA study comparing perindopril and placebo in patients with stable coronary disease and without heart failure reported similar findings.[91] However, a HOPE substudy has recently provided evidence that the observed event reduction may be ascribed to a larger than previously recognized decrease in the mean 24-hour blood pressure among those in the ramipril group.[92] In EUROPA, a 5/2 mm Hg blood pressure difference was reported between treatment groups and may account for much of the findings. No trial that has used an active control consisting of a blood pressure medication rather than placebo has convincingly demonstrated a superior clinical benefit of the newer agents in secondary prevention.[78] Even in the Losartan In**ver**vention for Endpoints (LIFE) study, atenolol and losartan were found to be equally effective among patients with established CVD.[93] Several ongoing studies with ACEIs and angiotensin receptor blockers in high-risk patients (eg, ONTARGET) should help to determine the clinical importance of the putative blood pressure-independent effects of these medications.

Goal blood pressure

The Hypertension Optimal Treatment (HOT) trial sought to determine the efficacy and safety of intensive versus usual blood pressure reduction. The study enrolled 3080 patients with established CVD.[94] The lowest incidence of major cardiovascular events occurred at a mean achieved diastolic pressure of 82.6 mm Hg. Only for MI was there a trend ($P = .05$) toward lower event rates at lower target blood pressures (a nonsignificant 25% event reduction in the target group ≤85 mm Hg and a 28% reduction in the target group ≤80 mm Hg, as compared with the target group ≤90 mm Hg). No effect on stroke incidence was observed. The HOT trial provided the first evidence from a randomized controlled trial that reduction in diastolic pressure below the usual target value of less than 90 mm Hg is safe (absence of a J-curve effect) and beneficial in certain subsets of high-risk patients. Aggressive treatment of diastolic pressure to the goal of less than 80 mm Hg cut the incidence of CVD events roughly in half in patients with diabetes mellitus.

Given the above, JNC-7 has recommended certain goal blood pressures, including:

- Less than 140 mm Hg systolic and less than 90 mm Hg diastolic in uncomplicated hypertensive patients, including those with prior CVD
- Less than 130 mm Hg systolic and less than 80 mm Hg diastolic for those with diabetes or chronic renal insufficiency

It is possible that the clinical event reductions observed in the HOPE[88] and EUROPA[91] trials actually represent the benefits of aggressive blood pressure lowering per se (even when patients start with levels <140/90 mm Hg) in high-risk patients with atherosclerosis. Whether more aggressive blood pressure lowering to less than 130/80 mm Hg reduces (recurrent) CVD events in high-risk patients without diabetes and/or renal disease remains to be clarified.

National guidelines and clinical recommendations for treatment of hypertension in secondary prevention

The Seventh Report of the Joint National Committee on Prevention, Detection, Evaluation, and Treatment of High Blood Pressure (JNC-7) published guidelines for the treatment of hypertension.[14] Included in this consensus statement is the recommended treatment of patients with established CVD.

Compelling indications are given for: use of beta blockers and ACEIs after MI; use of beta blockers and ACEIs in patients with CVD and compromised left ventricular function; and addition of aldosterone blockers with systolic dysfunction if tolerated (eg, EPHESUS study results[95]).

Angiotensin receptor blockers could be used in place of ACEIs in heart failure for intolerant patients (not equivalent to an ACE-I in the OPTIMAAL study[96] using losartan). In the recent CHARM study, however, candesartan was found to be equally efficacious in ACEI-intolerant heart failure patients[97] and to have additive benefits in patients continuing ACEI therapy.[98]

Diabetic patients, particularly those with albuminuria or renal insufficiency, should be on either an ACEI or angiotensin receptor blocker. The goal blood pressure of less than 130/80 mm Hg in diabetics usually requires three to four medications to achieve (eg, RENAAL study[99]).

In all other high-risk patients, any class (and combination) of antihypertensive drugs is acceptable.[14] The role of even newer medications, such as endothelin receptor blockers, and the use of combined ACEI and angiotensin receptor blockers in patients with heart failure, atherosclerosis, and/or diabetes (albuminuria) require more investigation. A suggested algorithm is presented in Fig. 23-4.

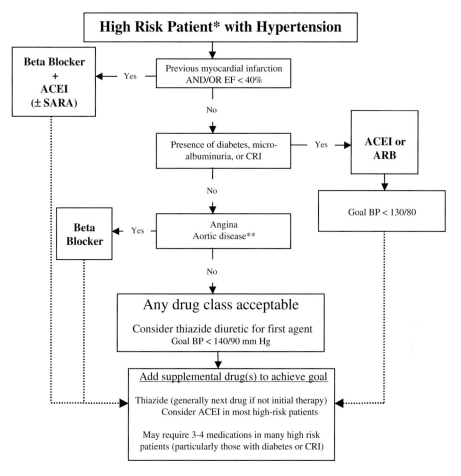

FIGURE 23-4 Algorithm for hypertension therapy in high-risk patients. ACEI, Angiotensin converting enyzme inhibitor; ARB, angiotensin receptor blocker; BP, blood pressure; SARA, selective aldosterone receptor antagonist; CRI, chronic renal insufficiency.

HEMOSTASIS AS A RISK FACTOR AND ANTIPLATELET THERAPY

Thrombosis and coagulation contribute to the occurrence of acute cardiovascular events, as well as to atherosclerosis itself. Measurements of fibrinogen,[100] platelet aggregability and counts,[101] and tissue plasminogen activator levels[102] have been associated with increases in CVD risk. Trials to date have not focused on manipulation of single elements in the cascade, but rather on therapy that affects the entire process of hemostasis.

The most recent meta-analysis performed by the Antiplatelet Trialists' Collaboration confirmed that therapy with antiplatelet agents in the secondary prevention of CVD is effective.[103] In more than 200,000 high-risk patients from 287 studies, antiplatelet medications were shown to reduce any serious vascular event and stroke by one quarter and nonfatal MI by one third. There was no evidence that high-dose aspirin (>325 mg/d) is more effective than low- to medium-strength doses (75–150 mg/d). The effect of doses less than 75 mg/d remains uncertain. There was also little evidence to suggest that other antiplatelet agents and/or combinations of medications are more efficacious. In most high-risk patients, the benefits of daily low-dose aspirin in preventing CVD events markedly outweigh the small excess risk in serious bleeding.

In a few studies, the adenosine diphosphate receptor antagonist clopidogrel has been compared, alone or in combination with aspirin, to traditional aspirin therapy. In the Clopidogrel versus Aspirin in Patients at Risk of Ischemic Events (CAPRIE) trial, there was a significant 8.7% relative risk reduction compared with aspirin in the clopidogrel group for the combined occurrence of stroke, MI, or vascular death.[104] Side effect profiles were similar in the two treatment groups. Because of the much lower cost of aspirin, and the relatively small additional benefit attributable to clopidogrel, low-dose aspirin therapy remains the medication of choice in secondary prevention for most patients. In high-risk diabetics,[105] and those with peripheral vascular disease,[104,106] studies have suggested that the benefits of clopidogrel over aspirin may be more pronounced.

More recently, the Clopidogrel in Unstable Angina to Prevent Recurrent Events (CURE) study tested the clinical efficacy of combined clopidogrel and aspirin versus aspirin alone in 12,562 patients immediately after an acute coronary event.[107] After a mean of 9 months, the combination medication group had a relative risk of 0.80 ($P < .001$) for recurrent CVD events compared with aspirin alone. These benefits were observed across all groups of patients. In a substudy (PCI-CURE), the proven effectiveness of the same combination therapy was extended to patients who also underwent a percutaneous coronary intervention.[108] Patients who received combined therapy for 1 year had a relative risk of 0.70 ($P = .03$) compared with standard therapy (aspirin + a thienopyridine for 4 weeks).[109] Although the largest salutary effects occur rapidly (within 24 hours), the benefits of combination therapy have been shown to extend and widen for up to 1 year after a coronary event.[110] Not unexpected, a significant excess risk of major bleeding (2.7% vs 3.7%, $P = .003$) was also observed in the clopidogrel + aspirin cohort. Ongoing studies will further investigate the role of combination antiplatelet strategies in CVD prevention.

Anticoagulation with warfarin after a coronary event may also be beneficial in secondary prevention as seen in early trials.[111] Initial studies demonstrated that warfarin alone, or in combination[112] with aspirin while maintaining subtherapeutic anticoagulation (INR 1.2–1.8), was not superior to aspirin alone. Most recently, the Warfarin, Aspirin, or Both after Myocardial Infarction study published discordant findings.[113] In 3630 patients, aspirin (75 mg/d) + warfarin (mean INR 2.2) was compared with warfarin alone (mean INR 2.8) and with aspirin alone (160 mg/d). The combination therapy group had a significant 29% relative risk reduction in composite CVD events compared with the group that took aspirin alone after 4 years. Warfarin alone lowered subsequent events by 19% compared with aspirin monotherapy. The major benefit seen in the warfarin groups was a reduction in nonfatal reinfarctions and thromboembolic strokes.

As anticipated, the incidence of minor and major bleeding episodes was four times higher in patients who received warfarin. No study to date has investigated the effectiveness of clopidogrel alone or in combination with aspirin plus systemic anticoagulation in reducing CVD events. However, the recently completed ESTEEM study demonstrated that the new direct thrombin inhibitor (ximelagatran) plus aspirin was more effective in preventing recurrent events than aspirin alone (hazard ratio = 0.76). Further studies are ongoing to investigate novel anticoagulant therapies.[114]

Management guidelines for antiplatelet therapy

The use of lifelong low-dose aspirin (75–160 mg/d) by all high-risk patients (including those with CVD risk equivalents and/or established CVD) is widely recommended in secondary prevention protocols.[2,11] Although the "optimal dose" is uncertain, doses in the range 75 to 160 mg/d appear to provide equal benefit, with a lower risk of bleeding, than higher doses. Aspirin is recommended as the primary therapy because of its low cost and safety and because other agents are at most marginally superior. Clopidogrel 75 mg/d or warfarin (INR 2.0–3.0) is recommended for patients who cannot tolerate aspirin.[11] Warfarin may also be a valuable substitute in post-MI patients with left ventricular dysfunction at risk for arterial embolization. Combination aspirin + clopidogrel therapy should be considered for selected very high-risk patients, and for at least 1 year after an acute coronary event and/or after percutaneous coronary interventions. The optimal duration of combination therapy in these settings remains to be determined. Figure 23-5 outlines a suggested algorithm for antiplatelet and anticoagulation therapy in high-risk patients.

TOBACCO SMOKING

Both active and passive tobacco smoking increase CVD risk. Cigarette smoking worsens CVD by several mechanisms. Angiographic studies have revealed that smoking is associated with the progression of atherosclerosis. Smoking induces an increase in fibrinogen levels, platelet activity, and blood viscosity. Vascular tone is enhanced and endothelial dysfunction occurs. HDL-C levels are lowered, while more LDL-C is oxidized. Blood pressure, heart rate, and sympathetic tone are also increased in response to cigarette smoking.[115]

There are no randomized controlled trials in the secondary prevention of CVD using smoking cessation. However, observational evidence overwhelmingly supports the need for smoking cessation in secondary prevention. One such analysis was performed in patients from the Coronary Artery Surgery Study (CASS) with

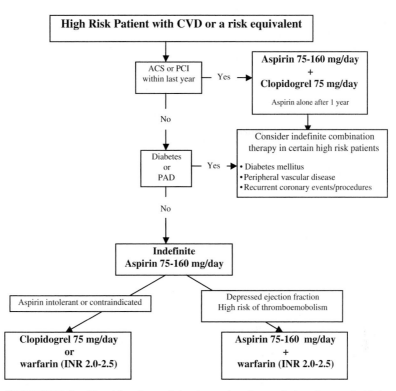

FIGURE 23-5   Algorithm for antiplatelet and anticoagulation therapy in high-risk patients. ACS, acute coronary syndrome; PCI, percutaneous coronary intervention; PAD, peripheral artery disease.

angiographically documented atherosclerosis.[116] In the total CASS cohort, patients who continued to smoke had a statistically higher adjusted relative risk (RR) of death than did patients who quit (RR = 1.7, 95% CI = 1.4–2.0, $P <$ .001). The RR of MI was also higher in those who continued to smoke (RR = 1.5, 95% CI = 1.2–1.7, $P =$ .001). Subgroup analyses in CASS showed that elderly patients and women benefited from smoking cessation, as did younger people and men. Also, patients at all levels of coronary risk (assessed by risk scores) benefited from smoking cessation. The CASS data confirmed results of earlier studies that smoking cessation reduces both cardiovascular events and total mortality in all groups of patients with established CVD.[117]

In a more recent study of 2619 patients who survived a MI, smoking status and risk for recurrent CVD events were investigated.[118] Continued active smokers maintained a RR of 1.51 for subsequent events. For those who quit smoking the relative risk declined with the duration of cessation from 1.62 (0–6 months), to 1.60 (6–18 months), to 1.48 (18–36 months), to essentially a baseline risk of 1.02 after 36 months or longer. This study suggests that the risk for recurrent vascular events

approaches the level of nonsmokers by 3 years of cessation.

The most comprehensive analytical review of the health effects of smoking in patients with CHD also strongly supports the benefit of smoking cessation.[119] Data derived from 20 studies revealed that patients who quit smoking had a 36% RR reduction in mortality compared with those who continued to smoke. Various patient demographics, age, gender, ethnicity, and medication usage did not alter the benefits derived from smoking cessation. The authors commented that the health impact is similar to or greater than that derived from all the modern medications used in secondary prevention.

Based on the strength of evidence, complete smoking cessation should be strongly advocated, especially to high-risk patients and those with documented CVD. Medications, nicotine replacement therapies, and formal cessation counseling should be used as required to achieve total abstinence. The ACC/AHA guidelines further recommend that family members of a patient with CVD should be urged to discontinue smoking to eliminate the known detrimental effects of secondhand tobacco smoke exposure.[11]

THERAPEUTIC LIFESTYLE CHANGES: DIETARY THERAPY AND EXERCISE

The benefits of different dietary therapies have been studied in patients with existing CVD. Several trials have shown a modest positive impact of dietary modifications in patients with established heart disease.[120–125] The largest comprehensive analysis of 147 publications suggested that three types of diets are likely to prevent CVD[126]:

1. Substitution of nonhydrogenated unsaturated fats for saturated/*trans*-fats
2. Increased consumption of omega-3 fats from fish, fish oil supplements, or plant sources of omega-3 fats (α-linolenic acid)
3. A diet high in fruits, vegetables, nuts, and whole grains and low in refined grain products

The present analysis suggests that simply lowering the percentage of energy from total fat in the diet does not improve CVD outcome. This conclusion was corroborated by a systematic review that revealed only modest benefits from a strictly low-fat diet.[127] In contrast, earlier studies of very low fat diets coupled with other lifestyle changes demonstrated some success in coronary risk reduction.[124,125] In a recent study of 409 patients with CVD, those who followed "maximal" treatment consisting of a very low fat diet (<10 g/d) plus aggressive cholesterol-lowering medication attained the greatest reduction in recurrent events.[128] The "maximal" treatment group had a 6.6% coronary event rate over 5 years, compared with 20.3% in patients on either medications or the AHA Step 2 diet alone. These results suggest an additive benefit of a very low fat diet on cholesterol-lowering medications. Therefore, the efficacy of a low-fat diet alone is uncertain. Current AHA guidelines for therapeutic lifestyle changes during secondary prevention recommend that all patients start a low-fat Step 2 AHA diet.[11]

Various studies that involved increasing the amount of omega-3 fats in the diet have demonstrated cardiovascular benefits. These include the Diet and Reinfarction Trial, the Indian Experiment of Infarct Survival, and the Lyon Diet Heart Study.[129] The most compelling evidence comes from the large GISSI-3 Prevention study[130] of 11,324 patients with established coronary disease. The daily supplementation of a capsule containing 1 g of total omega-3 fats reduced the composite endpoint of CVD events by 15% in patients already on standard cardioprotective medication therapy. The majority of the benefit was derived from a 53% reduction in sudden death within 4 months of initiating therapy[131]; no reduction in nonfatal MI was seen during the study, suggesting that fish oil prevents cardiac mortality primarily

by an antiarrhythmic mechanism. Evidence supporting the long-term (>1 year) use of fish oil post-MI is less compelling than that for short-term use.[132] With these aggregate findings in mind, the most recent AHA statement promotes the use of 1 g of omega-3 fats per day in patients with CVD.[126] Supplementation from oily fish is preferred; however concentrated omega-3 capsules are an acceptable alternative. Whether a Mediterranean-type diet rich in omega-3 fats is superior to the traditional AHA Step 2 diet in preventing CVD is unknown. Some investigators have called for such a trial[133]; however, due to logistical difficulties this seems unlikely.

Exercise capacity is one of the strongest predictors of long-term clinical outcomes in both healthy and high-risk patients with established CVD.[134,135] For example, among 3679 patients with an abnormal stress test or known CVD, the peak metabolic equivalent capacity was shown to be the single best predictor of subsequent death.[131] Each 1-metabolic equivalent greater exercise capacity improved survival by 12%. Exercise and cardiac rehabilitation in post-MI patients have also been demonstrated to reduce recurrent cardiovascular events. The most recent meta-analysis of exercise rehabilitation programs, including 8440 patients, demonstrated improved outcomes after an average of 2.4 years.[136] Total and CVD mortality were reduced by 27 and 31%, respectively, by 2 to 6 months of supervised exercise. Nonfatal MI was not decreased, suggesting a clinical benefit derived from an antiarrhythmic effect or via ischemic preconditioning. Cardiac rehabilitation also results in considerable improvements in cardiac symptoms and other measures of quality of life.[137–139] Formal guided exercise programs should be part of all secondary prevention and cardiac rehabilitation programs in patients with known CVD and those post-MI.[140]

RISK FACTOR MODIFICATIONS OF PROBABLE OR POSSIBLE BENEFIT

Diabetes mellitus

Diabetes conveys an increased risk of cardiovascular events and mortality in patients with CVD.[21] It is associated with a worse prognosis in women and, in some studies, is associated with a greater risk for coronary events than established CVD.[141] Limited data exist specifically in regard to blood glucose control and cardiovascular endpoints in secondary prevention. A small study from Europe using insulin-based therapy demonstrated a 29% reduction in mortality in patients post- MI with a hemoglobin A_{1c} of 7.1% versus 7.6%.[142] The modest reduction in macrovascular events seen in large primary prevention trials by intensive glucose control,[143,144] particularly with metformin usage in overweight patients,[145] may also apply to patients with established disease. Most recently, a trial of 1429 patients with impaired glucose tolerance treated with acarbose to lower postprandial glycemia demonstrated a marked reduction (49% relative risk) in CVD events in the active treatment group versus the placebo group.[146] Roughly 4.8% of patients had established CVD on study initiation. Although this study was not designed a priori to detect alterations in coronary events, these results are intriguing and may warrant further investigation. Ongoing studies using a variety of agents are currently investigating the ability of newer oral hypoglycemic medications, such as the thioglitazones, to reduce clinical CVD events.

Perhaps more importantly, subgroup analyses of large clinical trials demonstrate that control of all other risk factors in patients with established CVD, including the use of antiplatelet agents and ACEIs, is at least as effective in reducing CVD events in diabetics as in nondiabetics. A recent study of 80 diabetic patients confirmed the importance of aggressive multiple risk factor treatment. Intensive therapy reduced CVD complications by 53% compared with usual care.[147] Whether these results apply to patients with diabetes and established CVD remains to be determined.

EMERGING RISK FACTORS

Table 23-6 provides a partial list of the emerging CVD risk factors and putative therapies identified to date. An enormous number of clinical trials are ongoing or in the planning stage regarding treatment of some of these factors. At present, no recommendations exist regarding their management in secondary prevention. However,

TABLE 23-6   Emerging Cardiovascular Risk Factors and Therapies

Lipoproteins and Related Factors
Lipoprotein (a)
LDL and HDL particle size distributions
Remnant lipoproteins
Postprandial lipemia
Apolipoproteins CIII, apoE4, ApoA1/ApoB100
Free fatty acid levels
Hepatic lipase and lipoprotein lipase activities
Endogenous omega-3 fatty acid cell membrane content
Lipoprotein associated phospholipase A_2

Coagulation Factors
Plasminogen activator inhibitor 1
Fibrinogen
Multiple determinants of hypercoagulability
Tissue factor
Platelet count/aggregability
Aspirin resistance

Inflammation and Oxidative Stress
C-reactive protein
Asymmetric dimethyl arginine
Pro-inflammatory cytokines
Poor dental hygiene
Infectious agents (eg, *Chlamydia pneumoniae*)
Heat shock proteins
Low levels of anti-inflammatory cytokines
CD40 ligand
Circulating adhesion molecules (ICAM, VCAM, P-selectin)
Elevated free radicals (eg, superoxide, nitrotyrosine)
Low antioxidants (eg, extracellular superoxide dismutase)
White blood cell count
Uric acid level
Myeloperoxidase

Matrix metalloproteinase levels (MMP-9)
Activation of transcription factors (eg, nuclear factor κb)

Metabolic Factors
Homocysteine, cysteine, and folic acid status
Obesity and visceral fat (body fat distribution)
Insulin and tissue sensitivity
Leptin levels and tissue sensitivity
Postprandial glycemia

Social and Environmental Factors
Air pollution
Depression and anger
Neighborhood of residence
Socioeconomic status, spouse education level

Miscellaneous
Multiple genetic polymorphisms in blood pressure, coagulation, inflammation regulation (eg, ACE DD)
Activity of the renin–angiotensin system (levels of renin, angiotensinogen, aldosterone)
Sympathetic and autonomic tone (heart rate variability)
Circulating endothelial progenitor cell levels

Putative Therapies
Folic acid, B vitamins
Tetrahydabiopterin
L-Arginine
Antioxidant combinations
Selective estrogen receptor agonists
Antidepressant medications
Antibiotics versus infectious agents (macrolides)
Combination ACEI + ARB therapy (+ anti-aldosterone drugs)
New lipid medications (eg, cholesterol ester transfer protein inhibitors, liver X receptor agonists)
Herbal remedies (eg, gugulipid, policosanol)

*HDL, high-density lipoprotein; LDL, low-density lipoprotein; ARB, angiotensin receptor blocker.

homocysteine and antibiotic therapy deserve emphasis as preliminary trial data have become available during the past few years on these two novel risk factors.

Elevated levels of homocysteine have been linked to excess morbidity and mortality among patients with established CVD.[148] Whether homocysteine per se or other related factors (eg, total cysteine, folic acid status, tetrahydrobiopterin, methyl tetrahydrofolate reductase) are mechanistically responsible remains a matter of debate. Thus far, the results from completed studies using folic acid and B vitamins remains mixed. Two trials have demonstrated a reduction in coronary restenosis and requirement for revascularization procedures after percutaneous coronary interventions.[149,150] However, in a study of 593 patients with stable CAD, a reduction in homocysteine by folic acid therapy was unsuccessful in reducing clinical CVD events during 2 years of secondary prevention.[151] The most recent AHA Science Advisory statement considers treatment of an elevated homocysteine with supplemental vitamins experimental.[152]

In a similar fashion, available results from trials of antibiotics in secondary prevention are mixed. The largest and most recent studies of azithromycin in 1439 patients with CHD[153] and roxithromycin in 872 patients after an acute MI[154] failed to demonstrate a benefit of macrolide therapy. These antibiotics are presumably targeted against latent or persistent infection in the vasculature with *Chlamydia pneumoniae*. However, these trials may have prescribed the antibiotics for too limited a duration (few days to weeks rather than several months to a year).[155] In the Weekly Intervention with Zithromax for Atherosclerosis and Its Related Disorder (WIZARD), the macrolide was taken for a course of 3 months in stable post-MI patients. At present, no recommendations exist for prescribing antibiotics in patients with established CVD.

INTERVENTIONS OF NO PROVEN BENEFIT

Hormone replacement therapy

Despite epidemiologic evidence,[156,157] clinical trials to date do not demonstrate any cardiovascular benefit of hormone replacement therapy. The Heart and Estrogen/Progestin Replacement Study (HERS) results represented the first data from a large randomized clinical trial on the effect of hormone replacement therapy in women with preexisting heart disease.[92] The HERS trial found that in 4 years of follow-up in postmenopausal women with a uterus, the use of estrogen (as conjugated equine estrogen) and progestin (as continuous daily medroxyprogesterone acetate) did not prevent further heart attacks or death from CVD. Although the cardiovascular event rate was substantially higher in the ini-

tial year, there appeared to be a trend toward benefit in latter years; however, continued open-label follow-up of this cohort showed no benefit in prevention of recurrent CVD events over the long term. In agreement with the lack of clinical benefit, various estrogens, either alone or in combination with progesterone, have failed to significantly inhibit the progression of coronary atherosclerosis.[158] Large primary prevention outcome trials of estrogen replacement therapies have reported similarly negative results.[159] The most recent AHA statement therefore does not support the use of routine hormone replacement therapy for postmenopausal women to prevent CVD in either the primary or secondary prevention setting.[160]

Antioxidants

Despite the initial excitement over earlier trials, the most recent meta-analysis including patients with and without CVD[161] failed to demonstrate any mortality reduction following vitamin E (odds ratio = 1.02, 95% CI = 0.98–1.06, $P = .42$) or vitamin C supplementation. β-carotene use actually led to a slight increase in mortality (odds ratio = 1.07, 95% CI = 1.02–1.11, $P = .003$).[161] In addition, no reduction in any CVD endpoint was observed.[161] Several large secondary prevention studies have also demonstrated a lack of benefit from combined antioxidant therapy. In the large Heart Protection Study, daily antioxidant supplementation (vitamin E 600 mg, vitamin C 250 mg, β-carotene 20 mg) did not reduce all-cause morality, vascular deaths, nonfatal MI, coronary death, stroke, or revascularization.[162] Furthermore, recent evidence from HATS demonstrates that combination antioxidant use may blunt the HDL-C-raising ability of simvastatin–niacin treatment.[71] The authors suggest that this explains the blunted clinical benefit in their patients taking antioxidants plus lipid-lowering therapy versus those on simvastatin–niacin alone. Based on the lack of proven benefit, a recent American Heart Association science advisory does not recommend the use of antioxidants for either the primary or secondary prevention of CVD.[166] However, many issues remain to be clarified such as optimal dosing, patient selection, and timing of antioxidant supplementation (eg, supplementation in patients without heart disease or very early in the atherosclerotic process). Ongoing studies may provide further evidence about any potential benefit of antioxidant therapy.

CONCLUSIONS

Patients with established heart disease or CVD risk equivalents are at high risk for acute coronary events (from 2 to 5% per year). It may be helpful to further risk-stratify individuals, not only on the basis of functional test results, but also by information provided from physical examination and the individual risk factors obtained during office visits. The robust clinical benefits derived from global risk factor modification during secondary prevention are now proven beyond doubt. Comprehensive, aggressive treatment of all established risk factors should be initiated for most high-risk patients without delay. In particular, attention should be focused on control of LDL-C, HDL-C, and blood pressure by use of medications and therapeutic lifestyle therapies as required. Complete smoking cessation, administration of antiplatelet therapy, and prescription of appropriate dietary modifications and aerobic physical activity are also mandated. Close monitoring to ensure patient compliance to prescribed therapies and lifestyle modifications is vital to the success of secondary prevention strategies. Many ongoing trials due to be completed over the next few years will provide further insight into the potential incremental benefits of treating several emerging CVD risk factors.

REFERENCES

1. Rossouw JE, Lewis B, Rifkind BM. The value of lowering cholesterol after myocardial infarction. *N Engl J Med* 1990;323:1112–1119.

2. Califf RM, Armstrong PW, Carver JR, et al. 27th Bethesda Conference: matching the intensity of risk factor management with the hazard for coronary disease events. Task Force 5. Stratification of patients into high, medium, and low risk subgroups for purposes of risk factor management. *J Am Coll Cardiol* 1996;27:1007–1019.

3. Law LR, Watt HC, Wald NJ. The underlying risk of death after myocardial infarction in the absence of treatment. *Arch Intern Med* 2002;162:2405–2410.

4. Executive Summary of the Third Report of the National Cholesterol Education Program (NCEP) Expert Panel on Detection, Evaluation, and Treatment of High Blood Cholesterol in Adults (Adult Treatment Panel III). *JAMA* 2001;285:2486–2497.

5. Sarnak MJ, Levey AS, Schoolwerth AC, et al. Kidney disease as a risk factor for development of cardiovascular disease: a statement from the American Heart Association Councils on Kidney in Cardiovascular Disease, High Blood Pressure Research, Clinical Cardiology, and Epidemiology and Prevention. *Circulation* 2003;108:2154–2169.

6. Greenland P, Abrams J, Aurigemma GP, et al, for Writing Group III. Prevention Conference V: Beyond secondary prevention: identifying the high-risk patient for primary prevention: noninvasive tests of atherosclerotic burden. *Circulation* 2000;101:E16–E22.

7. Pearson TA, Mensah GA, Alexander RW, et al. Markers of inflammation and cardiovascular disease application to clinical and public health practices: a statement for healthcare professionals from the Centers for Disease Control and Prevention and the American Heart Association. *Circulation* 2003;107:499–511.

8. Greenland P, Gaziano JM. Clinical practice: selecting asymptomatic patients for coronary computed tomography or electrocardiographic exercise testing. *N Engl J Med* 2003;349:465–473.

9. Hiatt WR. Medical treatment of peripheral arterial disease and claudication. *N Engl J Med* 2001;344:1608–1621.

10. Simon A, Geriepy J, Chironi G, et al. Intima-media thickness: a new tool for diagnosis and treatment of cardiovascular risk. *J Hypertens* 2002;20:159–169.

11. Smith SC Jr, Blair SN, Bonow RO, et al. AHA/ACC guidelines for preventing heart attack and death in patients with atherosclerotic cardiovascular disease: 2001 update: a statement for healthcare professionals from the American Heart Association and the American College of Cardiology. *Circulation* 2001;104:1577–1579.

12. Pyorala K, De Backer G, Graham I, et al. Prevention of coronary heart disease in clinical practice: recommendations of the Task Force of the European Society of Cardiology, European Atherosclerosis Society and European Society of Hypertension. *Atherosclerosis* 1994;110:121–161.

13. Law MR, Wald NJ. Risk factor thresholds; their existence under scrutiny. *BMJ* 2002;324:1570–1576.

14. Chobanian AV, Bakris GL, Black HR, et al, for the National Heart, Lung, and Blood Institute Joint National Committee on Prevention, Detection, Evaluation, and Treatment of High Blood Pressure, National High Blood Pressure Education Program Coordinating Committee. The Seventh Report of the Joint National Committee on Prevention, Detection, Evaluation, and Treatment of High Blood Pressure: the JNC 7 report [published erratum appears in *JAMA* 2003;290:197]. *JAMA* 2003;289:2560–2572.

15. Magnus P, Beaglehole R. The real contribution of the major risk factors to the coronary epidemics: time to end the "only-50%" myth. *Arch Intern Med* 2001;161:2657–2660.

16. Wald NJ, Law MR. A strategy to reduce cardiovascular disease by more than 80% [published erratum appears in *BMJ*;327:586]. *BMJ* 2003;326:1419.

17. Smith LR, Harrell FE Jr, Rankin JS, et al. Determinants of early versus late cardiac death in patients undergoing coronary artery bypass graft surgery. *Circulation* 1991; 84(5, suppl):III245–III253.

18. Singh M, Reeder GS, Jacobsen SJ, et al. Scores for post-myocardial infarction risk stratification in the community. *Circulation* 2002;106:2309–2314.

19. Salazar HP, Raggi P. Usefulness of electron-beam computed tomography. *Am J Cardiol* 2002;89:17B–22B.

20. Quyyumi AA. Prognostic value of endothelial function. *Am J Cardiol* 2003;91:19H–24H.

21. Wong ND, Cupples LA, Ostfeld AM, et al. Risk factors for long-term coronary prognosis after initial myocardial infarction: the Framingham study. *Am J Epidemiol* 1989;130:469–480.

22. Dankner R, Goldbourt U, Boyko V, Reicher-Reiss H. Predictors of cardiac and noncardiac mortality among 14,697 patients with coronary heart disease. *Am J Cardiol* 2003;91:121–127.

23. Vittinghoff E, Shlipak MG, Varosy PD, et al. Risk factors and secondary prevention in women with heart disease: the Heart and Estrogen/Progestin Replacement Study. *Ann Intern Med* 2003 18;81–89.

24. Wong ND, Wilson PW, Kannel WB. Serum cholesterol as a prognostic factor after myocardial infarction: the Framingham Study. *Ann Intern Med* 1991;115:687–693.

25. Pekkanen J, Linn S, Heiss G, et al. Ten-year mortality from cardiovascular disease in relation to cholesterol level among men with and without preexisting cardiovascular disease. *N Engl J Med* 1990;322:1700–1707.

26. Pedersen TR, Olsson AG, Faergeman O, et al. Lipoprotein changes and reduction in the incidence of major coronary heart disease events in the Scandinavian Simvastatin Survival Study (4S). *Circulation* 1998;97:1453–1460.

27. Long-Term Intervention with Pravastatin in Ischemic Disease (LIPID) Study Group. Prevention of cardiovascular events and death with pravastatin in patients with coronary heart disease and a broad range of initial cholesterol levels. *N Engl J Med* 1998;339:1349–1357.

28. Sniderman AD, Furberg CD, Keech A, et al. Apolipoproteins versus lipids as indices of coronary risk and as targets for statin treatment. *Lancet* 2003;361:777–780.

29. Canner PL, Halperin M, for the Coronary Drug Project Research Group. Implications of findings in the coronary drug project for secondary prevention trials in coronary heart disease. *Circulation* 1981;63:1342–1350.

30. Law MR, Wald NJ, Rudnicka AR. Quantifying effect of statin on low density lipoprotein cholesterol, ischaemic heart disease, and stroke: systematic review and meta-analysis. *BMJ* 2003;326:1423.

31. Shepard J, Blauw GJ, Murphy MB, et al, for the PROSPER Study Group. PROspective Study of Pravastin in the Elderly at Risk. Pravastatin in elderly individuals at risk of vascular disease (PROSPER): a randomised controlled trial. *Lancet* 2002;360:1623–1630.

32. Collins R, Armitage J, Parish S, et al, for the Heart Protection Study Collaborative Group. MRC/BHF Heart Protection Study of cholesterol-lowering with simvastatin in 5963 people with diabetes: a randomized placebo-controlled trial. *Lancet* 2003;361:2005–2016.

33. Tonelli M, Moye L, Sacks FM, et al, for the Cholesterol and Recurrent Events (CARE) Trial Investigators. Pravastatin for secondary prevention of cardiovascular events in person with mild chronic renal insufficiency. *Ann Intern Med* 2003;138:98–104.

34. Takemoto M, Liao JK. Pleiotropic effects of 3-hydroxy-3-methylglutaryl coenzyme A reductase inhibitors. *Arterioscler Thromb Vasc Biol* 2001;21:1712–1719.

35. Pedersen TR, Kjekshus J, Pyorala K, et al. Effect of simvastatin on ischemic signs and symptoms in the Scandinavian Simvastatin Survival Study (4S). *Am J Cardiol* 1998;81:333–335.

36. Fathi R, Haluska B, Short L, Marwick TH. A randomized trial of aggressive lipid reduction for improvement of myocardial ischemia, symptom status, and vascular function in patients with coronary artery disease not amenable to intervention. *Am J Med* 2003;114:445–453.

37. Ray JG, Mamdani M, Tsuyuki RT, Anderson DR. Use of statins and the subsequent development of deep vein thrombosis. *Arch Intern Med* 2001;161:1405–1410.

38. Mehra MR, Uber PA, Vive Kananthan K, et al. Comparative beneficial effects of simvastatin and pravastatin on cardiac allograft rejection and survival. *J Am Coll Cardiol* 2002;40:1609–1614.

39. Bellamy MF, Pellikka PA, Klarich KW, et al. Association of cholesterol levels, hydroxymethylglutaryl coenzyme-A reductase inhibitor treatment, and progression of aortic stenosis in the community. *J Am Coll Cardiol* 2002;40:1723–1730.

40. Mitchell LB, Powell JL, Gillis AM, et al, for the AVID Investigators. Are lipid-lowering drugs also antiarrhythmic drugs? An analysis of the Antiarrhythmics versus Implantable Defibrillators (AVID) trial. *J Am Coll Cardiol* 2003;42:81–87.

41. Fried LF, Orchard TJ, Kasiske BL. Effect of lipid reduction on the progression of renal disease: a meta-analysis. *Kidney Int* 2001;59:260–269.

42. Glorioso N, Troffa C, Filigheddu F, et al. Effect of the HMG-CoA reductase inhibitors on blood pressure in patients with essential hypertension and primary hypercholesterolemia. *Hypertension* 1999;34:1281–1286.

43. The ALLHAT Officers and Coordinator for the ALLHAT Collaborative Research Group. Major outcomes in moderately hypercholesterolemic, hypertensive patients randomized to pravastatin vs usual care: the Antihypertensive and Lipid-Lowering Treatment to Prevent Heart Attack Trial (ALLHAT-LLT). *JAMA* 2002;288:2998–3007.

44. Jackevicius CA, Mamdani M, Tu JV. Adherence with statin therapy in elderly patients with and without acute coronary syndromes. *JAMA* 2002;288:462–466.

45. Sacks FM, Moye LA, Davis BR, et al. Relationship between plasma LDL-C concentrations during treatment with pravastatin and recurrent coronary events in the Cholesterol and Recurrent Events Trial. *Circulation* 1998;97:1446–1452.

46. Heart Protection Study Collaborative Group. MRC/BHF Heart Protection Study of cholesterol lowering with simvastatin in 20536 high-risk individuals: a randomised placebo-controlled trial. *Lancet* 2002;360:7–22.

47. Taylor AJ, Kent SM, Flaherty PJ, et al. ARBITER: Arterial Biology for the Investigation of the Treatment Effects of Reducing Cholesterol: a randomized trial comparing the effects of atrovastatin and pravastatin on carotid intima medial thickness. *Circulation* 2002;106:2055–2060.

48. Schartl M, Bocksch W, Koschyk DH, et al. Use of intravascular ultrasound to compare effects of different strategies of lipid-lowering therapy on plaque volume and composition in patients with coronary artery disease. *Circulation* 2001;104:387–392.

49. Van Wissen S, Trip MD, Smilde TJ, et al. Differential hs-CRP reduction in patients with familial hypercholesterolemia treated with aggressive or conventional statin therapy. *Atherosclerosis* 2002;165:361–366.

50. Hecht HS, Harman SM. Relation of aggressiveness of lipid-lowering treatment to changes in calcified plaque burden by electron beam tomography. *Am J Cardiol* 2003;92:334–336.

51. Budoff MJ, Raggi P. Coronary artery disease progression assessed by electron-beam computed tomography. *Am J Cardiol* 2001;88(2A):46E–50E.

52. Nissen SE, Tuzcu EM, Schoenhagen P, et al. Effect of intensive compared to moderate lipid-lowering therapy on progression of coronary atherosclerosis. A randomized controlled trial. *JAMA* 2004;291:1071–1080.

53. Cannon CP, Braunwald E, McCabe CH, et al. Comparison of intensive and moderate lipid lowering with statins after acute coronary syndromes. *N Engl J Med* 2003;350:1495–1504.

54. Arntz HR, Agrawal R, Wunderlich W, et al. Beneficial effects of pravastatin (+/−colestyramine/niacin) initiated immediately after a coronary event (the randomized Lipid-Coronary Artery Disease [L-CAD] Study). *Am J Cardiol* 2000;86:1293–1298.

55. Wright RS, Murphy JG, Bybee KA, et al. Statin lipid-lowering therapy for acute myocardial infarction and unstable angina: efficacy and mechanism of benefit. *Mayo Clin Proc* 2002; 77:1085–1092.

56. Schwartz GG, Olsson AG, Ezekowitz MD, et al, for the Myocardial Ischemia Reduction with Aggressive Cholesterol Lowering (MIRACL) Study Investigators. Effects of atorvastatin on early recurrent ischemic events in acute coronary syndromes: the MIRACL study: a randomized controlled trial. *JAMA* 2001;285:1711–1718.

57. Serruys PW, de Feyter P, Macaya C, et al, for the Lescol Intervention Prevention Study (LIPS) Investigators. Fluvastatin for prevention of cardiac events following successful first percutaneous coronary intervention: a randomized controlled trial. *JAMA* 2002;287:3215–3522.

58. Stenestrand U, Wallentin L, for the Swedish Register of Cardiac Intensive Care (RIKS-HIA). Early statin treatment following acute myocardial infacrction and 1-year survival. *JAMA* 2001;285:430–436.

59. Aronow HD, Topol EJ, Roe MT, et al. Effect of lipid-lowering therapy on early mortality after acute coronary syndromes: an observational study. *Lancet* 2001;357:1063–1068.

60. Newby LK, Kristinsson A, Bhapkar MV, et al, for the SYMPHONY and 2ND SYMPHONY Investigators. Early statin initiation and outcomes in patients with acute coronary syndromes. *JAMA* 2002;287:3087–3095.

61. Fonarow GC, Gawlinski A, Moughrabi S, Tillisch JH. Improved treatment of coronary heart disease by implementation of cardiac hospitalization atherosclerosis management program (CHAMP). *Am J Cardiol* 2001;87:819–822.

62. Braunwald E, Antman EM, Beasley JW, et al, for the American College of Cardiology/American Heart Association Task Force on Practice Guidelines (Committee on the Management of Patients with Unstable Angina). ACC/AHA guideline update for the management of patients with unstable angina and non-ST-segment elevation myocardial infarction—2002: summary article: a report of the American College of Cardiology/American Heart Association Task Force on Practice Guidelines (Committee on the Management of Patients with Unstable Angina). *Circulation* 2002;1893–1900.

63. Reaven G. Metabolic syndrome: pathophysiology and implications for management of cardiovascular disease. *Circulation* 2002;106:286–288.

64. Ford ES, Giles WH, Dietz WH. Prevalence of the metabolic syndrome among US adults: findings from the third National Health and Nutrition Examination Survey. *JAMA* 2002;287:356–359.

65. Lakka HM, Laaksonen DE, Lakka T, et al. The metabolic syndrome and total and cardiovascular disease mortality in middle-aged men. *JAMA* 2002;288;2709–2716.

66. Eberly LE, Stamler J, Neaton JD, for the Multiple Risk Factor Intervention Trial Research Group. Relation of triglyceride levels, fasting and nonfasting, to fatal and nonfatal coronary heart disease. *Arch Intern Med* 2003;163:1077–1083.

67. Sacks FM, for the Expert Group on HDL-C. The role of high-density lipoprotein (HDL) cholesterol in the prevention and treatment of coronary heart disease: expert group recommendations. *Am J Cardiol* 2002;90:139–143.

68. Rubins HB, Robins SJ, Collins D, et al. Gemfibrozil for the secondary prevention of coronary heart disease in men with low levels of high-density lipoprotein cholesterol. *N Engl J Med* 1999;341:410–418.

69. Bloomfield-Rubins HB, Davenport J, Babikian V, et al, for the VA-HIT Study Group. Reduction in stroke with gemfibrozil in men with coronary heart disease and low HDL-C: the Veterans Affairs HDL-C Intervention Trial (VA-HIT). *Circulation* 2001;103:2828–2833.

70. BIP Study Group. Secondary prevention by raising HDL-C and reducing triglycerides in patients with coronary artery disease: the Benzafibrate Infarction Prevention (BIP) Study. *Circulation* 2000;102:21–27.

71. Brown BG, Zhzo XQ, Chait A, et al. Simvastatin and niacin, antioxidant vitamins, or combination for the prevention of coronary disease. *N Engl J Med* 2001;245:1583–1592.

72. Grundy SM, Cleeman JI, Merz CN, et al. Implications of recent clinical trials for the National Cholesterol Education Program Adult Treatment Panel III guidelines. *Circulation* 2004;110: 227–239.

73. Cui Y, Blumenthal RS, Flaws JA, et al. Non-high density lipoprotein cholesterol level as a predictor of cardiovascular disease mortality. *Arch Intern Med* 2001;161:1413–1419.

74. Hirsch GA, Blumenthal RS. Usefulness of non-high-density lipoprotein cholesterol determinations in the diagnosis and treatment of dyslipidemia. *Am J Cardiol* 2003;91:827–830.

75. Stamler J, Stamler R, Neaton JD. Blood pressure, systolic and diastolic, and cardiovascular risks: U.S. population data. *Arch Intern Med* 1993;153:598–615.

76. MacMahon S, Peto R, Cutler J, et al. Blood pressure, stroke, and coronary heart disease: Part 1. Prolonged differences in blood pressure: prospective observational studies corrected for the regression dilution bias. *Lancet* 1990;335:765–774.

77. Kannel WB, Sorlie P, Castelli WP, McGee D. Blood pressure and survival after myocardial infarction: the Framingham study. *Am J Cardiol* 1980;45:326–30.

78. Staessen JA, Wang J, Thijs L. Cardiovascular prevention and blood pressure reduction: a quantitative overview updated until 1 March 2003. *J Hypertens* 2003;21:1055–1076.

79. PROGRESS Collaborative Group. Randomised trial of a perindopril-based blood-pressure-lowering regimen among 6105 individuals with previous stroke or transient ischaemic attack. *Lancet* 2001;358:1033–1041.

80. Gottlieb SS, McCarter RJ, Vogel RA. Effect of beta-blockade on mortality among high-risk and low-risk patients after myocardial infarction. *N Engl J Med* 1998;339:489–497.

81. Freemantle N, Cleland J, Young P, et al. Beta blockade after myocardial infarction: systematic review and meta regression analysis. *BMJ* 1999;318:1730–1737.

82. Flather MD, Yusuf S, Kober L, et al, for the ACE-Inhibitor Myocardial Infarction Collaborative Group. Long-term ACE-inhibitor therapy in patients with heart failure or left-ventricular dysfunction: a systematic overview of data from individual patients. *Lancet* 2000;355:1575–1581.

83. Langford HG, Stamler J, Wassertheil-Smoller S, Prineas RJ. All-cause mortality in the Hypertension Detection and Follow-up Program: findings for the whole cohort and for persons with less severe hypertension, with and without other traits related to risk for mortality. *Prog Cardiovasc Dis* 1986;29(3, suppl 1): 29–54.

84. ALLHAT Officers and Coordinators for the ALLHAT Collaborative Research Group. Major outcomes in high-risk hypertensive patients randomized to angiotensin-converting enzyme inhibitor or calcium channel blocker vs diuretic: the Antihypertensive and Lipid-Lowering Treatment to Prevent Heart Attack Trial (ALLHAT). *JAMA* 2002;288:2981–2997.

85. Wing LM, Reid CM, Ryan P, et al, for the Second Australian National Blood Pressure Study Group. A comparison of outcomes with angiotensin-converting-enzyme inhibitors and diuretics for hypertension in the elderly. *N Engl J Med* 2003;348:583–592.

86. Dzau VJ, Bernstein K, Celermajer D, et al, for the Working Group on Tissue Angiotensin-Converting Enzyme, International Society of Cardiovascular Pharmacotherapy. The relevance of tissue angiotensin-converting enzyme: manifestations in mechanistic and endpoint data. *Am J Cardiol* 2001;88(9, suppl):1L–20L.

87. Jacoby DS, Rader DJ. Renin–angiotensin system and atherothrombotic disease: from genes to treatment. *Arch Intern Med* 2003;163:1155–1164.

88. Yusuf S, Sleight P, Pogue J, et al, for the Heart Outcomes Prevention Evaluation Study Investigators. Effects of an angiotensin-converting-enzyme inhibitor, ramipril, on cardiovascular events in high-risk patient [published erratum appears in *N Engl J Med* 2000;342:1376]. *N Engl J Med* 2000;342:145–153.

89. Dagenais GR, Yusuf S, Bourassa MG, et al, for the HOPE Investigators. Effects of ramipril on coronary events in high-risk persons: results of the Heart Outcomes Prevention Evaluation Study. *Circulation* 2001;104:522–526.

90. Yusuf S, Gerstein H, Hoggwerf B, et al, for the HOPE Study Investigators. Ramipril and the development of diabetes. *JAMA* 2001;286:1882–1885.

91. Fox KM, for the European Trial on Reduction of Cardiac Events with Perindopril in Stable Coronary Artery Disease Investigators. Efficacy of perindopril in reduction of cardiovascular events among patients with stable coronary artery disease: randomised double-blind, placebo-controlled, multicentre trial (the EUROPA study). *Lancet* 2003;362:782–788.

92. Svensson P, de Faire U, Sleight P, et al. Comparative effects of ramipril on ambulatory and office blood pressures: a HOPE substudy. *Hypertension* 2001;38:e28–e32.

93. Devereux RB, Dahlof B, Kjeldsen SE, et al, for the LIFE Study Group. Effects of losartan or atenolol in hypertensive patients without clinically evident vascular disease: a substudy of the LIFE randomized trial. *Ann Intern Med* 2003;139:169–177.

94. Hansson L, Zanchetti A, Carruthers SG, et al. Effects of intensive blood-pressure lowering and low-dose aspirin in patients with hypertension: principal results of the Hypertension Optimal Treatment (HOT) randomised trial. HOT Study Group. *Lancet* 1998;351:1755–1762.

95. Pitt B, Remme W, Zannad F, et al, for the Eplerenone Post-Acute Myocardial Infarction Heart Failure Efficacy and Survival Study Investigators. Eplerenone, a selective aldosterone blocker, in patients with left ventricular dysfunction after myocardial infarction. *N Engl J Med* 2003;348:1309–1321.

96. Dickstein K, Kjekshus J, for the OPTIMAAL Steering Committee of the OPTIMAL Study Group. Effects of losartan and captopril on mortality and morbidity in high-risk patients after acute myocardial infarction: the OPTIMAAL randomised trial. *Lancet* 2002;360:752–760.

97. Granger DB, McMurray JJ, Yusuf S, et al, for the CHARM Investigators and Committees. Effects of candesartan in patients with chronic heart failure and reduced left-ventricular systolic function intolerant to angiotensin-converting-enzyme inhibitors: the CHARM-alternative trial. *Lancet* 2003;362:772–776.

98. McMurray JJ, Ostergren J, Swedberg K, et al, for the CHARM Investigators and Committees. Effects of candesartan in patients with chronic heart failure and reduced left-ventricular systolic function taking angiotensin-converting-enzyme-inhibitors: the CHARM-Added trial. *Lancet* 2003;362:767–771.

99. Brenner BM, Cooper ME, de Zeeuw D, et al, for the RENAAL Study Investigators. Effects of losartan on renal and cardiovascular outcomes in patients with type 2 diabetes and nephropathy. *N Engl J Med* 2001;345:861–869.

100. Yang XC, Jing TY, Resnick LM, Phillips GB. Relation of hemostatic risk factors to other risk factors for coronary heart disease and to sex hormones in men. *Arterioscler Thromb* 1993;13:467–471.

101. Trip MD, Cats VM, van Capelle FJ, Vreeken J. Platelet hyperreactivity and prognosis in survivors of myocardial infarction. *N Engl J Med* 1990;322:1549–1554.

102. Ridker PM, Vaughan DE, Stampfer MJ, et al. Endogenous tissue-type plasminogen activator and risk of myocardial infarction. *Lancet* 1993;341:1165–1168.

103. Antithrombotic Trialists' Collaboration. Collaborative meta-analysis of randomised trials of antiplatelet therapy for prevention of death, myocardial infarction, and stroke in the high risk patients. *BMJ* 2002;324:71–86.

104. CAPRIE Steering Committee. A randomized, blinded, trial of clopidogrel versus aspirin in patients at risk of ischaemic events (CAPRIE). *Lancet* 1996;348:1329–1339.

105. Bhatt DL, Marso SP, Hirsch AT, et al. Amplified benefit of clopidogrel versus aspirin in patients with diabetes mellitus. *Am J Cardiol* 2002;90:625–628.

106. Jneid H, Bhatt D, Corti R, et al. Aspirin and clopidogrel in acute coronary syndromes, therapeutic insights from the CURE study. *Arch Intern Med* 2003;163:1145–1153.

107. Yusuf S, Zhao F, Mehta SR, et al, for the Clopidogrel in Unstable Angina to Prevent Recurrent Events Trial Investigators. Effects of clopidogrel in addition to aspirin in patients with acute coronary syndromes without ST-segment elevation. *N Engl J Med* 2001;345:494–502.

108. Mehta SR, Yusuf S, Peters RJ, et al. Clopidogrel in Unstable angina to prevent Recurrent Events trial (CURE) Investigators. Effects of pretreatment with clopidogrel and aspirin followed by long-term therapy in patients undergoing percutaneous coronary intervention: the PCI-CURE study. *Lancet* 2001;358:527–533.

109. Steinhubl SR, Berger PB, Mann JT 3rd, et al, for the CREDO Investigators. Clopidogrel for the Reduction of Events During Observation: early and sustained dual oral antiplatelet therapy following percutaneous coronary intervention, a randomized controlled trial. *JAMA* 2002;288:2411–2420.

110. Yusuf S, Mehta SR, Zhao F, et al. Early and late effects of clopidogrel in patients with acute coronary syndromes. *Circulation* 2003;107:966–972.

111. Smith P, Arnesen H, Holme I. The effect of warfarin on mortality and reinfarction after myocardial infarction. *N Engl J Med* 1990;323:147–152.

112. Coumadin Aspirin Reinfarction Study (CARS) Investigators. Randomised double-blind trial of fixed low-dose warfarin with aspirin after myocardial infarction. *Lancet* 1997;350:389–396.

113. Hurlen M, Abdelnoor M, Smith P, et al. Warfarin, aspirin, or both after myocardial infarction. *N Engl J Med* 2002;347:969–974.

114. Wallentin L, Wilcox RG, Weaver WD, et al, for the ESTEEM Investigators. Oral ximelagatran for secondary prophylaxis after myocardial infarction: the ESTEEM randomized controlled trial. *Lancet* 2003;362:789–797.

115. Fuster V, Gotto AM, Libby P, et al. 27th Bethesda Conference: matching the intensity of risk factor management with the hazard for coronary disease events. Task Force 1. Pathogenesis of coronary disease: the biologic role of risk factors. *J Am Coll Cardiol* 1996;27:964–976.

116. Hermanson B, Omenn GS, Kronmal RA, Gersh BJ. Beneficial six-year outcome of smoking cessation in older men and women with coronary artery disease: results from the CASS registry. *N Engl J Med* 1988;319:1365–1369.

117. Coronary Drug Project Research Group. Cigarette smoking as a risk factor in men with a prior history of myocardial infarction. *J Chronic Dis* 1979;32:415–425.

118. Rea TD, Heckbert SR, Kaplan RC, et al. Smoking status and risk for recurrent coronary events after myocardial infarction. *Ann Intern Med* 2002;137:494–500.

119. Critchley JA, Capewell S. Mortality risk reduction associated with smoking cessation in patients with coronary heart disease: a systematic review. *JAMA* 2003;290:86–97.

120. de Lorgeril M, Renaud S, Mamelle N, et al. Mediterranean alpha-linolenic acid-rich diet in secondary prevention of coronary heart disease [published erratum appears in *Lancet* 1995;345:738]. *Lancet* 1994;343:1454–1459.

121. Burr ML, Fehily AM, Gilbert JF, et al. Effects of changes in fat, fish, and fibre intakes on death and myocardial reinfarction: diet and reinfarction trial (DART). *Lancet* 1989;2:757–761.

122. Singh RB, Rastogi SS, Verma R, et al. Randomised controlled trial of cardioprotective diet in patients with recent acute myocardial infarction: results of one year follow up. *BMJ* 1992;304:1015–1019.

123. Watts GF, Lewis B, Brunt JN, et al. Effects on coronary artery disease of lipid-lowering diet, or diet plus cholestyramine, in the St Thomas' Atherosclerosis Regression Study (STARS). *Lancet* 1992;339:563–569.

124. Ornish D, Brown SE, Scherwitz LW, et al. Can lifestyle changes reverse coronary heart disease? The Lifestyle Heart Trial. *Lancet* 1990;336:129–133.

125. Shuler G, Hambrecht R, Schlierf G, et al. Regular physical exercise and low-fat diet: effects on progression of coronary artery disease. *Circulation* 1992;86:1–11.

126. Hu FB, Willett WC. Optimal diets for prevention of coronary heart disease. *JAMA* 2002;288:2569–2578.

127. Hooper L, Summerbell CD, Higgins JP, et al. Dietary fat intake and prevention of cardiovascular disease: systematic review. *BMJ* 2001;322:757–763.

128. Sdringola S, Nakagawa K, Nakagawa Y, et al. Combined intense lifestyle and pharmacologic lipid treatment further reduce coronary events and myocardial perfusion abnormalities compared with usual-care cholesterol-lowering drugs in coronary artery disease. *J Am Coll Cardiol* 2003;41:263–272.

129. Kris-Etherton PM, Harris WS, Appel LJ, for the American Heart Association Nutrition Committee. Fish consumption, fish oil, omega-3 fatty acids, and cardiovascular disease [published erratum appears in *Circulation* 2003;107:512]. *Circulation* 2002;106:2747–2757.

130. Gruppo Italiano per lo Studio della Sopravvivenza nell'Infarto miocardico. Dietary supplementation with *n*-3 polyunsaturated fatty acids and vitamin E after myocardial infarction: results of the GISSI-Prevenzione trial [published erratum appears in *Lancet* 2001;357:642]. *Lancet* 1999;354:447–455.

131. Marchioli R, Barzi F, Bomba E, et al. Early protection sudden death by *n*-3 polyunsaturated fatty acids after myocardial infarction: time course analysis of the results of the Gruppo Italiano per lo Studio della Sopravvivenza nell'Infarto Miocardico (GISSI)—Prevenzione. *Circulation* 2002;105:1897–903.

132. Grundy SM. *n*-3 fatty acids: priority for post-myocardial infarction clinical trials. *Circulation* 2003;107:1834–1836.

133. Yancy WS Jr, Westman EC, French PA, Califf RM. Diets and clinical coronary events: the truth is out there. *Circulation* 2003;107:10–16.

134. Myers J, Prakash M, Froelicher V, et al. Exercise capacity and mortality among men referred for exercise testing. *N Engl J Med* 2002;346:793–801.

135. Kavanagh T, Mertens DJ, Hamm LF, et al. Prediction of long-term prognosis in 12,169 men referred for cardiac rehabilitation. *Circulation* 2002;106:666–671.

136. Jolliffee JA, Rees K, Taylor RS, et al. Exercise-based rehabilitation for coronary heart disease. *Cochrane Database Syst Rev* 2001;1:CD001800.

137. Wenger NK, Froelicher ES, Smith LK, et al, for the Agency for Health Care Policy and Research and National Heart, Lung, and Blood Institute. Cardiac rehabilitation as secondary prevention. *Clin Pract Guide Quick Ref Guide Clin* 1995;17:1–23.

138. Cardiac rehabilitation programs: a statement for healthcare professionals from the American Heart Association. *Circulation* 1994;90:1602–1610.

139. Greenland P, Chu JS. Efficacy of cardiac rehabilitation services—with emphasis on patients after myocardial infarction. *Ann Intern Med* 1988;109:650–663.

140. Thompson PD, Buchner D, Pina IL, et al. Exercise and physical activity in the prevention and treatment of atherosclerotic cardiovascular disease: a statement from the Council on Clinical Cardiology (Subcommittee on Exercise, Rehabilitation, and Prevention) and the Council on Nutrition, Physical Activity, and Metabolism (Subcommittee on Physical Activity). *Circulation* 2003;107:3109–3116.

141. Natarajan S, Liao Y, Cao G, et al. Sex differences in risk for coronary heart disease mortality associated with diabetes and established coronary heart disease. *Arch Intern Med* 2003;163:1735–1740.

142. Malmberg K, Ryden L, Efendic S, et al. Randomized trial of insulin–glucose infusion followed by subcutaneous insulin treatment in diabetic patients with acute myocardial infarction (DIGAMI Study): effects on mortality at 1 year. *J Am Coll Cardiol* 1995;26:57–65.

143. Diabetes Control and Complications Trial Group. Effect of intensive diabetes management on macrovascular events and risk factors in the Diabetes Control and Complications Trial. *Am J Cardiol* 1995;75:894–903.

144. UK Prospective Diabetes Study (UKPDS) Group. Intensive blood-glucose control with sulphonylureas or insulin compared with conventional treatment and risk of complications in patients with type 2 diabetes (UKPDS 33). *Lancet* 1998;352:837–853.

145. UK Prospective Diabetes Study (UKPDS) Group. Effect of intensive blood-glucose control with metformin on complications in overweight patients with type 2 diabetes (UKPDS 34) [published erratum appears in *Lancet* 1998;352:1557]. *Lancet* 1998;352:854–865.

146. Chiasson JL, Josse RG, Gomis R, et al. Acarbose treatment and the risk of cardiovascular disease and hypertension in patients with impaired glucose tolerance: the STOP-NIDDM trial. *JAMA* 2003;290:486–494.

147. Gaede P, Vedel P, Larsen N, et al. Multifactorial intervention and cardiovascular disease in patients with type 2 diabetes. *N Engl J Med* 2003;348:383–393.

148. Omland T, Sammuelsson A, Hartford M, et al. Serum homocysteine concentration as an indicator of survival in patients with acute coronary syndromes. *Arch Intern Med* 2000;160:1834–1840.

149. Schnyder G, Roffi M, Flammer Y, et al. Effect of homocysteine-lowering therapy with folic acid, vitamin B_{12} and vitamin B_6 on clinical outcome after percutaneous coronary intervention: the Swiss Heart Study: a randomized controlled trial. *JAMA* 2002;288:973–979.

150. Schnyder G, Roffi M, Pin R, et al. Decreased rate of coronary restenosis after lowering of plasma homocysteine levels. *N Engl J Med* 2001;345:1593–1600.

151. Leim A, Reynierse-Buitenwerf GH, Zwinderman AH, et al. Secondary prevention with folic acid: effects on clinical outcomes. *J Am Coll Cardiol* 2003;41:2105–2113.

152. Malinow MR, Bostom AG, Krauss RM. Homocyst(e)ine, diet, and cardiovascular diseases: a statement for healthcare professionals from the Nutrition Committee, American Heart Association. *Circulation* 1999;99:178–182.

153. Cercek B, Shah PK, Noc M, et al, for the AZACS Investigators. Effect of short-term treatment with azithromycin on recurrent ischaemic events in patients with acute coronary syndrome in the Azithromycin in Acute Coronary Syndrome (AZACS) trial: a randomised controlled trial. *Lancet* 2003;361:809–813.

154. Zahn R, Schneider S, Frilling B, et al, for the Working Group of Leading Hospital Cardiologists. Antibiotic therapy after acute myocardial infarction: a prospective randomized study. *Circulation* 2003;107:1253–1259.

155. Grayston JT. Antibiotic treatment of atherosclerotic cardiovascular disease. *Circulation* 2003;107:1228–1230.

156. Grodstein F, Stampfer MJ, Colditz GA, et al. Postmenopausal hormone therapy and mortality. *N Engl J Med* 1997;336:1769–1775.

157. Writing Group for the PEPI Trial. Effects of estrogen or estrogen/progestin regimens on heart disease risk factors in postmenopausal women: the Postmenopausal Estrogen/Progestin Interventions (PEPI) trial. *JAMA* 1995;273:199–208.

158. Hodis HN, Mack WJ, Azen SP, et al, for the Women's Estrogen-Progestin Lipid-Lowering Hormone Atherosclerosis Regression Trial Research Group. Hormone therapy and the progression of coronary-artery atherosclerosis in postmenopausal women. *N Engl J Med* 2003;349:535–545.

159. Manson JE, Hsia J, Johnson KC, et al, for the Women's Health Initiative Investigators. Estrogen plus progestin and the risk of coronary heart disease. *N Engl J Med* 2003;349:523–534.

160. Mosca L, Collins P, Herrington DM, et al. Hormone replacement therapy and cardiovascular disease: a statement for the healthcare professionals from the American Heart Association. *Circulation* 2001;104:499–503.

161. Vivekananthan D, Penn M, Sapp S, et al. Use of antioxidant vitamins for the prevention of cardiovascular disease: meta-analysis of randomized trials. *Lancet* 2003;361:2017–2023.

162. Heart Protection Study Collaborative Group. MRC/BHF Heart Protection Study of antioxidant vitamin supplementation in 20536 high-risk individuals: a randomized placebo-controlled trial. *Lancet* 2002;360:23–33.

163. Sacks FM, Pfeffer MA, Moye LA, et al, for the Cholesterol and Recurrent Events Trial Investigators. The effect of pravastatin on coronary events after myocardial infarction in patients with average cholesterol levels. *N Engl J Med* 1996;335:1001–1009.

164. Knatterud GL, Rosenberg Y, Campeau L, et al, for the Post-CABG Investigators. Long-term effects on clinical outcomes of aggressive lowering of low-density lipoprotein cholesterol levels and low-dose anticoagulation in the Post-Coronary Artery Bypass Graft Trial. *Circulation* 2000;102:157–165.

165. Athyros VG, Papageorgiou AA, Mercouris BR, et al. Treatment with atorvastatin to the National Cholesterol Educational Program goal versus 'usual' care in secondary coronary heart disease prevention: the Greek Atorvastatin and Coronary-Heart-Disease Evaluation (GREACE) Study. *Curr Med Res Opin* 2002;18:220–228.

166. Kris-Etherton PM, Lichtenstein AH, Howard BV, et al. Antioxidant vitamin supplements and cardiovascular disease. *Circulation* 2004;110:637–641.

Naturoceuticals and other complementary therapies in the prevention of cardiovascular disease

24

Denise D. Hermann

KEY POINTS

- *There is significant contemporary interest in the utilization of complementary and alternative medicine practices for the prevention of cardiovascular disease among the Western public and health care practitioners.*

- *Currently, complementary and alternative medicine therapies are divided into five categories to facilitate research, and to inform the public and health professionals about the results of research studies. Naturoceutical dietary supplement research falls under the domains of alternative medical systems and biologically based therapies.*

- *For the prevention of cardiovascular disease, naturoceutical supplements are commonly employed for the treatment of traditional cardiovascular disease risk factors including hypertension, hyperlipidemia, diabetes, and obesity, with variable efficacy.*

- *Naturoceutical supplement consumption is generally safe, but not without risk in certain individuals. The potential for herb–drug interactions or naturoceutical-related alterations of anticoagulation and hemostasis must be considered.*

- *Mind–body medicine therapies such as meditation, biofeedback, yoga, and Tai Chi are also being evaluated for effectiveness in modifying risk factors for cardiovascular disease.*

- *Current research in alternative medical systems such as acupuncture, traditional Chinese medicine and Ayurvedic practices may yield new therapies for the treatment of hypertension and established symptomatic cardiovascular disease.*

- *For the prevention and treatment of cardiovascular disease, safe and effective complementary and alternative medical practices should be integrated into contemporary medical therapy.*

INTRODUCTION

Complementary and alternative medicine (CAM) practices and products are increasingly being used in the West for purposes ranging from health promotion or health maintenance to the prevention and/or treatment of specific diseases or conditions. Essentially, *complementary therapies* are more common and are those used in combination with conventional medicine, whereas *alternative practices* are used instead of conventional medicine. The National Center for Complementary and Alternative Medicine (NCCAM) classifies these therapies into five domains, although therapies can be listed under multiple categories.[1] The five domains of CAM therapy are:

- Alternative medical systems (eg, homeopathic or naturopathic medicine, traditional Chinese medicine including acupuncture, and Ayurvedic practices)
- Mind–body interventions (eg, meditation, prayer, guided imagery)
- Biologically based therapies (dietary supplements, natural therapies)
- Manipulative and body-based therapies (eg, chiropractic or osteopathic manipulation, massage)
- Energy field therapies (eg, magnets, Reiki, therapeutic touch).

A strong and growing contemporary interest in CAM practices as applicable to the practice of cardiovascular medicine is reflected by the formation of a special task force by the American College of Cardiology (ACC). The panel has produced an expert clinical consensus document regarding the effectiveness of CAM therapies and their potential for integration into traditional care.[2]

The most popular subset of CAM practices in the United States today involves consumer "self-prescription" of over-the-counter dietary supplements (naturoceuticals) for the prevention and/or treatment of cardiovascular disease (CVD). This practice falls under the category of biologically based therapies. However, the same compound(s) or combinations thereof might also be recommended and prescribed by alternative medical system practitioners, or used as an adjunctive measure in other CAM practices.

Naturoceutical products are compounds or isolated ingredients originally found in nature that can be identified, extracted, purified, or synthesized and/or combined and otherwise manufactured, marketed, or recommended to consumers as concentrated dietary supplements with potential health benefits. *Naturoceuticals* are defined as high-dose vitamins, herbal products, or any other dietary supplement consumed specifically to prevent or provide symptomatic relief from disease or alleviate subjective physical or psychologic complaints.[3] Synonymous terms for naturoceutical supplements are listed in Table 24-1.[3–5] A *nutraceutical* has been more specifically defined as a "food product consumed or administered enterally, under medical supervision based on medical evaluation of specific dietary management of a disease."[4] The term *naturoceutical* seems more appropriate based on observable consumer habits, as it connotes self-prescription of a presumed nature-derived product with a specific "pharmaceutical intention to treat." The majority of supplement users do not seek the recommendation or supervision of either a physician or CAM provider before using naturoceuticals. Similarly, in most population surveys, large proportions of naturoceutical users fail to report supplement use to their

TABLE 24-1 Synonymous Terms for Dietary Supplements

Naturoceutical
Megavitamin
Nutriceutical
Nutraceutic, nutraceutical
Medicinal herb, herbal medicinal
Medicinal botanical product
Phytochemical, phytomedicinal, phytotherapeutic agent
Chemopreventive agent

physicians.[3,6–12] Sales of megavitamin, herbal, and other supplement products involved more than 160 million consumers and more than $17 billion in the year 2000, with an annual industry growth rate exceeding 10%.[13,14] More than half the American adult population surveyed reported using a self-prescribed herbal product between the years 1999 and 2000, and up to two thirds reported using these products on a regular basis.[7] *Prevention* magazine reported that one in three habitual supplement users acknowledged their intention was to prevent or treat a specific serious or life-threatening condition.[6,8] Of these conditions, CVD ranked highest, with any/all cancers rated second.

In the scope of traditional Western medicine, nutritional or dietary supplementation was originally promoted as indicated for the prevention or treatment of specific dietary deficiencies known to cause well-defined syndromes such as scurvy, beri-beri, and rickets. Dietary manipulation and/or supplementation are also routinely prescribed to mitigate or compensate for identifiable inborn errors of metabolism, enabling normal growth and development. Because of advances in medicine, agriculture, and other factors, the average life expectancy in developed countries increased dramatically in the twentieth century. This was followed by an increased incidence of chronic, age-related diseases including CVD. Observational studies of the incidence of CVD among world populations noted favorable and unfavorable associations with regional or cultural diets or dietary ingredients. In contrast, for health promotion or maintenance in contemporary Western cultures, patients are now typically advised to restrict their diet (in terms of dietary fat, cholesterol, salt, simple sugars, and calories) rather than supplement it. The role of these and other dietary factors in CVD risk factors is reviewed extensively in Chapter 11.

This chapter summarizes available data regarding naturoceutical products commonly used specifically for cardiac risk factor modification and CVD prevention. The evidence base for CAM therapies in CVD prevention is sparse and underpowered from a statistical perspective in comparison to traditional pharmacologic therapy. Clinical trials currently evaluating the safety and efficacy of certain naturoceuticals and other CAM therapies in CVD prevention are highlighted, and the risks and benefits of naturoceutical consumption are discussed.

NATUROCEUTICALS FOR SPECIFIC CARDIAC RISK FACTOR REDUCTION

Both traditional medicine and CAM therapies have addressed each major modifiable risk factor for the development of CVD. The two major "prescribing" guides for herbal therapies are the German Commission E monographs and the *PDR for Herbal Medicines*.[15,16] A recommendation for use by the German Commission E is officially recognized by the German government and approved for clinical applications. In the 1998 Monographs, there were a total of 260 approved and 127 unapproved herbs, fixed herbal combinations, or component characteristics.

It is important to note the frequent coexistence of cardiovascular risk factors, such as obesity with hypertension, hyperlipidemia, and diabetes. Many CAM treatments are derived from historical use or cultural tradition for health promotion and/or relief of a constellation of common symptoms. It is therefore not unexpected to find several naturoceutical products listed as potentially useful for any/all of these (and other) conditions. This purported plurality of health benefit further enhances the popularity of naturoceuticals among consumers, in contrast to prescribed pharmaceuticals that typically treat only one disorder. *Panax ginseng*, for example, has at least 15 indications for use within folk, Chinese, and homeopathic medicine practices.[15,16] The nomenclature of the genus *Panax* derives from the Greek *panacea*, meaning "cure-all."

Hypertension

Table 24-2 is a comprehensive list of herbal and other naturoceutical products reported to reduce blood pressure.[3,15–30] The most commonly consumed and most researched agent for this physiologic intention is garlic. Given the multiple proposed benefits of garlic and conflicting study results, the NCCAM requested a systematic review of the available evidence base performed by the Agency for Healthcare Research and Quality (AHRQ).

TABLE 24-2 Naturoceutical Products Used for Blood Pressure Reduction

Alpine ragwort (*Senicio nemorensis*)	Larch (*Larix decidua*)
Amino acids: arginine, taurine*	Lemon Balm (*Melissa officinalis*)
Bear's garlic (*Allium ursinum*)	*Linguisticum wallichii* (TCM)
Behen (*Moringa oleifera*)	Lycium bark (*Lycium chinense*)
Black cumin seed (*Nigella sativa*)	**Minerals: magnesium, potassium**
Brown kelp (*Macrocystis pyrifera*)	Noni (*Morinda citrifolia*)
Camphor (*Cinnamomum camphora*)	Olive leaf (*Olea africana, O. europa*)
Celandine (*Chelidonium majus*)	Onion (*Allium cepa*)
Centaury (*Centaurium erythraea*)	Plantain (*Musa paradisiaca*)
Cheken (*Eugenia chequen*)	Rosemary (*Rosmarius officinalis*)
Coenzyme Q-10 (ubiquinone)	Rust red rhododendron (*Rhododendron ferrugineum*)
Common stonecrop (*Sedum acre*)	Scotch broom (*Cyitsus scoparius*)‡
Digitalis (*Digitalis purpurea*)	Scotch pine (*Pinus* species)
English hawthorne (*Crataegus laevigata*)	Stevia (*Stevia rebaudiana*)
European mistletoe (*Viscum album*)	***Stephania tetrandra***
Evodia rutaecarpa (TCM†)	Strophanthus (*Strophanthus konbe'*)
Forskolin (*Coleus forshkohlii*)	Surinam cherry (*Eugenia uniflora*)
Garlic (*Allium sativum*)	*Uncarium rhynchophylla* (TCM)
Gotu Kola (*Centella asiatica*)	Wood sage (*Teucrium scorodonia*)
Hawthorne (*Crataegus oxycantha, C. monogyna*)	Whey protein extracts
Hellbore (*Veratrum* species)	Vitamin C (ascorbic acid)
Hwema bark (*Coynanthe pachyceras*)	Vitamin E (α-tocopherol)
Indian snakeroot (*Rauwolfia serpentina*)	Yarrow (*Achillea whilhemlsii*)

*Entries in boldface refer to agents discussed in the text.
†TCM, traditional Chinese medicine.
‡Recommended by German Commission E.
SOURCE: References 3, 15–30.

As reported in 2002, the AHRQ reviewed 27 small, randomized, placebo-controlled, short-duration trials using various garlic preparations. The majority of trials detected no significant difference in blood pressure outcomes between garlic supplementation and placebo, and in those studies reporting a favorable response, the clinical effect was small.[17] Other cardiovascular protectant qualities have been attributed to garlic as well. The active ingredients (sulfides) derived from allicin and alliin have been shown to inhibit platelet aggregation, enhance fibrinolysis, prolong bleeding and clotting times, and block prostaglandin production via lipoxygenase and cycloxygenase inhibition.[18] There are no published clinical trials evaluating cardiovascular outcomes using garlic as a preventative intervention.

Other popular supplements for reducing hypertension are magnesium and potassium.[20] There remains debate about the relative equivalency of minerals and other nutrients derived from their original dietary source versus isolated individual supplements. The Dietary Approaches to Stop Hypertension (DASH) diet combination determined most effective in reducing both systolic and diastolic blood pressure was a salt-restricted, low-saturated fat diet excluding red meat and sugar, with increased proportions of legumes, fish, and soy products, along with fruits, nuts, and vegetables providing complex carbohydrates.[21] Many of the recommended foods were otherwise rich in potassium, magnesium, and calcium. Whether healthy persons consuming a varied diet benefit from mineral supplementation is unclear, although magnesium toxicity is a health risk predominantly in the elderly and persons with renal insufficiency.[22] However, the evidence base regarding magnesium and hypertension was considered sufficient for the Joint National Committee on the Prevention, Detection, Evaluation, and Treatment of High Blood Pressure (JNC) to recommend maintaining an adequate magnesium intake as a positive lifestyle modification.[23]

Diets enriched with the amino acids L-arginine and taurine have been reported to have mild antihypertensive effects.[3,20,24] L-Arginine is the precursor molecule from which the potent endogenous vasodilator nitric oxide (NO), or endothelium-derived relaxing factor, is synthesized. In the presence of healthy endothelium, NO induces vascular smooth muscle relaxation. Taurine is reported to reduce plasma epinephrine levels in hypertensive persons and, through this mechanism, induce blood vessel relaxation along with enhanced endorphin production. There is insufficient evidence to recommend routine supplementation of either compound for the prevention or treatment of hypertension.[20] L-Arginine supplementation may be useful in treating claudication related to peripheral arterial disease (PAD).[3,24]

Interestingly, up to 30% of isolates from both traditional Indian and Chinese herbal remedies and other naturally occurring botanicals have been found to contain tannins, lactokinins, and other compounds with physiologically relevant angiotensin 1-converting enzyme (ACE) inhibitory activity.[25–28]

Hyperlipidemia

Naturoceutical products that are considered by CAM practitioners to reduce cholesterol levels are listed in Table 24-3.[3,15,16,29,31–52] The list of the most popular naturoceutical agents used for lipid-lowering and antiatherosclerotic effects again includes garlic. However, with respect to efficacy in reducing serum cholesterol levels, individual human population studies and meta-analyses have been as often neutral as favorable.[3,17] A recent well-designed study using a relatively high-dose, steam distillate of garlic, after controlling for body weight and dietary habits, found no evidence of benefit to the human lipid profile.[31] This study also demonstrated that the absorption of cholesterol in humans is unaffected by garlic. Garlic is theoretically appealing for this purpose, presumably for beneficial effects on lipid peroxidation, free radical scavenging activity, and endothelial health. The AHRQ summary stated that garlic preparations "may have small, positive short-term effects on lipids," but questioned sustainability beyond 3 months.[17] The range of average pooled reductions in total cholesterol (TC) at 3 months was 12.4 to 25.4 mg/dL; in low-density lipoprotein cholesterol (LDL-C), 0 to 13.5 mg/dL; and in triglycerides (TGs), 7.6 to 34 mg/dL. A recent review of garlic's antioxidant potential reveals the complexity of merely "supplementing" the diet with a random garlic preparation, and illustrates the difficulty in evaluating comparative trials.[32] The antioxidant activity of garlic varies greatly according to the organosulfur metabolites generated in the preparation process. The latter range from raw garlic homogenates, to heat-treated preparations, powder, aged extracts, steam oil distillates, and oil-macerated ether-extracted oils. In fact, pro-oxidant activity was observed in some instances.

On the basis of epidemiologic data on Greenland Eskimos from the 1970s, and from observational data in other countries where fatty fish are eaten, fish oil has been well studied with respect to lipid metabolism and the risk of coronary heart disease.[33] Omega-3 fatty acid preparations, including α-linolenic acid, are available to consumers over-the-counter and by prescription, when indicated. By inhibiting hepatic synthesis, fish oil is efficacious in lowering serum very low density lipoproteins (VLDLs) and TG concentrations in the range 20 to 33%; the higher end of the range is reached when supplementation is combined with exercise. The effective dose appears to be 4 g/d, ranging from 1 to10 g/d, with the maximum tolerated dose being 0.3 g/kg/d fish oil capsules. In contrast to recommending encapsulated

TABLE 24-3 Naturoceutical Products Used for Cholesterol Reduction

Artichoke leaf
Bilberry (*Vaccinium myrtillus*)
Buckwheat (*Fagopyrum esculentum*)*
Cayenne ((*Capsicum annuum*)*
Coenzyme Q-10 (ubiquinone)
Copper
Cotton (*Gossypium hirsutum*)
European mistletoe (*Viscum album*)*
Evening primrose (*Oenothera biennis*)
Garlic (*Allium sativum*)[†,‡]
Ginger root (*Zingiberis rhizoma*)
Green tea (*Camellia sinensis*)
Guar gum (*Cyamopsis tetragonoloba*)
Gugulipid (*Commiphora mukul*)
Fenugreek (*Trigonella foenum graecum*)
Fish oils
Olive oil polyphenols
Peanut (*Arachis hypogaea*)
Perilla (*Perilla fructescens*)
Plant stenol esters (benechol)
Policosanol
Psyllium (*Plantago ovata, P. afra, P. indica,* or *P. asiatica*)[†]
Red yeast rice extract (*Monascus purpureus*)
Safflower (*Carthamus tinctorius*)
Soybean protein (*Glycine soja*)[†]
Soy lecithin[†]
Soy phospholipid[†]
Strophanthus (*Strophanthus gratus*)
Surinam cherry (*Eugenia unifloria*)
Vitamin E (α-tocopherol) with or without vitamin C

*Use recommended for arteriosclerosis prophylaxis by German Commission E.
[†]Recommended by German Commission E.
Entries in boldface refer to agents discussed in the text.
SOURCE: References 3,15,16,29, 31–52.

supplements, both the American Heart Association and the American Diabetes Association recommend two servings of fish per week to confer cardioprotective effects, although the level of evidence for this recommendation is considered to be level C (based on expert opinion).[34,35] The National Cholesterol Education Program states that higher intake of omega-3 fatty acids "may" reduce the risk for coronary events.[34]

In India and Asia, gugulipid resin extract is commonly used to treat hypercholesterolemia. It received regulatory approval in India in 1987, although its medicinal use dates back to 600 BC[3,16,29,36] as a widely used agent within India's ancient Ayurvedic medical system. Plant sterols have been postulated to have favorable effects on bile acid regulation, hepatic LDL-C uptak, and cholesterol metabolism, with some evidence of mild hydroxymethylglutaryl coenzyme A (HMGCoA) reductase inhibition. However, in the only double-blind, randomized, placebo-controlled trial (using "standard" doses) in patients with moderate hypercholesterolemia eating a Western diet, investigators found a significant (net 9–10%) dose-related *increase* in LDL-C levels.[36] In addition, 9% of the treated population developed a dermatologic hypersensitivity reaction.

The medicinal use of red yeast fermented rice extract to promote blood circulation dates back to the Ming Dynasty (AD1368–1644). Reductions in plasma TC and LDL-C levels of up to 23 and 31%, respectively, were reported with a standardized extract containing nine different compounds with HMGCoA reductase inhibitory activity.[3,37–39] Furthermore, TG levels fell by 34% and HDL-C rose by 20%.[37] In fact, a major isolate was named monacolin K, or mevinolin, the synthetic form of which is available by prescription today as lovastatin. Red yeast rice extract appears to improve the lipid profile to a greater degree than predicted by its dose equivalent of lovastatin, approximately 5 mg/d. Human trials have not demonstrated toxicity, such as hepatic or renal impairment or rhabdomyolysis, but these risks should not be overlooked in patients taking the naturoceutical product, especially if taken in combination with other medications.[39]

The soybean is the world's oldest recorded food crop, and regular intake has been demonstrated to reduce plasma lipid concentrations both experimentally and clinically in dose-dependent fashion.[43,44] TC and LDL-C levels are reduced by 6 to 9% and 7 to 13%, respectively, with 25 g/d soy protein. The US Food and Drug Administration (FDA) approved use of the health claim "Diets low in saturated fat and cholesterol that include 25 g of soy protein may reduce the risk of heart disease" on soy product labels.[45] The relative benefits of soy isoflavones (phytoestrogens), saponins, soy phospholipid, and soy lecithin are unknown. Whether synthetic isoflavones and other derivatives are equally effective as a natural source of soy remains a matter of substantial debate.

Policosanol is a phytochemical drug consisting of a mixture of primary aliphatic alcohols purified from sugar cane wax (*Saccharum officinarum L.*). Drug development and the majority of human studies (involving more than 3000 patients in more than 60 clinical trials) were conducted in Cuba.[47,48] Regulatory approval for use in Cuba was granted in 1991, and policosanol is available for

TABLE 24-4 Selected Naturoceutical Products Used for Improving Glycemic Control in Diabetes

Alfalfa (*Medicago sativa*)	Greek sage (*Salvia triloba*)
Aloe vera	Guar gum (*Cyamopsis tetragonoloba*)
Alpine ragwort (*Senecio nemorensis*)	Holy fruit tree (*Aegle marmelose*)
Bean pod (*Phaseolus vulgaris*)	Ivy guard coccinia (*Coccinia indica*)
Beet (*Beta vulgaris*)	Indian gum tree (*Acacia arabica*)
Behen (*Moringa oleifera*)	Jabolan (*Syzygium cumini*)
Betelnut (*Areca catechu*)	Mountain ash berry (*Sorbus aucuparia*)
Bilberry (*Vaccinium myrtillus*)	Niacinamide
Bitter melon or gourd (*Momordica charantia*)	Noni (*Morinda citrifolia*)
Black catnip (*Phyllanthus amarus*)	Oats (*Avena sativa*)
Centaury (*Centaurium erythraea*)	**Onion (*Allium cepa*)**
Chromium	**Periploca of the woods (*Gymnema sylvestre*)**
Cocoa (*Theobroma cacao*)	Plantain (*Musa paradisiaca*)
Curry leaf tree (*Murraya koeingii*)	Pomegranate (*Punica granatum*)
Dandelion (*Taraxacum officinale*)	Reed herb (*Phragmites communis*)
Divi-Divi (*Caesalpinia bunducella*)	Salt bush (*Atriplex halimus*)
Eucalyptus (*Eucalyptus globulus*)	Stevia (*Stevia rebaudiana*)
European golden rod (*Solidago virguaurea*)	Stinging nettle (*Urtica dioica*)
Fenugreek (*Trigonella foenum graecum*)	Triticum (*Agropyron repens*)
Garlic (*Allium sativum*)	Wild service tree (*Sorbus torminalis*)
German sarsaparilla (*Carex arenaria*)	Vanadium
Ginseng (*Panax ginseng, P. quinquefolius*)	Zinc
Goat's rue, or French lilac (*Galega officinalis*)	

Entries in boldface refer to agents discussed in the text.
SOURCE: References 3,15,16,29,53–64.

prescription in more than 25 countries. In the United States, however, policosanol-containing products are sold as dietary supplements and may be derived from beeswax, for few data are available regarding product efficacy.[49] At a dose range of 5 to 20 mg daily, the drug policosanol appears to be effective in reducing elevated LDL-C and TC levels in combination with dietary therapy in patients with hypercholesterolemia.[47,48] TG levels are unaffected. In comparative trials in varied populations, policosanol improved lipid profiles to an extent statistically equal to or greater than that of simvastatin, pravastatin, lovastatin, probucol, or acipimox, with no difference in side effect profiles noted between the groups.[47,48,50] Animal studies suggest that LDL-C catabolism is enhanced, yet unlike statin drugs, policosanol does not competitively or noncompetitively inhibit HMGCoA reductase.[47,48] The precise mechanism of action in decreasing cholesterol synthesis is unknown. Policosanol has additional ancillary properties including reduced smooth muscle cell proliferation, inhibition of platelet aggregation, and reduced LDL-C peroxidation.[47,48] These properties are beneficial in CVD, including coronary, cerebrovascular, and peripheral vascular disease. Smaller studies suggest policosanol reduces angina, coronary ischemic burden, and claudication symptoms.[47,50] However, long-term efficacy as defined by a reduction in traditional clinical endpoints of CVD events, morbidity, and mortality have not been conducted.

Diabetes

Herbal and other naturoceutical agents that have been used to improve glycemic control in diabetes patients are listed in Table 24-4.[3,15,16,29,53–64] Few have strong scientific evidence to support their use. The most widely used and studied mineral supplement is chromium picolinate.[53,55–58] The rationale for supplementing chromium in both type 1 and type 2 diabetes mellitus relates to the fact that chromium is an essential cofactor in insulin binding and cellular glucose uptake. Diabetics exhibit increased urinary chromium excretion, which is considered to contribute to insulin resistance. Small studies have also demonstrated worsening of impaired glucose tolerance in borderline diabetics on a low-chromium diet. Diets high in simple sugars have also been shown to increase urinary chromium loss.[56] Prospective studies have not shown consistently positive results, although most suggest potential benefit from supplementation, as well as direct dose and treatment duration effects.[55–58] The Dietary Reference value for chromium considered to be an adequate intake for adults ranges between 20 and 35 μg/d.[59]

The recommended dose of chromium picolinate is a minimum of 200 μg/d to improve glucose tolerance.[55–58] Dietary sources include brewer's yeast and barley flour.

Worldwide, more than 1000 plants and herbs have been reported to induce hypoglycemic responses, but few have been extensively studied in large human populations.[60–64] Plant medicinals have been used to treat diabetes in Ayurvedic and Chinese medicine since at least the fourth to fifth centuries BC. The development of metformin, a third-generation synthetic biguanidine derivative, traces its "roots" back to the investigation of the traditional use of *Galega officinalis* to treat diabetes. The use of Goat's rue (*G. officinalis*) for this purpose dates back to medieval Europe.[60] The plant source contains guanidine, although this parent compound was found to be toxic in clinical use. It is highly likely that other plant sources will lead to the development of additional oral hypoglycemic agents in the future.[60,62–64]

Ginseng root has consistently been among the top 10 selling herbal naturoceutical products in the United States for its reported wide range of health-enhancing properties. Animal data support the contention that both Asian (*Panax ginseng*) and American (*Panax quinquefolius*) ginseng have hypoglycemic activity.[55,60,62] One small, but placebo-controlled trial in 9 type 2 diabetics and 10 nondiabetic subjects reported a significant reduction in the area under the postprandial blood glucose curve when 3 g American ginseng was given 40 minutes prior to an oral glucose challenge.[62] The results were reproducible, with each subject receiving 2 treatments each of ginseng versus placebo in random order. The mechanism is unclear, but is felt to relate to a beneficial effect on nitric oxide-mediated glucose transport or insulin secretion.[55,60,62] Although the incidence of adverse effects is low, serious side effects and drug interactions have been noted with chronic ingestion.[3] In addition, among commercial products, the chemical composition of ginseng products and relative potency of ginsenosides are highly variable and dangerous contaminants have been noted.[3,55]

Bitter melon or gourd (*Momordica charantia*) is a very common folklore remedy for diabetes and is widely cultivated across Asia, Africa, and South America. Research on animal models has shown it to have substantial antidiabetic activity, sometimes with a prolonged duration of action on blood glucose, along with modest cholesterol-lowering effects.[55,60,64] The mechanism of action is unknown, but it appears to involve hepatic mediation. Data regarding dose safety and efficacy in diabetic patients are sparse, but suggest improved glucose tolerance with daily ingestion of 15 to 50 mL/d of the extracted juice. However, its bitter taste is often prohibitive to compliance.

Fenugreek (*Trigonella foenum graecum*) is a plant that grows wild in northern India; its hypoglycemic activity is attributed to the defatted seed, which contains nicotinic acid, coumarin, and the alkaloid trigonelline and is 50% fiber. Improvement in fasting blood sugar and postprandial glucose tolerance and reduced glucosuria have been described within 10 days of treatment in type 1 diabetics given 50 g fenugreek seed powder with lunch and dinner.[62] In type 2 diabetics, doses of 15 g have been reported as efficacious in reducing the area under the postprandial blood glucose curve.[55] Antioxidant and lipid-lowering activity has also been observed in animal models.[55,62] Plant extracts appear to have a direct effect on islet cell glucose-dependent insulin release in animal models.[55,62] At a 1 g/kg dose, activity of hexokinase, glucokinase and phosphofructokinase was enhanced toward normal in type 2 diabetics.[63] The powdered seed fiber content is also thought be beneficial in humans.[55,62,63]

Other plants with some evidence for efficacy from adequately designed, randomized, controlled trials include ivy guard (*Coccinia indica*) and *Gymnema sylvestre*.[55,62–64] *Coccinia indica* appears to inhibit gluconeogenesis by reducing glucose-6-phosphatase activity. *Gymnema sylvestre* is another plant native to India and appears to enhance endogenous insulin production and potentiate the activity of pharmacologic oral hypoglycemic drugs in type 2 diabetics. Further, both onion (*Allium cepa*) and garlic (*Allium sativum*) extracts appear to reduce blood sugar in a dose-dependent manner; this is related to competition of derived disulfide compounds with insulin (another disulfide) for insulin-activating sites in the liver.[55,60]

Obesity

Overweight and obesity are increasingly prevalent in Western countries, and represent a serious cardiovascular health hazard. On the basis of initial successful results, there was enthusiastic prescription of the combination of phentermine and fenfluramine as an appetite-suppressing weight loss adjunct. However, the resultant recall of fenfluramine and an enormous class action lawsuit for drug-associated heart valve degeneration made national headlines. Despite this, there remains a large consumer demand for weight reduction aids, and naturoceutical supplement sales for weight loss, appetite suppression, and energy enhancement have steadily increased. Although not legally marketed with the following drug claim, "herbal phen-fen" naturoceutical products generally contain combinations of St. John's wort, ma huang, caffeine or its derivatives, and other ingredients. Other natural weight loss-enhancing products exist, as listed in Table 24-5.[3,15,16,53,65–68] Available evidence does not support a formal recommendation for their use.

TABLE 24-5 Naturoceutical Products Used for Weight Reduction

Brown kelp (*Macrocystis pyrifera*) (contains iodine)
Cola (*Cola acuminata*) (contains caffeine)
Dwarf elder (*Sambucus ebulus*) (via cathartic effect)
Gamboge (*Garcinia hanburyi*) (via cathartic effect)
Garcinia cambogia
Ginseng (*Panax ginseng*)
Guarana (*Paullinia cupana*) (contains caffeine, theophylline, and theobromine)
Guggul gum, gugulipid (*Commiphora mukul*)
Ma huang (*Ephedra sinica*) (ephedrine source)
Pineapple bran (*Ananas comosus*)

Entries in boldface refer to agents discussed in the text.

SOURCE: References 3,15,16,53,65–68.

Ma huang (*Ephedra sinica*) is found in many Chinese medicine preparations and represents a natural source of ephedrine, although there are approximately 40 plant species that contain ephedrine-like compounds. Ephedrine is similar in structure to amphetamines and can increase heart rate and blood pressure in susceptible individuals. Many ergogenic or energy-enhancing products contain ephedrine and caffeine derivatives in various amounts. The combination can clearly precipitate a hypertensive crisis in susceptible individuals; the effects on heart rate and blood pressure in normal individuals are often unpredictable.[15,16,65–67,72] Reported cardiovascular adverse effects seen with ma huang were not restricted to ingestion of large doses, nor was there a prerequisite for underlying CVD.[67]

The Department of Health and Human Services (DHHS) requested a review of the available literature regarding the efficacy and safety of ephedra to aid in determining the risk/benefit ratio of these products. This followed the receipt of more than 5000 reports of possible adverse effects related to these and other dietary supplements containing ephedra derivatives between 1995 and 2000. The resultant meta-analysis of weight loss trials evaluated 52 trials including 1706 patients.[65] Trials that assessed weight loss showed that ephedrine promoted weight loss of 0.6 kg/mo compared with placebo (95% confidence interval = 0.2–1.0), with a pooled average weight loss of 11% at 4 months. The authors concluded that products containing ephedrine and ephedra promote a 0.6 to 1.0 kg/mo weight loss over 2 to 6 months. However, when only studies of moderate or high quality were included, this estimate decreased to 0.2 kg/mo. No trials assessed weight loss beyond 6 months. In studies that have been conducted on ephedra-containing products for weight loss, the total amount of ephedrine ingested per day has ranged between 60 and 75 mg (usually in three divided doses of 20–25 mg/dose).

The FDA subsequently recommended that ephedrine consumption be limited to less than 24 mg/d and that dietary supplements contain no more than 8 mg per serving of ephedrine or related alkaloids. However, after receiving additional reports of serious adverse events, the FDA issued a consumer alert on December 20, 2003, advising the immediate discontinuation of use of any supplement product containing ephedra.[72] On February 6, 2004, the FDA subsequently issued a regulation prohibiting the sale of dietary supplements containing ephedrine alkaloids, citing that such supplements present an unreasonable risk of significant adverse health outcomes, including heart attach and stroke, to the consumer. Ephedra is listed as contraindicated for use only by persons with hypertension in the German Commission E Monographs.[15] However, ephedrine is on the list of substances banned by the International Olympic Committee and the National Collegiate Athletic Association.

The fruit of the green or bitter orange plant (*Citrus aurantium*) is also used in traditional Chinese medicine for weight loss or energy supplementation.[68] Its active ingredients include synephrine, tyramine, and octopamine, and each of these compounds can increase blood pressure. There are serious and valid concerns about the quality control of Chinese medicines imported into the United States, as ingredient substitution or omission, adulterants, and contaminants have been reported.[73] Combinations of Chinese herbal products for weight loss were also implicated in an outbreak of rapidly progressive renal failure, or Chinese herb nephropathy. This was later ascribed to substitution of *Aristolochia fangchi* for *Stephania tetrandra*. Exposure to aristocholic acid from any *Aristolochia* species is associated with the development of renal interstitial fibrosis (also termed *Chinese herbal nephropathy*) as well as urothelial cancer in humans.[29,74]

Hydroxycitric acid (HCA) is the active ingredient extracted from the rind of a small pumpkin-like fruit, *Garcinia cambogia* found primarily in India and Southeast Asia. Dietary supplements and a wide variety of weight loss formulas contain *Garcinia* extract. HCA appears to inhibit fat synthesis by blocking the enzymatic conversion of citrate into acetyl coenzyme A, and suppresses appetite in animal models.[41] The studies in humans are variable in quality and their results often controversial.[68] More research is needed to confirm the degree of weight loss that can be expected from regular HCA supplementation. Some have proposed that HCA may be most effective as an aid to preventing weight regain, rather than as an approach to stimulating significant fat loss (which is best achieved by lifestyle modifications in diet, behavior, and exercise patterns).

Antioxidants and vitamins/minerals for CVD prophylaxis

Vitamin supplementation, particularly with vitamins C and/or E, remains popular as a potential means to help reduce the risk of CVD and/or cancer. The Heart Outcomes Prevention Evaluation Study (HOPE) evaluated nearly 4800 patients over the age of 55 years randomized to receive 400 IU of vitamin E versus placebo over 4.5 years.[40] Supplementation had no protective effect on the occurrence of myocardial infarction, stroke, or death from all CVD. Controversy remained, as the theoretical and demonstrable benefits of α-tocopherol (vitamin E) on LDL-C oxidation, atherosclerotic plaque stabilization, and other effects are numerous, and perhaps more significant particularly in combination with ascorbic acid (vitamin C).

A much larger trial was conducted by the Heart Protection Study Collaborative Group.[41] More than 20,500 patients at high risk for cardiovascular events were given combined antioxidant supplementation with vitamin E (600 mg), vitamin C (250 mg), and β-carotene (20 mg) versus placebo over a 5-year period. The supplemented regimen increased blood concentrations of all vitamins, but there were also small, but highly significant increases in measured plasma TC, LDL-C, and TGs among those receiving the vitamin therapy. Overall there was no significant reduction (or increase) in the all-cause 5-year mortality rate or in death from or the incidence of adverse cardiovascular events or cancer.[40] The US Preventive Services Task Force under the direction of the AHRQ reviewed the entire body of scientific evidence regarding routine vitamin supplementation in the prevention of CVD (primarily atherosclerotic) and cancer.[42] They found a paucity of evidence to determine whether supplementation reduces these risks, and concluded the evidence was insufficient to recommend for or against the use of vitamin A, E, or C or antioxidant combinations for this therapeutic intent. They did recommend against the use of β-carotene supplements alone or in combination. With the exception of β-carotene (in smokers), there appears to be little harm in dietary supplementation (as long as Dietary Reference Intake doses are not significantly exceeded). No mortality benefit can be ascribed to this therapy, however.[3,42]

Folic acid supplementation, alone or in combination with vitamins B_6 and B_{12}, has been hypothesized to reduce the risk of CVD for certain persons.[69,70] In population-based studies, an elevated blood homocysteine concentration is an independent marker for the development of atherosclerotic CVD, presumably related to increased oxidative activity. Observational data suggest an inverse relationship between the plasma concentration of homocysteine and those of folate, vitamin B_6,

and vitamin B_{12}. Further, a reduction in homocysteine level is observed with supplementation of these compounds. A meta-analysis of 12 trials inclusive of more than 1100 patients determined that daily supplementation with 0.5 to 5.0 mg folate produced a 25% reduction in homocysteine concentration. Adding 0.5 mg of vitamin B_{12} reduced homocysteine levels by another 7%, with no further benefit with additional supplementation with vitamin B_6.[69] Whether the reduction in plasma homocysteine is sustainable with ongoing supplementation is uncertain There are no prospective data demonstrating improved survival or clinical outcomes (reduced rates of infarction, stroke, or other CVD events) with folate, vitamin B_6, or vitamin B_{12} supplementation.

Coenzyme Q-10 (CoQ-10), or ubiquinone, is a fat-soluble endogenous antioxidant structurally similar to vitamins E and K. CoQ-10 is an essential cofactor in mitochondrial adenosine triphosphate production present in all tissues dependent on oxidative phosphorylation. The highest concentrations are found in the heart, liver, and pancreas. Patients with various forms of CVD have been noted to have lower plasma levels of CoQ-10 that can be increased with exogenous supplementation.[38,49,70,71] Thus dietary supplementation with CoQ-10 has been theorized as beneficial in conditions that manifest oxidative endothelial dysfunction including hypertension, hyperlipidemia, diabetes, coronary artery disease, cardiomyopathy, and heart failure. However, a thorough literature review of more than 780 articles relating to CVD and ubiquinone revealed few trials reporting relevant clinical outcomes or using a double-blind, placebo-controlled format.[71] There remains debate whether the administration of certain statin-type medications for hypercholesterolemia reduces endogenous CoQ-10 levels. Contemporary clinical practice guidelines for the treatment of CVD do not recommend routine supplementation with CoQ-10 for the prevention or treatment of CVD.[2,35]

NATUROCEUTICALS FOR SPECIFIC CARDIOVASCULAR DISORDERS

Although CVD is fundamentally a preventable condition, the prevalence of chronic CVD states remains substantial, with high associated cost, morbidity, and mortality. In parallel to specific traditional medical therapies employed for the treatment of these conditions, it readily follows that there are CAM therapies, including naturoceuticals, used for the treatment of ischemic heart disease and heart failure, as well as peripheral arterial and cerebrovascular disease. Several of the naturoceutical products discussed in this chapter as CVD preventive measures are also used in the treatment of manifest CVD, perhaps with the implicit goal of "secondary" prevention. Many other naturoceuticals are employed for the treatment of CVD symptoms such as angina, heart failure, arrhythmia, intermittent claudication, and cerebral dysfunction. The reader is referred to reviews and other resources on the use of naturoceutical agents for the management of manifest CVD.[2,3,15,16,38,71]

THE RISKS OF NATUROCEUTICAL THERAPY

Naturoceutical supplements can be generally thought of as safe and, perhaps, effective for the condition or purpose of use. Vitamin supplements taken in excess have known toxic effects only at relatively high intake levels.[3] It is important, however, to realize that herbal and plant-derived products may have significant intrinsic biologic activity and therefore carry the risk of toxicity. Plant-derived naturoceuticals can have wide source- and processing-dependent variation in component content, relative potency, purity, and bioavailability of the presumed or unknown "active" ingredient.[3,75–78] Significant numbers of dietary supplement manufacturers lack adequate quality control in assuring the consumer consistency of product composition across lots and lack of adulterants or contaminants.[3,73]

Herbal naturoceuticals may contain multiple pharmacologically active phytochemicals or metabolites.[54] Two such products possessing significant vasoactive pharmacologic activity include Indian snakeroot (*Rauwolfia*) and *Stephania tetrandra*. Snakeroot is the natural source of the alkaloid reserpine, one of the first drugs used to treat hypertension.[20,29] Pharmacologic reserpine has multiple contraindications and is now rarely prescribed in modern clinical practice given its irreversible sympatholytic effects and side effect profile and the availability of many alternative efficacious agents. The maximal daily dose of reserpine is 0.25 mg; the equivalent powdered whole root equivalent dose is between 100 and 150 mg. Tetrandrine is an extract of *Stephania tetrandra*, an herb used in traditional Chinese medicine.[29] It has calcium channel antagonistic activity similar to that of verapamil, and suppresses the production of aldosterone, but not plasma renin activity. Risks of hepatotoxicity and myocardial depression have been observed, and no safe dose has been determined in human.[15,16,29]

A valid concern about naturoceutical consumption is that of a serious drug interaction in the patient taking prescription medications.[3,75–78] The route of metabolism, pharmacokinetics, and mode of excretion of most herbal naturoceutical products are typically unknown. A well-recognized potential drug interaction involves agents processed by the hepatic cytochrome P450 enzyme complex (CYP), representing up to 80% of pharmaceutical products and an unknown number of naturoceuticals. For example, grapefruit juice is a well-known inhibitor of CYP3A4, whereas St. John's wort appears to be a potent inducer. Red yeast rice extract with intrinsic HMGCoA reductase activity has the same potential adverse drug interactions as do the "statin" class of drugs. There is ongoing research funded by the NCCAM evaluating assays of herbal products with in vitro CYP enzyme-specific activity substrate probes.[3]

A related concern is that of naturoceutical-induced alterations in anticoagulation and hemostasis. Many naturoceutical products have antiplatelet activity or the potential for an interaction with warfarin. This has been highlighted by increasing recognition of anesthetic or surgical complications from preoperative naturoceutical use, particularly ginseng, garlic, *Gingko biloba*, and CoQ-10.[3,29,75–77]

OTHER CAM THERAPIES FOR PREVENTION OF CVD

Mind–body medicine

Psychosocial stress appears to contribute to CVD morbidity and mortality. Additional psychologic factors such as depression, personality profile, and intrinsic hostility also play an important role in the development or progression of CVD. There is fairly good evidence that adding behavioral therapy and stress management techniques to cardiac rehabilitation or other lifestyle modifications improves clinical outcome and survival in the setting of coronary artery disease and after myocardial infarction.[78,79] Thus, nonpharmacologic techniques for stress reduction and mood enhancement may also be useful for CVD prevention. Although these techniques are classified under the mind–body domain of CAM therapies, they are also frequently an integral part of alternative medical systems, or manipulative medical therapies. Common mind–body therapies (MBTs) are listed in Table 24-6, and were the subject of a recent comprehensive review.[78] The authors point out that there are no large-scale trials directly comparing MBTs with aggressive traditional lifestyle interventions, including exercise, weight loss, and dietary modification, with self-monitoring of ambulatory blood pressure.

TABLE 24-6 Categories of Therapy in the Domain of Mind–Body Medicine

Relaxation techniques
Meditation
Guided imagery
Hypnosis
Biofeedback
Cognitive behavioral therapy
Psychoeducational approaches

Meditation has been defined as the "intentional self-regulation of attention," and reflects a directed and systematic mental focus on particular aspects of the individual's internal and/or external experiences.[79] The two most extensively researched forms are transcendental meditation (TM) and mindfulness meditation (MM). Most meditation practices were developed within a religious or spiritual context with the desired goal being spiritual growth, personal transformation, or transcendental experience. In TM, subjects repeat a silent word or phrase (a mantra) with the goal of ultimately transcending their internal stream of thoughts and mental dialogue. In MM, practitioners quietly observe or attend to their various thoughts, emotions, sensations, and perceptions as they arise in their field of awareness, in a nonjudgmental, detached, and objective fashion.

As applied to treatment of hypertension as a primary cardiovascular risk factor, TM and MM have each shown promise as MBTs.[20,78,79,81–85] The most positive data come from a trial conducted in 127 hypertensive older African-Americans. Patients were randomized to a 3-month trial of TM or an educational control group practicing muscle relaxation techniques. The TM group showed significant 10.7 and 6.4 mm Hg reductions in systolic and diastolic pressures, respectively. However, as pointed out by both MBT advocates and critics, no trial has been conducted evaluating outcome assessment as a primary intervention, and most trials have methodologic limitations that limit the strength and credibility of the data.[78,79,84,85]

Biofeedback techniques were developed in the 1960s and involve the use of devices that amplify physiologic processes such as blood pressure, heart rate, and muscle activity. Participants are typically guided through relaxation and imagery exercises and instructed to alter their physiologic processes using as a guide the provided biofeedback (typically visual or auditory).[86,87] Biofeedback training using the delay from the electrocardiographic R wave to the pulse interval as a measure of pulse wave velocity was effective in producing significant reductions in systolic and diastolic blood pressure of 15.3 and 17.8 mm Hg, respectively.[86] However, the study group had only mild hypertension, averaging 143 ± 14 and 99 ± 12 mm Hg, respectively, and maintenance of long-term effect was not assessed.

A meta-analysis of 26 studies of hypertension control through cognitive or behavioral modifications included such techniques as stress reduction, progressive relaxation, and biofeedback or meditation.[88] The authors concluded that cognitive techniques were superior to no therapy, but not to ambulatory self-monitoring as a sole approach. In addition, neither the National High Blood Pressure Education Program Working Group Report on Primary Prevention of Hypertension, nor the Seventh Report of the Joint National Committee on Prevention, Detection, Evaluation and Treatment of High Blood Pressure (JNC-7) recommendations include mention of relaxation techniques for the prevention of hypertension.[23,89]

Yoga and Tai Chi

Yoga and Tai Chi are widely practiced in the United States both as a form of exercise for enhancing fitness and for stress reduction. There are no large case–control, cohort, or randomized clinical trials evaluating evidence of the benefit of these approaches for preventing CVD or improving the risk factor profile. Yet, the availability of some controlled research and the minimal risk involved in performing these practices warrant further investigation.[90–93] Both yoga and Tai Chi have been used in the elderly and as an adjunct to cardiac rehabilitation with favorable results, and appear to have positive psychophysiologic effects. Whether potential benefits on well-being, blood pressure, or heart rate derive from nonspecific exercise conditioning, the mind–body connection made during the practice, or both is unknown.

Acupuncture

Acupuncture is a widely practiced therapeutic intervention for a vast range of conditions symptoms and disorders.[94–97] Areas of CVD for which acupuncture may eventually be indicated include ischemic CVD, hypertension, heart failure, and arrhythmias.[2] Reports have documented beneficial effects of acupuncture on patients with severe stable angina and, in an experimental model, on demand-induced myocardial ischemia.[98,99] Several small studies have suggested possible effects of acupuncture on lowering blood pressure in the range of 5 to 10 mm Hg; however, there are no published randomized trials demonstrating unequivocal efficacy in treating or preventing hypertension.[2] Acupuncture is an incredibly multifaceted intervention, and this intrinsic complexity makes designing clinical trials more difficult.[97] The number and length of treatments and the specific acupuncture points used frequently vary among patients and during the course of treatment. Many small case–control studies have reported evidence of the potential usefulness of acupuncture in treating hypertension, but other studies have yielded equivocal results because of trial design flaws, low sample size, and other factors.[93–97] The proposed mechanisms of action are multifactorial, including positive effects from release of endorphins and endogenous opiates, reduced plasma renin concentration, and increased endothelial nitric oxide production or responsiveness.[97] Currently, a National Institutes of Health-funded randomized, double-blind crossover clinical trial is investigating the sustainability of the effects of low-frequency electroacupuncture on 24-hour ambulatory blood pressure among 18- to 65-year-old adults.

INTEGRATIVE MEDICINE: A MODERN MANDATE

The National Center for Complementary and Alternative Medicine has defined *integrative medicine* as treatment combining mainstream medical and CAM therapies for which there exists some high-quality scientific evidence of safety and effectiveness.[3,78,97,100] Thus, what may be considered "complementary" or "alternative" today may be considered "integrative" or "standard" therapy tomorrow. This evolution or integration will be fostered by the strength of the evidence base supporting the individual therapy, although a number of general and perceptual barriers exist.[100–103]

Enormous consumer popularity of herbal and other naturoceutical products has drawn significant attention to this form of CAM and has stimulated NCCAM-funded fundamental mechanistic research along with improved clinical trial design and oversight. Because of the potential risk of serious herb–drug interactions, more research is needed to provide reliable patient safety information. Most naturoceutical products are generally safe, however, and some have reasonable evidence of efficacy in the treatment of hypertension, hypercholesterolemia, and diabetes. The link between cardiovascular risk factor profile improvement due to naturoceutical therapy and primary CVD prevention has yet to be demonstrated. At present, neither the American College of Cardiology nor the American Heart Association recommends the use of most naturoceuticals for the prevention or treatment of CVD, although healthy dietary recommendations frequently include components that can be provided and consumed in supplement form.

Physicians are advised to be objective and communicative with their patients about CAM therapies, including supplement use.[3,100–103] Care providers should document their patients' naturoceutical product list in the medical record as they do with pharmaceutical products and over-the-counter medications. Given the rapidly growing public interest in CAM, integrating CAM education into medical school curricula and seeking continuing medical education about CAM therapies are advisable.

REFERENCES

1. National Center for Complementary and Alternative Medicine. What is Complementary and Alternative Medicine? Available at: http://nccam.nih.gov/health/whatiscam/. Accessed September 1, 2003.

2. Vogel JHK, Bolling SF, Costello RB, et al. ACC clinical expert consensus document on alternative medicine: a report of the American College of Cardiology Task Force on Clinical Expert Consensus Documents (ACC Committee to Develop an Expert Consensus Document on Alternative Medicine). *J Am Coll Cardiol* 2004 (in press).

3. Hermann DD. Naturoceutical agents in the management of cardiovascular disease. *Am J Cardiovasc Drugs* 2002;2:173.

4. Hardy G: Nutraceuticals and functional foods: introduction and meaning. *Nutrition* 2000;16:688.

5. Ferrari CKB, Torres EAFS. Biochemical pharmacology of functional food and prevention of chronic diseases of aging. *Biomed Pharmacother* 2003;57:251.

6. *Prevention Magazine's Survey of Consumer Use of Dietary Supplements.* New York: Rodale Press; 1999/2000:1–79.

7. Greger JL. Dietary supplement use: consumer characteristics and interests. *J Nutr* 2001;131:1339S.

8. *Prevention's International Survey on Wellness and Consumer Reaction to Direct- to-Consumer Advertising of Prescription Medicines.* New York: Rodale Press; 2000/2001:1–71.

9. Eisenberg DM, Davis RB, Ettner SL, et al. Trends in alternative medicine in the United States, 1990–1997. Results of a follow-up national survey. *JAMA* 1998;280:1569.

10. Wootton JC, Sparber A. Surveys of complementary and alternative medicine: Part I. General trends and demographic groups. *J Altern Complementary Med* 2001;7:195.

11. Kessler RC, Davis RB, Foster DF, et al. Long-term trends in the use of complementary and alternative medical therapies in the United States. *Ann Intern Med* 2001;135:262.

12. Eisenberg DM, Kessler RC, Van Rompay MI, et al. Perceptions about complementary therapies relative to conventional therapies among adults who use both: results from a national survey. *Ann Intern Med* 2001;135:344.

13. *The Consumer Market for Heart Health Benefits.* 2001 Health-Focus Specialty Market Research Report. Atlanta, Ga: Health-Focus International; 2001.

14. Lennie TA. Influence of market forces on nutraceutical research: role of the academic researcher. *Nutrition* 2001;17:423.

15. Blumenthal M, Busse WR, Goldberg A, et al, eds. *The Complete German Commission E Monographs: Therapeutic Guide to Herbal Medicines.* Austin, Tex: American Botanical Council; 1998.

16. *PDR for Herbal Medicines.* 2nd ed. Montvale, NJ: Medical Economics; 2000.

17. *Garlic: Effects on Cardiovascular Risks and Disease, Protective Effects Against Cancer, and Clinical Adverse Effects.* Summary, Evidence Report/Technology Assessment: 20. AHRQ Publication 01-E022. Rockville, Md: Agency for Healthcare Research and Quality; October 2000. Available at: http://www.ahrq.gov/clinic/epcsums/garlicsum.htm. Accessed September 1, 2003.

18. Bordia A, Verma SK, Srivastava KC. Effect of garlic (*Allium sativum*) on blood lipids, blood sugar, fibrinogen and fibrinolytic activity in patients with coronary artery disease. *Prostaglandins Leukotrienes Essential Fatty Acids* 1998; 58:257.

19. Sato T, Miyata G. The nutraceutical benefit: Part IV. Garlic. *Nutrition* 2000;16:787.

20. Khosh F, Khosh M. Natural approaches to hypertension. *Altern Med Rev* 2001;6:590–600.

21. Conlin PR, Chow D, Miller ER 3rd, et al. The effect of dietary patterns on blood pressure control in hypertensive patients: results from the Dietary Approaches to Stop Hypertension (DASH) trial. *Am J Hypertens* 2000;13:949.

22. Office of Dietary Supplements, National Institutes of Health. *Facts About Magnesium.* Available at: http://www.cc.nih.gov/ccc/supplements/magn.html. Accessed September 1, 2003.

23. Chobanian AV, Bakris GL, Black HR, et al. The Seventh Report of the Joint National Committee on Prevention, Detection, Evaluation, and Treatment of High Blood Pressure: the JNC 7 report. *JAMA* 2003;289:2560.

24. Appleton J. Arginine: clinical potential of a semi-essential amino. *Altern Med Rev* 2002;7:512–522.

25. Black HR, Ming S, Poll DS, et al. A comparison of the treatment of hypertension with Chinese herbal and Western medication. *J Clin Hypertens* 1996;24:371.

26. Somanadhan B, Varughese G, Palpu P, et al. An ethnopharmacological survey for potential angiotensin converting enzyme inhibitors from Indian medicinal plants. *J Ethnopharmacol* 1999;65:103.

27. Liu JC, Hsu FL, Tsai JC, et al. Antihypertensive effects of tannins isolated from traditional Chinese herbs as nonspecific inhibitors of angiotensin converting enzyme. *Life Sci* 2003;73:1543.

28. FitzGerald RJ, Meisel H. Lactokinins: whey protein-derived ACE inhibitory peptides. *Nahrung* 1999;43:165.

29. Mashour NH, Lin GI, Frishman WH. Herbal medicine for the treatment of cardiovascular disease: clinical considerations. *Arch Intern Med* 1998;158:2225.

30. Duffy SJ, Gokce N, Holbrook, et al. Treatment of hypertension with ascorbic acid. *Lancet* 1999;354:2038.

31. Berthold HK, Sudhop T, von Bergmann K. Effect of a garlic oil preparation on serum lipoproteins and cholesterol metabolism. *JAMA* 1998;179:1900.

32. Banerjee SK, Mukherjee PK, Maulik SK. Garlic as an antioxidant: the good, the bad, and the ugly. *Phytotherapy* 2003;17:97–106.

33. Fish oil [monograph]. *Altern Med Rev* 2000;5:576.

34. Franz MJ. So many nutrition recommendations: contradictory or compatible? *Diabetes Spectrum* 2000;16:56.

35. Krauss RM, Eckel RH, Howard B, et al. AHA Dietary Guidelines. Revision 2000: a statement for healthcare professionals from the nutrition committee of the American Heart Association. *Circulation* 2000;102:2284.

36. Szapary PO, Wolfe ML, Bloedon LT, et al. Guggulipid for the treatment of hypercholesterolemia: a randomized controlled trial. *JAMA* 2003;290:765.

37. Heber D, Yip I Ashley JM, et al. Cholesterol-lowering effects of a proprietary Chinese red-yeast-rice dietary supplement. *Am J Clin Nutr* 1999;69:231.

38. Morelli V, Zoorob RJ. Alternative therapies: Part II. Congestive heart failure and hypercholesterolemia. *Am Fam Physician* 2000;62:1325.

39. Patrick L, Uzick M. Cardiovascular disease: C-reactive protein and the inflammatory disease paradigm: HMG-Co-A reductase inhibitors, alpha-tocopherol, red yeast rice, and olive oil polyphenols: a review of the literature. *Altern Med Rev* 2001; 6:248.

40. Yusuf S, Dagenais G, Pogue J, et al, for the Heart Outcomes Prevention Evaluation (HOPE) Study Investigators. Vitamin E supplementation and cardiovascular events in high-risk patients. *N Engl J Med* 2000;342:154.

41. Heart Protection Study Collaborative Group. MRC/BHF Heart Protection Study of antioxidant vitamin supplementation in 20536 high-risk individuals: a randomised placebo-controlled trial. *Lancet* 2002;360:23.

42. US Preventive Services Task Force. Routine vitamin supplementation to prevent cancer and cardiovascular disease: recommendations and rationale. Rockville, Md: Agency for Healthcare Research and Quality; June 2003. Available at: http://www.ahrq.gov/clinic/3rduspstf/vitamins/vitaminsrr.htm. Accessed July 29, 2003.

43. Howard BV, Kritchevsky D. Phytochemicals and cardiovascular disease: a statement for healthcare professionals from the American Heart Association. *Circulation* 1997;95:2591.

44. Erdman JW Jr. AHA Science Advisory: soy protein and cardiovascular disease: a statement for healthcare professionals from the Nutrition Committee of the AHA. *Circulation* 2000;102:2555.

45. Anderson JW, Johnstone BM, Cook-Newell ME. Meta-analysis of the effects of soy protein on serum lipids. *N Engl J Med* 1995;333:276.

46. Sato T, Miyata G. The nutraceutical benefit: Part I. Green tea. *Nutrition* 2000;16:315.

47. Janikula M. Policosanol: a new treatment for cardiovascular disease? *Altern Med Rev* 2002;7:203.

48. Gouni-Berthold I, Berthold HK. Policosanol: clinical pharmacology and therapeutic significance of a new lipid-lowering. *Am Heart J* 2002;143:356.

49. A close look at coenzyme Q10 and policosanol. *Harv Heart Lett* 2002;13:i4, p0.

50. Castano G, Mas R, Fernandez L, et al. Effects of policosanol and lovastatin in patients with intermittent claudication: a double-blind comparative pilot study. *Angiology* 2003; 54:25.

51. Klevay LM, Bazzano L, He J. Copper in legumes may lower heart disease risk. *Arch Intern Med* 2002;162:1780.

52. Pittler MH, Thompson Coon J, Ernst E. Artichoke leaf extract for treating hypercholesterolaemia [Cochrane Review]. In: *The Cochrane Library,* Issue 3. Oxford: Update Software; 2003.

53. Morelli V, Zoorob RJ. Alternative therapies: Part I. Depression, diabetes, obesity. *Am Fam Physician* 2000;62:1051.

54. Goldman P. Herbal medicines today and the roots of modern pharmacology. *Ann Intern Med* 2001;135:594.

55. Dey L, Attele AS, Yuan C. Alternative therapies for type 2 diabetes. *Altern Med Rev* 2002;7:45.

56. Lamson DS, Plaza SM. The safety and efficacy of high-dose chromium. *Altern Med Rev* 2002;7:218.

57. Anderson RA. Chromium, glucose intolerance and diabetes. *J Am Coll Nutr* 1998;17:548.

58. Cunningham JJ. Micronutrients as nutriceutical interventions in diabetes mellitus. *J Am Coll Nutr* 1998;17:7.

59. Trumbo P, Yates AA, Schlicker S, et al. Dietary Reference Intakes: vitamin A, vitamin K, arsenic, boron, chromium, copper, iodine, iron, manganese, molybdenum, nickel, silicon, vanadium, and zinc. *J Am Diet Assoc* 2001;101:294n.

60. Grover JK, Yadav, S, Vats V. Medicinal plants of India with anti-diabetic potential. *J Ethnopharmacol* 2002;81:81.

61. Oubre' AY, Carlson TJ, Reaven GM. From plant to patient: an ethnomedical approach to the identification of new drugs for the treatment of NIDDM. *Diabetologia* 1997; 40:614.

62. Vuksan V, Sievenpiper JL, Koo VYY, et al. American gingseng (*Panax quinquefolius* L) reduces postprandial glycemia in non-diabetic subjects and subjects with type 2 diabetes mellitus. *Arch Intern Med* 2000;160:1009.

63. Vats V, Yadav SP, Grover JK. Effect of *T. foenum-graecum* on glycogen content of tissues and the key enyzymes of carbohydrate metabolism. *J Ethnopharmacol* 2003;85:237.

64. Yeh GY, Eisenberg DM, Kaptchuk TJ, et al. Systematic review of herbs and dietary supplements for glycemic control in diabetes. *Diabetes Care* 2003;26:1277.

65. Shekelle PG, Hardy ML, Morton SC, et al. Efficacy and safety of ephedra and ephedrine for weight loss and athletic performance: a meta-analysis. *JAMA* 2003;289:1537.

66. *Ephedra and Ephedrine for Weight Loss and Athletic Performance Enhancement: Clinical Efficacy and Side Effects.* File Inventory, Evidence Report/Technology Assessment 76. AHRQ Publication 03-E022. Rockville, Md: Agency for Healthcare Research and Quality; March 2003.

67. Samenuk DL, Homoud MS, Contreras MK, et al. Adverse cardiovascular events temporally associated with ma huang, an herbal source of ephedrine. *Mayo Clin Proc* 2002;77: 12–16.

68. Heymsfield SB, Allison DB, Vasselli JR, et al. *Garcinia cambogia* (hydroxycitric acid) as a potential antiobesity agent: a randomized controlled trial. *JAMA* 1998;280: 1596.

69. Homocysteine Lowering Trialists' Collaboration. Lowering blood homocysteine with folic acid based supplements: meta-analysis of randomised trials. *BMJ* 1998;316:894.

70. Wald DS, Bishop L, Wald NJ et al. Randomised trial of folic acid supplementation and serum homocysteine levels. *Arch Intern Med* 2001;161:695.

71. Gundling K, Ernst E. Complementary and alternative medicine in cardiovascular disease: what is the evidence it works? *West J Med* 1999;171:191.

72. Federal Register. Rules and regulations. Final rule declaring dietary supplements containing ephedrine alkaloids adulterated because they present an unreasonable risk. February 11, 2004; volume 69, number 28:6787–6854. Available at: http://www.fda.gov/OHRMS/DOCKETS/98fr/04-2912.htm. Accessed June 17, 2004.

73. Ko R. Adulterants in Asian patent medicines. *N Engl J Med* 1998;339:847.

74. Nortier JL, Vanherweghem JL. Renal interstitial fibrosis and urothelial carcinoma associated with the use of a Chinese herb (*Aristolochia fangchi*). *Toxicology* 2002;27:181.

75. Valli G, Giardina EGV. Benefits, adverse effects and drug interactions of herbal therapies with cardiovascular effects. *J Am Coll Cardiol* 2002;39:1083.

76. Dasgupta A. Review of abnormal laboratory test results and toxic effects due to use of herbal medicines. *Am J Clin Pathol* 2003;120:127.

77. Ko R. Adverse reactions to watch for in patients using herbal remedies. *West J Med* 1999;17:181.

78. Astin JA, Shapiro SL, Eisenberg DE, et al. Mind–body medicine: state of the science, implications for practice. *J Am Board Fam Pract* 2003;16:131.

79. Astin JA, Shapiro SL, Schwartz GE. Meditation. In: Novey D, ed. *Clinicans' Rapid Access Guide to Complementary and Alternative Medicine*. St. Louis: Mosby; 2000.

80. Lin MC, Nahin R, Gershwin ME, et al. State of complementary and alternative medicine in cardiovascular, lung, and blood research: executive summary of a workshop. *Circulation* 2001;103:2038.

81. Schneider RH, Castillo-Richmond A, Alexander CN, et al. Behavioral treatment of hypertensive heart disease in African Americans: rationale and design of a randomized controlled trial. *Behav Med* 2001;27:83.

82. King MS, Carr T, D'Cruz C. Transcendental meditation, hypertension and heart disease. *Aust Fam Physician* 2002; 31:164.

83. Fields JZ, Walton KG, Schneider RH, et al. Effect of a multimodality natural medicine program on carotid atherosclerosis in older subjects: a pilot trial of Maharishi Vedic medicine. *Am J Cardiol* 2002;89:952.

84. Schneider RH, Staggers F, Alexander CN, et al. A randomized controlled trial of stress reduction for hypertension in older African Americans. *Hypertension* 1995;26:820.

85. Canter PH. The therapeutic effects of meditation: the conditions treated are stress related, and the evidence is weak. *BMJ* 2003;326:1049.

86. Rau H, Bührer M, Weitkunat R. Biofeedback of r-wave-to-pulse interval normalizes blood pressure. *Appl Psychophysiol Biofeedback* 2003;28:37.

87. Lee MS, Kim BG, Huh HJ, et al. Effect of Qi-training on blood pressure, heart rate and respiration rate. *Clin Physiol* 2000;3:173.

88. Eisenberg DM, Delbanco TL, Berkey CS, et al. Cognitive behavioral techniques for hypertension: are they effective? *Ann Intern Med* 1993;118:964.

89. *Primary Prevention of Hypertension.* Clinical and Public Health Advisory from the National High Blood Pressure Education Program. NIH Publication 02-5076, 2002. Available at http://www.nhlbi.nih.gov/health/prof/heart/hbp/pphbp.htm. Accessed October 6, 2003.

90. Labarthe D, Ayala C. Nondrug interventions in hypertension prevention and control *Cardiol Clin* 2002;20:249.

91. Taylor-Piliae RE. Tai Chi as an adjunct to cardiac rehabilitation exercise training. *J Cardiopulm Rehabil* 2003; 23:90.

92. Wang J, Lan C, Wong M. Tai Chi Chuan training to enhance microcirculatory function in healthy elderly men. *Arch Phys Med Rehabil* 2001;82:1176.

93. Raub JA. Psychophysiologic effects of Hatha yoga on musculoskeletal and cardiopulmonary function: a literature review. *J Altern Complementary Med* 2003;8:797.

94. Guo W, Ni G. The effects of acupuncture on blood pressure in different patients. *J Tradit Chin Med* 2003;23:49.

95. Townsend RR. Acupuncture in hypertension. *J Clin Hypertens* 2002;4:229.

96. Chiu YJ, Chi A, Reid IA. Cardiovascular and endocrine effects of acupuncture in hypertensive patients. *Clin Exp Hypertens* 1997;19:1047.

97. National Institute of Health Consensus Development Conference Statement 107. *Acupuncture* 1997;15:1. Available at:

http://odp.od.nih.gov/consensus/cons/107/107_statement.htm. Accessed September 3, 2003.

98. Richter A, Herlitz J, Hjalmarson A. Effect of acupuncture in patients with angina pectoris. *Eur Heart J* 1991;12:175.

99. Li P, Pitsillides KF, Rendig SV, et al. Reversal of reflex-induced myocardial ischemic by median nerve stimulation: a feline model of electroacupuncture. *Circulation* 1998; 97:1186.

100. Wetzel, SM, Kaptchuk TJ, Haramati A, et al. Complementary and alternative medical therapies: Implications for medical education. *Ann Intern Med* 2003;138:191.

101. Torpy JM. Integrating complementary therapy into care. *JAMA* 2002;287:306.

102. Barrett B. Alternative, complementary, and conventional medicine: is integration upon us? *J Altern Complementary Med* 2003;9:417.

103. Eisenberg DM. Advising patients who seek alternative medical therapies. *Ann Intern Med* 1997;127:61.

Establishing a preventive cardiology program

25

Nathan D. Wong
Mahtab Jafari
Julius M. Gardin
Henry R. Black

KEY POINTS

- *A multidisciplinary team effort is essential for successful implementation of preventive cardiology services.*

- *Recommended components of a successful clinical program in preventive cardiology include: (1) lifestyle and cardiovascular risk assessment, (2) behavioral change, (3) education, (4) family-based intervention, (5) risk factor management, and (6) screening of first-degree relatives.*

- *Priority for services should be reserved for those with established coronary heart disease or other atherosclerotic disease and for those who are at high risk of developing such diseases in the future.*

- *A system of preventive cardiology services can be implemented by solo practitioners, small*

group practices, and hospital-based or other clinics, as well as by managed care and governmental organizations. The role of the pharmacist or nurse/nurse practitioner has also been expanded to provide a wide range of preventive services.*

- *A number of barriers—patient, physician, and external—have been identified that can affect delivery of, and compliance with, preventive services.*

- *An active preventive cardiology program is often engaged in research—basic, epidemiologic, and/or clinical—as well as in professional and community educational programs and outreach.*

INTRODUCTION

To be effective in reducing the burden due to atherosclerotic coronary heart disease (CHD), both community and academic medical care facilities need to have an appropriate infrastructure for providing preventive cardiology services. Although many health care facilities do have active cardiac rehabilitation programs, effective programs for evaluating and treating high-risk persons without preexisting CHD and for long-term secondary prevention are too frequently lacking. Appropriate services for the screening and identification of those at risk and for the management of cardiovascular risk factors are the cornerstones of such a preventive cardiology program. However, a well-rounded program will also provide professional and community education opportunities and, as well as a research component. Consensus-based statements for both primary[1] and secondary[2] prevention, as well as guidelines for the identification and management of major coronary risk factors,[3–5] are available. The fact that these are often inadequately implemented in a general practice setting[6–8] provides a basis and rationale for preventive cardiology programs.

In this chapter, the components of preventive cardiology services, as well as the resources needed and challenges faced in developing such office- and clinic-based approaches, are described. In addition, barriers to the implementation of preventive services are discussed, as are the needs for professional and community education, community services, and research. This chapter is intended to provide a general overview and foundation for the development of such a program that will be applicable to many health care settings.

PRIORITIES FOR PREVENTIVE CARDIOLOGY SERVICES

No single structure will necessarily satisfy all the needs of all preventive cardiology programs. Often, a combination of approaches, integrated into the health care system, are needed to optimize the effectiveness of the program. What is necessary is close cooperation and communication among a wide range of physician and nonphysician health care specialists, who have in common the mission to deliver an effective, efficient, and cost-effective service. Screening (or identification of patients at risk), treatment, follow-up, and ongoing professional and patient education are crucial components of an effective program. Components recommended by the Second Joint Task Force of European and Other Societies on Coronary Prevention[9] include: (1) lifestyle and cardiovascular risk assessment, (2) behavioral change, (3) education, (4) family-based intervention, (5) risk factor management, and (6) screening of first-degree relatives.

PRIORITIZATION OF PATIENTS

Priority for services should be reserved for those with established CHD or other atherosclerotic disease and for those who are at high risk of developing such diseases in the future, those with high absolute risk.[9,10] Table 25–1 lists priorities regarding types of patients that should be considered for preventive strategies. In addition to patients with established CHD, CHD risk equivalents (including >20% 10-year risk), or those with significant subclinical atherosclerosis, priority patients include those with familial hyperlipidemias, a strong family history of premature CHD, diabetes mellitus, other lipid profile abnormalities, hypertension, obesity, and unhealthful lifestyle practices such as a high-fat diet and cigarette smoking.[10] The probability of future events is usually very high in such individuals, particularly if multiple risk factors are present. By dealing first with those at highest absolute risk, the service will prevent the most events per dollar spent and thus be

TABLE 25-1 Priorities of Coronary Heart Disease Prevention in Clinical Practice

1. Patients with established CHD or other atherosclerotic vascular disease, CHD risk equivalents (including >20% 10-year risk), or those with significant subclinical atherosclerosis
2. Asymptomatic subjects with particularly high risk (subjects with severe hypercholesterolemia or other forms of dyslipidemia, diabetes, or hypertension; subjects with the metabolic syndrome)
3. Close relatives of patients with early-onset CHD or other atherosclerotic vascular disease
4. Other subjects encountered in connection with ordinary clinical practice who are identified or reported to have one or more CHD risk factors

SOURCE: Modified, with permission, from Swan et al.[10]

more justifiable from cost–effectiveness and cost–benefit perspectives.

IDENTIFICATION OF PATIENTS AT RISK

Many key candidates for risk factor modification are not currently being identified, because of failure of physicians to request the appropriate tests (eg, lipid profiles in patients with established CHD, or blood pressure follow-up of those with high normal blood pressure or with hypertension) or the inability of health care systems to adequately identify patients needing such tests. The current reimbursement environment provides few, if any, incentives to follow these individuals aggressively. Partly because of the failure to identify adequately those with risk factors that warrant treatment, risk factor management is often lacking, even among patients with preexisting CHD (Table 25–2).[6,11–13] A recent chart audit of nearly 50,000 patients in the United States with CHD showed only 445 to have annual diagnostic testing of low-density

TABLE 25-2 Estimated Compliance with Secondary Prevention Measures of Patients Surviving Myocardial Infarction

Referral to a cardiac rehabilitation program	<5%
Smoking cessation counseling	20%
Lipid-lowering drug therapy	25%
Beta blocker therapy	40%
Angiotensin-converting enzyme inhibitor therapy (for reduced left ventricular ejection fraction)	60%
Aspirin	70%

SOURCE: Adapted, with permission, from Pearson et al.[11]

lipoprotein cholesterol (LDL-C); and, of those tested, only 25% reached the target goal of 100 mg/dL or less. Only 39% were on lipid-lowering therapy.[6] The lack of patient adherence to lipid-lowering therapy was also demonstrated in a study in which, of the patients in whom it was actually prescribed, only 50% continued to take it for 6 months and less than 40% continued therapy for 12 months.[13] Also, a European survey among 4863 patients with CHD showed that 53% still had elevated blood pressure and 44% had elevated cholesterol. Of those receiving blood pressure- or lipid-lowering drugs, approximately half were not adequately controlled, and only 2% reported being advised to have their relatives screened for coronary risk factors.[12] There are many reasons why preventive cardiology care is inadequate. The patients' perception that physicians spend relatively little time explaining the different aspects of cardiovascular disease (CVD) and the efficacy of cholesterol reduction in preventing a cardiovascular event in the future may contribute to the lack of compliance with therapy.[14]

The components and examples of questionnaires and tools used for cardiovascular risk assessment are discussed in earlier chapters in this book dealing with primary (Chapter 22) and secondary (Chapter 23) prevention, physical activity (Chapter 12), nutrition (Chapter 11), and psychosocial characteristics (Chapter 14). Chapter 1 contains key algorithms based on levels of major risk factors, for determining the probability of experiencing CHD, stroke, or intermittent claudication.

Accurate risk assessment begins with ensuring that the appropriate patients receive the necessary tests. At a minimum, a physician's list of patients should be reviewed to ensure the performance of certain tests, where clearly indicated (eg, lipid profiles for all patients with CHD). Although this can be done manually by a member of the physician's office staff, computerized patient-tracking databases can streamline the process. Moreover, global risk assessment algorithms, such as the Framingham risk score determination recommended by the National Cholesterol Education Program[3] can be downloaded into PDAs or office computers and used as an educational tool during the patient visit. Interrelated databases, for example, electronic medical records with patient diagnoses, laboratory data, and pharmacy prescriptions, are rapidly becoming a standard for larger health care organizations. Computer identification of abnormal cholesterol values is more likely to lead to preventive or follow-up treatment,[15] as are reminder checklists attached to outpatient records[16] or computer or nurse-generated preventive care reminders.[16–18] Others have also shown a significant increase in physician compliance with treatment guidelines prompted by a structured message pasted on patients' charts summarizing their risk and the appropriate guideline recommendations.[19]

QUALITY OF CARE AND PERFORMANCE MONITORING

Quality assurance programs should include risk factor management as a key indicator of quality of care and performance monitoring. Ten key measures (Table 25–3)[12] has been proposed as a starting point, and may be modified as new risk factors, and the efficacy of interventions designed to decrease or reverse them, become established. Reliable mechanisms to monitor the level to which clinical guidelines, practice standards, and other goals in preventive cardiology are being carried out should be developed and implemented. With the advent of new Health Employer Data Information Set (HEDIS) measures from the National Committee on Quality Assurance (NCQA) mandating evidence of LDL-C screening and control (to <130 mg/dL within 1 year of discharge) for patients with established CVD and of the rates of control of hypertension, the motivation for developing these systems becomes even stronger.

Preventive care can also be enhanced with varying degrees of success by using computer-based clinical support systems.[18] Monitoring systems can provide data for individual and organizational feedback,[20] as in a "report card" format, facilitating quality assurance efforts to provide performance data and reinforcement of organizational and provider behavior.[11] Such systems should ideally be able to provide physician-specific lists of names and contact information on patients who, for example, have CHD or diabetes (as identified by the appropriate ICD-9-CM codes) and for whom a lipid profile has not been performed in the last year. For those for whom a recent lipid profile is available, a list of patients whose LDL-C levels are above a specified target level for treatment and who are on cholesterol-lowering treatment (if any) can be generated.

ORGANIZATIONAL STRUCTURES FOR PREVENTIVE CARDIOLOGY SERVICES

A system of preventive cardiology services can be implemented by solo practitioners, small group practices, and hospital-based or other clinics, as well as by large providers, such as managed care and governmental organizations (such as the Department of Veterans Affairs).[10] However, clinical preventive services cannot be effectively implemented unless clinicians accept responsibility for providing and directing them. If physicians have limited time to provide these services, they can design the system, determine the indications for such services, and delegate the implementation to colleagues. However, they must provide staff implementing these services with the necessary direction, resources, and unambiguous support for the concept.[22]

TABLE 25-3   Key Measures of Quality of Preventive Care*

1. Smoking status should be documented in all patients with coronary or other vascular disease.

2. Organizations should have a smoking cessation program suitable for the smoking patient and his or her family.

3. All eligible patients hospitalized with coronary or other vascular disease should be offered, as documented in the medical record, physician advice and self-help materials to stop smoking.

4. All patients with coronary or other vascular disease should have a fasting lipoprotein profile documented at the appropriate time within the first 3 months of onset of disease if the patients are deemed appropriate for diet or pharmacologic intervention.

5. All patients with coronary or other vascular disease should be offered, as documented in the medical record, nutritional evaluation and counseling at the time of diagnosis.

6. All patients with coronary or other vascular disease who have a LDL-C level ≥ 100 should be prescribed, as documented in the record, lipid-lowering pharmacologic therapy if the patients are deemed appropriate for intervention.

7. All patients with coronary or other vascular disease should be assessed and provided with exercise counseling/prescription at the time of diagnosis if the patients are deemed appropriate for intervention.

8. Aspirin therapy should be offered to all patients eligible at the time of diagnosis of coronary or other atherosclerotic disease. If aspirin therapy is contraindicated, the contraindication should be documented in the medical record.

9. All patients with coronary or other vascular disease should have a blood pressure measurement documented at every visit.

10. If the average of three blood pressure measurements is equal to or greater than 140 mm Hg systolic or 90 mm Hg diastolic, lifestyle and pharmacologic treatment plans should be offered and documented at the time of diagnosis. In certain patients, such as diabetics, lower blood pressure levels are appropriate to initiate treatment (≥ 130/80 mm Hg).

*As endorsed by the American Heart Association and American College of Cardiology to be implemented in patients with established CVD. Some of these strategies can be used to create performance monitoring measures to assess quality of care.

SOURCE: Reproduced, with permission, from Pearson et al.[11]

OFFICE-BASED APPROACH

In many cases, risk factor identification and management are the responsibility of the primary health care provider, with intervention accomplished one patient at a time.[22] In this model, there may be multiple (perhaps hundreds of) primary care physicians within a given health care organization serving as a focal point for prevention efforts for a given panel of patients.

The vast majority of uncomplicated cases of dyslipidemia, hypertension, diabetes, and individuals with other risk factors are currently managed through relatively short office-based visits. During such visits, the physician can be most effective in explaining the clinical significance of the problem and the necessity for the patient to comply with prescribed lifestyle modifications and, when necessary, pharmacologic therapy. Increased efforts in this regard are particularly needed, as surveys suggest that after 1 year, up to half of patients stop prescribed preventive therapy, such as cholesterol-lowering drugs.[24] Reasons for this lapse in compliance are numerous, but include: (1) the failure of the medical care profession to agree on appropriate strategies, (2) the failure of physicians to implement risk reduction therapies, (3) poor patient adherence to such therapies, (4) patient-presumed adverse reactions to the treatment, and (5) lack of reimbursement for such therapies.[18] For many of these issues, the physician is in the best position to ensure that they do not become barriers to patient compliance. Practice models for incorporating CHD prevention strategies, including educational and counseling components, have been developed.[25]

As the office-based approach provides limited opportunity for adequate patient education, a responsible prevention program entails recommendations (or "prescriptions") to obtain needed education for risk factor management from other members of the health care team, including nurses, dietitians, exercise specialists, pharmacists, psychologists, and, if necessary, vocational staff (Table 25–4).[9] The management of risk factors is a complex process, involving not only educating patients, but also teaching them the skills to change and maintain healthful behaviors and to adhere to prescribed regimens.[11] This may involve establishing appointments or referrals with a dietitian with expertise in cardiovascular nutrition, a clinical psychologist, and/or an exercise physiologist as needed.

Protocols should be developed for the type of specialty services each team member will provide, which patients are to receive them, and to what extent and in what format (eg, initial group sessions followed by individualized counseling sessions to address individual needs, and so on). As is often the case, however, the physician may bear the burden of much of this education about

TABLE 25-4   Recommended Resources for Cardiac Prevention and Rehabilitation Programs

Physicians
Cardiologists and other physicians in the hospital and in the community have a central role to play because of their professional relationship with the patient, and are ultimately responsible for all aspects of a patient's care. They need to give leadership to the organization of such a service, ensuring that it becomes an integral part of the health care delivery system. They must unambiguously endorse prevention.
Nurses/Nurse Practitioners
Specially trained cardiac nurses or nurse practitioners can help recruit patients and organize lifestyle assessments, risk factor screening, and health promotion sessions. Training in models of behavioral change, health promotion, and psychosomatic aspects of disease is essential.
Dietitians
Dietitians provide important management and professional advice for assessment and recommendation of dietary changes that need to be made. Most nurses and doctors have not received any formal training in this area, and if professional dietitian staff are not available, such training needs to be provided on key aspects of nutrition using well-written educational materials.
Exercise Specialists
Exercise evaluation and prescriptions are important for all patients and for those with CHD; supervised exercise is an important component of patient management.
Pharmacists (or PhD lipid specialists)
The role of pharmacists may vary from direct patient care and consultation to education in relation to the use of drugs, their clinical indications, mode of action, side effects, and benefits. The increasing role of pharmacists (or PhD lipid specialists) in providing general health education necessary for successful risk reduction is also recognized.
Psychologists
Mental health staff, including psychologists, psychiatrists, and other qualified staff, can design necessary programs and inform patients about how to address the psychologic consequences of developing CHD, including how to cope with and manage stress. This can have an important impact on the patient's quality of life and improve compliance to achieve other goals in the program, such as weight loss and smoking cessation. By helping patients to understand and manage their emotions and reactions to stress, psychologists can also help to increase their motivation to make and sustain appropriate lifestyle changes, as well as to return to a full and active role in the community.
Vocational Support
Adequate assistance may be needed by some patients to help them return to work or find more suitable alternative employment.
Facilities
These should include office space for staff, an area for individual and family lifestyle and risk factor assessment, a private area for counseling, and an area for group activities, including education and health promotion sessions and supervised physical activity.

SOURCE: Adapted, with permission, from the Second Joint Task Force of European and Other Societies on Coronary Prevention.[9]

risk factors and, if so, should have had the training (or use appropriate team members within the office visit) to provide such education. For instance, a 15-minute physician office visit may need to be extended to 30 minutes to provide appropriate dietary advice, and perhaps 40 to 45 minutes to provide appropriate consultation on physical activity and/or stress management. The constraints on physician time in the managed care era make this unrealistic in many cases, but physicians should spend the time that is needed to provide the best care for patients. Unambiguous endorsement of prevention by the physician is critical if CVD is to be effectively prevented.

Finally, a key to the success of this model for preventive services lies in the ability to provide—and ensure—that preventive services personnel obtain appropriate training,

so that there is some standard (ideally based on nationally recognized and agreed-on guidelines) for the management strategies that are being prescribed. For more complicated risk factor management needs, referral is recommended to a specialty physician provider, for example, a cardiologist, endocrinologist, lipid specialist, or hypertension specialist.[4] In addition, the general internist might have an arrangement with an appropriate specialist for periodic review of evaluation and treatment plans.[10]

A schedule should be developed for regular follow-up visits by patients to the primary care physician, with appointments scheduled in advance, if possible. At these visits, progress made in controlling risk factors should be reviewed and appointments with the above-recommended specialists should be scheduled as necessary. The provider should have a system implemented to remind patients of their visits to promote better compliance.

MULTIDISCIPLINARY COLLABORATIVE PROGRAMS

The hallmark of a preventive cardiology program is often a specialty multidisciplinary clinic, such as a "risk reduction" or "prevention and reversal" clinic. Such clinics can be particularly attractive from a marketing standpoint, potentially offering a unique program that appeals to the public. In many regions, except for certain well-known medical centers and clinics, some of which have been involved in this specialty for more than a decade, such clinics are still relatively uncommon. Some health care facilities have become aggressive at providing a heart disease prevention and reversal program, with an educational program for the public (a "cardiac college") directed toward reducing suffering and death due to heart disease.[26]

A preventive cardiology clinic in the academic setting might have as its focus the management of a particular disorder, such as dyslipidemia or hypertension, by virtue of its physician director having a particular academic expertise. Ideally, however, the clinic should provide services for managing multiple risk factors, including smoking, obesity, and physical inactivity, as most of the patients seen are likely to exhibit multiple risk factors. As diabetes programs normally exist at major hospitals, these specialty programs will normally receive the referrals for many of the diabetic patients. As the need to manage cardiovascular disease in high-risk individuals becomes more urgent, it is hoped that the currently existing "silos" of care will break down.

A preventive cardiology clinic should be prepared to handle more difficult-to-manage cases of dyslipidemia and hypertension, as well as problems related to obesity and tobacco use. The initial visit normally requires a comprehensive medical history and physical examination (Appendix 25–1). Frequently, it is desirable to conduct a battery of assessment tests, including a blood chemistry and fasting lipid profile, urinanalyses with attention to microalbuminuria, and, in those at intermediate risk (eg, two or more risk factors or 10–20% 10-year calculated risk of CHD), a measurement of high-sensitivity C-reactive protein, a nutritional and exercise inventory, and a behavioral health survey, and have them completed prior to the initial physician visit. Assessment for subclinical atherosclerosis (eg, from carotid ultrasound or coronary calcium screening) may also be ordered by the physician (Chaps. 3 and 4) in those at intermediate risk. These results should be made available to the physician in advance of the patient visit, so that a preliminary review and initial plan (see Appendix 25–1) can be drafted and, if necessary, modified at the initial visit. Forms for a sample progress note and follow-up plan are also provided in Appendix 25-1.

A single physician director and, if necessary, other trained health care providers (ie, pharmacists, PhD lipid specialists, nurse practitioners) with expertise in the major risk factor therapeutic areas usually provide medical supervision for the program. In a pharmacist-managed lipid clinic that was initiated within a private cardiology group, after 6 months, 69% of patients reached the National Cholesterol Education Program (NCEP) LDL-C goals compared with only 50% of the patients in a control clinic group ($P < .0001$).[27]

In a multidisciplinary, collaborative practice lipid clinic, after four clinic visits, patients were four times more likely than patients in traditional physician-based clinics to reach the NCEP LDL-C goal. This clinic team, which was led by a clinical nurse, included a clinical pharmacist, a nurse practitioner, a dietitian, and a clinical psychologist. A consultant cardiologist reviewed all laboratory tests and confirmed all therapeutic decisions prior to each clinic visit.[28] In some cases, there is a research or administrative director responsible for research operations or general management. A nurse or other allied health care provider, such as a clinical pharmacist, is frequently employed as a clinic manager for the facility, and additional nurses and administrative staff provide the needed support services.

As in the office-based approach, access is needed to a specialized team of allied health care providers, including dietitians, exercise physiologists, psychologists, and other personnel (see Table 25–4).[9] For the specialty clinic, such individuals are ideally on staff, either part- or full-time and dedicated to providing the highest quality of care. Patients should normally be able to receive "one-stop" preventive care for CVD, with most services available in a single facility.

PHARMACIST AND NURSE/NURSE PRACTITIONER CASE MANAGEMENT APPROACHES

In an increasing number of health care settings, particularly within managed care, the role of the pharmacist or nurse/nurse practitioner has been expanded to provide a wide range of preventive services. One scenario is the operation of a lipid or hypertension clinic using a case management approach. Although a physician usually oversees such a clinic, the nurse or pharmacist may be the focal point of care. A pharmacist-coordinated clinic may be appropriate where multiple or complex medication algorithms need to be followed and where the patient can benefit from advice on how best to comply with prescribed medications. The important role of the pharmacist to improve the care of patients with myocardial infarction was confirmed by the Centers for Medicare and Medicaid Services (CMS). The CMS Acute Myocardial Infarction Project, which also focuses on preventive therapeutic interventions, includes representation from internal medicine, cardiology, emergency medicine, and pharmacy.[29]

In a program that involved medical record review and written coronary risk assessment and recommendations by a pharmacist, both the secondary and primary prevention groups experienced significant decreases in LDL-C (26 and 27%, respectively, $P < .0001$) compared with their baseline.[30] In this study, the LDL-C reduction was achieved through the medical records with minimal interaction between the pharmacist and the patient. In the secondary and primary prevention groups, the percentage of patients reaching their NCEP LDL-C goal increased from 6 to 27% ($P < .04$) and from 20 to 51% ($P < .006$), respectively.

Protocols for pharmacotherapy of lipid disorders (and/or hypertension) can be developed and followed closely by the pharmacist in conjunction with the physician, who approves all prescriptions. This type of setting can be successful in managing thousands of patients in a given facility who attend follow-up visits with staff within a pharmacist-based clinic. The pharmacist is well prepared to provide patient education, particularly with respect to information about cardiovascular risk factors and their control, and to ensure compliance with the prescribed medication regimen. One study demonstrated a community pharmacy to be an easily accessible, well-accepted, and effective site for cholesterol screenings, with a high degree of follow-up of abnormal results.[31]

Case management systems for risk factor modification, such as those operated by trained nurses, can not only be more efficacious, but are often more cost-effective than physician-staffed risk factor modification approaches. This is true partly because of the full-time, dedicated staff often involved and the reliance by some systems on phone and mail contact, rather than face-to-face visits. Nurses can be hired and trained to devote their time completely to such an activity, whereas physicians must often divide their efforts among numerous responsibilities. Patient satisfaction and convenience are often enhanced by such approaches.

A nurse-based case management system may be most useful for more general risk factor reduction or lifestyle modification efforts. Ultimately, available resources are an important factor in determining the precise administrative structure. A nurse/nurse practitioner case management approach has been shown to be effective in the management of hypertension,[32] diabetes,[33] smoking cessation,[34] and hyperlipidemia.[35] Among patients with CHD, a physician-directed, nurse-managed, home-based case management system for coronary risk factor modification had, compared with usual care, a significantly greater confirmed smoking cessation rate (70% vs 53%, respectively), better LDL-C control (107 mg/dL vs 132 mg/dL), and improved functional capacity (9.3 metabolic units [METs] vs 8.4 METs).[36] A recently published trial of 19 nurse-run general practice clinics involving 1173 patients with CHD demonstrated, after 1 year, significant improvements in aspirin use, blood pressure control, lipid management, physical activity, and diet modification, but not smoking cessation.[37]

A case management approach such as that offered by a dedicated pharmacist or nurse can improve the efficacy of risk factor modification because three important objectives are achieved: (1) patients can be encouraged to adhere to drug and diet regimens; (2) patients can be instructed in the self-monitoring of weight, blood pressure, blood glucose, and be trained to cope with a smoking relapse; and (3) patients can be taught to take appropriate action in response to new or worsening symptoms. Such a system can be integrated into the usual care of patients with the use of existing facilities (hospital or outpatient clinics) and convenient channels of communication (telephone, mail, and even the Internet).[10] Physicians can be kept apprised of patients' progress, and be involved in approving prescriptions and management strategies.

APPROACH TO PREVENTIVE CARE

The approach to delivering preventive cardiology services begins with the traditional workup by medical history and physical examination, as in a traditional practice. The clinical and laboratory findings should then be summarized and related to a general level of CHD risk, as by using a health appraisal or Framingham-type risk algorithm (such as presented in Chapter 1). The risk level should be linked to the patient's personal behavior and genetic makeup, as well as family and social behaviors. Smoking, eating, physical activity, and weight change should be reviewed and possible causes of excess risk discussed. The entire family should be engaged in making healthy lifestyle choices, reducing risk if it is high, and preventing increases in risk at all ages. The patient should be encouraged to set goals and be given guidance on how to reach them. Progress should be reviewed at each visit and there should be a focus on success rather than failure. Whether a patient is at low, medium, or high risk based on the evaluation, positive messages related to preventive strategies should be given.[38]

BARRIERS TO IMPLEMENTATION OF PREVENTIVE SERVICES

A number of barriers—patient, physician, and external—have been identified that can affect delivery of, and compliance with, preventive services.

Patient factors may involve lack of knowledge and motivation, lack of access to care, cultural factors, and social factors. Physicians frequently perceive patients as unmotivated or noncompliant, but patients indicate preventive services as a high priority in their health care and frequently cite physicians' failure to order certain tests or communicate results of such tests.[11,22] Physician barriers to implementing preventive services may include their fundamental focus on, and increasing time commitment to, acute care, often including noninvasive and invasive procedures. In addition, the pressures of the managed care environment have tended to result in shorter patient visits. Also, although reimbursement for acute interventions is frequently perceived as acceptable, it remains generally poor for risk factor interventions,[11] particularly dietary and other ancillary services, a major reason for their not being appropriately used. Risk factor interventions may also be accompanied by patient complaints of side effects. Finally, lack of training or confidence in implementing risk reduction strategies, such as smoking cessation, dietary counseling, and even treatment with cholesterol-lowering medications, is cited by a substantial proportion of primary care physicians as an important barrier to the delivery of preventive services. Cardiologists do not fare much better in terms of reporting adequate training and confidence in applying preventive strategies. This is not surprising, given that most cardiology programs do not have specialists in the treatment of lipid disorders or risk factor management, resulting in inadequate training in preventive cardiology.[11,40]

Although physicians and other health care providers may be ready and able to provide preventive services, hospitals often create obstacles to their implementation. Often, the focus of care in secondary and tertiary care hospitals is on acute conditions that prompt hospital admission. Furthermore, once the patient is hospitalized, there is frequently limited time to interact with (and educate) the patient because of the pressure for early discharge.[11] In addition, patients are not necessarily in the best condition to discuss nutrition, exercise, or other preventive strategies. However, while they are in the acute care setting, they are often highly impressionable and can be encouraged to make such changes. Unfortunately, there is frequently a lack of infrastructure or resources, including facilities and staffing, to allow health care professionals to focus on risk factor management. Staff nurses are often trained to deal with acute management issues, and neither physicians nor nurses have undergone formal training in the behavioral aspects of risk factor modification. Finally, most hospitals do not ensure adequate continuity of care after the hospitalization, making long-term risk factor modification difficult to ensure.[11]

EDUCATIONAL PROGRAMS
Professional education

Although postgraduate continuing medical education programs frequently provide courses and symposia directed at cardiovascular risk reduction, few physician training programs (eg, internal medicine residencies or cardiology fellowships) provide sufficient background in preventive cardiology. Subspecialty training programs should include requirements for adequate instruction on: (1) the pathophysiologic roles of risk factors, and epidemiologic and clinical trial evidence supporting the efficacy of treatment in reducing the risk of cardiovascular disease; (2) comprehensive assessment of individual risk factors and overall risk; and (3) techniques to modify risk factors using both lifestyle and pharmacologic interventions.[41,42] It is also important that training take place in an academic medical center or institution with a strong commitment to academic training and appropriate certification. Trainees in adult cardiology training programs should have adequate preparation in the biologic, physical, and epidemiologic sciences basic to medicine.[42] The American College of Cardiology has proposed content for such a training program at three levels (Table 25–5).[42]

Family practice physicians frequently see patients with major coronary risk factors; they should be able to assess an individual patient's overall risk and provide advice and counseling to reduce that risk. Teaching-consultation clinics have been developed where family practice residents learn from knowledgeable faculty with expertise in preventive cardiology how to assess cardiac risk in the general patient and develop counseling skills to manage that risk.[43]

Once a preventive cardiology clinic is established, mechanisms for integrating participation in the clinic by cardiology fellows, internal medicine residents, and medical, pharmacy, and nursing students should be developed. These programs serve as outstanding ways for health care providers from different backgrounds to learn the value of working together toward a common goal and to learn what each provides to patient care. In addition, opportunities should be provided to enhance training of dietetic, exercise physiology, and behavioral medicine interns as members of the preventive cardiology health care team. Patient conferences reviewing specific cases and involving input from all members of the team can be an invaluable educational experience while also enhancing the quality of patient care by obtaining input from multiple disciplines simultaneously.

Community education

Educational programs on preventing heart disease aimed at the community can potentially provide information of interest and relevance to most lay attendees. Participating physicians, dietitians, and other members of the health care team should conduct community outreach seminars on such popular topics as: (1) how to optimize cholesterol and blood pressure control, (2) nutritional strategies

TABLE 25-5 Recommended Content for Training in Preventive Cardiovascular Medicine

Level 1

This includes training that should be part of the knowledge base of all clinical cardiologists and includes exposure to the following general and specific areas.

General content:

1. Vascular biology of the heart and blood vessels (It is important for cardiovascular medicine trainees to understand the language of molecular biology, as well to continue self-study and critical review of published medical reports.)
2. Clinical epidemiology and biostatistics
3. Principles of clinical trials and outcomes research
4. Principles of clinical pharmacology

Specific content:

1. Diagnosis and treatment of primary and secondary hypertension
2. Diagnosis and treatment of primary and secondary dyslipidemias
3. Diagnosis and treatment of thrombosis and hypercoagulable states
4. Management of smoking cessation and nicotine addiction
5. Cardiac rehabilitation
6. Exercise physiology
7. Nutrition and its effects on the cardiovascular system
8. Psychosocial and behavioral aspects of cardiovascular disease
9. Diagnosis and treatment of peripheral vascular disease

Training in these areas should be integrated into consultative, inpatient, and outpatient rotations and into didactic components of the core cardiovascular medicine programs. The time allotted should be equivalent to 1 month of full-time training. Alternatively, this goal could be met by 1 month of block time followed by experience in continuity clinics.

Level 2

Level 2 training should achieve a level of expertise for the cardiovascular specialist so that the trainee could serve as an independent consultant to other cardiovascular practitioners in the management of cardiovascular risk factors. This should involve 6 to 12 months of training within the 36 months of a cardiovascular training program and include block time for direct evaluation of patients with advanced atherosclerosis, resistant hypertension or hyperlipidemia, or recurrent thrombosis.

This could involve block time in hypertension and lipid clinics or services, or both, coagulation laboratories, peripheral vascular laboratories, clinical and cardiac rehabilitation services, and additional exposure to behavioral medicine, exercise physiology, clinical epidemiology, outcomes research, and vascular biology.

The clinical application of information contributed by newly emerging fields, such as vascular biology and medicine, lends itself to the development of the clinician/scientist and the expert teacher/clinician.

Level 3

Level 3 requires advanced training to qualify as a director of a clinical service or research program, or both. Examples include director of a preventive cardiology, hypertension, or lipid service; director of a cardiac rehabilitation program; director of a vascular biology laboratory; and a trainee who obtains a Master of Public Health degree in clinical epidemiology, outcomes research, or both.

Training to this level would require at least 1 year of a 36-month program. Alternatively, 2 to 3 years in a vascular biology laboratory or health services outcome research/clinical epidemiology program would be required to attain expertise in these fields, possibly leading to an advanced degree.

SOURCE: Reproduced, with permission, from Sullivan et al.[42]

for preventing heart disease and stroke, (3) preventing heart disease in women, and (4) preventing heart disease in the elderly. The public is eager to learn all they can about how to prevent a disease that has likely affected many of their friends, if not themselves. They are often anxious, whether in a lecture or small group setting, to obtain informed advice from professionals specializing in the topic that is being addressed—information that they frequently are unable to obtain from the limited contact with their primary health care provider. Often, such talks are an integral part of community education programs offered by senior centers, corporations, local hospitals, and organizations such as the American Heart Association. Physicians and other health care personnel with the appropriate expertise should be encouraged to participate on community education speaker bureaus.

Educational community outreach programs are especially needed for minority and underserved communities.

An example is the National Heart Lung and Blood Institute (NHLBI) Latino Community Cardiovascular Disease Prevention and Outreach Initiative, Salud para su Corazon. This heart disease prevention and education campaign addresses language preferences and cultural values by developing educational materials and interventions targeting the Latino community.[44]

RESEARCH

An active preventive cardiology program is often engaged in basic, epidemiologic, and/or clinical research—investigation aimed at elucidating mechanisms of atherosclerosis development or plaque stabilization, epidemiologic projects studying newer risk factors or subclinical disease assessment, or clinical trials testing the efficacy of newer pharmacologic agents for risk factor reduction. Such research, particularly projects that have national recognition or those that offer unique treatments or services, can help to establish the program as a center of excellence, enhancing its reputation in the community. Furthermore, patients are often interested (sometimes because of financial need) in participating in ongoing clinical trials, such as those testing new cholesterol-lowering agents, that provide them with free medications, limited risk factor evaluation, and consultative services to which they may not otherwise have access.

CONCLUSIONS

Although the provision of preventive services can be challenging in the current health care environment, most providers express a desire to implement such services, and a large proportion of the public expects such services and is willing to pay for them.[10] A team and multidisciplinary effort to implementing preventive cardiology services and a process of continuous quality improvement will promote the delivery of high-quality preventive services.[10] Physicians and other health care providers must reflect on the strengths, limitations, resources, and goals at hand and settle on the systematic practice of preventive cardiology as a routine component of medical care.[38] Physicians and all health care providers must decide themselves to implement the lessons learned regarding the value of prevention. All people would prefer to prevent their own heart attack or stroke rather than join a rehabilitation program and relearn how to speak or walk. This message should be emphasized to patients and colleagues whenever and wherever possible.

REFERENCES

1. Pearson TA, Blair SN, Daniels SR, et al. AHA Guidelines for Primary Prevention of Cardiovascular Disease and Stroke: 2002 update: Consensus Panel Guide to Comprehensive Risk Reduction for Adult Patients Without Coronary or Other Atherosclerotic Vascular Diseases. American Heart Association Science Advisory and Coordinating Committee. *Circulation* 2002;106:388–391.

2. Smith SC, Blair SN, Bonow RO, et al. AHA/ACC Scientific Statement: AHA/ACC guidelines for preventing heart attack and death in patients with atherosclerotic cardiovascular disease: 2001 update: A statement for healthcare professionals from the American Heart Association and the American College of Cardiology. *Circulation* 2001;104:1577–1579.

3. Expert Panel on Detection, Evaluation, and Treatment of High Blood Cholesterol in Adults. Executive Summary of the Third Report of he National Cholesterol Education Program (NCEP) Expert Panel on Detection, Evaluation, and Treatment of High Blood Cholesterol in Adults (Adult Treatment Panel III). *JAMA* 2001;285:2486–2497.

4. Chobanian AV, Bakris GL, Black HR, et al. The seventh report of the Joint National Committee on Prevention, Detection, Evaluation, and Treatment of High Blood Pressure: The JNC 7 report. *JAMA* 2003;289:2560–2572.

5. National Institutes of Health, National Heart, Lung, and Blood Institute: *Clinical Guidelines on the Identification, Evaluation, and Treatment of Overweight and Obesity in Adults: The Evidence Report.* Washington, DC: U.S. Department of Health and Human Services; 1998.

6. Sueta CA, Chowdhury M, Boccuzzi SJ, et al. Analysis of the degree of undertreatment of hyperlipidemia and congestive heart failure secondary to coronary artery disease. *Am J Cardiol* 1999;83:1303–1307.

7. Burt VL, Cutler JA, Higgins M, et al. Trends in the prevalence, awareness, treatment, and control of hypertension in the adult U.S. population: data from the health examination surveys, 1960 to 1991. *Hypertension* 1995;26:60–69.

8. Abrams J. Reporting of coronary risk factors. *Am J Cardiol* 1995;75:716–717.

9. Joint Task Force of European and Other Societies on Coronary Prevention. Prevention of coronary heart disease in clinical practice. *Eur Heart J* 1998;19:1434–1503.

10. Swan HJC, Gersh BJ, Graboys TB, Ullyot DJ (Task Force 7). 27th Bethesda Conference: matching the intensity of risk factor management with the hazard for coronary disease events: Task Force 7. Evaluation and management of risk factors for the individual patient (case management). *J Am Coll Cardiol* 1996;27:1030–1039.

11. Pearson TA, McBride PE, Miller NH, Smith SC (Task Force 8). 27th Bethesda Conference: matching the intensity of risk factor management with the hazard for coronary disease events: Task Force 8: Organization of a preventive cardiology service. *J Am Coll Cardiol* 1996;27:1039–1047.

12. EUROASPIRE Study Group. A European Society of Cardiology survey of secondary prevention of coronary heart disease: principal results: European Action on Secondary Prevention through Intervention to Reduce Events. *Eur Heart J* 1997;10:1569–1582.

13. Simons LA, Levis G, Simons J. Apparent discontinuation rates in patients prescribed lipid-lowering drugs. *Med J Aust* 1996;164:208–211.

14. Kiortsis DN, Viral P, Bruckert E, et al. Factors associated with low compliance with lipid-lowering drugs in hyperlipidemic patients. *J Clin Pharmacol Ther* 2000;25:445–451.

15. Reed RG, Jenkins PL, Pearson TA. Laboratory's manner of reporting serum cholesterol affects clinical care. *Clin Chem* 1994;40:847–848.

16. Williams BJ. Efficacy of a checklist to promote a preventive medicine approach. *J Tenn Med Assoc* 1981;74:489–491.

17. McDonald CJ. Protocol-based computer reminders, the quality of care and the nonperfectibility of man. *N Engl J Med* 1976;295:1351–1355.

18. Davidson RA, Fletcher SW, Retchin S, Duh S. A nurse-initiated reminder system for the periodic health examination: implementation and evaluation. *Arch Intern Med* 1984;144:2167–2170.

19. Weingarten SR, Riedinger MS, Conner L, et al. Practice guidelines and reminders to reduce duration of hospital stay for patients with chest pain: an interventional trial. *Ann Intern Med* 1994;120:257–263.

20. Johnston ME, Langton KB, Haynes RB, Mathieu A. Effects of computer-based clinical decision support systems on clinician performance and patient outcome: a critical appraisal of research. *Ann Intern Med* 1994;120:135–142.

21. Vuori HV. *Public Health in Europe, 1982.* Copenhagen: World Health Organization; 1982.

22. Kottke TE, Brekke ML, Solberg LI. Making time for preventive services. *Mayo Clin Proc* 1993;68:785–791.

23. Smith SC. The challenge of risk reducing therapy for cardiovascular disease. *Am Fam Physician* 1997;55:491–500.

24. Smith SC. The need for broad preventive therapies in the new millenium: a challenge to change. Lecture delivered at: Reducing Cardiovascular Risk in the New Millennium: One Heart at a Time; June 5, 1999; Leesburg, Va [personal communication].

25. Makrides L, Veinot PL, Richard J, Allen MJ. Primary care physicians and coronary heart disease prevention: a practice model. *Patient Educ Counsel* 1997;32:207–217.

26. Reddell JR. Expansion of an existing program for the prevention and reversal of heart disease. *J Cardiovasc Manage* 1997;8:33–35.

27. Bozovich M, Rubino CM, Edmunds J. Effect of a clinical pharmacist-managed lipid clinic on achieving National Cholesterol Education Program low-density lipoprotein goals. *Pharmacotherapy* 2000;20:1375–1383.

28. Shaffer J and Wexler LF. Reducing low-density lipoprotein cholesterol levels in an ambulatory care system. *Arch Intern Med* 1995;155:2330–2335.

29. Stringer KA, Lopez L, Talbert RL. A call for pharmacists to improve the care of patients with myocardial infarction. *Pharmacotherapy* 2001;21:1317–1319.

30. Carson JJ. Pharmacist-coordinated program to improve use of pharmacotherapies for reducing risk of coronary artery disease in low-income adults. *Am J Health-Syst Pharm* 1999;56:2319–2324.

31. Madejski RM, Madejski TJ. Cholesterol screening in a community pharmacy. *J Am Pharm Assoc* 1996;NS36:243–248.

32. Reichgott MJ, Pearson S, Hill MN. The nurse practitioner's role in complex patient management: hypertension. *J Natl Med Assoc* 1983;75:1197–1204.

33. Weinberger M, Kirkman MS, Samsa GP, et al. A nurse-coordinated intervention for primary care patients with non-insulin-dependent diabetes mellitus: impact on glycemic control and health-related quality of life. *J Gen Intern Med* 1995;10:59–66.

34. Taylor CB, Houston-Miller N, Killen JD, DeBusk RF. Smoking cessation after acute myocardial infarction: effects of a nurse-managed intervention. *Ann Intern Med* 1990;113:118–123.

35. Blair TP, Bryant FJ, Bocuzzi S. Treatment of hypercholesterolemia by a clinical nurse using a stepped-care protocol in a nonvolunteer population. *Arch Intern Med* 1988;148:1046–1048.

36. DeBusk RF, Miller NH, Superko HR, et al. A case-management system for coronary risk factor modification after acute myocardial infarction. *Ann Intern Med* 1994;120:721–729.

37. Campbell NC, Ritchie LD, Thain J, et al. Secondary prevention in coronary heart disease: a randomised trial of nurse led clinics in primary care. *Heart* 1998;80:447–452.

38. Kottke TE, Blackburn H, Brekke ML, Solberg LI. The systematic practice of preventive cardiology. *Am J Cardiol* 1987;59:690–694.

39. Shea S, Gemson DH, Mossel P. Management of high blood cholesterol by primary care physicians: diffusion of the National Cholesterol Education Program Adult Treatment Panel guidelines. *J Gen Intern Med* 1990;5:327–334.

40. Roberts WC. Getting cardiologists interested in lipids. *Am J Cardiol* 1993;72:744–745.

41. 25th Bethesda Conference: future personnel needs for cardiovascular health care, Nov. 15–16, 1993. *J Am Coll Cardiol* 1994;24:275–328.

42. Sullivan JM, Frohlich ED, Lewis RP, Pasternak RC. Guidelines for training in adult cardiovascular medicine: Core Cardiology Training Symposium (COCATS). Task Force 10: training in preventive cardiovascular medicine. *J Am Coll Cardiol* 1995;25:33–34.

43. Cable TA, Delaney MJ. Teaching preventive cardiology: the consultation clinic. *Am J Prev Med* 1996;12:161–164.

44. Moreno C, Alvarado M, Balcazar H, et al. Heart disease education and prevention program targeting immigrant Latinos: using focus group responses to develop effective interventions. *J Commun Health* 1997;22:435–450.

APPENDIX 25-1   SAMPLE CLINIC FORMS FOR INITIAL ASSESSMENT, INITIAL PLAN, PHYSICAL EXAMINATION, PERSONAL MEDICAL HISTORY, PROGRESS, AND FOLLOW-UP

Initial Assessment

Date of Services _____

Referral: ☐ self   ☐ send copy to Dr. _____

Summary: _____ year old (Cauc Hisp Black Oriental Am. Indian) M / F   for (evaluation   treatment) of

_____

_____

_____

_____

_____

_____

_____

_____

_____

_____

_____

#1   **Hyperlipidemia Dx:** Heterozygous / Homozygous Familial Hypercholesterolemia (FH)   definite / probable
Familial Defective Apo B (apo B_{3500} or FDB) polygenic   Other IIa _____
Familial Combined Hyperlipidemia (FCHL) type IIb   type III   type IV   LPL deficiency   type I/V   low HDL   high
Lp(a)   other _____

_____

_____

Molecular Defect(s) (if known): _____

Contributing cause(s): overweight   inactivity   smoking   diabetes   menopause   estrogen   hypothyroidism

hepatic disease   renal disease   alcohol   other _____

_____

_____

Risk for pancreatitis (trig): ☐ minimal (<1000 mg/dL) ☐ moderate (1000-2000 mg/dL) ☐ high (>2000 mg/dL)

Current diet: ☐ poor ("typical" American)   ☐ fair (step1)   ☐ good (step 2)   ☐ excellent (step 3)
☐ vegetarian with very low saturated fat _____

_____
_____

Medications (indications / rationale): _____

_____
_____
_____

Additional indicated Rx: control 2° cause   diet   weight loss   exercise   sugar control   added fiber
fish   fish oil   alcohol restriction   modest alcohol OK   estrogen replacement   decrease estrogen
change to estrogen patch   antioxidants (Vit E, Vit C)   vitamin therapy for high homocysteine

_____
_____
_____

#2   **Coronary Artery Disease:** ☐ none suggested   ☐ possible   ☐ probable   ☐ needs evaluation
☐ definite (prior Dx): Events (ages): MI _____   CABG _____   PTCA _____
Chest pain: none   nonanginal   old / new   angina (atypical   definite   unstable) _____

_____
_____

Physiology: CHF (mild   moderate   severe)   EF _____%   Arrhythmias _____
_____

Other CAD risk reduction indicated: ☐ ASA ☐ β blocker ☐ ACE inhibitor ☐ Cardiac rehab ☐ other (describe):

_____
_____

#3   **Other Cardiovascular Disease:** ☐ TIA (age of onset) _____   (most recent) _____
☐ Stroke (ages) _____   [thrombotic / embolic (source) _____ / hemorrhagic]

_____

☐ Peripheral vascular disease _____

☐ Hypertension _____
_____
_____
_____

#4   **Other CV Risk Factors:** +FHx   smoking   diabetes   overweight   high homocysteine   other

_____
_____
_____
_____
_____
_____

From Cardiovascular Genetics Research. University of Utah, Salt Lake City, UT, with permission.

Initial Plan

Date of Services _____

1. Diet & Exercise Therapy: *(in all cases a diet low in saturated fat and cholesterol is strongly encouraged)*
   ☐ Meet with dietitian   ☐ Diet classes   ☐ Controlled sugar   ☐ Added fiber   ☐ Encourage fish
   ☐ Fish oil (dose) _____   ☐ Antioxidants (Vit E 400-800 IU qd   Vit C 250-500 mg qd)
   ☐ Very low fat diet (≤10% calories fat) _____
   ☐ Vitamin therapy for high homocysteine _____
   ☐ Weight loss _____
   ☐ Exercise _____
   ☐ Other _____
   _____

2. Lipid Meds: ☐ Continue current therapy   ☐ Discontinue _____
   ☐ Add / Change _____
   _____
   _____

   ☐ Information sheet(s) given: statins   resins   niacin   gemfibrozil   antioxidants   high homocysteine   weight loss
   _____

3. Other Medications: ☐ ASA _____ mg qd _____
   _____
   _____
   _____

4. Initial Labs: <u>Date</u>_____ ☐ Extended lipid panel (circle method: ultracentrifugation / direct LDL)
   ☐ Coronary risk (total cholesterol, triglycerides, HDL, calculated LDL)   ☐ Lp(a)   ☐ apo E genotype
   ☐ Liver panel (Alk Phos, ALT, AST, GGT, bilirubin total & direct)   ☐ CK (total)   ☐ T4   ☐ TSH
   ☐ Chemistry panel (glucose, uric acid, creatinine, BUN, albumin)   ☐ Electrolytes (Na, K, Cl, Bicarb, Ca)
   ☐ Homocysteine   ☐ Hgb$_{A1c}$ ☐ CBC with auto diff   ☐ urinalysis (blood, protein, sugar)   ☐ other (describe):
   _____
   _____

   Other Labs: _____ ☐ Extended Lipid Panel (circle method: ultracentrifugation / direct LDL)
   ☐ Coronary Risk (total cholesterol, triglycerides, HDL, calculated LDL)   ☐ Lp(a)   ☐ apo E genotype
   ☐ Liver panel (Alk Phos, ALT, AST, GGT, bilirubin total & direct)   ☐ CK (total)   ☐ T4   ☐ TSH
   ☐ Chemistry panel (glucose, uric acid, creatinine, BUN, albumin)   ☐ Electrolytes (Na, K, Cl, Bicarb, Ca)
   ☐ Homocysteine   ☐ Hgb$_{A1c}$ ☐ CBC with auto diff   ☐ urinalysis (blood, protein, sugar)   ☐ other (describe):
   _____

5. Return to clinic in _____ Consider: _____

FLC 7/5-98 uucvg   Resident/Fellow _____ Clinic Physician _____

Initial Physical Exam

Date of Services _____

(See reverse side for additional narrative history)   M.D. Initials _____

☐ *performed*   ☐ *deferred*   *(Underline heading if examined and normal, circle and describe abnormalities)*

Vital signs: Height _____ (in / cm)   Weight _____ (lbs / kg)   BMI _____ (kg/m^2)

    sitting-BP: R _____ / _____   L _____ / _____   Heart Rate _____ bpm (reg / irreg)

    Orthostatics: lying BP _____ / _____ HR _____   standing BP _____ / _____ HR _____

    Temp _____ ° C / F   Resp _____   Comments: _____

_____

General appearance: overweight (central / diffuse   mild / moderate / morbid)   Cushingoid   acromegaly (pos / def)

_____

Head, neck, lymphatics: thyroid   earlobe crease present   lymph nodes _____

_____

Eyes: arcus (partial / complete)   xanthelasma   lipemia retinalis   definite arteriolar narrowing   wiring (silver / copper)

    A-V nicking   hemorrhages   exudates   microaneurysms   neovascularization _____

_____

Chest: crackles   wheezes   rhonchi   expiratory delay   diminished sounds   dullness _____

_____

Cardiovascular: elevated JVP _____   enlarged heart   S1 (increased / decreased)   S2 (paradoxical split / S2>S1 apex)

    S3   S4   mid-systolic click   Murmurs: systolic ejection (likely innocent / likely pathological / uncertain)

    holosystolic   late systolic   diastolic   Pulses: decreased (R / L carotid   R / L radial   R / L femoral   R / L PT

    R / L DP) Osler's nodes bruit (R / L carotid   sys / dia aortic   R / L renal   R / L femoral)   abdominal aneurysm

    Doppler: Arm systolic: R _____ L _____   Ankle systolic: R _____ L _____   Ankle/Arm index _____

_____

_____

Abdomen: R / L enlarged kidney   hepatomegaly   splenomegaly   ascites _____

_____

_____

Extremities & neurological: edema   xanthomas   reflexes (unequal   delayed relaxation)   Babinski   Gait   Other

_____

_____

Other findings and comments: _____

_____

FLC 11/5-98 uucvg   Intern/Resident _____ Clinic Physician _____

Personal Medical History

Name _____

Age _____   Birthdate _____   Date filled out this form _____

Referred by: _____   Address _____

Primary care physician: _____   Address _____

Main reason you are seeking help at this time: _____

_____

_____

Current Medications *(List all medicines and supplements you are currently taking.)*

Medication or supplement name (include aspirin, etc.)	Pill size or dose	Times taken per day	Date started (approximate)	Why started, any problems
Example - Lovastatin	20 mg	2	9/89	High cholesterol

Current Medical Problems *(Describe any active problems you are currently being seen for)*

_____

_____

_____

_____

_____

_____

Allergies *(also note reaction to each)*

Food: _____

_____

Medications: _____

_____

Other (such as hay fever): _____

_____

Past Medical Problems *(please circle if you have ever been diagnosed with any of the following problems. If none, check "none")*

Head and Eye Problems: None ☐

head injuries frequent headaches migraines glaucoma cataracts macular degeneration serious eye injury
serious eye infection

Other: _____

Ear, Nose and Throat Problems: None ☐

hearing loss vertigo chronic sinusitis nasal polyps frequent nose bleeds recurrent throat infections

Other: _____

Respiratory Problems: None ☐

asthma   chronic obstructive pulmonary disease (COPD) emphysema   pulmonary embolism   sleep apnea

Other: _____

Cardiovascular Problems: None ☐

Heart attack(s) (date, age, hospital): _____

_____

_____

_____

Angioplasty or atherectomy (date, age, hospital): _____

_____

_____

_____

Coronary bypass surgery (date, age, hospital): _____

_____

_____

_____

Angina (duration, severity): _____

_____

_____

_____

Most recent angiogram or treadmill (date, results): _____

_____

_____

_____

Arrhythmias, valvular or other heart disease: _____

_____

_____

Stroke or transient ischemic attack (age, hospital): _____

_____

_____

Claudication or aortic aneurysm (age of onset, surgeries):

_____

_____

Venous thrombosis (date or age, hospital): _____

_____

_____

Varicose veins (any surgeries, procedures): _____

_____

Other: _____

_____

_____

Gastrointestinal Problems *(circle)*:   None ☐
esophageal spasm   esophagitis   acid reflux   hiatal hernia ulcer (stomach or duodenal)   gastritis
liver cirrhosis hepatitis: (type _____) pancreatitis (age _____)   irritable bowel   diverticulosis   diverticulitis   colitis
Other: _____

Genitourinary Problems *(circle)*:   None ☐
frequent bladder infections   urethritis   prostatitis
glomerulonephritis   nephrotic syndrome   kidney stones   vaginitis   Candida infections   renal vascular disease
Other: _____

Nervous System Problems: None ☐
Alzheimer's   multiple sclerosis   peripheral neuropathy
Other: _____

Blood and Lymph Problems: None ☐
Anemia (low blood count)   Clotting disorder   lymphoma
Other: _____

Cancer *(give age, therapy, and outcome)*:   None ☐
breast   lung   colon   prostate   cervix   uterus   blood melanoma   other skin (type)
Other: _____

_____

_____

_____

Endocrine & Metabolic Problems: None ☐
high cholesterol   high triglycerides   low HDL   diabetes   low thyroid (hypothyroidism)   high thyroid   Grave's   gout
severe obesity   Cushing's   pituitary insufficiency
Other: _____

Muscle, Bone, Joint Problems: None ☐
low back pain   osteoarthritis   rheumatoid arthritis   osteoporosis   systemic lupus erythematosus
Other: _____

Skin and Hair Problems: None ☐
severe acne   psoriasis   alopecia   severe skin infections

Other: _____

Emotional Problems: None ☐

depression   anxiety   panic attacks   schizophrenia

Other: _____

_____

Surgeries *(list age and type of surgery)*

_____

_____

_____

_____

_____

_____

_____

_____

_____

Risk Factors *(check all that apply)*

Blood Pressure

My last blood pressure check was (date) _____. Results: systolic _____ / diastolic _____

Was this result typical? (Circle) yes / no   If not, what is your usual blood pressure? _____ / _____.

☐   I was never told that my blood pressure was high.

☐   I am currently taking medications for high blood pressure. First started medications age _____.

☐   My blood pressure was borderline/high in the past but is now normal without special treatment.

☐   My blood pressure was borderline/high in the past but is well controlled with diet and/or exercise.

☐   I have been told I have borderline or high blood pressure but it was **never treated**.

☐   My blood pressure increased in **pregnancy** to a degree that my physician(s) was/(were) concerned, or I had **toxemia**.

List any blood pressure medications you have had in the past and why you stopped taking them (side effects, etc):

_____

_____

_____

Diabetes

☐   I have never been told that I have diabetes.

☐   I have had diabetes since (age) _____.

☐   My diabetes is controlled with weight loss and diet.

☐   I take oral medication for my diabetes (yrs _____).

☐   I take insulin for my diabetes (yrs _____).

☐   I check my blood sugar levels at home regularly.

Prior diabetes medications: _____

_____

Exercise

☐ I do not exercise regularly.

☐ I walk for _____ minutes _____ times per week.

☐ I do other moderate exercise (gardening, playing tennis, etc.) 3 or more times each week but do not keep track of my pulse rate.

☐ I engage in vigorous exercise 3 or more times each week which raises my heart rate to a good training level (about 75% of my maximum) for at least 20 minutes without interruption.

☐ I engage in vigorous sports (basketball, racquetball, soccer, other) _____ times each week.

☐ I engage in weight training or resistance exercises.

☐ I am not able to exercise because of pain or limitation (specify):

_____

_____

Tobacco

☐ I have never smoked cigarettes

☐ I smoked cigarettes in the past but have quit:

Number of years since quit: _____

Average packs per day while smoking _____

Total number of years smoked: _____

☐ I currently smoke cigarettes:

Average packs per day: _____

Total number of years smoked: _____

☐ I smoke a pipe. # per day _____ for _____ yrs

☐ I smoke cigars. # per day _____ for _____ yrs

☐ I use snuff or chew tobacco.

Alcohol

☐ I never drink alcoholic beverages (skip to the next section)

☐ I have less than one drink per week (skip to the next section)

☐ I have one or more drinks per week (list amounts):

_____ cans of beer

_____ glasses of wine

_____ shots of whiskey, vodka, rum, etc.

☐ I have felt a need to cut down on my drinking.

☐ I have sometimes felt annoyed by criticism about my drinking.

☐ I have felt guilty at times about drinking.

☐ I sometimes have a morning "eye-opener."

Serum Cholesterol History *(**Please** call your physician's office for past results if you do not have them.)*

Date	Weight	Total Cholesterol	Serum Trigl	HDL Chol	LDL Chol	Treatment for cholesterol at the time of other test results, comments
_____	_____	_____	_____	_____	_____	_____
_____	_____	_____	_____	_____	_____	_____

___	___	___	___	___	___	_____
___	___	___	___	___	___	_____
___	___	___	___	___	___	_____
___	___	___	___	___	___	_____
___	___	___	___	___	___	_____
___	___	___	___	___	___	_____

List below any cholesterol or triglyceride lowering drugs you have tried or that were prescribed for you in the past (including niacin and fish oil) and any adverse effects you may have experienced while using them:

_____

_____

_____

Caffeine Intake *list cups or cans per day of:*

Caffeinated coffee: _____ Decaffeinated coffee: _____

Regular tea: _____ Caffeinated soda pop: _____

Sleep

Usual number of hours of sleep: _____

Heavy snoring? Y / N Sleep apnea? Y / N

Other sleep problems: _____

_____

Vaccinations *(list approximate year of most recent)*

Tetanus and diphtheria _____

Pneumovax (pneumococcal vaccine) _____

Flu _____ Hepatitis B _____

Measles _____ Mumps _____ Rubella _____

Social History

Circle: Single Married Divorced Spouse deceased

Number in household (include self) _____

Number of close friends or relatives near you: _____

Are you active in a religious or social group? Y / N

Years of education (12 = high school grad.) _____

Occupation: _____

Occupational Exposures *(circle):* None ☐

loud noise paints solvents dyes mineral dust organic dust (hay, flour, etc.)

Other: _____

Seat belts worn in the car: always sometimes never

For Women

Age when period first started _____

Number of live births _____ Miscarriages _____

Age at first pregnancy _____ Complications? Y / N

_____

Passed <u>menopause</u>? Y / N   Age at menopause _____

Bleeding problems/spotting? Y / N _____

_____

<u>Hysterectomy</u>? (Age) _____ Ovaries removed? Y / N

Birth control pills ever? Y / N   Years since used _____

Last breast exam _____ Mammogram _____

Any problems noted? _____

Last PAP smear _____ Normal? Y / N

<u>Estrogen replacement therapy</u>: Age started _____

Age stopped _____ Problems? : _____

_____

From Cardiovascular Genetics Research. University of Utah, Salt Lake City, UT, with permission.

Progress Note

Date of Services_____

Referral: ☐ self ☐ send copy to Dr. _____

HISTORICAL (include current diet compliance):- _____
_____
_____
_____
_____
_____
_____
_____
_____
_____
_____

Medications, Dose	Compliance (%)	Side Effects, Other Problems, Changes, Comments
	( )	
	( )	
	( )	
	( )	
	( )	
	( )	
	( )	
	( )	

Exercise Level/Tolerance: _____
_____

Other CV Risk Factors: smoking hypertension diabetes overweight high homocysteine _____
_____
_____

Cardiovascular Symptoms/Events/Procedures Update: _____
_____

☐ definite CHD (ages): MI _____ CABG _____ PTCA _____ Other _____
☐ CVD (ages): stroke: _____ TIA_____ ☐ PVD _____

From Cardiovascular Genetics Research. University of Utah, Salt Lake City, UT, with permission.

OBSERVATIONS: Height _____ in   Weight _____ lbs   BP _____

Physical Exam: ☐ deferred   ☐ performed   Findings (include xanthoma changes): _____

_____

Labs: Date_____   Chol _____   Trig _____   HDL _____   LDL (calc / meas) _____

meas VLDL _____   meas VLDL / Trig _____   Estimated $_\beta$-VLDL Chol _____   Apo E _____

Lp(a) _____   Homocysteine _____   Glucose_____   T4 _____   TSH _____

Abnormal LFT's / Renal / Uric Acid/Other Labs: _____

_____

ASSESSMENT

#1   Hyperlipidemia: Dx & contributing cause(s): _____

_____

Risk for pancreatitis (triglycerides): ☐ minimal (<1000 mg/dL)   ☐ moderate (1000-2000 mg/dL)   ☐ high (>2000 mg/dL)

Diet assessment: ☐ poor ("typical" American)   ☐ fair (step1)   ☐ good (step 2)   ☐ excellent (step 3+)

Medications (indications / rationale): _____

_____

_____

_____

Additional indicated Rx: control 2° cause   diet   weight loss   exercise   sugar control   added fiber

fish   fish oil   alcohol restriction   modest alcohol OK   estrogen replacement   decrease estrogen

change to estrogen patch   antioxidants (Vit E, Vit C)   vitamin therapy for high homocysteine

_____

_____

#2   Coronary Artery Disease: ☐ none suggested   ☐ possible   ☐ probable   ☐ definite (prior Dx)

Chest pain: none   nonanginal   old / new angina (atypical   definite   unstable)   ☐ needs evaluation

Other CAD risk reduction indicated: ☐ ASA   ☐ β blocker   ☐ ACE inhibitor   ☐ Cardiac rehab

_____

_____

_____

_____

_____

_____

_____

_____

Follow-up Plan

Date of Services _____

1. Diet & Exercise Therapy: *(in all cases a diet low in saturated fat and cholesterol is strongly encouraged)*

    ☐ Meet with dietitian   ☐ Diet classes   ☐ Controlled sugar   ☐ Added fiber   ☐ Encourage fish

    ☐ Fish oil (dose) _____   ☐ Antioxidants (Vit E 400-800 IU qd   Vit C 250-500 mg qd)

    ☐ Very low fat diet (≤10% calories fat) _____

    ☐ Vitamin therapy for high homocysteine _____

    ☐ Weight loss _____

    ☐ Exercise _____

    ☐ Other _____

    _____

2. Lipid Meds: ☐ Continue current therapy   ☐ Discontinue _____

    ☐ Add / Change _____

    _____

    _____

    ☐ Information sheet(s) given: statins resins niacin gemfibrozil anti-oxidants high homocysteine weight loss

    _____

3. Other Medications: ☐ ASA _____ mg qd _____

    _____

    _____

    _____

4. Next Labs: Date _____ ☐ Extended lipid panel (circle method: ultracentrifugation / direct LDL)

    ☐ Coronary risk (total cholesterol, triglycerides, HDL, calculated LDL)   ☐ Lp(a)   ☐ apo E genotype

    ☐ Liver panel (Alk Phos, ALT, AST, GGT, bilirubin total & direct)   ☐ CK (total)   ☐ T4   ☐ TSH

    ☐ Chemistry panel (glucose, uric acid, creatinine, BUN, albumin)   ☐ Electrolytes (Na, K, Cl, Bicarb, Ca)

    ☐ Homocysteine   ☐ Hgb$_{A1c}$ ☐ CBC with auto diff   ☐ urinalysis (blood, protein, sugar)   ☐ other (describe):

    _____

    Other Labs: _____ ☐ Extended lipid panel (circle method: ultracentrifugation / direct LDL)

    ☐ Coronary Risk (total cholesterol, triglycerides, HDL, calculated LDL)   ☐ Lp(a)   ☐ apo E genotype

    ☐ Liver panel (Alk Phos, ALT, AST, GGT, bilirubin total & direct)   ☐ CK (total)   ☐ T4   ☐ TSH

    ☐ Chemistry panel (glucose, uric acid, creatinine, BUN, albumin)   ☐ Electrolytes (Na, K, Cl, Bicarb, Ca)

    ☐ Homocysteine   ☐ Hgb$_{A1c}$ ☐ CBC with auto diff   ☐ urinalysis (blood, protein, sugar)   ☐ other (describe):

5. Return to clinic in _____   Consider: _____

    _____

    Resident/Fellow _____   Attending Physician _____

From Cardiovascular Genetics Research. University of Utah, Salt Lake City, UT, with permission.

Implementation of preventive cardiology guidelines

26

Gregg C. Fonarow

KEY POINTS

- *Despite compelling scientific evidence of the benefits of secondary prevention therapies in patients with atherosclerotic vascular disease or similar risk, a substantial proportion of patients are not on treatment with evidence-based, guideline-recommended therapies.*

- *Applying hospital-based systems to ensure initiation of lipid-lowering and other cardiovascular protective therapies has been demonstrated to improve treatment rates, long-term patient compliance, and clinical outcomes.*

- *The national guidelines have been revised to recommend that, in addition to smoking cessation and diet and exercise counseling, key cardiovas-cular protective medications be initiated prior to hospital discharge in patients hospitalized with a cardiovascular event.*

- *By initiating cardiovascular protective medications and patient education in-hospital as part of an effective management plan, physicians and nurses can make a vital contribution to the elimination of the "treatment gap" and dramatically reduce the death and disability caused by atherosclerotic vascular disease.*

- *Increased efforts to develop and apply effective strategies to improve use of and adherence with primary prevention therapies are clearly needed.*

INTRODUCTION

There is consistent and compelling scientific evidence that lipid-lowering therapy, other cardiovascular protective therapies, and therapeutic lifestyle changes reduce the risk of cardiovascular events and improve survival in patients with atherosclerotic vascular disease (secondary prevention).[1,2] The benefits of cardiovascular protective therapies are cumulative, and as a result, substantial risk reduction occurs when evidence-based, guideline-recommended therapies are applied in clinical practice. Similar potential benefits exist for risk reduction in patients without established coronary heart disease (CHD) (primary prevention).[3] Clinical trials demonstrate that significant cardiovascular risk reduction can be achieved by aggressive reduction of risk factors in high-risk patients who have not yet manifested CHD.

However, the risk status of persons without CHD varies greatly, and this variability mandates a range in the intensity of interventions.[3] Effective primary prevention thus requires an assessment of risk to categorize patients for selection of appropriate interventions.

The scientific evidence for primary and secondary prevention has served as the basis for preventive cardiology guidelines from the National Cholesterol Educational Program (NCEP), the American Heart Association (AHA), and the American College of Cardiology (ACC).[2–4] These guidelines aim to provide health care professionals with a comprehensive approach to reducing the cardiovascular risks of patients across a wide spectrum of risk and multiple cardiovascular risk factors. These guidelines have focused on primary as well as secondary prevention. The incorporation of these guidelines into routine clinical practice would be expected to result in major reductions in cardiovascular morbidity and mortality.

While the various preventive cardiology guidelines have the potential to improve the primary and secondary prevention of CHD, the reality of undertreatment has greatly limited their impact. Indeed, recent studies in both the United States and Europe have highlighted a significant "treatment gap" between the risk-reducing objectives published in international and national guidelines and current clinical practice.[5–7]

This chapter provides a brief overview of current preventive guidelines and reviews the studies documenting the underuse of guideline-recommended risk-reducing therapy in conventional practice. Effective strategies and systems to improve evidence-based, guideline-recommended treatment implementation are discussed, highlighting successful programs that have been demonstrated to improve treatment rates and clinical outcomes in different patient risk groups. Other strategies to facilitate treating risk factors to goal levels and new therapies in clinical development are also reviewed. This chapter also aims to illustrate the important role that health care professionals can play in bridging the "treatment gap" and allowing the guidelines to fulfill their potential.

PREVENTIVE CARDIOLOGY GUIDELINES

Primary prevention guidelines

Primary prevention guidelines, revised in 2002, highlight effective strategies for reducing first cardiovascular events.[4] These include discussion of recommendations for smoking cessation, blood pressure control, lipid management, physical activity, and weight management. These interventions and the importance of population-based interventions as a critical component of primary prevention are described in detail in Chapter 22.

AHA/ACC secondary prevention guidelines

The AHA/ACC guidelines for comprehensive risk reduction in patients with coronary and other vascular disease provide a concise summary of the recommendations of evidence-based risk-reducing therapies for secondary prevention (see Chapter 23). These guidelines were first released in 1995 and then revised in 2001.[1,2] These guidelines support aggressive risk reduction in patients with established atherosclerosis using a multifaceted approach with cardiovascular protective medications, risk factor control, and lifestyle modification.[1,2] The components of comprehensive secondary prevention include exercise, smoking cessation, and management of dyslipidemia, hypertension, diabetes, and weight.[2] Goals for frequency of exercise, body mass index, blood pressure, and lipid levels

are provided for patients with documented atherosclerosis. Combinations of cardiovascular protective medications are recommended in appropriate patients without contraindications or documented intolerance.[2] These recommended cardiovascular medications include aspirin, beta blockers, angiotensin-converting enzyme inhibitors (ACEIs), and lipid-lowering medications.[2]

Cardiovascular risk reduction is far more effective when the multitude of independent modifiable risk factors are addressed and a combination of cardiovascular protective medications are used, rather than when the focus is on single elements of care.

NCEP ATP-III guidelines

Since publication of the updated guidelines on CHD risk management compiled by the NCEP Adult Treatment Panel (NCEP ATP-III),[3] the attention of the health care community has become refocused on the importance of providing effective lipid-lowering strategies. Although several key revisions differentiate the current guidelines from previous versions (as discussed in Chapter 8), the reduction of elevated levels of plasma low-density lipoprotein cholesterol (LDL-C) remains the main focus.

One of the fundamental changes made to the NCEP ATP-III guidelines is the inclusion within the secondary prevention category of a wider range of individuals who may be at risk of developing cardiovascular events within the next 10 years.[3] In addition to those with preexisting CHD, patients with other forms of atherosclerotic vascular disease such as peripheral arterial disease and symptomatic carotid arterial disease are considered CHD risk equivalents. This also includes persons with diabetes mellitus but without established CHD, as these individuals have a high risk of developing macrovascular disease if left untreated.[8] The additional inclusion in this group of those with a calculated 10-year global risk exceeding 20% from the presence of multiple risk factors presents a new challenge for health care providers to identify and aggressively treat this new group of individuals. Furthermore, the lowest limit for reduced high-density lipoprotein cholesterol (HDL-C) has been raised from less than 35 mg/dL in ATP-II to less than 40 mg/dL in both men and women in ATP-III.[3,9] This change is warranted, as low HDL-C is a strong independent risk factor for the development of CHD.[10] While the NCEP ATP-III guidelines recommend initiating LDL-C-lowering medications in patients whose baseline LDL-C is 100 mg/dL or greater, a recent update considers initiating therapy at LDL-C levels <100 mg/dL to be optional. And while a goal for an LDL-C of <100 mg/dL is now standard, an LDL-C goal of <70 mg/dL is considered an option for those patients at *very high risk* (eg, recent acute coronary syndromes or CVD plus diabetes).[11]

JNC-7 guidelines for high blood pressure

The Seventh Report of the Joint National Committee on Prevention, Detection, Evaluation, and Treatment of High Blood Pressure (JNC-7)[12] has provided updated guidelines that simplify the classification and revise the nomenclature of blood pressure categories in an effort to achieve better population levels of blood pressure. Whereas the prior version of the guidelines incorporated optimal, normal, and high-normal for those below levels defining hypertension, normal is now defined as less than 120/80 mm Hg and the previously defined normal and high-normal levels are now combined into a category called "prehypertension" (120–139 mHg systolic or 80–89 mm Hg diastolic). This latter revision is an effort to bring to the attention of the large number of persons in this category the importance of lifestyle management to prevent the likely progression of blood pressure to hypertensive levels. Further, the previously defined stages 2 and 3 are now combined into a single stage 2 to reflect those with significant hypertension (≥ 160 mm Hg systolic or ≥ 100 mm Hg diastolic). Those with target organ damage are classified as high risk for more intensive blood pressure lowering (to <130/80 mm Hg) below the customary nominal treatment goal of less than 140/90 mm Hg.

THE GAP IN APPLYING GUIDELINE-RECOMMENDED CARE

Use of lipid-lowering treatment

There is overwhelming scientific evidence that LDL-C reduction with statin therapy reduces the risk of recurrent cardiovascular events and improves survival in patients after an acute coronary event.[13–16] The benefits of lipid-lowering medications have been proven to apply to men and women, patients older and younger than 65 years of age, and diabetics and nondiabetics.[17–28] The magnitude of benefit with statin therapy matches or exceeds the benefits seen with other secondary prevention medications such as aspirin, beta blockers, and ACEIs in the patient after an acute coronary event.[2]

Recently, data from the Heart Protection Study suggest that lipid-lowering therapy may provide clinical benefit to a greater number of patients than previously thought.[16] During this study, treatment of high-risk patients (documented atherosclerosis and/or diabetes) with simvastatin 40 mg/d reduced the occurrence of cardiovascular events irrespective of the individual's age, gender, or baseline LDL-C level. The cohort with the lowest cardiovascular risk were patients with on-treatment LDL-C levels of 50 to 70 mg/dL. The benefits seen with LDL-C lowering in patients with baseline LDL-C below 100 mg/dL may reflect that levels of LDL-C in the range 80 to 100 mg/dL are still causative or

permissive of atherosclerotic vascular disease.[22] Alternately non-LDL-C effects of the statins have been postulated to account for these benefits. Thus, virtually all patients with atherosclerosis, in the absence of contraindications or intolerance, would be expected to be appropriate candidates for lipid-lowering medical therapy.[22] It is likely that the Heart Protection Study data will impact future treatment guidelines, as this study provides compelling evidence that patients with atherosclerosis and/or diabetes in whom the baseline LDL-C is less than 100 mg/dL derive significant benefit from statin treatment. As a result, the number of patients eligible for lipid-lowering treatment is further expanded. Despite the effectiveness of lipid-lowering therapy in altering subsequent cardiovascular mortality and the widespread dissemination of national treatment guidelines, a number of studies show relatively low treatment rates in patients with established coronary artery disease, including high-risk patients after acute coronary events.[5–7,25–27]

Recent US physician practice regarding prescribing lipid-lowering medication to patients hospitalized for acute myocardial infarction was assessed in an analysis of 138,001 patients from 1470 hospitals in the National Registry of Myocardial Infarction 3 from July 1998 to June 1999.[25] This study revealed that only 31.7% of patients hospitalized with an acute myocardial infarction were discharged on a lipid-lowering medication. Among patients with prior history of coronary artery disease, revascularization procedure, or diabetes, less than half were discharged on treatment. Elderly patients, independent of associated comorbidities, were at increased risk for being discharged without lipid-lowering therapy. Women were also less likely to be treated with lipid-lowering medications, with 34.8% of men discharged on lipid-lowering therapy as compared with 26.8% of the women ($P < .0001$).[25] A variety of other clinical, demographic, treatment, and process of care factors that significantly influenced treatment utilization of lipid-lowering medications were also identified.

Other studies have shown similar underutilization of lipid-lowering therapy in high-risk hospitalized patients. Among the 20,809 patients hospitalized with an acute coronary syndrome and enrolled in the Platelet Glycoprotein IIb/IIIa in Unstable Angina: Receptor Suppression Using Integrilin Therapy (PURSUIT) trial or Global Use of Streptokinase or t-PA for Occluded Coronary Arteries (GUSTO) IIb trial, only 3653 patients (17.6%) were discharged on lipid-lowering therapy.[26] In a study of 19,599 acute myocardial infarction patients hospitalized at 58 Swedish Hospitals, only 28.2% of patients younger than 80 were discharged on statins.[28] Among 12,365 patients with acute coronary syndromes enrolled in the Sibrafiban vs. Aspirin to Yield Maximum Protection from Ischemic Heart Events Post-Acute Coronary Syndromes (SYMPHONY) I and II trials who

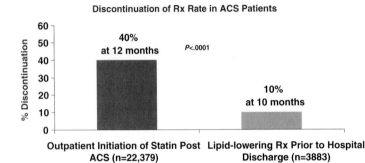

FIGURE 26-1 Impact of in-hospital initiation of statin therapy on adherence. Rates of discontinuation of statin therapy from two studies of statin use in patients with acute coronary syndromes are illustrated. The first study followed 22,379 acute coronary syndrome patients 66 years or older newly started on statin therapy as outpatients.[31] The second study followed 3883 acute coronary syndrome patients discharged from the hospital on statin therapy.[53]

were not previously treated with statin therapy prior to their index hospitalization, only 32% were started on statin therapy.[29]

In the outpatient setting, this treatment gap for statin therapy in post-acute coronary syndrome patients persists. The Quality Assurance Project (QAP) analyzed treatment rates in 48,586 outpatients with documented CHD (29% with prior history of myocardial infarction) from 140 medical practices (80% cardiology).[6] Only 39% of these patients were treated with lipid-lowering medications and only 11% were documented to have a LDL-C of 100 mg/dL or lower. In the third National Health and Nutrition Examination Survey (NHANES-III), lipid-lowering medication was used in only an estimated 11% of participants with a history of myocardial infarction.[30] In the Lipid Treatment Assessment in Practice (L-TAP) study, only 18% of outpatients with CHD treated for hyperlipidemia had a LDL-C level below 100 mg/dL.[7] This was not due to a lack of provider knowledge, as 95% of the surveyed physicians reported that they were knowledgeable of NCEP guidelines and 65% reported they follow the guidelines on most patients.[7] The ACC Evaluation of Preventive Therapeutics (ACCEPT) study, which evaluated 6875 patients from 55 US centers, demonstrated that at 6 months after cardiac hospitalization, despite prospective monitoring, only 28% of patients were at goal for LDL-C.[27] A significant treatment gap for statin therapy use in patients after cardiovascular hospitalization has also been documented in 47 centers in 15 European countries that participated in the European Action on Secondary Prevention through Intervention to Reduce Events (EUROASPIRE) II study.[5]

The documented treatment gap is accounted for by physicians not initiating statin therapy in appropriate patients. When statin therapy is initiated on an outpatient basis after an acute coronary event, studies have shown that the rate of adherence to statin treatment is remarkably poor. Among 22,379 patients receiving a statin prescription on an outpatient basis after an acute coronary

syndrome, the 2-year adherence rate to statin therapy was only 40.1% (Fig. 26-1).[31]. Other studies have also shown that when initiation of therapy is delayed until after hospital discharge. the rate of adherence to statin therapy is poor.[32] This low rate of patient adherence to therapy undoubtedly is a significant contributor to the large number of patients not being treated with this evidence-based therapy on an outpatient basis.

Together, these studies demonstrate that under conventionally guided management, regardless of the health care delivery system, an unacceptably large number of atherosclerotic vascular disease patients are left untreated and undertreated with lipid-lowering therapy. The underuse of lipid-lowering therapy in patients with atherosclerotic vascular disease represents a major clinical practice and pubic health issue.[25,33] Given the substantial number of patients at risk and the benefits of therapy, there is an urgent need to adopt effective strategies that will improve the number of CHD and CHD risk-equivalent patients who are being effectively treated with statins and other lipid-lowering therapy.[33]

Use of hypertension treatment and awareness of guidelines

Despite significant evidence regarding the efficacy of hypertension treatment in prevention of cardiovascular events, there still remains a significant gap between the guidelines and actual practice. Although targets for blood pressure control as set by the 7th Joint National Committee on the Prevention, Detection, Evaluation, and Treatment of High Blood Pressure (JNC-7) for uncomplicated patients or those with diabetes or decreased renal function have existed for several years, only about one fourth of hypertensive patients and an estimated 11% of diabetic patients and 3 to 5% of those with decreased renal function achieved adequate blood pressure control.[34] Data from NHANES show that from 1988–1991 to 1999–2000, treatment rates among those with hypertension remained inadequate, improving only in men (from 44.5 to 54.3%, $P < .001$), but not in women (60.1 to 62.0%, $P = .24$).[35] Rates of treatment have improved significantly in non-Hispanic whites and non-Hispanic African-Americans, but only marginally in Mexican-Americans, during this period. Significant improvement in control of hypertension, both among those treated and among all with hypertension, has also been observed in men, but not in women, during this period. In 1999–2000, approximately 60% of men being treated had their hypertension controlled to less than 140/90 mm Hg, compared with less than 50% of women. The improvement in control rates for men was due exclusively to substantial improvements in control in non-Hispanic white men, without any significant change in men of other race/ethnic groups.[35] Data from a practice-based setting, in particular a specialty hypertension clinic, demonstrate achievement of systolic and diastolic blood pressure goals of below 140 mm Hg and below 90 mm Hg, respectively, to be 59% overall, but lower in those with diabetes, particularly if more stringent goals are imposed (52% had control to <140/90 mm Hg, but only 22% reached <130/85 mm Hg and 15% reached <130/80 mm Hg).[34]

A report of randomly selected records of Medicaid recipients without hospitalization who had a diagnosis of hypertension showed in 1999 that the combined use of ACEIs and calcium channel blockers accounted for greater than 65% of all single-drug therapy, and that 48% of all patients received therapy not in compliance with JNC recommendations (eg, use of diuretic or beta blockers as first-line agents).[36] Also, in an Italian study examining 228 consecutive patients with recently diagnosed hypertension, during a specialist visit, 71% were on treatment, but only 19% were controlled to a blood pressure below 140/90 mm Hg. A complete clinical and laboratory evaluation as suggested by the guidelines had been carried out in only 10% of the patients; most laboratory assessments were done only about half the time.[37] Finally, in an analysis of 11,547 returned questionnaires (out of nearly 25,000 surveyed) given to German physicians conducted in a national survey, only 24% of the physicians who returned questionnaires (ranging from 19% of general practitioners to 37% of cardiologists) were adequately aware of the German Hypertension Society guidelines, indicating the impact of hypertension guidelines on actual medical knowledge to be only modest.[38] With respect to patient-related reasons for noncompliance, a study examining patient-perceived problems and outcomes of hypertension treatment revealed that two thirds of respondents suffered from one or more problems, most commonly symptoms and adverse drug effects. Those with three or more problems were nearly five times more likely to have modified their dosage instructions and twice as likely not to achieve goal blood pressure levels.[39]

Compliance to diabetes guidelines

Treatment of three clinical indicators—hemoglobin A_{1c}, blood pressure, and LDL-C—has been shown to reduce the morbidity and mortality associated with type 2 diabetes. In an evaluation of compliance with clinical practice guidelines for patients with type 2 diabetes, data from 368 patients in northern Alberta, Canada, were collected from patient interviews, drug histories, physical and laboratory assessments, and other sources. Although overall hemoglobin A_{1c} levels averaged 7.25%, blood pressure 131.7/76.2 mm Hg, and LDL-C 105.2 mg/dL, only 10% of patients reached targets for all three recommended measures. and of those not at target levels, 14, 28, and 87% of those patients reported receiving no therapy for hyperglycemia, hypertension, and dyslipidemia, respectively. Also, only 22% were taking aspirin. These findings indicated the existence of significant treatment gaps.[40] In a retrospective review of charts among diabetic patients in a university-based family medicine teaching practice, 58% of patients met NCEP-II goals for LDL-C (but which were <130 mg/dL for primary prevention and <100 mg/dL for secondary prevention), 38% were in compliance with standards for systolic and diastolic blood pressure, and only 22% had hemoglobin A_{1c} levels below 7%, suggesting more aggressive therapy is needed to achieve optimal compliance with treatment goals.[41]

Compliance with smoking cessation

Insufficient documentation of tobacco use and advice for quitting in the medical record remains a major problem in cardiovascular guideline compliance. In a study conducted at HealthPartners, a large network-model health plan in Minnesota, records of nearly 15,000 ambulatory adult patients from 1996 to 1999 indicated that over this period, identification of overall tobacco use increased from 49 to 73%, and advice to smokers to quit increased from 32 to 53% (both $P < .01$), but still only a small proportion of medical groups achieved the benchmark of identifying tobacco status in more than 80% of visits and providing advice to quit to more than 80% of tobacco users.[42]

Compliance with acute coronary syndrome/myocardial infarction guidelines

Quebec administrative data on all elderly survivors of acute myocardial infarction over a 3-year period (1996–1998) revealed rates of discharge medications were 65% for aspirin, 54% for beta blockers, 45% for ACEIs, and only 21% for lipid-lowering drugs. Although these discharge levels were suboptimal, 1-year compliance and persistence rates were high, with approximately three fourths or more of patients remaining on each of the therapies.[43] Compliance with these therapies administered in other programs is discussed below in the section on in-hospital initiation of preventive therapies.

BARRIERS TO TREATMENT AND CONTRIBUTING FACTORS

A number of barriers to implementing risk factor modification, including lipid-lowering therapy, in patients with CHD were highlighted at the 27th American College of Cardiology Bethesda Conference.[44] These included physicians' focus on acute problems, time constraints and lack of incentives, lack of training, and limited resources and outpatient facilities (Table 26-1). It has more recently been recognized that the setting in which treatment is initiated may be a very important factor influencing treatment rates.[45] Early treatment guidelines and algorithms such as NCEP ATP-I and NCEP ATP-II, had recommended delaying baseline lipid assessment and lipid-lowering treatment until 6 weeks after acute coronary event presentation. This recommendation was made because it was recognized that the acute phase response triggered by acute myocardial infarction and coronary artery bypass grafting can substantially lower total cholesterol and LDL-C levels.[9] As a result, the first opportunity for initiating lipid-lowering medications was delayed to a time when the patient may no longer feel he or she is at risk for recurrent events. The failure of cardiologists and other inpatient physicians to initiate lipid-lowering therapy during the period of hospitalization may inadvertently have been perceived by patients, their family members, and primary care physicians as a lack of endorse-

TABLE 26-1 Barriers to Implementing Lipid-Lowering Therapy in Patients after Acute Coronary Events

- Focus of physicians on acute problems
- Time constraints and lack of incentives, including lack of reimbursement
- Lack of physician training, including inadequate knowledge of benefits and lack of prescription experience
- Lack of resources and facilities
- Lack of specialist–generalist communication, passing on responsibility
- Costs of therapy, inadequate prescription medication benefits, restrictive formularies
- Guidelines that call for delaying initiation of therapy and for multiple steps, time points, and treatment options

ment of this risk-lowering therapy.[46] Frequently fewer resources are available in the outpatient as opposed to the inpatient setting, and coordination of care between cardiologists and generalists may be more difficult.

The studies assessing use of lipid-lowering therapy in patients after acute coronary events have consistently identified a variety of clinical, demographic, treatment, and process of care factors that significantly influence use of lipid-lowering medications.[6,28] This would seem to indicate that lipid-lowering therapy use is impacted by physician education and the process of care in place within the health care delivery system and, thus, could be favorably impacted by educational initiatives, quality improvement programs, and treatment systems.

IMPACT OF IN-HOSPITAL INITIATION OF PREVENTIVE THERAPIES

Institution of lipid-lowering therapy in the inpatient setting for patients hospitalized with acute coronary events and/or for a cardiovascular procedure has a number of advantages.[45] Measurement of baseline lipid levels can be systematically integrated into the diagnostic testing performed during cardiovascular hospitalization through the use of preprinted orders and care maps. The finding that lipid panels obtained in the first 12 to 24 hours of hospital admission reasonably reflect steady-state lipid levels at 6 weeks removes a perceived barrier to initiating lipid-lowering medications in the hospital setting.[46,47] The structured setting within the hospital can facilitate the initiation of lipid-lowering medications though the use of physician prompts and reminders such as preprinted order sets, discharge forms, and involvement of other health care professionals.[22] Hospital-based initiation of therapy may help to alleviate patient concerns regarding medication tolerability and side effects. Linking the initiation of lipid-lowering therapy and other secondary prevention measures to the patient's cardiovascular hospitalization conveys the message that this therapy is essential for the prevention of recurrent events and is an essential part of the patient's long-term treatment.[48]

Other evidence provides support to the concept that in-hospital of initiation of lipid-lowering medications could be a more effective way of ensuring treatment is started and continued. Studies in other patient populations, such as those with heart failure, have demonstrated that initiation of ACEIs at the time of hospitalization as part of a disease management program results in higher utilization rates at 6 months as compared with treatment utilization rates in conventionally managed outpatients.[49] Initiation of interventions for smoking cessation while patients are hospitalized with

UCLA Healthcare

CHAMP Discharge Checklist

	Agent	Dose	Indications
☐	**Aspirin**	81-325 mg qd	All patients with atherosclerosis, unless containdicated, indefinitely Clopidigrel in ASA allergic/intolerant
☐	**Beta Blocker**	Target Dose	All patients with AMI, UA, angina, heart failure. First line for HTN Diabetes, mild asthma, COPD are not contraindications, indefinitely
☐	**ACE Inhibitor**	Target Dose	All patients with atherosclerosis or diabetes. Start in AMI 12-24 hrs First line for HTN, indefinitely
☐	**Statin**	Dose to achieve LDL < 100 mg/dl	All patients with atherosclerosis or diabetes, regardless of baseline LDL, indefinitely
☐	**Exercise**	Individualize Aim, 5-7 × week 30-45 min	All patients with atherosclerosis, once stabilized, home based or cardiac rehab
☐	**Diet**	Step II AHA	All patients with atherosclerosis, started in conjunction with statin Rx
☐	**Smoking Cessation**		All patients who smoke

FIGURE 26-2 Discharge treatment checklist used in the Cardiac Hospitalization Atherosclerosis Management Program (CHAMP). (Reproduced, with permission, from Greg Fonarow.)

acute myocardial infarction has been shown to result in higher cessation rates than interventions initiated in the outpatient setting.[50] Utilization rates 1 year after hospital discharge are substantially higher for therapies, such as aspirin and beta blockers, that are initiated prior to hospital discharge than for therapies, such as lipid-lowering medications, that are conventionally initiated on an outpatient basis.[51]

Proof of concept that in-hospital initiation of lipid-lowering therapy and other secondary prevention measures improves treatment rates and long-term patient compliance was provided by the University of California, Los Angeles Cardiovascular Hospitalization Atherosclerosis Management Program (CHAMP).[51] This program, started in a university hospital setting in 1994, focused on initiation of aspirin, statin (irrespective of baseline LDL-C, dosed to achieve LDL-C < 100 mg/dL), beta blocker, and ACEI therapy in conjunction with dietary and exercise counseling in patients with established CHD prior to hospital discharge. Preprinted admission orders, critical pathways, discharge forms, physician/nursing education, and treatment utilization reports were employed to facilitate program implementation (Fig. 26-2).[22] Algorithms for both hospitalization and outpatient phases of care were used (Fig. 26-3). Statin therapy use at the time of discharge increased from 6% before initiation of the program to 86% immediately after implementation of CHAMP ($P < .001$). Improved use of aspirin, beta blockers, and ACEIs was also observed. Importantly, the in-hospital initiation of statin therapy had a dramatic effect on long-term treatment rates and patient compliance.[51] With CHAMP, 1 year after hospital discharge, 91% of CHD patients were treated with statins and 58% were documented to have LDL-C levels below 100 mg/dL, compared with 10 and 6%, respectively, of patients who received conventional management before CHAMP was implemented ($P < .01$) (Table 26-2). Whereas use of aspirin prior to CHAMP was 68% and use of beta blockers and ACEIs was less than 20%, after CHAMP, aspirin use increased to more 90% and use of beta blockers and ACEIs to approximately 60%. This improved use of statin therapy, along with other

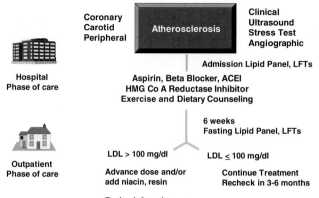

FIGURE 26-3 Hospitalization and outpatient care algorithms provided as part of the Cardiac Hospitalization Atherosclerosis Management Program (CHAMP). (Reproduced, with permission, from Fonarow and Gawlinski.[22])

cardiovascular protective therapies, was associated with a significant reduction in clinical events the first year after discharge: the rate of death and nonfatal myocardial infarction decreased from 14.8 to 6.4% (odds ratio = 0.43, $P < .01$) (Fig. 26-4).[51] These improved treatment rates have been sustained since the inception of the program (Fig. 26-5).

More recently, other studies have demonstrated that a high rate of lipid-lowering medication initiation can be achieved with hospital-based systems. A pharmacy-based program that included placing lipid treatment reminders on charts of patients hospitalized with CHD demonstrated an increase in treatment rates to 77% at the time of discharge.[52] Of the 10,288 patients in the Oral Glycoprotein IIb/IIIa Inhibition with Orbofiban in Patients with Unstable Coronary Syndromes (OPUS-TIMI-16) trial hospitalized with an acute coronary syndrome, 90% of patients who were started on statin treatment in the hospital remained on therapy at 10 months.[53]

In another systemwide approach to management of acute myocardial infarction (MI), implementation of protocols for each phase of MI management with clinical care paths developed for accountability showed, at the end of a 4-year period in 1999, rates of prescriptions for secondary prevention were 92% for aspirin and beta blockers and 97% for smoking cessation, demonstrating that recommendations set forth by the ACC and AHA are realistic and achievable and do not require additional resources.[54]

The AHA recently launched a national program called Get With The Guidelines, based in part on the UCLA CHAMP program.[55] This program uses an Internet-based interactive patient management tool. The GWTG program is implemented by AHA volunteers working in conjunction with hospital teams, using a collaborative implementation model. Within the hospital, following identification of a health care provider to champion implementation of the program, a feedback system of continuous quality improvement, including a cycling of stages of assessment of treatment rates, evaluation, protocol refinement, and implementation of a refined protocol occur to encourage the best outcomes (Fig. 26-6). Program implementation is facilitated by interactive conferences, teleconferences, and hospital tools including preprinted orders sets and a web-based tool that allows for recording of treatments prescribed at discharge (Fig. 26-7). In a pilot phase conducted in 24 New England Hospitals in the year 2000, the use of

TABLE 26-2 Treatment Rates at Hospital Discharge and at 1-Year Follow-up with the Cardiovascular Hospitalization Atherosclerosis Management Program (CHAMP)[51]

Therapy	Pre-CHAMP (n = 256)		Post-CHAMP (n = 302)	
	Discharge	**1 Year**	**Discharge**	**1 Year**
Aspirin	78%	68%	92%	94%
Beta blocker	12%	18%	61%	57%
ACEI	4%	16%	56%	48%
Statin	6%	10%	86%	91%
LDL-C < 100 mg/dL	—	6%	—	58%

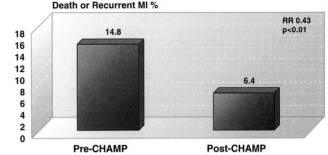

FIGURE 26-4   Impact on clinical outcomes in the first year post-hospital discharge of the Cardiac Hospitalization Atherosclerosis Management Program (CHAMP). (Reproduced, with permission, from Fonarow et al.[51])

256 AMI pts discharged in 92/93 pre-CHAMP compared to 302 pts in 94/95 post-CHAMP
ASA 78% vs 92%; Beta Blocker 12% vs 61%; ACEI 4% vs 56%; Statin 6% vs 86%
Fonarow Am J Cardiol 2001;87:819-822

lipid-lowering therapy increased from 54% pre-intervention to 78% postintervention ($P < .01$).[55] More than 250 hospitals are currently participating in Get With The Guidelines. In the ACC's Guideline Application into Practice (GAP) project performed in 10 hospitals in Michigan, the use of lipid-lowering therapy in ideal candidates increased from 68% pre-intervention to 92% postintervention in the subgroup of hospitals that were documented to be using the program's tool kit.[56] Thus, hospital-based systems for implementing lipid-lowering and other cardiovascular protective therapy have been demonstrated to be successful in the university and community, teaching and nonteaching, and urban and rural settings. These and other studies demonstrate that programs for in-hospital initiation of lipid-lowering and other cardiovascular protective medications can substan-

tially improve treatment rates in patients with atherosclerotic vascular disease.

Potential early benefits of statin treatment

Beyond the long-term benefits and improved treatment rates with statins, in-hospital initiation of statin therapy may also be associated with an early benefit in reducing cardiovascular events, one that could be missed if therapy is delayed. In the Myocardial Ischemia Reduction with Aggressive Cholesterol Lowering (MIRACL) study, 3086 patients hospitalized for unstable angina or non-Q-wave MI were randomized within 24 to 96 hours of admission to receive atorvastatin 80 mg or placebo; after a brief follow-up of only 4 months, there was a 16% relative risk reduction in cumulative ischemic events (14.8%

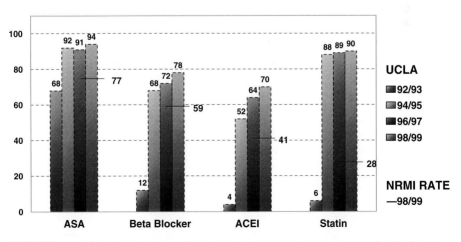

FIGURE 26-5   Sustained impact of treatment rates over a 6-year period in the Cardiac Hospitalization Atherosclerosis Management Program (CHAMP). (Reproduced, with permission, from Greg Fonarow.) NRMI, National Registry of Myocardial Infarction.

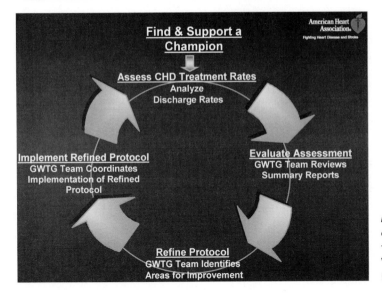

FIGURE 26-6 System of continuous quality improvement as implemented by the American Heart Association's Get With The Guidelines program (American Heart Association, Dallas, TX).

vs 17.4%, $P = .048$), with the majority of benefit due to a reduction in worsening angina with new objective evidence of ischemia requiring urgent rehospitalization (6.2% vs. 8.4%, $P = .02$).[57] Other trials involving enrollment of acute coronary syndrome patients, including one with fluvastatin[58] and pravastatin,[59] have failed to demonstrate beneficial effects on reducing recurrent event rates.

A number of observational studies assessing statin use prior to hospital discharge after acute coronary syndromes have shown a significantly lower mortality rate at 30 days, 90 days, and 1 year of follow-up.[29,31] But other observational studies have found no relationship between early statin initiation and improved outcomes.[32] Studies have also suggested that withdrawal of statin therapy during an acute coronary event may be associated with increased risk. A retrospective analysis of the Platelet Receptor in Ischemic Syndrome Management (PRISM) study reported that the withdrawal of statin treatment immediately after hospitalization for an acute coronary syndrome

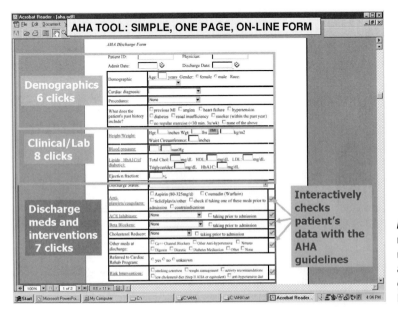

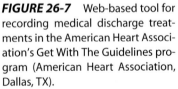

FIGURE 26-7 Web-based tool for recording medical discharge treatments in the American Heart Association's Get With The Guidelines program (American Heart Association, Dallas, TX).

was associated with an increase in the 30-day event rate, compared with patients who remained on statins.[60]

Postulated biologic mechanisms for early cardiovascular event reductions in acute coronary syndromes with statins include effects on the inflammatory response, endothelial function, platelet aggregation, endothelial nitric oxide, metalloproteinases, plasminogen activator inhibitor, and free radical production.[61,62] The molecular mechanisms of cholesterol-independent effects of statins may involve inhibition of the isoprenoid intermediates of the cholesterol pathway, essential for the function of signal transduction molecules of the *Rho* family.[62] Whether these so-called pleiotropic effects of statin therapy demonstrated experimentally are clinically relevant remains to be determined.

The early benefit of intensive lipid-lowering remains an area of active investigation and recently published clinical trials point toward the continued importance of this regimen. The recently published Pravastatin or Atorvastatin Evaluation and Infection Therapy (PROVE-IT) study[63] showed that among 4162 patients hospitalized for acute coronary syndrome that intensive therapy with atorvastatin 80 mg/d which resulted in lowering the LDL-C to a mean of 62 mg/dL, versus standard therapy with pravastatin 40 mg/d, resulted in a 16% lower risk for the composite endpoint of total mortality, myocardial infarction, unstable angine requiring hospitalization, revascularization, or stroke. More recently, intensive LDL-C reduction to 79 mg/dL (compared with usual care achieving a mean LDL-C of 110 mg/dL) resulted in less plaque progression as assessed by intravascular ultrasound.[64]

Potential concerns regarding in-hospital initiation of statin therapy

Arguments against early statin initiation include the question of early benefit, increased potential for adverse events in "unstable" patients, and the premature treatment of patients who could benefit solely from lifestyle interventions. These concerns are largely unfounded, as no significant adverse events were reported for patients receiving aggressive statin therapy during the MIRACL study, or in any of the other clinical trials involving thousands of patients, or in any of the observational studies involving tens of thousands of patients. Statins have now been shown to benefit patients with atherosclerosis, irrespective of baseline LDL-C. Also, because statin drug therapy is initiated concurrently with lifestyle interventions, the option remains for a subsequent reduction in statin dose if the patient achieves an exceptional reduction in LDL-C level.[33]

Many inpatient physicians may be reluctant to initiate statin therapy during patient hospitalization as they will not be following the patient longer term; however, the

evidence from several studies provides a compelling argument in favor of in-hospital drug initiation. By implementing statin therapy while the patient is in the hospital setting, inpatient physicians and nurses can play a pivotal role in ensuring not only that the individual's short-term management needs are met, but also that long-term risk factor therapy is effectively established.[33] Delaying initiation of statin therapy until after the patient is discharged is associated with lower treatment rates, higher rates of drug discontinuations, fewer patients at LDL-C goal, and higher clinical event rates.[34,35]

In-hospital initiation of statin therapy: new standard of care

Hence, although further research is needed to address the question of early cardiovascular event reduction, the benefits associated with in-hospital initiation of statin therapy, such as improved compliance and long-term clinical benefit, are compelling enough to establish this as the standard of care (Table 26-3).[33] In this regard, the new NCEP ATP-III guidelines, the AHA/ACC Secondary Prevention Guidelines 2001, and the ACC/AHA Acute Coronary Syndrome Guidelines 2002 have all endorsed this approach, recommending the initiation of lipid-lowering medications prior to discharge in patients hospitalized with atherosclerotic vascular disease.[2,3,65] The compelling data from the Heart Protection Study may allow these guidelines to be further revised to include recommendations for in-hospital initiation of statin therapy in all cardiovascular event patients, irrespective of baseline LDL-C. An essential element of the new AHA program Get With The Guidelines is the use of protocols and a web-based discharge tool to encourage in-hospital initiation of statin therapy and other secondary prevention measures proven to save lives in patients hospitalized with CHD.

TABLE 26-3   Benefits of In-Hospital Initiation of Statin Therapy

- Therapy is more likely to be initiated by physicians.
- Therapy is more likely to be continued by physicians long-term.
- Patients are more likely to view therapy as essential (heart medication).
- Patients are less likely to be concerned about side effects and monitoring.
- Patients are more likely to be compliant (lower discontinuation rates).
- Patients are more likely to achieve LDL-C goals.
- Early event reduction (if present) is not missed.

OPTIMIZING LIPID AND OTHER CARDIOVASCULAR PREVENTIVE THERAPY MANAGEMENT

Although relatively fixed dosing of statins as tested in the major clinical outcome trials has proved effective at reducing the risk of CHD, optimization of LDL-C levels would be expected to further improve patient outcome. Studies such as L-TAP have shown that even in patients on statin therapy, the LDL-C level often remains above the recommended goal of less than 100 mg/dL.[7] In the CHAMP study, even though 91% of patients were treated with lipid-lowering therapy, 1 year after discharge, only 58% had a documented LDL-C level below 100 mg/dL.[45] The majority of patients who were not at goal were still being treated with the same dose of statin on which they had been discharged home. Thus, in addition to the treatment gap, there remains a significant lipid-lowering therapy titration gap. Strategies for treating more patients to target may include initiation of the currently available statins at higher dosing levels, implementation of effective outpatient systems for adjusting dosing, development of more efficacious statins, development of additional lipid-lowering therapies, and combination of statins with other agents to maximize the effect on the lipid profile (Table 26-4).

Initiating higher does of currently available statins may help to bridge the outpatient titration gap by achieving LDL-C levels less than 100 mg/dL in a greater percentage of patients without the need for further dose titration.[36] The MIRACL trial demonstrated the short-term safety of starting patients hospitalized with acute coronary syndromes on a dose of atorvastatin of 80 mg/d (mean LDL-C achieved at 16 weeks was 72 mg/dL), with a withdrawal rate similar to that of placebo.[57] The Heart Protection Study demonstrated the long-term safety of starting and maintaining a dose of simvastatin 40 mg/d over 5 years in more than 10,000 CVD patients, including a large number of patients older than 75.[16] This approach also can help to minimize the number of laboratory tests (lipid panels and liver function tests) required for the patient to achieve goal levels. In the occasional patient with an exceptional reduction in LDL-C level, there is always the option for a subsequent reduction in medication dosing.

OUTPATIENT SYSTEMS TO IMPROVE GUIDELINE IMPLEMENTATION

Outpatient disease management and preventive cardiology programs have also been shown to facilitate lipid treatment. Various clinic-based systems have been developed to provide cardiovascular risk reduction services in both primary and secondary prevention.[66] Many of these programs have employed nurses to coordinate the services of a multidisciplinary team (Table 26-5). The program teams frequently include dietitians, pharmacists, social workers, exercise physiologists, and psychologists. The success of these programs is attributed largely to the availability of defined protocols for management of medications, development of comprehensive well-defined treatment plans, weekly team meetings, individualized education of patients, and coordinated care (eg., pre-appointment reminders, use of home health agencies).[66] Improving adherence often requires addressing psychosocial problems and coordinating a multitude of other comorbidities and medical problems.

A physician-directed nurse-managed home-based case management system has been shown to result achievement of a lower LDL-C level (107 mg/dL vs. 132 mg/dL) as compared with usual care in patients discharged post-MI.[24] The need to hire additional medical personnel, that is, specialty trained nurses, may limit the application of this type of system outside of health maintenance organizations. The use of an electronic medical record system to create a virtual lipid clinic in a large community outpatient cardiology practice setting increased the percentage of CHD patients with LDL-C levels below 100 mg/dL from 22% at baseline to 65% postintervention.[67] Other studies have demonstrated improved treatment-to-goal rates in specialty lipid clinics, pharmacist-guided interventions, and cardiac rehabilitation programs.[45,68,69] Some of these programs have been associated with improved patient outcomes. However, little research has been done in evaluating the cost-effectiveness of the various type of outpatient programs.[70] Despite the reported success of these programs, the vast majority of patients with atherosclerosis are not referred to such programs. Thus, hospital based systems for in-hospital initiation of lipid-lowering therapy

TABLE 26-4 Strategies for Initiating and Optimizing Lipid-Lowering Therapies in Patients with Atherosclerosis

- In-hospital initiation of lipid-lowering therapy
- Hospital-based performance improvement systems
- Nurse- or pharmacist-managed outpatient disease management programs
- Preventive cardiology and cardiac rehabilitative programs
- Virtual lipid clinics using electronic medical record systems
- Initiation of higher doses of currently available statins
- Combination of lipid-lowering therapies
- Development of new, more efficacious lipid-lowering therapies

TABLE 26-5 Primary/Secondary Medical Models for Cardiovascular Disease Prevention

Reference	Population and study design	Intervention	Components of intervention	Outcomes
Shaffer and Wexler, 1995	• Convenience sample • High-risk dyslipidemic patients • Comparison of lipid team vs general internal medicine • N = 120 • Mean age = 61 y, F/U = 18 mo	• Lipid intervention team led by RN (pharmacist, NP, dietitian, clinical psychologist) (lipid management)	• Clinic visit by RN, including health and physical exam, review of lipid profile, and secondary causes. Referral to endocrinologist as needed. • Dietary counseling by dietitian (all patients) • Screening by health psychologist for behavioral barriers to lifestyle changes. • Printed health education materials and individualized treatment plan. • F/U visits every 3 months (RN and dietitian)	• At 18 mo, reduction in total cholesterol (19% INT vs 10% UC, P = .02) and LDL-C (26% INT vs 8% UC, P < .01) • No significant change in TGs or HDL-C between groups
Aubert et al., 1998	• RCT in 138 type 1 (n = 17) and type 2 (n = 121) patients • Mean age = 54, F/U = 12 mo	• Nurse case management (patients recruited from 2 large primary care clinics) (diabetes management)	• Care provided by nurse case manager • Treatment algorithms developed by multidisciplinary team • Baseline visit with RN (45 min) and 2-week F/U (glucose mon., med adj. meal planning) • Referral to 5 weeks, 12-week diabetes education program (dietitian, exercise psychologist) • Quarterly F/U visits (RN) • Biweekly telephone contacts for review of glucose logs and medication adjustment	• At 12 mo, change in hemoglobin A_{1c} of 1.7 ($9.0 \rightarrow 7.3$) (INT) compared with 0.6 ($8.9 \rightarrow 8.3$) (UC), P < .01 • Change in fasting glucose: −48.3 ($194 \rightarrow 146$ mg/dL INT) vs −14.5 ($191 \rightarrow 176$ mg/dl UC) (P = .003) • Improved perception of health status at 12 mo in INT patients (P = .02)
Taylor et al., 1990	• RCT in 173 post-MI males • Mean age = 54, F/U = 12 mo	• Nurse case management (patients recruited from large staff model HMO) (smoking cessation)	• Behavioral counseling for smoking cessation at bedside by RN (30 min) • Health education pamphlet/audiotape • Nicotine replacement therapy as needed • F/U telephone contacts (10 min) at 48 h, 21 d, and monthly through 6 mo	• At 12 mo, biochemically documented smoking cessation 71% (INT) vs 45% (UC), P = .003

(continued)

TABLE 26-5 (Continued)

Reference	Population and study design	Intervention	Components of intervention	Outcomes
DeBusk et al., 1994	• RCT in 585 post-MI patients • Mean age = 57, F/U = 12 mo	• Nurse case management/liaison cardiologist (patients recruited from large staff model HMO) (multiple risk factor interventions)	• In-hospital baseline/education visit by RN • Behavioral education/counseling for diet, exercise, and smoking primarily by telephone (11 telephone contacts over 12 mo • Protocol-driven medical algorithms for lipid management • Referral to other health disciplines as needed (dietitian, psychologist)	• At 12 mo, mean exercise capacity (METs) 8.6 → 10.3 (INT) vs 9.1 → 9.9 (UC), $P = 0.01$. • LDL-C 107 mg/dL (INT) vs 132 mg/dL (UC), $P = .001$ • Smoking rate 70% (INT) vs 53% (UC), $P = .03$
Haskell et al., 1994	• RCT in 300 patients with documented CAD • Mean age = 57, F/U = 4 y	• Clinic-based intervention team (RN, MD, psychologist, dietitian) and nurse case management (multiple risk factor interventions)	• Baseline visit by nurse and dietitian • Risk reduction goals including written health educations, materials • Individual F/U via phone/mail by nurses about patient progress • Lipid-lowering medications provided under protocol • Clinical visits every 2–3 mo with project staff (5–7 visits/y)	• Significant 4-y improvements in risk factors: LDL-C (22%) ↓, HDL-C (12%) ↑, TGs (20%) ↓, exercise capacity (20%) ↑, diet fat (24%) ↓, diet cholesterol (40%) ↓, body weight (4%) ↓ • Significant (47%) ↓ in narrowing of diseased coronary artery segments vs UC • Reduction in clinical cardiac events (25 INT vs 44 UC, $P = .05$)

*RCT, randomized clinical trial; TGs, triglyceride levels; INT, intervention; F/U, follow-up; UC, usual care.

remain an important means of ensuring risk reduction is provided.

Collectively, these data show that initiating higher doses of currently available statins, using more efficacious statins if they are proven to be safe and effective, and combining currently available statins with other lipid-modifying agents will enable a larger percentage of individuals to reach their NCEP ATP-III goal—if treatment is initiated early and continued long term. Clinicians should endeavor to maximize the success of these treatment regimens through effective follow-up.

Compliance with other therapies

Although antihypertensive treatment has been shown to be highly effective in reducing cardiovascular morbidity, high rates of noncompliance still exist and may contribute to poorer outcomes. In a large retrospective cohort study of 4068 elderly enrollees of the New Jersey Medicaid program, patients filled prescriptions about half the prescribed duration (179 of 365 days) on average. Good compliance ($\geq$80%) was associated with advanced age and white race, but not gender.[71] Researchers have shown that monitoring compliance by use of electronic pill dispensers may result in improved compliance as seen by lower blood pressure levels.[72] Data from a German multicenter study revealed that the predominant reasons for noncompliance, as assessed by patients, were forgetfulness (40%), followed by adverse effects (9.6%) and irregular lifestyle (6.5%). Doctors noted changes in therapy were due primarily to inadequate blood pressure control, followed by adverse effects, patient dissatisfaction, and noncompliance. Although cost was not a major issue in this study, it may be a significant problem in the United States.[73]

In one study addressing the improvement of acute MI discharge treatments, use of an acute MI discharge worksheet designed to educate patients, prompt caregivers, and provide chart documentation regarding evidence-based therapies post-MI resulted in greater documentation of secondary prevention indicators and a higher "discharge score," a sum of the number of quality treatment indicators documented at discharge.[74]

In the case of diabetes preventive care guidelines, implementation of a computer-generated reminder system in a randomized controlled study in outpatient clinics serving internal medicine residents at the University of Utah and Salt Lake Veterans Affairs hospitals showed that after a 6-month period, both computerized patient-specific and nonspecific reports resulted in significantly greater improvements in compliance with guidelines.[75]

Finally, in a survey examining physician characteristics associated with compliance with adult preventive care guidelines, factors which independently predicted compliance included female physician gender, knowledge about preventive care guidelines, and perceived effectiveness in changing patient behavior. After controlling for these factors, other variables including lack of time, lack of reminder systems, attitudes about prevention, and amount of formal preventive care education were not related to self-reported compliance with guidelines.[76]

PRIMARY PREVENTION APPROACHES

The imperative to prevent the first episode of coronary disease or stroke or the development of peripheral arterial disease is strong because of the high rate of first cardiovascular events that are fatal or disabling.[4] The evidence that most CVD is preventable continues to grow. Clearly, the majority of the causes of CVD are known and modifiable. Preventive efforts are most effective when targeting each major cardiovascular risk factor.[4] The major and independent risk factors for CHD are cigarette smoking of any amount, elevated blood pressure, elevated serum total cholesterol and LDL-C, low serum HDL-C, diabetes mellitus, and advancing age. The quantitative relationship between these risk factors and CHD risk has been elucidated by the Framingham Heart Study and other studies.[10] These studies show that the major risk factors are additive in predictive power. Any major risk factor, if left untreated for many years, has the potential to produce CVD. The summation of contributions of individual risk factors can be a valuable first step in planning a risk reduction strategy for individual patients.[4]

Clinical trials demonstrate that significant risk reduction can be achieved by aggressive reduction of risk factors in high-risk patients.[13,14] Clinical trials have shown that excess risk can be reduced by approximately 33 to 50% in 5 years.[4] This is particularly the case when risk reduction strategies use lipid-lowering medications, antihypertensives-, aspirin, and smoking cessation. The gap between which evidence-based primary prevention interventions are recommended and what is actualized in routine clinical practice remains large.[7] Preventive cardiology guidelines, even when based on the best available scientific evidence from randomized, placebo-controlled clinical trials, cannot be successfully implemented without acceptance by the entire health care team, including physicians, nurses, and other health care professionals. A lasting health care provider–patient partnership should be created. A global risk assessment should be performed and carefully communicated to the patient.[4] Together with the patient, a preventive action plan should be developed. A variety of tools for providers are available to foster this partnership, such as the AHA's Health Profilers information for the public on CVD and stroke risk factors on the AHA's web site.

The challenge for health care professionals is to engage greater numbers of patients, at an earlier stage of their disease, in comprehensive cardiovascular risk reduction with the use of interventions that are designed to circumvent or alleviate barriers to participation and adherence, so that many more individuals may realize the benefits primary prevention can provide. It has been recommended that the health care professional create an environment supportive of risk factor change, including long-term reinforcement of adherence to lifestyle and drug interventions.[4] Practice-based systems for risk factor monitoring, reminders, and support services need to be established, reimbursed, and otherwise supported by managed care organizations and third-party payers. Primary prevention, by its very nature, requires a lifetime of interactions that virtually define successful provider–patient relationships.[4]

PERFORMANCE MEASURES

Performance measures are increasingly employed to quantify the quality of care being provided in the inpatient and outpatient settings. These measures allow comparison of individual providers and different health care delivery systems. Disease management programs frequently integrate the monitoring of quality-of-care measures into their formal structure. Performance measures are the discrete parameters for structure, process, or outcome, the attainment of which defines good quality care.[70] Important attributes for performance measures include the following:

1. The performance measure must be meaningful. Any potential performance measure must either be a meaningful outcome to patients or be closely linked to such an outcome.

2. The measure must be valid and reliable. For health care quality to be successfully quantified, it must be possible to reliably and accurately measure the structure, process, or outcome of interest.

3. The measure can account for patient variability. Although more relevant to process and outcome measures, it is important that the results of potential performance measures may be adjusted so that differences observed among providers are attributable to the care provided rather than to the patients treated.

4. The measure can be modified by improvements in the health care system. To be useful for facilitating change, performance measures must be amenable to improvement by motivated providers. This requires that the potential measure have variability (ie, some systems do well when judged by the measure, and others do not) and that evidence supports the feasibility of institutions or practitioners improving their performance over time.

5. The measure is feasible. Quantifying health care quality can be complex and costly. Proposed performance measures should be sensitive to the logistical and fiscal implications of assessing quality.[70] Measurement of treatment rates with lipid-lowering therapy in patients with atherosclerosis or diabetes is increasingly being viewed as an appropriate quality-of-care performance indicator.[70] Frequency of lipid measurement and treatment to goal in patients hospitalized with an acute coronary event and/or for a revascularization procedure were added to the Health Plan Employer and Data Information Set (HEDIS) 2000 quality-of-care measures.[77]

POTENTIAL IMPACT OF OPTIMAL CARDIOVASCULAR PREVENTION

As reviewed in this chapter, it has been clearly documented that not enough has been done to ensure the use of statin therapy in patients after an acute coronary event. Projecting available data nationwide, in the year 2002, more than 3 million potentially eligible patients were discharged home without one or more indicated cardiovascular protective medications after being hospitalized with an acute coronary event or for a cardiovascular procedure.[23,33] A review of the evidence from recent trials and clinical studies provides a compelling argument for implementing lipid-lowering and other cardiovascular protective medications in-hospital as part of a systematic approach to addressing the patient's underlying atherosclerotic disease process.[33] With optimal use of lipid-lowering and other cardiovascular protective medications in the patient with CHD, as many as 83,000 additional lives could be saved each and every year.[33] Even more impressive event reductions would be achieved with ideal implementation of primary prevention strategies.

REFERENCES

1. Smith SCJ, Blair SN, Criqui MH, et al. AHA/ACC Guidelines for Preventing Heart Attack and Death in Patients with Atherosclerotic Cardiovascular Disease. *Circulation* 1995;92:2–4.

2. Smith SCJ, Blair SN, Bono RO, et al. AHA/ACC Guidelines for Preventing Heart Attack and Death in Patients with Atherosclerotic Cardiovascular Disease: 2001 update. *Circulation* 2001;104:1577–1579.

3. Executive summary of the third report of the National Cholesterol Education Program (NCEP) Expert Panel on Detection, Evaluation, and Treatment of High Blood Cholesterol in Adults (Adult Treatment Panel III). *JAMA* 2001;285:2486–2497.

4. Pearson TA, Blair SN, Daniels SR, et al. AHA Guidelines for Primary Prevention of Cardiovascular Disease and Stroke: 2002 Update: Consensus Panel Guide to Comprehensive Risk Reduction for Adult Patients Without Coronary or Other Atherosclerotic Vascular Diseases. American Heart Association Science Advisory and Coordinating Committee. *Circulation* 2002;106:388–391.

5. EUROASPIRE II Study Group. Lifestyle and risk factor management and use of drug therapies in coronary patients from

15 countries: principal results from EUROASPIRE II Euro Heart Survey Program. *Eur Heart J* 2001;22:554–572.

6. Sueta CA, Chowdhury M, Boccuzzi SJ, et al. Analysis of the degree of undertreatment of hyperlipidemia and congestive heart failure secondary to coronary artery disease. *Am J Cardiol* 1999;83:1303–1307.

7. Pearson TA, Laurora I, Chu H, Kafonek S. The Lipid Treatment Assessment Project (L-TAP): a multicenter survey to evaluate the percentages of dyslipidemic patients receiving lipid-lowering therapy and achieving low-density lipoprotein cholesterol goals. *Arch Intern Med* 2000;160:459–467.

8. Haffner SM, Lehto S, Ronnemaa T, et al. Mortality from coronary heart disease in subjects with type 2 diabetes and in nondiabetic subjects with and without prior myocardial infarction. *N Engl J Med* 1998;339:229–234.

9. Second report of the National Cholesterol Education Program Expert Panel on Detection, Evaluation, and Treatment of High Blood Cholesterol in Adults (Adult Treatment Panel II). *Circulation* 1994;89:1329–445.

10. Castelli WP, Garrison RJ, Wilson PWF, et al. Incidence of coronary heart disease and lipoprotein cholesterol levels: the Framingham Study. *JAMA* 1986;256:2835–2838.

11. Grundy SM, Cleeman JI, Merz CN, et al. Implications of recent clinical trials for the National Cholesterol Education Program Adult Treatment Panel III guidelines. *Circulation* 2004;110:227–239.

12. Chobanian AV, Bakris GL, Black HR, et al. The seventh report of the Joint National Committee on Prevention, Detection, Evaluation, and Treatment of High Blood Pressure: the JNC 7 Report. *JAMA* 2003;289:2560–2572.

13. Scandinavian Simvastatin Survival Study Group. Randomised trial of cholesterol lowering in 4444 patients with coronary heart disease: the Scandinavian Simvastatin Survival Study (4S). *Lancet* 1994;344:1383–1389.

14. Sacks FM, Pfeffer MA, Moye LA et al, for the Cholesterol and Recurrent Events Trial Investigators. The effect of pravastatin on coronary events after myocardial infarction in patients with average cholesterol levels. *N Engl J Med* 1996;335:1001–1009.

15. The Long-Term Intervention with Pravastatin in Ischaemic Disease (LIPID) Study Group. Prevention of cardiovascular events and death with pravastatin in patients with coronary heart disease and a broad range of initial cholesterol levels. *N Engl J Med* 1998;339:1349–1357.

16. Heart Protection Study Collaborative Group. MRC/BHF Heart Protection Study of cholesterol lowering with simvastatin in 20536 high-risk individuals: a randomised placebo-controlled trial. *Lancet* 2002;360:7–22.

17. Grundy SM, Cleeman JI, Rifkind BM, et al. Cholesterol lowering in the elderly population. *Arch Intern Med* 1999;159:1670–1678.

18. Mosca L, Grundy SM, Judelson D, et al. Guide to Preventive Cardiology for Women. AHA/ACC Scientific Statement Consensus panel statement. *Circulation* 1999;99:2480–2484.

19. Grundy SM, Benjamin IJ, Burke GL, et al. Diabetes and cardiovascular disease. a statement for healthcare professionals from the American Heart Association. *Circulation* 1999;100:1134–1146.

20. Hunninghake DB, Stein EA, Dujovne CA, et al. The efficacy of intensive dietary therapy alone or combined with lovastatin in outpatients with hypercholesterolemia. *N Engl J Med* 1993;328:1213–1219.

21. Debusk RF, Miller NH, Superko HR, et al. A case-management system for coronary risk factor modification after acute myocardial infarction. *Ann Intern Med* 1994;120:721–729.

22. Fonarow GC, Gawlinski A. Rationale and design of the Cardiac Hospitalization Atherosclerosis Management Program at the University of California Los Angeles. Am J Cardiol 2000;85:10A–17A.

23. *2003 Heart and Stroke Statistical Update*. Dallas Tex: American Heart Association; 2002.

24. Murray CL, Lopez AD, eds. *The Global Burden of Disease*. Vol 1. Cambridge, MA: Harvard University Press; 1996:325–396.

25. Fonarow GC, French WJ, Parsons LS, et al. Use of lipid-lowering medications at discharge in patients with acute myocardial infarction: data from the National Registry of Myocardial Infarction 3. *Circulation* 2001;103:38–44.

26. Aronow HD, Topol EJ, Roe MT, et al. Effect of lipid-lowering therapy on early mortality after acute coronary syndromes: an observational study. *Lancet* 2001;357:1063–1068.

27. Pearson TA, Peters TD, Feury D, et al. The American College of Cardiology Evaluation of Preventative Therapeutics (ACCEPT) study: attainment of goals for comprehensive risk reduction in patients with coronary disease in the US. *J Am Coll Cardiol* 1998;31:186A.

28. Stenestrand U, Wallentin L, for the Swedish Register of Cardiac Intensive Care (RIKS-HIA). Early statin treatment following acute myocardial infarction and 1-year survival. *JAMA* 2001;285:430–436.

29. Newby LK, Kristinsson A, Bhapkar MV, et al. Early statin initiation and outcomes in patients with acute coronary syndromes. *JAMA* 2002;287:3087–3095.

30. Jacobson TA, Griffiths GG, Varas C, et al. Impact of evidence-based "clinical judgment" on the number of American adults requiring lipid-lowering drug therapy based on updated NHANES III data. *Arch Intern Med* 2000;160:1361–1369.

31. Jackevicius CA, Mamdani M, Tu JV. Adherence with statin therapy in elderly patients with and without acute coronary syndromes. *JAMA* 2002;288:462–467.

32. Muhlestein JB, Horne BD, Bair TL, et al. Usefulness of in-hospital prescription of statin agents after angiographic diagnosis of coronary artery disease in improving continued compliance and reduced mortality. *Am J Cardiol* 2001; 87:257–261.

33. Fonarow GC. Treating to goal: new strategies for initiating and optimizing lipid-lowering therapies in patients with atherosclerosis. *Vasc Med* 2002;7:187–194.

34. Singer GM, Izhar M, Black HR. Guidelines for hypertension: are quality-assurance measures on target? *Hypertension* 2004;43: 198–202.

35. Hajjar I, Kotchen TA. Trends in prevalence, awareness, treatment, and control of hypertension in the United States, 1988–2000. *JAMA* 2003;290:199–206.

36. Clause SL, Hamilton RA. Medicaid prescriber compliance with Joint National Committee VI hypertension treatment guidelines. *Ann Pharmacother* 2002;36:1501–1511.

37. Cuspidi C, Michev I, Lonati L, et al. Compliance to hypertension guidelines in clinical practice: a multicenter pilot study in Italy. *J Hum Hypertens* 2002;16:699–703.

38. Hagemeister J, Schneider CA, Barabas S, et al. Hypertension guidelines and their limitations: the impact of physicians'

compliance as evaluated by guideline awareness. *J Hypertens* 2001;19: 2079–2086.

39. Enlund H, Jokisalo E, Wallenius S. Patient-perceived problems, compliance, and the outcome of hypertension treatment. *Pharm World Sci* 2001;23:60–64.

40. Toth EL, Majumdar SR, Guirguios LM, et al. Compliance with clinical practice guidelines for type 2 diabetes in rural patients: treatment gaps and opportunities for improvement. *Pharmacotherapy* 2003;23:659–665.

41. Kirk JK, Poirier JE, Mattox MG, et al. Compliance with national guidelines in patients with diabetes in a family practice clinic. *Pharmacotherapy* 2002;22:1541–1546.

42. Amundson G, Solberg LI, Reed M, et al. Paying for quality improvement: compliance with tobacco cessation guidelines. *Jt Comm J Qual Saf* 2003;29:59–65.

43. Simpson E, Beck C, Richard H, et al. Drug prescriptions after acute myocardial infarction: dosage, compliance, and persistence. *Am Heart J* 2003;145:438–444.

44. Pearson TA, McBride PE, Miller NH, et al. 27th Bethesda Conference: matching the intensity of risk factor management with the hazard for coronary disease events. Task Force 8. Organization of preventive cardiology service. *J Am Coll Cardiol* 1996;27:1039–1047.

45. Fonarow GC, Ballantyne CM. In-hospital initiation of lipid-lowering therapy for patients with coronary heart disease: the time is now. *Circulation* 2001;103:2768–2770.

46. McCall M, Elmfeldt D, Vedin A, et al. Influence of a myocardial infarction on blood pressure and serum cholesterol. *Acta Med Scand* 1979;206:477–481.

47. Rosenson RS. Myocardial injury: the acute phase response and lipoprotein metabolism. *J Am Coll Cardiol* 1993;22:933–940.

48. Fonarow GC, Stevenson LW, Walden JA, et al. Impact of a comprehensive heart failure management program on hospital readmission and functional status of patients with advanced heart failure. *J Am Coll Cardiol* 1997;30:725–732.

49. Taylor CB, Houston-Miller N, Killen JD, et al. Smoking cessation after acute myocardial infarction: effects of a nurse-managed intervention. *Ann Intern Med* 1990;113:118–123.

50. Marciniak TA, Ellerbeck EF, Radford MJ, et al. Improving the quality of care for Medicare patients with acute myocardial infarction: results from the Cooperative Cardiovascular Project. *JAMA* 1998;279:1351–1357.

51. Fonarow GC, Gawlinski A, Moughrabi S, Tillisch JH. Improved treatment of coronary heart disease by implementation of a Cardiac Hospitalisation Atherosclerosis Management Program (CHAMP). *Am J Cardiol* 2001;87:819–822.

52. Birtcher KK, Bowden C, Ballantyne CM, et al. Strategies for implementing lipid-lowering therapy: pharmacy-based approach. *Am J Cardiol* 2000;85:30A–35A.

53. Cannon CP, McCabe CH, Bentley J, et al. Early statin therapy is associated with markedly lower mortality in patients with acute coronary syndromes: observations from OPUS-TIMI-16. *J Am Coll Cardiol* 2001;37:334A.

54. Akosah KO, Larson DE, Brown WM, et al. *Jt Comm J Qual Saf* 2003;29:248–259.

55. McCarthy M. US heart-guidelines program makes a promising start. *Lancet* 2001;358:1618.

56. Mehta RH, Montoye CK, Gollogly M, et al. Improving quality of care for acute myocardial infarction: the guidelines ap-plied into practice (GAP) initiative. *JAMA* 2002;287:1269–1276.

57. Schwartz GG, Olsson AG, Ezekowitz MD, et al. Effects of atorvastatin on early recurrent ischemic events in acute coronary syndromes: the MIRACL study: a randomized controlled trial. *JAMA* 2001;285:1711–1718.

58. Liem AH, van Boven AJ, Veeger NJ, et al. Effect of fluvastatin on ischaemia following acute myocardial infarction: a randomized trial. *Eur Heart J* 2002;23:1931–1937.

59. Thompson PL, Amerena J, Campbell TJ, et al, for the PACT Investigators. Presented at: World Congress of Cardiology; May 2002; Sydney.

60. Heeschen C, Hamm CW, Laufs U, et al. Withdrawal of statins increases event rates in patients with acute coronary syndromes. *Circulation* 2002;105:1446–1452.

61. Rosenson RS, Tangney CC. Antiatherothrombotic properties of statins: implications for cardiovascular event reduction. *JAMA* 1998;279:1643–1650.

62. Kwak B, Mulhaupt F, Myit S, et al. Statins as a newly recognized type of immunomodulator. *Nat Med* 2000;6:1399–1402.

63. Cannon CP, Braunwald E, McCabe CH, et al. Comparison of intensive and moderate lipid lowring with statins after acute coronary syndromes. *N Engl J Med* 2003;350:1495–1504.

64. Nissen SE, Tuzcu EM, Schoenhagen P, et al. Effect of intensive compared with moderate lipid-lowering therapy on progression of coronary atherosclerosis: a randomized controlled trial. *JAMA* 2004;291:1071–1081.

65. Braunwald E, Antman EM, Beasley JW, et al. ACC/AHA guideline update for the management of patients with unstable angina and non-ST-segment elevation myocardial infarction—2002: summary article: a report of the American College of Cardiology/American Heart Association Task Force on Practice Guidelines. *Circulation* 2002;106:1893–1900.

66. Ades PA, Kottke TE, Miller NH, et al. 33rd Bethesda Conference: Task force 3. Getting results: who, where, and how? *J Am Coll Cardiol* 2002;40:615–630.

67. Kinn JW, Brown AS. Cardiovascular risk management in clinical practice: the midwest heart specialists experience. *Am J Cardiol* 2002;89(suppl):23C–29C.

68. Haskell WL, Alderman EL, Fair JM, et al. Effects of intensive multiple risk factor reduction on coronary atherosclerosis and clinical cardiac events in men and women with coronary artery disease: the Stanford Coronary Risk Intervention Project (SCRIP). *Circulation* 1994;89:975–990.

69. Blair TP, Bryant FJ, Bocuzzi S. Treatment of hypercholesterolemia by a clinical nurse using a stepped-care protocol in a nonvolunteer population. *Arch Intern Med* 1988;148:1046–1048.

70. Challenges and opportunities in quantifying the quality of care for acute myocardial infarction: summary from the Acute Myocardial Infarction Working Group of the American Heart Association/American College of Cardiology First Scientific Forum on Quality of Care and Outcomes Research in Cardiovascular Disease and Stroke. *Circulation* 2003;107:1681–1691.

71. Monana M, Bohn RL, Gurwitz JH. Compliance with antihypertensive therapy among elderly Medicaid enrollees: the roles of age, gender, and race. *Am J Public Health* 1996;86:1805–1808.

72. Waeber B, Vetter W, Darioli R, et al. Improved blood pressure control by monitoring compliance with antihypertensive therapy. *Int J Clin Pract* 1999;53:37–38.

73. Dusing R, Weisser B, Mengden T, Vetter H. Changes in anti-hypertensive therapy: the role of adverse effects and compliance. *Blood Pressure* 1998;7:313–315.

74. Nori D, Johnson J, Kapke A, et al. Use of a discharge worksheet enhances compliance with evidence-based myocardial infarction care. *J Thromb Thrombolysis* 2002;14:43–49.

75. Nilasena DS, Lincoln MJ. A computer-generated reminder system improves physician compliance with diabetes preventive care guidelines. *Proc Annu Symp Comput Appl Med Care* 1995:640–645.

76. Ely JW, Goerdt CJ, Bergus GR, et al. The effect of physician characteristics on compliance with adult preventive care guidelines. *Fam Med* 1998;30:34–39.

77. Lee TH, Cleeman JI, Grundy SM, et al. Clinical goals and performance measures for cholesterol management in secondary prevention of coronary heart disease. *JAMA* 2000;283:94–98.

Index

Note: Page numbers followed by a *t* indicate tables; numbers followed by an *f* indicate figures.